Handbook
of Population

Handbooks of Sociology and Social Research

Series Editor:
Howard B. Kaplan, *Texas A&M University, College Station, Texas*

HANDBOOK OF COMMUNITY MOVEMENTS AND LOCAL ORGANIZATIONS
Edited by Ram A. Cnaan and Carl Milofsky

HANDBOOK OF DISASTER RESEARCH
Edited by Havidán Rodríguez, Enrico L. Quarantelli, and Russell Dynes

HANDBOOK OF DRUG ABUSE PREVENTION
Theory, Science and Prevention
Edited by Zili Sloboda and William J. Bukoski

HANDBOOK OF THE LIFE COURSE
Edited by Jeylan T. Mortimer and Michael J. Shanahan

HANDBOOK OF POPULATION
Edited by Dudley L. Poston and Michael Micklin

HANDBOOK OF RELIGION AND SOCIAL INSTITUTIONS
Edited by Helen Rose Ebaugh

HANDBOOK OF SOCIAL PSYCHOLOGY
Edited by John Delamater

HANDBOOK OF SOCIOLOGICAL THEORY
Edited by Jonathan H. Turner

HANDBOOK OF THE SOCIOLOGY OF EDUCATION
Edited by Maureen T. Hallinan

HANDBOOK OF THE SOCIOLOGY OF EMOTIONS
Edited by Jan E. Stets and Jonathan H. Turner

HANDBOOK OF THE SOCIOLOGY OF GENDER
Edited by Janet Saltzman Chafetz

HANDBOOK OF THE SOCIOLOGY OF MENTAL HEALTH
Edited by Carol S. Aneshensel and Jo C. Phelan

HANDBOOK OF THE SOCIOLOGY OF THE MILITARY
Edited by Giuseppe Caforio

Handbook of Population

Edited by

Dudley L. Poston

*Texas A&M University, College Station,
Texas, USA*

Michael Micklin

*National Institutes of Health, Bethesda,
Maryland, USA*

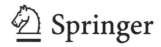 Springer

Library of Congress Cataloging-in-Publication Data
A C.I.P. Catalogue record for this book is available from the Library of Congress.

ISBN 0-306-47768-8   e-ISBN 0-387-23106-4   Printed on acid-free paper.

Printed in the United States of America.

9 8 7 6 5 4 3

springer.com

Preface

Completion of this *Handbook* would not have been possible without the generous and dedicated assistance of numerous people. Several years ago Howard Kaplan, Editor of the Kluwer/Plenum *Handbooks of Sociology and Social Research*, asked Dudley Poston to edit a *Handbook of Population*. Poston then asked his long-time collaborator and fellow demographer, Michael Micklin, to join him as co-editor. Poston and Micklin next assembled a list of chapter topics and possible authors. We endeavored to shape the contributions to the *Handbook* in two ways: We wished to parallel in many ways the outline of *The Study of Population*, edited by Philip M. Hauser and Otis Dudley Duncan, and published in 1959. The Hauser and Duncan volume was the key compendium and inventory of the state of demography; one had not been published since. In shaping this *Handbook* we also took into account the increased scope of demography, its development in other social science areas, and its application outside the academy.

In the subsequent development of this *Handbook*, we worked closely with Teresa Kraus, our editor at Springer, and also received advice from Howard Kaplan. Poston and Micklin read and edited each of the *Handbook* chapters and then sent them back to the authors for their revisions. We appreciate their timely responses to our requests for revisions. All the chapters were then copy edited at Texas A&M University by Amanda K. Baumle, who then discussed and reviewed the final changes and edits with Poston.

We dedicate this *Handbook* to our dear friend and fellow demographer, the late William R. Serow, formerly of Florida State University. Bill was to have written one of the chapters of this *Handbook*. Unfortunately, he passed away suddenly and unexpectedly in early November of 2003 at age 57. We will miss his scholarly contributions to this *Handbook*. We already miss his laughter and friendship in our lives.

Dudley L. Poston, Jr.
College Station, Texas
Michael Micklin
Bethesda, Maryland

Contributors

Amanda K. Baumle is a Ph.D. Candidate in Sociology and Demography at Texas A&M University, College Station, Texas 77843.

Frank D. Bean is Professor of Sociology, and Codirector of the Center for Research on Immigration, Population and Public Policy, at the University of California, Irvine, Irvine, California 92717.

Susan K. Brown is Assistant Professor of Sociology at the University of California, Irvine, Irvine, California 92717.

James R. Carey is Professor of Entomology and Program Director, Biodemographic Determinants of Life Span, at the University of California, Davis, Davis, California 95616.

Glenn R. Carroll is the Laurence W. Lane Professor of Organizations and (by courtesy) Professor of Sociology at Stanford University, Stanford, California 94305.

Mark A. Fossett is Professor of Sociology at Texas A&M University, College Station, Texas 77843.

W. Parker Frisbie is Professor of Sociology and Research Associate of the Population Research Center at the University of Texas at Austin, Austin, Texas 78712.

Avery M. Guest is Professor of Sociology at the University of Washington, Seattle, Washington 98195.

Kellie J. Hagewen is a Ph.D. Candidate and NIA predoctoral trainee in sociology at Duke University, Durham, North Carolina 27708.

Mark D. Hayward is Distinguished Professor of Sociology and Demography and Director, Center on Population Health and Aging, at Penn State University, University Park, Pennsylvania 16802.

Charles Hirschman is Boeing Professor of Sociology and Public Affairs at the University of Washington, Seattle, Washington 98195.

Robert A. Hummer is Professor of Sociology and Director, Population Research Center, at the University of Texas at Austin, Austin, Texas 78712.

Ichiro Kawachi is Professor of Social Epidemiology and Director of the Center for Society and Health at Harvard University, Boston, Massachusetts 02115.

David I. Kertzer is the Paul Dupee University Professor of Social Science and Professor of Anthropology and Italian Studies at Brown University, Providence, Rhode Island 02912.

Olga M. Khessina is an Assistant Professor of Strategy, Economics, Ethics and Public Policy at Georgetown University, Washington, D.C. 20057.

Patrick M. Krueger is a Robert Wood Johnson Health and Society Scholar at the University of Pennsylvania, Philadelphia, Pennsylvania 19104.

Kenneth C. Land is the John Franklin Crowell Professor of Sociology and Demographic Studies at Duke University, Durham, North Carolina 27708.

David P. Lindstrom is Associate Professor of Sociology and Faculty Associate of the Population Studies and Training Center at Brown University, Providence, Rhode Island 02912.

Andrew Mason is Professor of Economics at the University of Hawaii at Manoa and Senior Fellow at the East-West Center, Honolulu, Hawaii 96822.

John F. May is a Senior Population Specialist, Human Development II, Africa Region, at The World Bank, Washington, D.C., 20433.

Michael Micklin is Chief of the Risk, Prevention, and Health Behavior Integrated Review Group, Center for Scientific Review, National Institutes of Health, Bethesda, Maryland 20892. Dr. Micklin contributed to this volume in his personal capacity. The views expressed are his own and do not necessarily represent the views of the National Institutes of Health or the United States Government.

M. Cristina Morales is Assistant Professor of Sociology at the University of Nevada–Las Vegas, Las Vegas, Nevada 89154.

S. Philip Morgan is Professor of Sociology and Chair of the Department at Duke University, Durham, North Carolina 27708.

Peter A. Morrison is Founding Director of the Population Research Center at The RAND Corporation, Santa Monica, California 90407.

Axel I. Mundigo is Director of International Programs at the Center for Health and Social Policy, San Francisco, California 94121.

Daniel A. Powers is Associate Professor of Sociology and Research Associate of the Population Research Center at the University of Texas at Austin, Austin, Texas 78712.

Dudley L. Poston, Jr., is Professor of Sociology and Holder of the George T. and Gladys H. Abell Endowed Professorship in Liberal Arts at Texas A&M University, College Station, Texas 77843.

Joseph E. Potter is Professor of Sociology and Training Director, Population Research Center, at the University of Texas at Austin, Austin, Texas 78712.

Nancy E. Riley is Professor of Sociology at Bowdoin College, Brunswick, Maine 04011.

Richard G. Rogers is Professor of Sociology and Director of the Population Program at the University of Colorado, Boulder, Colorado 80309.

Rogelio Saenz is Professor of Sociology and Head of the Department at Texas A&M University, College Station, Texas 77843.

Arthur Sakamoto is Associate Professor of Sociology and Research Associate of the Population Research Center at the University of Texas at Austin, Austin, Texas 78712.

Stanley K. Smith is Professor of Economics and Director of the Bureau of Economic and Business Research at the University of Florida, Gainesville, Florida 32611.

S. V. Subramanian is Assistant Professor of Society, Human Development, and Health at Harvard University, Boston, Massachusetts 02115.

Teresa A. Sullivan is Executive Vice Chancellor, University of Texas System, and Professor of Sociology and Research Associate of the Population Research Center at the University of Texas at Austin, Austin, Texas 78701.

Michael S. Teitelbaum is Program Director at the Alfred P. Sloan Foundation, New York, New York 10111.

Stewart Tolnay is Professor of Sociology and Chair of the Department at the University of Washington, Seattle, Washington 98195.

Peter Uhlenberg is Professor of Sociology at The University of North Carolina, Chapel Hill, North Carolina 27599.

Etienne van de Walle is Emeritus Professor of Demography and Associate Member of the Population Studies Center at the University of Pennsylvania, Philadelphia, Pennsylvania 19104.

James W. Vaupel is Founding Director of the Max Planck Institute for Demographic Research, Rostock, Germany.

Linda J. Waite is Lucy Flower Professor of Sociology, Director of the Center on Aging, and Co-Director of the Alfred P. Sloan Center on Parents, Children and Work at the University of Chicago, Chicago, Illinois 60637.

David Warner is a Postdoctoral Fellow at the Carolina Population Center, University of North Carolina, Chapel Hill, Chapel Hill, North Carolina 27516.

Michael J. White is Professor of Sociology and Faculty Associate of the Population Studies and Training Center at Brown University, Providence, Rhode Island 02912.

Yang Yang is a Ph.D. Candidate in Sociology and Demography and a Fellow of Program for Advanced Research in the Social Sciences at Duke University, Durham, North Carolina, 27708.

Yi Zeng is Research Professor, Center for Demographic Studies and Department of Sociology, at Duke University, Durham, North Carolina 27708.

Contents

Prologue: The Demographer's Ken: 50 Years of Growth
and Change 1
Michael Micklin and Dudley L. Poston, Jr.

I.   **Population Structure** 17

1.   **Age and Sex** 19
     Dudley L. Poston, Jr.

2.   **Population Distribution and Suburbanization** 59
     Avery M. Guest and Susan K. Brown

3.   **Marriage and Family** 87
     Linda J. Waite

4.   **Demography of Gender** 109
     Nancy E. Riley

5.   **Demography of Aging** 143
     Peter Uhlenberg

6.   **Demography of Race and Ethnicity** 169
     Rogelio Saenz and M. Cristina Morales

7.   **Labor Force** 209
     Teresa A. Sullivan

II. Population Processes 227

 8. Fertility 229
     S. Philip Morgan and Kellie J. Hagewen

 9. Infant Mortality 251
     W. Parker Frisbie

10. Adult Mortality 283
     Richard G. Rogers, Robert A. Hummer and Patrick M. Krueger

11. Internal Migration 311
     Michael J. White and David P. Lindstrom

12. International Migration 347
     Susan K. Brown and Frank D. Bean

13. Demography of Social Stratification 383
     Arthur Sakamoto and Daniel A. Powers

III. Population and the Social Sciences 417

14. Social Demography 419
     Charles Hirschman and Stewart E. Tolnay

15. Organizational and Corporate Demography 451
     Glenn R. Carroll and Olga M. Khessina

16. Urban and Spatial Demography 479
     Mark Fossett

17. Anthropological Demography 525
     David I. Kertzer

18. Economic Demography 549
     Andrew Mason

19. Historical Demography 577
     Etienne Van de Walle

20. Ecological Demography 601
     Dudley L. Poston, Jr., and W. Parker Frisbie

21. Biodemography 625
     James R. Carey and James W. Vaupel

22. Mathematical Demography 659
     Kenneth C. Land, Yang Yang, and Zeng Yi

23. **Political Demography** 719
     Michael S. Teitelbaum

IV. **Applied Demography** 731

24. **Fertility Planning** 733
     Joseph E. Potter and Axel I. Mundigo

25. **Small-Area and Business Demography** 761
     Stanley K. Smith and Peter A. Morrison

26. **Health Demography** 787
     Ichiro Kawachi and S. V. Subramanian

27. **The Demography of Population Health** 809
     Mark D. Hayward and David F. Warner

28. **Population Policy** 827
     John F. May

Epilogue: **Needed Research in Demography** 853
           Dudley L. Poston, Jr., Amanda K. Baumle, and Michael Micklin

Name Index 883

Subject Index 903

Prologue:

The Demographer's Ken: 50 Years of Growth and Change[1]

MICHAEL MICKLIN AND DUDLEY L. POSTON, JR.

INTRODUCTION

The field of demography (also referred to as population studies) has evolved significantly since the mid-twentieth Century. A useful benchmark for gauging the nature and extent of change of the field is Hauser and Duncan's landmark work, *The Study of Population: An Inventory and Appraisal*, published in 1959. The 33 chapters contained in that volume were grouped into four sections. Part I, *Demography as a Science*, contained four chapters laying out the substantive, methodological, epistemological, and organizational foundations of the discipline (Hauser and Duncan 1959a, 1959b, 1959c, 1959d). Part II, *Development and Current Status of Demography*, offered eight chapters portraying the origins and practice of demography in selected nations, along with an insightful overview of disciplinary history (Lorimer 1959). Part III, *Elements of Demography*, included a dozen chapters covering elements of the demographic equation[2] (structure and components of change), as well as assessments of demographic data. Finally, Part IV, *Population Studies in Various Disciplines*, contained seven chapters discussing common interests of demography and selected disciplines, including

---

[1] The notion of the demographer's ken is borrowed from Ryder (1964).
[2] See Davis (1948, pp. 551–594) for the original elaboration of this concept.

sociology (Moore 1959), economics (Spengler 1959), and human ecology (Duncan 1959). See the Epilogue to this *Handbook* by Poston, Baumle, and Micklin for more discussion.

Not surprisingly, this *Handbook* covers many of the same topics as *The Study of Population*, but they are organized a little differently to reflect the evolution of population studies. This Prologue highlights the principal developments in the field during the past 45 years and thus serves at least three purposes. First, it provides an account, albeit abbreviated, of the significant ways in which the demography of today differs from the field on which *The Study of Population* was based—substantively, methodologically, and in terms of its use for public policy guidance. Second, it illustrates how demographic science has expanded to incorporate portions of heretofore peripheral disciplines, resulting in much wider recognition of the significance and impacts of demographic phenomena. Third, it shows how changes in population studies over the past five decades have been influenced by the expansion of the infrastructure on which modern scientific disciplines depend, namely, information, technology, and organizational structures.

THE EVOLUTION OF DEMOGRAPHY:
CA. 1950–2000

A commonly recognized definition of *demography* is "the study of the size, territorial distribution, and composition of population, changes therein, and the components of such changes, ... [namely], natality, mortality, territorial movement, and social mobility [change of status]" (Hauser and Duncan 1959d).[3] How this activity, the study of population, is carried out, and the results it produces, depend on a set of disciplinary resources.[4]

Demographic theories and models are statements of the evident or hypothesized course, causes, and/or consequences of these phenomena at varying levels of aggregation (Coale and Trussell 1996; Coleman and Schofield 1986; Hauser and Duncan 1959b).

Demographic methods comprise a body of procedures and techniques for collecting, evaluating, adjusting, estimating, and analyzing demographic data, while d*emographic materials* consist of the sources of raw data such as censuses, vital registration systems, population registers, and sample surveys (Hauser and Duncan 1959a; also see Siegel and Swanson 2004).

The *infrastructure of demography* consists of the professional organizations, modes of disseminating ideas and research findings, and institutional sources of research support that influence the kinds of work done under the banner of the discipline and how the results are portrayed and received.

Finally, *demographic praxis* refers to the use of demographic data and research findings by governments, businesses, and other organizations for predicting, planning, monitoring, and evaluating a wide range of demographic and nondemographic conditions, events, and trends (Siegel 2002).

---

[3] As of 2004, the front cover of the journal *Demography*, the official journal of the Population Association of America, offers a concise definition: "the statistical study of human populations."

[4] The resources listed are probably important for the operation of most, if not all, disciplines, but do not exhaust the class of resources that might be mentioned. For an interesting discussion of the context and social structure of scientific disciplines see Abbott, 2001, Chapter 5, though he is more interested in relations among disciplines than in the kinds of resources that make disciplinary activity possible.

The Trend of Population Parameters

One approach to understanding the changes that have taken place in the field of demography over the past half century is to consider the differences in major demographic indicators between then and now. This strategy is based on the assumption that one factor underlying shifts of disciplinary research emphasis is the evolution of important population parameters. Selected demographic indicators for the world, the more developed and less developed regions, and the least developed nations, are shown in Table 1.

Several conclusions may be drawn. Over the past five decades the population of the world increased by about 150%. The bulk of the change was concentrated in the less developed regions, with the greatest proportional increase in the poorest nations. Nonetheless, there was a significant reduction in the annual rate of population growth, particularly in the more developed regions. Only the least developed countries showed an increase in the population growth rate during this period, surpassing that for the less developed regions as a whole.

These changes in population size and growth parameters were due largely to shifts in the two principal components of growth, i.e., fertility and mortality. Between 1950 and the turn of the century the total fertility rate showed a marked decrease at the global level and for both the more and less developed regions, and a decrease of about half that amount in the least developed countries. The infant mortality rate, often used as a key indicator of the well-being of a population, showed a sizeable decline in all the major regions, though the more developed region versus less developed region differential remains substantial. Life expectancy at birth, another commonly used index of social well-being, showed substantial progress, particularly in the less developed regions. These trends in fertility and mortality combined to produce a clear trend of population aging. The median age increased in all but the least developed countries, with a sharp increase evident in the more developed regions.

Finally, significant changes are evident in two indicators of population distribution. The percentage of population living in urban localities increased considerably, especially in the less developed regions, though the overall proportion of population that is urban is still substantially higher in the more developed regions. Not surprisingly, population density also increased, with the proportional increase and the absolute level highest in the less developed regions.

These trends and differentials suggest that while some contemporary demographers have continued to focus on the issues that concerned their predecessors in the 1950s, namely, the description and explanation of fertility, mortality, and migration differentials, between and within population aggregates, the contours of demographic science have probably shifted as a consequence of emerging population patterns. One would expect that concerns related to population conditions and trends in the developing world, particularly in the least developed nations, grew over the past half century. Increased size, density, and urban concentration constitute population problems that require increased demographic understanding and, moreover, call for the use of demographic knowledge to formulate remedial actions. The observed demographic trends in the more developed regions also point to emerging topics for demographic research, e.g., population aging and its consequences.

In short, global, regional, and national demographic conditions have changed substantially since the publication of *The Study of Population*. A reassessment of the

TABLE 1. Selected Demographic Indicators by Aggregated Areas, Ca. 1950 and 2003[1]

Indicators and Areas	Ca. 1950	Ca. 2003	Percent Change, Ca. 1950–2003
Total Population[2]			
World	2519	6301	150
MDRs[3]	813	1203	48
LDRs[4]	1706	5098	199
Least DCs[5]	200	851	326
Population Growth[6]			
World	1.8	1.2	−22
MDRs	1.2	0.2	−83
LDRs	2.0	1.5	−25
Least DCs	1.9	2.4	26
TFR[7]			
World	5.0	2.7	−46
MDRs	2.8	1.6	−43
LDRs	6.1	2.9	−52
Least DCs	6.6	5.1	−23
IMR[8]			
World	156	55	−65
MDRs	59	7	−88
LDRs	179	61	−66
Least DCs	194	**[9]	**
Life Expectancy[10]			
World	46	65	41
MDRs	66	76	15
LDRs	41	63	54
Least DCs	36	50	39
Median Age			
World	24	26	8
MDRs	29	37	28
LDRs	21	24	14
Least DCs	19	18	−5
Percent Urban[11]			
World	30	47	57
MDRs	55	75	36
LDRs	18	40	122
Least DCs	**	**	**
Population Density[12]			
World	19	46	142
MDRs	15	23	53
LDRs	21	62	195
Least DCs	10	35	250

[1] *Sources*: United Nations, *World Population Prospects: The 1994 Revision*, Appendix II; United Nations, *World Population Prospects: The 2002 Revision*, Annex Tables; United Nations, *World Urbanization Prospects: The 2001 Revision*, Annex Tables; Population Reference Bureau, *2003 World Population Data Sheet*.
[2] In thousands.
[3] More Developed Regions.
[4] Less Developed Regions.
[5] Least Developed Countries.
[6] Annual percent change, 1950–1955 and 2000–2003.
[7] Total fertility rate per woman, 1950–1955 and 2000–2003.
[8] Infant mortality rate, 1950–1955 and 2000–2005.
[9] Not reported.
[10] Life expectancy at birth, both sexes, 1950–1955 and 2000–2003.
[11] 1950 and 2000.
[12] Per square kilometer.

state of demographic knowledge and research trends is long overdue. This a principal objective of the chapters that follow in this *Handbook*.

The Development of Disciplinary Resources

The progress of any scientific discipline depends on the adequacy of its fundamental resources: theories, methods, and data.[5] Theories provide the basis for selection of research topics and statement of hypotheses to be tested. Methods encompass a set of standardized procedures for the collection and analysis of data, thus increasing confidence in the validity and reliability of research findings. Data are the raw materials of scientific inquiry, the observations and indicators of conditions, trends, and differentials in the empirical world. The past 50 years of demographic science show significant, though probably uneven, progress in each of these basic disciplinary resources.

DEMOGRAPHIC THEORIES AND MODELS.   The period surrounding the publication of *The Study of Population* produced a variety of views on the status of population theory. In 1952 Rupert Vance, in his presidential address to the Population Association of America, lamented the "poverty" of high theory in demography (Vance 1952). Only a decade later Robert Gutman wrote "in defense" of population theory, contending that "demography ... continues to offer illuminating theoretical statements which organize knowledge, lead to the acquisition of new knowledge, and help in the solution of population problems" (Gutman 1960). Hauser and Duncan (1959b: 89–102) identified several important population theories, including those derived from Malthus, optimum population theory, demographic transition theory, and psychosocial theories of fertility. Nonetheless, they concluded their discussion by stating that "demographers in general may have much to gain from additional allocation of energy to deliberate efforts directed toward theory-construction in conjunction with the conduct of empirical research (1959b: 104).

Recent assessments of the discipline of demography show similar ambivalence about the adequacy of population theories. Writing in 1979, Charles Nam argued "the issues of demographic journals today are replete with theoretically based articles, in stark contrast to those of the past. We no longer fall behind our fellow disciplines in theoretical development, and a merging of lower-order propositions into a theoretical whole is now as conceivable in demography as in any of the social sciences."

Yet, a decade and a half later Eileen Crimmins (1993: 587) stated that "although our theoretical approaches are considerably more complex now than in the past, demography still has highly developed theories in only a few areas. Fertility behavior is the exception."[6] Other population scientists point to demographic transition theory as the theoretical staple of the discipline (Caldwell 1997; Kirk 1996; Lee 2003).

It is the opinion of the authors of this Prologue that on the one hand, although a variety of new or reformulated population theories have been proposed over the past half century, their clarification and evaluation remain a challenge for the field. On the

---

[5] Dudley Kirk (1960, p. 309) wrote that "The study of population is at once a body of data, a methodology, and a bundle of generalizations concerning the causes and consequences of demographic phenomena."

[6] Note, however, that there is no consensus on the adequacy of fertility theory. See, for example, Stolnitz, 1983; Mason, 1993; Hirschman, 1994; Szreter, 1994; van de Kaa, 1996; and Caldwell, 1997.

other hand, demography has such an abundance of both formal theory and discursive theory that its theoretical accomplishments rival those of any of the other social sciences. Regarding formal theory, one need only consider, for instance, the richness and precision of stable population theory. Regarding discursive theory, there are few social sciences that may claim as much discursive theory as one finds in, say, the demographic study of fertility. Prominent theories to explain fertility behavior include demographic transition theory, wealth flows theory, human ecological theory, political economic theory, feminist theory, proximate determinants theory, biosocial theory, relative income theory, and diffusion theory. The view among nondemographers 50 years ago that demography is void of theory was incorrect then and is incorrect today.

DEMOGRAPHIC METHODS. There is agreement among demographers about the significant advances that have occurred in the past 50 years in methods of data collection and analysis. Hauser and Duncan (1959a) covered standard census procedures, vital registration systems, the sample survey, rudimentary data processing, and several types of administrative record systems. They also discussed techniques for evaluating, adjusting, estimating, and analyzing demographic data.

Each of the techniques covered in *The Study of Population* has been improved, partly through the application of advances in electronic information systems. National census taking is increasingly based on statistical sampling theory and techniques, particularly in the more developed nations, resulting in more efficient and accurate data collection. Perhaps due to the importance of demographic data for administrative decisions, there have also been improvements in collection procedures in the less developed countries (Cleland 1996).

Over the past five decades the uncertain quality and availability of demographic data have led to development of a variety of techniques for evaluating, adjusting, estimating, and projecting population parameters (Ahlburg and Lutz 1998; Ahlburg, Lutz, and Vaupel 1998; Brass 1996; Coale and Demeny 1968; Keyfitz 1975; Keyfitz 1981; Siegel and Swanson 2004). Although the results of many of these exercises, particularly population forecasts, are notoriously inaccurate, their use continues. As an example, one need only to recall that in 2003 the United Nations issued to significant acclaim a set of global and regional population projections to the year 2300.

DEMOGRAPHIC MATERIALS. This set of basic disciplinary resources can be divided into *primary data sources* and *data compendia*, e.g., data banks. The most comprehensive and generalizable primary data source is the national population census. National census coverage has improved considerably since the end of World War II, largely through assistance provided to developing country governments by the United Nations and a few other organizations such as the U.S. Census Bureau. Among 94 developing countries with a population of at least one million, only 49 conducted a national population census in the decade of the 1950s; by the 1990s that figure had risen to 71 countries (Cleland 1996).[7]

---

[7] The decade with the largest number of censuses conducted in these countries was the 1980s, with a total of 79.

The content, completeness, and accuracy of information collected through the census method continue to vary widely from one country to the next. Overall, however, the situation has surely improved worldwide.

Another important source of information is the civil registration system, which typically collects information on demographic events such as births, deaths, and changes of civil status as they occur. Though not 100% accurate and complete, vital registration in the more developed nations is far better than in the poor nations. Cleland (1996: 435) contends that although civil registration systems in developing countries are "seriously defective, it would not be correct that the data are of little value to demographers." Techniques have been developed for data adjustment and analysis, yielding a rough notion of trends and differentials in vital events.

Beginning in the 1970s, coordinated cross-national surveys emerged as an important source of demographic information. Between 1974 and 1986 sample surveys of reproductive behavior and related social and psychological indicators were conducted in 62 countries, representing 40 percent of the world's population, under the auspices of the World Fertility Survey (Cleland and Hobcroft 1985; Cleland and Scott 1987). This effort was succeeded by another coordinated international program of research, the Demographic and Health Surveys, with 170 sample surveys carried out in 69 developing countries between 1986 and 2003. The obvious advantage of these survey programs was the opportunity for comparative analysis and generalization of findings beyond a single population.

Less ambitious demographic surveys, typically focusing on a single country or community, have been a part of the demographer's repertoire for many decades. Early studies included the Indianapolis study (Kiser 1953; Kiser and Whelpton 1953), the Princeton study (Westoff, Potter, and Sagi 1963; Westoff et al. 1961), and surveys of family and reproductive behavior carried out in Puerto Rico (Hill, Stycos, and Back 1959; Stycos 1955). The number of demographic surveys has grown steadily over the years. Examples in the United States include the monthly Current Population Survey, the weekly health interview survey, and the various rounds of the National Survey of Family Growth carried out by the National Center for Health Statistics. Another important source of demographic information is the Adolescent Health Survey, begun in the early 1990s by the Carolina Population Center.

In short, over the past 50 years there has been an enormous increase in the availability of primary demographic data. The data quality of various sources differs somewhat, but the trend has been toward better coverage and reduced error in census enumeration and collection of survey data. Moreover, the development of techniques to estimate missing values or reduce measurement error has increased the utility of these sources of demographic information.

Another welcome addition to the disciplinary resources of demography is the growing availability of repositories for demographic data. Some of these collections are long-standing, such as the *Demographic Yearbook* published by the United Nations since 1948. Over the years the U.N. Population Division has increased its publication and distribution of very useful demographic information. The currently recurring population publications include *World Population Prospects, World Urbanization Prospects, World Contraceptive Use, The State of World Population,* and *National Population Policies.* A variety of other organizations, some part of the U.N., also provide recurring population-related data sets, including *HIV/AIDS Epidemic Update* (UNAIDS), *Human Development Report* (United Nations Development Programme), *Global Environmental*

Outlook (United Nations Environment Programme), *State of the World's Children* (UNICEF), *The State of Food and Agriculture* (Food and Agriculture Organization), the *Yearbook of Labour Statistics* (International Labour Organization), *World Development Report* (World Bank), and *World Health Report* (World Health Organization). Collectively, these publications offer a wide range of global, regional, and national demographic and population-related statistics covering at least several decades. Of course, the user must pay close attention to definitions, units of coverage, and specific measures, and the fact that they frequently vary from one publication to another.

In addition, there are a number of other organizations that provide comparable data sets. The International Division of the U.S. Bureau of the Census offers the International Data Base, an on-line data bank of country-level demographic information covering a range of years. The Population Reference Bureau publishes an annual *World Population Data Sheet*. And the World Resources Institute issues a biennial *World Resources* report containing a wealth of global, regional, and national environmental data.

A very important source of national census microsurveys via the Internet is the Integrated Public Use Microdata Series (IPUMS), created at the University of Minnesota in October 1997. As of the writing of this Prologue (June 2004), the U.S.–IPUMS consists of 27 high-precision samples of the American population drawn from 14 U.S. censuses that span the censuses of 1850 to 2000. U.S. American Community Survey microfiles and U.S. Current Population Survey microfiles are also accessible. In 2002 the IPUMS was expanded to include census microfiles from other countries. Currently available are data from censuses from many countries of the world for several census rounds. The U.S. and international microsurveys are easily accessible on the Internet via the IPUMS web page. The ease and speed with which the census microdata are available from IPUMS have truly revolutionized demographic research, particularly for researchers not located in the half dozen or so large demography centers. IPUMS has provided virtually all demographers the opportunity to participate in "big science" demographic research.

Overall, the volume of demographic and population-related information resources has grown dramatically during the past half century, particularly over the last two decades. The research-oriented demographer has virtually unlimited access to multiple data banks and statistical yearbooks, many of them via the Internet (see below). Used judiciously, this rapidly increasing set of resources provides a means of examining linkages between population conditions and trends and a wide range of societal phenomena.

The Infrastructure of Demography

Development of any scientific discipline depends to an increasing extent on its organizational infrastructure, which includes several components. In the case of demography these are the following: (1) professional and affiliated organizations, (2) professional journals that serve as outlets for results of demographic research; and, most recently, (3) Internet sites that facilitate communication among demographers, access to research ideas and reports, and retrieval of demographic data; and (4) the application of knowledge produced to resolve societal problems. Each of these infrastructure components has shown dramatic development since the publication 45 years ago of *The Study of Population*.

PROFESSIONAL ORGANIZATIONS. The oldest professional association of population scientists is the International Union for the Study of Population (IUSSP).[8] The Union was founded officially in Paris in 1928, following the 1927 International Population Conference in Geneva. In 1947 the IUSSP was reorganized as an association of 147 individual members representing 32 countries. By 1994 the IUSSP had grown to more than 2,000 members, an increasing number of them from developing nations. The IUSSP represents itself as a purely scientific organization; it does not hold particular points of view on population issues and does not lobby on behalf of specific population policies (Mertens 1994: 1). The basic organizational unit of the IUSSP is the research committee, of which there may be 10 to 15 at a given time, each devoted to a substantive demographic research topic. The IUSSP publishes a set of monographs covering diverse topics related to population; many are the result of scientific meetings sponsored by the IUSSP. The full meetings of the IUSSP are held every four years.

Shortly after the launch of the IUSSP, the Population Association of America (PAA) was organized in 1931 with 38 original members.[9] By 1955 membership numbered 430, and at the date of the 68th annual meeting in 2003 the organization had nearly 3,000 members. Annual meetings of the PAA are devoted to presentation and discussion of research reports and theoretical papers, some of which are published in the PAA's official quarterly journal, *Demography*.

In 1983 the European Association for Population Studies (EAPS) was founded.[10] EAPS is an international, interdisciplinary forum for population studies, with a special focus on Europe's population, and is affiliated with the IUSSP and the Committee for International Cooperation in National Research in Demography (CICRED). It organizes conferences, seminars, and workshops, and disseminates population-related information. EAPS publishes the *European Journal of Population*.

The Southern Demographic Association is a scientific and educational corporation of the Commonwealth of Virginia.[11] Organized in 1971 as the Southern Regional Demographic Group, the SDA has approximately 200 members. The group's research interests are national and international in scope. The SDA also encourages the demographic study of the Southern United States and also provides a forum for the discussion and presentation of issues of state and local demography. The SDA publishes a journal, *Population Research and Policy Review*.

The professional associations listed above certainly do not exhaust those that exist worldwide. These descriptions are intended to illustrate the variety of activities undertaken by such organizations and to suggest that while not as large as many scientific disciplines, demography is a viable and flourishing profession.

AFFILIATED ORGANIZATIONS. More or less loosely linked with the professional demographic organizations, and with the discipline as a whole, are various organizations that perform one or more functions that contribute to the activities of demographers. These functions include (1) funding demographic research, (2) public advocacy of important demographic and population-related issues and/or policy concerns, (3) dissemination of

---

[8] This information is taken from Mertens, 1994.
[9] Information about the PAA is provided on the organization's website.
[10] Information about the EAPS is provided on the organization's website.
[11] Information about the SDA is provided on the organization's website.

demographic data and research findings, (4) population education, and (5) delivery of services to address population problems and improve population health.

For nearly 75 years the Population Reference Bureau (PRB) in Washington, D.C. has been providing information and support for population activities.[12] Currently, PRB's principal efforts include (1) publishing, disseminating, and promoting print and electronic materials on population issues, (2) collaborating with other organizations to develop and implement strategies for communicating with policy makers, (3) conducting training on policy communications and Internet use, and (4) collaborating with journalists to expand the coverage of population, health, and environmental subjects. The PRB quarterly *Population Bulletin* has been published for nearly 60 years, with each issue devoted to the analysis of a timely demographic issue.

The Population Council in New York City was established in 1952 with the objective of developing a better understanding of population problems.[13] The Council contains three research divisions: the Center for Biomedical Research, the International Programs Division, and the Policy Research Division. Branch offices are located in 19 countries, and Council research is conducted in another 51 countries. The Council's research efforts are concentrated in three areas: biomedical science, social science, and public health. In 1975 the organization launched a new journal, the *Population and Development Review*, now recognized as the premier periodical in the field of population studies. The Population Council also publishes the quarterly *Studies in Family Planning*.

The International Planned Parenthood Federation (IPPF) in London is an umbrella organization, founded in Bombay in 1952, linking autonomous national family planning associations in more than 180 countries.[14] IPPF activities focus on (1) meeting the family planning service needs of families around the world, (2) promoting sexual and reproductive health, (3) eliminating unsafe abortion, (4) promoting equality and empowerment for women, (5) helping youth understand their sexuality and providing them with needed services, and (6) maintaining high standards of care throughout the Federation.

Another organization, the Alan Guttmacher Institute (AGI) in Washington, D.C., focuses on research on sexual and reproductive health in the United States and other countries.[15] Founded in 1968, AGI's programs encompass social science research, policy analysis, and public education. AGI publishes two widely circulated journals, *Perspectives on Sexual and Reproductive Health* (formerly *Family Planning Perspectives*) and *International Family Planning Perspectives*.

An alternative type of population-affiliated organization is seen in Population Action International (PAI), an independent policy advocacy group working to strengthen public awareness of population issues and promote political and financial support worldwide for population programs.[16] PAI activities concentrate on advancing universal access to family planning programs through an integrated program of research, advocacy, and communications.

There are many other organizations that fit this category. The number has increased substantially over the past three decades. The information provided on the small sample described above illustrates the variety of functions they provide to

[12] Information about PRB is provided at the organization's website.
[13] Information about the Population Council is provided at the organization's website.
[14] Information about the IPPF is provided at the organization's website.
[15] Information about AGI is provided at the organization's website.
[16] Information about PAI is provided at the organization's website.

demographers and the discipline of demography. In short, these affiliated organizations constitute a significant portion of the social infrastructure of demography, which is much more obvious today than 50 years ago.

DEMOGRAPHIC PERIODICALS.   In the 1950s demographers had few specialized periodical outlets for their work. Most demographic research was published in journals of sociology and economics. The only demographic journals available were the Italian journal *Genus* (1934), the *Population Index* (1935)[17] (which was devoted primarily to bibliographic references), the Population Reference Bureau's *Population Bulletin* (1945), the British journal *Population Studies* (1947), and the Indian journal *Population Review* (1957). There was a slow but steady increase in the 1960s in periodicals devoted to population studies. *Studies in Family Planning*, published by the Population Council, made its appearance in 1963. A year later the first issue of the official journal of the Population Association of America, *Demography*, appeared along with initial publication of the *International Migration Review*. In 1969 the Alan Guttmacher Institute issued the first volume of *Family Planning Perspectives* and followed it in 1975 with the *International Family Planning Digest* (which would soon be called *International Family Planning Perspectives*). The Population Council's creation of the *Population and Development Review* in 1975 was a major addition to demography's journal repertoire. Later debuts of demographic journals included *Population and Environment* (1978), *Population Research and Policy Review* (1981), the *European Journal of Population* (1985), *Journal of Population* Economics (1987), the English edition of the French journal *Population* (1989), *Demographic Research* (1999) and *Applied Population and Policy* (2004). Clearly, demographers of today have more opportunities to publish results of their research in discipline-friendly periodicals.

DEMOGRAPHY AND THE INTERNET.   A recent review of the social implications of the Internet overlooks its effects on the evolution of scientific disciplines (DiMaggio et al. 2001). Considering the case of demography, one cannot help but be impressed with changes in the infrastructure of the discipline resulting from Internet access. A recent article by Thomas Gryn (1997) reviews Internet resources available to demographers. However, given the rate of change of web addresses and the addition of new sites, the sources listed cannot be up-to-date. Accordingly, it would be futile to devote a great deal of space here to site reference[18]—except for the following useful sites, which are likely to remain stable.

The United Nations operates a Population Information Network (POPIN) at *http://www.un.org/popin/*. POPIN includes a list of relevant publications from UN and affiliated organizations, as well as a list of journals and newsletters that contain population content. The Population Reference Bureau operates a site (POPNET) *http://www.popnet.org/* that includes links to a wealth of organizational sources (international, nongovernmental, university centers, associations, directories, listservs, and databases). The Office of Population Research of Princeton University provides access

---

[17] The figure in parentheses is the year of initial publication. The *Population Index* was known as *Population Literature* until 1937.
[18] However, Gryn mentions a supplementary web site for the paper at http://members.tripod.com/~tgryn/demog.html.

to its *Population Index site (http://popindex.princeton.edu/index.html)* with regular coverage of 400 journals. Finally, the Committee for International Cooperation in National Research in Demography (CICRED) offers access to a wide range of information.

Demographic Praxis

The Study of Population makes little reference to applications of demographic knowledge. Over the past half century, however, circumstances have changed dramatically. Applied demography is a thriving enterprise, providing employment for a sizeable number of demographers (Micklin 1992; Siegel 2002). Three varieties of applied demographic activity will be mentioned here.

First, demographers have served as advisors, witnesses, and technicians on matters of political redistricting. Over time, populations become redistributed within political jurisdictions. Periodically, the decision is made to reassess the correspondence between population distribution and voting districts. In such cases, demographic expertise is invaluable.

Second, increased size and rate of population growth as well as population density have been linked to environmental deterioration, particularly in less developed nations. Demographers are frequently called to participate in multidisciplinary teams and given the responsibility of developing a plan to halt the environmental damage.

Third, demographers are often asked to provide various types of population forecasts in conjunction with community development programs. Large-scale expansion of transportation facilities and construction of residential structures are likely to change patterns of population growth, distribution, and perhaps composition. Officials need research to estimate the extent of disruption that will occur.

AN ASSESSMENT OF THE PROGRESS OF DEMOGRAPHY

There can be little doubt that the field of demography has changed since *The Study of Population* was published 45 years ago. One difference, and not a trivial one, is that many more people are trained in, and practicing, demography than there were in 1959. That fact, combined with the significant increase in opportunities to offer demographic conclusions and advice, means that people generally are more familiar with demographic issues and presumed problems.

Second, demographic issues are found today in a much wider range of disciplines. In 1959, demographic training was largely limited to sociologists and economists. Today, demographic expertise is found among many social and behavioral science disciplines, e.g., political science, anthropology, urban planning, psychology, public health, and environmental science. The 10 chapters in Part III of this *Handbook* on "Population and the Social Sciences" are a testament to the diffusion of demography throughout the social sciences in the past half century.

Third, the tools of the discipline, namely, the techniques for collecting and analyzing data, are much more precise, complex, and powerful than in the past. Before the 1970s, demographers were restricted to a few focused demographic methods texts, including Cox's *Demography*, first published 1950 with a fifth and final edition published in 1976 (Cox 1976), Spiegelman's *Introduction to Demography*, first published in 1955 with a revised edition published in 1968 (Spiegelman 1968), and Barclay's *Techniques of Population Analysis* (Barclay 1958). The publication in 1971 of the comprehensive two-volume edition of *The Methods and Materials of Demography* (Shryock and Siegel and Associates 1971) was heralded by demographers and social scientists. A one-volume condensed edition of "*M&M*" was published in 1976 (Shryock and Siegel and Associates 1976). Almost 30 years later the second edition of this masterpiece was published (Siegel and Swanson 2004). In the meanwhile, in 1981, Pollard, Yusuf, and Pollard's (1981) *Demographic Techniques* was published, followed by two editions, with the third published in 1990. Important demographic methods texts published in the 1990s and later include Smith's (1992) *Formal Demography*, Halli and Rao's (1992) *Advanced Techniques of Population Analysis*, Hinde's (1998) *Demographic Methods*, Preston, Heuveline, and Guillot's (2001) *Demography: Measuring and Modeling Population Processes*, and Rowland's (2003) *Demographic Methods*.

Fourth, the volume and variety of demographic and related data available are far greater than ever before. This situation is both an opportunity and a danger, calling for the careful assessment of data quality. Finally, the principal issues calling for demographic analysis have changed. Population aging, effects of population change on the natural environment, and persisting social and economic inequalities related to population size and growth are the demographic issues of import for today. Many of these are addressed in various chapters in this *Handbook*.

REFERENCES

Abbott, A. 2001. *Chaos of disciplines*. Chicago: University of Chicago Press.

Ahlburg, D. A., and W. Lutz. 1998. Introduction: The need to rethink approaches to population forecasts. *Population and Development Review* 24(Supplement: Frontiers of Population Forecasting): 1–14.

Ahlburg, D. A., W. Lutz, and J. W. Vaupel. 1998. Ways to improve population forecasting: What should be done differently in the future? *Population and Development Review* 24(Supplement: Frontiers of population forecasting): 191–198.

Barclay, G. W. 1958. *Techniques of population analysis*. New York: John Wiley.

Brass, W. 1996. Demographic data analysis in less developed countries, 1946–1996. *Population Studies* 50(3):451–467.

Caldwell, J. C. 1997. The global fertility transition: The need for a unifying theory. *Population and Development Review* 23(4):803–812.

Cleland, J. 1996. Demographic data collection in less developed countries, 1946–1996. *Population Studies* 50(3):433–450.

Cleland, J., and J. Hobcroft. 1985. Reproductive change in developing countries: Insights from the world fertility survey. New York: Oxford University Press.

Cleland, J., and C. Scott. 1987. The world fertility survey: An assessment. New York: Oxford University Press.

Coale, A. J., and P. Demeny. 1968. *Methods of evaluating basic demographic measures from limited and defective data*. New York: United Nations.

Coale, A. J., and J. Trussell. 1996. The development and use of demographic models. *Population Studies* 50(3):469–484.

Coleman, D., and R. Schofield. 1986. *The state of population theory: Forward from Malthus*. Oxford: Basil Blackwell.

Cox, P. R. 1976. *Demography*. 5th ed. New York: Cambridge University Press.

Crimmins, E. M. 1993. Demography: The past 30 years, the present, and the future. *Demography* 30(4):579–591.

Davis, K. 1948. *Human society*. New York: Macmillan.

DiMaggio, P., E. Hargittai, W. R. Neuman, and J. P. Robinson. 2001. Social implications of the Internet. *Annual Review of Sociology* 27:307–336.

Duncan, O. D. 1959. Human ecology and population studies. In *The study of population: An inventory and appraisal*, edited by P. M. Hauser and O. D. Duncan, 678–716. Chicago: University of Chicago Press.

Gryn, T. A. 1997. Internet resources for demographers. *Population Index* 63(2):189–204.

Gutman, R. 1960. In defense of population theory. *American Sociological Review* 25(3):325–333.

Halli, S. S., and K. V. Rao. 1992. *Advanced Techniques of Population Analysis*. New York: Plenum Press.

Hauser, P. M., and O. D. Duncan. 1959a. The data and methods. In *The study of population: An inventory and appraisal*, edited by P. M. Hauser and O. D. Duncan, 45–75. Chicago: University of Chicago Press.

Hauser, P. M., and O. D. Duncan. 1959b. Demography as a body of knowledge. In *The study of population: An inventory and appraisal*, edited by P. M. Hauser and O. D. Duncan, 76–105. Chicago: University of Chicago Press.

Hauser, P. M., and O. D. Duncan. 1959c. Demography as a profession. In *The study of population: An inventory and appraisal*, edited by P. M. Hauser and O. D. Duncan. Chicago: University of Chicago Press.

Hauser, P. M., and O. D. Duncan. 1959d. The nature of demography. In *The study of population: An inventory and appraisal*, edited by P. M. Hauser and O. D. Duncan, 29–44. Chicago: University of Chicago Press.

Hill, R., J. M. Stycos, and K. Back. 1959. *The family and population control: A Puerto Rican experiment in social change*. Chapel Hill: University of North Carolina Press.

Hinde, A. 1998. *Demographic methods*. New York: Edward Arnold Publishers.

Hirschman, C. 1994. Why fertility changes. *Annual Review of Sociology* 20:203–233.

Keyfitz, N. 1975. How do we know the facts of demography? *Population and Development Review* 1(2):267–288.

Keyfitz, N. 1981. The limits of population forecasting. *Population and Development Review* 7(4):579–593.

Kirk, D. 1960. Some reflections on American demography in the nineteen sixties. *Population Index* 26(4):305–310.

Kirk, D. 1996. Demographic transition theory. *Population Studies* 50(3):361–387.

Kiser, C. V. 1953. The Indianapolis fertility study—an example of planned observational research. *Public Opinion Quarterly* 17(4):496–510.

Kiser, C. V., and P. K. Whelpton. 1953. Resume of the Indianapolis study of social and psychological factors affecting fertility. *Population Studies* 7(2):95–110.

Lee, R. 2003. The demographic transition: Three centuries of fundamental change. *Journal of Economic Perspectives* 17(4):167–190.

Lorimer, F. 1959. The development of demography. In *The study of population: An inventory and appraisal*, edited by P. M. Hauser and O. D. Duncan, 124–179. Chicago: University of Chicago Press.

Mason, K. O. 1997. Explaining fertility transitions. *Demography* 34(4):443–454.

Mertens, W. 1994. The context of IUSSP contribution to the International Conference on Population and Development, 1–14. Liége, Belgium: International Union for the Scientific Study of Population.

Micklin, M. 1992. LDC population policies: A challenge for applied demography. *Journal of Applied Sociology* 9(1):45–63.

Moore, W. E. 1959. Sociology and demography. In *The study of population: An inventory and appraisal*, edited by P. M. Hauser and O. D. Duncan, 832–851. Chicago: University of Chicago Press.

Nam, C. B. 1979. The progress of demography as a scientific discipline. *Demography* 16(4):485–492.

Pollard, A. H., F. Yusuf, and G. N. Pollard. 1981. Demographic Techniques. New York: Pergamon.

Preston, S., P. Heuveline, and M. Guillot. 2001. *Demography: Measuring and modeling population processes*. Malden, Mass.: Blackwell Publishers.

Rowland, D. T. 2003. Demographic methods and concepts. New York: Oxford University Press.

Shryock, H. S., J. S. Siegel, and Associates. 1971. *The methods and materials of demography*. 2 vols: Washington, D.C.: U.S. Government Printing Office.

Shryock, H. S., J. S. Siegel, and Associates. 1976. *The methods and materials of demography*. Condensed ed. by E. G. Stockwell. New York: Academic Press.

Siegel, J. S. 2002. *Applied demography: Applications to business, government, law and public policy*. San Diego: Academic Press.

Siegel, J. S., and D. Swanson. 2004. *The methods and materials of demography*. 2d ed. Boston: Academic Press.

Smith, D. P. 1992. *Formal demography*. New York: Plenum Press.

Spengler, J. J. 1959. Economics and demography. In *The study of population: An inventory and appraisal*, edited by P. M. Hauser and O. D. Duncan, 791–851. Chicago: University of Chicago Press.

Spiegelman, M. 1968. *Introduction to demography*. Rev. ed. Cambridge, Mass.: Harvard University Press.

Stolnitz, G. J. 1983. Three to five main challenges to demographic research. *Demography* 20(4):415–432.

Stycos, J. M. 1955. *Family and fertility in Puerto Rico: A study of the lower income group.* New York: Columbia University Press.

Szreter, S. 1993. The idea of demographic transition and the study of fertility change—a critical intellectual history. *Population and Development Review* 19(4):659–701.

van de Kaa, D. J. 1996. Anchored narratives: The story and findings of half a century of research into the determinants of fertility. *Population Studies* 50(3):389–432.

Vance, R. B. 1952. Is theory for demographers? *Social Forces* 31(1):9–13.

Westoff, C. F., J. Potter, and P. Sagi. 1963. *The third child: A study in the prediction of fertility.* Princeton, N.J.: Princeton University Press.

Westoff, C. F., J. Potter, P. Sagi, and E. G. Mishler. 1961. *Family growth in metropolitan America.* Princeton, N.J.: Princeton University Press.

PART I

POPULATION STRUCTURE

The basic population model, according to Ryder (1964), consists of a "...web of structures and processes." The first section of this *Handbook* is devoted to the topic of population structure, which encompasses population size, composition, and distribution.

The notion of "structure" is a fundamental element of all efforts to formulate a science of human society, extending from the nineteenth century ideas of Spencer, Marx, Durkheim, and Simmel (Turner 1975, 1984, 1985, 1998) to contemporary theories of societal organization (Blau 1974, 1977, 1994, 2001; Giddens 1984; Mark 1998). The central idea underlying theories of social and demographic structure is that the number, types, and relative proportion of parameters forming the structural context provide both constraints and opportunities that affect individual and collective action. For example, it has been argued that a high rate of female employment reduces the amount of time and other resources women can devote to maternal activities, one consequence of which is a lower fertility rate (Bernhardt 1993; Mason and Palan 1981; Standing 1978). Another theory suggests that "the strength of ethnically based organizations is...an especially powerful determinant of the likelihood of ethnic collective action" (Hechter, Friedman and Appelbaum 1982). Generally, the full range of indicators of demographic structure—size, composition (e.g., age, sex, civil status, household structure, race and ethnicity, employment, income and education), and distribution—are important considerations for the assessment of human needs and the explanation of individual and collective behavior.

The Study of Population contains four chapters clearly devoted to demographic structure. They include general assessments of population composition (Hawley 1959) and population distribution (Bogue 1959) as well as the consideration of selected dimensions of labor force (Jaffe 1959), and family structure (Glick 1959).

This *Handbook* offers seven chapters devoted to population structure. In chapter 1, Poston covers age and sex composition, dimensions that many social scientists believe to be the most elementary basis of societal organization (e.g., Davis 1948: 98–110). In chapter 2, Guest and Brown review developments in the study of population distribution, with an emphasis on suburban structure. Waite provides in chapter 3 an overview of the growing field of family and household demography, and Riley focuses in chapter 4 on the related topic of gender roles. In chapter 5 Uhlenberg addresses population aging, believed by many demographers to be among the most significant forces for demographic and social change in recent decades. In chapter 6 Saenz and Morales examine recent work reflecting the longstanding concern with consequences of variation in the racial and ethnic composition of populations. Finally, Part I concludes with Sullivan's examination in chapter 7 of population structure in terms of labor force participation and employment status.

These seven chapters do not, of course, cover the full range of issues pertaining to population structure. Nonetheless, the authors provide thought provoking analyses of the results and implications of research on seven fundamental dimensions of demographic organization.

REFERENCES

Bernhardt, E. M. 1993. "Fertility and Employment." *European Sociological Review* 9(1): 25–42.

Blau, P. M. 1974. "Presidential Address: Parameters of Social Structure." *American Sociological Review* 39(5):615–635.

——. 1977. *Inequality and Heterogeneity: A Primitive Theory of Social Structure*. New York: The Free Press.

——. 1994. *Structural Contexts of Opportunities*. Chicago: University of Chicago Press.

——. 2001. "Macrostructural Theory." pp. 343–352 in *Handbook of Sociological Theory*, edited by J. H. Turner. New York: Klewer Academic/Plenum Publishers.

Bogue, D. J. 1959. "Population Distribution." pp. 383–399 in *The Study of Population: An Inventory and Appraisal*, edited by P. M. Hauser and O. D. Duncan. Chicago: University of Chicago Press.

Davis, K. 1948. *Human Society*. New York: Macmillan Co.

Giddens, A. 1984. *The Constitution of Society: Outline of a Theory of Structuration*. Berkeley, CA: University of California Press.

Glick, P. C. 1959. "Family Statistics." pp. 576–603 in *The Study of Population: An Inventory and Appraisal*, edited by P. M. Hauser and O. D. Duncan. Chicago: University of Chicago Press.

Hawley, A. H. 1959. "Population Composition." pp. 361–382 in *The Study of Population: An Inventory and Appraisal*, edited by P. M. Hauser and O. D. Duncan. Chicago: University of Chicago Press.

Hechter, M., D. Friedman, and M. Appelbaum. 1982. "A Theory of Ethnic Collective Action." *International Migration Review* 16 (2, Special Issue: Theory and Methods in Migration and Ethnic Research):412–434.

Jaffe, A. J. 1959. "Working Force." pp. 604–620 in *The Study of Population: An Inventory and Appraisal*, edited by P. M. Hauser and O. D. Duncan. Chicago: University of Chicago Press.

Mark, N. 1998. "Beyond Individual Differences: Social Differentiation from First Principles." *American Sociological Review* 63(3):309–330.

Mason, K. O. and V. T. Palan. 1981. "Female Employment and Fertility in Peninsular Malaysia: The Maternal Role Incompatibility Hypothesis Reconsidered." *Demography* 18(4):549–575.

Ryder, N. B. 1964. "Notes on the Concept of a Population." *American Journal of Sociology* 69(5):447–463.

Standing, G. 1978. *Labor Force Participation and Development*. Geneva: International Labour Office.

Turner, J. H. 1975. "Marx and Simmel Revisited: Reassessing the Foundations of Conflict Theory." *Social Forces* 53(4):618–627.

——. 1984. "Durkheim's and Spencer's Principles of Social Organization." *Sociological Perspectives* 27(1):21–32.

——. 1985. *Herbert Spencer: A Renewed Appreciation*. Newbury Park, CA: Sage.

——. 1998. *The Structure of Sociological Theory*. Belmont, CA: Wadsworth Publishing Company.

CHAPTER 1

Age and Sex

Dudley L. Poston, Jr.

Of all the characteristics of human populations, age and sex are arguably the most important and relevant for demographers. So important are they for demographic analysis that they are referred to as "the demographic variables" (Bogue 1969: 147). Their importance lies in the fact that the interaction of the demographic processes produces a population's age and sex structure (Horiuchi and Preston 1988), and the demographic processes are themselves affected by the age and sex structure. This reciprocal set of relationships constitutes a major component of demography (Weeks 2002: 294).

But the importance of age and sex extends beyond demography. The division of labor in traditional societies is based almost entirely on age and sex. Indeed age and sex differentiation of one form or another is found in all known human societies (Davis 1949: chapter 4; Murdock 1949: chapters 1 and 8).

Changes in the age distribution of a population have consequences for educational, political, and economic life (Keyfitz and Flieger 1971: chapter 2). A society's age and sex distribution has important implications for socioeconomic and demographic development (Keyfitz 1965), as well as for labor force participation and gender relations (South and Trent 1988). Indeed "almost any measurement that can be taken of human beings, or of groups of human beings, will show substantial variation by sex and age" (Bogue 1969: 147).

In Hauser and Duncan's *The Study of Population* (1959), the topic of age and sex received only minimal treatment. In a chapter on "Population Composition" by Amos Hawley (1959: 361–382), the discussion of age and sex was limited to fewer than four pages. In the present *Handbook*, age and sex composition is the subject of this chapter.

Also, in this *Handbook*, Nancy Riley discusses the broader topic of the "Demography of Gender," and Peter Uhlenberg does the same for the "Demography of Ageing."

In this chapter the topic of age and sex is placed into context by focusing on its conceptualization, substantive concerns, and relevance. Next, some of the theoretical issues in demography dealing with age and sex structure are reviewed; these pertain principally to stable population theory. The major part of the chapter covers methodological issues dealing with age and sex structure. Research dealing with the age and sex structure of the Republic of Korea (Poston et al. 2000; Poston et al. 2003) is used to illustrate some of the major methodological tools available to the demographer for the analysis of age and sex. Key empirical findings dealing with age and sex are integrated with the methodological presentations. Finally, the chapter concludes with discussions of two key areas of age and sex structure in which future research should be concentrated.

SUBSTANTIVE CONCERNS

Age and sex are two central features of a population. Populations are not homogeneous units. They differ by age, sex, race/ethnicity, marital status, and a host of other characteristics. Accordingly, the study of population composition receives considerable attention in demography. In his chapter in *The Study of Population*, Hawley (1959) mentions four objectives that are served by the study of population composition (also see Namboodiri 1996: chapter 7):

1. Data on composition make possible an elaboration of the description of a population and therefore permit detailed interpopulation comparisons.
2. Such data also constitute an inventory of the human resources of a society.
3. The data describe the variables essential for analyzing the demographic processes, e.g., birth, death, migration, growth. In the absence of direct information on demographic processes, composition data, particularly age and sex data, provide a means for estimating the incidence of birth and death.
4. Demographic variables, together with population size, are important conditions affecting the formation and change of social structure (Hawley 1959: 361).

Age and sex are arguably the most important of the many characteristics of human populations. Weeks (2002: 294) writes that "it would not be exaggerating too much to say that changes in the age and sex structure affect virtually all social institutions." The demographic processes of fertility, mortality, and migration are all affected directly by factors of age and sex, and these influences can be via biological, psychological, cultural, and social variables (Palmore 1978; Halli and Rao 1992).

Age and sex are defined more straightforwardly than most demographic variables. Age is an ascribed, yet changeable, characteristic. It is typically defined in population censuses in terms of the age of the person at last birthday. The United Nations (1998: 69) defines age as "the estimated or calculated interval of time between the date of birth and the date of the census, expressed in complete solar years" (see also Hobbs 2004). In most censuses, the respondent is asked to give his/her current age as well as the date of birth. Adjustments are then usually introduced by census officials if the respondent's current age does not correspond to the age denoted by the date of birth. This tends to minimize the phenomenon of age heaping, an issue discussed later in this chapter.

Sex is also an ascribed characteristic, yet for the most part unchangeable. With but a few exceptions, it is fixed at birth. When a baby is born, its sex is determined on the basis of the newborn's genital tubercle. On average, boys are born with penises ranging in length from 2.9 to 4.5 cm (Flatau et al. 1975). For girls, clitoral length at birth ranges from 0.2 to 0.85 cm (Fausto-Sterling 2000: 60; Sane and Pescovitz 1992). When the length of the tubercle is between these two average ranges, sex determination is open for discussion and decision making by the parents and medical workers. But even in such extreme situations (one or two cases per 1,000 live births), sex assignment is usually made soon after birth, and most often is permanent (Money 1988). The census definition of sex therefore is usually not problematic because everyone knows his or her sex, and it is easily ascertainable.

It has already been noted that sex is an ascribed variable whose designation (male or female) is based on biology. In the social sciences, therefore, the concept of *sex* is used when discussing biological differences between males and females, e.g., fertility and mortality differences. The concept of *gender* is used when discussing nonbiological differences between males and females, e.g., differences in socioeconomic status. However, demographers use the term *sex* in the context of both biological and nonbiological differences owing, perhaps, to demography's major focus on fertility and mortality. This is not to say that demographers are uninterested in nonbiological differences between the sexes. Differences between males and females in migration, marriage and divorce, and labor force participation, to name but a few, are nonbiological differences of significant interest to demographers. But even when demographers study these nonbiological behaviors, they retain the use of *sex*. (For a broader discussion, see chapter 4, "Demography of Gender.")

The classification, definition, and enumeration of persons by age and sex are more straightforward than classifications of most other characteristics of human populations. This is so "because . . . [the other characteristics] involve numerous categories and are subject to alternative formulation as a result of cultural differences, differences in the uses to which the data will be put, and differences in the interpretations of respondents and enumerators" (Shryock and Siegel 1976: 105). Consider, for instance, the debates and extensive discussion in recent years about how to classify, define, and count persons according to race and ethnicity and how this far from simple conceptual and methodological matter is further complicated when the population includes multiracial individuals (see Perlmann and Waters 2002; Kertzer and Arel 2002; also see chapter 6 in this *Handbook* by Saenz and Morales).

The age and sex structure of a population is an important piece of information because in many ways it can be viewed as a map of the demographic history of the population. Persons of the same age constitute a cohort of people who were born during the same period; they therefore have been exposed to similar historical facts and conditions. These experiences may also differ according to sex. For instance, military personnel who participate in wars are usually restricted to a narrow age range and are males. For decades after the cessation of fighting, one will observe heavier attrition among the male cohorts owing to war casualties. Later in this chapter, population pyramids for South Korea will be presented. The heavier attrition due to war casualties among South Korean males born between 1920 and 1930 compared to females born in the same period, or to males and females born in other periods, will be noticeable. Major events in a population's immediate history, say those that occurred within the past eight decades, are easily recognized when examining only the population's current data on age and sex.

Social scientists in particular are interested in the age and sex composition of populations. The numerical balance between the sexes affects many social and economic relationships, not the least of which is marriage. Later in this chapter it will be shown how the severely imbalanced sex ratios at birth in China, South Korea, and Taiwan since the mid-1980s are affecting and will continue to affect the marriage markets in these countries for the next few decades.

Age is of equal importance. As Bogue (1985: 42) notes, "almost any aspect of human behavior, from states of subjective feeling and attitudes to objective characteristics such as income, home ownership, occupation, or group membership, may be expected to vary with age." Populations with large proportions of young members may be expected to differ in many ways from those with large proportions of elders. Also considered later in this chapter are some of the major changes that may be expected in China, South Korea, and Taiwan in the next four to five decades as a consequence of the rapid ageing of these countries.

The demographic processes themselves vary significantly by age and sex. With regard to fertility, more males are born than females, usually around 105 males for every 100 females. The fecundity, and hence the childbearing years, of females and males occurs within certain ages, for females between 15 and 49 and, for males, usually between 15 and 79. This is "usually" the situation for males because while "in polygamous populations a man's fertility can remain high well into his fifties and sixties,... in controlled fertility societies, it peaks... with a mode in the mid-twenties" (Coleman 2000: 41). This is due in part to low fertility norms in Western societies, as well as to a small average age difference of about two to three years between men and women in first marriages (Poston and Chang 2005).

Regarding mortality, females have lower death rates than males at every age of life. Death rates are high in the first year of life and then drop to very low levels. In modern populations they do not again attain the level reached in the first year of life for another five to six decades. Also, cause-specific mortality is often age related. For instance, causes of "mortality such as infanticide, parricide and suicide are... age (and sex) related" (Goldscheider 1971: 227). Shryock and Siegel thus state that "in view of the very close relation between age and the risk of death, age may be considered the most important demographic variable in the analysis of mortality" (1976: 224).

Migration also differs by age and sex. Traditionally, males and females have not migrated to the same places in equal numbers. Long-distance migration has tended to favor males; short-distance migration, females. This has been especially the case in developing countries. However, with increases in the degree of gender equity in a society, migration rates of females tend to approximate those of males. Migration is also age-selective, with the largest numbers of migrants found among young adults (Stone 1978; Tobler 1995). "Age is an important determinant of migration because it is related to life-cycle changes that affect most humans in most societies" (Weeks 2002: 255). Goldscheider notes that "given different political, social, economic, cultural and demographic contexts, age remains as a critical differentiation of migration... [These contexts] determine the specifics of age and mobility" (1971: 311).

Finally, the age and sex structure of human populations sets important limits on sustenance organization. The two characteristics of age and sex define a biological entity to which the population's sustenance organization is or must be adapted. Hawley notes that the demographic structure (of age and sex) contains the possibilities and sets the limits of organized group life (1950: 78). The age and sex structure of a population at "any given time constitutes a limiting factor on the kinds of collective activities (it) may engage in. . . . In effect, the organization of relationships in a population is an adaptation to its demographic (i.e., age and sex) structure. And to the extent that the (sustenance organization) is differentiated, the adaptation to its demographic features must be precise" (Hawley 1950: 144). The degree to which a population's age and sex structure limits the kinds and varieties of sustenance activities in which the collectivity may be engaged is an important analytical issue but one not well explored or understood.

The next section of the chapter is devoted to a brief statement of some formal theoretical issues in demography that pertain directly to age and sex.

THEORETICAL ISSUES

In demography discursive theory dealing with age and sex structure is not abundant. Instead, demographers are best known for formal theory and have developed some of the most mathematically elegant formal theories in the social sciences. Age and sex, particularly age, are the centerpiece of most formal theory in demography. Examples of formal age models include Coale's (1971) development of marriage patterns by age, Rogers' (1975) elaborate presentation of migration patterns by age, and Henry's (1961) delineation of fertility patterns by age in the absence of voluntary fertility control. But the most powerful and elegant formal mathematical theory in demography that incorporates a population's age and sex structure, particularly age, is stable population theory, which many believe to be the most important theorem in the mathematics of population (Pollard et al. 1990: 104).

The concept of a stable population was first set forth by Euler (1760 [1970]), but its current development stems from the work of Alfred J. Lotka, who first introduced the concept in a brief note in 1907. Later, Sharpe and Lotka (1911) proved mathematically that if a population that is closed to migration experiences constant schedules of age-specific fertility and mortality rates, it will develop a constant age distribution and will grow at a constant rate, irrespective of its initial age distribution. The mathematical bases and foundation of stable population theory are laid out and discussed in many places, one of the better expositions being Coale's masterpiece, *The Growth and Structure of Human Populations* (1972) (see also, Keyfitz 1977: chapter 4; Schoen 1988: chapter 3; Pollard et al. 1990: chapter 7; Preston et al. 2001: chapter 7).

A stable population has certain characteristics. Pollard and his associates (1990: 105) write that even though the age distribution is constant, "the total population is increasing at a rate r% per year." This means that everything else is also increasing at a rate of r% per year, e.g., the total number of births, "the number of births to mothers of a given age," and number of deaths in each age group. The demographic "parameters of the population (i.e., the birth and death rates, the expectation of life, the average age at death, the average age of mothers at the birth of their daughters, the average number of children to a mother, etc.) remain unchanged, but the absolute numbers in each category increase at a rate of r% per year."

The age distribution of the stable population depends on two items, namely, the underlying age-specific mortality rates and the rate of growth r. "The higher the mortality, the more rapidly the age distribution falls with increasing age; and also the higher the rate of growth, the more rapidly the age distribution falls with age" (Pollard et al. 1990: 106).

The phenomenon of a population that is closed to migration and experiencing constant schedules of age-specific fertility and mortality rates and eventually developing a constant age distribution is referred to as ergodicity, and the theorem just stated is known as the strong ergodic theorem (Lopez 1967; Coale 1987; Namboodiri 1991; Hinde 1998: 167–170). Coale (1968) has studied the amount of time that it would take a population with a given age distribution to achieve stability. Since under the conditions of strong ergodicity, a stable population converges to a constant age distribution irrespective of the age distribution with which it began, this has led to the statement that stable populations forget their past. In other words, when fixed fertility and mortality rates have prevailed, a stable population will attain an unchanging age structure that will be completely independent of its form at any earlier time.

Pollard and his colleagues (1990: 104–105) present an instructive figure (see Figure 7.1) which makes the above point graphically and informatively. They show the gradual development of a stable age distribution for two populations with markedly different initial age distributions, but experiencing stable schedules of fertility and mortality. Initial "gashes" in their population pyramids, likely occurring during wars or other periods of abnormally low births, decade by decade work their way up the pyramids until they leave through the top. When the "gashes" on the female side of the pyramid pass through the reproductive years, fewer births result in a less pronounced "gash" about 30 years later, "but eventually these will all disappear and the stable age structure will be established." Hence a population forgets its past.

Actually, Ansley Coale has demonstrated that all human populations, not just stable populations, forget their pasts (Coale 1957). For instance, he writes that the "age distribution of France is no longer much affected by the excess mortality and reduced numbers of births experienced during the Napoleonic wars, and the age distribution of Greece is no longer affected at all by the Peloponnesian Wars" (Coale 1987: 466). Obviously when fertility and mortality schedules constantly change, the age structure constantly changes. This "independence of a changing age distribution from long past influences is called 'weak ergodicity' " (Coale 1987: 466). Thus, following Coale, it may be stated that all populations, whether or not stable, have forgotten the past. But the stable population, in addition, has a fixed form and fixed birth and death rates.

The "weak ergodicity" theorem is illustrated nicely in van de Walle and Knodel's (1970) "The Case of Women's Island." This is a demographic simulation exercise and shows quantitatively the "story" of 1,000 young women marooned with five men on an island that is forever closed to migration. After 100 years have elapsed (via simulation), "one cannot find any evidence that the initial population (of the island was so)...distorted in both its (initial) age and sex composition" (van de Walle and Knodel 1970: 436). This is a superb demonstration of "weak ergodicity": a population, stable or not, "forgets" its past and "stabilizes itself in due time with a structure that is entirely dependent on fertility and mortality levels" (van de Walle and Knodel 1970: 436).

Stable population theory has many implications for age and sex distribution. One is that changes and fluctuations in fertility cause far greater change in a population's age distribution than do changes and fluctuations in mortality. Coale and Demeny (1983) have shown that populations closed to migration that have near stable fertility rates but differ only in their mortality schedules will have similar age and sex structures (see also Pollard et al. 1990: chapter 7; and Hinde 1998: chapter 13).

This section has discussed briefly one of the most elegant mathematical models in the social sciences, stable population theory, and has shown some of the implications of this theory for age and sex structure. (See further discussions in chapter 22, "Mathematical Demography.")

METHODS, MEASURES, AND EMPIRICAL FINDINGS

The age and sex structure of a population can be examined and portrayed along several dimensions. The two structures may be analyzed separately, and a summary evaluation may be conducted of age cross-classified by sex. In this section methods are reviewed that describe the age and sex structure of a population and also evaluate its patterns and quality.

The Population Pyramid

The age and sex structure of a population at a given moment of time may be viewed as an aggregation of cohorts born in different years. A popular graphic representation of the age-sex structure of the population is the "Age-sex Pyramid," or "Population Pyramid"; it shows for a specific point in time the different surviving cohorts of persons of each sex. A population pyramid is one of the most elegant ways of presenting age and sex distribution data graphically, but it is used strictly for descriptive purposes. It does not enable the analyst to examine directly the quality of the population's age and sex data.

A population pyramid is nothing more than two ordinary histograms, representing the male and female populations in, usually, five-year age categories placed on their sides and back to back (see the interesting and instructive presentation and discussion of "death" pyramids in chapter 10, "Adult Mortality").

Figure 1.1 is a population pyramid for the Republic of Korea (ROK) for 1970; it shows, for instance, that more than 21% of Korea's total population in 1970 was male aged 0 to 14, and just under 20% was female aged 0 to 14. Figure 1.1 also shows the high attrition of males aged 40 to 49 in 1970 (aged 20 to 29 in 1950), due most likely to Korean war casualties 20 years earlier; females aged 40 to 49 did not experience as much attrition due to the war. Higher female than male life expectancy is the main cause of the larger numbers of women at the oldest ages.

Figure 1.2 is a pyramid for the ROK in 1995. The bottom bars show the effects of the fertility reduction in Korea that has occurred since the 1970s. In 1995 less than 12% of Korea's population was male aged 0 to 14 (compared to more than 21% in 1970), and also less than 12% was female aged 0 to 14. The lower bars of Figure 1.2 also indicate the much larger number of males, compared to females, which have been born in Korea since the mid-1980s. The lowest two bars of the pyramid in Figure 1.2 indicate that the sex ratio for Koreans in 1995 in the age group 0 to 4 is 113.4; this suggests a much higher sex ratio at birth than that regulated by biology, and likely is evidence of son preference (see Zeng et al. 1993; Poston et al. 1997; Poston, Chu et al. 2000; Poston 2002; Poston, et al. 2003, for more discussion). Also, in the 1995 pyramid the men who suffered the most in the Korean War are now between the ages of 65 and 74. There are even fewer of them in 1995, compared to females of the same age; war casualties along with higher female life expectation are the causes of the differential.

In some subnational populations, usually counties, states, or provinces, the sustenance and livelihood base is so restrictive in terms of persons of one sex, or of just one or

Dudley L. Poston, Jr.

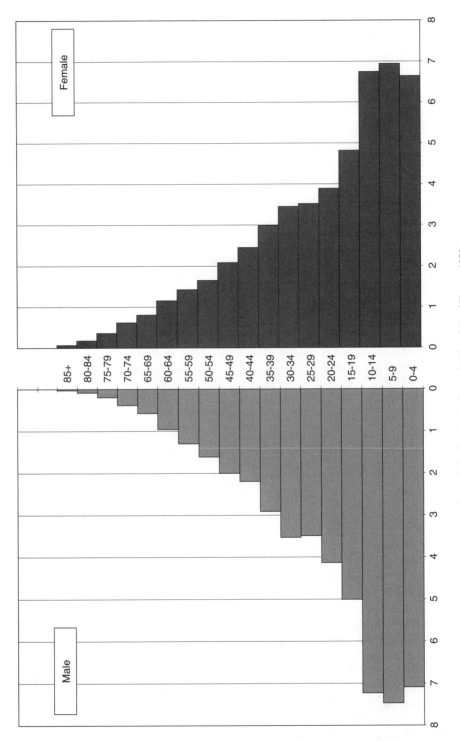

FIGURE 1.1. Population Pyramid, Republic of Korea: 1970.

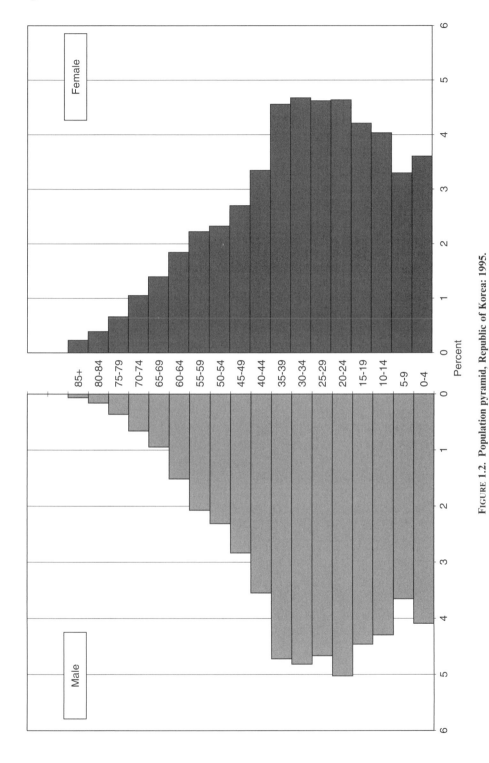

FIGURE 1.2. Population pyramid, Republic of Korea: 1995.

a few age groups, that they overwhelm the area's demography. Often their principal ecological organization and function may be inferred by viewing their population pyramid. Figures 1.3 to 1.6 are pyramids for four counties in Texas in 2000, namely, Llano County, Coryell County, Walker County, and Brazos County.

Llano County (Figure 1.3), located in the Highland Lakes area of central Texas, is demographically an extremely old county, with almost 40% of its population aged 60 or more. It is a prime destination of inter- and intrastate elderly migrants and is demo-graphically top-heavy because elderly people have moved into the county, and young people have moved out. Llano County's population pyramid is typical of the pyramids of the so-called "retirement" counties in such states as Texas, Florida, Arizona, and California.

Coryell County (Figure 1.4) is the home of Fort Hood, the largest U.S. Army installation in the United States. It is also the home of five female prison units (Texas Department of Criminal Justice 2000). More than 28% of the county's male population, and almost 15% of the total population, is male aged 20 to 29. There are also large numbers of females in the county in their 20s and early 30s who are either prisoners, military personnel, or the wives of male military. Since the nonmilitary and nonprisoner population of the county is predominantly white, a population pyramid for Coryell County's black population is even more exaggerated with respect to the bars portraying the male and female populations aged 20 to 29.

Over 30% of Walker County's (Figure 1.5) population is comprised of males aged 20 to 44. The major sustenance activities of the county are higher education and male prisons. In Walker County there are six male prison units and one prison transfer facility in Walker County, including the state's large death row unit (Texas Department of Criminal Justice 2000). There are more male prisoners in Walker County than in almost any other county in the United States. Walker County is also the home of Sam Houston State University. The male and female college students are mainly in the 20 to 24 age group, and their presence in Walker County's pyramid, especially that of the females, is palpable. But the prisoners in Walker County predominate in the age groups 20 to 44.

The major sustenance activity of Brazos County (Figure 1.6) is higher education. Texas A&M University, with a student body population of over 45,000, is located in Brazos County and is the fifth largest institution of higher learning in the United States. Also located in Brazos County is Blinn College, a community college with a student body population of over 8,200. Since most of the students attending Texas A&M and Blinn live in Brazos County, they overwhelm the county's demog-raphy. Almost one-quarter of the county's population is in the age group 20 to 24, the ages of most of the Texas A&M and Blinn students. Younger A&M and Blinn undergraduates comprise a part of the preceding age group 15 to 19, which is almost 13% of the county's population. And many of the around 7,000 A&M graduate students are in the 25 to 29 age group, which comprises over 8% of the county's population.

Despite their descriptive utility, however, population pyramids do not provide the analyst with direct empirical information on data quality. They only give a graphic representation of age and sex structure at a particular point in time. Issues of data quality require more specific considerations. Presented next is a discussion of indexes that may be used to examine patterns of age data, patterns of sex data, and patterns of age and sex data considered together.

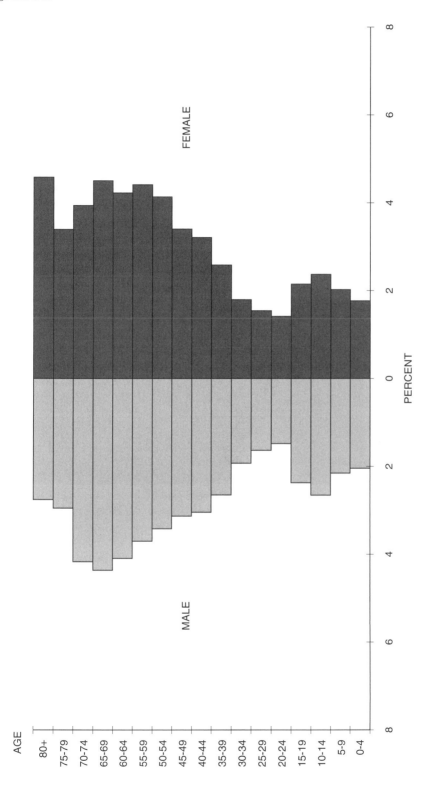

FIGURE 1.3. Population by age and sex: Llano Country, Texas, 2000.

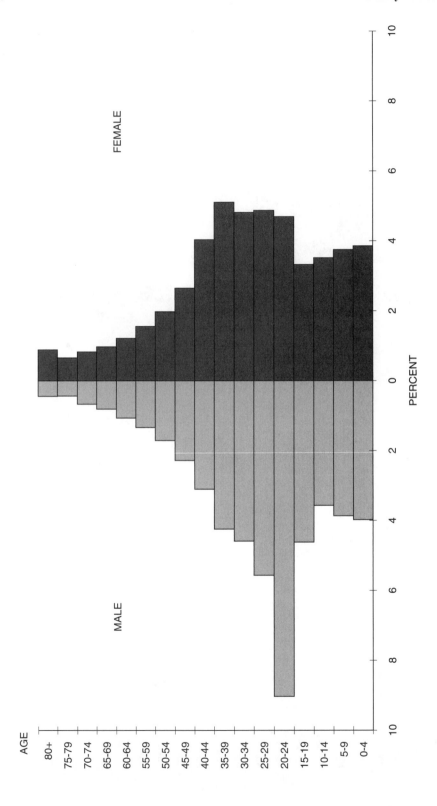

FIGURE 1.4. Population by age and sex: Coryell Country, Texas, 2000.

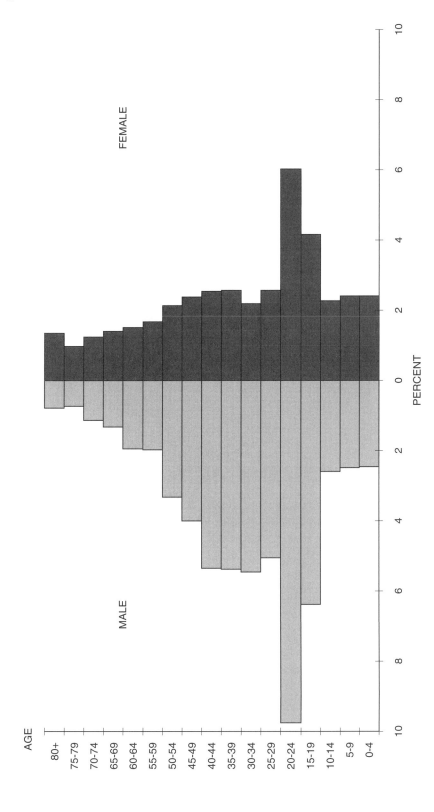

FIGURE 1.5. Population by age and sex: Walker County, Texas, 2000.

Dudley L. Poston, Jr.

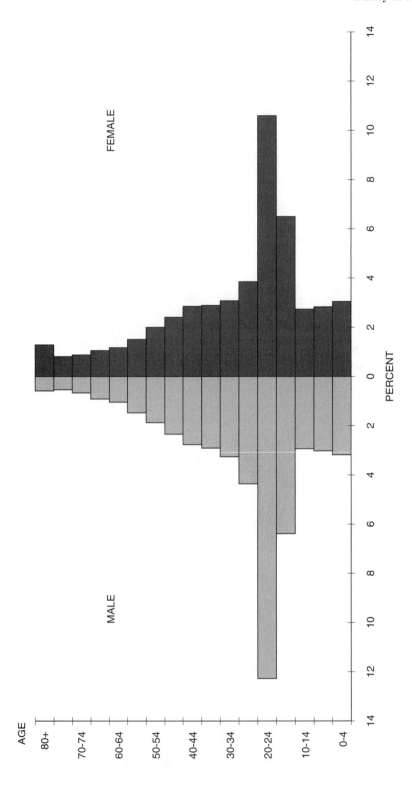

FIGURE 1.6. Population by age and sex: Brazos County, Texas, 2000.

Evaluation of Patterns of Age Dependency

Shryock and Siegel (1976: 115) have noted that errors in the reporting of age have been examined more thoroughly and intensively by demographers than reporting errors for any other question in population censuses. There are several reasons for this, two of which are that the "errors are readily apparent, and that measurement techniques can be more easily developed for age data" (Shryock and Siegel 1976: 115).

One may analyze the age distribution of a population in many ways (cf., Shryock and Siegel 1976: chapter 8; Arriaga and Associates 1994: chapter 2; Hobbs 2004: chapter 7). A popular measure of age structure is the dependency ratio (DR). The DR is the ratio of the dependent-age population (both young [persons 0 to 14 years old] and old [persons 65 years of age and older]) to the working-age population (persons 15 to 64 years old). The DR is usually multiplied by 100. The higher the ratio, the more people each worker has to support; the lower the DR the fewer the number of dependents. The DR may be split into the Youth–DR and the Old Age–DR; both have the same denominator, viz., the population aged 15 to 64. The numerator of the Youth–DR is the population 0 to 14; and the numerator of the Old Age–DR is the population 65+. The Youth–DR plus the Old Age–DR equals the DR.

An index somewhat analogous to the Old Age–Dependency ratio is a United Nations–developed measure of elderly support known as the Potential Support Ratio (PSR). It represents "the extent that persons of working age (15 to 64) can be seen as supporting the older population (65 years or older), and is the ratio between the two" (United Nations, 2001: 7). The PSR value represents the number of persons in the population who "support" every one old person in the population. Later in this chapter the PSR will be illustrated.

Presented in Table 1.1 are values of the Youth–DR, Old Age–DR, and Total DR for 13 countries of the world. These countries were chosen because they have low or high values of the Total DR and low or high values of the component DRs. South Korea and China have Total DRs that are among the lowest in the world. For every 100 persons in the economically producing ages (15 to 64) in South Korea and China, there

TABLE 1.1. **Values of Youth-Dependency Ratio, Old Age–Dependency Ratio, and Total Dependency Ratio, Selected Countries of the World, 2001**

Country	Youth–DR	Old Age–DR	Total DR
South Korea	31.0	9.9	40.9
China	32.9	10.0	42.9
Italy	20.6	26.5	47.1
Spain	22.1	25.0	47.1
Japan	22.1	25.0	47.1
United States	31.8	19.7	51.5
Yugoslavia	31.8	19.7	51.5
Sweden	29.7	26.6	56.3
Mexico	55.7	8.2	63.9
Nigeria	83.0	5.7	88.7
Yemen	98.0	6.1	104.1
Niger	104.2	4.2	108.4
Uganda	108.5	4.3	112.8

Data Source: Population Reference Bureau, 2001.

are 41 and 43 persons, respectively, in the dependent ages that the producers must support; and more than three-fourths of these dependents are young people (under age 15). Compare this situation with that in Italy, Spain, and Japan, countries with only slightly higher Total DRs (47.1 in all three countries), but where just over two-fifths are young dependents. Persons in the producing ages in Italy, Spain, and Japan have about the same dependency burden as producers in South Korea and China, but they have twice the proportion of elderly dependents. At the other extreme are Yemen, Niger, and Uganda, with Total DRs that are the highest in the world. For every 100 persons in the economically producing ages in Yemen, Niger, and Japan, there are 104, 108, and 113 persons, respectively, in the dependent ages that the producers must support; and virtually all these dependents are young people. The producers in these three countries are supporting more than twice as many dependents as in the five countries mentioned above. Weeks (2002: 305) notes that the DR "does not capture all the intricacies of the age structure, but it is a useful indicator of the burden (or lack thereof) that some age structures place on a population."

Evaluation of Patterns of Age Structure Based on Single Year of Age Data

In the analysis of single years of age data, if there are no irregularities, the counts for adjacent ages should be similar. Examples of irregularities are digit preference and avoidance. If a population tends to report certain ages (say, those ending in 0 or 5) at the expense of other ages, this is known as *age heaping*. *Digit preference*, an analogous concept, carries the added feature of respondents having a preference for various ages having the same terminal digit. *Digit avoidance* refers to the opposite.

Age heaping tends to be more pronounced among populations or population subgroups with low levels of education. "The causes and patterns of age or digit preference vary from one culture to culture, but preference for ages ending in '0' and in '5' is quite widespread" (Shryock and Siegel 1976: 115; Hobbs 2004), especially in the Western world. In Korea, China, and some other countries in East Asia, there is sometimes a preference for ages ending in the numeral 3 because it sounds like the word or character for life. In some cultures certain numbers and digits are avoided, e.g., 13 is frequently avoided in the West because it is considered unlucky. The numeral 4 is avoided in Korea and in China because it has the same sound as the word or character for death.

Heaping, i.e., digit preference, or the lack of heaping, i.e., digit avoidance, are the major forms of error typically found in single-year-of-age data. Irregularities in reporting single years of age can be detected using graphs and indices. Both will be considered.

Figure 1.7 is a graph of single years of age for females in South Korea in 1995. Aside from some heaping on ages 43, 53, and 63, there is little evidence elsewhere of age heaping. Compare the situation in South Korea with that of males in Pakistan in 1981 (Figure 1.8). In Pakistan there is an astounding amount of age heaping on ages ending in zero.

Age heaping and digit preference may be ascertained more precisely with indices. Indices of digit preference assume that the true figures are rectangularly distributed over an n-year age range that is centered on the specific age being examined. If the index equals 100, there is no age heaping on the age being examined. The greater the value above 100, the greater the concentration on this age. The lower the value from 100, the greater the avoidance of the age being examined.

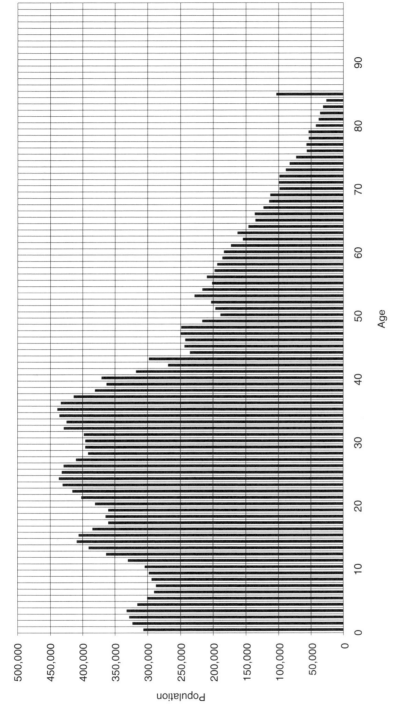

FIGURE 1.7. Single years of age, female population, Republic of Korea, 1995.

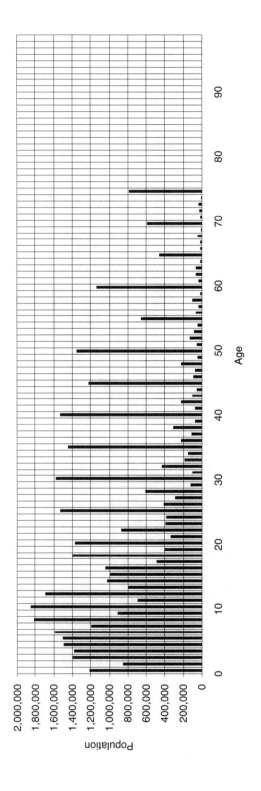

FIGURE 1.8. Single years of age, male population, Pakistan, 1981.

One of the most popular rectangular-type age-heaping methods is Whipple's Method (WM), an index designed to reflect preference for the terminal digits of 0 and 5, usually in the age range 23 to 62 (cf., Hobbs 2004). WM varies from 0 (when the digits 0 and 5 are not reported in the census data) to 100 (when there is no preference for 0 or 5 in the census data) to a maximum of 500 (when only the digits 0 and 5 are reported in the census data). The United Nations (1990) states that if the values of Whipple's Index are less than 105, then the age distribution data are deemed to be "highly accurate." If the WM values are between 105 and 109.9, they are "fairly accurate"; if between 110 and 124.9, "approximate"; if between 125 and 174.9, "rough"; and if 175 or more, "very rough" (United Nations 1990: 18–19). WM is calculated as follows (Shryock and Siegel 1976: 116):

$$WM = \frac{\sum (P_{25} + P_{30} + \ldots + P_{55} + P_{60})}{1/5 \sum (P_{23} + P_{24} + P_{25} \ldots P_{60} + P_{61} + P_{62})} * 100$$

The United Nations notes that "although Whipple's Index measures only the effects of preferences for ages ending in 5 and 0, it can be assumed that such digit preference is usually connected with other sources of inaccuracy in age statements, and the indexes can be accepted as a fair measure of the general reliability of the age distribution" (United Nations 1990: 20).

The decision in the Whipple's Index to focus on the age range of 23 to 62 is an arbitrary one. The ages of early childhood and old age are excluded since, frequently, they are more influenced by other types of errors and issues than digit preference; also, "the assumption of equal decrements from age to age is less applicable" at the older ages (Shryock and Siegel 1976: 117; Hobbs 2004).

The WM value for South Korean females in 1995 (as in Figure 1.7) is 100.1; the WM value for Pakistani males in 1981 (as in Figure 1.8) is 330.8. Among Korean females, the WM index indicates virtually no age heaping on digits ending in 0 and 5. The WM figure may be interpreted as indicating that in South Korea the numbers of females counted in 1995 at ages ending in 0 and 5 overstate an unbiased population (that is, one in which there is no age heaping on 0 or 5) by 0.1% (cf., Shryock and Siegel 1976: 117). Conversely, in Pakistan in 1981 males counted at ages ending in 0 and 5 overstate an unbiased population by almost 231%.

WM scores for three more developed countries, namely, Japan in 1985, Denmark in 1988, and Hong Kong in 1995; and for two more developing countries, namely, Iran and Mexico in 1988, are Japan (98.4), Denmark (101.5), and Hong Kong (101.7) versus Iran (122.7) and Mexico (133.4). The WM values for the developed countries, as expected, are lower and closer to 100 than those for the developing countries.

Given the presumed tendency for Koreans and Chinese to heap around ages ending in the numeral 3 (see earlier discussion), Poston and his students (Poston, et al., 2000; 2003) have developed a Whipple-type index to reflect only the degree of heaping on age 3 for the ages between 23 and 53. The index, referred to here as Whipple-3 (W-3) is:

$$W - 3 = \frac{\sum (P23 + P33 + P43 + P53)}{\frac{1}{10} \sum (P23 + P24 + P25 \ldots P60 + P61 + P62)} * 100$$

The values of W–3 for males and females in the ROK in 1970 are 118.9 and 115.2, and an overall W–3 measure (without regard to sex) is 117.0. In 1995 the corresponding W–3 values are 115.2, 112.6, and 114.0. These W–3 scores indicate a more than insignificant amount of heaping on digits ending in 3 among Korean males and females in 1970 and in 1995. In 1970 and in 1995, the number of South Koreans counted at ages 23, 33, 43, and 53 overstate an unbiased population by 17% and 14%, respectively. Korean males overstate on these ages more so than Korean females.

Another popular index of digit preference is the Myers Blended Method (MBM) (Myers 1940). MBM avoids the possible bias in indices like the WM that is likely due to the fact that "numbers ending in '0' [are normally] larger than the following numbers ending in '1' to '9' because of the effect of mortality" (Shryock and Siegel 1976: 117; also see Spiegelman 1969: 70–75). The MBM is also preferred because of its low bias and the fact that it tests for preference and avoidance of all digits (Smith 1992: 35).

For each terminal digit MBM yields an index of preference, or deviation from 10%, of the proportion of the total population reporting the given digit. An overall or summary index for all terminal digits is derived as "one-half the sum of the deviations from 10 percent, each taken without regard to sign" (Shryock and Siegel 1976: 118). If there is no age heaping, MBM will be zero. The theoretical maximum of MBM is 90, which would result if the entire population reported ages ending in the same digit.

Figure 1.9 is a histogram showing values of MBM for each of the 10 terminal digits for the male and female populations of South Korea in 1995. There is a preference for the terminal digit 3, with the preference level for males only slightly greater than that for females. There is an avoidance of ages ending in 0 and in 1, with females avoiding these digits much more than males.

Summary values of MBM are calculated by taking one-half of the sum of the absolute deviations of each terminal digit from 10%. MBM summary values for South Korean males and females in 1995 are 1.6 and 2.6, for an overall MBM value of 2.1, indicating very little evidence among Koreans in 1995 of preference or avoidance of terminal age digits. The MBM values for males and females combined from the other three developed countries mentioned above, i.e., Japan, Denmark, and Hong Kong, are also very low, ranging from 3.4 for Japan to 1.8 for Hong Kong. In contrast the MBM values for males and females in Pakistan are 69.8 and 72.3. An MBM value of 90, the maximum, would mean that all persons report an age with the same terminal digit. Pakistani males and females overwhelmingly prefer ages ending in 0.

Several other summary indices of digit preference have been developed by Bachi (1951), by Carrier (1959), and by Ramachandran (1967). According to Shryock and Siegel (1976) and Hobbs (2004), these "have some theoretical advantages over the Whipple and Myers indexes" (Shryock and Siegel 1976: 118), but they differ little from them as general indicators of heaping.

Evaluation of Patterns of Age Structure Based on five-Year Group Data

The age structure of a population may also be examined by using age data grouped in five-year categories, and calculating Age Ratios for the five-year age groups (United Nations 1955). In populations with no major fluctuations in fertility and with insignificant levels of migration, age ratios should be fairly similar across the age categories (Arriaga and Associates 1994: 19). An age ratio for any five-year age category is the population in the age group multiplied by 200, divided by the sum of the populations in the adjacent (preceding and following) age groups (United Nations 1952; Arriaga and Associates 1994). Shryock and Siegel (1976: 124) note that "barring extreme fluctu-

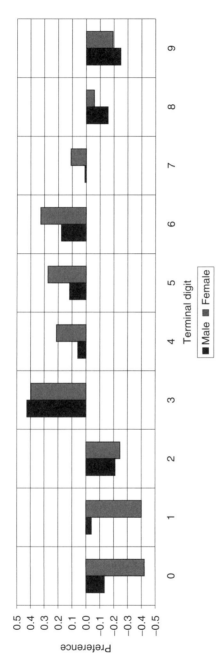

FIGURE 1.9. Values of Myers Blended Method, ten terminal digits, males and females, Republic of Korea, 1995.

ations in past births, deaths, or migration, the three age groups should form a nearly linear series. Age ratios should...approximate 100.0, even though actual historical variations in these factors would produce deviations from 100.0 in the age ratio for most ages." However, it must be remembered that owing to fluctuations over the years in one or more of the demographic processes in the country or region being examined, age ratios for some age groups could well deviate quite a bit from 100.0, while maintaining a relatively high overall quality of age reporting.

Figure 1.10 is a graph of the age ratios for males and females for each of the five-year age groups of 5 to 9 through 70 to 74 for South Korea in 1970. The age ratio for males in the age group five to nine is 104.3. The highest age ratio shown in Figure 1.10 is 116.0 for males in age group 10 to 14. The largest negative age ratios are 85.7 for males in age group 65 to 69 and 89 for males in the age group 40 to 44. The value of 89 for age group 40 to 44 means that there are 11% fewer males in the age group 40 to 44 than the sum of the numbers of persons in the two age groups that are adjacent to age group 40 to 44. These low values could reflect age misreporting, but there are also substantive reasons for the low values. For instance, there is good reason to expect many fewer males in 1970 in the 40 to 44 age group: this is one of the age groups that suffered a large number of soldier casualties in the Korean War.

Age ratios "serve primarily as measures of net age misreporting, not net census error, and they should not be taken as valid indicators of error for particular age groups" (Shryock and Siegel 1976: 125). Consequently, an overall appraisal of age data is desirable, rather than reliance on a schedule of age ratios for the entire age distribution. For each sex, an Age-Ratio Score (ARS) may be calculated by summing the differences of each age ratio from 100, without regard to sign, and then taking the mean of these differences. The resulting ARS represents the mean deviation for males (or for females) from 100 of the age ratios for each age group.

According to the United Nations, the ARS has an "advantage over the methods of Whipple, Myers and [others because] the index which is obtained is affected by differential omission of persons in various age groups from the census count and by tendentious age misstatement as well as by digit-preference and is therefore more truly a reflection of the general accuracy of the age statistics" (United Nations 1955: 42).

The simple average of the male and female age ratio scores is a measure of the overall accuracy of the age data across the two sexes and may be referred to as an Age-Accuracy Index (AAI). Smith (1992) notes, however, that the title of this index is a misnomer because deviations in the age ratios, and hence high AAI values, could result at least in part from other than inaccurate statements of age: the AAI "measures accuracy of age reporting only to the extent that the irregularities it identifies are not present in the true age distribution" (Smith 1992: 34).

In Table 1.2, AAI values for the year 2000 are presented for 42 developing and developed countries from all the major areas of the world. The lowest AAI values are for Syria, South Korea, the West Bank, Ireland, Kenya, South Africa, and Sri Lanka; these low values indicate relatively good-quality age data and/or relatively stable demographic dynamics. The highest AAI values, representing a poorer quality of age reporting and/or changes and fluctuations in the demographic processes, are found in the United Arab Emirates, Russia, China, and Macau. To a degree the AAI values are related negatively with the general development level of the country, but they also reflect the degree of stability in the demographic processes. The more stable the processes, the lower the AAI values.

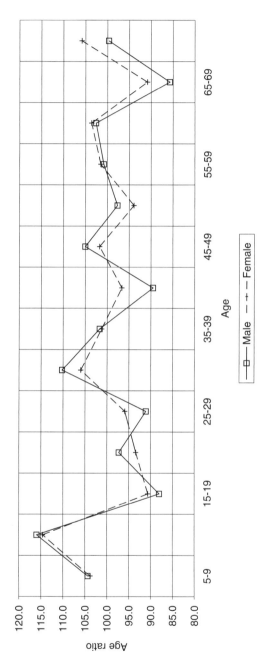

FIGURE 1.10. Age ratios by sex for five-year age groups, Republic of Korea, 1970.

TABLE 1.2. Values of Age Accuracy Index (Ranked from High to Low) for 42 Countries of the World in 2000.

Country	Age Accuracy Index
United Arab Emirates	14.9
Russia	14.6
China	8.9
Macau S.A.R.	8.8
North Korea	7.7
Germany	7.3
Bahrain	7.2
Iraq	6.7
Bangladesh	6.7
South Korea	6.4
Sweden	6.3
Taiwan	6.2
Finland	6.0
Yugoslavia	6.0
Hong Kong S. A. R.	6.0
Somalia	5.9
Singapore	5.8
Vietnam	5.5
Italy	5.0
Yemen	5.0
Japan	5.0
Kuwait	5.0
France	4.8
Iran	4.8
Spain	4.8
United Kingdom	4.8
Indonesia	4.2
Saudi Arabia	4.0
Gaza Strip	3.9
Liberia	3.7
Israel	3.7
Uganda	3.5
Jordan	3.4
United States	3.4
Thailand	3.3
Zambia	3.3
Syria	3.2
West Bank	3.1
Ireland	3.0
Kenya	2.7
Sri Lanka	2.6
South Africa	1.7

Data Source: U.S. Bureau of the Census, 2002.
S.A.R = Special Administration Region.

Evaluation of Patterns of Sex Structure

Only a few methods used in demography index sex composition: (1) the masculinity proportion, (2) the ratio of the excess or deficit of males to the total population, and (3) the sex ratio. The masculinity proportion is commonly used in nontechnical discussions of sex composition (Shryock and Siegel 1976: 106) and is calculated by dividing the number of males in the population by the number of males and females and multiplying the result by 100.

The ratio of the excess, or deficit, of males to the total population is obtained by subtracting the number of females from the number of males, dividing by the total number in the population, and multiplying by 100.

The sex ratio (SR) is the most popular index of sex composition in demographic and other scholarly analyses. It is usually defined as the number of males per 100 females:

$$SR = \frac{P_m}{P_f} * 100$$

A sex ratio above 100 indicates an excess of males, and an SR below 100 an excess of females. In some Eastern European countries and in India, Iran, Pakistan, Saudi Arabia, and a few other countries, the sex ratio is calculated as the number of females per 100 males. But the first SR definition above, namely the number of males per 100 females, is used by most demographers and by international bodies such as the United Nations.

In general, "national sex ratios tend to fall in the narrow range from about 95 to 102, barring special circumstances, such as a history of heavy war losses (less males), or heavy immigration (more males); national sex ratios outside the range of 90 to 105 should be viewed as extreme" (Shryock and Siegel 1976: 107). And as is the situation with age ratios, the greater the abrupt deviation or departure of age-specific sex ratios from 100, the greater the potential for errors in the data. This statement also assumes, of course, that the deviations are not caused by fluctuations in the demographic processes.

Most societies have sex ratios at birth (SRBs) between 104 and 106, i.e., 104 to 106 boys are born for every 100 girls. This so-called biologically normal SRB is likely an evolutionary adaptation to the fact that females have higher survival probabilities than males (see Clarke 2000, for another discussion). Since at every year of life males have higher age-specific death rates than females, slightly more males than females are required at birth for there to be around equal numbers of males and females when the groups reach their marriageable ages. Biology thus dictates that the age-specific SR will be highest at the very young ages, starting around 104 to 106 at age 0, and should then decline with age, attaining a value of around 100 for persons in their late 20s and continuing to decline to levels around 50 or 60 in the oldest ages.

Barring extreme forms of human intervention and disturbance, these kinds of SR patterns by age should occur in most populations. One such intervention would be a major war, such as the Korean War, which would reduce significantly the numbers of males in their 20s and 30s. Another would be high amounts of immigration or emigration. International migration is usually driven economically when, typically, males depart one country and enter another in search of employment. Such disturbances in some countries can be extreme, as will be shown below for some of the oil-producing countries in the Middle East. Still another intervention would be female-specific abortion, resulting in an SR at birth well above 105.

An easy way to evaluate the quality of data on sex composition by age, as well as the extent to which human interventions have disturbed these patterns, is to calculate sex ratios for each five-year age group, and then to calculate for each age group the Sex Ratio Difference (SRD), that is, the difference between the SR for the age group and the

SR for the previous age group. Then, for the population as a whole, the Sex-Ratio Score (SRS) may be calculated by taking the mean difference of the SRDs, without regard to sign (Arriaga and Associates 1994: 20).

Figure 1.11 is a graph of the sex ratios by age for South Korea in 1970. The SRs in the younger ages are about normal, at levels between 103 and 107 males per 100 females. The SR for age group 40 to 44 is lower than it should be and is likely due to war casualties to men who were in their 20s during the Korean War. The Sex Ratio Score for the ROK for 1970 is 5.3. This means that the average deviation of an age-specific SR from the SR of the preceding age group in the ROK in 1970 is 5.3 persons per 100.

Figure 1.12 is a graph of the age-specific sex ratios for South Korea in 1995. The figure shows sex ratios at very young ages that are much higher than would be expected biologically. These are likely the result of human interventions, namely, prenatal sex identification, followed by female-specific abortion. The SRs for age groups 0 to 4 and 5 to 9 are 113.4 and 110.6. Other than the higher than expected SRs at the very young ages, the declining trend in SRs in 1995 shown in Figure 1.12 for the remaining ages is pretty much as expected. The Sex Ratio Score for the ROK in 1995 is 4.7.

In Table 1.3, the Sex Ratio Scores for South Korea in 1970 and 1995 may be compared and contrasted with those of 41 developing and developed countries of the world for the year of 2000. Observe, first, that very high SRS values are shown for four countries: the United Arab Emirates, Saudi Arabia, Bahrain, and Kuwait, all above 16.0. These high values are due mainly to the large numbers of foreign-born males between the ages of 20 and 55 who have migrated to these countries as temporary laborers. To illustrate, the sex ratios of 35 to 39 and 40 to 44 year olds in Kuwait are 241 and 242, respectively; that is, there are 241 males aged 35 to 39 in Kuwait for every 100 females in the same age group. Second, it is likely that these very high values do not reflect the gross underenumeration, misreporting, or neglect of females. Indeed, the sex ratios for these countries for persons under age 20 are all slightly above 100, the values that would be expected under a situation of equal treatment of the sexes.

South Korea's SRS values of 5.3 in 1970 and 4.7 in 1995 are not that different from those of most of the countries shown in Table 1.3. South Korea's slightly higher SRS in 1970 is due largely to military casualties during the Korean War, and its slightly higher value in 1995 is due to the experience in the country since the mid-1980s of higher than normal sex ratios at birth. The next section analyzes age and sex structure considered together.

Evaluation of Overall Patterns of Age and Sex Structure

The overall picture of the age and sex structure of a population may be determined by calculating the Age-Sex Accuracy Index (ASAI) developed by the United Nations (1955). The ASAI is the sum of the Age Ratio Score for males, the Age Ratio Score for females, and three times the Sex Ratio Score (Shryock and Siegel 1976: 126). The assumption underlying the ASAI is that "accurate" age data are rectangularly distributed and that age-specific sex ratios decline over the life cycle in an even manner. Departures from these patterns will result in "inaccurate" data patterns. Of course, departures from rectangular age distributions and from declining sex ratios over the life course may also be due to variations and changes in the demographic processes. Thus,

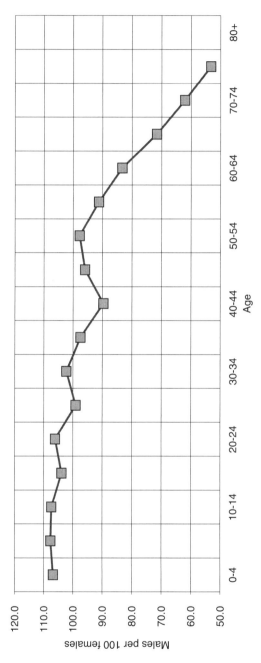

FIGURE 1.11. Sex ratios by age group, Republic of Korea, 1970.

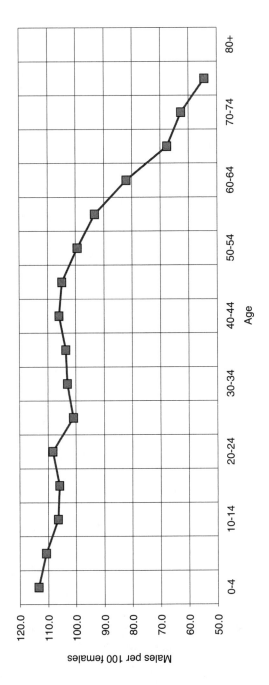

FIGURE 1.12. Sex ratios by age group, Republic of Korea, 1995.

TABLE 1.3. Values of Sex Ratio Score (Ranked from High to Low) for South Korea in 1970 and 1995 and for 41 Countries of the World in 2000.

Country	Sex Ratio Score
United Arab Emirates	26.9
Saudi Arabia	18.2
Bahrain	16.8
Kuwait	16.1
Macau S.A.R.	9.6
Hong Kong S.A.R.	7.6
Somalia	5.7
South Korea (1970)	5.3
North Korea	4.7
South Korea (1995)	4.7
Zambia	4.6
Liberia	4.2
Jordan	4.1
Singapore	4.0
Russia	3.9
Yemen	3.9
Gaza Strip	3.7
Taiwan	3.3
Yugoslavia	3.1
Uganda	3.0
Bangladesh	2.8
Iraq	2.7
Ireland	2.7
West Bank	2.7
Germany	2.5
Finland	2.5
South Africa	2.4
France	2.3
Israel	2.3
Italy	2.2
Vietnam	2.1
China	2.0
Kenya	2.0
Sweden	2.0
United States	2.0
Spain	1.9
Indonesia	1.8
Japan	1.7
Sri Lanka	1.7
United Kingdom	1.7
Iran	1.4
Thailand	1.4
Syria	1.3

Data Source: U.S. Bureau of the Census, 2002.

Smith's (1992) contention (cited above) that the title of the Age Accuracy Index is a misnomer can also be applied to the Age-Sex Accuracy Index.

The ASAI has other limitations as a summary measure of age and sex data. Among them are the "failure to take account of the expected decline in the SR with increasing age, and of real irregularities in age distribution due to migration, wars, and epidemics, as well as normal fluctuations of births and deaths; ... also, the considerable weight given to the sex ratio component in the formula" [namely, three times the SRS] (Shryock and Siegel 1976: 126; Hobbs 2004).

Values of the ASAI for 42 developed and developing countries in 2000 are shown in Table 1.4. Given the fact that the value of a country's Sex Ratio Score figures heavily in the calculation of the ASAI, it is no surprise to see a similarity in the way the countries are distributed on ASAI values (Table 1.4) and the way they are distributed on Sex Ratio Scores (Table 1.3). The major reasons for the ASAI distribution are very similar, if not largely the same as, the reasons for the distribution of Sex Ratio Scores.

Owing to the above-mentioned limitations of the ASAI, the index is only useful for making rough comparisons and distinctions between and among populations regarding the accuracy in the censuses of reporting age by sex (Shryock and Siegel 1976: 126; Hobbs 2004). Its major function, to be sure, is its ability to flag extreme values, which often are not due necessarily to underenumeration and misreporting but to fluctuations in the demographic processes.

This section has discussed in some detail major methods of analyzing age and sex structure and principal findings. These are essentially the same kinds of approaches and methods that were used to analyze age and sex when Hauser and Duncan's *The Study of Population* was written in 1959. Indeed the Whipple and Myers' indices of age heaping and digit preference were in use prior to the 1950s, and the methods for analyzing age and sex structure were developed by the United Nations in the 1950s. Alterations of, and improvements to, some of these methods have been made (see, for instance, Ramachandran's [1967] work on digit preference). But for the most part since the publication of *The Study of Population*, there have been few major breakthroughs in approaches for analyzing age and sex structure.

RESEARCH DIRECTIONS

This final section considers two directions where age and sex research should be focused. The first has to do with the unbalanced sex ratios at birth now being experienced in China, South Korea, Taiwan, and a few other countries such as India. These unbalanced sex ratios at birth will have important societal implications when the excess males are adults. The second research direction has to do with the process of demographic ageing being experienced by many countries around the world. Considered here specifically is the ageing of the Chinese, South Korean, and Taiwanese populations and its implications for the provision of elderly care that will be required over the next few decades. These are important, relevant, and challenging research areas in the study of age and sex.

Sex Ratio at Birth

Most societies have sex ratios at birth (SRBs) of around 105; that is, 105 boys are born for every 100 girls. This so-called biologically normal level of about 105 is likely an evolutionary adaptation to the fact that females have higher survival probabilities than males. Since at every year of life males have higher age-specific death rates than females, around 105 or so males are required at birth for every 100 females for there to be about equal numbers of males and females when the groups reach marriageable age.

TABLE 1.4. **Values of Age Sex Accuracy Index (Ranked from High to Low) for 42 Countries of the World in 2000.**

Country	Age Sex Accuracy Index
United Arab Emirates	110.4
Bahrain	64.8
Saudi Arabia	62.7
Kuwait	58.1
Macau S.A.R.	46.5
Russia	40.9
Hong Kong S.A.R.	34.6
North Korea	29.6
South Korea	29.2
Somalia	29.0
China	23.9
Singapore	23.5
Taiwan	22.2
Germany	22.1
Yemen	21.7
Yugoslavia	21.4
Bangladesh	21.3
Iraq	21.3
Zambia	20.3
Liberia	20.1
Finland	19.4
Jordan	19.1
Gaza Strip	18.8
Sweden	18.3
Vietnam	17.2
France	16.6
Italy	16.5
Uganda	15.9
Spain	15.4
Japan	15.0
United Kingdom	14.6
Ireland	14.1
West Bank	14.1
Israel	14.0
Indonesia	13.9
Iran	13.8
United States	12.8
Kenya	11.5
Thailand	10.9
South Africa	10.7
Syria	10.4
Sri Lanka	10.3

Data source: U.S. Bureau of the Census, 2002.

Figure 1.13 shows time-series data for the sex ratio at birth for China, South Korea, Taiwan, and the United States from 1980 to 2001. The U.S. shows an invariant pattern, with an SRB of just about 105 for every year. This kind of stability over time at around 105 is what one should see if no human interventions disturb the biology. In contrast, whereas in 1980 China had an SRB only slightly above 107, it began to increase in the late 1980s, reaching a value of 115 by 1990. By the year of 2000, the

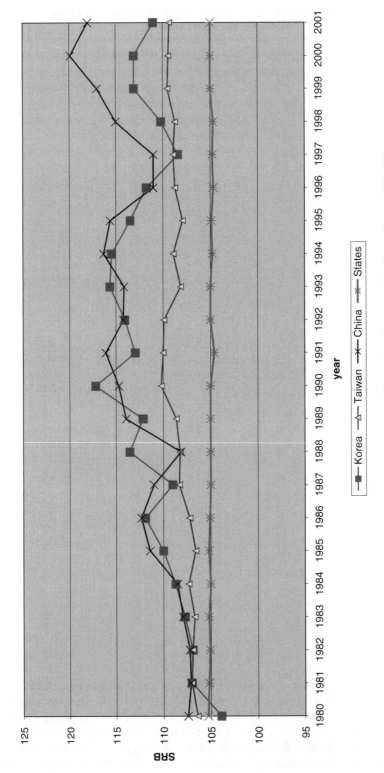

FIGURE 1.13. Sex ratio at birth: Taiwan, mainland China, South Korea, and the United States, 1980–2001.

China SRB was just under 120; the SRBs for South Korea and Taiwan are only slightly lower. Since the early 1980s, the SRBs for all three countries have been significantly above normal levels.

The sex ratio at birth (the SRB), referred to as the secondary sex ratio, may be distinguished from the sex ratio at conception (the SRC), referred to as the primary sex ratio. If there are no human interferences with biological processes, the SRB depends on the factors that produce the SRC. However, if human activities such as sex-selective abortion are introduced, these are interventions that will influence only the SRB and not the SRC. What is known about these sorts of interventions?

China, Taiwan, South Korea, and a few other countries have been reporting abnormally high SRBs since the 1980s (Arnold and Liu 1986; Gu and Roy 1995; Goodkind 1996; 2002; Poston et al. 1997; Eberstadt 2000; Poston and Glover 2005). Research indicates that the SRBs are even higher for higher-order parities (Arnold and Liu 1986; Poston et al. 1997). In South Korea, for instance, "high sex ratios at birth keep growing unacceptably as birth order progresses" (Kim 1997: 20–27).

What are the immediate causes of these abnormally high SRBs? The three East Asian countries under review are all showing, in varying degrees of importance, the same kinds of intervention leading to abnormally high SRBs, namely, prenatal sex identification followed by gender-specific abortion (Hull 1990; Johansson and Nygren 1991; Chu 2001; Banister 2002). All three countries have experienced very rapid fertility declines from around six children per woman in the 1950s to fewer than two children per woman in the 1980s. All three countries have a Confucian patriarchal tradition where son preference is strong and pervasive (Arnold and Liu 1986; Gu and Roy 1995; Kim 1997; Park and Cho 1995; Poston et al. 1997). When birth rates are low or are on the decline, and "where a strong preference for sons over daughters is already part of the culture, SRBs tend to be higher" (Poston et al. 1997: 59).

Birth planning policies, as well as social, economic, and industrial transformations, have been responsible for the fact that the number of babies born per woman in China, South Korea, and Taiwan has fallen to below replacement levels and has done so quickly (Poston 2000, 2002). Couples now have fewer children than they had just a couple of decades ago because of fertility policies and newly emerging social norms and mores. However, the deeply rooted cultural influences of son preference still make it important for many families to have at least one son. Therefore, strategies and interventions are sought by many to ensure that they will have a son (Gu and Roy 1995; Zeng et al. 1993).

In China, South Korea, and Taiwan since the late 1980s, ultrasound technology enabling the prenatal determination of sex has been widely available. There is little evidence of female infanticide causing the high SRBs (Zeng et al. 1993; Eberstadt 2000: 228; Chu 2001; Banister 2002). These human interventions that disturb the SRB, it is hypothesized, are mainly due to norms and traditions among Chinese and Korean families to have sons—within a changing context where fertility policies and social norms encourage fewer births.

How many excess boys will there be in China, South Korea, and Taiwan who will be unable to find brides from their countries? For every year from 1978 to 2001, Poston and Glover (2005) have taken data on China's, South Korea's, and Taiwan's total population size, crude birth rate, and sex ratio at birth and have calculated the numbers of males and females born every year. Using "l(x)" data from life tables for the three countries, they next survived the boys born each year to the ages of 26 and the girls to the ages of 24, which are, or are near, the average ages boys and girls marry. They estimated that there will be around 23 million surplus boys in China, over 1 million surplus boys in South Korea, and over 200,000 surplus boys in Taiwan, all of whom will be looking for wives between the years of 2005 and 2025. And there will not be enough Chinese, Korean, and Taiwanese women in the marriage market for them to marry. What will these many millions of young men do when they cannot find brides? Here are some speculations.

While it is true that throughout history, especially in Western Europe, "bachelor-hood was an acceptable social role, and the incidence of never-marrying bachelors in the total population was high" (Eberstadt 2000: 230; Hajnal 1965), China, South Korea, and Taiwan throughout their thousands of years of history have never been so characterized. Unless in the next few decades these three countries are "swept by a truly radical change in cultural and social attitudes toward marriage . . . they are poised to experience an increasingly intense, and perhaps desperate, competition among young men for the nation's limited supply of brides" (Eberstadt 2000: 230.)

The three countries could well turn to more authoritarian forms of government in order to better control the bachelors. In such a scenario, the countries' progress toward democracy could be stalled if not halted. The countries could modify the magnitude of the potential unrest of these millions of unmarried young men by dispatching them to public works projects thousands of miles away from the big cities. In China, for instance, there are several huge construction projects currently underway, all of which could benefit from a young male labor force.

When confronted with large numbers of excess males during the Middle Ages, Portugal sent them off to wars in North Africa. With many millions of bachelors in the big cities, all within 20 years of age, bellicose Chinese leaders might be tempted to "kill two birds with one stone": they could reduce the tensions caused by bachelors in the cities by sending the excess manpower to pick a fight with, or participate in an invasion of, another country. And what better country with which to engage in such activities than their "renegade province," Taiwan, located less than 100 miles across the Taiwan Straits from the southern province of Fujian. Bellicose leaders in South Korea might send their bachelors to fights in North Korea, where, by the way, there is a balanced sex ratio at birth (Goodkind 1999).

One solution to the problem would be the immigration to the country of Chinese or Korean brides from other countries. This would be very likely in the case of South Korea and Taiwan, but not at all likely for China. China is a poor country, and most of its bachelors will likely be poor rural workers unable to afford "mail order brides" (Eberstadt 2000). In South Korea and Taiwan men will be able to afford mail order brides. If this kind of marriage immigration were to occur, it would need to be of a substantial magnitude to even begin to offset the gender imbalances of marriage-age males that are expected in the first two decades of this new century. And, of course, if this immigration did occur, it would cause shortages of many millions of females in the areas of origin. So if a country gains brides, other countries would lose them.

Polyandry would be another possibility (see Cassidy and Lee 1989). Although some might think this to be an unlikely scenario, there is limited evidence of its existence in China among some of the country's minority populations (Zhang 1997; Johnson and Zhang 1991), but no evidence of it in South Korea or Taiwan. However, this alternative is probably unlikely.

An even less likely solution would be increased homosexuality. This is an unlikely alternative because most scientific evidence on the origins of homosexuality argues in favor of a biological foundation, that is, persons are born with a homosexual orientation (LeVay 1991, 1996; also see Murray [2000] for other views and arguments). It is not at all likely that when Chinese and Korean males are unable to find females to marry they will turn to homosexual relationships as an alternative to (heterosexual) marriage. On the other hand, homosexual behavior in China, South Korea, and Taiwan could well become more acceptable, so that closeted homosexuals will be freer to openly declare their orientation.

The most likely possibility, of course, is that these Chinese and Korean and Taiwanese bachelors will never marry and will have no other choice but to develop their own lives and livelihoods. They will resettle with one another in "bachelor ghettos" in Beijing, Shanghai, Tianjin, Seoul, Pusan, Taipei, and other big cities, where commercial sex outlets would likely be prevalent. The possible implications of large numbers of bachelors using commercial sex workers need also to be addressed, particularly with regard to the worldwide AIDS epidemic.

There is some historical precedent for an expected growth of bachelor ghettos. In the 19th century many thousands of young Chinese men immigrated to the United States to work in the gold mines and help build the railroads. When the work projects were completed, many stayed in the U.S. and resettled in Chinese bachelor ghetto areas in New York, San Francisco, and a few other large U.S. cities (Kwong 1988; Zhou 1992). The sex ratios of the Chinese in these areas were extraordinarily high.

If these Chinese, Korean, and Taiwanese men do not marry, research suggests that they will be more prone to crime than if they married (Sampson and Laub 1990). This possibility has alerted some to the potential increases in crime in China's, South Korea's, and Taiwan's future, perhaps with political ramifications (Hudson and Den Boer 2002).

No one, of course, knows what this excess number of young Chinese, South Korean, and Taiwanese males will do. Several possibilities have been entertained. The only certainty is that there are already many, many millions more baby boys than there will be girls for them to marry in these three countries. This issue needs the immediate research attention of scholars and policymakers.

Demographic Ageing

The second area where research on age and sex needs to be directed pertains to the process of demographic ageing (see Poston and Duan 2000; Poston 2002). Although the ageing phenomenon in China, South Korea, and Taiwan will be mainly considered here, much of what is reported also applies to other countries in Asia and Latin America.

Since the early 1960s, China, South Korea, and Taiwan have experienced dramatic declines in fertility. These fertility reductions are striking and will greatly increase the proportions of elderly in this new century. The data in Table 1.5 indicate that in the year 2000, the total populations of China, South Korea, and Taiwan numbered over 1.26 billion, 47.5 million, and 22.0 million, respectively. But of even greater interest is the size of the older and oldest old populations, defined as persons aged 60 and over, and persons aged 80 and over, respectively (Velkoff and Lawson 1998).

TABLE 1.5. **Elderly Populations: China, South Korea, and Taiwan: 2000, 2020, and 2050.**

Country	Year	Total	Older	Oldest	PSR
China	2000	1,262,474,301	116,344,118	11,778,971	9.78
	2020	1,424,064,346	213,171,750	28,919,295	5.81
	2050	1,417,630,630	337,319,304	115,167,938	2.47
South Korea	2000	47,470,969	5,143,263	459,815	10.26
	2020	52,977,940	10,548,043	1,512,950	5.12
	2050	51,147,663	16,804,119	4,959,824	1.96
Taiwan	2000	22,009,588	2,611,221	284,464	8.11
	2020	24,977,303	5,168,915	801,959	4.74
	2050	24,596,527	8,204,089	2,378,365	1.94

Data source: U.S. Bureau of the Census, 2002.

In 2000, China had 116 million older persons and 11.8 million oldest old; South Korea had 5.1 million older persons and under 500 thousand oldest old; and in Taiwan in 2000, there were 2.6 million older persons and 284 thousand oldest old. These are but small fractions of the total number of older and oldest old persons in the world in 2000.

Table 1.5 shows projections for the total population, the older population, and the oldest old population for the years of 2020 and 2050 (Bureau of the Census 2002). By the midpoint of this new century, there are projected to be over 337 million older persons in China and 115 million oldest old. In South Korea the numbers are projected to be 16.8 million older persons and 4.96 million oldest old. Taiwan is projected to have 8.2 million older persons and 2.4 million oldest old.

There will be almost three times as many older persons in China in 2050 than in 2000 and more than three times as many older persons in South Korea and in Taiwan than in 2000. In China in the year 2050, there are projected to be almost 10 times as many oldest old as in 2000; in South Korea in 2050 the projections indicate that will be almost 11 times as many oldest old as in 2000; and in Taiwan there are projected to be over eight times as many oldest old as there were in 2000.

These population projections indicate that the absolute and relative numbers of the older and oldest old populations in China, South Korea, and Taiwan will increase tremendously in the years of this new century. By 2050 these three countries are projected to have made the transition to demographically very old countries. What are some of the implications of the ageing of these populations?

One effect of the ageing is the tremendous change that will occur in the extent to which the older population will be able to be supported economically and emotionally by the younger members. The United Nations has developed a measure of elderly support, known as the "potential support ratio" (PSR); it represents "the extent that persons of working age (15 to 64) can be seen as supporting the older population (65 years or older), and is the ratio between the two" (United Nations 2001: 7). The PSR value represents the number of persons in the population who "support" every one old person in the population.

In 2000 in China, there were 855,614,459 persons aged 15 to 64, and there were 87,396,780 persons aged 65+. Dividing the former by the latter indicates the number of persons in the population who are available to "support" every one old person. In 2000 in China the PSR was 9.78 producers for every one elderly dependent. The corresponding PSR values for 2000 for South Korea and Taiwan were 10.26 and 8.11, respectively (see Table 1.5).

In the last few decades in these countries, the fertility rates have decreased dramatically, and levels of life expectancy at birth for both sexes have increased remarkably. These two rapid changes in fertility and mortality have resulted in the pace of population ageing in China, South Korea, and Taiwan being among the fastest in the world.

The PSRs for the three countries are projected to drop between the years of 2000 and 2050 from 9.78 to 2.47 (China), from 10.26 to 1.96 (South Korea), and from 8.11 to 1.94 (Taiwan). These are dramatic reductions in the ratios of persons in the supporting ages to persons in the elderly dependent ages.

The United States is also projected to have a low PSR in the year 2050, a PSR of 2.8, just slightly above that of China. But the U.S. had a PSR in 2000 of 5.3, a much lower level of elderly support than in the three East Asian countries under review. The process of population ageing in the U.S. has been much less rapid than in China, South Korea, and Taiwan. The U.S. population has had much more time to adjust to the increased proportions of elderly.

The provision of eldercare in these three East Asian countries will be a major concern in the years of the 21st century. The three societies will have to adjust and make many changes demographically and economically. To offset demographically these dramatic declines in the support ratio, they would need either to turn to international migration for demographic replacement or to increase the upper limits of the working-age population. These and related issues associated with demographic ageing need the attention of researchers and policy makers.

There are likely other issues pertaining to age and sex structure that have not been mentioned in this concluding section but that also need attention. The two that have been addressed, namely, the sex ratio at birth and demographic ageing, require the consideration and reflection of demographers and other social scientists. Both situations result from declining fertility rates and, in the case of population ageing, increases in life expectancy. In many ways, these demographic processes have interacted with the age and sex structures of the countries and have determined their destinies. Finally, although the focus here has been on the three countries of China, South Korea, and Taiwan, much of the discussion applies to other countries in similar situations, e.g., India.

REFERENCES

Arnold, F., and Z. Liu. 1986. Sex preference, fertility, and family planning in China. *Population and Development Review* 12:221–246.

Arriaga, E. E., et al. 1994. *Population Analysis with Microcomputers.* Vol. 1, *Presentation of techniques.* Washington, D.C.: U.S. Bureau of the Census.

Bachi, R. 1951. The tendency to round off age returns: Measurement and correction. *Bulletin of the International Statistical Institute (Proceedings of the 27th Session, Calcutta)* 33:195–221.

Banister, J. 2002. Recent population trends and issues in China. Paper presented at the annual meetings of the Australian Population Association, Sydney, October.

Bogue, D. J. 1969. *Principles of demography.* New York: John Wiley.

Bogue, D. J. 1985. *The population of the United States.* New York: The Free Press.

Carrier, N. H. 1959. A note on the measurement of digital preference in age recordings. *Journal of the Institute of Actuaries* 85:71–85.

Cassidy, M. L., and G. R. Lee. 1989. The study of polyandry: A critique and synthesis. *Journal of Comparative Family Studies* 20:1–11.

Chu, J. 2001. Prenatal sex determination and sex-selective abortion in rural central China. *Population and Development Review* 27:259–281.

Clarke, J. I. 2000. *The human dichotomy: The changing numbers of males and females.* Amsterdam: Pergamon.

Coale, A. J. 1957. How the distribution of human population is determined. *Cold Spring Harbor Symposium on Quantitative Biology* 22:83–89.

Coale, A. J. 1968. Convergence of a human population to a stable form. *Journal of the American Statistical Association* 63:395–435.

Coale, A. J. 1971. Age patterns of marriage. *Population Studies* 25:193–214.

Coale, A. J. 1972. *The growth and structure of human populations.* Princeton, N.J.: Princeton University Press.

Coale, A. J. 1987. Stable populations. In *The new Palgrave: A dictionary of economics*, Vol. 4, edited by J. Eatwell, M. Milgate, and P. K. Newman, 466–469. London: Macmillan.

Coale, A. J., and P. Demeny. 1983. *Regional model life tables and stable populations*, 2nd ed. New York: Academic Press.

Coleman, D. A. 2000. Male fertility trends in industrial countries: Theories in search of some evidence. In *Fertility and the Male Life-Cycle in the Era of Fertility Decline*, edited by C. Bledsoe, S. Lerner, and J. I. Guyer. New York: Oxford University Press.

Davis, K. 1949. *Human society.* New York: Macmillan.

Eberstadt, N. 2000. *Prosperous paupers & other population problems.* New Brunswick, N.J.: Transaction Publishers.

Euler, L. 1760 [1970]. General research on mortality and multiplication. *Memoires de l'Academie Royale des Sciences et Belles Lettres* 16:144–164 (in French), translated by N. Keyfitz and B. Keyfitz, *Theoretical Population Biology* 1:307–314.

Fausto-Sterling, A. 2000. *Sexing the body: Gender politics and the construction of sexuality.* New York: Basic Books.

Flatau, E., Z. Josefsberg, S. H. Reisner, O. Bialik, and Z. Laron. 1975. Penis size in the newborn infant. *Journal of Pediatrics* 87:663–664.

Goldscheider, C. 1971. *Population, Modernization and Social Structure.* Boston: Little, Brown.

Goodkind, D. 1996. On substituting sex preference strategies in East Asia: Does prenatal sex selection reduce postnatal discrimination? *Population Research and Policy Review* 22:111–125.

Goodkind, D. 1999. Do parents prefer sons in North Korea? *Studies in Family Planning* 30:212–218.

Goodkind, D. 2002. Recent trends in the sex ratio at birth in East Asia. Paper presented at Conference on Chinese Populations and Socioeconomic Studies: Utilizing the 2000/2001 Round Census Data. Hong Kong: Hong Kong University of Science and Technology, June 19–21.

Gu, B., and K. Roy. 1995. Sex ratio at birth in China, with reference to other areas in East Asia: What we know. *Asia-Pacific Population Journal.* 10(3):17–42.

Hajnal, J. 1965. European marriage patterns in perspective. In *Population in history*, edited by D. V. Glass and D. E. C. Eversley, 101–143. London: Edward Arnold.

Halli, S. S., and K. V. Rao. 1992. *Advanced techniques of population analysis.* New York: Plenum Press.

Hauser, P. M., and O. D. Duncan, (eds.). 1959. *The study of population: An inventory and appraisal.* Chicago: The University of Chicago Press.

Hawley, A. H. 1950. *Human ecology: A theory of community structure.* New York: The Ronald Press.

Hawley, A. H. 1959. Population composition. Chapter 16 in Philip M. Hauser and Otis Dudley Duncan (editors), *The Study of Population: An Inventory and Appraisal.* Chicago: The University of Chicago Press.

Henry, L. 1961. Some Data on Natural Fertility. *Eugenics Quarterly* 8:81–91.

Hinde, A. 1998. *Demographic Methods.* London: Arnold.

Hobbs, F. 2004. Age and sex composition. In *The methods and materials of demography*, 2nd ed., edited by J. S. Siegel and D. A. Swanson, Chapter 7. San Diego: Elsevier Academic Press.

Horiuchi, S., and S. H. Preston. 1988. Age-specific growth rates: The legacy of past population dynamics. *Demography* 25:429–441.

Hudson, V. M., and A. Den Boer. 2002. A surplus of men, a deficit of peace. *International Security* 26:5–38.

Hull, T. H. 1990. Recent trends in sex ratios at birth in China. *Population and Development Review* 16:63–83.

Johansson, S., and O. Nygren. 1991. The missing girls of China: A new demographic account. *Population and Development Review* 17:35–51.

Johnson, N. E., and K. Zhang. 1991. Matriarchy, polyandry, and fertility amongst the Mosuos in China. *Journal of Biosocial Science* 23:499–505.

Kertzer, D. I., and D. Arel, eds. 2002. *Census and identity: The politics of race, ethnicity, and language in national censuses.* New York: Cambridge University Press.

Keyfitz, N. 1965. Age distribution as a challenge to development. *American Journal of Sociology* 70:659–668.

Keyfitz, N. 1977. *Applied mathematical demography.* New York: John Wiley.

Keyfitz, N., and W. Flieger. 1971. *Population: Facts and methods of demography.* San Francisco: W. H. Freeman.

Kim, D. 1997. The pattern of changing trends and the regional difference in the sex ratio at birth: Evidence from Korea and Jilin Province, China. *Korea Journal of Population and Development* 26:19–44.

Kwong, P. 1988. *The new Chinatown.* New York: Hill and Wang.

LeVay, S. 1991. A difference in hypothalamic structure between heterosexual and homosexual men. *Science* 252:1034–1037.

LeVay, S. 1996. *Queer science: The use and abuse of research into homosexuality.* Cambridge, Mass.: MIT Press.

Lopez, A. 1967. Asymptotic properties of a human age distribution under a continuous net maternity function. *Demography* 4:680–687.

Lotka, A. J. 1907. Relation between birth rates and death rates. *Science*, New Series 26 (653):21–22.

Money, J. 1988. *Gay, straight, and in-between: The sexology of erotic orientation.* New York: Oxford University Press.

Murdock, G. P. 1949. *Social structure.* New York: Macmillan.

Murray, S. O. 2000. *Homosexualities.* Chicago: University of Chicago Press.

Myers, R. J. 1940. Errors and bias in the reporting of ages in census data. *Transactions of the Actuarial Society of America* 41 (Part 2):411–415.

Namboodiri, K. 1991. *Demographic analysis: A stochastic approach.* New York: Academic Press.

Namboodiri, K. 1996. A Primer of Population Dynamics.

Palmore, E. 1978. When can age, period, and cohort be separated? *Social Forces* 57:282–295.

Park, C. B., and N. Cho. 1995. Consequences of son preference in a low-fertility society: Imbalance of the sex ratio at birth in Korea. *Population and Development Review* 21:59–84.

Perlmann, J., and M. C. Waters, eds. 2002. *The new race question: How the census counts multiracial individuals.* New York: Russell Sage Foundation.

Pollard, A. H., F. Yusuf, and G. N. Pollard. 1990. *Demographic techniques*, 3rd ed. Sydney, Australia: Pergamon Press.

Population Reference Bureau. 2001. *2001 World Population Data Sheet.* Washington, D.C.: Population Reference Bureau.

Poston, D. L., Jr. 2000. Social and economic development and the fertility transitions in mainland China and Taiwan. *Population and Development Review* 26 (Supplement): 40–60.

Poston, D. L., Jr. 2002. South Korea's demographic destiny: Marriage market and elderly support implications for the 21st century. In *International Conference on the Longevity and Social, Medical Environment of the Elderly*, 69–83. Taegu, South Korea: Institute of Gerontology, Yeungnam University.

Poston, D. L., Jr., and C. Chang. 2005. Bringing males in: A critical demographic plea for incorporating males in methodological and theoretical analyses of human fertility. *Critical Demography*, forthcoming.

Poston, D. L., Jr., and C. C. Duan. 2000. The current and projected distribution of the elderly and eldercare in the People's Republic of China. *Journal of Family Issues* 21:714–732.

Poston, D. L., Jr., and K. S. Glover. 2005. China's demographic destiny: Marriage market implications for the 21st century. In *Fertility, family planning and population policy in China*, edited by D. L. Poston, Jr., C. F. Lee, C. Chang, S. L. McKibben, and C. S. Walther. London: Routledge Publishers, forthcoming.

Poston, D. L., Jr., B. Gu, P. P. Liu, and T. McDaniel. 1997. Son preference and the sex ratio at birth in China: A provincial level analysis. *Social Biology* 44:55–76.

Poston, D. L., Jr., I. H. J. Chu, J. M. Ginn, G. Jin-Kai Li, C. Hong Vo, C. S. Walther, P. Wang, J. J. Wu, and M. M. Yuan. 2000. The quality of the age and sex data of the Republic of Korea and its provinces, 1970 and 1995. *The Journal of Gerontology* 4:85–126.

Poston, D. L., Jr., C. S. Walther, I. H. J. Chu, J. M. Ginn, G. J. Li, C. H. Vo, P. Wang, J. J. Wu, and M. M. Yuan. 2003. The age and sex composition of the Republic of Korea and its provinces, 1970 and 1995. *Genus* 59:113–139.

Preston, S. H., P. Heuveline, and M. Guillot. 2001. *Demography: Measuring and modeling population processes.* Malden, Mass.: Blackwell Publishers.

Ramachandran, K. V. 1967. An index to measure digit preference error in age data. *World Population Conference, 1965, Belgrade* Vol. III: 202–203.

Rogers, A. 1975. *Introduction to multiregional mathematical demography.* London: Wiley.

Sampson, R. J., and J. H. Laub. 1990. Crime and deviance over the life course: The salience of adult social bonds. *American Sociological Review* 55:609–627.

Sane, K., and O. H. Pescovitz. 1992. The clitoral index: A determination of clitoral size in normal girls and in girls with abnormal sexual development. *Journal of Pediatrics* 120:264–266.

Schoen, R. 1988. *Modeling multigroup populations*. New York: Plenum Press.

Sharpe, F. R., and A. J. Lotka. 1911. A problem in age distribution. *Philosophical Magazine* 21:435–438.

Shryock, H. S., J. S. Siegel, and Associates. 1976. *The methods and materials of demography*, condensed ed. by Edward G. Stockwell. New York: Academic Press.

Smith, D. P. 1992. *Formal demography*. New York: Plenum Press.

South, S. J. and K. Trent. 1988. Sex ratios and women's roles: A cross-national analysis. *American Journal of Sociology* 93:1096–1115.

Spiegelman, M. 1969. *Introduction to demography*, rev. ed. Cambridge, Mass.: Harvard University Press.

Stone, L. O. 1978. *The frequency of geographic mobility in the population of Canada*. Ottawa: Statistics Canada.

Texas Department of Criminal Justice. 2000. *Statistical Report, Fiscal Year 2000*. Huntsville, Texas: Texas Department of Criminal Justice.

Tobler, W. 1995. Migration: Ravenstein, Thornthwaite, and Beyond. *Urban Geography* 16:327–343.

United Nations. 1952. Accuracy tests for census age distributions tabulated in five-year and ten-year groups. *Population Bulletin* 2:59–79.

United Nations. 1955. *Methods of appraisal of quality of basic data for population estimate*s. Manual II, Series A, Population Studies No 23. New York: United Nations.

United Nations. 1990. *1988 Demographic Yearboo*k. New York: United Nations.

United Nations. 1998. Principles and recommendations for population and housing censuses, rev. 1. *Statistical Papers* Series M, No. 67/Rev. 1. New York: United Nations.

United Nations. 2001. *Replacement migration: Is it a solution to declining and ageing populations?* New York: United Nations.

U.S. Bureau of the Census. 2002. *Census Bureau International Data Base*. Available at http://www.census.gov (Accessed 12/20/2002.)

van de Walle, E., and J. Knodel. 1970. Teaching population dynamics with a simulation exercise. *Demography* 7:433–448.

Velkoff, V. A., and V. A. Lawson. 1998. Gender and aging caregiving. *International Brief*, IB/98–3 (December). Washington, D.C.; U.S. Bureau of the Census.

Weeks, J. R. 2002. *Population: An introduction to concepts and issues*, 8th ed. Belmont, Calif.: Wadsworth/Thomson.

Zeng, Y., P. Tu, B. Gu, Y. Xu, B. Li, and Y Li. 1993. Causes and implications of the recent increase in the reported sex ratio at birth in China. *Population and Development Review* 19:283–302.

Zhang, T. 1997. Marriage and family patterns in Tibet. *China Population Today* 14:9–12.

Zhou, M. 1992. *Chinatown: The socioeconomic potential of an urban enclave*. Philadelphia: Temple University Press.

CHAPTER 2

Population Distribution and Suburbanization

AVERY M. GUEST AND SUSAN K. BROWN

Much of contemporary demographic research focuses on population groups that are geographically defined by a single areal universe, such as the United States or the world. Population research has gained much of its impetus in the past few decades from the effort to understand the unparalleled growth of many of these aggregates—what has been termed the *population explosion.*

Geographically defined aggregates may be further divided by their distribution according to specific territorial subdivisions such as regions, metropolitan areas, cities, and neighborhoods. Often the patterns for a country in terms of population size and growth have only a weak relationship to those reported for the subdistricts. Indeed, many national populations are characterized by such incredibly diverse patterns of internal change among their subdistricts that the interpretation of "average" patterns for a population universe may have little practical meaning. Thus, in some countries, specific territories are growing at rates of 10% or more per year while others are declining. To illustrate, in the United States, the Las Vegas metropolitan area tripled its population between 1980 and 2000, while 46 of the 53 counties in the state of North Dakota lost population.

For those who study population distribution, a key term is *population implosion,* which is the dramatic, growing tendency for human populations to be disproportionately concentrated in large urban agglomerations. In other words, high proportions of the population are found in a small number of communities, occupying generally low proportions of national territories. In effect, the population implosion represents urbanization, but in its current manifestation also includes the idea of megacities (Zwingle

2002), where literally millions of people are concentrated together within one part of a nation's territory.

One consequence of the population implosion is a growing inequality in population distribution within societies, a trend that will likely continue for a number of decades. Societies may need, as in recent decades, to develop bipolar social policies toward their parts: for the large agglomerations, the problem will be providing enough new infra-structure (roads, highways, and services) so that the community may function smoothly; for the small agglomerations, the problem will be providing enough services to cushion the ill effects of the decreasing opportunities for their residents.

Historically, the implosion of populations occurred in a relatively finite geograph-ical space so that cities emphasized upward growth of densities to accommodate increasing numbers. But in recent decades, territorial distribution has been character-ized by a new pattern of outward spread into surrounding areas that were once lightly settled, areas commonly called suburbs. This suburbanization process is especially evident in highly developed societies such as the United States but is also occurring in many other societies around the world with lower standards of material living.

While this chapter provides a general overview of major trends in population redistribution in the world, it devotes special attention to suburbanization. In particu-lar, it analyzes the case of the United States, where suburbanization has been particu-larly important. This chapter documents some of the principal trends of the past few decades and then uses the results of the 2000 U.S. census to chart the major dimensions of recent change.

THE WORLDWIDE IMPLOSION

For most of human history, aggregate populations were relatively small and mobile. Limited human technology made it difficult for most communities to produce goods and services beyond very basic needs. Many groups knew so little about the techniques of sedentary agriculture that they roamed or foraged to find adequate food. Most agriculturalists lacked the knowledge and tools to produce a food surplus that would support large numbers of individuals in nonagricultural places (Sjoberg 1960).

During the past several thousand years, this situation gradually changed, and urban agglomerations slowly began to develop. Even in 1800, only 2% of the world's population lived in agglomerations of 20,000 or more (Davis 1955). Since 1800, the percentage of the world's population living in dense concentrations of this size has doubled about every 50 years or so. According to the United Nations (2004: Table 3), almost one-half of the world's population lived in urban agglomerations, as defined by member countries in 2000, in comparison to about one-third in 1950.

Interestingly, while national populations differ greatly in their population distribu-tions, they have all had major increases in population concentration. Almost all parts of the world have higher levels of urbanization today than were found 200 years ago. Even the continent of Africa, which has an unusually high proportion of very poor countries, was more than 37% urban in 2000, according to the United Nations (2004: Table 8).

One social science approach to the study of population issues is that of human ecology (see chapter 20, "Ecological Demography," in this *Handbook*). A central interest of human ecology is how population growth and change respond to the level and complexity of technology, to the ways that societies and communities organize their productive and political activities, and to the social and physical environment (Hawley 1986; Namboodiri 1988). Human ecologists study various levels of population aggregation, including regions, cities, and neighborhoods, but tend to eschew individuals as units of analysis.

From the human ecological perspective, the simultaneous emergence of the population explosion and implosion is understandable. As technological knowledge has increased, it has been possible to improve dramatically the living conditions of populations, setting off declines in mortality and increasing overall population growth. At the same time, as the general level of technological knowledge has increased, individual agriculturalists have developed techniques to raise more food than they need and, consequently, support large numbers of nonagriculturists in concentrated communities. In addition, both population explosion and implosion have resulted from the increasing complexity and sophistication of human social organization. For instance, contemporary societies often have highly organized and relatively efficient health care services that enhance the health and well-being of their population and, in the process, encourage high population growth due to low mortality rates. At the same time, the development of organized government bureaucracies has permitted the planning and coordination that are necessary to sustain the spatial concentration of thousands, even millions, of diverse individuals.

THE IMPLOSION MOVES OUTWARD

For most of human history, population implosion involved concentration within small geographical areas. Urban agglomerations generally had only, at most, a few thousand residents (Davis 1955; Winsborough 1963). In addition, transportation, communication, and building construction were relatively primitive by standards of recent decades. Most movement was by foot, and most communication occurred by face-to-face contact. Given the primitive development of transportation and communication, most interrelated activities such as workplace and home had to be located in proximity. The problem of accommodating populations was complicated by the fact that primitive methods of building construction facilitated only small structures that were rarely more than two to four stories in height. The result was a cluttered and spatially delimited community at points of population concentration.

This situation changed greatly after about 1880 in societies such as the United States, resulting in an expansion of the population boundaries of many territories. One fundamental development was the electric streetcar/railway in the very late 1800s, which generally emanated from the center of cities on fixed radial lines (Ward 1971; Warner 1972). Given its relatively rapid speed, this development permitted the outward dispersal of activities, both workplaces and residences, but especially residences, since many individuals wanted to reside outside the congestion of the center. In addition, activities within the metropolis began to separate spatially into various subdistricts because they no longer required physical proximity. Clearly delineated areas of the rich and poor, of residences and workplaces, began to appear. The electric streetcar, with its orientation to transportation points at the center of the urban core, also had what might be considered the paradoxical effect of increasing the concentration of activities there that especially depended on proximity to the whole region (such as government offices and retail department stores).

Perhaps a more important transportation development was the mass production of the motor vehicle, which spread throughout the population, particularly the economically stable working and middle social classes, in the period after 1920, that is, roughly the years after World War I (Hawley 1978). Individuals and families could now live at some distance from various activities but be within reasonable commuting distance. While the streetcar oriented many activities to the downtown, the motor vehicle with its more flexible routes encouraged the development of numerous subcenters outside the traditional downtown.

Historically, much of the outward physical movement of Americans from traditional urban concentrations occurred via the political annexation of territories by the central cities, leading to a situation in which the social, physical, and political cities were largely coterminous. However, in the period after 1920, populations in many of the newer outer areas rejected the political dominance of the central cores and began forming numerous legally recognized communities. In general, political jurisdictions that were the traditional growth nodes of urban agglomerations became known as central cities, and the more peripheral communities were known as *suburbs*. This division and specialization of parts between the politically defined central city and the suburban ring became known as the metropolitan community (Schnore 1959).

The most dramatic outward expansion of urban concentrations occurred after World War II ended (Guest 1975; Hawley 1978; Tobin 1976). Furthermore, growth was sprawling, creating extensive geographical regions where much of the population lived at low densities. Even in comparison to the 1920s and 1930s, automobile ownership increased greatly in importance, influenced partly by the merchandising of auto manufacturers and by the development of high-speed, limited-access highways. In addition, affluence grew greatly in American society, especially in comparison to the economically depressed years of the 1930s. As a result, families sought larger and lower-density living units. The federal government also played an important role by encouraging and offering low-interest loans for persons buying homes on the periphery.

A primary historical factor in the clustering of population within small areas was the need for direct face-to-face interaction. This changed some in the post-1920 period with the development of community telephone systems (Fischer 1992), but the electronic revolution of the past few decades has undoubtedly had an even greater impact. In the past two decades, computer technology has permitted electronic workplaces in which individuals communicate actively with each other but at some physical distance. Individuals can work and live well beyond the conventional spatial limits of metropolitan areas, and many workplaces such as banks can spin off auxiliary operations like record keeping to remote locations where they are linked electronically with central offices.

Without doubt, the outward spread of population in American urban concentrations during the early post–World War II period had many ill effects on the older central core areas. Downtowns suffered precipitous declines in many types of employment, especially in retailing, as peripheral auto-oriented shopping malls developed for the first time in American history (Sternlieb 1971). A number of central neighborhoods experienced significant population declines (Price-Spratlen and Guest 2002), and, unlike the early part of the 20th century, few population groups were available to serve as replacements. Immigration from abroad had declined to a trickle, and the major in-migration group to urban cores was comprised of African Americans (Taeuber and Taeuber 1965). As the demand for centrally located housing became low, the surviving residents lacked the resources and the social incentive to maintain the quality of many areas. Central city governments, while aggressively confronting their social ills, developed many financial problems as they tried to deal with an eroding tax base, due to factors such as population loss.

The tremendous redistribution of population within the United States is indicated in recent data from the U.S. Census Bureau. Counties have been divided by the Census Bureau into those that are considered part of metropolitan areas and those that are not. The metropolitan counties themselves have been divided into their central cities, or historic centers, and the remaining parts of the metropolitan areas, i.e., the suburbs. The Census Bureau reports (Hobbs and Stoops 2002: 33) that in 2000, for the first time in American history, at least half of the U.S. population lived in suburbs. This represents an incredible change since 1950, the midpoint of the 20th century, when for the first time at least half (56.1%) the U.S. population lived in metropolitan areas, whether central cities or suburbs. In 1950, only about one-quarter of the American population lived in what were considered suburbs, and the number of central city residents outnumbered suburbanites by almost 10 million. Yet even the 1950 pattern represented a dramatic change from 1910, in which only 7% of the U.S. total population lived in suburban areas.

Since 1970, in several time periods, nonmetropolitan areas have grown at faster rates than metropolitan areas, and, overall, metropolitan and nonmetropolitan growth rates have not differed strikingly (Fuguitt and Brown 1990; Wardwell 1980). It turns out that much of the nonmetropolitan growth in these periods has occurred in territories that are physically close to the suburbs of conventional metropolitan areas. Apparently, the borderline between territories of heavy population concentration and those of low population concentration is becoming blurred, so that the "real" boundaries of metropolitan agglomerations are increasingly difficult to define.

The influence of the metropolis now extends to long distances from the traditional centers. On the metropolitan periphery, previously independent communities such as agricultural service centers are increasingly housing residents who work elsewhere in the metropolis. In addition, new communities, sometimes called exurbs, are being created from scratch by developers. These communities are often detached physically from the expanding crest of suburban development.

CHANGING SUBURBAN DEVELOPMENT

Much of our understanding of suburbs rests on the literature and observations of the middle part of the 20th century. However, new social forces have emerged in recent decades, and the major dimensions of the suburban community demand charting. What are the key questions and the possible answers about changing suburban development?

One set of questions deals with the *degree* to which suburbs continue to grow rapidly in population, especially relative to their central cities. No one doubts that suburban rings continue to grow more rapidly, in an absolute sense, than their central cities. But what is the emerging balance of growth between central cities and suburbs?

Certainly, many central cities have emerged from their depressed years in the early post–World War II period. The 2000 census shows that a number of central cities, especially older places in the Northeast and Midwest, experienced patterns of population increase (albeit often small) in the 1990s compared to the 1980s (*New York Times* 2001c, 2001d). A number of central city downtown areas have begun to prosper as they have assumed important roles in specialized employment niches such as convention centers and government/legal services for extensive surrounding territories. These downtown industries have undoubtedly attracted many individuals (often characterized by at least moderate socioeconomic status) to live nearby, and one can point to a number of gentrifying neighborhoods in central cities (London et al. 1986).

Few could doubt that many central cities have shown recent sparks of vitality and that some suburbs face central city–like problems, but one should be cautious about downgrading the importance of suburbs as growth centers in American society. Many central cities have limited physical space in which to expand, while suburban rings continue to offer extensive undeveloped land. Indeed, the persistence of massive suburban growth is suggested by the growing political issue of suburban sprawl (Squires 2002). Many individuals dislike the formless, haphazard nature of peripheral metropolitan development and fear that highly valued land that might be used for recreation and nonresidential activities will be lost forever (Lindstrom and Hartling 2003).

Another important factor in considering suburban versus central city growth is the explosive development of diverse employment activities in suburban rings (Bourne 1996). Whereas early post–World War II suburbanization heavily involved residences that were tied to central city workplaces, more recent years have seen the creation of major peripheral employment centers. This has involved high rates of job relocation from central cities to suburbs and the creation of many new job opportunities, as in the computer industry. Examples that come to mind are Silicon Valley in the San Francisco metropolitan region and Redmond, outside Seattle. This growth of employment, both the amount and the diversity of activity, has created a need to house increasingly diverse workforces, a factor that would encourage growing diversity in the age and family structure of suburbs.

Many metropolitan dwellers now work and live in suburban rings and have little contact with central cities. Some (Leinberger and Lockwood 1986) have even argued that communities in the suburban rings are becoming "urban villages," characterized by self-sustaining autonomous mixes of employment and residence. Garreau (1991) has described such self-sustaining settlements as "edge cities," since they are often on the suburban outskirts.

A second set of questions deals with the universality of the suburban movement across metropolitan areas in the United States. Historically, older metropolitan areas, disproportionately concentrated in the Northeast and Midwest, have experienced the greatest loss of population from their central core cities (Schnore 1957, 1959). This may partially reflect the fact that they often have congested and unattractive neighborhoods in their centers, providing an incentive for the residential population to move elsewhere. At the same time, newer metropolitan areas may still have some open space for development in their central cities. In addition, central cities in newer metropolitan areas may also have an unusual propensity to grow by political annexation of potentially suburban territory. Older central cities tend to be hemmed in by already incorporated suburbs, and new central cities can often exert political leverage over surrounding territories by exercising control of amenities such as water rights.

Yet, as has been pointed out, a number of older central cities apparently resumed population growth in the 1990s after experiencing decline for several decades. Perhaps old and new metropolitan areas are converging into a common pattern of suburbanization.

A third set of questions deals with the emerging population composition of various parts of suburbia. In comparison to their central cities, suburban rings have traditionally had adult residents with above-average incomes, a disproportionate number of whom were married with children. Today, however, there is a great deal of population diversity within suburbs. Although perhaps the most striking traditional characteristic of suburbia is the overwhelming dominance of persons from European ancestries (Guest 1980), these patterns are changing. Indeed, a dominant theme in recent research about suburbia is its growing diversity (Bourne 1996, Frey 2003). Allegedly, suburbs have become less homogeneous over time. It is increasingly difficult to distinguish a suburban neighborhood from a central city neighborhood. People of African, Asian, and Hispanic ancestry are increasingly represented, although not in proportions equivalent to their representation in the larger metropolitan population (Frey 2003). Poverty is evident in many suburban rings, and the increasing diversity of American family structure is also represented in many suburbs.

A primary task in the study of territorial distribution in relationship to suburbs is charting the variations in composition but, just as importantly, understanding why they occur. According to the human ecological perspective, such factors as the spatial position of the community in the metropolis and the overall density of the population should affect the characteristics of the types of persons who live there. The following sections of this chapter deal with each of these questions.

SUBURBAN GROWTH: SLOWING OR ROARING?

To chart the general dimensions of suburban growth in the last part of the 20th century, designated central cities are compared with their total suburban rings for metropolitan areas in each decade between 1960 and 2000. While some of the analysis in this chapter concentrates on the period since 1970, inclusion of 1960 in the analysis of growth provides some comparative perspective with the heyday of post–World War II suburbanization. The data focus on the census-designated Metropolitan Statistical Areas (MSAs) with total populations of at least 250,000 in 2000, an admittedly arbitrary threshold but one suggesting large-scale urbanization. While 163 such areas were recognized in the 2000 census, two could not be included because they lacked the requisite data for 1960.

Since the development of the census-designated metropolitan area in the 1940s, numerous changes in the specific definitions and their parts have occurred, although many of the basic conceptions remained fixed. Literal use of central city designations in 2000 would be a mistake. In earlier censuses, central city designations were generally limited to one or two places per metropolitan area and were restricted primarily to places with over 50,000 population. However, by 2000, the number of central cities "exploded" in census reports. By then, many MSAs contained "central cities" of less than 50,000 population, and many of the designated central cities could hardly be considered original growth centers for their regions. For instance, the Seattle-Bellevue-Everett MSA includes Seattle, clearly the original growth center for the region and the dominant community in terms of population; Bellevue, which now has over 100,000 population but which developed as a residential suburb near Seattle in the period after World War II; and Everett, a peripheral, small lumber mill city that was the hometown for Henry "Scoop" Jackson, Washington's powerful senator at the time Everett was designated as a "central city."

This chapter treats as central cities those census-designated places that have at least 50,000 population and are the largest designated central city in the MSA. In addition, to recognize the very real possibility of dual central cities, census-designated central cities of 50,000 population that are at least half the size of the largest recognized central city are also included.

The stupendous dimensions of suburbanization since 1960 are suggested by Figure 2.1, which shows the total numbers of persons living in the central cities and suburban rings of the 161 profile areas. In 1960, 61.9 million persons lived in the suburban rings, while 124.8 million lived in the rings in 2000. Some observers of the suburban scene (Jackson 1985: 297) have argued that suburbanization would slow down in the late 20th century due to such checks as the high costs of transportation fuel and new land. But the most noteworthy aspect of the figure is the virtually linear, continuous increase in the suburban population, regardless of decade. The data suggest that suburbanization, as measured by raw numbers, is on an upward, endless trajectory. The figure shows that the absolute number of new suburbanites has grown by a constant number each decade, although the percentage growth rate is higher in earlier decades because the base number of suburbanites was smaller.

In contrast, central cities have also shown some overall growth, but the pattern is much less dramatic and more erratic. Interestingly, in the 1970s, the average central city actually declined slightly in population size, yet the 1990s were characterized by the most positive growth of any decade, gaining 5.3 million residents. In addition, the 1980s also showed overall positive central city growth, but at a lower rate. Apparently, the 1970s involved the "dog days" of central cities in the United States, when their problems and outmoded land uses resulted in little attraction for population growth.

However, one should be cautious about emphasizing the rebound of central cities from their losses in the 1970s. Even in the 1990s, suburban growth was strikingly higher than central city growth, and there is little evidence that any central cities have moved from dramatic patterns of population decline to dramatic patterns of population increase. The so-called rebound of central cities is but a "blip" in the larger pattern of continuing, massive suburbanization. For instance, Chicago, the third largest U.S. central city, grew in the 1990s by 112,290 to a population of 2,896,016 in 2000. However, given previous losses, Chicago's population size in 2000 was still 109,662 less than in 1980, and 470,941 less than in 1970.

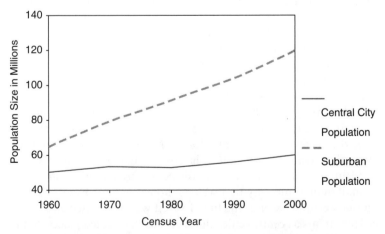

FIGURE 2.1. Persons (in millions) in U.S. central cities and suburban rings.

While the differences in central city growth across decades are socially significant, one should be cautious in interpreting the data. As Frey and Berube (2003: 264) show for large metropolitan areas, the 1970s involved substantial growth in the numbers of households in many central cities, but the shrinkage in the average household size had major effects in producing overall population decline. The depressed period of central cities in the 1970s is not as evident if one compares growth in the number of central city households in the 1970s with the 1990s.

SUBURBAN GROWTH: OLD VERSUS NEW METROPOLITAN AREAS

While the overall degree of suburbanization is impressive, patterns may differ significantly over metropolitan areas. How important is this variation? As suggested earlier, metropolitan age or the major period of development of central cities is important for distinguishing the growth of central cities from their suburban rings. Age is defined by the census year in which the central city (or cities) first achieved a population of at least 50,000. The figure of 50,000 is important because it has historically been used to define the existence of central cities within metropolitan regions (Schnore 1959). Age thus indicates the rough time period in which population size grew large enough to foster a metropolitan region.

In this chapter, metropolitan areas are divided into three age groups that are roughly defined by major changes in the nature of urban transportation. Pre-1890 metropolitan areas developed their large sizes when most movement occurred by foot or horse and were characterized, at the time, by high-density central development. Metro areas that developed between 1890 and 1910 were heavily influenced by the more rapid electric streetcar, which encouraged some physical expansion of the metropolitan territory. Finally, post-1910 metropolitan areas became important in the era of the motor vehicle.

Figure 2.2 illustrates three different aspects of growth in the 161 metropolitan areas when they are divided by their age. The first panel depicts the percentage of central city agglomerations, by age group, that showed any population growth at all during each decade. The second panel illustrates similar information for the suburban rings of the same central cities. Since suburban ring growth occurs ubiquitously across metropolitan areas, suburban rings are distinguished by whether they grew at a high rate (by at least 20% in each decade) or at a relatively low rate (less than 20%). The third panel presents, for the same age groups of metropolitan areas, the relative percentage of all metropolitan dwellers that live in the suburban rings (as opposed to central cities) at each point in time.

Panel 1 of the figure shows quite strong differences in central city growth by age, regardless of time period. Clearly, the existence of central city population decline is most evident in the oldest metropolitan areas having central cities which were originally developed in a period of slower transportation. Less than 40% of central cities in the oldest metropolitan areas (pre-1890) grow in any decade. In contrast, the newest metropolitan areas are characterized by positive growth of central cities, regardless of decade. In each decade, at least 80% of central cities that came of age in 1910 or later show population growth.

The data do suggest, nevertheless, that the gap in central city growth between new and old metropolitan areas has declined. In the 1970s, a quite striking gap was evident

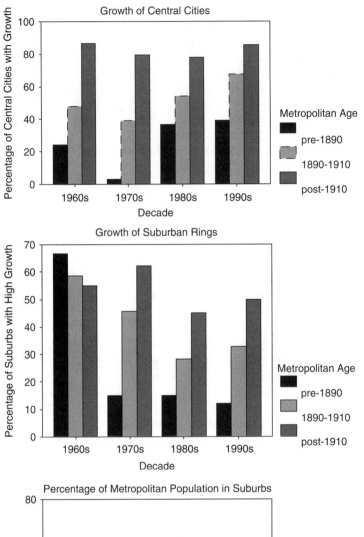

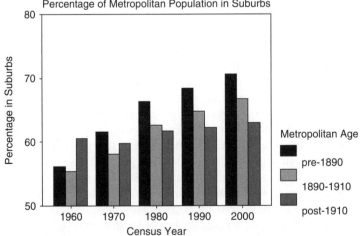

FIGURE 2.2. Growth patterns, 1960 to 2000, by age of metropolitan area.

with hardly any of the old metropolitan areas showing positive central city growth. By the 1990s, the percentage of growing central cities among the oldest metropolitan agglomerations was the highest in the decades. Yet, the "rebound" pattern was limited, with only 39% of the central city agglomerations of old metropolitan areas growing in the 1990s.

Perhaps surprisingly, the second panel shows that the same general metropolitan age effects characterize suburban rings. Suburban rings of older metropolitan agglomerations have quite low percentages growing by 20%, except during the 1960s. Suburban rings of the newest metropolitan areas show higher percentages with at least 20% growth in each decade.

The age variation in suburban growth, similar to the central city variation, partially reflects the fact that older metropolitan areas in the United States have been less attractive for overall population growth than newer metropolitan areas, which tend to be concentrated in the southern and western regions, where the population is shifting. In other words, older metropolitan areas have less overall population growth than new metropolitan areas, and both their central cities and suburban rings have less chance of longitudinal growth. However, this finding must be interpreted cautiously because suburban rings are less differentiated by age in growth pattern than central cities. In other words, high suburban ring growth is a more universal characteristic of metropolitan areas than changes in central city populations.

The fate of the older central cities relative to their suburban rings is more starkly delineated in the third panel of Figure 2.2. This panel shows how the percentage of MSA residents living in suburban rings has changed over the decades. The major finding is that old and new metropolitan areas are becoming increasingly differentiated in the degree of population suburbanization. In 1960 and 1970, *both* the oldest and the newest metropolitan areas have the highest suburban percentages. By 2000, all types of metropolitan areas show an increasing percentage of population in the suburban ring. Yet by 2000, the oldest metropolitan areas clearly have the highest percentage living in the suburban ring. This is a product of the newest metropolitan areas showing little change in their suburbanization of population, while the oldest metropolitan areas have lost relative shares of population to the suburban ring.

The march toward a suburb-dominated society thus seems evident, at least superficially, in the oldest and medium-aged metropolitan regions. But, almost paradoxically, suburban rings are growing less rapidly in absolute numbers in the older metropolitan regions than in newer regions. The reason for these different patterns is that overall metropolitan growth in newer metropolitan areas fuels both the central cities and suburban rings, while the lower overall growth in the older metropolitan areas is disproportionately oriented toward the suburban ring. This is a pattern that slowed down in the 1990s but still continues. Even the so-called "rebound" growth pattern of central cities in the 1990s did not slow what appears to be an inevitable march toward increasing suburban proportions of older metropolitan populations. In other words, the rebound of old central cities in the 1990s is only a blip in the long-term historical redistribution of population.

Why is suburbanization, at least in terms of share of the total metropolitan population, more evident in the oldest metropolitan areas? For the oldest metropolitan areas, this reflects partially their undesirability for residential living. But it also reflects the fact that central cities are largely hemmed in by incorporated suburbs and have difficulty expanding their geographical area. Newer central cities benefit from residential desirability, but another important factor is the ability of central cities in the newer metropolitan regions to annex what had been suburban territory. In these regions, suburban areas less often have incorporated city governments to resist annexation, or, if incorporated, they have shorter-term traditions of community sentiment that would encourage them to remain independent.

While longitudinal 1960 to 2000 data on populations in annexed areas are unavailable, the geographical size of central cities may be compared. For the oldest metropolitan regions, the 1960 areas of their central cities are over 90% of the size of their 2000 central city areas. At the other extreme, in the newest metropolitan regions, the 2000 areas of central cities are typically at least twice the size of the 1960 areas of their central cities. However, this apparently dramatic change for new metropolitan areas must be tempered by the knowledge that the average is heavily influenced by a few extreme cases of massive growth of central city areas.

In some statistical analyses, patterns of change between 1960 and 2000 in the percentage of population in the suburban ring showed little variation by age of the central city among metropolitan areas that had relatively fixed central city borders. To an important degree, then, peripheral population redistribution occurs in all metropolitan regions, but central cities in newer metropolitan regions have retained their viability at the expense of the suburbs on their peripheries.

Clearly, more needs to be known about the relative effects of annexation versus actual living conditions of central cities in producing differential patterns of suburbanization. For some previous research on this topic, see Klaff and Fuguitt 1978.

POPULATION DECLINE AMIDST SUBURBAN GROWTH

Since the suburban rings are growing so dramatically over time, one might superficially assume that nearly all parts of the suburban ring are also growing. This need not be true. As previously pointed out, urban centers before the late 1800s accommodated population growth by increasingly concentrating residents in relatively fixed areas. But the development of high-speed transportation and communication permits the well-known phenomenon of sprawl, where new territories are continually developed at low densities. Once communities are built up, there is little reason to develop them more intensely because builders can simply move on or leapfrog to new territory. Many suburbs, of course, will continue to grow over time, but one should anticipate that a sizable number of suburbs will also experience population decline. So it is worthwhile to ask, among individual suburban places, how universal is growth? What are the major spatial, social, and economic characteristics of individual suburbs that continue to predict their growth?

Guest's (1979) research on population loss for individual suburbs in the three time periods of 1950 to 1960, 1960 to 1970, and 1970 to 1975 serves as a model for analyzing recent decades. He found a dramatic temporal increase in the number of suburbs that lost population; consistent with early post–World War II images of suburbia, loss was quite rare in the 1950s and 1960s, but by the 1970s occurred in about one-third of the suburban communities.

Historically, analysts have used a "life-cycle" perspective in analyzing the relative growth rates of various parts of metropolitan areas. According to this view, parts of the metropolis pass through a regular cycle of population growth and decline as a consequence of spatial position. The cycle involves an initial period of rapid residential growth, the achievement of a slower rate of change with the aging and building up of the community, and finally population decline (Hoover and Vernon 1962). The alleged mechanisms are severalfold. For instance, areas that are close to the metropolitan center are desired for commercial and industrial activities, and residential uses may be pre-empted. Furthermore, many older, central parts of the metropolis have achieved high levels of residential development and have little land left for residential development. In addition, many of the existing older residential structures, linked to low socioeconomic status, are undesirable for occupancy.

Researchers (Duncan, Sabagh, and Van Arsdol 1962; Price-Spratlen and Guest 2002) have applied the life-cycle perspective to parts of the central city and inner suburbs, showing that some of the very oldest parts of the central city experience population declines after periods of growth. Indeed, the life-cycle perspective helps address the question of why many central cities have population declines, especially those in older metropolitan areas. The answer is that many central city neighborhoods are too dense and the housing is too outmoded.

The general life-cycle idea has been applied to suburbs (Jackson 1985: 301–302; Orfield 1997). Research suggests that the inner suburbs of many metropolitan areas are especially experiencing population decline and an associated economic decline because they are considered unattractive for residential living.

Guest's (1979) study of suburban growth between 1950 and 1975 provides support for the life-cycle perspective. Population loss was most evident in suburbs that had borders touching their central cities, although loss was not as great as for the central cities. Guest found, furthermore, a dramatic increase over these time periods in population loss in the inner suburbs, relative to more peripheral areas. This pattern could have reflected a tendency for decline to be evident in communities that were at advanced stages in the life cycle.

Guest's study of suburban growth between 1950 and 1975 also investigated population change in the most peripheral communities. This was an attempt to test whether the outward expansion of the suburban ring was relatively boundless or had distinct constraints based on distance of the community from its central city. He found that those suburbs more than 20 miles from central city borders (a substantial distance) were more likely to experience population loss in the 1950 to 1960, 1960 to 1970, and 1970 to 1975 periods than suburbs between 10 and 20 miles from the central city. This pattern showed little change over the three time periods. However, population loss was still most characteristic of inner suburbs, those with borders touching the central city, rather than the most peripheral communities.

Guest's study ended in 1975. It could well have limited implications for more recent time periods, especially in light of what has been found about broad patterns of central city and suburban growth in the 1990s. As noted, some central cities, especially in the oldest metropolitan areas, have shown some rebound from previous population declines. Presumably inner suburbs in older metropolitan areas would benefit from this pattern, also showing some rebounds. Indeed, the increasing ability of developers to leapfrog already existing patterns of suburban development may mean that the life-cycle theory is less useful now for studying the growth patterns of individual suburbs.

To analyze these issues for the last part of the 20th century, Guest's sample of suburbs for the 1950 to 1975 time periods is used. His basic sample included 3,282 suburban places of at least 2,500 population in the metropolitan areas, as defined in

1970. All census-designated urban places in the metropolitan counties are called suburban except the census-designated central cities in 1970. The 1970 cutoff of 2,500 population was necessary since the census data on a variety of social and economic characteristics are reported only for communities of this size. The longitudinal parts of this analysis include only the 3,061 suburbs, from the 1970 sample, that could be traced over time, both backward and forward. Most of the omitted suburbs were likely annexed or consolidated with other communities, although they could have disappeared for other reasons such as major name changes.

Census definitions of metropolitan area have changed over time, and it is impossible to identify a constant set of "suburbs" over various time periods. In this longitudinal analysis, suburbs will be defined on the basis of the 1970 metropolitan area definition. There is a high overlap over time in the counties that are included in metropolitan areas, but in general the number of metropolitan areas and the number of counties in them have expanded. In particular, peripheral counties have tended to be added to metropolitan areas, and as a result, the sample underrepresents the most peripheral suburban communities, using the metropolitan area definitions of 1990 and 2000.

The 1970 definition of metropolitan area also differs in other ways from more contemporary definitions. One important virtue of the 1970 definition is its more exclusive definition of central city, generally only identifying places that were the "original" growth centers of their metropolitan regions. Another difference is that 1970 metropolitan areas are treated as all being at one hierarchical level, rather than differentiated into various complicated tiers of metropolitan types on the basis of population size. Thus, the 1970 definition has the virtue of simplicity, if not necessarily the analytical neatness of later definitions.

Suburbs are categorized by four distance zones, measuring from the nearest suburban community border to the nearest central city border as of 1970: (1)borders touch, (2)within 10 miles, (3)between 10 and 20 miles, and (4)more than 20 miles. The crude nature of the categories is necessitated by the often unusual and elongated shapes of some communities. This distance categorization does not account for central city and suburban boundary change before or since 1970 but should provide a crude approximation of suburban proximity to central cities.

TEMPORAL DISTANCE TRENDS

The percentage of central cities and suburbs in each distance zone that gained (as opposed to lost) population is shown for each of the three time periods in Figure 2.3. Even though the longitudinal analysis of individual suburbs involves a slightly different definition of metropolitan area than the central city–suburban ring comparisons, there is a great overlap in the growth patterns for the central cities. As Figure 2.3 shows, the 1970s and 1980s involved dramatic patterns of population loss for many central cities, but these had become somewhat less evident with the rebound in the 1990s.

Many suburbs also lost population in the three time periods. Only 57.8% of suburbs in the sample grew in the 1970s compared to 69.2% in the 1990s. A sample that included brand new or recently developed suburbs would show higher percentages of positive growth, but still it is striking that over 30% of this sample of suburbs was losing population in the 1990s.

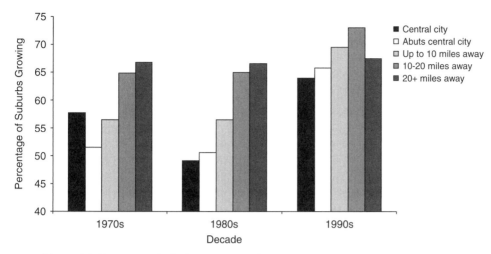

FIGURE 2.3. Percentage of suburbs that are growing, by decade and distance from central city.

Among the individual suburbs, consistent with the life-cycle perspective, the areas adjoining central cities have lower percentages growing, compared to the other groups of suburbs, regardless of time period. Also noteworthy is the pattern of growth of the most distant suburbs. In a metropolis where the constraints of transportation and communication place few limits on the outward spread of population, the most peripheral communities might be expected to have the greatest population growth. However, in the 1990s, the most peripheral suburbs are actually less likely to grow in population than those located 10 to 20 miles from central city borders. This does not indicate that the metropolis has stopped expanding outward, but only that distance from the center of the metropolis still constrains growth possibilities.

Variations across time in patterns of growth within the suburban ring are related to the patterns that are evident among the central cities. In the 1970s and 1980s, patterns of population growth are least pronounced in the inner suburbs, just as they were in the central cities. However, just as the 1990s represented a rebound for central cities, the same pattern is evident in the inner suburbs.

The net result of the growth renewal in the inner suburbs is that suburban growth patterns in the 1990s tend to have little overall relationship with centrality in the metropolis. Thus, growth has a much more formless character than in the previous time periods. The dominant view of community growth, the life-cycle perspective, receives limited support in the 1990s.

ALTERNATE GROWTH PERSPECTIVES

With the declining usefulness of the community life-cycle perspective, new major correlates of suburban growth should be identified. Figures 2.4 and 2.5 consider a few other suburban characteristics that may play crucial roles in emerging suburban growth and development patterns. The figures show how characteristics of suburbs at the initial point in time, 1970 or 1990, are related to population growth in the subsequent decade.

Of particular importance in understanding recent suburban growth is the influence of immigration. As noted earlier, the amount of immigration to the United States changed greatly between the 1970s and 1990s (Smith and Edmonston 1997). In the 1970s, immigration to the U.S. was low compared to earlier and later decades in the 20th century. In such a situation, communities with high proportions of the foreign born would exert little attraction for an overwhelmingly native-born population. In contrast, the 1990s involved heavy immigration to American society, and communities of the foreign born have exerted an attraction for the large numbers of individuals seeking new residences. For instance, in the New York metropolitan region, communities of the foreign born were growth centers of the suburban ring relative to communities with smaller percentages of the foreign born (*New York Times* 2001a, 2001b).

The data are presented in a series of bar graphs. In Figure 2.4, the darkest bars indicate the suburbs in the 1970s. The lighter bars refer to the same suburbs in the 1990s. The height of the bars indicates the percentage of suburbs growing in that category of

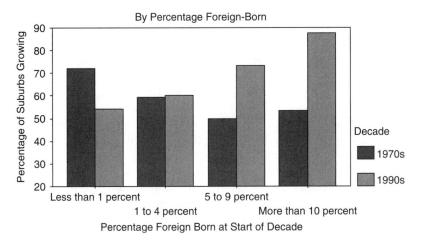

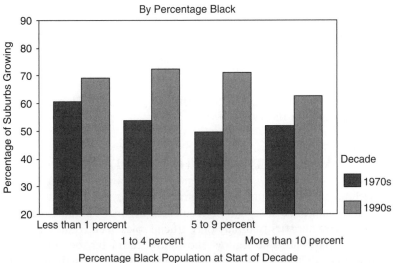

FIGURE 2.4. Changes in patterns of suburban growth, 1970 to 2000.

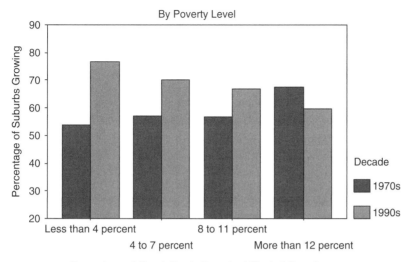

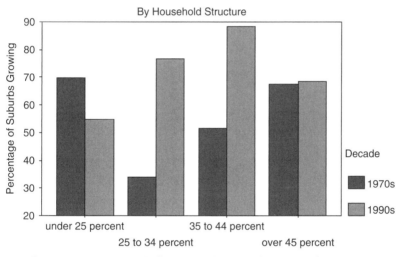

FIGURE 2.4. (*continued*)

the population characteristic. Thus, note that population growth occurred among about 70% of the suburbs in the 1970s with less than 1% foreign born, while only slightly more than 50% grew in the 1990s with the same low percentage foreign born.

The graph in the first panel of Figure 2.4 supports the point that population growth has shifted to the suburbs with high percentages of foreign born. As the percentage foreign born increases in 1970, the percentage of growing suburbs generally declines (the bars are lower in height). As the percentage foreign born increases in 1990, the percentage of growing suburbs sharply increases. Now a strong positive gradient occurs with regard to population growth. Note, for instance, that only slightly more than 50% of suburbs with hardly any foreign born grew in the 1990s, while over 80% of suburbs grew with at least 10% foreign born.

Black population composition of suburbs should also be considered. Historically, the black population has had limited housing opportunities in suburbia, a manifestation primarily of their general difficulties in finding housing in nonblack parts of the metropolis. Greater representation in suburbs could have two possible conflicting influences. On the one hand, their presence might lead nonblacks to flee or avoid living in the community, depressing population growth. On the other hand, their presence could attract other minorities, previously excluded from suburban areas. This might enhance community growth. However, little association occurs in either decade between the percentage of black residents and community growth (see second panel of Figure 2.4).

Consideration should be given to other characteristics that have traditionally been identified with the suburbanites: their economic status and the traditional suburban family, that is, married couples with children under 18.

Past research has shown that a community's socioeconomic status is related to its population growth, with well-off areas having higher population growth (Guest 1978). Not surprisingly, families would prefer to locate in communities where the population is affluent. In fact, some research (Price-Spratlen and Guest 2002) finds that socioeconomic status is increasingly correlated with neighborhood growth in central cities. Using poverty status as a measure of community socioeconomic position, the data do not show much of a systematic relationship of poverty status to growth, either in the 1970s or the 1990s (see third panel of Figure 2.4). Nevertheless, the relationship of socioeconomic status to population growth shows a systematically stronger pattern in the 1990s with poor communities having lower growth than other communities.

Given the past identification of suburbs with familism, one might expect, especially in the 1970s, for this factor to be related positively with population growth. Family status is measured as the percentage of all households that include married couples with children under 18. In both decades, population diversity is a strong correlate of population growth but in somewhat unusual ways (see the fourth panel of Figure 2.4). In the 1970s, the communities with the fewest and the most married couples with children were the most likely to grow, but in the 1990s, these were the communities that were most likely to experience population decline. Another way to put this is that diversity in family structure has emerged as an important positive predictor of community growth. Within the context of growing diversity in the organization of American families, the suburbs that represent this diversity tend to have the greatest growth.

Environmental characteristics also need to be considered in an explanation of recent population growth. One such factor is whether the suburb possesses extensive workplace activity. Historically, manufacturing activity has had a reputation as being incompatible with the location of residences, since the production facilities are often polluting and visually unattractive (Logan and Golden 1986). Thus, suburbs with high amounts of manufacturing might be characterized by population decline. However, manufacturing has been in a process of change. Environmental regulations increasingly regulate the nature of manufacturing sites, and new clean manufacturing industries such as those developing computer software have emerged. As a consequence, the location of manufacturing may not deter growth as it did in past decades. Furthermore, a noticeable trend of recent decades has been the relocation of workplace activities to the suburban rings. The location of workplaces could encourage residential development for workers who wish to live nearby.

Manufacturing censuses are not taken in the same year as the population census, but it is possible to link data from the 1967 and 1987 manufacturing censuses with data on community growth in the subsequent decade. Consistent with the traditional view of manufacturing, its presence was associated in the 1970s with population decline, but its later presence in the 1990s was actually associated with population growth (see the top panel of Figure 2.5).

Although the distance of the suburb from its central city had little relationship to population growth in the 1990s, a correlated factor, the already existing population density of the community, should be considered. High-density communities usually have less room to grow than low-density communities. In fact, the life-cycle perspective implies that a major reason for the disproportionate negative growth in inner suburbs is the high levels of population density that restrict the possibilities of growth. Consistent with the patterns for distance from the central city, high density is associated with negative growth in the 1970s but has a much weaker relationship in the 1990s. This is especially true for the highest-density suburbs. High density in 1970 was associated with population decline, but this pattern changed noticeably by the 1990s (see the bottom

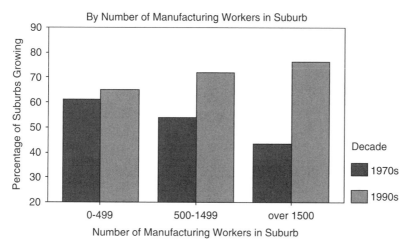

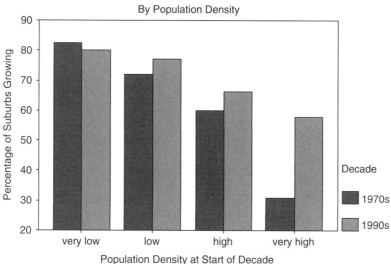

FIGURE 2.5. Changes in patterns of suburban growth, 1970 to 2000.

panel of Figure 2.5). Apparently, pre-existing intensity of settlement has decreased as a constraint on population growth.

A noteworthy trend of suburban growth research has been the development of political economy perspectives (Baldassare and Protash 1982; Logan and Zhou 1989; see also Chapter 16, "Urban and Spatial Demography," in this *Handbook*). Such perspectives view the suburb's growth as somewhat indifferent to its general environmental context and, rather, emphasize the role of community elites (primarily business interests and the wealthy) in encouraging or discouraging growth through a variety of mechanisms, including planning and zoning requirements. Consistent with the political economy view, community growth should be less related to traditional life-cycle predictors such as distance from the central city and population density, which presumably reflect the intensity of development. But the suburb's environmental characteristics still tend to maintain an importance, as indicated by factors such as the presence of workplaces and the immigrant composition of the population. More research is definitely needed to better understand these changing patterns of central city and suburban growth. Certainly, the life-cycle perspective is decreasingly useful for interpreting growth among suburbs.

HOW SUBURBS EVOLVE IN STATUS

Space does not permit an extensive analysis of the substantial diversity of population composition among suburbs. To provide a flavor of some of the issues and trends, this section focuses on variations in poverty rates across suburban communities. Of particular interest is the issue of whether neighborhood life-cycle theory may be applied to the socioeconomic status of communities. As the community develops high density land uses, experiences older and outmoded housing, and becomes attractive to nonresidential uses, the theory argues (Hoover and Vernon 1962), the relatively poor will increasingly become the only economic group that is willing to occupy the area.

This issue may be appraised empirically with the sample of Guest's suburban communities that were previously traced, using the 1970 metropolitan definition. One important pattern shown in the data is the substantial stability in economic status. Among the continuously existing suburbs, there is a .71 correlation between the 1970 and 2000 levels of poverty. This means that about half of the variance in suburban status in 2000 is a function of the status 30 years earlier. Indeed, the correlation of 1990 and 2000 status is .90, indicating that one will do well predicting 2000 status simply by knowing 1990 status level. Yet the data also suggest that the socioeconomic status of suburbs is not totally inflexible. These high correlations, by the way, represent the continuation of a pattern that was also evident for the 1950 to 1970 period (Guest 1978; Farley 1964).

Figure 2.6 shows how poverty rates of suburbs vary by distance from the central city over the three decades from 1970 to 2000. Regardless of date, there is a curvilinear relationship between distance and economic status, with the lowest-status suburbs being located the most centrally and peripherally. Yet the highest poverty rates occur at the greatest distances from the central city (more than 20 miles), presumably areas that are beyond the normal commuting range and are characterized disproportionately by nonurban work activities such as agriculture, forestry, and mining, which tend to pay low wages. While the most proximate areas to the central city are not the highest in poverty, a very slight longitudinal trend indicates that poverty has increased over time in these areas.

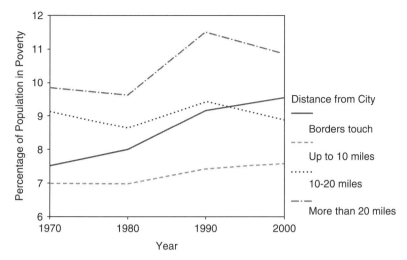

FIGURE 2.6. Suburban poverty levels by distance from central city, 1970 to 2000.

Even though the finding is consistent with the idea that central city problems are being transposed to the inner suburbs, a suburb's level of poverty in relationship to its distance from the central city remains amazingly constant over time. The upward trend in poverty among the central suburbs is real but relatively unimportant.

Some support for the life-cycle theory is evident if changes are analyzed in the poverty rates of the sample of suburbs in the two time periods, the 1970s and the 1990s. A straightforward measure of how the status of the population changed in each time period is whether the poverty rate at the second time point is higher than at the first time point. In Figure 2.7, bar graphs show the percent of suburbs, separately for the 1970s and the 1990s, that have increasing percentages in poverty by the distance of the suburb from its central city. In addition, the patterns are shown by level of population density at the initial point of the decade. In general, the more dense suburbs should be more advanced in the neighborhood life cycle. As expected, the figure shows that poverty rates increased in both decades in the relatively central suburbs, but, consistent with Figure 2.6, most of the differences are not large. A stronger pattern is found when population density is considered. It is especially noteworthy that over two-thirds of the very-high-density suburbs had increasing poverty rates in the 1990s compared to only slightly more than 40% of the very-low-density suburbs. But again these patterns indicate a wide variation in the experience of suburbs, even with the same characteristics.

An alternate perspective on the evolution of suburban economic levels is that they are being influenced noticeably by their changing population composition. Given that immigration had become an important determinant of population growth patterns among suburbs, it is reasonable to expect that immigration may also affect the status levels of suburban communities, especially since significant shares of the immigrant population experience low wages.

Immigration is having a major impact on poverty rates within the suburban ring. Figure 2.8 shows that while communities of the foreign born had only a tendency for economic decline in the 1970s, the relationship emerges as quite strong in the 1990s. Almost three-quarters of the 1990 communities with the highest percentage of foreign born showed an increase in poverty in comparison to only about 30% of the

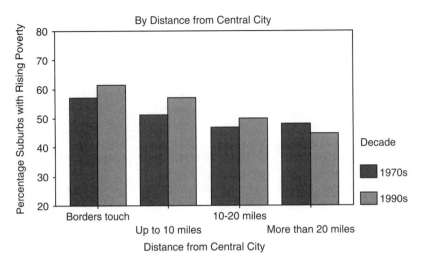

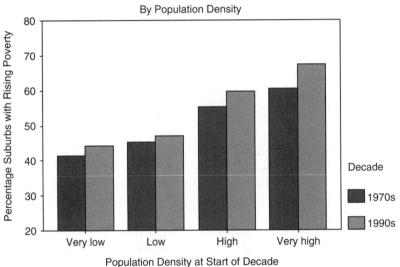

FIGURE 2.7. Changes in suburban poverty levels, 1970 to 2000.

communities with the lowest representation of the foreign born. The differences are greater than those found for the life-cycle variables.

Although immigration has emerged as a strong correlate of poverty problems in the suburbs, the in-movement of blacks to suburbs, another important social trend, seems to have had little direct relationship with changes in poverty rates. The patterns in Figure 2.8 show little consistent relationship between the presence of African Americans in 1970 or in 1990 and increasing rates of poverty in the subsequent decade.

CROSS-CULTURAL PERSPECTIVES

Compared to many other economically developed societies (especially those in Europe), urban agglomerations in the United States are relatively young. They thus represent an

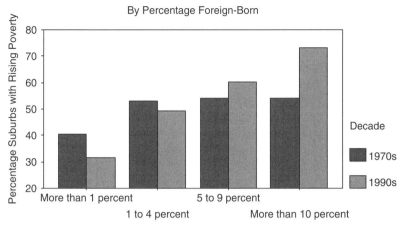

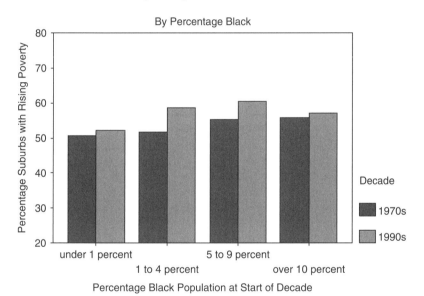

FIGURE 2.8. **Changes in suburban poverty levels, 1970 to 2000.**

essentially "pure" case of how cities have developed under capitalistic/industrial economic structures. Land use allocation has primarily occurred through competition among numerous individuals and organizations (such as realtors, corporations, and neighborhood associations). European cities have long histories under various political and economic systems such as monarchies and socialism that have influenced their basic patterns of land use and the spatial relationship of different activities.

In addition, American metropolitan areas have not experienced much centralized planning of their overall development. Rather, the political jurisdictions, both the central cities and their suburbs in each metropolitan area, have tended to compete with each other, although cooperation has been possible when the various interests benefit. In Europe, coordinating power over the character of population distribution is typically more vested in the national state or at least with regional authorities. National policies are frequently promulgated to direct overall metropolitan development (Summers et al. 1999).

Since the 1930s, the U.S. national government has had a major influence on metropolitan development through extensive housing, land clearance, and neighborhood renewal programs. There is little doubt that these programs increasingly affect the nature of population concentrations, including suburbanization, but they are less oriented toward a comprehensive program of planning than in the European case.

Even though the control of suburbanization differs between the United States and many European countries, suburbanization as a large-scale movement from central cities is also important in many European societies, both in size and date of major development. In the United Kingdom, population loss in such central core areas as Liverpool, London, and Manchester began in the 1960s, and 89% of the urban core areas (equivalent to central cities) lost population between 1981 and 1991 (Summers et al. 1999). Interestingly, the efforts of national and metropolitan authorities in the United Kingdom to control suburban growth have had mixed effects (Cohen 1994; Harper 1987). During the past few decades, greenbelts as wide as 25 km have been built around the original settled core areas of major metropolitan areas, with major restrictions on the density and type of development. These areas were intended to provide high-quality suburban environments, but the restrictions on development were also intended to encourage the continued growth of core areas. However, in practice, there has been extensive pressure to develop the greenbelts beyond the original plans, and suburban development has tended to leapfrog the original greenbelts, producing even more sprawling suburbanization.

The rate of urban growth is unprecedented in world history in parts of the developing world, mainly Africa, Asia, and Latin America. This primarily occurs due to the unprecedented population explosions of these societies, as a function of the gap between declining mortality and still high fertility. While historically most of the largest urban agglomerations were in Europe, they are now becoming dominant among countries in the developing world.

Urban concentrations differ greatly within and across continents, and it is not easy to develop simple generalizations. As an example, Malawi's leading urban center, Blantyre (with a population of over 500,000), is best described as a mélange of little villages in close proximity. The villages, many with thatched huts and shacks, are spread at relatively low density over many square miles and differ little between the center of the metropolis and its suburban ring. In contrast, Kenya's Nairobi (with a population of over 1.8 million) has a well-developed central business district with tall buildings and varied residential neighborhoods.

Unfortunately, while there is substantial literature on the overall population implosion in the developing world, there is little literature on patterns of suburbanization, except to recognize its importance (Kasarda and Crenshaw 1991; Lowry 1990). Nevertheless, it is clear that the outward deconcentration of traditional cores is probably important in developing countries, just as in the United States and Europe. Much of the outward spread of population likely began in the period after 1950 or 1960. In one sense, this should hardly be surprising, given that most developing countries have been heavily impacted by worldwide revolutions in technology and communications and organizational complexity. In a typical developing country, many individuals own automobiles, and a segment of the population has the income that is necessary to support a lifestyle with a low-density, single-family dwelling. Yet incomes in many developing countries are often maldistributed, with a large proportion of the population in poverty. One consequence is that land, regardless of whether it is suburban, is often as maldistributed as income, so that a small proportion of the population lives on a high proportion of the land (Griffin and Ford 1980).

Suburbanization is also encouraged in many developing societies by factors that are not as important in highly developed societies (Hackenberg 1980). Due to their explosive overall growth, many urban agglomerations lack space in central areas for new employment activities such as manufacturing goods for foreign corporations; these activities have hence been forced to relocate to the outskirts. Their employees often congregate in suburban areas to be near their workplaces. In addition, many dwellers in the major urban centers often maintain strong family, social, and employment ties with the rural areas from where they originated. Being located in the suburban region maximizes physical access to the rural areas.

A major issue about suburbanization in the developing world is whether it will eventually assume the same spatial form as suburbanization in a country such as the United States. Some (Schnore 1965) have suggested the possibility of a universal "evolutionary" pattern for metropolitan areas in which suburbanization occurs at a high rate, with disproportionate selectivity of high-status households in the outskirts, as occurred in the United States. This, of course, is a variation of the traditional neighborhood life-cycle perspective. Indeed, in many suburban rings of developing societies, one finds relatively new neighborhoods that are similar to the single-family tracts of the prosperous working and middle classes in the United States. However, others (Griffin and Ford 1980) challenge the generality of this idea, arguing that historical and cultural differences among countries are too great to indicate a convergence of suburban form in the near future. Many low-income persons in developing societies lack the resources to buy or build "nice" homes. As a result, they gravitate to undeveloped land on the urban outskirts where they "squat" at little or no cost. They construct cheap dwellings out of available materials, and then upgrade to the degree that improved economic resources permit.

SUBURBAN FUTURES

Suburbanization seems here to stay, whether in the United States or in the world as a whole. Indeed, almost all available evidence suggests that the redistribution of population outward within areas of population concentration will be one of the great demographic trends of the 21st century. The most fundamental factors are twofold. First, transportation technology increasingly makes it possible to travel over long distances in short time spans, although traffic congestion in cities such as Chicago, Los Angeles, New York, and Seattle imposes constraints. Second, improvements in electronic communications decreasingly make it necessary for interacting individuals and activities to be in physical proximity. One of the traditionally important advantages of central core areas should thus continue to decrease in importance.

Of course, one should not just assume the position of a technological determinist. Clearly the way of life in contemporary society is affected increasingly by large governmental organizations, large corporations, and large organized interest groups of citizenry. Powerful organizations will exert important influences in fostering or discouraging suburbanization and may be especially crucial in understanding differences across societies. Yet given the sweeping power of broad societal forces such as technology, it is difficult to envision much slowing of the outward spread of urban agglomerations.

Many societies will continue their population explosions, although at lower levels than in recent history due to declines in fertility. For many societies, there will be little choice except to tolerate or encourage further suburbanization.

As this chapter has suggested, an important goal for researchers will be the development of more sophisticated models that explain suburbanization rates across metropolitan areas and countries. Some ambiguity continues on whether suburbanization is an essentially ubiquitous phenomenon in which individual characteristics of places have little differential effect. Clearly, researchers need to undertake more research in which they separate the influence of changing physical boundaries as opposed to inherently attractive community qualities in the ability of central core areas to retain their populations.

A major goal for population researchers should also be understanding the internal spatial organization of the suburban community and how central core areas differ from their suburban rings. A sizable empirical literature on suburbanization exists for the United States, but recently it has tended to have a somewhat specialized focus, for instance, on the ethnic composition of suburbs. Research should compare suburban rings with their central cities and suburbs with each other on a number of dimensions of population composition and land use.

While simple ideas such as the neighborhood life-cycle theory may have an intrinsic appeal, it appears that they are decreasingly useful for understanding suburban differences in both cross-sectional and longitudinal population patterns. In contrast, international immigration has become a major determinant of the fate of many suburbs. Since immigration flows to the United States show no indication of declining, this factor will undoubtedly continue to influence suburban development.

In addition, there is a great need to relate the employment base of suburbs to the types of residents and to their growth patterns. Traditional assembly-line manufacturing is on the decline, and as suggested, the presence of manufacturing workplaces no longer has the same consequences for community character that it once did. It is important to recognize, however, the influence on communities of the dramatic growth of human service industries such as government, health care, retirement services, finance, and real estate. These are undoubtedly having major consequences for the types of persons and families who live in the surrounding areas.

REFERENCES

Baldassare, M., and W. Protash. 1982. Growth controls, population growth and community satisfaction. *American Sociological Review* 47:339–1346.

Bourne, L. S. 1996. Reinventing the suburbs: Old myths and new realities. *Progress in Planning* 46:141–194.

Cohen, S. E. 1994. Greenbelts in London and Jerusalem. *Geographical Review* 84:74–89.

Davis, K. 1955. The Origin and growth of urbanization in the world. *American Journal of Sociology* 60:429–437.

Duncan, B., G. Sabagh, and M. Van Arsdol, Jr. 1962. Patterns of city growth. *American Journal of Sociology* 67:418–429.

Farley, R. 1964. Suburban persistence. *American Sociological Review* 29:38–47.

Fischer, C. 1992. *America calling : A social history of the telephone to 1940*. Berkeley: University of California Press.

Frey, W. H. 2003. Melting pot suburbs: A study of suburban diversity. In *Redefining urban and suburban America*. Vol I, edited by B. Katz and R. E. Land, 155–179. Washington, D.C.: Brookings Institution Press.

Frey, W. H., and A. Berube. 2003. City families and suburban singles: An emerging household story. In *Redefining urban and suburban America*. Vol I, edited by B. Katz and R. E. Land, 257–259. Washington, D.C.: Brookings Institution Press.

Fuguitt, G. V., and D. L. Brown. 1990. Residential preferences and population redistribution: 1972–1988. *Demography* 27:589–600.

Garreau, J. 1991. *Edge city*. New York: Doubleday.

Griffin, E., and L. Ford. 1980. A model of Latin American city structure. *Geographical Review* 70:397–422.

Guest, A. M. 1975. Population suburbanization in American metropolitan areas, 1940–1970. *Geographical Analysis* 7:267–283.

Guest, A. M. 1978. Suburban social status: Evolution or persistence? *American Sociological Review* 43:251–264.

Guest, A. M. 1979. Patterns of suburban growth, 1970–75. *Demography* 16:401–415.

Guest, A. M. 1980. The suburbanization of ethnic groups. *Sociology and Social Research* 64:458–513.

Hackenberg, R. 1980. New patterns of urbanization in southeast Asia: An assessment. *Population and Development Review* 6:391–419.

Harper, S. 1987. The rural-urban interface in England: A framework for analysis. *Transactions of the Institute of British Geographers*, New Series. 12:284–302.

Hawley, A. 1978. Urbanization as process. In *Handbook of Contemporary Urban Life*, edited by D. Street, 3–26. San Francisco: Jossey-Bass.

Hawley, A. 1986. *Human ecology: A theoretical essay*. Chicago: University of Chicago Press.

Hobbs, F., and N. Stoops (U.S. Census Bureau). 2002. Census 2000 Special Reports, Series CENSR-4, *Demographic trends in the 20th century*. Washington, D.C.: U.S. Government Printing Office.

Hoover, E. M., and R. Vernon. 1962. Anatomy of a metropolis: The changing distribution of people and jobs within the New York metropolitan region. New York: Anchor/Doubleday.

Jackson, K. T. 1985. *Crabgrass frontier: The suburbanization of the United States*. New York: Oxford University Press.

Kasarda, J. D., and E. Crenshaw. 1991. Third world urbanization: Dimensions, theories, and determinants. *Annual Review of Sociology* 17:467–501.

Klaff, V. Z. and G. V. Fuguitt. 1978. Annexation as a factor in the growth of U.S. cities, 1950–1960 and 1960–1970. *Demography* 15:1–12.

Leinberger, C. B., and C. Lockwood. 1986. How business is reshaping America. *Atlantic Monthly* 258:43–52.

Lindstrom, M. J., and H. Hartling, eds. 2003. *Suburban sprawl: Culture, theory, and politics*. Lanham, Md: Rowman & Littlefield.

Logan, J. , and R. M. Golden. 1986. Suburbs and satellites: Two decades of change. *American Sociological Review* 51:430–437.

Logan, J., and M. Zhou. 1989. Do suburban growth controls control growth? *American Sociological Review* 54:461–71.

London, B., B. A. Lee, and S. G. Lipton. 1986. The determinants of gentrification in the United States: A city-level analysis. *Urban Affairs Quarterly* 21:369–387.

Lowry, I. S. 1990. World urbanization in perspective. *Population and Development Review* 16 (Supplement):148–176.

Namboodiri, K. 1988. Ecological demography: Its place in sociology. *American Sociological Review* 53:619–633.

New York Times. 2001a. Minorities changing landscape of New Jersey. March 9.

New York Times. 2001b. Newest immigrants head straight to New Jersey's suburbs. March 10.

New York Times. 2001c. Chicago reverses 50 years of declining population. March 19.

New York Times. 2001d. Most cities in U.S. expanded rapidly over last decade. May 6.

Orfield, M. 1997. *Metropolitics: A regional agenda for community and stability*. Washington, D.C.: Brookings Institution Press.

Price-Spratlen, T., and A. M. Guest. 2002. Race and population change: A longitudinal look at Cleveland neighborhoods. *Sociological Forum* 17:105–136.

Schnore, L. F. 1957. Metropolitan growth and decentralization. *American Journal of Sociology* 63:171–180.

Schnore, L. F. 1959. The timing of metropolitan decentralization: A contribution to the debate. *Journal of the American Institute of Planners* 15:200–206.

Schnore, L. F. 1965. On the spatial structure of cities in the two Americas. In *The study of urbanization*, edited by P. M. Hauser and L. F. Schnore, 347–398. New York: John Wiley and Sons.

Sjoberg, G. 1960. *The preindustrial city, past and present*. Glencoe, Ill.: Free Press.

Smith, J. P., and B. Edmonston. 1997. *The new Americans: Economic, demographic, and fiscal effects of immigration*. Washington, D.C.: National Academy Press.

Squires, G. D., ed. 2002. *Urban sprawl: Causes, consequences, and policy responses*. Washington, D.C.: Urban Institute Press.

Sternlieb, G. 1971. The city as a sandbox. *The Public Interest* 25:14–21.

Summers, A. A., P. C. Cheshire, and L. Senn, eds. 1999. *Urban change in the United States and western Europe: Comparative analysis and policy*. Washington, D.C.: Urban Institute Press.

Taeuber, K. E., and A. F. Taeuber. 1965. *Negroes in cities: Residential segregation and neighborhood change*. Chicago: Aldine.

Tobin, G. A. 1976. Suburbanization and the development of motor transportation: Transportation technology and the suburbanization process. In *The changing faces of the suburbs*, edited by B. Schwartz, 95–111. Chicago: University of Chicago Press.

United Nations. 2004. *World urbanization prospects: The 2003 revision*. New York: United Nations.

Ward, D. 1971. *Cities and immigrants: A geography of change in nineteenth-century America*. New York: Oxford University Press.

Wardwell, J. M. 1980. Toward a theory of urban-rural migration in the developed world. In *New directions in urban-rural migration: The population turnaround in rural America*, edited by D. L. Brown and J. M. Wardwell, 71–114. New York: Academic Press.

Warner, S. B. 1972. *The urban wilderness: A history of the American city*. New York: Harper & Row.

Winsborough, H. H. 1963. An ecological approach to the theory of suburbanization. *American Journal of Sociology* 68:565–570.

Zwingle, E. 2002. Cities. *National Geographic* 203:75–99.

CHAPTER 3

Marriage and Family

Linda J. Waite

SUBSTANTIVE CONCERNS

The family is one of the foundational social institutions in all societies, although the definition of *the family* varies from place to place and from time to time. The married couple generally forms the nucleus of the family. This chapter defines the family and locates this definition broadly in time and space. It examines marriage as a social institution and the role of marriage in the family. It assesses the ways that families have changed and examines contemporary variations in family forms and functions. Finally, it addresses some of the alternatives to the married couple family, including gay and lesbian couples and cohabiting couples.

THEORETICAL ISSUES

This section discusses key theoretical issues in studies of marriage and the family. It begins with problems that arise in attempting to define the family. It discusses the family mode of social organization, which is an important organizing concept. Next, it describes the social institution of marriage, its legal structure, and key features of the institution, including the benefits it confers, on average. Then, marriage is compared to cohabitation, in its characteristics, causes, and consequences. Finally, current issues surrounding gay and lesbian families are presented.

Defining the Family

Thornton and Fricke's (1989: 130) inclusive definition of the family provides a good starting point: The "family [is] a social network, not necessarily localized, that is based on culturally recognized biological and marital relationships." In most times and places, families were responsible for the production, distribution, and consumption of commodities, for reproduction and socialization of the next generation, and for coresidence and transmission of property. Families generally still are. Theoretically, however, the rise of alternative family structures, including gay and lesbian partnerships and cohabiting couples, sometimes including children, raises the question of whether a family must have a culturally recognized biological or marital relationship, which is unclear for such groups. In most current cultural schemas, a cohabiting couple living with their own child would constitute a family. But what of a woman, her child, and her cohabiting boyfriend? Does the family consist of the woman and the child, or does it include the boyfriend, who has no marital, legal, or biological relationship to either one? Since many stepfamilies are formed by cohabitation and then proceed to marriage, this is an important question for definitions of the family. The answer turns on the extent to which the cohabiting couple is culturally recognized as a family. Marriage would move this social group located at the outer boundaries of the family securely into a recognized stepfamily, with all the attendant rights and responsibilities, until and unless the marriage is dissolved. In such cases, social and legal issues arise about the continued rights and responsibilities of the former spouse and stepfather, who is not biologically related to the child, although the social, emotional, and financial ties between them may well be strong.

Family Mode of Social Organization

Under the family mode of social organization, kin groups tend to pool resources (including their labor), specialize in particular tasks, coordinate their activities, and connect to the larger community as a unit. This family mode of social organization is often associated with agricultural production, but it appears in a wide range of economic environments (Thornton and Fricke 1989).

The family mode of social organization has been altered with other, far-reaching social changes, including the rise of the market economy, vast increases in productivity with concomitant increases in real income (Fogel 2000), urbanization, changes in ideology toward greater individualization (Lesthaeghe 1983), and changes in the structure of education. All of these changes have shifted decision making and social control away from the family and toward the individual or other social institutions. As families have less control over the time and resources of children, they are less able to influence marriage choices—whether, when, and whom to wed. As more people support themselves through wage-based employment rather than through work on a family farm or small business, families have less stake in the property and family connections that a potential marriage partner brings, and accordingly, young adults acquire more autonomy in marriage choices (Caldwell, Reddy, and Caldwell 1983). Urbanization and electronic communication have made the family a less important source of companionship and entertainment now than when most people lived on farms or in villages (Burch and Matthews 1987).

In developed industrial societies such as the U.S., the family retains responsibility for reproduction, socialization, coresidence, and the transmission of property across generations. It is the main unit of consumption and often also produces considerable amounts of goods and services. Families provide care and support for both the young and the old. Although older adults receive financial transfers and access to medical care from the government in many societies, family members still provide most of their help and support (Logan and Spitze 1996), and children depend almost entirely on their families for financial, emotional, and instrumental support.

Marriage

Marriage is a legal contract between two individuals to form a sexual, productive, and reproductive union. Through the marriage, this union is recognized by family, society, religious institutions, and the legal system. Marriage defines the relationship of the two individuals to each other, to any children they might have, to their extended families, to shared property and assets, and to society generally. It also defines the relationship of others, including social institutions, toward the married couple.

The key features of marriage include a legally binding, long-term contract; sexual exclusivity; coresidence; shared resources; and joint production. Spouses acquire rights and responsibilities with marriage, enforceable through both the legal systems and through social expectations and social pressure.

LEGAL ASPECTS OF MARRIAGE.   "Marriage" differs from other, less formal, relationships primarily in its legal status. Marriage is a legally binding contract. As such, the treatment of marriage in the law shapes the institution, and recent changes in family law appear to have made marriage less stable. Historically, in the U.S. and many other countries, both secular and religious law generally viewed marriage vows as binding and permanent. The marriage contract could only be broken if one spouse violated the most basic obligations to the other and could be judged "at fault" in the breakdown of the marriage (Regan 1996).

Beginning in the mid-1960s, however, states in the U.S. substantially liberalized and simplified their divorce laws. One of the key features of these changes was a shift from divorce based on fault or mutual consent to unilateral divorce, which required the willingness of only one spouse to end the marriage. Most states also adopted some form of "no-fault" divorce, which eliminated the need for one spouse to demonstrate a violation of the marriage contract by the other. The shift to unilateral or no-fault divorce laws was accompanied by a surge in divorce rates in the U.S. At least some of the increase in divorce rates appears to have resulted directly from the shift in the legal environment in which couples marry and decide to remain married or in which they divorce (Friedberg 1998). The link between divorce rates and laws that permit unilateral divorce has led several states to develop alternative, more binding, marriage contracts, such as *covenant marriage*.

KEY FEATURES OF THE INSTITUTION OF MARRIAGE.   Permanence, joint production, coresidence, and the social recognition of a sexual and childrearing union are, perhaps, the most important characteristics of the institution of marriage (Waite and Gallagher

2000). These features lead to some of the other defining characteristics of marriage. Because two adults make a legally binding promise to live and work together for their joint well-being and to do so, ideally, for the rest of their lives, they tend to *specialize*, dividing between them the labor required to maintain the family. This specialization allows married men and women to produce more than they would if they did not specialize. The coresidence and resource sharing of married couples lead to substantial economies of scale; at any standard of living it costs much less for people to live together than it would if they lived separately. These economies of scale and the specialization of spouses both tend to increase the economic well-being of family members living together.

The institution of marriage assumes the sharing of economic and social resources and *coinsurance*. Spouses act as a small insurance pool against life's uncertainties, reducing their need to protect themselves against unexpected events. Marriage also connects spouses and family members to a larger network of help, support, and obligation through their extended family, friends, and others. The insurance function of marriage increases the economic well-being of family members. The support function of marriage improves their emotional well-being.

The institution of marriage also builds on and fosters *trust*. Since spouses share social and economic resources, and expect to do so over the long term, both gain when the family unit gains. This reduces the need for family members to monitor the behavior of other members, increasing efficiency (Becker 1981).

THE BENEFITS OF MARRIAGE.   As a result of the features just discussed, marriage changes the behavior of spouses and thereby their well-being. The specialization, economies of scale, and insurance functions of marriage all increase the economic well-being of family members, and the increase is typically quite substantial. Generally, married people produce more and accumulate more assets than unmarried people (Lupton and Smith 2003). Married people also tend to have better physical and emotional health than single people, at least in part because they are married (Mirowsky and Ross 1989; Waite and Gallagher 2000). The social support provided by a spouse, combined with the economic resources produced by the marriage, facilitate both the production and maintenance of health.

In most societies, marriage circumscribes a large majority of sexual relationships. Data from the U.S. show that almost all married men and women are sexually active and almost all have only one sex partner—their spouse. Unmarried men and women have much lower levels of sexual activity than the married, in part because a substantial minority have no sex partner at all. (Just under a quarter of unmarried men and a third of unmarried women who were not cohabiting at the time of the survey had no sex partner in the previous year.) Men and women who are cohabiting are at least as sexually active as those who are married but are less likely to be sexually exclusive (Laumann et al. 1994).

A key function of marriage is the bearing and raising of children. The institution of marriage directs the resources of the spouses and their extended families toward the couple's children, increasing child well-being.

Current theoretical issues surrounding marriage focus on the elasticity of the definition: Must marriage, by definition, include only adults of opposite sexes? Is it possible for two men to marry? Two women? An adult and a child? Two children? Clearly, in some societies, a husband may have more than one wife, although the reverse is rarely true (Daly and Wilson 2000). And, theoretically, in countries such as Norway and Sweden in which the legal distinction between cohabiting and married couples has shrunken to the point of vanishing, have cohabiting couples become "married?" Is this just a return to the common-law marriages of the past, or is it something different?

Cohabitation

Many contemporary couples begin their life together not in a marriage but when they begin sharing a residence. In some countries, cohabitation is a socially recognized form of partnership that is quite stable and is a permanent alternative to marriage. In other countries, cohabitation appears to be more like a stage in the courtship process. In the United States, unmarried heterosexual cohabitation has become so common that the majority of marriages and remarriages are preceded by cohabitation, and most young adults cohabit at some point in their lives.

The similarity between cohabitation and marriage is apparent: they are both romantic coresidential unions. Many marriages, especially remarriages, begin as cohabitations. Cohabitation differs from marriage in requiring no formal, socially recognized, legally enforceable commitment for the long term. Couples begin a cohabitation when they begin to share a residence; most also share a sexual relationship. But they need share little else. Cohabiting couples are much less likely than married couples to commingle financial resources (Brines and Joyner 1999); less likely to be sexually exclusive (Treas and Giesen 2000); less likely to share leisure time and a social life (Clarkberg, Stolzenberg, and Waite 1995); less likely to have children (Bachrach 1987); and less likely to remain together (Smock 2000).

Cohabitation and marriage are different social institutions, according to some scholars. Nock (1995) has argued that cohabitation is much less *institutionalized* than marriage, at least in the United States and other countries in which it has become common relatively recently, because it is not covered by clear expectations or norms, and the legal rights and responsibilities of cohabiting partners have not been established. The requirements for establishing or ending a cohabiting union are minimal, with no legal or religious or community formalities involved. There is ambiguity about what it means to be a cohabiting partner, to the members of the couple themselves, their families and friends, their community, and to children belonging to one or both of them. The uncertainty about the nature of the relationship and its future seems to lead to lower levels of commitment, lower levels of relationship happiness (Brown and Booth 1996), and lower levels of emotional well-being, especially for cohabiting women with children (Brown 2000). Cohabiting couples with plans to marry show few of these poor outcomes (Brown and Booth 1996), especially if neither has been married before and neither brings children to the relationship, perhaps because these couples are clear about their future together (Brown 2000).

Some explanations for the dramatic increase in cohabitation in many societies over the last several decades focus on long-term social change, including rising individualism and secularism (Lesthaeghe 1983); economic change, especially women's increasing labor force participation; liberalization of attitudes toward gender roles (McLanahan and Casper 1995); and the sexual revolution (Bumpass 1990). Together, these changes have shifted attitudes and values away from responsibility to others and toward individual goal attainment, away from patriarchal authority toward egalitarianism, away from stigmatization of sexual activity outside of marriage (at least if both parties were unmarried—attitudes toward extramarital sex have remained generally disapproving), and toward acceptance of sexual activity in other relationships, including cohabitation. Individuals may find cohabitation attractive because it allows them to lead a different sort of life than marriage, within an intimate union.

Cohabitation may act as an alternative to being single (Rindfuss and VandenHeuvel 1990), as a step in the courtship process, or as an alternative to marriage. Cohabitation plays a different role in peoples' lives, depending on economic and social circumstances, age of the cohabitors, or previous martial status. When couples select cohabitation at the beginning of their relationship and rarely make the transition from cohabitation to marriage, when cohabitions are about as stable as marriages, when cohabiting couples are socially recognized as a couple and treated as married, and when childbearing takes place in cohabiting relationships at about the same rate as in marriage, then we can argue that cohabitation is an alternative to marriage. This seems to be the case in the Nordic countries, where cohabitation has much the same legal and social status as marriage (Kiernan 2000b) and among Puerto Ricans in the United States (Landale and Fennelly 1992), although not all the above conditions apply. In the Nordic countries cohabiting relationships are less stable than marriages (Kiernan 1999), and among mainland Puerto Ricans, fathers in cohabiting couples with children are less likely to provide financial support to the family and are less involved in child care than fathers in married-parent families (Landale and Oropesa 2001).

The behavioral link between cohabitation, marriage, and childbearing can also tell us something about the nature and meaning of cohabitation. In the U.S., never-married cohabiting women show high levels of contraceptive usage and are much less likely than married women to expect a birth in the near future, whereas previously married cohabitors resemble married women in their contraceptive behavior and birth expectations (Bachrach 1987). This suggests that cohabitation may have a different meaning in the process of initial union formation than in the process of union re-formation.

The relationship between cohabitation, childbearing, and marriage also appears to differ by racial and ethnic group, at least in the contemporary U.S., which suggests that the meaning of cohabitation is not the same for these groups. Cohabitation increases the chances of conception more for white women than for black women. An unmarried conception increases the chances of marriage quite substantially for white women and modestly for black women (Brien, Lillard, and Waite 1999; Manning 1993). And a birth while single increases the chances of entering a cohabitation up to the date of the birth for white women and for the four years following the birth for black women (Brien, Lillard, and Waite 1999). A general consensus has emerged that cohabitation acts primarily as an alternative to marriage for black and mainland Puerto Rican women in the U.S. and as a step in the courtship process for non-Latino white women (see Smock 2000 for a summary of this literature.) It is important to keep in mind that these findings refer to specific cohorts of women, in a particular social and economic context, and there is no reason to think they apply in other times, cultures, or contexts.

Gay and Lesbian Families

Historically and traditionally, a *family* consisted of people related by blood or marriage in a culturally recognized social network of biological and marital relationships (Thornton and Fricke 1989). *Marriage* is a legal relationship between an adult man and an adult woman to form a new family. Gay and lesbian families, sometimes based on a socially recognized and/or legally recognized relationship, challenge these definitions. Attitudes toward sex between two adults of the same sex have become substantially more accepting in the U.S. over the past several decades (Smith 1994). Extension of the definition of *family* and *marriage* to same-sex couples has been hotly contested and fiercely debated. In the United States, many attempts to extend access to marriage and family rights to same-sex couples have been turned back by legislators or voters, with some notable exceptions. Several European countries have moved furthest on these issues. France now allows same-sex couples to register their partnerships, Denmark has extended child custody rights to same-sex couples, and the state supreme courts in Ontario, Canada, and Vermont have both ruled that same-sex couples are entitled to full and equal family rights. In 2003, the Massachusets Supreme Court ruled that the state constitution requires the state to give same-sex couples marriage rights equal to those of opposite-sex couples. And, perhaps most definitively, the Netherlands has granted same-sex couples full and equal rights to marriage (Stacey and Biblarz 2001).

METHODS AND MEASURES

Data

Data for the study of marriage and family come from a wide variety of sources—from surveys of the general population or special populations, to historical records, vital records, ethnographic research, and intensive interviews. Unfortunately, in the U.S. a number of key sources of data on marriage, divorce, and family have been discontinued, leaving at best a patchwork system of collecting information on these important dimensions of life. The U.S. Bureau of the Census collected a marital history supplement to the June Current Population Survey every five years in 1980, 1985, 1990, and 1995 but no longer does so. Until 1995, the National Center for Health Statistics (NCHS) Vital Statistics program compiled marriage and divorce registration data obtained from states into reports for the nation. Since 1995 only annual total counts of marriages and divorces have been produced by NCHS, with no information on the characteristics of those marrying or divorcing. The loss of these sources of data on marriage, divorce, and the family has limited research on these important topics in the United States, forcing scholars, policy makers, and journalists to rely on less-representative data or on data that are increasingly out of date.

SAMPLE SURVEYS.   One common method for studying families involves collecting data through a *survey* of a sample of the population of interest. Survey methods allow a large number of people to provide information in response to standardized questions asked in a consistent way. Survey methods are particularly well-suited for tracking trends in behaviors such as unemployment and in attitudes such as consumer confidence (Bradburn and Sudman 1988).

Scholars, policy makers, and government statistical agencies frequently use survey methods for describing and studying marriage and the family. In the U.S. and other countries, household surveys obtain information about current marital status, marital history, fertility, household composition, family-related attitudes and plans, and, more recently, cohabitational status and cohabitation history, sexual activity, sexual partnerships and sexual networking, and gay and lesbian relationships. Important federal government surveys on the family include marriage and fertility supplements to the Current Population Survey, the National Survey of Family Growth, the decennial Census of Population, and the Census Bureau's Survey of Income and Program Participation (SIPP). In Europe, a series of Eurobarometer Surveys carried out by numerous members of the European Community in various years provide comparative data on marriage, cohabitation, and other family behaviors (Kiernan 2000a).

VITAL REGISTRATION.   Data on key family events, including marriage, divorce, and births, have been collected through the registration of these events with religious institutions or government agencies. Historical data on family status or family events often appear in parish registers, in tax rolls, census documents, or township records of property ownership. In the U.S., the registration of vital events has been the responsibility of state departments of health. The United States did not gather vital statistics on marriage until relatively late in its history, with information compiled from state marriage certificates beginning in 1920. Differences between states in the information collected make these data less than ideal for studying marriage, and since 1990, the National Center for Health Statistics has published no statistics on marriage except raw counts of the monthly number of marriages by state (Fitch and Ruggles 2000).

LIFE/NEIGHBORHOOD HISTORY CALENDAR.   The Life History Calendar was developed to assist in the collection of retrospective accounts of life experiences. The LHC usually consists of a chart that combines the records of a number of event histories, for example, labor force participation, migration, education, marriage, cohabitation, and fertility. One format places calendar year in the columns of the chart and events in the rows. The cells might contain information on a specific transition, with a horizontal line indicating an ongoing state, such as an intact marriage, school enrollment, or employment. Use of a life history calendar improves respondent recall through a number of processes. First, the calendar instrument allows the respondent to see the sequence of events on paper and to place events along one dimension in relation to those along another. Respondents can use memorable events such as marriage or school graduation to fix the timing of other events or transitions. A respondent might use the date of marriage to recall changes in living arrangements or the date of graduation from school to recall the timing of changes in labor force participation. Second, the use of a calendar seems to improve the interviewers' ability to obtain complete and accurate data across domains by making gaps and inconsistencies readily apparent (Freedman et al. 1988).

The Neighborhood History Calendar extends the Life History Calendar to the local environment, allowing researchers to collect contextual event-history data. This method allows the direct collection of measures of the local context and changes in it, which permits researchers to distinguish among contexts that may have similar characteristics at one point but arrived at by different pathways. The resulting contextual event–history can be linked to individual life histories and the two can be analyzed together (Axinn, Barber, and Ghimire 1997).

VIGNETTES. The factorial survey approach, exemplified in *Of Human Bonding: Parent-Child Relations Across the Life Course* (Rossi and Rossi 1990), allows researchers to measure the normative structure underlying family relationships. The result is an empirical picture of of this normative structure, including the strength of felt obligation to kin of various levels of and types of relationship, the degree of consensus about these obligations, and the importance of the nature of the obligation. The method involves the creation of vignettes that describe a situation involving a specific type of kin, such as cousin, stepdaughter, or sibling. Each vignette differs along a number of dimensions, including kin relationship, gender and marital status, 1 of 11 "crisis" or "celebratory" events, and type of obligation. A computer randomly generated a set of 32 vignettes, each of which respondents rated on how strongly compelled they would feel to offer a given type of support. The greatest advantage of the factorial survey approach is its efficiency: the combination of respondents' ratings provides data on all unique vignettes and allows the researcher to quantify the relative strength of felt obligation to close and more distant relatives. Sometimes, however, certain dimensions cannot be integrated into the vignettes; the framework of Rossi and Rossi's factorial survey could not accommodate spouses, a centrally important kin category. The vignette technique captures reports of kinship ties in a hypothetical situation but offers no information on past or current behavior toward kin.

ETHNOGRAPHIC METHODS. Survey research, vital statistics, and historical data all paint a general picture of families and their members but do not uncover much detail about daily lives in families, decision making, and interactions between family members or the relationship between members. The complexity of families, their members, and their lives together is often studied using ethnographic methods, in which a research or team of researchers interviews family members using a general guide rather than structured questionnaires. Often these interviews are lengthy and repeated, covering multiple members of the family. Ethnographic methods allow scholars to place families in a cultural, social, economic, and community context; to uncover and incorporate complex or unusual family characteristics, experiences or situations; and to examine values, hidden assumptions, and values or behavior that might not be revealed in another context. Ethnographic methods allow research subjects to speak with their own voices and to tell their own stories. The volume of information about each family in ethnographic research generally restricts the researcher to a relatively small sample and does not support a great deal of generalization. Strengths of ethnographic methods include the richness of the information and the vividness of the picture of family life that can be obtained (Rubin 1994; Stacey 1990).

HISTORICAL METHODS. Historical studies of marriage rely on parish records, vital registration, tax records or, sometimes, literary documents. For the United States, data for the colonial period are not sufficient enough or reliable enough to allow researchers to calculate age at first marriage or proportions never marrying with any degree of confidence. Scattered data exist on marriage age from particular communities, mainly in New England, that allow the calculation of some key statistics (Wells 1992; Haines 1996).

Recent advances have made high-quality data for earlier periods available for the United States. The Integrated Public Use Microdata Series (IPUMS) consists of individual-level national samples of census data from 1850 to 1990 (with the exception of 1890). These data allow researchers to examine the demographic characteristics of the American population in detail and with a variety of measures, greatly increasing our understanding of marriage behavior over the last 150 years (Fitch and Ruggles 2000).

Researchers using historical methods must rely on information collected and recorded long ago, often incompletely or for purposes other than recording population characteristics carefully and completely. For example, in 1850, 1860, and 1870 the census did not inquire about marital status. Using individual records from decennial censuses, Fitch and Ruggles (2000) used other information about the individual and household to create measures of family relationships using a probabilistic approach, although they could not identify all those who had been married but were not married at the time of the census. Emigh (1998) studied the relationship between household structure and sharecropping in 15th-century Tuscany using data from the *Catasto* of 1427—fiscal documents from 15th-century Tuscany used to assess taxes. Documentary evidence of this sort "makes sampling by households virtually impossible" and makes it difficult to gather variables for large numbers of cases (Emigh 1999). A small number of cases, in turn, makes generalization difficult. The data, with these limitations, provide a view into family and household not possible in any other way.

BIOMARKERS. As theoretical perspectives on human behavior expand to include evolutionary biology, biodemography, and biopsychology, it becomes important to measure biological characteristics of respondents in household surveys and other social science research. These biomarkers often include DNA sampling, obtained from cheek swabs, blood samples, and other sources, performance testing, such as lung capacity or handgrip strength, and environmental measures to characterize the local environments of subjects (Finch and Vaupel 2001). They may include measures of physiological functioning, such as blood pressure, endocrine or immune function, or physiological symptoms of disease such as blood sugar. The collection of these data serves at least three important purposes: (1) detection of common undiagnosed or subclinical diseases such as hypertension and diabetes that plausibly exert major influence on biophysiological aspects of function; (2) provision of objective direct and indirect measures of physiological function or conditions that can be compared to self-reports and that influence social behavior (e.g., height, weight, vision, hearing, sense of taste and smell, libido, depression, cognition); (3) determination of prevalence of diseases that may affect behavior. Biomarkers are essential in "explicating pathways and elaborating causal linkages between social environment and health" (Weinstein and Willis 2001). More specifically, DNA samples can help identify "demogenes," genes with noticeable effects at the population level, in addition to environmental factors that interact with particular genes to produce harmful traits or behaviors (Ewbank 2001).

Serious theoretical and practical concerns accompany research that involves biomarkers. Among the ethical issues of genetic research are privacy, psychological effects associated with providing genetic information to participants, and ownership of and access to genetic materials and information (Durfy 2001). Difficulties also arise in the collection, storage, and analyses of biological specimens: they can be expensive and logistically challenging, and they require training new and existing personnel (Wallace 2001). But the availability of biomarkers allows researchers to examine a wide range of relationships between biological and social characteristics (see chapter 21, "Biodemography," in this *Handbook* on more general issues of biodemography.)

Measures

RATES.   Two basic measures of marriage and divorce are based on events occurring in a calendar year as captured by vital statistics. The marriage rate is measured as the number of marriages in a year per 1,000 population. The divorce rate is measured as the number of divorces in a year per 1,000 population. These rates present snapshots of marital events, which can be compared across years to see if the events of marriage and divorce are taking place at a faster or slower rate than in the past and compared across countries to answer the same questions. These crude rates are sensitive to differences in the characteristics of the populations being compared, which limits their utility.

SINGULATE MEAN AGE AT MARRIAGE.   The $SMAM$ is the mean age at first marriage for a cohort of women or men who marry by age 50, which can be computed from information on current marital status in a single census or survey. It requires only a census tabulation of marital status by age, making it the only measure of marriage age available in many historical populations. The $SMAM$ calculated in this way assumes that marriage rates have been constant over time and that only negligible differences exist in mortality or migration rates by marital status. In situations in which these assumptions seem reasonable, the $SMAM$ offers an acceptable summary measure of marriage age (Preston, Heuveline, and Guillot 2001). It is analogous in concept and methodology to the total fertility rate.

MARITAL HISTORY LIFE TABLES.   Marriage and divorce can be studied using life table techniques (Preston, Heuveline, and Guillot 2001). If research questions are addressed to surviving members of a cohort, first marriage can be treated as a single-decrement process, with marriage the only mode of leaving the never-married state. Similar life tables can be created for all married members of a cohort, with marital disruption as the only mode of leaving the married state. If surviving members of a cohort faced different probabilities of marriage (or divorce) than those who died, these life-table estimates would not represent the experience of all members of a cohort that began life at age zero, or of all who survived to age 20, or of all whom ever married. For many purposes, the biases are small and unavoidable, since the only information available comes from retrospective reports from surviving members of the cohort (Preston, Heuveline, and Guillot, 2001).

PROBABILITY OF MARRIAGE AND DIVORCE.   Annual rates tell us little about the chances that a person will marry eventually or the chances that a person who marries will divorce or separate. Estimates of lifetime chances, if estimated directly from the experiences of members of a birth cohort, require longitudinal data covering many years, which are rarely available and are out of date by the time they are available. For these reasons, estimates of the lifetime probability of marriage or divorce usually rely upon life-table methods and retrospective information on marital histories, often from a single survey. Martin and Bumpass (1989) used these methods to estimate the proportion of women in various marriage cohorts who will divorce or separate within 40 years of the marriage. They estimated period rates of disruption by using the most recent marriage cohort to complete a given year of duration since marriage as of the survey date. This provided observations of the risk of marital disruption at each marital duration for each year between the wedding and the 40th anniversary, conditional on being married at the start of the specific duration. These duration-specific rates were then combined using life-table methods to give the cumulative proportion of marriages expected to remain intact to specific durations. Martin and Bumpass (1989) estimated these survival rates separately for first, second, and third marriages. Goldstein and Kenney (2001) used forecasting models developed by Coale and McNeil (1972) and by Hernes (1972) to estimate the proportion of birth cohorts of women who will eventually marry by education and race.

EMPIRICAL FINDINGS

The next section of this chapter paints an empirical picture of marriage and the family using current research findings. First, changes in the structure of the family are summarized. Then, this section reviews changes in age at marriage, proportions married, and cohabitation from an international perspective. Next, patterns of union formation, marital disruption, and union dissolution are described. Finally, this section discusses alternative family forms.

Structure of the Family

In the U.S. and many industrialized societies, the structure of the family looks quite different than it did a half a century ago. In fact, fewer people live in *families* as traditionally defined and more live in nonfamily households. The rise in nonfamily living can be traced to earlier nest-leaving by young adults (Goldscheider, Thornton, and Young-DeMarco 1993), to delayed marriage and to nonmarriage, to continued high rates of marital disruption with lower rates of remarriage (Cherlin 1992), and to increases in independent living at older ages (Michael, Fuchs, and Scott 1980). In 1998, 15% of all people lived in nonfamily households, 10% alone (U. S. Bureau of the Census 1999: Table 16), compared to 6% in nonfamily households in 1950 (U.S Bureau of the Census 1955).

Marriage

AGE AT MARRIAGE.   Age at marriage generally declined in the first half of this century, but then rose dramatically. Both men and women in the United States and many European countries are now marrying later than at any other time in past decades (Fitch and Ruggles 2000; Kiernan 2000b). Between 1970 and 2000 the median age of first marriage for women increased by almost five years, from 20.8 to 25.1, and for men the median age increased by almost four years, from 23.2 to 26.8 (Fields and Casper 2001). In this same time period, the proportion of women who had never been married increased from 36% to 73% among those 20 to 24 years old and from 6% to 22% among those 30 to 34 years old. Similar increases occurred for men (Fields and Casper 2001).

For African Americans, the delay in first marriage has been especially striking. The median age at first marriage increased to 28.6 for African-American men, and 27.3

for African-American women (Fitch and Ruggles 2000). This represents a six-year delay for African-American men and a seven-year delay for African-American women since the 1960s. And, in 2000 among those 30 to 34 years old, 44% of African-American women and 46% of African-American men had never married (Fields and Casper 2001).

Similar changes in marriage patterns have taken place in most European countries; recent cohorts are marrying at older ages and over a wider range of ages than in the past. In addition, European countries differ substantially in marriage ages. The Nordic countries of Sweden, Denmark, and Iceland show the highest average ages at marriage for women (around age 29) and the Eastern European countries of Bulgaria, the Czech Republic, Hungary, and Poland, the lowest (around age 22). Since societies with a relatively high age at marriage also tend to be those in which many people never marry, this diversity suggests that marriage is a more salient component of the family in some European countries than others (Kiernan 2000b).

Marriage typically takes place at substantially younger ages in Africa, Asia, and Latin America than in North America and Europe. The average mean age at marriage among countries in the developed regions is almost 28 for men and 25 for women, compared to 25 for men and 21 for women in the less developed regions of the world. Young average ages at marriage are common in some parts of Africa, in countries like Uganda, Chad, and Burkina Faso; in some parts of Asia, in countries such as India, Nepal, and Indonesia; in the Middle East; and in Eastern Europe. Within regions of the world, women and men in developed countries tend to marry at older ages than those living in less developed countries. For example, in Southeast Asia women's age at first marriage is about 27 in Singapore and about 22 in Indonesia. Men tend to marry at older ages than women, but the gap in average age at marriage varies quite substantially both within and between regions. The gap tends to be the largest where women marry relatively early (United Nations 2000).

PROPORTION MARRIED.   Age at marriage has risen substantially, divorce rates are high and stable, and rates of remarriage have fallen, so a larger proportion of adults are unmarried now than in the past. In 1970, unmarried people in the U.S. made up 28% of the adult population. In 2000, 46% of all adults were unmarried. In fact, the shift away from marriage has been so dramatic for blacks that in 2000, only 39% of black men and 31% of black women were married, compared to 59% of white men and 56% of white women (Fields and Casper 2001: Table A1).

Countries in Europe also show a great deal of variation in the proportion of women in marital unions. Marriage is most common in Greece and Portugal, where over 60% of women ages 25 to 29 are married, and least common in the Nordic countries, Italy, and Spain, where a third or fewer are married (Kiernan 2000b).

In spite of increases in the age at first marriage in some countries, the vast majority of adults marry at some time in their lives, with the proportion ever married by age 50 reaching more than 95% of both men and women. Relatively high proportions of men and women have not married by their late 40s in the Nordic countries, where cohabitation is common, and in Caribbean countries such as Jamaica and Barbados, countries characterized by a long history of visiting relationships. In Sweden, for example, 76% of men and 84% of women in their late 40s had ever married, whereas in Jamaica, 52% of men and 54% of women had never married by these ages (United Nations 2000).

Cohabitation

Increasingly, couples form intimate unions by *cohabiting,* with marriage following at some later point unless the relationship dissolves. Since cohabitations tend to be relatively short-lived in the U.S., the proportion currently cohabiting is only about 10% among women ages 20 to 29, compared to 27% to 53% currently married. At older and younger ages, fewer than 1 woman in 10 is currently cohabiting. However, in the U.S. cohabitation has become an increasingly common step in the courtship process; only 7% of the women born in the late 1940s cohabited before age 25 compared to 55% among those born in the late 1960s (Raley 2000). The percentage of marriages preceded by cohabitation increased from about 10% for those marrying between 1965 and 1974 to more than 50% of those marrying between 1990 and 1994 (Bumpass and Lu 2000). Cohabitation is especially common for those whose first marriage dissolved (Brien, Lillard, and Waite 1999).

Although a number of European countries have experienced similar increases in cohabitation, some have experienced much more and some much less. Cohabitation is strikingly common in the Nordic countries of Denmark, Sweden, and Finland. France also shows fairly high levels, with about 30% of the women ages 25 to 29 in cohabiting unions. A group of countries including the Netherlands, Belgium, Great Britain, Germany, and Austria shows moderate levels of cohabitation—from 8% to 16% of women 25 to 29 are in this type of union. In the southern European countries and in Ireland cohabitation is rare, with less than 3% cohabiting among women 25 to 29 (Kiernan 2000b).

In the United States, cohabiting relationships are typically short-lived, with most either transformed into marriages or dissolved within a few years. The most recent estimates for the United States suggest that about 55% of cohabiting couples marry and 40% end their relationship within five years of moving in together. Only about one-sixth of cohabitations last *as cohabitations* for at least three years and only 1 in 10 last for five years or more (Bumpass and Lu 2000). Similar patterns appear for cohabiting relationships in Canada (Wu and Balakrishnan 1995), although in the Nordic countries, cohabitation seems to function more as an alternative to marriage than a substitute for it, so that both the proportion of women currently cohabiting and the length of cohabitations are relatively high (Kiernan 2000b).

It is important to assess the stability of relationships regardless of their form, so cohabitations that make the transition to marriage and then disrupt should be included in measures of union disruption. In the U.S., the probability that a first cohabitation dissolves within three years is 39%, and within five years is 49%. Differentials in the chances that a first cohabitation will dissolve mirror the chances of disruption of a first marriage: black women face higher risks of disruption than white or Hispanic women; women who were younger than 25 at the start of the cohabitation are more likely to disrupt than older women. And recent evidence suggests that women who have ever been forced to have intercourse at some time before the cohabitation are more likely to dissolve their relationship than other women, as are women who have ever had Generalized Anxiety Disorder (Bramlett and Mosher 2002).

The rise of cohabitation has meant, among other changes, that more children are spending time in a cohabiting union, either because their parents cohabit or, more commonly, because their mother lives with a man who is not their biological father.

The most recent estimates for the United States suggest that about 40% of children born to unmarried mothers are born into cohabiting unions, including over half of white and Hispanic births to unmarried mothers and a quarter of black births to unmarried mothers (Bumpass and Lu 2000). For children born into cohabiting unions, Bumpass and Lu (2000) have estimated that about a quarter of their childhood years will be spent in a cohabiting union, about one-half in a married-couple family, and about one quarter with a single mother.

Couples who cohabit and then marry show higher chances of marital disruption than couples who marry without living together first, even in countries like Sweden, where cohabitation is socially and legally supported (Bennett, Blanc, and Bloom 1988). Explanations suggested include the relatively "poor marital quality" of those who cohabit, including personality problems, alcohol or drug abuse, financial irresponsibility, or unstable employment patterns, all of which tend to increase the chances of divorce (Booth and Johnson 1988). Cohabitation appears to select individuals who are relatively approving of divorce as a solution to marital problems (Axinn and Thornton 1992) and those who are not committed to the institution of marriage (Bennett, Blanc, and Bloom 1988). And the experience of cohabiting may cause changes in individual's attitudes and values toward individualism (Waite, Goldscheider, and Witsberger 1986), toward more acceptance of divorce (Axinn and Thornton 1992), thereby increasing chances of marital disruption.

Union Formation

In the United States and similar countries, many couples begin their intimate life together by cohabiting rather than by marrying, so that the form of the union has changed more than its existence. But even when we consider both marriage and cohabitation, young adults are less likely to have formed a union now than in the past. Among young women born in the early 1950s, about one-quarter had not formed a union by age 25, compared to one-third of those born in the late 1960s (Raley 2000).

In many European countries, women typically are in either cohabitational or marital unions by their mid-to-late 20s. However, over 60% of Italian women and 50% of Spanish women are single—neither cohabiting nor married at these ages, compared to around one in three Portuguese and Greek women. In the Nordic countries and France, about one-third of women ages 25 to 29 are cohabiting, one-third are married, and one-third are single. Marriage is much more common than cohabitation in all other European countries (Kiernan 2000b).

Those who choose to cohabit as a first union, some research suggests, seek an alternative to marriage not only because it is a tentative, nonlegal form of a coresidential union but, more broadly, because it accommodates a very different style of life. For couples who eventually marry, cohabitation allows them to delay rather than avoid the assumption of marital roles and to gather information about the quality of the match. Men who prefer to avoid the breadwinner role are more likely to choose cohabitation for a first union, as are women who value money and career success for themselves (Clarkberg, Stolzenberg, and Waite 1995).

Economic considerations are important for formation and stability of intimate unions and for transitions between them. Both men and women who enter cohabitations tend to have more unstable job histories than those who marry, but cohabiting women earn more than either single or married women, suggesting that cohabitation is both similar to and different from marriage in key ways (Clarkberg 1999). And the chances that a cohabiting couple makes the transition to marriage increases with the *man's* but not the woman's earnings and education, whereas the chances of separation are lower for men who are employed full-time compared to those employed part-time or not at all (Smock and Manning 1997).

Marital Disruption and Union Dissolution

A substantial proportion of all marriages end in divorce or separation due to marital discord. The divorce rate, which reflects the number of divorces in a year relative to the number of married people, rose continuously for more than a century in the U.S. and many similar industrialized countries, then leveled off at a fairly high level in about 1980 (Goldstein 1999). In the U.S., the best estimates suggest that around one-half of all marriages will end in separation or divorce rather than in the death of one of the partners (Martin and Bumpass 1989). Recent data for the U.S. show that after five years, 20% of all first marriages have disrupted through separation or divorce. By 10 years after the wedding, 32% of white women's first marriages, 34% of Hispanic women's first marriages, and 47% of black women's first marriages have dissolved. Asian women show the lowest levels of marital disruption; after 10 years only 20% have divorced or separated. The marriages most likely to end include those with no children, with children from a previous union, or with older children (Waite and Lillard 1991), marriages begun at a young age, and marriages between partners with relatively low levels of education (Martin and Bumpass 1989). Black women are more likely to experience the disruption of their first marriage and any subsequent remarriage than are white or Hispanic women. Those raised by one parent or by others during childhood are more likely to divorce later, as are women who had a child prior to marriage. Women whose religion is not important to them are more likely to divorce than women for whom religion is somewhat or very important (Bramlett and Mosher 2002). Couples who share the same religion at marriage show a substantially lower likelihood of disruption than couples with different religious faiths. The destabilizing effects of religious intermarriage decrease with the increasing similarity of the beliefs and practices of the two religions and with the mutual tolerance embodied in their doctrines (Lehrer and Chiswick 1993).

Although high divorce rates make marriages seem unstable, other types of unions are much more likely to dissolve. Cohabitational unions have high chances of disruption, with one-quarter ending in separation within three to four years compared to only 5% of marriages, according to one study (Wu and Balakrishnan 1995). In the U.S., the probability that a first premarital cohabitation will break up is higher for black than for white or Hispanic women and is higher among younger than older women. Cohabiting women are more likely to experience the end of their relationship the more economically disadvantaged the community in which they live, the higher the level of male unemployment, the higher the rates of poverty, and the higher the level of receipt of welfare (Bramlett and Mosher 2002). Many cohabitations become marriages, but these show a lower stability than marriages not preceded by cohabitation (Lillard, Brien, and Waite 1995).

Alternative Family Structures

The married, two-parent family has been the most common family form in the U.S. and other industrialized countries for some centuries. But even at the height of the married-couple family era, many people lived in other types, most often due to the death of one member of the couple before all the children were grown (Watkins, Menken, and Bongaarts 1987). When death ended many marriages relatively early in life, remarriage and stepfamilies were common, as were single-parent families caused by widowhood. High rates of divorce combined with relatively low rates of remarriage, especially for women with children, have been shown to lead to sizable proportions of families with a divorced single mother. The rise of cohabitation and nonmarital childbearing has meant that unmarried-couple families and never-married mother families are now common alternative family forms.

In the U.S., families consisting of a married couple with children fell from 87% in 1970 to 69% in 2000. The percent of single-mother families rose from 12% to 26%, and that of single-father families rose from 1% to 5%.

One alternative family form consists of two adults of the same sex, sometimes raising children. About 2.4% of men and 1.3% of women in the U.S. identify themselves as homosexual or bisexual and have same-gender partners (Laumann et al. 1994). Although information on the number and characteristics of gay and lesbian couples has not generally been available, in the U.S., one estimate suggests that in 1990 fewer than 1% of adult men lived with a male partner and about the same percentage of adult women lived with a lesbian partner (Black et al. 2000). These estimates are based on responses to the "unmarried partner" question in the U.S. census and are thus thought to be conservative estimates of the numbers of same-sex cohabitors. This is the case because some of those living in gay and lesbian couples do not identify as such in survey and other data. Legal and social recognition of these unions as "marriages" is generally not available in the United States.

Gay and lesbian families may, of course, include children, either born to one member of the couple or adopted by the couple. Black and his colleagues (2000) constructed estimates of the presence of children in families headed by gay and lesbian couples, using data from several sources. They estimated that 22% of partnered lesbians and 5% of partnered gays currently have children present in the home, about three-quarters of whom are under age 18. Some gays and lesbians are single parents and some are in heterosexual marriages. Including these families in the estimates suggests that over 14% of gays and over 28% of lesbians have children in the household. Black and associates (2000) have estimated that about 25% of gay men and 40% of lesbian women are married or previously were married.

Sex

In spite of the sexual revolution, marriage circumscribes most sexual relationships. Almost all married men and women are sexually active, and almost all have only one sex partner—their spouse. Unmarried men and women have much lower levels of sexual activity than the married, and frequently have no sex partner at all. Cohabiting couples are at least as sexually active as married couples, but are much less likely to be sexually exclusive (Laumann et al. 1994). Thus, the married couple remains the locus of most sexual activity.

RESEARCH DIRECTIONS

Rapid changes in family processes in many postindustrial societies such as the U.S. mean that researchers studying cohabitation, marriage, or even the family are aiming at a moving target. Defining each of these is both crucial and difficult. Must families be related by blood or marriage? If so, does a cohabiting couple constitute a family? Clearly not, under the current definition, because they share neither a blood nor legal tie. What if they have a child? Blood ties exist between the mother and the child and between the father and the child, so each of these constitutes a family. It becomes difficult to argue that this triad consists of two separate families and much easier to argue that they form a single family, although the adults do not share a blood or legal tie.

What about a cohabiting couple with a child belonging only to the woman? The mother and child constitute a family, but does it include the man who lives with them but shares no blood or legal ties to either? It is difficult to say. The man has no legal responsibilities to either the woman or her child and no legal rights as a husband or father. But the three may share powerful social, financial, and emotional bonds.

A central question becomes, What *is* cohabitation? Nock (1995) has argued that cohabitation is incompletely institutionalized, leaving partners, their families, and others unsure about the nature of the relationship. Brown and Booth (1996) and Brown (2000) have suggested that cohabitation may be *several* institutions, with distinct characteristics. One consists of couples who are engaged, have no children and no previous marriages. These couples appear to be similar to married couples in their behavior and relationship outcomes. Another type of cohabitation includes couples with no plans to marry, with children—generally from a previous relationship, and at least one divorced partner. These couples seem to differ in important ways from more committed cohabitors and from married couples. So, scholars must ask, and continue asking, What kind of a relationship is this? What are the rules under which the partners are operating? How does the relationship affect choices made by the members and by others? How does the existence of the relationship and its form affect the well-being of the individuals involved?

Family scholars face as many questions about marriage. What are the irreducible characteristics of "marriage"? In the United States, same-sex couples are forbidden to "marry," although in a few places they may register a "domestic partnership." Opponents of granting same-sex couples access to "marriage" argue that, by definition, marriage must involve a man and a woman (Wardle 2001). Supporters argue that if marriage provides a wide variety of important benefits to participants, it is discriminatory to deny these to same-sex couples. Does a registered domestic partnership provide same-sex couples with the same benefits as marriage provides heterosexual couples? What *is* marriage?

Perhaps the most perplexing issue facing family researchers in the U.S. revolves around the rapid and dramatic divergence of family patterns and processes between whites and blacks. In about 1950, the proportions of black and white adults who were married was quite similar. Black men and women show little evidence of the substantial decline in age at marriage that characterized the Baby Boom of the 1950s and early 1960s for whites in the U.S. and a much more rapid rise in age at marriage since that time (Fitch and Ruggles 2000). Currently, almost twice as many black men as white men are not married (Waite 1995), with a similar differential for women. Goldstein and Kenney (2001) have found a dramatic decline in the proportion of black women predicted to ever marry, especially among those who are not college graduates, whereas marriage remains virtually universal among whites. The proportion of births to unmarried women is three times as high for blacks as for whites (Martin et al. 2002). Although numerous hypotheses for this divergence have been put forward, none explains more than a small portion of the racial gap in family patterns.

The forms and patterns of family life have shifted, quite noticeably in some countries and among some groups. But *Homo sapiens* developed as a species in conjunction with the development of the family. Our future and the future of the family are inextricably intertwined and always will be.

REFERENCES

Axinn, W. G., J. S. Barber, and D. J. Ghimire. 1997. The neighborhood history calendar: A data collection method designed for dynamic multilevel modeling. In *Sociological methodology*, Vol. 27. Edited by A. E. Raftery, 355–392. Boston: Blackwell.

Axinn, W. G., and A. Thornton. 1992. The relationship between cohabitation and divorce: Selectivity or causal influence? *Demography* 29:357–374.

Bachrach, C. 1987. Cohabitation and reproductive behavior in the U. S. *Demography* 24:623–637.

Becker, G. S. 1981. *A treatise on the family*. Chicago: University of Chicago Press.

Bennett, N. G., A. K. Blanc, and D. E. Bloom. 1988. Commitment and the modern union: Assessing the link between premarital cohabitation and subsequent marital stability. *American Sociological Review* 53:127–138.

Black, D., G. Gates, S. Sanders, and L. Taylor. 2000. Demographics of the gay and lesbian population in the United States: Evidence from available systematic data sources. *Demography* 37:139–154.

Booth, A., and D. Johnson. 1988. Premarital cohabitation and marital success. *Journal of Family Issues* 9:255–272.

Bradburn, N. M., and S. Sudman. 1988. *Polls and surveys: Understanding what they tell us*. San Francisco: Jossey-Bass.

Bramlett, M. D., and W. Mosher. 2002. Cohabitation, marriage, divorce and remarriage in the United States. National Center for Health Statistics. Vital and Health Statistics 23(22).

Brien, M., L. A. Lillard, and L. J. Waite. 1999. Interrelated family-building behaviors: Cohabitation, marriage, and non-marital conception. *Demography* 36:535–552.

Brines, J., and K. Joyner. 1999. Ties that bind: Commitment and stability in the modern union. *American Sociological Review* 64:333–356.

Brown, S. L. 2000. The effects of union type on psychological well-being: Depression among cohabitors versus marrieds. *Journal of Health and Social Behavior* 41:241–255.

Brown, S. L., and A. Booth. 1996. Cohabitation versus marriage: A comparison of relationship quality. *Journal of Marriage and the Family* 58:668–678.

Bumpass, L. 1990. What's happening to the family? Interaction between demographic and institutional change. *Demography* 27:483–498.

Bumpass, L., and Hsien-Hen Lu. 2000. Trends in cohabitation and implications for children's family contexts in the United States. *Population Studies* 54:29–41.

Burch, T. K., and B. J. Matthews. 1987. Household formation in developed societies. *Population and Development Review* 13(3):495–511.

Caldwell, J. C., P. H. Reddy, and P. Caldwell. 1983. The causes of marriage change in south Asia. *Population Studies* 37:343–361.

Cherlin, A. J. 1992. *Marriage, divorce and remarriage*. Cambridge, Mass.: Cherlin, Harvard.

Clarkberg, M. 1999. The price of partnering: The role of economic well-being in young adults' first union experiences. *Social Forces* 77:945–968.

Clarkberg, M., R. M. Stolzenberg, and L. J. Waite. 1995. Attitudes, values and entrance into cohabitational versus marital unions. *Social Forces*. 74(2):609–634.

Coale, A. J., and D. R. McNeil. 1972. The distribution of age at first marriage in a female cohort. *Journal of the American Statistical Association* 67:743–749.

Daly, M., and M. I. Wilson. 2000. The evolutionary psychology of marriage and divorce. In *Ties that bind: Perspectives on marriage and cohabitation*. Edited by L. Waite, C. Bachrach, M. Hindin, E. Thomson and A. Thornton, 91–110. New York: Aldine de Gruyter.

Durfy, S. J. 2001. Ethical and social issues in incorporating genetic research into survey studies. In *Cells and surveys: Should biological measures be included in social science research?* Edited by C. E. Finch, J. W. Vaupel, and K. Kinsella, 303–328. Washington, D.C.: National Academy Press.

Emigh, R. J. 1998. Labor use and landlord control: Sharecropping and household structure in fifteenth-century Tuscany. *Journal of Historical Sociology* 11:37–73.

Emigh, R. J. 1999. Means and measures: Property rights, political economy, and productivity in fifteenth-century Tuscany. *Social Forces* 78(2):461–491.

Ewbank, D. 2001. Demography in the age of genomics: A first look at the prospects. In *Cells and surveys: Should biological measures be included in social science research?* Edited by C. E. Finch, J. W. Vaupel, and K. Kinsella, 64–109. Washington, D.C.: National Academy Press.

Fields, J., and L. M. Casper. 2001. *America's families and living arrangements: March 2000*. Current Population Reports, P20–537. Washington, D.C.: U.S. Census Bureau.

Finch, C. E., and J. W. Vaupel. 2001. Collecting biological indicators in household surveys. In *Cells and surveys: Should biological measures be included in social science research?* Edited by C. E. Finch, J. W. Vaupel, and K. Kinsella, 1–8. Washington, D.C.: National Academy Press.

Fitch, C. A., and S. Ruggles. 2000. Historical trends in marriage formation: The United States 1850–1990. In *Ties that bind: Perspectives on marriage and cohabitation*. Edited by L. Waite, C. Bachrach, M. Hindin, E. Thomson, and A. Thornton, 59–90. New York: Aldine de Gruyter.

Fogel, R. W. 2000. *The fourth great awakening and the future of egalitarianism*. Chicago: University of Chicago Press.

Freedman, D., A. Thornton, D. Camburn, D. Alwin, and L. Young-DeMarco. 1988. The life history calendar: A technique for collecting retrospective data. In *Sociological Methodology 1988*. Edited by C. C. Clogg, 27–68. Washington, D.C.: American Sociological Association.

Friedberg, L. 1998. Did unilateral divorce raise divorce rates? Evidence from panel data. *American Economic Review* 88:608–627.

Goldscheider, F., A. Thornton, and L. Young-DeMarco. 1993. A portrait of the nest-leaving process in early adulthood. *Demography* 30:683–699.

Goldstein, J. R. 1999. The leveling of divorce in the United States. *Demography* 36:409–414.

Goldstein, J. R., and C. T. Kenney. 2001. Marriage delayed or marriage forgone? New cohort forecasts of first marriage for U.S. women. *American Sociological Review* 66:506–519.

Haines, M. R. 1996. Long-term marriage patterns in the United States from colonial times to the present. *The History of the Family* 1:15–39.

Hernes, G. 1972. The process of entry into first marriage. *American Sociological Review* 37:173–182.

Kiernan, K. 1999. Cohabitation in western Europe. *Population Trends* 96:25–32.

Kiernan, K. 2000a. Cohabitation in western Europe: Trends, issues and implications. In *Just living together: Implications of cohabitation for children, families, and social policy* (3–31). Mahwah, NJ: Lawrence Erlbaum.

Kiernan, K. 2000b. European perspectives on union formation. In *Ties that bind: Perspectives on marriage and cohabitation*. Edited by L. Waite, C. Bachrach, M. Hindin, E. Thomson, and A. Thornton, 40–58. New York: Aldine de Gruyter.

Landale, N. S., and K. Fennelly. 1992. Informal unions among mainland Puerto Ricans: Cohabitation or an alternative to legal marriage? *Journal of Marriage and the Family* 54:269–280.

Landale, N. S., and R. S. Oropesa. 2001. Father involvement in the lives of mainland Puerto Rican children: Contributions of nonresident, cohabiting and married fathers. *Social Forces* 79:945–968.

Laumann, E. O., J. H. Gagnon, R. T. Michael, and S. Michaels. 1994. *The social organization of sexuality*. Chicago: University of Chicago Press.

Lehrer, E., and C. U. Chiswick. 1993. Religion as a determinant of marital stability. *Demography* 30:385–404.

Lesthaeghe, R. 1983. A century of demographic and cultural change in western Europe: An exploration of underlying dimensions. *Population and Development Review* 9(3):411–435.

Lillard, L. A., M. J. Brien, and L. J. Waite. 1995. Pre-marital cohabitation and subsequent marital dissolution: Is it self-selection? *Demography* 32:437–458.

Logan, J. R., and G. D. Spitze. 1996. *Family ties: Enduring relations between parents and their grown children*. Philadelphia: Temple University Press.

Lupton, J., and J. P. Smith. 2003. Marriage, assets, and savings. *Marriage and the economy: Theory and evidence from advanced industrial societies*. S. Grossbard-Shechtman, 129–152. Cambridge: Cambridge University Press.

Manning, W. D. 1993. Marriage and cohabitation following premarital conception. *Journal of Marriage and the Family* 55:839–850.

Martin, J. A., B. E. Hamilton, S. J. Ventura, F. Menacker, and M. M. Park. 2002. Births: Final data for 2000. *National Vital Statistics Reports*. Vol. 50, No. 5. Hyattsville, Md: National Center for Health Statistics.

Martin, T. C., and L. L. Bumpass. 1989. Recent trends in marital disruption. *Demography* 32:509–520.

McLanahan, S., and L. Casper. 1995. Growing diversity and inequality in the American family. In *State of the union: America in the 1990s.*, Vol. 2. Social trends. Edited by R. Farley, 1–46. New York: Russell Sage.

Michael, R. T., V. R. Fuchs, and S. R. Scott. 1980. Changes in the propensity to live alone: 1950–1976. *Demography* 17(1):39–56.

Mirowsky, J., and C. E. Ross. 1989. *Social causes of psychological distress*. New York: Aldine de Gruyter.

Nock, S. L. 1995. A comparison of marriages and cohabiting relationships. *Journal of Family Issues* 16:53–76.

Preston, S. H., P. Heuveline, and M. Guillot. 2001. *Demography: Measuring and modeling population processes*. Oxford: Blackwell.

Raley, R. K. 2000. Recent trends in marriage and cohabitation. In *Ties that bind: Perspectives on marriage and cohabitation*, Edited by L. Waite, C. Bachrach, M. Hindin, E. Thomson, and A. Thornton, 19–39. New York: Aldine de Gruyter.

Regan, M. C., Jr. 1996. Postmodern family law: Toward a new model of status. In *Promises to keep: Decline and renewal of marriage in America*. Edited by D. Popenoe, J. B. Elshtain, and D. Blankenhorn, 157–186. Lanham, Maryland: Rowman and Littlefield Publishers.

Rindfuss, R. R., and A. VandenHeuvel. 1990. Cohabitation: Precursor to marriage or alternative to being single? *Population and Development Review* 16:703–726.

Rossi, A. S., and P. H. Rossi. 1990. *Of human bonding: Parent-child relations across the life course*. New York: Aldine de Gruyter.

Rubin, L. B. 1994. *Families on the fault line: America's working class speaks about the family, the economy, race, and ethnicity*. New York: HarperCollins.

Smith, T. W. 1994. Attitudes toward sexual permissiveness: Trends, correlates, and behavioral connections. In *Sexuality across the life course*. Edited by A. S. Rossi, 63–97. Chicago, University of Chicago Press.

Smock, P. J., and W. D. Manning. 1997. Cohabiting partners' economic circumstances and marriage. *Demography* 34:334–341.

Smock, P. J. 2000. Cohabitation in the United States: An appraisal of research themes, findings, and implications. In *Annual Review of Sociology*, Vol. 26, Annual Reviews, 1–20.

Stacey, J. 1990. *Brave new families*. New York: Basic Books.

Stacey, J., and T. J. Biblarz. 2001. (How) Does the sexual orientation of parents matter? *American Sociological Review* 66:159–183.

Thornton, A., and T. E. Fricke. 1989. Social change and the family: Comparative perspectives from the West, China and South Asia. In *Demography as an interdiscipline*. Edited by J. Mayone Stycos, 128–161. New Brunswick, N.J.: Transaction.

Treas, J., and D. Giesen. 2000. Sexual infidelity among married and cohabiting Americans. *Journal of Marriage and the Family* 62:48–60.

United Nations. *http://www.un.org/english/*2000.

U.S. Bureau of the Census. 1955. Household and family characteristics: March 1954. *Current population report, P20–55*. Washington, D.C.: U.S. Government Printing Office.

U.S. Bureau of the Census. 1999. Household and family characteristics: March 1998 (update). *Current population report, P20–515*. Washington, D.C.: U.S. Government Printing Office.

Waite, L. J. 1995. Does marriage matter? *Demography* 32:483–508.

Waite, L., and M. Gallagher. 2000. *The case for marriage*. New York: Doubleday.

Waite, L. J., and L. A. Lillard. 1991. Children and marital disruption. *American Journal of Sociology* 96:930–953.

Waite, L. J., Frances K. Goldscheider, and Christina Witsberger. 1986. Nonfamily Living and the Erosion of Traditional Family Orientations Among Young Adults. *American Sociological Review* 51: 541–554.

Wallace, R. B. 2001. Applying genetic study designs to social and behavioral population surveys. In *Cells and surveys: Should biological measures be included in social science research?* Edited by C. E. Finch, J. W. Vaupel, and K. Kinsella, 229–249. Washington, D.C.: National Academy Press.

Wardle, L. 2001. "Multiply and replenish": Considering same-sex marriage in light of state interests in marital procreation. *Harvard Journal of Law and Public Policy* 24:771–814.

Watkins, S. C., J. A. Menken, and J. Bongaarts. 1987. Demographic foundations of family change. *American Sociological Review* 52:346–358.

Weinstein, M., and R. J. Willis. 2001. Stretching social surveys to include bioindicators: Possibilities for the health and retirement study, experience from the Taiwan study of the elderly. In *Cells and surveys: Should biological measures be included in social science research?* Edited by C. E. Finch, J. W. Vaupel, and K. Kinsella, 250–275. Washington, D.C.: National Academy Press.

Wells, R. V. 1992. The population of England's colonies in America: Old English or New Americans? *Population Studies* 46:85–102.

Wu, Z., and T. R. Balakrishnan. 1995. Dissolution of premarital cohabitation in Canada. *Demography* 32(4):521–532.

CHAPTER 4

Demography of Gender

Nancy E. Riley

Over the last two decades, there has been a major shift in the way demographers think about issues of gender. In published accounts, the field has gone from a seeming lack of awareness that many demographic events are closely connected to gender to a nearly required nod to the relevance of gender. So have we broken through the barrier that has kept gender out of demography for so long? This chapter will argue that we have not completely removed the barriers to demographic work on gender but that headway is being made. This is a case of the half-empty and half-full glass. Depending on the angle from which we approach the issue, we can argue that things have changed radically in demography and that our knowledge of gender's role in demographic events has grown quickly and broadly over the last couple decades. Or we can point to the continuing weaknesses in the area of gender and demography.

This chapter will attempt to demonstrate that both perspectives have merit. It will draw on work from mainstream demography to demonstrate the progress that the field has made, both in understanding the importance of gender and in developing empirical support for the role of gender in demographic processes. The chapter will also discuss work from outside mainstream demography in order to suggest the paths and kinds of thinking that have yet to influence the field and which, if borrowed, might enrich demography's understanding of gender. The aim of this chapter is not to cover all the work on gender in demography but rather to illustrate and discuss how gender is studied and understood by demographers. To that end, it will illustrate arguments with relevant research and cover the types of work currently taking place. This chapter will focus on the issues of fertility and mortality; gender is equally important in migration, but space limitations and the different issues involved in that area of work necessitate separating these processes.

INTRODUCTION

Interest in gender has grown for a number of reasons. In some ways, interest has arisen in demography as it has in other disciplines and reflects a recognition of the importance of gender as an organizing principle of society. Thus to study nearly any social behavior requires some attention to gender. But attention to gender has also emerged for its potential ability to rescue the theory of demographic transition theory, which has been criticized and critiqued for its weaknesses in understanding and explaining cross-cultural demographic change (Greenhalgh 1996; Hirschman 1994; Szreter 1993). Increasingly, demographers argue that "women's position," or something like it, is a contributing factor in demographic change. Several scholars (Caldwell 1982; Cleland and Wilson 1987) connect women's position to demographic transition, either in the past or future. Although the empirical evidence has been insufficient to allow specific connections between fertility decline and women's position, there is nevertheless a continued belief that, if properly measured, understanding gender might contribute to demographers' understanding of the pattern of demographic transition.

Defining Gender

Gender can be defined as a pervasive system of patterned inequality. Gender operates on several levels across any society and plays a role in all aspects of social life, particularly because gender is an organizing principle in all societies. While most social scientists emphasize the social constructedness of gender, biology also plays a role (Udry 1994). Particularly important are reproduction and the differing roles that reproductive processes have played in women's and men's lives. The terms *sex*, denoting biological, and *gender*, denoting social, are often used to emphasize the different influences on gender, but most social scientists understand that such a seemingly simple dichotomy is more complicated than can be captured by such terminology. Even our definitions and understandings of sex and biology are socially constructed and, on the other side, the biological differences between women and men have been important to the ways that the social world is organized (see Riley 2003; Tuana 1983; Birke and Vines 1987). In addition, it is often difficult to separate biological and social aspects of human behavior, or to point to distinct biological and social influences on the differences between women and men. Real and perceived physical differences between women and men are often part of the meaning and organization of gender.[1]

While differences between individuals are important, as Chapter 1, "Age and Sex," illustrates, social scientists increasingly emphasize a broader definition of gender, which focuses on the ways societies are organized rather than on the attributes of individuals (Ferree, Lorber, and Hess 1999). From this perspective, the differences between women and men are of less central concern than the role that gender plays as a social institution. Like any other social institution such as social class, family, or economy, gender is a set of social and cultural practices that influences the lives of all women and men in the way that

---

[1] In his Presidential Address to the Population Association of America, Richard Udry (Udry 1994) emphasized and attempted to trace the biological origins of some gender differences. This chapter will focus on gender as a social construction, even while recognizing the obvious biological influences on human behavior.

it organizes society and interacts with other social institutions. Thus, gender helps to define and shape other social institutions but is also, in turn, defined and shaped by them. From this perspective, gender refers not just to differences between women and men but to the multiple levels at which gender operates, the ways those differences create and are created by societal and cultural norms, expectations, patterns of behavior and ideology, and the inequalities that result (Scott 1986). Gender operates in all spheres of society, from the economy, to education, to art and law (Marshall 2000). Family and marriage practices are also central pieces of the gender system that relate to demographic events, of course. In social systems where women marry early, where marriage is patrilocal, and where lineage is traced through the patriline, women seem to fare less well than in other social systems. As discussed later, in these kinds of systems, women may have a smaller voice in decisions that relate to illness, death, birth, or contraception.

There are no universal rules or patterns that allow us to know what kinds of societies or communities are likely to have more or less equitable gender systems (Yanagisako and Collier 1987). Women seem to fare better in communities where their traditional spheres of work are valued, even if those differ from men's. But it is also true that women's access to and control over those resources of the society considered most valuable—such things as land, money, steady work, political power, or time—influence their status and gender equality. Thus, while it is certainly important whether or not women have choices in their own lives, gender's more pervasive influence is probably not at this individual level but through its influences on the social, economic, and political contexts in which individuals live, make decisions, have children, and die.

Gender in Demography: Increasing Attention

How do we measure the amount and extent of scholarship on gender in demography? There are a number of signposts, and most suggest that work on gender has increased significantly over the last 15 years or so. Perhaps the best illustration of the recency of demography's attention to gender is the direct involvement of the International Union for the Scientific Study of Population (IUSSP) in issues of gender (see Federici, Mason, and Sogner 1993). Early discussions in IUSSP led to a 1988 conference on "Women's Position and Demographic Change" and the establishment of a Gender Committee in 1990. Through a series of conferences on various topics related to gender, with many of the conference papers later published in volumes (Federici, Mason, and Sogner 1993; Mason and Jensen 1995; Presser and Sen 2000), IUSSP has provided a space for study and discussion of ways that gender is involved in demographic processes. This is not to say there had been no work on gender in demography before 1988, but it was at this time that more systematic and collaborative work began on this issue.

Whereas 20 years ago sessions directly related to gender were nearly absent from the Population Association of America's (PAA) annual meetings, now there are several sessions directly focused on gender at any annual PAA, dealing with a number of gender issues: from measurement of gender equality to gender influence on some demographic outcome to larger issues that certainly come from interests in gender, such as issues of domestic violence. In addition, questions related to or informed by gender research are integrated in additional PAA sessions, from those about teenage fertility in the United States to sessions on the impact of AIDS in Africa.

Another indicator of the attention to gender is the new interest in documenting the role of men in demographic outcomes, particularly in fertility outcomes. Men's roles in reproduction have long been ignored in most demographic projects. Even now, "most family demographic research on men has concentrated on the absence more than the presence of men in families" (Bianchi 1998: 133). In their examination of men's roles in fertility in western societies, Goldscheider and Kaufman (1996: 88) find that "the level of commitment between men and women is the key variable missing in the current study of fertility." Greene and Biddlecom (2000) suggest more serious and extensive over-sights, however, when they argue that demographic models and assumptions do not permit the easy inclusion of men in our understanding of fertility outcomes. This is due in part to the fact, as Poston and Chang (2003) have observed, that fertility rates calculated for females need not be, and seldom are, the same as fertility rates calculated for males. Even as men continue to be missing from most demographic analyses, there is larger agreement on the importance of including men in the assessment of demographic change and an increasing amount of research is being undertaken in this area (see also Bawah et al. 1999).

Attention to gender has also come from reproductive rights activists. Although such perspectives have been present for some time (Freedman and Isaacs 1993; Cook 1993; Dixon-Mueller 1993; Kabeer 1994), their voices were especially heard during and after the 1994 International Conference on Population and Development in Cairo. This conference, and the discussions surrounding it, put scholars and activists interested in gender, especially those from the Third World, onto the radar screen of demographers. Even in the disagreement of some mainstream demographers and in their concern of what was removed from the population agenda to make room for issues of women and gender (McIntosh and Finkle 1995), we see a new way of dealing with the issues surrounding gender. One of the most important contributions of the reproductive health activists has been the attention given to feminist projects. Feminist research is necessarily political, and the activist work relating to the Cairo conference made clear the connections among research, policy, and women's lives and encouraged those interested in gender to consider these connections (Petchesky 1997, 2000; El Dawla 2000; Desai 2000). While much of this work came from outside mainstream academic demography, it nevertheless has had an impact on the field. It has been influential in linking researchers and family planning practitioners, and has brought to demograph-ers' attention feedback from actual users of contraceptives and family planning pro-grams. Coming perhaps most forcefully from Third World feminists and practioners in health programs, these discussions have often been controversial, with parties from many sectors deeply engaged in the issues. These have not been merely ideological debates (see Presser 1997). Rather, while such discussions do continue, many have tried to incorporate the thinking and findings from the discussions into both research and health delivery programs. Thus, many of the recent changes in many family planning programs, from the dismantling of family planning targets in India to the role of the state in China, invoke, if they did not arise out of, discussions about reproductive rights.

Just how pervasive attention to gender has become is also seen in the way that issues of gender have become part of data collection projects. For example, the largest data collection project in demography, the Demographic and Health Surveys (DHS), seeks to collect information on gender in a variety of ways. In addition to several questions on the standard DHS questionnaire, there are now separate modules on women's status, on domestic violence, and modules for male respondents. While such modules are used only in selected countries, their development and use in such a large-scale survey endeavor are indicative of the understanding of the ways that gender is central in demographic change. In addition to the inclusion of these questions and modules, the researchers at DHS and its affiliates have focused on gender in their analyses and reports. For example, researchers at DHS (Blanc et al. 1996) reported on an experimental survey designed to measure the strategies and negotiations that women in Uganda use to achieve their reproductive goals. Using data from a DHS module on women's status in Egypt, Kishor (1994) reported on both the strengths and weaknesses of the survey measures and the survey's findings.

Also promising for the future of demographic work on gender is the number of new and younger scholars who have been working in this area to develop new techniques and theories to address old and new questions. At any large professional meeting of demographers, there are reports from new scholars who are working through some of these difficult questions. All indications, therefore, suggest that work on gender continues to draw significant interest and attention from demographers.

SUBSTANTIVE CONCERNS

The most important and extensive contribution of recent work on gender is the way that gender issues have been regularly brought in to demographic inquiry; gender is now something that most demographers consider as they think about demographic behavior (see also Bachrach 2001). The significance of this cannot be overstated. As already noted, this attention and recognition may be traced through a variety of means, especially the way that gender appears in so many pieces of demographic research, is the subject of many panels at demography conferences, and is the theme of some smaller conferences. But in addition to putting gender on the map in demographic research, this new research has also raised a number of related substantive concerns. They will now be briefly mentioned, and then in later sections of the chapter further elaborated.

One area that has received sustained attention is measurement. Once we recognize that gender is a significant factor in social and demographic processes, its measurement becomes paramount. Measurement of gender has been difficult and not always successful. But the problems with measurement connect to issues of epistemology (what counts as knowledge or evidence and how we use that knowledge) and methodology (theory about how we acquire that knowledge). Thus, some researchers are wrestling with how to expand the models we use to measure demographic processes so they may better evaluate gender's role; others talk about abandoning those models and developing new ones. If we continue with old models, what aspects of gender do we want to measure and why? Are there better models to be found to examine gender and its role in demographic processes? These questions are at the core of much of the gender research currently underway in demography. Most demographers recognize that there are gaps in our knowledge in this area but differ in their suggestions and plans to fill those gaps. In addition, while most recognize the role of gender as both an independent and dependent variable, work has been much more focused on the former than the latter. All of these issues and questions underscore the complexities, difficulties, and importance of continuing work on gender in demography.

METHODS AND MEASURES

As in early work in other social science fields, the earliest demographic work on gender—which is still ongoing—documents differences between women and men. Differences in mortality and morbidity rates, educational attainment, or labor force participation have all been measured and documented. These data have contributed to our understanding of the different lives of women and men across the world, as many of the chapters in the *Handbook* demonstrate. While these findings are important, of course, they often do not go beyond the mapping of sex differences and do not capture the full impact of gender.

In recent years, demographers have been eager to find more comprehensive measures of gender. While women's labor force participation and education have regularly been used as "proxies" for gender, many demographers understand that these measures do not, in fact, represent the depth or scope of gender inequality in any society, and some have attempted to develop new measures. Balk (1994), for example, examined four different aspects of women's position in two villages in Bangladesh; she distinguished among mobility (how freely women move about in public), leniency (a woman's perception about what her family permits her to do), authority (women's participation in household decisions), and attitudes (a woman's opinions about women's rights in Bangladesh). She found that where women's autonomy is high, women's mobility and their household authority go far in explaining variance in total number of children ever born. "Thus," she concludes, "models of fertility that rely solely on proxy measures of women's status [such as education] will be underspecified" (Balk 1994: 1). Balk's research speaks to the complexity and necessity of understanding and measuring gender in new ways, well beyond the use of education and work. However, as will be clear in the next sections on empirical findings, it is easier to collect and explain measures of women's work or education than it is to work with other measures, ones that might give us a deeper understanding of how gender operates. For this reason and others, these measures constitute a large proportion of work which purports to understand the role of gender in demographic change.

One of the difficulties in measuring gender is trying to measure gender's effect at multiple levels (Smith 1989). Early on, Mason (1993: 24) identified the heart of the problem, and demographers have yet to solve this difficulty (see also Cain 1993). Mason argues that in societies which are relatively culturally homogeneous:

> an individual-level analysis cannot reveal anything about the impact on demographic change of women's position *as it is determined by the social institutions of gender*, unless the analysis covers a period during which these institutions have changed significantly. Cross-national or cross-cultural analyses conducted wholly at the aggregate level (for example, those in which countries are used as the units of analysis) avoid this problem, but often suffer from other shortcomings, for example, the problem of making inferences about individual behavior from correlations computed at the aggregate level (emphasis in original).

The availability of appropriate data is key, as Dixon-Mueller and Germain make clear. They have written that:

> National-level surveys such as the DHS, as valuable as they are for many purposes, tell us little about the social context of sexual and reproductive decision-making or women's empowerment. One needs more than statistical correlations to understand contexts. One needs to understand where the individual fits in larger configurations of individuals, couples, households, kin and peer groups, and communities—and in social structures marked by hierarchies of prestige, power, and wealth (Dixon-Mueller and Germain 2000: 72).

The above are examples of the kind of work that is more likely to address more central (and thornier) issues of gender. Further difficulties of capturing the central issues of gender are reflected in the debates and struggles in the demographic community over definitions and uses of concepts such as autonomy, empowerment, or women's status. Scholars are asking if gender is about power and inequality, how may power be measured? Autonomy, empowerment, or women's status each measures some aspect of power but is also problematic in some way. The discussions over the terms may be as valuable as the actual results and further underscore the very difficult task of trying to measure gender. While it is impossible to discuss all the measures that have been tested or used to measure gender, a sampling of some of the research and discussion shows the range, depth, and disagreements among these efforts (see also Kishor 1994; Balk 1994, 1997; Malhotra, Vanneman, and Kishor 1995; Kabeer 1999). As Mason (1993) argues, one of the major problems in the empirical literature on "women's position" is the varying terms and meanings of those terms to describe women's position and the ways that some authors do not make clear their definition or methods of measurement of this concept. Mason notes that two of the most important aspects of women's position are "women's control over resources compared to that of men [and] the degree of their autonomy from men's control" (Mason 1993: 19).

Nawar, Lloyd, and Ibrahim (1995) used data from two surveys from Egypt to flesh out measures of autonomy. They sought to measure how and to what extent women were able to make independent decisions regarding social activities, participation in the public sphere, and health-seeking behavior. While some characteristics such as urban residence, high levels of education, and some aspects of socioeconomic status are positively correlated with autonomy, the authors found that women from across social and economic categories were both restricted in their independence in decision making and at the same time had some control over those areas of their lives deemed most relevant to women, particularly in family planning and child rearing.

While these findings are interesting, particularly salient for this review are the ways the authors discuss the complexities of defining and measuring autonomy. The authors remind us that human behavior is not only influenced at the individual level, but is "embedded in economic and institutional systems, social norms and influence, and personal interconnection" (Nawar, Lloyd, and Ibrahim 1995: 152). They also point out that autonomy is influenced by the way that "the very definitions of appropriate gender behavior proscribe or encourage autonomy...[and how] women are socialized to express lower levels of autonomy than men, even when their actual behavior suggests otherwise" (Nawar, Lloyd, and Ibrahim 1995: 52). One of the most important points they make is how "cultures differ in the extent to which autonomy is valued and sought as a social 'good.' Contemporary Western societies may equate autonomy with power, independence, and privacy, all of which are highly valued. Non-Western societies often place higher value on social interdependence and the support and status achieved from belonging to a group" (Nawar, Lloyd, and Ibrahim 1995: 152–153).

Writing from the perspective of Southeast Asia, Errington (1990) makes a similar argument when she describes economic control as a manifestation of power in western societies but not a key aspect of power in many Southeast Asian societies; in such situations, she (Errington 1990: 7) argues, women's "economic 'power,' may be the opposite of the kind of 'power' or spiritual potency that brings the greatest prestige" (see also Riley 1997a, 1999). The ramifications of these societal differences for the study of gender are enormous and are often overlooked in much demographic literature on gender. Even Nawar and her coauthors focus on absolute autonomy, not women's autonomy relative to that of men; without a larger sense of the overall gender system in Egypt, their measures are not able to capture some of the key issues of gender, which, as discussed above, relate to power and inequality between and among women and men.

In other work, scholars have attempted the further elaboration of women's autonomy. A very interesting analysis by Ghuman, Lee, and Smith (2001), for example, used results from a study conducted in five Asian countries. They examined the validity and reliability of measures of women's autonomy through an investigation of the sometimes contradictory responses of wives and husbands on questions related to women's independence and autonomy. They attempted to understand the relationships among the different responses but for the most part were not able to do so. They came to the conclusion that we cannot be confident that measures—including women's power to make economic decisions, their freedom of movement, their control over household resources, and attitudes about gender equality—capture gender and gender equality. They were struck by the instability of the measures, between wives and husbands, within the communities, and across different societies. Their research underscores a dilemma for those working on issues of gender in demography; while we may find associations between some of the measures and demographic outcomes, we must still be concerned with the validity of the measures as representative of gender. Thus we remain in the early stages of truly assessing gender's role in demographic outcomes.

Given the difficulties of capturing gender and its role in demographic outcomes using conventional demographic methodologies, qualitative approaches might provide useful alternative or complementary information. But there has been little discussion of the different value of qualitative and quantitative methods for assessing gender's effects in demography compared to that in neighboring fields, particularly women's studies (see Lather 1991; Jayaratne and Stewart 1991; Barrett and Phillips 1992; Fonow and Cook 1991; Maynard and Purvis 1994; Reinharz 1992; Riley 1999). It may be the predominance of quantitative work and the general preference for quantitative methods in demography (see Riley and McCarthy, 2003) that have resulted in relatively little attention to discussions of methodological strengths and weaknesses.

Nevertheless, as some have argued (Greenhalgh 1990; Scheper-Hughes 1997), qualitative methods might deepen our understandings of gender and other complex social processes; they are more likely to capture the messiness of social life than are the more parsimonious quantitative models. Qualitative methodologies, with their interpretive frameworks and underlying arguments against universalizing, may also be more likely to capture the shifting and varying notions of gender across national and cultural borders and ethnic and age groups. Related to these issues, qualitative approaches tend to be more constructionist than positivist (Warren 2002), thus following an epistemology that matches much theorizing on gender (Keller 1989). But these issues of epistemology and methodology are more complex than implied by a simple focus on the qualitative/quantitative divide, as we will discuss later in this chapter (see also Maynard 1994).

The importance of these discussions and issues becomes clearer when we examine the empirical evidence on gender and demographic change, and observe the successes, as well as the presence and extent of continuing gaps, in our understanding.

EMPIRICAL FINDINGS

The volume of empirical findings about the role of gender in demographic processes has increased noticeably in recent years. Since 1993, when Watkins summarized the extent of our knowledge about gender as "a great deal about a limited range of women's activities and characteristics" (Watkins 1993: 553), progress has been made. Some of these findings are better characterized as sex differences (which Poston discusses in Chapter 1): women and men have different demographic outcomes, as do boys and girls. But here is where the distinction between gender and sex becomes important, and where the central issues of gender are key: the role of power, the socially constructed nature of gender, and the way that gender is a force at more than the individual level. While demographers are examining gender's effects in many areas of demography, we are probably more confident in our understanding of the role of gender in mortality than in our understanding of its role in fertility.

Morbidity and Mortality

As chapter 10, "Adult Mortality," makes clear, there is wide agreement that gender affects morbidity and mortality. As will become evident below, however, some of this agreement may be premature, as scholars are beginning to unravel some of the apparent connections between gender and mortality outcomes; while there may be clear and strong statistical associations between certain aspects of women's lives, it is not as clear how well these proxies accurately represent gender inequality or even women's empowerment—or what the pathways of influence are. The two areas that have received the most attention are maternal health and infant and child health. Maternal health has obvious connections to women's position in society. We know that women and men have different mortality and morbidity rates (see Chapter 10); we are now trying to understand the causes of those differentials and the role that gender inequalities play. It is also probable that gender affects child and infant health outcomes. Presumably, mothers will have a greater impact on their children's health and survival than will other family members, and mothers' position in the society may influence that impact.

MATERNAL HEALTH.   Much of the research on women's health concerns maternal health—the health of women before, during, and after pregnancy. Maternal mortality is a very serious issue in some societies, where rates can be as much as 100 times the rates in industrialized countries with the lowest maternal mortality rates (McCarthy and Maine 1992). To some extent, maternal mortality is another aspect of sex-differentiated mortality outcomes: women are exposed to the risks of pregnancy, and men are not. But differences in women's and men's health are not only about exposure to risk; gender is also involved in the kinds of access women have to health services and in the ways that health care is structured and supported in any society or community.
    Several studies (Santow 1995; Obermeyer 1993; Dixon-Mueller and Germain 2000; Sen and Batliwala 2000) have found that the more independence women have, especially the more freedom they have to move about the community, the more likely it is they will seek health care for themselves. The pathways of influence seem clear in most instances: when women have access to and the skills to understand health provision, they are more

likely to use it and use it effectively. In her study of Morocco and Tunisia, for example, Obermeyer (1993) found that in both countries, women who have higher education and are from a higher socioeconomic class are more likely to have received maternal care. As discussed below, Obermeyer argues that while these findings represent an argument for the positive influence of education on women's use of health care, education does not simply translate into better maternal care. The surrounding society and norms, particularly gender norms, also play a role.

An analysis undertaken in North India deepens our understanding of how women's roles and positions can influence their health. Consistent with the findings of other researchers, Bloom and colleagues (2001) found that women's autonomy (particularly their freedom of movement) is an important factor in health care utilization among poor and middle income women and that this impact is independent of other social and demographic factors such as education or number of children. The authors highlight the role of family structures and practices in these processes. They argue that in North India, "because women's lives are rooted in the domestic sphere, family and kinship are the key factors defining the parameters of their autonomy" (Bloom, Wypij, and Das Gupta 2001: 68). Women with closer natal ties are more likely to have greater freedom of movement, which in turn translates into greater use of prenatal care; the importance of this relationship is further underscored in the way that it explains the differences found between Hindus and Muslims. The authors argue that in this area of India, the key issue is not whether women can move about alone, but whether they can move about when and where they wish; contact with natal kin allows women to move about in the company of others, and it is this contact which seems to be an important part of health care utilization.

While maternal mortality is as obviously influenced by gender inequality as is overall maternal health, in many ways maternal mortality involves different pathways of influence. In some respects, we can see the handling of maternal mortality and morbidity risk as reflecting the seriousness that the health network of any society places on women's health and lives. Most pregnancy-related deaths cannot be reduced by some of the other interventions often promoted to improve the lives of people, especially women and children, in poorer countries. While access to better nutrition, prenatal and postnatal care, and primary health services have many benefits for women (and others), they are not the surest routes to lower maternal mortality rates. Such medical crises require more sophisticated and on-the-spot services such as surgical intervention, blood transfusions, and well-trained health personnel. Thus, to reduce maternal mortality and morbidity, health facilities must be established to deal with the needs of pregnant women (Maine and Rosenfield 1999; McCarthy and Maine 1992; Ward and Maine 1994). Communities and health systems thus need to make special and directed efforts toward reducing maternal mortality in order to produce effective results.

Of course, maternal mortality is also, at least indirectly, related to the overall role of women through other pathways. If women are restricted in the roles they play in society, they may be more likely to have a higher number of pregnancies, putting them at increased risk for pregnancy complications. Thus maternal mortality is the immediate outcome of a lack of attention at the time of a pregnancy crisis, an outcome that many argue is preventable if health and government officials understand and take the issue seriously (Yamin and Maine 1999). But a further influence relates to the overall roles and options of women and the pressure they face to fill particular maternal roles.

INFANT AND CHILD MORBIDITY AND MORTALITY.   We know that along with its effect on women, gender also shapes the processes surrounding the morbidity and mortality of the children women care for. Work in this area of demography has been long-standing, and while some early findings have been revised or even challenged, many early findings have held up to later scrutiny. Mosley and Chen's (1984) model depicting the pathways of influence on infant and child mortality points to several places where gender, and women's position in particular, play potentially key roles. Mothers are usually the family members most involved with children and their health concerns and so their position in the family, the community, and the society at large often acts as a mediating influence on children.

Other research has corroborated the influence of women's position on child health. For example, in an article published as early as 1986, Caldwell argued that women's status is a major factor in the reduction of infant and child mortality in many societies. He compared countries' economic status with the level of infant mortality and found that women's status helped to explain those places where the direction of the relationship was unexpected (that is, higher mortality in wealthier countries or lower mortality in poorer countries). In places such as Sri Lanka or Kerala, the lower-than-expected infant mortality rates can be explained by norms which allow girls to go to and stay in school and allow women access to the public sphere without sanction. In societies such as Oman or Morocco, the higher-than-expected rates could be attributed to limitations on women's movement and schooling imposed at the societal level.

But as others have pointed out, this connection between gender and mortality might be better characterized as one between mother's education and mortality outcomes (Mason 1995; Desai and Alva 1998). Research has consistently shown a strong link between mother's education and child health outcomes and has specified the possible pathways at both the individual and societal or community levels (Cleland and van Ginneken 1988; Kaufmann and Cleland 1994; Mosley and Chen 1984). Most have argued that because mothers are more likely to be closely involved in child care than are other family members, it is their behavior that will influence child health outcomes. Women who have freedom of movement, who have had schooling that allows them to read, who are confident in their ability to work with and through the health system, and who are self-assertive will be more likely to translate these characteristics into improved health of their children (Mosley and Chen 1984; Caldwell 1979; Caldwell 1986).

In spite of these apparent and quite reasonable-sounding connections, however, recent research has questioned the strength and pervasiveness of the relationship. Desai and Alva (1998), for example, analyzed DHS results for 22 countries and found that while a mother's education is significantly correlated with child immunization, even controlling only for household socioeconomic status and community of residence[2] reduces the connection between infant mortality and mother's education and is significant only in a few countries. Their work suggests that the role of maternal education in infant health is not as clear, consistent, or as strong as once believed (Caldwell 1994; Mason 1995), nor is it easily separated from other measures of socioeconomic status.

---

[2] The authors argued that had they been able to control other key variables such as race/ethnicity and income, the relationship would have been further weakened.

Other research has tried to move beyond using the proxies of education (or work) to understand how women's position is related to infant and child health. Two pieces of research illustrate this line of inquiry (see also Desai and Jain 1994; Kishor 1993). Using DHS data from Egypt, including a specific module on women's status, Kishor (2000) examined influences on infant health and survival. She identified 32 indicators of women's "empowerment" and divided these into three groups: indicators of *evidence* of, *sources* of, and *setting* for women's empowerment, each of which can play a part in gender's role in child outcomes. Her analysis led her to conclude that certain family structures that give women decision-making control have the largest effect on infant health and survival. But perhaps her major contribution was her evidence demonstrating the many facets of women's position that can influence child outcomes and the contradictory effects of those facets. Her work underscores the difficulty of capturing gender's effects and the dangers of trying to do so in models which work best with a limited number of variables.

Durrant and Sathar (2000) conducted an investigation to identify the aspects of women's status that are most likely to influence investment in children, particularly those related to infant survival and children's schooling. They explored and elaborated on the conflicting findings from other studies (e.g., Kishor and Parasuraman 1998; Basu and Basu 1991) that suggested that women's work outside the home affects child and infant survival. They argued that these studies support an understanding of women's status as "elusive, multidimensional, and hard to measure" (Durrant and Sathar 2000: 10). They then broke down the concept *women's status* into independent- and community-level components (including such variables as women's ability to move about outside the house, women's fear of their husbands, decision making regarding children's lives, and access to resources). They sought to determine which of them influence child health and schooling outcomes.

They found that higher female status at the individual level, as measured by less physical abuse by husbands, greater access to financial resources in the household, and fewer restrictions regarding purdah, was negatively associated with infant mortality. But children's schooling, particularly that of girls, was less subject to women's status at the individual level. In this case, mothers' individual situations have less of an effect than do community-level measures of women's status, most notably higher mean levels of women's mobility and a lower percentage of women in the community who fear to disagree with their husbands. Durrant and Sathar's findings are important not only because of the obvious policy implications but also because they underscore the ways that women's status is multidimensional and the ways these different measures (at both individual and community levels) differently affect various demographic outcomes. Community-level aspects of gender interact with—attenuating or enhancing—individual aspects of gender. Further, these influences and interactions are likely to vary by context.

From some provocative and important research (Jejeebhoy 1998; Rao and Bloch 1993), there is increasing evidence that violence against women is not only widespread in some societies and obviously connected to women's physical survival and well-being but also has significant ramifications for infant and fetal health and death. Jejeebhoy's (1998) analysis connects women's higher rates of infant and fetal mortality with wife beating. She argues that there are two reasons for the connection: a pregnant woman who is beaten is more likely to experience a miscarriage and those who are beaten are less likely to have the kind of power that they might use to further their own or their infants' health and well-being. "As a consequence, their health-care seeking and nutrition are compromised, and they are more likely than other women to experience fetal mortality, to deliver babies of low birth weight whose survival is generally uncertain, and to have less decision-making authority or confidence in caring for their infants" (Jejeebhoy 1998: 305).

An interesting finding in this study is that the relationship between women's experience of being beaten and fetal and infant loss remains statistically significant and strong even after introducing controls for age, education, economic status, and indices of a woman's autonomy. While this relationship holds in both the North Indian state of Uttar Pradesh and the southern state of Tamil Nadu, it is stronger in the north, where women have less power than do those in the south. This research is strong evidence of the way that gender—here evidenced in physical threats to women's lives and health—has long-term and far-reaching consequences, for women themselves as well as their children.[3]

From these and other studies on gender and mortality, it has become evident that gender's role in mortality and morbidity outcomes is not as clear-cut as once thought. Gender plays a role in child health even before birth in the ways that pregnant women are treated and have access to health care. As we have seen here and in other chapters in this *Handbook*, girls and boys often have different health and survival outcomes, and many of them are socially induced. Maternal health and mortality are also outcomes of gender's influence, again at different points in women's lives. But as complex as are the relationships between gender and mortality and morbidity, these relationships are nevertheless better understood than is gender's role in fertility (Mason 1993; Durrant and Sathar 2000).

Gender and Fertility

The connections between gender and fertility at the community/societal level are clearly strong but complicated. Mason (1993: 30ff) has hypothesized seven major links between women's position and fertility. These include the ways that women's economic and social independence might delay age at marriage and how women's access to knowledge and technology can influence women's "innovative behavior," including fertility regulation. A series of potential links revolves around the way that women's position in society can influence motivations to limit fertility within marriage. Women will be less interested in limiting the number of children when their roles, status, and respect derive particularly from their position as mothers and when they are dependent on males (husbands and sons).

Several scholars (Bloom, Wypij, and Das Gupta 2001) have suggested that family structure—whether it is patriarchal, patrilocal, and/or patrilineal—and the kind of contact women have with their natal family will also affect fertility. In families organized around and traced through men, the material rewards of childbearing accrue to men more than to women, while women bear the physical burdens. In such situations, where women do not often have as much voice in childbearing decisions, family patriarchs do not support fertility limitation (Caldwell 1982; Folbre 1994). But evidence also shows that women, too, have reason for wanting children in such family structures. Evidence from

---

[3] Violence against women has drawn increasing attention from demographers, as a recent Population Reports testifies (Heise, Ellsberg, and Gottemoeller 1999).

China (Wolf 1972) and India (Cain 1991; Cain, Khanam, and Nahar 1979) indicates that women's vulnerable position in these families and households makes them highly dependent on males. Creating a "uterine family" (Wolf 1972) consisting of daughters and, especially, sons, will give them love and support that help to counteract their disadvantaged position, especially if they become widowed (Cain 1991).

Related to these issues is another: what women do when they have a voice in fertility outcomes. While some presume that women want fewer children than do their husbands, the evidence for this is not consistent across social settings. Mason and Taj (1987), for example, reviewed studies conducted in many social settings and found that there was no strong or consistent evidence for women preferring fewer children than men. This finding is consistent with that of other studies. In their study of Nepal, Morgan and Niraula (1995) found that women do not want more children than men, and in a study of five Asian countries, Mason and Smith (2000: 308) found "no evidence that gender stratification influences spouses' agreement about whether to stop having children."

THE ROLE OF EDUCATION.   As in the area of mortality, we are more certain about the links between certain variables, such as women's education or women's labor force participation, and fertility outcomes. And although these variables do not cover or even represent the full range of gender influences, the connections are important to our understanding of fertility, fertility differentials, and fertility change.

In a review of recent findings, Castro Martin (1995) used DHS data for 26 countries to demonstrate both the connections between women's education and fertility and the complexities and variability in this relationship. Her findings are consistent with previous studies (Cochrane 1979, 1983; Cleland and Rodriguez 1988) that found that while education had a generally negative relationship with fertility, the magnitude and direction of the effect of education also differed depending on the economic development of the country. Castro Martin found that in virtually all societies, women with the most formal education have the lowest levels of fertility.

However, the magnitude of difference between those with the least and most education varied widely across societies. The largest differences were found in Latin America. She related this gap to "a highly polarized social structure, in which the living standards of the upper social strata contrast sharply with those of the lower strata" (Castro Martin 1995: 190). In sub-Saharan Africa, in contrast, education has a weaker effect on fertility; in some countries in the region, fertility is actually higher among women with some schooling than among those with no schooling, although Jejeebhoy (1995) has observed that in most places, this pattern does not hold true for more highly educated women. Researchers have pointed to the ways that education might affect fertility: delayed marriage, changed fertility preferences, and increasing contraceptive (particularly modern) use all are potential results of women's education (Castro Martin 1995; Jejeebhoy 1995; Weinberger, Lloyd, and Blane 1989; Cleland and Rodriguez 1988; Sathar, et al. 1988).

THE ROLE OF WORK.   The connections between women's work and fertility outcomes are even more complex and difficult to disentangle than those related to education; while giving us important information about fertility, they are not necessarily fully informative about the role of gender in fertility outcomes. For some years, drawing from the experience of western societies, demographers believed that fertility had a linear and negative relationship to women's work. Indeed, that relationship was consistent across many industrialized societies (Singh and Casterline 1985) and, partly based on that information, the same relationship was assumed to hold in other places. In fact, in less industrialized societies this relationship is sometimes evident. Results from DHS surveys, for example, show that across many societies, women who work for cash have lower fertility rates than those who do not work for cash. This relationship is evident in places as diverse as Botswana, Bolivia, and Kenya (Muhuri, Blanc, and Rutstein 1994: 10). But the connections between fertility and women's work are complex. Even in industrialized countries, scholars point out, ideological change seems to have as large a role as work in changing fertility levels (Chafetz 1995; Mason and Jensen 1995).

Widely used cross-national surveys such as the WFS and DHS have not always been useful for untangling the complex relationships. In her assessment of World Fertility Survey results and their strengths and weaknesses in helping us understand the fertility/work connection, Lloyd (1991) argues that while these surveys offer important descriptive evidence of differing relationships between fertility and women's work, "these cross-sectional fertility and family planning surveys have taught us very little about the causal mechanisms underlying work-fertility relationships. The challenges and frustrations of working with these data have sharpened our understanding of the strengths and limitations of large-scale cross-national surveys" (Lloyd 1991: 157).

One of the major difficulties in understanding the relationship between work and fertility is connected to the problems of measurement of women's work (Dixon 1982; Oppong 1994; Anker 1994). When women work full-time throughout the year, information on their participation in the paid labor force is relatively easy to gather. However, throughout the world, women—more often than men—work part-time, part of the year, and in the informal sectors of the economy. Unpaid work also influences demographic outcomes (Desai and Jain 1994). These aspects of women's work undoubtedly influence all aspects of women's lives in some ways, including childbirth, but are difficult to measure accurately. And even if we have accurate measures of work, we know that the reasons that women work differ from setting to setting, and from woman to woman, and these differences underscore the different meanings of work. Thus, although whether women work (for wages or not) is an important piece of information, for the purposes of understanding its use in measuring gender, it is necessary to know a great deal more about that work, including its meaning to a woman, her family, and her community (for a fuller discussion of these issues, see Riley 1998).

What do these findings about the connections between education and work on the one hand and mortality and fertility on the other suggest about gender? Because of their relative ease of collection, education and work have been widely used as proxies for gender, empowerment, and women's status in demographic research. That use has strengths and weaknesses. In the details of the pathways of influence of education or work on fertility and mortality, we can see possible linkages. For example, paralleling Caldwell's arguments about infant mortality (noted earlier), Castro Martin (1995) has argued that the overall level of education in a community may have a larger effect on fertility levels than does average length of schooling among individuals who have attended school. While community educational resources are related to overall community resources, we can expect gender to play a role in the differential access of women and men which results in different levels of school attendance and graduation rates. Jejeebhoy (1995) has further argued that in highly gender-stratified communities, women's education does not necessarily translate into social or economic self-reliance, even though it may have an influence on fertility outcomes.

Similarly, women's access to work is not universally interpretable as representing increased status or power. While in some cases, women's access to labor force participation may increase their independence from family resources, it is also true that labor force participation and education, no matter how strongly linked to fertility or mortality outcomes, do not in themselves capture the role of gender. Folbre (2001), for example, discusses how gender ideologies and inequalities are part of social and legal institutions in industrialized societies and remain potent influences in the organization of family and work life. She argues that this influence has contributed to the low fertility trends seen across the western world. How these differences might or might not be related to gender or differential power is a separate question. In different contexts, education and work have different meanings and different uses. As will be detailed below, it is the meaning of the behavior, meaning that arises from the social, economic, and cultural context, that is likely to give us clues to gender's influence (for empirical work on this issue, see Kishor 1993).

Increasingly, demographers are moving to other means to try to understand the role of gender in demographic outcomes. Many have attempted to understand gender as a complex issue and have tried to capture its influence through various methodologies. Some research has focused on power and empowerment as key ways to understand gender; others have looked at resistance to policies and norms to understand gender's role. Several scholars have examined the way that gender's role in institutions such as the economy or state has been linked to demographic outcomes. I will examine some of the strands of this work here and discuss it and other perspectives on gender in the next section.

RESEARCH FINDINGS: NEW ISSUES AND METHODOLOGIES

Power and Empowerment

Recently, demographers interested in understanding gender's role in fertility and mortality have focused on the issues of power and empowerment. While not all agree that this is the best way to understand gender's role in demographic behavior, this work has nevertheless produced insights into these issues, as suggested above in our discussions of Balk (1994) and Durrant and Sathar (2000). Discussion of a few pieces of research cannot do justice to all that is being done but will give the flavor and general direction of the field. In research on the determinants of contraceptive behavior in Ethiopia, Hogan, Berhanu, and Hailemariam (1999) relied heavily on conventional measures of women's position, including literacy, women's work, and age differences between spouses. They found that literacy, in particular, influences women's knowledge of and use of contraception. Those measures, as we have seen, are not particularly useful proxies of women's position, even though they help to explain contraceptive behavior. But these researchers have also included a measure that more directly gauges women's position: their involvement in household decisions. They found that rural women who are highly involved in household decisions are 36% more likely to use a contraceptive than are those who are less involved. While the mechanisms of this relationship are not fully spelled out, this research and others like it suggest that women's contraceptive and fertility behavior is linked to their role in their households.

Other researchers have delved further into the issue of women's power, either at the community or the household level, to examine the relationship between power and demographic outcomes. Unequal structures of power are present at many, and often several, layers of society, as these examples indicate. Browner's (1986) work on an indigenous community in Mexico has demonstrated how women's inability to resist community expectations of fertility can result in their having more children than they prefer. While the Mexican government pressured women to limit their births, many in their own community believed that high fertility would help to stave off ethnic elimination. In this situation, women were caught between two conflicting pressures. Even those who wanted to limit their fertility were unable to realize their desires. Not only did they have to negotiate these competing pressures, but their unequal access to decision-making power relative to village men also played a role. In this village, then, women's difficulty in navigating both the larger political tensions and structures and the household dynamics meant that fertility remained high despite government efforts and women's desires.

Kerala, India, has often been used as an example of a place where women's status has had a strong negative correlation with fertility. Many have argued that women's high levels of education are influential in Kerala's low fertility rates. Using Kerala Fertility Survey data from three Kerala districts, Rajan, Ramanathan, and Mishra (1996) found that the pathways of influence are more complicated than this simple correlation might indicate. They argue that the increase in female literacy and the rise in women's age at marriage were actually the outcome of other processes. With increases in male schooling came an increased demand for brides with higher levels of schooling. Parents were thus compelled to educate their daughters to make them more eligible marriage partners. Women's increased levels of schooling, in turn, meant later age at marriage.

Their results suggest that gender's role is best understood by examining not only women's behavior and characteristics but men's as well. They found, for example, that although higher education is associated with greater autonomy for women (defined through a series of measures related to sources of income, buying power, and independence in seeking health services for their children), Keralan women, in general, do not have a high level of autonomy. Most women do not retain control of their income or property, and most women have to seek their husband's permission when they want to make purchases. Thus, while the relationship between women's education and fertility remains robust, Rajan and colleagues concluded that, given the pathway of influence, it is better characterized as the effect of the wife's *and* husband's education on fertility outcome.

Marriage timing is also a key issue in recent fertility in Japan: delayed marriage age has substantially influenced falling fertility rates in that country. Here again, changes in women's position have been central to these demographic changes. Tsuya (2000) has examined marriage behavior of young Japanese women and has argued that women view marriage more negatively than do men, and unmarried women residing with their parents are particularly likely to see the negative consequences (both psychological and material) of marriage. The subordination of and constraints placed on women within marriage makes these issues particularly salient. As Tsuya has phrased it, "the institution of marriage is not serving the needs and desires of adult Japanese, especially

Japanese women, well" (Tsuya 2000: 343). She argued that marriage delay thus can be seen as evidence of young Japanese women's empowerment; they use their education, jobs, and living situations (often with their parents) to postpone marriage and remain independent as long as possible.

A study done in Nigeria takes a different perspective on how gender might influence demographic outcomes—in this case fertility. Renne (1993) has asked, Why do beliefs about women and men and their place in society affect decisions about reproduction? She found that men continue to dominate in most areas of this Yoruba village; men are the property owners, families are patrilineal, and "the husband is the head of the wife," (Renne 1993: 346) as one respondent stated. But even within this male-dominated setting, women (and men) find strategies to obtain their reproductive goals. Renne argued that now that women are receiving more education, there has been an ideational shift in that women feel an enhanced self-worth that allows them to argue that they should take part in reproductive decisions. They are more likely to discuss contraceptive use and reproductive goals with their husbands and to assert their own ideas and goals in this area of family life. Here, then, women's increased power has not resulted in changes in overall male dominance but has given women new strategies to achieve their own goals in this one important area of their lives.

Thus, in these studies we can see how gender influences demographic outcomes through women's use of power in smaller or larger areas of their lives. While researchers are still endeavoring to measure women's power and status in ways that truly capture what is happening in their lives, this research has underscored the importance of power in understanding gender's role.

Identifying Resistance

Research that has sought out and analyzed incidents of resistance has also contributed to the understanding of gender's role in demographic change. Resistance, of course, comes in many shapes and has any number of directions or targets. Women or men might resist their proscribed roles as wives, husbands, fathers, or mothers; they can resist those who keep them from their own goals; they might resist policies (pronatalist or antinatalist policies, for example); or they could resist something even less tangible, such as new changes that influence their lives. Resistance may be overt and direct, like the collective protests over abortion and abortion rights in the United States (Ginsburg 1989; Luker 1985) or it may consist of small, hidden acts that may be difficult to identify as resistance (Scott 1990; see Kligman 1998 on Romania's population policies and resistance to them).

We have already seen evidence of resistance in some of the literature discussed above. For example, young women in Japan are resisting by postponing marriage. In that case, they are resisting the expected roles of adult women. While the motivation of such resistance may be individual (women are not taking to the streets as a group to protest marriage), the outcome may have effects well beyond the individual level. As Tsuya argues, the resistance exhibited by young women suggests that in order to stop or reverse the fertility decline and other societal changes caused at least partly by this marriage delay, large societal changes might be necessary. In particular, she argues that "we need to make the gender system more equitable by bringing about changes in different spheres of the society...home, market, and government" (Tsuya 2000: 344).

In this case, then, we have an example of how gender relations in the society affect demographic changes which may in turn affect gender relations.

A similar case of individual resistance culminating in changes in gender relations at the societal level can be seen in China, although in a significantly different way. As Greenhalgh (1994), White (2000), and others have reported, women in rural China often resist the birth planning policy that limits their fertility, but that resistance is often hidden from others. Thus, some women who are pregnant with an "out-of-quota" (thus illegal) child hide from authorities (and others) until the birth; other women quietly remove IUDs that have been inserted during official birth control campaigns; still others resort to the abortion of female fetuses or the abandonment of girl infants. These resistances suggest a way that women assert their own goals and mechanisms to achieve a more desirable family size or structure. These actions testify to both women's disagreement with the policy and the "influence of traditional patriarchal culture... which... places family loyalty and filial obligation, not socialist ethics, at the center of the childbearing calculus" (White 2000: 111).

Although women's actions in these situations are not the kind commonly referred to when we talk about "empowerment," they are nevertheless acts of assertion of power. As Scott (1990) has reminded us, we have to look for these kinds of "hidden transcripts" of resistance in the actions of those outside the realm of formal power, in this case village women who are subject to official birth planning policy. The irony is that as women in China resist the birth planning policy, they are also accommodating to societal and family norms that value males over females (White 2000). Thus, sex-selective abortions and the abandonment or outright killing of girl babies has resulted in an alarming number of "missing girls," a very unbalanced sex ratio at birth, with other serious consequences for the future, including the numbers of men who will not be able to find women to marry. As Greenhalgh has argued, when the state accommodated peasants' desire for sons by allowing those with only a daughter to try to have a boy, it was evidence of the state's public recognition of "the unequal value of daughters and sons... Thus... son preference... [was] incorporated into the formal population policy of the province" (Greenhalgh and Li 1995: 625, 627).

We see another kind of resistance in Kenya. There, among the Luo, women's use of contraceptives may be undermining men's control over their families. In that setting, men's dominance has rested on their ability to control important material and symbolic wealth and the connections those various components of wealth and prestige could bring: "Cattle were used primarily as bridewealth, which legitimated control over the women who would produce the children that would perpetuate the husband's lineage" (Watkins, Rutenberg, and Wilkinson 1997: 216). While men continue their economic control and domination today, they have not been able to control women's reproduction in the same way. Watkins and her colleagues attribute this change to the new family planning programs, introduced by outsiders to the culture, which have made contraception easy to obtain. Consequently, Luo women have been able to make decisions about contraception and reproduction that their husbands may disagree with. While most women do not use birth control secretly, the fact that some do, or that it is clearly a possibility, has undermined a vital aspect of men's dominance in the family and society. This contraception availability is "a... fundamental challenge to the fulfilment of what men traditionally considered to be one of the major elements, if not *the* major element, of the good life: children that will in turn produce cattle that can be exchanged for wives who will bear more children" (Watkins, Rutenberg, and Wilkinson 1997: 239). In this setting, women's position in the society, particularly vis-à-vis their husbands, has been influenced by the introduction and spread of fertility control measures.

Gender Change Out of Demographic Change

In all of these cases of resistance, we can see another way of viewing the relationship between gender and demographic behavior: the way that the direction of influence can vary. In Kenya, increased access to contraceptives has given women new space to negotiate their relationships to men. In Japan, lower fertility and delayed marriage may lead to changes in women's and men's lives that will result in increased opportunities for women outside the home and/or more shared responsibility by men for home and child care tasks. In China, lower fertility has come with high sex ratios at birth and new dangers to girls and women living under two competing pressures from the state and the family. While there are many ways that demographic change could influence gender relations and hierarchies in a society, this is not an area that has received a lot of attention. The work above speaks to the importance of this aspect of demographic change. Perhaps the bulk of research in this area has been done in industrialized settings. There, where fertility has dropped to low levels, there is considerable evidence that this change has contributed to changes in women's position in the society. For example, Rindfuss and Brewster (1996) found strong evidence for the way that fertility desires and outcomes in industrialized countries are influenced by the organization of work and the availability of child care. The diversity in fertility rates across industrialized countries can be partly explained by the ease or difficulty women face in trying to combine work and family roles (see also Chesnais 1996; Pinnelli 1995; Folbre 1994). This work and the research reported above in Japan, China, and Kenya speak to other ways that demographic change can influence women's position in society and the kinds of research focuses that are possible in this area.

Toward Broader Thinking about Gender

Most recently, we have witnessed the beginning of even broader thinking about gender and its role in demographic change. As illustrations of the contributions that such work can make, two pieces of such work, both on the issue of Islam and women, will be mentioned. They underscore the difficulty of doing this kind of work in demography and lead to a discussion of the theoretical issues in the study of gender in demography, the focus of the following next section. Obermeyer (1992) and Jejeebhoy and Sathar (2001) have tackled the relationships among gender, Islam, and demographic processes. Obermeyer (1992: 34) examined "the 'fateful triangle' model that sees a pernicious association between Islam, women, and demographic outcomes." She argued for disentangling these elements of social behavior and for a recognition of the wide variation with Arab countries on each of them. Women's status, however measured, varies enormously from one culture to another, as do fertility and mortality rates. Obermeyer makes a strong argument for the importance of understanding the cultural and social underpinnings of those differences and of the ways that Islam both shapes and is interpreted in different cultural and economic settings. Thus, we cannot assume a simple causal relationship between Islam and women's status or demographic outcomes;

rather, research "must include in-depth investigations of the context in which decisions about fertility and health are made" (Obermeyer 1992: 50).

Jejeebhoy and Sathar (2001) were also concerned with the ways that Islam is assumed to affect women's status and fertility. Using data collected in South Asia, they were able to look at regional and religious influence across several settings. Their data include information from both Muslim and Hindus in three different regions: Punjab Province, Pakistan; Uttar Pradesh in North India; and Tamil Nadu in South India. By comparing the many permutations of religion, region, and economic setting, they were able to demonstrate that many of the assumptions about Islam and women's position are not supportable with these kinds of data. By many measures, women in Punjab and Uttar Pradesh—both Hindu and Muslim—are more constrained and have less access to resources than do women—again both Hindu and Muslim—in Tamil Nadu. Thus, they argue, their "findings clearly suggest that differences between Indian and Pakistani women can be attributed neither to nationality nor to religion. Rather, after controlling for the effect of a host of sociocultural factors, every indicator of autonomy remained strongly conditioned by region within the subcontinent, with Tamilian women (representing women from the south) experiencing significantly greater autonomy than women from either Uttar Pradesh or Punjab (jointly representing women from the north)" (Jejeebhoy and Sathar 2001: 706).

Further, they found that the levels and determinants of women's autonomy vary widely among the settings. Whereas in the south, education enhances women's position, higher autonomy for women in the north seems to come from "traditional factors conferring authority on women—age, marital duration, number of surviving sons, nuclear family residence and dowry" (Jejeebhoy and Sathar 2001: 704). These projects and others underscore the importance of context in understanding even those seemingly common elements of different societies and the dangers of assuming or attempting to measure what appear to be universal characteristics across settings, such as religion or women's status. In this research, both Islam and women's status vary and interact differently, depending on context, reminding us of how complex gender can be.

THEORETICAL ISSUES

While demography has begun to wrestle with the larger meanings of gender and its broader relationships with demographic behavior, it is particularly from the perspective of theory that we can best see the gaps in our knowledge on these issues and some of the reasons why these gaps remain. The best way to recognize potential contributions to understanding gender's role in demographic change is to step back from demography, look at what is happening and is being discussed about gender in other social sciences, and then see how those insights and perspectives might be used in demography.[4] Theory holds a very important place in gender studies. Theory has been central to the growth and depth of gender studies over the last couple decades. Work has focused both on critiquing and " 'destabil[izing]' the founding assumptions of modern theory" (Barrett and Phillips 1992:1) and creating new theory that speaks to the role of women, men,

---

[4] For more discussion on this issue, see Riley and McCarthy, 2003; Riley 1997b; Riley 1998; Greenhalgh and Li 1995.

and gender in the social world (see Evans 1997; Barrett and Phillips 1992; Scott 1988a, 1988b; Hirsh and Keller 1990). Among the areas potentially relevant for demographic inquiry have been theoretical developments concerning the role of the state (Brown 1995; Foucault 1980); the connections between the "private" and the "public" (Ginsberg 1989; Rich 1979, 1980; Tilly and Scott 1987; Kelly 1986); work on the body (Martin 1989; Rothman 2000; Gordon 1977); the place and understanding of difference (Mohanty 1991; Moore 1994; Spelman 1988; Higginbotham 1992); the role of gender in relations among nations (McClintock 1995); and the gendered nature of knowledge production (Keller 1985, 1992; Harding 1986, 1991) One of the important pieces missing from demographic work on gender is a strong and consistent link to the key work of scholars of gender outside the field of demography (Bachrach 2001).

While this is not the place to discuss the wide-ranging work outside demography, it is useful to consider a few of the areas of work that might be particularly useful to demographers. As discussed above, an especially important understanding among feminist scholars is the way that gender operates on many levels in any society. To capture its effects, then, we have to recognize that "the gender perspective simultaneously emphasizes the symbolic and the structural, the ideological and the material, the interactional and the institutional levels of analysis" (Ferree 1990: 868). As we have seen, many demographers working on issues of gender have argued that proxies for gender inequality—education and work in particular—are inadequate for capturing gender's influence. But one of the major differences between work on gender inside and outside demography is that demographers usually approach the issue of gender in an attempt to explain some specific demographic outcome.

Research in this area rarely begins with a broad question about how best to understand gender; such a perspective would better allow us to consider—and then revise, pursue, or abandon—potential paths of inquiry. Because demographic research on gender often begins with an attempt to understand which aspect of women's lives influences demographic change, it is thus handicapped from the onset. When we start from that focus, we are easily neglectful of—and usually never even consider—other important aspects of gender, even within the specific area of work and women's position (Riley 1998).

Scott's plea for the need for the development of new theory speaks strongly to this issue. She argues that we need theory that can analyze the workings of patriarchy in all its manifestations—ideological, institutional, organizational, subjective—accounting not only for continuities but also for change over time. We need theory that will let us think in terms of pluralities and diversities rather than of unities and universals. We need theory that will break the conceptual hold, at least of those long traditions of (Western) philosophy that have systematically and repeatedly construed the world hierarchically in terms of masculine universals and feminine specificities. We need theory that will enable us to articulate alternative ways of thinking about (and thus acting upon) gender without simply reversing the old hierarchies or confirming them. And we need theory that will be useful and relevant for political practice (Scott 1988a: 33).

A second key area of work in feminist studies is epistemology. Scholars are examining what counts as knowledge and how we know what we know and the ways that gender has influenced our epistemological approaches. Discussions on these issues are ongoing and influential in many disciplines (Alcoff and Potter 1993; Harding 1991). Scholars have asked whether we can expand and deepen our understanding of gender using traditional epistemologies or whether these must be abandoned in order to do justice to these issues. In what ways might newer epistemological and methodological perspectives help to improve our understanding? In nearly all research on gender within demography, the answer to these questions seems to be that demography's long-standing epistemological and methodological frameworks are adequate, even if they need to be updated. Mason (1995: 4) has argued for retaining the "the dominant scientific standard in demography, which is quantitative and positivistic, and which therefore requires statistical or experimental proof of causality." She has thus suggested "leav[ing] intact much of scientists' and philosophers' conventional understanding of the principles of adequate scientific research" (Harding 1991: 113). Harding has pointed out that such an approach is appealing because "it conserves, preserves, and saves understandings of scientific inquiry that have been intellectually and politically powerful. It enables the results of feminist research to enter conventional bodies of knowledge and to encounter less resistance in doing so than if less conventional epistemologies were used to justify them" (Harding 1991: 113).

Thus, most of the work on gender reported on in this chapter works to bring gender into demography's existing models and assumptions, adding variables to demographic models that might allow us to better examine the role of women and gender and their effects on demographic behavior. Certainly, as is evidenced by the strides that demography has made in recognizing and understanding gender's role, this is a strong argument (see also Maynard 1994). By working from within the existing models, we expand their use and, when appropriate, make changes to the models and even methodologies to promote further understanding. Many demographers, for example, have called for combining quantitative and qualitative methods as a way of getting information on different elements of any demographic process.

As useful as this approach has been, Harding and others (Haraway 1988 and some within demography: see Greenhalgh 1994, 1995; Riley and McCarthy 2003) have argued that demographic understanding of both gender and other issues would be enhanced through an examination and expansion of methodologies and epistemologies. Greenhalgh (2001), for example, has argued for more attention to discourse among demographers. Discourse is "not a language or a text but a historically, socially, and institutionally specific structure of statements, terms, categories and beliefs" (Scott 1988b: 256–257). Discourse analysis focuses attention on the creation of categories such as *gender* but also on categories that are central to demographic work, such as "too high fertility," "overpopulation," and others (see Furedi 1997). The importance of discourse, and thus its analysis, is its connection to outcomes. "Once institutionalized, the discourses become attached to specific disciplinary practices, and techniques and tactics of control. Through institutionalization, gendered discourses on population produce material effects—including demographic effects" (Greenhalgh 2001:2).[5]

Thus, some interested in the role of gender in demographic change want better demography, but through retaining demography's methodologies and epistemologies. Others believe that new methodologies and epistemologies are necessary for understanding gender. Perhaps there is some middle ground here for pursuing an understanding of gender's role in demographic processes. Some demographers may continue to look for new directions outside of demography (Dixon-Mueller and Germain 2000; Riley and McCarthy 2003). If other demographers feel they need to retain their

---

[5] For examples of work on demographic events using discourse analysis, see Chatterjee and Riley 2001; Greene 1999; Greenhalgh 2001.

own methodologies and epistemologies, they can also borrow from the insights and work done in other fields, even if they do not choose to use those methodologies in their own work. Although there are many areas of work that could be mentioned, three will be discussed here: context, power, and the meaning of motherhood. In each, there has been significant work in other social science fields and each has important potential contributions to demographers' understanding of gender. These discussions will be necessarily brief but may indicate the kinds of connections between demography and other fields that could be made or strengthened.

Context

Perhaps the most central issue, both to the study of gender generally, and to what might be most useful to a field like demography with its focus on cross-setting comparisons, is the notion of gender as a social and cultural construction. This notion strongly argues that understanding any social behavior requires understanding the context in which it arises. Many demographers already know this, of course. In the literature on gender in demography, many have either warned about this aspect of gender or concluded that context is central to gender's effects. Obermeyer (1993: 361), for example, in her study of maternal care in Tunisia and Morocco, argues that we need to take seriously the importance of examining closely how "cultural norms relating to women are translated into reproductive outcomes." After looking at north-south comparisons of women's status and religion in South Asia, Jejeebhoy and Sathar (2001: 708) conclude that what is needed is "context-specific measures of women's autonomy."

But a deep understanding of cultural context requires commitments of time, language study, and cultural immersion that are not viewed as important by many quantitative demographers. Such training is, however, at the core of training in other disciplines, particularly anthropology. It is not surprising, then, that particularly from anthropologists we have access to studies of gender and other social institutions that provide depth and breadth and across-society perspectives that could give context to any focused study of demographic behavior. While we certainly should not abandon large quantitative surveys, the gaps in our knowledge of gender (and of many other aspects of social life) give weight to the arguments regarding the importance of combined methodological studies (see especially Kertzer and Fricke 1997 but also Greenhalgh 1997; Scheper-Hughes 1997). In her study of infant and child mortality in Northeast Brazil, Scheper-Hughes's (1992) rich descriptions of life in the poor shanty town provide the context that makes clear just how complex are the reasons that so many children die at young ages. While a quantitative survey might have assessed the extent of the poverty and mortality, and in-depth or focus-group interviews might have fleshed out some of the issues covered in the survey, these methods would not provide the depth that Scheper-Hughes does. Her study chronicles the reasons for the undercount of child deaths, the ways that gender construction plays a significant role in the kind of mothering that takes place in this shanty-town area, the connection between people who live in poverty and those who live much higher up on the socioeconomic index, both in Brazil and beyond, and the ways that researchers are involved in how information is collected and disseminated.

Again, while most demographers may not do this kind of ethnographic work, they can use the studies and perspectives that others outside the field have developed and read that work against what is being done within demography itself. Some have argued (Greenhalgh 1995; Kertzer and Fricke 1997) that the ethnographic and anthropological insights most easily adopted by demographers are depth and richness of context but that it is also possible to incorporate these insights into demographic research, thus creating new epistemological pathways for demography.

Power is at the heart of gender construction and inequality, reflecting the ways that gender is a hierarchical social division which awards more privileges and resources to men than to women. From this perspective, what is most important in gender is not the differences we find between women and men, but the meaning of those differences and the ways they reflect differences in power. Here again, demographers working on gender know the importance of power, as is clearly apparent in the way many researchers have been involved in discussions of empowerment: what it is, how to measure it, and how to decide about its importance. And demographers by no means have ignored the importance of women's power (or empowerment) in general, that is, its importance outside of any demographic change (for example, among many others, see Mason 1995: 22; Jejeebhoy and Sathar 2001: 709; Riley 1997a).

However, the conceptualization of power has been the subject of interesting and useful work well outside demography, and some of that is particularly useful for the study of gender's role in demographic processes (Foucault 1980; Gramsci 1971; Scott 1985, 1990). Gramsci, for example, has elaborated on hegemonic dominance, found and asserted particularly in social institutions, such as the economy or family. To identify this kind of power, we must look carefully at the social landscape. Scott has argued that one way to understand the extent of such power and the resistance to it (Foucault 1980) is to look for the "hidden transcripts" of the subordinate groups (Scott 1990; see also Scott 1985). Scott's work is useful for thinking about the different ways that subordinates work against and within hegemonic structures and the unusual and often hidden assertions of power. This perspective draws attention to sites of resistance and action outside the dominant discourse (see also de Certeau 1984).

In a situation where the dominant and subordinate are intimately connected, as are men and women, these hidden transcripts may be particularly difficult to untangle. Scott (1990: 136) has written that "most of political life of subordinate groups is to be found neither in overt collective defiance of powerholders nor in complete hegemonic compliance, but in the vast territory between these two polar opposites." To find the dissension or the resistance, then, we have to look in public transcripts too, but much of it will likely be very subtle, showing up as silence, as euphemisms, or grumbling. This research speaks to the enormous complexity of power and resistance and the ways that it is found in a myriad of sites and forms. Identifying and measuring this power, then, requires multiple methods and perspectives. As demographers go about trying to map power, resistance, empowerment, and other versions of these processes, they would do well to learn from those who are working to understand power at its many social, cultural, and political levels.

The Meaning of Motherhood

A very obvious area of research that would help inform demographers in their work on gender, particularly as it relates to fertility, is research on the meaning of motherhood. While demographers have already done research on the "value of children," there is an extensive and growing literature on what motherhood means, how it is shaped by the culture and by gendered social, political, and economic institutions, and how individuals interact with those meanings in their own lives. This literature spans many disciplines, from economics (Folbre 2001), to sociology (Hays 1996), to anthropology (Lewin 1994). These and other works (Jetter, Orleck, and Taylor 1997; O'Barr, Pope, and Wyer 1990; Glenn, Chang, and Forcey 1994) often fill out the ways that women and men negotiate through the tensions and expectations about children and parenting and the ways that daily lives reveal these tensions and expectations. Particularly interesting is recent work on childlessness and the new reproductive technologies. Both areas reveal the ways that reproduction is at the center of a society's values.

Inhorn's insights (1994, 1996) about childless women in urban Egypt is an example of research that is not part of mainstream demography but can inform demographic research. In this society, particularly among poor migrants who have moved from rural to urban centers, women's status and power are so powerfully tied to the bearing and raising of children that to be childless is a disaster. When these women moved to the city, they lost other sources of power, income, and even identity, and those losses made children even more important. Inhorn lived and talked with women who were searching for cures to their infertility and came to understand the cultural necessity of bearing children for women in this part of the world. She notes that "indeed, it is from the study of infertility that issues of pronatalism, or child desire, are perhaps best understood. Namely, those who are missing children and who therefore have had much cause to reflect on their object of desire are often in the best position to articulate why children are so very important on a number of levels, ranging from the personal to the political" (Inhorn 1996: 234).

She connects the attitudes of infertile women with the (often negative) responses to the government's family planning program, arguing that "such programs as state-sponsored population control in Egypt, which 'target' women, have literally operated in the dark with regard to the real knowledge, attitudes and practices of their female constituencies. Given this inattention to women's lives and desires (let alone the almost complete neglect of men in population discourse), it should come as no surprise that Egypt's population control efforts have been judged to be weak and ineffective" (Inhorn 1996: 236–237). Here, then, we have clues about the underlying reasons that women want children and how those reasons, and the social context generally, might derail or slow down the government's family planning efforts.

Another angle on the meaning of motherhood and the ways that it is written into policies, practices, and technologies comes from research on the new reproductive technologies. This research (Rapp 1990,1998; Hartouni 1997; Franklin 1995) suggests how "new technologies fall onto older cultural terrains, where women interpret their options in light of prior and contradictory meanings of pregnancy and childbearing" (Rapp 1990: 41). Hartouni (1997) argued that these technologies—with their different roles for biological mother, gestational mother, and social mother, for example—challenge definitions once thought stable. Called into question by this "radical transformation of reproductive practices and processes" (Hartouni 1997: 83) are "the social relations and practices that constitute what are called mother, father, and family" (Hartouni 1997: 83). This work on motherhood, pregnancy, childlessness, and families suggests ways of approaching questions of motherhood, fertility, and pregnancy from new angles in order to illuminate the ways that fertility and reproduction are negotiated and mediated by individuals, families, communities, and states.

All of these areas, and many more that have not been mentioned, suggest the possible contributions from this rich literature. Much of this research takes a step back from the usual goals of demography—of finding the way a particular behavior or status influences a particular demographic outcome. The focus, then, is often not on demographic processes but rather encompasses work that lies outside of demography's traditional scope. In that richness and scope—with its strong connections to demographic processes—lie its strong potential for enriching and enlarging our understandings of gender and demographic processes.

CONCLUSIONS

Examining the research on gender in demography makes clear that we work in a much more hopeful environment than existed just 10 years ago. We have accumulated a rich store of information on gender's connection to processes surrounding fertility and mortality. Perhaps the most positive sign is the sheer volume of work dealing with gender, and the ways that most demographers recognize gender's importance in all social processes. Gaps do remain in our understanding of gender and demographic behavior. It may be that the tools of demography are not geared to understanding the complexities of gender; more data may not necessarily give us more answers. But these gaps, then, are linked to the theoretical and methodological weaknesses in the field generally and the ways that much of the work on gender continues to follow the field instead of "imagining" something different (Dixon-Mueller and Germain 2000; see also Kertzer and Fricke 1997 and McNicoll 1992 on some of demography's other weaknesses).

That issue speaks to the ways that demography might expand its tools and outlook generally—by developing new epistemologies and methodologies or at least by borrowing the findings and insights of others who approach these topics from different perspectives. Our knowledge gaps, then, are not about the problem we used to have, when gender was barely recognized as important. It is clear we will continue to move forward in our understanding of gender; if we connect to work beyond demography, we will make even more progress in understanding the powerful role of gender in demographic change.

REFERENCES

Alcoff, L., and E. Potter, eds. 1993. *Feminist epistemologies.* New York: Routledge.

Anker, R. 1994. Measuring women's participation in the African labour force. In *Gender, work and population in sub-Saharan Africa.* Edited by A. Adepoju and C. Oppong, 64–75. London: James Currey, for ILO.

Bachrach, C. 2001. How can thinking about gender help us do better science? Presented at Population Association Annual Meeting. Washington, D.C., 29 March 2001.

Balk, D. 1994. Individual and community aspects of women's status and fertility in rural Bangladesh. *Population Studies* 48:21–45.

Balk, D. 1997. Defying gender norms in rural Bangladesh: A social demographic analysis. *Population Studies* 51:153–172.

Barrett, M., and A. Phillips, eds. 1992. Introduction. In *Destabilizing theory: Contemporary feminist debates.* Edited by M. Barrett and A. Phillips, 1–9. Stanford, Calif.: Stanford University Press.

Barrett, M., and A. Phillips, eds. 1992. *Destabilizing theory: Contemporary feminist debates.* Stanford, Calif.: Stanford University Press.

Basu, A., and K. Basu. 1991. Women's economic roles and child survival: The case of India. *Health Transition Review* 1:83–103.

Bawah, A., P. Akweongo, R. Simmons, and J. Phillips. 1999. Women's fears and men's anxieties: The impact of family planning on gender relations in northern Ghana. *Studies in Family Planning* 30:54–66.

Bianchi, S. 1998. Introduction to the special issue: Men in families. *Demography* 35:133.

Birke, L., and G. Vines. 1987. Beyond nature vs. nurture. *Women's Studies International Forum* 10:555–570.

Blanc, A., B. Wolff, A. Gage, A. Ezeh, S. Neema, and J. Ssekamatte-Ssebuliba. 1996. *Negotiating reproductive health outcomes in Uganda.* Calverton, Md: Macro International.

Bloom, S., D. Wypij, and M. Das Gupta. 2001. Dimensions of women's autonomy and the influence on maternal health care utilization in a North India city. *Demography* 38:67–78.

Brown, W. 1995. *States of injury.* Princeton, N.J.: Princeton University Press.

Browner, C. H. 1986. The politics of reproduction in a Mexican village. *Signs* 11:710–724.

Cain, M. 1991. Widows, sons and old-age security in rural Maharashtra. *Population Studies* 45:519–528.

Cain, M., S. Khanam, and S. Nahar. 1979. Class, patriarchy, and women's work in Bangladesh. *Population and Development Review* 5:405–438.

Cain, M. 1993. Patriachal structure and demographic change. In *Women's position and demographic change.* Edited by N. Federici, K. O. Mason, and S. Sogner, 43–60. Oxford: Clarendon Press.

Caldwell, J. 1979. Education as a factor in mortality decline: An examination of Nigerian data. *Population Studies* 33:395–413.

Caldwell, J. 1982. *Theory of fertility decline.* London: Academic Press.

Caldwell, J. 1986. Routes to low mortality in poor countries. *Population and Development Review* 12:171–220.

Caldwell, J. 1994. How is greater maternal education translated into lower child mortality? *Health Transition Review* 4:224–229.

Chafetz, J. S. 1995. Women's condition, low fertility, and emerging union patterns in Europe. In *Gender and Family Change in Industrialized Countries.* Edited by K. O. Mason and A. M. Jensen. Oxford: Clarendon Press.

Castro Martin, T. 1995. Women's education and fertility: Results from 26 demographic and health surveys, *Studies in Family Planning* 26:187–202.

Chatterjee, N., and N. E. Riley. 2001. Planning an Indian modernity: The gendered politics of fertility control. *Signs* 26:811–845.

Chesnais, J. 1996. Fertility, family, and social policy in contemporary Western Europe. *Population and Development Review* 22:729–39.

Cleland, J., and J. van Ginneken. 1988. Maternal education and child survival in developing countries: The search for pathways of influence. *Social Science Medicine* 27:1357–1368.

Cleland, J., and G. Rodriguez. 1988. The effect of parental education on marital fertility in developing countries. *Population Studies* 42:419–442.

Cleland, J., and C. Wilson. 1987. Demand theories of the fertility transition: An iconoclastic view. *Population Studies* 41:5–30.

Cochrane, S. 1979. *Fertility and education: What do we really know?* Baltimore, Md.: Johns Hopkins University Press.

Cochrane, S. 1983. Effects of education and urbanization on fertility. In *Determinants of fertility in developing countries* 2. Edited by R. Bulatao and R. Lee 587–626. New York: Academic Press.

Cook, R. 1993. International human rights and women's reproductive health. *Studies in Family Planning* 24:73–86.

de Certeau, M. 1984. *The practice of everyday life.* Berkeley, Calif.: University of California Press.

Desai, S. 2000. Maternal education and child health: A feminist dilemma. *Feminist Studies* 26:425–446.

Desai, S., and S. Alva 1998. Maternal education and child health: Is there a strong causal relationship? *Demography* 35:71–82.

Desai, S., and D. Jain. 1994. Maternal employment and family dynamics: The social context of women's work in rural South India. *Population and Development Review* 20 (1):115–136.

Dixon, R. 1982. Women in agriculture: Counting the labor force in developing countries. *Population and Development Review* 8:539–566.

Dixon-Mueller, R. 1993. *Population policy and women's rights: Transforming reproductive choice.* Westport, Conn.: Praeger.

Dixon-Mueller, R., and A. Germain. 2000. Reproductive health and the demographic imagination. In *Women's empowerment and demographic processes: Moving beyond Cairo.* Edited by H. Presser and G. Sen, 69–94. Oxford: Oxford University Press.

Durrant, V., and Z. Sathar. 2000. Greater investments in children through women's empowerment: A key to demographic change in Pakistan? New York: Population Council Policy Research Division Working Papers, No. 137.

El Dawla, A. S. 2000. Reproductive rights of Egyptian women: Issues for debate. *Reproductive Health Matters* 8(15):45–54.

Errington, S. 1990. Recasting sex, gender and power: A theoretical and regional overview. In *Power and difference: Gender in island southeast Asia*. Edited by J. Atkinson and S. Errington, 1–58. Palo Alto, Calif.: Stanford University Press.

Evans, M. 1997. *Introducing contemporary feminist thought*. Cambridge, Mass.: Polity Press.

Federici, N., K. O. Mason, and S. Sogner, eds. 1993. *Women's position and demographic change*. Oxford: Clarendon Press.

Ferree, M. M. 1990. Beyond separate spheres: Feminism and family history. *Journal of Marriage and the Family* 52:866–884.

Ferree, M. M., J. Lorber, and B. Hess. 1999. *Revisioning gender*. Thousand Oaks, Calif.: Sage Publications.

Folbre, N. 1994. *Who pays for the kids? Gender and the structures of constraint*. London: Routledge.

Folbre, N. 2001. *The invisible heart: Economics and family values*. New York: New Press.

Fonow, M., and J. Cook. 1991. *Beyond methodology: Feminist scholarship as lived research*. Bloomington, Ind.: Indiana University Press.

Foucault, M. 1980. *The history of sexuality*. New York: Vintage.

Franklin, S. 1995. Postmodern procreation: A cultural account of assisted reproduction. In *Conceiving the New World Order*. Edited by F. Ginsburg and R. Rapp, 323–345. Berkeley: University of California Press.

Freedman, L. P., and S. Isaacs. 1993. Human rights and reproductive choice. *Studies in Family Planning* 24(1):18–30.

Furedi, F. 1997. *Population and development: A critical introduction*. New York: St. Martin's Press.

Ghuman, S., H. Lee, and H. Smith. 2001. Measurement of female autonomy according to women and their husbands: Results from five Asian countries. Paper presented at the Population Association of America Annual Meetings, April 2001.

Ginsburg, F. D. 1989. *Contested lives: The abortion debate in an American community*. Berkeley, Calif.: University of California Press.

Glenn, E. N., G. Chang, and L. R. Forcey, eds. 1994. *Mothering: Ideology, experience, and agency*. New York: Routledge.

Goldscheider, F., and G. Kaufman. 1996. Fertility and commitment: Bringing men back in. *Population and Development Review* 22 Special Supplement to Vol. 22: Fertility in the United States: 87–99.

Gordon, L. 1977. *Woman's body, woman's right*. New York: Penguin.

Gramsci, A. 1971. *Selections from the prison notebooks*. New York: International Publishers.

Greene, M. E., and A. E. Biddlecom. 2000. Absent and problematic men: Demographic accounts of male reproductive roles. *Population and Development Review* 26(1):81–116.

Greene, R. 1999. *Malthusian worlds: US leadership and the governing of the population crisis*. Boulder, Colo.: Westview Press.

Greenhalgh, S. 1990. Toward a political economy of fertility: Anthropological contributions. *Population and Development Review* 16(1):85–106.

Greenhalgh, S. 1994. Controlling births and bodies in village China. *American Ethnologist* 21:3–30.

Greenhalgh, S. 1995. Anthropology theorizes reproduction: Integrating practice, political, economic, and feminist perspectives. In *Situating fertility: Anthropology and demographic inquiry*. Edited by S. Greenhalgh, 3–28. Cambridge: Cambridge University Press.

Greenhalgh, S. 1996. The social construction of population science: An intellectual, institutional, and political history of 20th century demography. *Comparative Studies in Society and History* 38(1):26–66.

Greenhalgh, S. 1997. Methods and meanings: Reflections on disciplinary difference. *Population and Development Review* 23(4):819–824.

Greenhalgh, S. 2001. The discursive turn in the study of gender and population. Population of Association Annual Meeting. March 2001. Panel presentation.

Greenhalgh, S., and J. Li. 1995. Engendering reproductive policy and practice in peasant China: For a feminist demography of reproduction. *Signs* 20(3):601–641.

Haraway, D. 1988. Situated knowledges: The science question in feminism and the privilege of partial perspective. *Feminist Studies* 14(3) (Fall): 575–600.

Harding, S. 1986. *The science question in feminism*. Ithaca, N.Y.: Cornell University Press.

Harding, S. 1987. Is there a feminist method? *Hypatia* 2(fall).

Harding, S. 1991. *Whose science? Whose knowledge? Thinking from women's lives*. Ithaca, N.Y.: Cornell University Press.

Hartouni, V. 1997. *Cultural conceptions: On reproductive technologies and the remaking of life*. Minneapolis: University of Minnesota Press.

Hays, S. 1996. *The cultural contradictions of motherhood*. New Haven, Conn.: Yale University Press.

Heise, L., M. Ellsberg, and M. Gottemoeller. 1999. *Ending violence against women*. Population Reports Series L, No. 11. Baltimore, Md.: Johns Hopkins Population Information Program.

Higginbotham, E. B. 1992. African-American women's history and the metalanguage of race. *Signs* 17(2):3–26.

Hirsh, M., and E. F. Keller, eds. 1990. *Conflicts in feminism*. New York: Routledge.

Hirschman, C. 1994. Why fertility changes. *Annual Review of Sociology* 20:203–233.

Hogan, D., B. Berhanu, and A. Hailemariam. 1999. Household organization, women's autonomy, and contraceptive behavior in southern Ethiopia. *Studies in Family Planning* 30(4):302–314.

Inhorn, M. 1994. *Quest for conception: Gender, infertility, and Egyptian medical traditions*. Philadelphia: University of Pennsylvania Press.

Inhorn, M. 1996. *Infertility and patriarchy: The cultural politics of gender and family life in Egypt*. Philadelphia: University of Pennsylvania Press.

Jayaratne, T., and A. Stewart. 1991. Quantitative and qualitative methods in the social sciences: Current feminist issues and practical strategies. In *Beyond methodology: Feminist scholarship as lived research*. Edited by M. Fonow and J. Cook, 85–106. Bloomington: Indiana University Press.

Jejeebhoy, S. 1995. *Women's education, autonomy, and reproductive behavior: Experience from developing countries*. Oxford: Clarendon Press.

Jejeebhoy, S. 1998. Associations between wife-beating and fetal and infant death: Impressions from a survey in rural India. *Studies in Family Planning* 29(3):300–308.

Jejeebhoy, S., and Z. A. Sathar. 2001. Women's autonomy in India and Pakistan: The influence of religion and region. *Population and Development Review* 27(4):687–712.

Jetter, A., A. Orleck, and D. Taylor, eds. 1997. *The politics of motherhood: Activist voices from left to right*. Hanover, N.H.: University Press of New England.

Kabeer, N. 1994. *Reversed realities*. London: Verso.

Kabeer, N. 1999. Resources, agency, achievement: Reflections on the measurement of women's empowerment. *Development and Change* 30:435–464.

Kaufmann, G., and J. Cleland. 1994. Maternal education and child survival: Anthropological responses to demographic evidence. *Health Transition Review* 4(2):196–199.

Keller, E. F. 1985. *Reflections on gender and science*. New Haven, Conn.: Yale University Press.

Keller, E. F. 1989. Just what is so difficult about the concept of gender as a social category? (Response to Richards and Schuster). *Social Studies of Science* 19:721–724.

Keller, E. F. 1992. *Secrets of life, secrets of death*. New York: Routledge.

Kelly, J. 1986. Family and society. In *Women, history, and theory: The essays of Joan Kelly*, 110–156. Chicago: University of Chicago Press.

Kertzer, D., and T. Fricke. 1997. Toward anthropological demography. In *Anthropological demography: Toward a new synthesis*. Edited by D. I. Kertzer and T. Fricke, 1–35. Chicago: University of Chicago Press.

Kishor, S. 1993. May God give sons to all: Gender and child mortality in India. *American Sociological Review* 58 (2):247–265.

Kishor, S. 1994. Autonomy and Egyptian Women: Findings from the 1988 Egypt demographic and health survey. Occasional Papers, No. 2. Demographic and Health Surveys, Calverton, Md.: Macro International.

Kishor, S. 2000. Empowerment of women in Egypt and links to the survival and health of their infants. In *Women's empowerment and demographic processes: Moving beyond Cairo*. Edited by H. Presser and G. Sen, 118–156. Oxford: Oxford University Press.

Kishor, S., and S. Parasuraman. 1998. Mother employment and infant and child mortality in India. National Family Health Survey Subject Reports. No. 8. Mumbai and Calverton, Md.: Institute for Population Sciences and Macro International.

Kligman, G. 1998. *The politics of duplicity: Controlling reproduction in Ceausescu's Romania*. Berkeley: University of California Press.

Lather, P. 1991. *Getting smart: Feminist research and pedagogy with/in the postmodern*. New York: Routledge.

Lewin, E. 1994. Negotiating lesbian motherhood: The dialectics of resistance and accommodation. In *Mothering: Ideology, experience, agency*. Edited by E. Glenn, G. Chang, and L. Forcey, 333–353. New York: Routledge.

Lloyd, C. 1991. The contribution of the world fertility surveys to an understanding of the relationship between women's work and fertility. *Studies in Family Planning* 22(3):144–161.

Luker, K. 1985. *Abortion and the politics of motherhood*. Berkeley: University of California Press.

Maine, D., and A. Rosenfield. 1999. The safe motherhood initiative: Why has it stalled? *American Journal of Public Health* 89:480–483.

Malhotra, A., R. Vanneman, and S. Kishor. 1995. Fertility, dimensions of patriarchy, and development in India. *Population and Development Review* 21:281–306.

Marshall, B. 2000. *Configuring gender: Explorations in theory and politics*. Toronto: Broadview Press.

Martin, E. 1989. *The woman in the body: A cultural analysis of reproduction*. Boston: Beacon Press.

Mason, K. O. 1993. The impact of women's position on demographic change during the course of development. In *Women's position and demographic change*. Edited by N. Federici, K. O. Mason, and S. Sogner. Oxford: Clarendon Press.

Mason, K. O. 1995. Gender and demographic change: What do we know? IUSSP Paper.

Mason, K. O., and A. Jensen, eds. 1995. In *Gender and family change in industrialized countries*. Oxford: Clarendon Press.

Mason, K. O., and H. L. Smith. 2000. Husbands' versus wives' fertility goals and use of contraception: The influence of gender context in five Asian countries. *Demography* 37:299–311.

Mason, K. O., and A. M. Taj. 1987. Differences between women's and men's reproductive goals in developing countries. *Population and Development Review* 13:611–638.

Maynard, M. 1994. Methods, practice, and epistemology: The debate about feminism and research. In *Researching women's lives from a feminist perspective*. Edited by M. Maynard and J. Purvis. New York: Taylor and Francis.

Maynard, M., and J. Purvis, eds. 1994. *Researching women's lives from a feminist perspective*. New York: Taylor and Francis.

McCarthy, J., and D. Maine. 1992. A framework for analyzing the determinants of maternal mortality. *Studies in Family Planning* 23:23–33.

McClintock, A. 1995. *Imperial leather: Race, gender, and sexuality in the colonial contest*. London: Routledge.

McIntosh, C. A., and J. Finkle. 1995. The Cairo Conference on Population and Development: A new paradigm? *Population and Development Review* 21:223–260.

McNicoll, G. 1992. The agenda of population studies: A commentary and complaint. *Population and Development Review* 18:399–420.

Mohanty, C. T. 1991. Under western eyes: Feminist scholarship and colonial discourses. In *Third world women and the politics of feminism*. Edited by C. Mohanty, A. Russo, and L. Torres, 51–80. Bloomington: Indiana University Press.

Moore, H. 1994. *A passion for difference: Essays in anthropology and gender*. Oxford: Polity Press (Blackwell).

Morgan, S. P., and B. B. Niraula. 1995. Gender inequality and fertility in two Nepali villages. *Population and Development Review* 21:541–562.

Mosley, W. H., and L. Chen. 1984. An analytical framework for the study of child survival in developing countries. *Population and Development Review* (Supplement to Vol. 10: Child Survival: Strategies for Research): 25–45.

Muhuri, P., A. Blanc, and S. Rutstein. 1994. *Socioeconomic differentials in fertility. Demographic and health surveys comparative studies No. 13*. Calverton, Md.: Macro International.

Nawar, L., C. Lloyd, and B. Ibrahim. 1995. Women's autonomy and gender roles in Egyptian families. In *Family, gender, and population in the Middle East: Policies in context*. Edited by C. Obermeyer, 147–178. Cairo: American University in Cairo Press.

O'Barr, J., D. Pope, and M. Wyer, eds. 1990. *Ties that bind: Essays on mothering and patriarchy*. Chicago: University of Chicago Press.

Obermeyer, C. M. 1992. Islam, women, and politics: The demography of Arab countries. *Population and Development Review* 18:33–60.

Obermeyer, C. M. 1993. Culture, maternal health care, and women's status: A comparison of Morocco and Tunisia. *Studies in Family Planning* 24:354–365.

Oppong, C. 1994. Introduction. In *Gender, work, and population in sub-Saharan Africa*. Edited by A. Adepoju and C. Oppong, 1–16. Geneva: International Labour Office, by James Currey.

Petchesky, R. P. 1997. Spiraling discourses of reproductive and sexual rights: A post-Beijing assessment of international politics. In *Women transforming politics*. Edited by C. Cohen, K. Jones, and J. Tronto, 569–587. New York: New York University Press.

Petchesky, R. P. 2000. Human rights, reproductive health and economic justice: Why they are indivisible. *Reproductive Health Matters* 8:12–17.

Pinnelli, A. 1995. Women's condition, low fertility and emerging union patterns in Europe. In *Gender and family change in industrialized countries*. Edited by K. O. Mason and A. M. Jensen, 82–101. Oxford: Clarendon Press.

Poston, D. L., Jr., and Chiung-Fang Chang. 2005. Bringing males in: A critical demographic plea for incorporating males in methodological and theoretical analyses of human fertility. *Critical Demography*, forthcoming.

Presser, H. B. 1997. Demography, feminism, and the science-policy nexus. *Population and Development Review* 23:295–332.

Presser, H., and G. Sen. 2000. Women's empowerment and demographic processes: Laying the groundwork. In *Women's empowerment and demographic processes: Moving beyond Cairo*. Edited by H. Presser and G. Sen, 3–14. Oxford: Oxford University Press.

Rajan, S. I., M. Ramanathan, and U. S. Mishra. 1996. Female autonomy and reproductive behaviour in Kerala: New evidence from the recent Kerala Fertility Survey. In *Girls' schooling, women's autonomy and fertility change in South Asia*. Edited by R. Jeffery and A. Basu, 268–287. New Delhi: Sage Publications.

Rao, V., and F. Bloch. 1993. Wife-beating, its causes and its implications for nutrition allocations to children: An economic and anthropological case study of a rural South Indian community. Washington, D.C.: World Bank, Policy Research Department.

Rapp, R. 1990. Constructing amniocentesis: Maternal and medical discourses. In *Uncertain terms: Negotiating gender in American culture*. Edited by F. Ginsburg and A. Tsing, 28–42. Boston: Beacon Press.

Rapp, R. 1998. Refusing prenatal diagnosis: The meanings of bioscience in a multicultural world. *Science, Technology and Human Values* 23:45–71.

Reinharz, S. 1992. *Feminist methods in social research*. New York: Oxford.

Renne, E. 1993. Gender ideology and fertility strategies in an Ekiti Yoruba village. *Studies in Family Planning* 24:343–353.

Rich, A. 1979. *Of woman born*. New York: W. W. Norton.

Rich, A. 1980. Compulsory heterosexuality and lesbian existence. *Signs* 5:631–660.

Riley, N. E. 2003. Gender. *Encyclopedia of Population*. New York: Macmillan Reference.

Riley, N. E. 1999. Challenging demography: Contributions from feminist theory. *Sociological Forum* 14:369–397.

Riley, N. E. 1998. Research on gender in demography: Limitations and constraints. *Population Research and Policy Review* 17:521–538.

Riley, N. E. 1997a. Gender, power and population change. *Population Bulletin* 52. Washington, D.C.: Population Reference Bureau.

Riley, N. E. 1997b. Similarities and differences: Anthropological and demographic perspectives on gender. In *Anthropological demography: Toward a new synthesis*. Edited by D. I. Kertzer and T. Fricke, 115–138. Chicago: University of Chicago Press.

Riley, N. E., and J. McCarthy. 2003. *Demography in the age of the postmodern*. Cambridge, Mass.: Cambridge University Press.

Rindfuss, R. R., and K. L. Brewster. 1996. Childrearing and Fertility. In *Fertility in the United States: New patterns, new theories*. Edited by J. Casterline, R. Lee, and K. Foote, 258–289.

Rosenfield, A., and D. Maine. 1985. Maternal mortality, a neglected tragedy: Where is the "M" in "MCH"? *Lancet* 2:83–85.

Rothman, B. K. 2000. *Recreating motherhood*. New Brunswick, N.J.: Rutgers University Press.

Santow, G. 1995. Social roles and physical health: The case of female disadvantage in poor countries. *Social Science and Medicine* 40:147–161.

Sathar, Z., N. Crook, C. Callum, and S. Kazi. 1988. Women's status and fertility change in Pakistan. *Population and Development Review* 14:415–432.

Scheper-Hughes, N. 1992. *Death without weeping: The violence of everyday life in Brazil*. Berkeley: University of California Press.

Scheper-Hughes, N. 1997. Demography without numbers. In *Anthropological demography: Toward a new synthesis*. Edited by D. I. Kertzer and T. Fricke, 201–222. Chicago: University of Chicago Press.

Scott, J. 1985. *Weapons of the weak: Everyday forms of peasant resistance.* New Haven, Conn.: Yale University Press.

Scott, J. 1990. *Domination and the arts of resistance: Hidden transcripts.* New Haven, Conn.: Yale University Press.

Scott, J. W. 1986. Gender: A useful category for historical analysis. *American Historical Review* 91:1053–1075.

Scott, J. W. 1988a. Deconstructing equality-vs-difference: Or, the uses of post-structuralist theory for feminism. *Feminist Studies* 14:33–50.

Scott, J. W. 1988b. *Gender and the politics of history.* New York: Columbia University Press.

Sen, G., and S. Batliwala. 2000. Empowering women for reproductive rights. In *Women's empowerment and demographic processes: Moving beyond Cairo.* Edited by H. Presser and G. Sen, 15–36. Oxford: Oxford University Press.

Singh, S., and J. Casterline. 1985. The socio-economic determinants of fertility. In *Reproductive change in developing countries: Insights from the world fertility survey.* Edited by J. Cleland and J. Hobcraft, 199–222. Oxford: Oxford University Press.

Smith, H. 1989. Integrating theory and research on the institutional determinants of fertility. *Demography* 26:171–183.

Spelman, E. 1988. *Inessential woman.* Boston: Beacon Press.

Szreter, S. 1993. The idea of demographic transition and the study of fertility: A critical intellectual history. *Population and Development Review* 19:659–701.

Tilly, L., and J. Scott. 1987. *Women, work, and family.* New York: Methuen.

Tsuya, N. 2000. Women's empowerment, marriage postponement, and gender relations in Japan: An intergenerational perspective. In *Women's empowerment and demographic processes: Moving beyond Cairo.* Edited by H. Presser and G. Sen, 318–348. Oxford: Oxford University Press.

Tuana, N. 1983. Re-fusing nature/nurture. *Women's Studies International Forum* 6:621–632.

Udry, J. R. 1994. The nature of gender. *Demography* 31:561–573.

Ward, V., and D. Maine. 1994. A strategy for the evaluation of activities to reduce maternal mortality in developing countries. *Evaluation Review* 18:438–458.

Warren, C. 2002. Qualitative interviewing. In *Handbook of interview research: Context and method.* Edited by J. Gubrium and J. Holstein, 83–102. Thousand Oaks, Calif.: Sage.

Watkins, S. 1993. If all we knew about women were what we read in *Demography*, what would we know? *Demography* 30:551–578.

Watkins, S. C., N. Rutenberg, and D. Wilkinson. 1997. Orderly theories, disorderly women. In *The continuing demographic transition.* Edited by G. W. Jones, R. M. Douglas, J. C. Caldwell, and R. M. D'Souza, 213–245. Oxford: Clarendon Press.

Weinberger, M. B., C. Lloyd, and A. Blanc. 1989. Women's education and fertility: A decade of change in four Latin American countries. *International Family Planning Perspectives* 15:4–14.

White, T. 2000. Domination, resistance, and accommodation in China's one child campaign. In *Chinese society: Change, conflict, and resistance.* Edited by E. Perry and M. Selden, 102–119. London and New York: Routledge.

Wolf, M. 1972. *Women and the family in rural Taiwan.* Palo Alto, Calif.: Stanford University Press.

Yamin, A. E., and D. Maine. 1999. Maternal mortality as a human rights issue: Measuring compliance with international treaty obligations. *Human Rights Quarterly* 21:563–607.

Yanagisako, S., and J. Collier. 1987. Toward a unified analysis of gender and kinship. In *Gender and kinship: Essays toward a unified analysis.* Edited by J. Collier and S. Yanagisako, 14–50. Polo Alfo, Calif.: Stanford University Press.

CHAPTER 5

Demography of Aging

PETER UHLENBERG

In the 1960s, the demographic phenomenon that received a great deal of both scholarly and popular attention was rapid population growth, popularly referred to as the population explosion. By the end of the 20th century, global population aging—the graying of the world (Peterson 1999)—was the demographic phenomenon receiving a great deal of attention. These demographic trends generated widespread alarm regarding the threat that each posed to the future social and economic well-being of societies. Interestingly, both are produced by the modernization of demographic behavior, or the demographic transition. Rapid population growth occurred as death rates declined rapidly, resulting in birth rates exceeding death rates. As birth rates subsequently declined around the world, population growth slowed and population aging began. In other words, population aging is the price paid for solving the challenge of population growth. There is, however, an important contrast between the issues of rapid population growth and population aging. Rapid population growth appears to be a short-term phenomenon, whereas the marked change in age composition resulting from population aging is unlikely to be reversed in the future.

This chapter begins by discussing the demographic determinants and global patterns of population aging and then explores a series of important issues related to population aging: How does migration affect population age composition? What are the implications of population aging for pension systems? How does population aging affect population health and health care? How does population aging affect kinship structures? Finally, it reviews methodological issues related to studying population aging and future research directions.

SUBSTANTIVE ISSUES

Demographic Determinants of Population Aging

Population aging is a basic demographic phenomenon, determined by a population's fertility, mortality, and migration patterns. Indeed, the age distribution of a population at any time is uniquely determined by its history of births and age-specific death and migration rates. Demographers have been able to carefully explicate how population aging occurs. Two approaches are especially useful in this type of demographic analysis: the stable population model and population projections.

THE STABLE POPULATION MODEL.   The use of the stable population model to examine population aging has been developed in several books on mathematical demography (Coale 1972; Keyfitz 1968; Preston, Heuveline, and Guillot 2001; also see chapter 22 in this *Handbook*). Discussions of the stable population model for population analysis begin by establishing that the age distribution of a closed population is determined by past fertility and mortality schedules. If age-specific fertility and mortality rates remain unchanged for a long time (a century is generally long enough), and no migration occurs, the population will have a unique and unchanging age distribution. That is, under these conditions the proportion of the population in any age category does not change from one year to the next. Because the age distribution is mathematically determined by age-specific birth and death rates in a stable population, it is possible to determine the effect of a change in the age-specific fertility and/or mortality rates on the age distributions of a stable population. This approach is called "comparative statics," indicating that it does not deal with the dynamics of the transition from one stable population to another but only with the comparison of a stable population after a change in vital rates to the initial stable population.

Using the stable population model, the effect of a change in fertility on the age composition of a population is found to be straightforward. A permanent shift to a lower fertility level, with no change in mortality rates, leads to an aging of the population. This result is not surprising, because it seems obvious that under similar mortality conditions, a population with lower fertility will have proportionately fewer children, and hence an older population, than one with higher fertility. Comparing stable populations with different fertility levels and similar levels of life expectancy shows the magnitude of the effect of a fertility decline. For example, in a stable population with life expectancy of 80 years, 11.9% of the population will be over age 65 if the gross reproduction rate (GRR) is 1.5, but 25.9% if the GRR is 0.8. Other comparisons of stable population age composition under differing fertility and mortality conditions can be made from data in Table 5.1. The effect of decreasing fertility can be seen by looking down columns in this table. Clearly, under any particular mortality condition, sustained low fertility leads to an older population than sustained high fertility.

Analyzing the stable population model shows that the effect of mortality change on population aging is not straightforward. The effect of a change in mortality depends on the specific ages at which mortality changes. Contrary to what most nondemographers assume, an increase in life expectancy (average years lived by a cohort) does *not* necessarily result in an aging of the population and may actually produce a younger population. The variable effect of changing mortality levels for the age distribution of a

TABLE **5.1. Percent over Age 65 in Stable Populations with Various Combinations of Fertility and Mortality.**

Gross Reproduction Rate	Expectation of Life (in years)					
	30	40	50	60	70	80
4.0	1.8	1.8	1.7	1.7	1.7	2.1
3.0	3.1	3.0	3.0	2.9	3.0	3.6
2.0	5.8	5.9	5.9	5.9	6.1	7.5
1.0	14.5	14.9	15.5	15.7	16.5	20.2
0.8	17.8	18.9	19.7	20.1	21.2	25.9

Source: Coale and Demeny 1983.

stable population can be seen by exploring several different causes of increasing life expectancy. For example, an increase in life expectancy that occurs only because of a decrease in infant mortality results in a younger population. Indeed, increasing the proportion of babies who survive would have the same long-term effect on population age composition as would an increase in the birth rate. On the other hand, an increase in life expectancy caused only by decreasing death rates in later life (among those over age 50 years, for example) would increase only the size of the older population and hence lead to population aging. A third scenario is one in which there is an equal absolute decline in death rates at all ages. Stable population analysis shows that this particular mortality decline has no effect on population age composition. Thus it turns out that, depending on the ages at which mortality declines, increasing life expectancy can lead to population aging, population "younging," or no change in age composition. Examples of these different possible outcomes can be seen by looking across rows in Table 5.1. Increasing life expectancy from 40 to 60 with a GRR of 3.0 decreases the proportion over age 65 in a population, but increasing life expectancy from 60 to 80 with a GRR of 1.0 produces a significant aging of the population. As discussed later, the actual effect of declining mortality on the age composition of a population depends primarily on what life expectancy is when the decline occurs.

POPULATION PROJECTIONS. Basically, a population projection begins with a baseline population and then, using some method, determines what size that population would be at some future date under a particular set of assumptions. Some methods make it possible to project not only the size but also the composition (age, sex, race, etc.) of a population into the future. Unless a calculation error is made, a projection is accurate— that is, under the given set of assumptions, the baseline population will change as expected. Of course, when a projection is used to forecast the future size and composition of a population, it may be totally wrong if the assumptions are not an accurate description of actual future demographic behavior. Population projections used as population forecasts are discussed below; here the interest is in using population projections to examine the determinants of population aging. What are the effects of alternative patterns of mortality, fertility, and migration on future population age composition?

A series of alternative projections of the United States population by the Census Bureau (Day 1996) can be used to illustrate how population projections aid our understanding of the determinants of population aging. The baseline for these particular projections is 1995, when 12.8% of the population was aged 65 years and over, the total fertility rate was 2.055, life expectancy was 75.9, and yearly net immigration was 820,000. Using various assumptions regarding fertility, mortality, and migration over the ensuing 55 years, the Census Bureau calculates what the size and age composition of the population would be in 2050. The alternative assumptions used for these calculations are shown in Table 5.2. Projections of the percent of the United States population over age 65 years in 2050 under differing sets of assumptions are shown in Table 5.3.

Following the middle series for all three demographic variables would lead to a population with 20.0% over age 65 in the year 2050. The other entries in Table 5.3 show the projected proportion of the old population (age 65 and over) when one of the variables follows either a higher or lower trajectory while the other two follow the middle series. This allows us to isolate the effect of alternative fertility, mortality, or migration scenarios on population aging. As expected from the discussion of the stable population model, a pattern of higher fertility would produce a younger population (17.6% over age 65 years) and a pattern of lower fertility would produce an older population (22.8% over age 65 years). The alternative mortality assumptions have an even larger consequence for population aging over this period than the alternative fertility assumptions. A large reduction in mortality results in the largest proportion over age 65 years of any of these scenarios (23.3%), while a slight increase in mortality results in the smallest proportion of the old of any scenario (16.5%).

Perhaps the most interesting finding revealed in these alternative projections is the relatively small effect of differing assumptions about future immigration levels on the future age distribution. Either increasing or decreasing the annual net flow of immigrants to the United States by half a million would change the proportion over age 65 years in the population by less than 1% from the middle series. Indeed, a projection

TABLE 5.2. Census Bureau Assumptions of Fertility, Mortality, and Migration for 2050.

Item	2050 Level Assumption			
	1995	Low	Middle	High
Fertility (GRR)	2.055	1.910	2.245	2.580
Life expectation (yrs)	75.9	74.8	82.0	89.4
Net immigration (000's)	820	300	820	1,370

TABLE 5.3. Percent of the United States Population Projected to be Over Age 65 years in 2050 Under Alternative Assumptions.

Assumptions[*]	% 65+
Middle series for fertility, mortality, and migration	20.0
Low fertility, middle mortality, and migration	22.8
High fertility, middle mortality, and migration	17.6
Low mortality, middle fertility, and migration	23.3
High mortality, middle fertility, and migration	16.5
High immigration, middle mortality, and fertility	19.4
Low immigration, middle mortality, and fertility	20.8
Zero immigration, middle mortality, and fertility	22.3

Source: Day 1996.
[*]See text for description of assumptions.

using the extreme assumption of zero future immigration results in an only a slightly older population (22.3% over age 65 years) in 2050 than the middle series with 820,000 net immigrants per year. The ineffectiveness of using immigration to slow population aging is discussed more fully below. A more thorough use of population projections to study determinants of population aging is possible by using various starting populations and a wider range of alternative assumptions about future fertility, mortality, and migration patterns.

Using either the stable population model or experimenting with alternative assumptions in making population projections leads to the same basic conclusions regarding the demographic determinants of population aging. A decline in fertility leads to population aging. A decline in mortality spread across all ages has little effect on the age composition of a population, but a decrease in mortality concentrated in later life can significantly increase population aging. And, within typical boundaries actually observed, immigration has only a small effect on population aging. Using this information helps us understand past trends in population aging and provides a basis for anticipating future trends.

Trajectories of Population Aging

From the perspective of the early 21st century one can see an amazing revolution of demographic behavior that began slowly in Europe in the 18th century and accelerated around the world in the 20th century. All populations before the demographic transition, as the revolution is generally called, had to contend with high death rates. When half or fewer of all babies survived to adulthood, fertility was necessarily high or a population would not survive. Under these conditions of high fertility and high mortality, all populations were young by contemporary standards, with no more than 3% or 4% of any population being over age 65 years. Without entering into the discussion (and debates) about the causal mechanisms involved (Casterline 2003; Chesnais 1992), the basic description of what happened can be simply noted. Death rates and birth rates in Europe, North America, and Australia declined drastically between 1850 and 2000. During this transition, populations in these areas grew significantly larger and became much older. Almost all other countries experienced significant declines in mortality and fertility rates beginning sometime in the 20th century, and consequently experienced rapid population growth and some population aging. But because the pattern and timing of the demographic transition has varied widely across countries, some countries are still at an early stage of the demographic transition and have yet to experience any population aging. Thus, as a consequence of differences in demographic behavior over the past century, in 2000 there were enormous variations across countries in the age composition of their populations.

The dimensions of global population aging, and issues related to it, received a great deal of attention at the beginning of the 21st century. Major reports on this topic were published by the Population Division of the United Nations (United Nations 2002), the United States Census Bureau (Kinsella and Velkoff 2001), and the National Academy of Sciences (National Research Council 2001). Each of these reports notes that societies around the world are now in the midst of a profound change in the age distribution of their populations. There is interest both in changes that have occurred, as well as those anticipated in coming decades. To describe these patterns of global population aging, it is useful to focus on the period 1950 to 2050. Data in Table 5.4 show percent over age 65 years and over age 80 for a variety of populations in 1950, 2000, and 2050. The data for 1950 and 2000 are based upon estimates from national censuses and surveys, and data for 2050 are projections based on certain assumptions regarding future demographic behavior. These particular populations are selected to illustrate the diversity in patterns of population aging, but there is also a degree of arbitrariness. The percent over age 80 years is included in this table because of the growing interest of social and health policy researchers in the "oldest-old" portion of the population.

The first comparison in Table 5.4 is between the more developed regions (Europe, Northern America, Japan, and Australia and New Zealand) and the less developed regions (Africa, Latin America, and Asia excluding Japan). In general, countries included in the "more developed" regions have had higher levels of income, higher life expectancy, and lower birth rates since 1950 than countries in the "less developed" category. Although this is a crude division of world societies, it is clear that it captures large differences in population aging. Between 1950 and 2000, population aging progressed much more rapidly in more developed areas, and the difference between more and less developed was marked in 2000 (14.3% over age 65 years in more developed, compared to 5.1% in less developed). Between 2000 and 2050 it is anticipated that the proportion of old will nearly double in developed regions (to 26.8%) and triple in less developed regions (to 14.0%). In 2050 the less developed regions will have populations as old as developed regions had in 2000, and developed regions will have historically unprecedented proportions of their populations over age 65 years. But, as shown by the next comparison, there is great variation within both more and less developed regions.

AFRICA, ASIA, AND LATIN AMERICA.   The pattern of population aging is very similar in Asia and Latin America over the 100 years between 1950 and 2050. In both regions, modest population aging occurred prior to 2000, but extremely rapid aging will occur

TABLE 5.4. **Percent of Population Over Age 65 years and 80 years for the World and Selected Areas, 1950, 2000, and 2050.**

Area	65 +			80 +		
	1950	2000	2050*	1950	2000	2050*
World	5.2	6.9	15.6	0.5	1.1	4.1
More developed countries	7.9	14.3	26.8	1.0	3.1	9.6
Less developed countries	3.9	5.1	14.0	0.3	0.7	3.3
Least developed countries	3.3	3.1	6.3	0.3	0.4	1.0
Africa	3.2	3.3	6.9	0.3	0.4	1.1
Asia	4.1	5.9	16.7	0.3	0.8	4.2
Europe	8.2	14.7	29.2	1.1	3.0	10.0
Latin America	3.7	5.4	16.9	0.4	0.9	4.1
Northern America	8.2	12.3	21.4	1.1	3.2	7.7
United States	8.3	12.3	21.1	1.1	3.2	7.6
China	4.5	6.9	22.7	0.3	0.9	6.8
France	11.4	16.0	26.7	1.7	3.7	10.4
Italy	8.3	18.1	35.9	1.1	3.9	14.1
Uganda	3.0	2.5	3.6	0.3	0.3	0.5

Source: United Nations 2002.
*"Medium projection" by The United Nations.

over the subsequent 50 years as the proportion of the population over age 65 years triples. The primary reason for anticipating rapid aging after 2000 is the sharp decline in birth rates that began in the last three decades of the 20th century in these regions. Before 1970 the total fertility rate in both Asia and Latin America was above 5.5, but by 1995 to 2000 it had fallen to just 2.7. Africa, in contrast, has yet to experience population aging, and only 3.3% of the population of Africa was over age 65 years in 2000. Birth rates in most of Africa remained high by world standards throughout the 20th century (the total fertility rate in Africa was 5.2 in 1995 to 2000), and life expectancy increased slowly compared to patterns in Asia and Latin America. With the HIV/AIDS epidemic in the 1990s, some African countries experienced large declines in life expectancy, and for the continent as a whole life expectancy was lower in 2000 than in 1990. Nevertheless, the United Nations population projections anticipate that Africa will experience a demographic transition in the 21st century, the total fertility declining to 2.4 by 2050. Under this scenario, the proportion of old in Africa's population will double between 2000 and 2050. However, the population of Africa in 2050 would still be younger than the population of the more developed regions was in 1950.

EUROPE AND NORTHERN AMERICA.   In both Europe and Northern America the proportion of old in 1950 (8.2% over age 65 years) was about double what it had been in 1900. Significant population aging continued in both areas in the second half of the 20th century as fertility declined to replacement level or below and mortality declines among the elderly persisted. Because fertility in Europe was consistently lower than in any other continent over this time period, Europe had the oldest population of any region in 2000. Rapid population aging in both Northern America and Europe is expected to continue for some decades into the 21st century, with Europe becoming even more distinctive as having the oldest population of any region. By 2050, almost 30% of the population of Europe is expected to be older than 65 years.

SELECTED COUNTRY COMPARISONS.   Table 5.4 contains data for five countries that are following distinctive patterns of population aging. France was characterized by relatively low fertility in the 19th century, and 7% of its population was over age 65 in 1865—the first time any country reached this level. Compared to countries where population aging started later, the process occurred slowly in France. It took 115 years, until 1980, for the proportion old in France to double to 14%. In Italy and Spain, where fertility decline began much later and then proceeded more rapidly than in France, it took only 45 years for the proportion old to double from 7% to 14%. An even more dramatic drop in fertility occurred in China, where the transition from 7% to 14% old is expected to take only 27 years (from 2000 to 2027).

Italy provides an example not only of a country with very rapid population aging, but also a country where fertility fell far below replacement level. The total fertility rate in Italy fell below 2.0 in the late 1970s, and then continued to decline to only 1.2 by 2000. As a result of this sustained low fertility, Italy had the oldest population of any country in 2000, with 18.1% over age 65 years. By 2050, the United Nations population shows about 36% of the population old in Italy, and this result depends on fertility increasing by 50% between 2000 and 2050. Should a fertility increase not occur in Italy, Italy's population would become even older than this United Nations projection.

If Italy has the oldest population of any country, the East African country of Uganda represents one of the youngest with only 2.5% over age 65 years in 2000. In fact, the proportion old in Uganda's population declined between 1950 and 2000. This "younging" of the population occurred because fertility remained at the same high level (total fertility rate over 7.0) over this time period, while the infant death rate declined by about 40% (from 160 to 90 per 1,000). Although the United Nations anticipates a significant decline in fertility and increase in life expectancy before 2050, the proportion old in Uganda is projected to increase to only 3.6% by 2050. The small number of older people expected in 2050 in Uganda is partially explained by the devastating effect of the AIDs epidemic on cohorts that will occupy the older age categories at that time (the cohorts in the young adult stage of life in the late 20th and early 21st centuries).

China had a larger absolute number of people over age 65 years in 2000 than any other country, and its lead in this category is expected to continue through 2050. At both dates, United Nations data show over one-fifth of the world's older population living in China. More significant for China than its absolute number of older people, however, is the extremely rapid pace of population aging that it will experience in the 21st century. In just 40 years, between 2000 and 2040, the proportion of the population over age 65 is expected to more than triple—from 6.8% to 21.8%. This dramatic shift in age composition is the result of the total fertility rate dropping from above 6 prior to 1970 to only 2.6 by the end of the 1970s, and then continuing to decline to below replacement level by 1990. In addition, declining mortality after 1965 is enabling most members of the large cohorts born in the two decades before 1970 to survive to old age. The demographic transition responsible for rapid population aging in China will also produce a marked shift in family composition, so that the older population in the future will have very few adult children compared to the historical situation (Zeng and George 2001).

UNITED STATES.   The long-term trend of population aging in the United States (from 4% over age 65 years in 1900 to 20% by 2030), as in other countries, is a consequence of the long-term trend from high fertility and mortality to low fertility and mortality. But the pathway to an older population is not smooth in the United States. Because the older population grew more rapidly than the nonold population over most of the 20th century, the proportion of the population over age 65 years increased steadily. But this trend was reversed between 1990 and 2000, as the proportion over age 65 years declined slightly—from 12.6% to 12.4% (United States Bureau of the Census 2001b). Census Bureau projections show slight population aging occurring again between 2005 and 2010, followed by very rapid aging between 2010 and 2030, with the percent over age 65 years growing from 13.2% to 20.0% over these two decades (Day 1996). The explanation for this irregular pattern of population aging can be traced to the postwar baby boom that lasted from the mid-1940s to the mid-1960s, and the baby bust of the late 1960s and 1970s. The large fluctuations in the total fertility rate, from 2.1 in 1936 to 3.7 in 1957 to 1.7 in 1976, resulted in cohorts differing widely in size. As the relatively small cohorts born in the 1930s entered old age around 2000, population aging briefly ceased. Then, as the baby boom cohorts enter old age between 2010 and 2030, rapid population aging will occur. Finally, as the baby bust cohorts enter old age after 2030, population aging will again almost cease for several decades.

THEORETICAL ISSUES

Migration and Population Aging

In-migration and out-migration do not necessarily alter the age distribution of a population. If migration rates did not vary by age, and if migrants experienced the same fertility and mortality levels as the population of interest, then migration would affect the size of the population but not the age composition. However, migration rates almost always do vary with age. Out-migration from an area is predictably higher for young people than for older people. Although some exceptions may be found, the tendency of young adults to migrate at higher rates than older people generally has been true across time and across cultures (Bean et al. 1994; also see chapter 11 in this *Handbook*). Despite the age selectivity of migrants, both analytic and empirical studies of the effect of migration on population aging have shown that migration generally has only a small effect on the age composition of a population. Further insight into the link between migration and population aging is gained through examination of two situations: internal migration in the United States as it affects regional differences in age composition and "replacement migration" as a solution to population aging in developed countries.

MIGRATION AND POPULATION AGING IN THE UNITED STATES.   At the state level, the proportion of the population over age 65 years in 2000 varied from a low of 5.7% in Alaska to a high of 17.6% in Florida. For the United States as a whole, 12.4% of the population was over age 65 in 2000. The extreme positions of these two states reflect their exceptional in-migration patterns—a disproportionate number of migrants to Alaska have been young and a disproportionate number to Florida have been old. Excluding the extremes, the proportion old in state populations ranged from 8.5% to 15.6%, and relatively clear patterns can be seen. All 14 states in which older people comprised less than 12% of the population were in the West and the South. Seven of the 10 oldest states were in the Northeast or Midwest. Why is it that although more old people move from colder to warmer climates than vice versa, the oldest regions are the Northeast and Midwest, and the youngest regions are the West and South?

The answer is that direction of migration is generally similar for older and younger people, and that the young are much more likely to move than the old. For example, between March of 1999 and March of 2000 someone aged 20 to 24 was eight times as likely to change place of residence as someone aged 65+ (35.2% versus 4.4%) (United States Bureau of the Census 2001a). Because of this age pattern of migration, states (or counties) in which out-migration exceeds in-migration over a sustained period of time have relatively old populations. Older people in these areas tend to "age in place," while a disproportionate number of younger people move out. In recent decades, the areas that have experienced substantial net out-migration have been concentrated in the farm states of the Midwest and the declining industrial states of the Northeast. These two regions, as noted above, are the regions with the highest concentration of older people. Using this reasoning, one should anticipate that areas with substantial net in-migration would tend to have relatively young populations. This is the general pattern and accounts for the below-average proportion old in the Sunbelt (which has gained population through migration in recent decades). Florida is simply an exception to this pattern—it has been such a magnet for older retirees moving out of the Northeast that its in-migration rate for older people has exceeded that of younger people.

Moving to areas smaller than states, even greater variations in age composition can be observed. Some counties might be classified as "gerontic enclaves." In two counties (one in Florida and one in North Dakota), over one-third of the population was over age 65 in 2000, and there were 57 counties in which over one-fourth of the population is old. Half of these very old counties were in Florida (reflecting a large in-migration of retirees) and in South Dakota and North Dakota (reflecting the large out-migration of young adults).

REPLACEMENT MIGRATION.   It was noted above that, within usual boundaries, immigration tends to have only a small long-term effect on a population's age distribution. It is useful, nevertheless, to see what volume of migration would be required to counter the population aging anticipated in developed countries. The United Nations (2000) provides this type of information for several countries and regions in a report titled *Replacement Migration: Is it a Solution to Declining and Ageing Populations*. Because the motivating concern for this report is the increased future burden on the working population to support the growing older, dependent population, the population indicator of interest in this report is the potential support ratio (PSR). The PSR is defined simply as the population aged 15 to 64 years divided by the population aged 65+ years. The basic question involves the relationship between PSRs in 2050 and alternative scenarios regarding the annual number of net migrants entering each population between 1995 and 2050. The analysis involves a straightforward comparison of the age distribution (PSR) resulting from projecting various populations using alternative assumptions regarding net immigration.

The results of this study are summarized in Table 5.5, where outcomes of several alternative population projections are reported for Japan, the European Union, and the United States (results for France, Germany, Italy, Republic of Korea, Russian Federation, United Kingdom, and Europe are also included in the United Nations report). For each country there is baseline information about the PSR in 1950 and 1995; then selected outcomes in 2050 are shown for each of four alternative projections. Each projection uses the medium variant fertility and mortality assumptions used in the standard United Nations population projections. The four migration alternatives are as follow: (1) migration as assumed in the medium variant projection, (2) zero migration, (3) migration required to keep PSR from falling below 3.0 before 2050, (4) migration required to keep PSR at the 2000 level. The outcomes for each projection are PSR in 2050, average annual number of migrants between 2000 and 2050, percent of the 2050 population that is comprised of post-2000 immigrants and their descendants, and the ratio of the population size in 2050 to that in 2000.

The PSR in Japan declined from 12 to 4 between 1950 and 2000 and is projected to decline further to 1.7 in 2050 under the medium assumptions of future demographic behavior. For Japan, where it is assumed that no migration will occur, the medium projection results in a population in 2050 that is almost 20% smaller than the population in 2000 and is unaffected by non-Japanese immigrants. If immigration were used to prevent the PSR from falling below 3.0, Japan would need to admit an average of nearly two million immigrants per year, and by 2050, 30% of the population would be of non-Japanese origin. The fourth scenario, maintaining the same PSR as 1995, shows that a

TABLE 5.5. **Population Indicator for Japan, European Union, and the United States in 2050 Under Alternative Demographic Scenarios**

Country & Indictor	1950	2000	2050[5]			
			Proj.1	Proj.2	Proj.3	Proj.4
Japan						
1. PSR[1]	12.1	4.0	1.7	1.7	3.0	4.8
2. Ave. Immig.[2]			0	0	1,897	10,471
3. % Immig.[3]			0	0	54.2	87.2
4. Pop. Incr.[4]			0.83	0.83	1.81	6.46
Unites States						
1. PSR[1]	7.8	5.3	2.8	2.6	3.0	5.2
2. Ave. immig.[2]			760	0	816	10,777
3. % immig.[3]			16.8	0	17.4	72.7
4. Pop. incr.[4]			1.25	1.04	1.26	3.83
European Union						
1. PSR[1]	7.0	4.1	2.0	1.9	3.0	4.3
2. Ave. immig.[2]			270	0	3,073	13,480
3. % immig.[3]			6.2	0	40.2	74.7
4. Pop. incr.[4]			0.88	0.83	1.39	3.27

Source: United Nations 2000.
[1] PSR = Potential Support Ratio ($^{pop.\ 15\text{-}64}/_{pop.\ 65+}$)
[2] Ave. immig. = Average annual volume of immigration in 1,000s, 2000–2050.
[3] % Immig. = Percent of population composed of post-2000 immigrants and their descendants.
[4] Pop. incr. = Ratio of total population to total population in 2000.
[5] Proj. 1 – Median variant
Proj. 2 – Median variant, except zero migration
Proj. 3 – Maintain PSR of 3.0
Proj. 4 – Maintain PSR existing in 1995

strategy for eliminating population aging through immigration is totally unrealistic. Preventing further population aging after 1995 through replacement migration would lead to a population in 2050 that was eight times larger than the 1995 population, and one in which 80% were non-Japanese.

Results of similar analyses for the European Union and the United States are shown in Table 5.5. In both cases, it is surprising how little difference the effect of anticipated migration has on population aging compared to a scenario of zero immigration. Also, in both cases the level of future immigration required to prevent any population aging after 1995 is wholly unrealistic, as was the case for Japan. The cost of trying to stop population aging via immigration would be a tremendous increase in population density and a transformation of the culture as most residents would be first- or second-generation immigrants. And, because populations cannot indefinitely grow at a rapid pace, this "solution" would only postpone the ultimate need to adapt to an older population. Because the United States is expected to maintain near-replacement-level fertility over the 21st century, the medium projection shows a PSR only slightly below 3.0 in 2050, so maintaining a PSR of 3.0 would require an average immigration level only 20% greater than the expected one. In contrast, the European Union would need an annual level of immigration three times greater than that occurring around 2000 to prevent the PSR from slipping below 3.0.

Efforts to use replacement migration to prevent population aging are not likely to gain significant political support. Greatly increasing the volume of immigration to developed countries would generate concerns about environmental consequences of population growth and cultural challenges of large immigrant populations (Grant 2001; Meyerson 2001). Furthermore, as shown by the study of replacement migration, the magnitude of immigration required to significantly alter future patterns of population aging is staggering. It seems that any country with low fertility and mortality must anticipate a future population that will be far older than any that have existed previously. This is not, of course, equivalent to saying that the social and economic challenges of an older population constitute a crisis. For perspective, it should be noted that the well-being of the older population increased remarkably between 1950 and 2000 as PSRs declined to unprecedented lows in developed countries (see Table 5.5).

Public Pension Programs

Almost all industrialized countries have established public pension programs that collect taxes from the current working population, often levied as a payroll tax, to provide benefits to the current retired population. An example of this approach is the Social Security program in the United States. This type of pension system is referred to as an unfunded pay-as-you-go (PAYG) pension, reflecting the fact that the contributions of current workers are not being invested in assets to be used to finance their own retirement. Rather, the current generation of workers is supporting current retirees, and the current generation will be dependent on contributions of future generations to support them in their old age. As currently designed, PAYG public pension programs in Europe, North America, and Japan will need to be altered significantly in order to achieve fiscal sustainability in coming decades (Disney 2000; World Bank 1994). An important reason why projections show that PAYG public pensions are headed toward fiscal imbalance is population aging.

The effect of population aging on PAYG pension systems is rather obvious, as can be seen by looking at the ratio of workers to pension beneficiaries. As a population ages, there is a decline in the relative number of workers available to support the expanding proportion of the population that is retired. The projected decrease in the support ratio over the first several decades of the 21st century is large for every developed country (see Table 5.5), creating fiscal imbalances in almost every public pension system. The challenge is greatest for nations that have the lowest projected support ratios (countries such as Japan and Italy), but is also substantial for the United States.

Problems in the long-term stability of PAYG pension systems as the demographic transition reached maturity might have been anticipated in their initial formulations (Disney 2000), but other developments have complicated the situation. First, across all developed countries the labor force participation rate of older men declined in the second half of the 20th century. Of course a major explanation for men leaving the labor force at younger ages over this time period was the growing availability of pensions (Wise 1997). The result, nevertheless, was to further reduce support ratios. Second, population forecasts available to those designing the major national pension schemes seriously underestimated the future decline in both death rates among the old and fertility rates among women. Consequently the pension programs as initially formulated did not anticipate the speed and extent of subsequent population aging. Third, for political reasons the generosity of pension benefits increased over time. Thus it is population aging, in combination with these other factors, that is forcing policy makers to decide among alternative reform options to stabilize public pensions in the near future.

Two basically different approaches to reforming public pensions are being debated (Disney 2000). The less radical approach, referred to as "parametric" reform (Chand and Jaeger 1996), argues that unfunded PAYG schemes can be brought into equilibrium by making changes in a few parameters. More money available for paying pension benefits could come from either increasing taxes on the workers or by increasing the proportion of the working age population that participates in the labor force. Pension expenditures could be reduced by decreasing benefits, either by directly cutting benefits or by increasing age for pension eligibility. The approach of increasing normal retirement age has received support from some demographers who point out that that increasing life expectancy and improving health of cohorts entering old age make a fixed retirement age (such as 60 or 65) increasingly obsolete (Chen 1994; Uhlenberg 1988). The general view of those favoring parametric reform is that by making moderate changes in several of the parameters (payroll tax, eligibility age, cost of living adjustment, means testing), existing public pension systems could be maintained as unfunded PAYG programs despite population aging (Kingson and Williamson 2001; Williamson 1997).

The alternative proposal argues that rather than "fixing" the existing programs, the required long-term solution is to move from unfunded to funded pensions. This approach is referred to as "paradigmatic" reform because it calls for a fundamental change away from the PAYG system. In a funded pension program the money collected from current workers and/or employers is invested in private sector equity markets (stocks, bonds), and these investment accounts are used to pay retiree benefits. This capital reserve–financing system could be operated as a public pension program. In the United States, for example, this would mean that the balance of funds in the Social Security Trust Fund would be invested in capital markets rather than in government bonds. Most often, however, plans for moving to funded pension plans expect that the transition would involve privatizing social security with a system of individual–based accounts. The most cited example of a country moving to a privatized social security plan is Chile (Edwards 1998), but there also are examples of partial privatization in several European countries (Feldstein and Siebert 2002).

The key difference between the two pension plans is that in a PAYG program retirees are dependent on current workers to support them, whereas in a funded program each generation funds its own retirement by accumulating capital. The relevance of this debate to population aging is obvious: population aging does not threaten the fiscal sustainability of funded pension plans. Other potential advantages of reforming public pension programs by moving to funded systems are often noted, such as the higher expected real rate of return on contributions and the contribution to development of financial markets (World Bank 1994). On the other hand, there are strong critics of paradigmatic pension reform who argue that this solution involves unfair transition costs, creates increasing inequality and greater individual risk, and threatens the viability of intergenerational solidarity in society (Walker 1999; Williamson 1997). Not surprisingly, many analysts suggest that a compromise of partial privatization of social security is a reasonable way to achieve the reform of public pensions required by population aging (Boldrin et al.1999).

Health and Health Care

Over the past two centuries all developed countries have experienced an epidemiological transition characterized by declining death rates and shifting cause-of-death patterns.

Before this transition most people died of infectious diseases (smallpox, scarlet fever, tuberculosis, influenza, and pneumonia, etc.), which affected all ages. The young were especially vulnerable, and most people did not survive to old age (Caldwell 2001; Riley 2001). With the conquest of infectious diseases, mortality is concentrated in the older ages, and the primary causes of death are chronic degenerative diseases (heart disease, cardiovascular disease, and cancer). Therefore, population aging may have significant implications for population health, as a growing proportion of the total population is comprised of older people with chronic diseases. Growth in the prevalence of chronic disease in a population raises concerns about declining vitality of its members, the overall burden of care for those with physical and cognitive limitations, and the health care costs to society. For example, the health care cost per capita is three to five times greater for the population over age 65 than for the population under age 65 in developed countries (CDC 2003).

In addition to possible effects of population aging on the burden of disease, it is also important to consider the impact of the aging of the older population. Aging of the older population can be measured as changes in the proportion of its members over age 80 or 85. At the global level around year 2000, the average annual growth rate of persons aged 80 and older was three times greater than the growth rate of the total population, and twice as high as the growth rate of the population over age 60 (United Nations 2001). Consequently, in the late 20th and early 21st centuries an increasing proportion of the total population and of the older population is in the "very old" category. The proportion of the elderly population in Europe that is 80 years and older is expected to grow from 20% in 2000 to over 35% by 2050, and 40% of Japan's elderly population is projected to be 80 years and older by 2030 (National Research Council 2001). In the United States, the proportion of the older population aged 85 and older is expected to double between 2000 and 2050, increasing from 12.6% to 23.6% (Federal Interagency Forum on Aging Related Statistics 2000).

The aging of the older population is significant for the health burden in a population because rates of disability and dependency increase rapidly at very old ages. Examples of differences in health problems and health costs for different segments of the older population in the United States are shown in Table 5.6. The contrast between the "youngest-old" (65 to 69) and the "oldest-old" (85+) tend to be striking. For example, compared to the youngest-old, the oldest-old are 16 times more likely to reside in nursing homes and 12 times more likely to have severe memory loss. Average per capita health care expenditures in 1999 increased from $6,711 for those aged 65 to 69 to $16,596 for those aged 85 or older. Thus one might anticipate that the challenge to provide adequate health care would grow in societies that are experiencing both population aging and aging of their older population. Indeed, assuming no future changes in age-specific rates of Alzheimer's disease and functional disabilities leads to alarming conclusions about the burden of disease and suggests that societies may become "global nursing homes" (Eberstadt 1997), where severe age-based health care rationing is inevitable (Peterson 1999).

In discussing the future of population health and health care expenditures, however, some writers argue that "demography is not destiny" (National Academy on an Aging Society 1999) and warn against alarmist forecasts based simply on demographic forces (Gee and Gutman 2000). The point of these arguments is that as a population ages, the composition and characteristics of the elderly population also are likely to change and the social policies and technology affecting the delivery of health care can change. Therefore,

TABLE 5.6. Health Indicators for the United States Older Population Around Year 2000, by Age.

Indicator	65–69	Age 70–74	75–79	80–84	85 +
Average per capita health expenditures (1998 $)	6,711	8,099	9,241	10,683	16,596
Nursing home	1.1[*]			4.3[**]	18.3
Severe memory impairment (%)	1.1	2.5	4.5	6.4[**]	12.9
Needing assistance (%)	8.1	10.5	16.9	34.9[***]	

Sources: Federal Interagency Forum on Aging Related Statistics 2000.
[*]Age category is 65–74.
[**]Age category is 75–84.
[***]Age category is 80+.

one cannot accurately forecast future health conditions and costs by assuming that the only thing that will change over time is the population age composition. One important source of support for this position is research in the United States that has found significant changes in age-specific disability rates among the elderly since 1990.

A widely debated research question related to increasing life expectancy has been whether the years added to life past age 65 are years lived with or without major disabilities. If extending life increases the burden of disease in a population by lengthening the time between onset of chronic disease and death, then population aging is likely to entail large increases in health expenditures. On the other hand, if the added years of life are disability-free years, population aging does not necessarily have a negative effect population health. An analysis of the empirical research on this topic conducted since 1990 finds strong support for the conclusion that there was a decline in prevalence of age-specific functional limitations among older Americans after 1982 (when reliable data were first collected) (Freedman, Martin, and Schoeni 2002). The most ambitious of these studies reports that rates of disability declined by 1.7% annually between 1982 and 1999 (Manton and Gu 2001). There is also evidence that severe cognitive impairments have been declining (Freedman, Aykan, and Martin 2001). Part of the explanation for these positive trends is that educational levels of older adults have been improving, and higher levels of education are associated with better physical and cognitive health (Freedman and Martin 1999). Further, it is clear that there remain significant aspects of lifestyle associated with disease and disability (smoking, obesity, exercise) where substantial improvement is possible for those who will reach old age in the future. In other words, it is possible that the potential increase in burden of disease associated with population aging could be averted, or partially averted, if trends toward increasing duration of disability-free aging past age 65 years continue.

Although it seems common sense to expect that population aging will result in higher societal per capita expenditures on health care, two types of research suggest that age structure is not an important determinant of health care spending. First, comparing per capita health care spending across a number of developed countries fails to find a statistically significant effect of demographic factors. Despite wide variations in both per capita health care spending and proportion old in the population across the 30 countries in the Organization for Economic Cooperation and Development (OECD), there is little relationship between the two (Reinhardt et al. 2002). Most striking is the United States, where the proportion of the population above age 65 is small relative to the OECD average, but per capita health spending was 134% higher than the OECD median in 2000 (Anderson et al. 2003). Despite the relatively high cost of health care in the United States, there is no evidence that Americans have better health or even utilize more health care services than the OECD median (Anderson et al. 2003). Second, population aging is estimated to contribute little to the projected growth of total spending on personal health in the United States or Canada in coming decades (Burner, Waldo, and McKusick 1992; Gee and Gutman 2000; Reinhardt 2003). These studies conclude that health care spending in the future is likely to be determined more by medical technology, health policy, and the organization of health care services than by population age structure.

Population Aging and Kinship Structure

The demographic forces responsible for population aging (declining fertility and declining mortality at older ages) have significant implications for the structure of kinship networks. Particularly relevant for the well-being of both older and younger people are changes in the structure of intergenerational relationships associated with an aging society. The basic relationship among fertility, mortality, and supply of intergenerational kin can be seen by thinking about extreme situations. In a society where everyone has a large number of children and few people survive to very old ages, grandparents would be in short supply for children, but individuals who survive to old age would tend to have many grandchildren. Similarly, most middle-aged adults would not have surviving parents, but individuals who survive to old age would typically have multiple children. This type of kinship structure is quite similar to the one existing in China before 1900. At the opposite extreme is the ideal expressed in contemporary Chinese society, where women would have only one child each and most adults survive past age 70 years. Under these conditions, children would have no siblings or cousins and would have the undivided attention of two sets of grandparents. Older people, however, would have a short supply of grandchildren, being forced to share their one grandchild with a competing set of grandparents. The parent-child relationship in later life in a low-mortality, one-child family society would be characterized by middle-aged adults having surviving parents who have no other child to depend upon for support. Although the above scenario is idealized, it correctly identifies the direction of change in intergenerational relationships that occurs as populations age.

The family and kinship implications of rapid population aging in Japan, China, and South Korea have received some attention (Jiang 1995; Martin 1990; Zeng and George 2001). In these countries, as well as in other Asian countries, the long tradition of elderly people coresiding with an adult child is being challenged by population aging. In Japan, for example, the proportion of people over age 65 who live with a child declined from 77% in 1970 to 52% in 1991 (Brown et al. 2002; Martin 1990). In countries where adult children have provided most of the care for dependent older people, the changing supply of children challenges existing caregiving arrangements. The average number of children available to provide care for parents aged 65 to 69 in urban areas of China will decline from 3.1 in 1990 to only 1.1 in 2030 (Jiang 1995). Changing intergenerational relationships related to population aging are also occurring in the United States and Europe.

PARENT-CHILD RELATIONSHIPS.   An aspect of the parent-child relationship that has received a great deal of research attention is the care that adult children provide for their aging parents who experience disabilities. It is now well established that adult children, especially daughters, provide a substantial proportion of the care required by older people with functional limitations (Rein and Salzman 1995; Stone 2000). Data from the 1993 study of Assets and Health Dynamics show that the largest category of caregivers for older people with limitations in activities of daily living in the United States is adult children, who comprise 42% of the total (spouses provide 25%) (Shirey and Summer 2000). The economic value of informal caregiving in the United States in 1997 was estimated to be 1.7 times the total national spending for paid home care and nursing home care (Arno, Levine, and Memmott 1999). This pattern of adult children providing much of the care required by their elderly parents is found across many, if not all, societies currently experiencing rapid population aging (Pickard et al. 2000; Schofield and Bloch 1998; Traphagan and Knight 2003). Thus changes in the supply of adult children available to provide informal care for the disabled older population have potentially significant social and economic implications for aging societies.

From the perspective of older people, the average number of living adult children was substantially smaller in 2000 than in 1900. For example, women around age 70 years in the United States had an average of more than five children each in 1900, compared to three in 2000 (Downs 2003; United States Bureau of the Census 1976). In terms of risk of not receiving caregiving from adult children, however, changes in average number of children is not as significant as changes in the proportion of old people who are childless or have only one child (Uhlenberg 1993). By this indicator, older people in the early 21st century are relatively advantaged, but conditions will be much less favorable by 2030. In the United States the average number of living children for people aged 70 to 85 years will fall below two by 2030 and the proportion who are childless will nearly double (Downs 2003; Wachter 1997). In Italy, microsimulation projections show mean number of children for women aged 75 to 84 years falling from 2.1 in 1994 to only 1.4 in 2050, and one-fourth of the older women in 2050 are expected to be childless (Tomassini and Wolf 2000). Similar decreases in the supply of adult children will occur in all aging societies, suggesting that informal care may play a smaller part in meeting the health care needs of the elderly in the future.

Wachter (1997) suggests that a growth in number of stepchildren might partially reduce the consequences of a declining number of biological children for older people. However, evidence thus far does not indicate that stepchildren provide the same level of care as biological children, and presence of a stepparent may have a negative effect on the child-parent relationship (Lye et al.1995; White 1994). One study finds partial empirical support for Wachter's hypothesis that remarriage, by generating more diverse kin ties, expands perceptions of total kinship support among the elderly, but it concludes:

> Since more people in the population are not marrying (or marrying later), and since more people divorce than remarry, it is hard to imagine that the next several cohorts of elderly people will be better off than the current cohort in terms of perceived social support from extended kin. The marital status changes are especially problematic for women ... (Curran et al. 2003:188).

Concern over future shifts in the ratio of adult daughters to older people does not focus only on the needs of older people. There is also a large literature on the burden that caring for parents places on middle-aged women (Schulz et al. 1990). Decreasing death rates among adults lead to an increasing likelihood over time that middle-aged women will have parents who are still living. Under fertility and mortality conditions existing in the late 20th century, a person could expect to spend more years living with parents over age 65 than with dependent children under age 18 (Watkins, Menken, and Bongaarts 1987). A trend toward an increasing number of years lived with a cosurviving old parent will continue if, as expected, death rates at older ages continue to decline. But when women born after the baby boom reach age 50 years, beginning around 2020, they will have significantly fewer siblings to share the task of caring for their parents, who will be living longer. Other social changes are expected to further increase the burden of caregiving for these women. A growing proportion of middle-aged women are expected to have careers that compete with caregiving for their time and energy (Doty, Jackson, and Crown 1998; Pavalko and Artis 1997), and a growing proportion will be divorced (Uhlenberg 1994). Also, a growing proportion of their older parents will be divorced and consequently will not have access to caregiving that a spouse might provide (Evandrou and Falkingham 2000). If current patterns of children providing informal care for their aging parents continue, the burden of caregiving among middle-aged women might be expected to increase significantly.

GRANDPARENT-GRANDCHILD RELATIONSHIPS.   Changes in the structure of grandparent-grandchild relationships in the United States associated with population aging over the 20th century have been studied (Uhlenberg and Kirby 1998; Uhlenberg 2005). In examining the effects of demographic change on this relationship, it is important to be clear regarding whose perspective is being taken. Declining adult mortality increased the supply of grandparents for children and young adults, while declining infant and child mortality affected the supply of grandchildren for older people. Decreasing fertility reduced the number of grandchildren for older people, while for young people it reduced the number of siblings and cousins who might compete for a grandparent's attention. Although the direction of these changes is obvious, the magnitude and timing of structural changes in grandparent-grandchild relations requires empirical investigation.

The declining death rates occurring throughout the 20th century meant that an ever-increasing proportion of those who bore children would survive long enough to experience the birth of grandchildren and great grandchildren. For example, the proportion of women that would survive from age 25 years to age 80 years under mortality conditions existing in 1900 was only 19%, compared to 59% under conditions existing in 2000. The proportion surviving between these ages is expected to continue to increase over the 21st century, reaching 70% by 2050 (Bell and Miller 2002). This remarkable mortality revolution produces large changes over time in the supply of grandparents. For example, the proportion of 10-year-olds with all four grandparents alive increased from about 6% in 1900 to 41% in 2000 and is projected to be 48% by 2020 (Uhlenberg 2005). Even more impressive was the increase in number of living grandparents among young adults. Based on estimates using life tables, the proportion of 30-year-olds with a grandparent alive more than tripled between 1900 and 2000—from 21% to 75%, and should grow to 82% by 2020 (Uhlenberg 2005). Thus, in an aging population, children grow up with access to an increasing number of grandparents, and most young adults will have grandparents living when they bear children.

The number of sets of grandchildren that an older person has is equal to the number of his or her children who have produced children. Thus in a society where low fertility has persisted over several generations, old people will have far fewer sets of grandchildren than in a high-fertility society. The transition to older people typically having few sets of grandchildren is not necessarily monotonic, however, as changes in the distribution of women in the United States aged 60 to 64 years by number of grandchild sets shows (Uhlenberg 2005). The baby boom and subsequent baby bust greatly affected the supply of grandchildren for people in different cohorts as they approached old age. Women aged 60 to 64 in 2000, who became mothers during the baby boom, had low rates (around 13%) of grandchildlessness, and 38% had three or more sets of grandchildren. Thus in the United States there was an increasing supply of grandchildren between 1950 and 2000, despite the aging of the population. By 2020, however, the proportion of older adults who are grandchildless will increase to 22%, and the proportion with more than two sets of grandchildren will be cut in half. After this date, the proportion of older people with more than two sets of grandchildren will remain low and probably decline further, unless there is a future increase in fertility. In Europe and Japan, where fertility has been much lower than in the United States, the supply of grandchildren for older people will be considerably smaller than in the United States. Unless there is drastic future decrease in the amount of time and energy that grandparents invest in grandchildren, children in aging societies will receive increasing attention from grandparents.

MEASURES AND METHODS

Measures

There are three basic approaches to measuring the age structure of a population. The most common measure, and the one most used in this chapter, is simply proportion of the total population that is over a fixed chronological age, usually 60 or 65 years. Although there is no chronological age that marks a universal transition in physical or social condition, social programs often use age 60 or 65 years as a criterion for entitlement. This measure provides a straightforward way to compare the relative number of older people in populations across time or across societies.

A second commonly used measure is the median age of a population—the age that divides the population into equal numbers of younger and older people. This measure does not focus specifically on the older population, but rather tracks broad patterns of population aging. In general, the indicators *percent old* and *median age* tell the same story about population aging, but they do not always move in the same direction over a short time period. For example, the aging of particularly small or large cohorts across certain age markers may produce unusually small or large changes in percent old over a short time period, while median age is changing quite smoothly. A good example of this is the aging of baby boom cohorts in the United States, in combination with the aging of the smaller cohorts that preceded and followed them. Between 1990 and 2000 the median age of the U.S. population increased from 32.8 to 35.3 years, but the percent over 65 declined slightly, from 12.6% to 12.4%. Over this time period the large baby boom cohorts grew older, but it was the relatively small cohorts born before the baby boom that entered old age. Between 2010 and 2030 the median will continue its gradual upward movement, going from 37.4 to 39.0 years, but the percent old will increase dramatically, from 13.2% to 20.0%, as baby boomers pass age 65 years.

The third measure of age distribution is the ratio of the size of two age categories. Measures of this type are used to focus on shifts in the age composition that are considered to have particular economic or social significance. Examples of these measures include the old age dependency ratio, the potential support ratio, and the aging index. The old age dependency ratio (population aged 65+ years/population aged 20 to 64 years) provides a rough index of the relative size of the retired population to the working-age population. Obviously this is only a crude indicator of the relative size of these two categories, because not all adults below age 65 years are in the labor force and not all over age 65 years are retired. The same issue of dependency of older people sometimes is discussed using the potential support ratio, which is simply the inverse of the old-age dependency ratio. The potential support ratio is useful to provide general audiences with a sense of the change that population aging produces in the number of workers available to support each older person. For example, this measure can be used to show the dramatic implications of population aging in Japan, where the potential support ratio is expected to drop from 12.1 in 1950 to 1.7 in 2050 (see Table 5.5). The aging index—(population aged 65+ years/population aged 0 to 14 years) X 100—is used to dramatize the shifting balance of young and old in populations that are aging. South Korea, where the aging index goes from 32 to 125 between 2000 and 2030, illustrates a country rapidly changing from one where children greatly outnumber old people to one where old outnumber young (Kinsella and Velkoff 2001).

PROJECTION UNCERTAINTIES.   The basic methods used to study determinants of population aging—the stable population model and population projections—are discussed at the beginning of this chapter. However, there is an issue related to the uncertainty of forecasts based on population projections that merits closer attention. A great deal of interest in the future financing of pensions and health care concerns the anticipated changes in the old-age dependency ratio. But how much confidence should be placed in the forecasts provided by the United Nations or the United States Census Bureau regarding future trends in population aging?

Demographers have given a great deal of attention in recent years to the accuracy of past population forecasts and to ways of improving forecasts (e.g., Lutz, Vaupel, and Ahlburg 1998; National Research Council 2000). These studies find that forecasting errors of 15% or more are common when predicting the size of the very old population in industrialized countries 15 years into the future (Keilman 1997). One thing learned from reviewing the errors in past forecasts, particularly with respect to the size of the older population, has been a tendency of demographers to underestimate future declines in adult mortality. Based on the argument that past gains in life expectancy could not be sustained once the unrepeatable transition to low infant and child mortality occurred, conventional wisdom suggested that life expectancy in the future would grow slowly as it approached a biological maximum (Olshansky and Carnes 2001). But an important study shows that maximum life expectancy in developed countries has been increasing at a steady rate of about 2.4 years per decade since 1840 (Oeppen and Vaupel 2002), and another study found a quite steady average increase of 2.1 years per decade for 21 industrialized countries between 1955 and 1995 (White 2002). Although past trends do not necessarily predict future trends, these findings suggest the possibility of life expectancy exceeding 100 by 2100. Should this level of mortality decline persist, populations in the future could be far older than any of the scenarios offered by existing official forecasts.

But it is not only future mortality trends that will determine future population age distributions. There is uncertainty regarding future fertility rates. The extremely low fertility experienced in Spain, Italy, and Japan at the beginning of the 21st century could rebound to replacement level or above, stay steady, or decline further (Vallin 2002). Future levels of international migration, dependent on economic, social, and political factors, are certainly unknown. Thus the future of population aging is really not known. The problem of uncertainty in forecasts is not large in the short-term but becomes greater the further the horizon of the forecast. Over 20 or 30 years, scenarios based on different plausible assumptions of vital rates do not differ greatly. However, when forecasts are made of conditions 50 or 100 years into the future, the results diverge so much that they are useless for planning. For example, using a probabilistic projection technique, one study provided confidence intervals for its projection of the proportion of Western Europe's population that would be over age 80 years in the future. It concluded, with 95% confidence, that between 3% and 43% would be aged 80+ years in 2100 (O'Neill and Lutz 2003). This level of uncertainty indicates that demographers do not have methods that provide meaningful answers to questions about long-term population patterns. Population experts may consider some scenarios as highly unlikely, but their past record of anticipating large changes is weak. Demographers did not predict the baby boom, nor did they predict that total fertility rates in some countries would fall below 1.2.

FUTURE RESEARCH DIRECTIONS

The ways in which fertility, mortality, and migration determine the pattern of population aging are well understood by demographers, but there are many opportunities for researchers to expand understanding of the social, economic, political, and health implications of population aging. A growing number of researchers from multiple disciplines and many countries are engaged in exploring diverse aspects of global population aging. Recognizing the value of coordinating some of the research on this topic, the National Research Council of the National Academy of Sciences commissioned a panel to examine existing data and knowledge regarding global population aging with the goal of identifying critical areas for future research. Results of this study were published in 2001 (National Research Council 2001), and these results guide much of the discussion on future research directions that follows.

First, there is an opportunity to expand multidisciplinary work that examines connections across domains. Currently there is a tendency for demographers to focus on population projections, sociologists to focus on family and kin ties, economists to focus on pension and work issues, and epidemiologists to focus on health and disability issues. But each of these domains is linked to the others, and none can adequately be understood in isolation from the others. By working together on research design, investigators from these various disciplines can develop measures and coordinate data collection so that linkages across domains can be studied. One goal would be that policy recommendations could reflect a more complete understanding of population aging that comes from recognizing that the experience of aging is multifaceted.

Second, there is growing recognition in the social sciences of the need to collect longitudinal microdata to improve our understanding of causal mechanisms. Nowhere is the need for these types of data greater than in the field of aging. Cross-sectional data are notoriously weak for drawing conclusions about aging because different age categories at a point in time represent different cohorts. A panel study with repeated observations over time is more useful for studying the dynamics of aging over the life course. But to be most useful, a panel study needs to continuously add new cohorts at the bottom in order to track how the experience of aging changes over time. This approach to data collection is both expensive and necessary for advances in research to match advances in conceptualization.

Third, the harmonization of research across countries has the potential of greatly expanding our understanding of aging. There is substantial variation across countries in population aging, welfare policies, family systems, health care organization, economic conditions, etc. These cross-country variations in societal and population conditions provide the possibility for exploring the consequences of aging in different macro contexts. For this possibility to be realized, multinational research teams might be assembled to standardize, or at least harmonize, data collected in multiple countries.

Fourth, existing computer technology is making it increasingly possible to create databases that link information from multiple sources. For example, data from administrative health records and social security files can be linked with survey information to provide a wealth of longitudinal information on individuals. In addition, geographical information on neighborhood and regional context could be added to individual records to allow cross-level analyses. It is clear that individuals do not age in isolation, but as members of households, communities, regions, and countries. Ethical concerns about assembling large and complex data files on individuals are obviously significant, but the potential availability of these types of data excites the research imagination.

A final note on directions of research concerns theoretical advances. If population aging progresses as expected, more than 30% of the population in some countries (Japan and Italy, for example) will be older than 65 years by 2050, and all developed countries will have an unprecedented proportion of old people. Assuming no changes in technology and social organization, one must conclude that this dramatic population aging would produce huge problems. Using the same logic, alarmists in the 1960s made forecasts of impending disasters that would result from rapid population growth. The point is, of course, that "other things" do not remain constant. Social organization changes in response to challenges. New technology alters the relationship between humans and the environment. Demographic behavior of people changes over time in response to changing social conditions. A challenge for researchers is to develop a better theoretical understanding of how societies adapt to changing social and demographic conditions. In particular, in what ways might societies change as their populations grow increasingly old?

REFERENCES

Anderson, G. F., U. E. Reinhardt, P. S. Hussey, and P. Varduhi. 2003. It's the price, stupid: Why the United States is so different from other countries. *Health Affairs* 22:89–105.

Arno, P. S., C. Levine, and M. M. Memmott. 1999. The economic value of informal caregiving. *Health Affairs* 18:182–188.

Bean, F. D., G. C. Myers, J. L. Angel, and O. R. Galle. 1994. Geographic concentration, migration, and population redistribution among the elderly. In *Demography of aging*. Edited by L. G. Martin and S. H. Preston, 319–351. Washington, D.C.: National Academy Press.

Bell, F. C., and M. L. Miller. 2002. *Life tables for the United States social security area 1900–2100* (Social Security Actuarial Study No. 116), Baltimore, Md.: Social Security Administration.

Boldrin, M., J. J. Dolado, J. F. Jimeno, and F. Peracchi. 1999. The future of pensions in Europe. *Economic Policy* 29:287–320.

Brown, J. W., J. Liang, N. Krause, H. Akiyama, H. Sugisawa, and T. Fukaya. 2002. Transitions in living arrangements among elders in Japan: Does health make a difference? *Journal of Gerontology: Social Sciences* 57B: S209–S220.

Burner, S. T., D. R. Waldo, and D. R. McKusick. 1992. National health expenditures through 2030. *Health Care Financing Review* 14:1–29.

Caldwell, J. C. 2001. Population health in transition. *Bulletin of the World Health Organization* 70:159–160.

Casterline, J. B. 2003. Demographic transition. In *Encyclopedia of Population*. Edited by P. Demeny and G. McNicoll 210–216. New York: Macmillan Reference USA.

Centers for Disease Control and Prevention (CDC). 2003. Public health and aging: Trends in aging—United States and worldwide. *MMWR* 52:101–106.

Chand, S. K. and A. Jaeger. 1996. Aging populations and public pension schemes. *Occasional Paper No. 147, International Monetary Fund.*

Chen, Y. P. 1994. Equivalent retirement ages and their implications for Social Security and Medicare financing. *The Gerontologist* 34:731–735.

Chesnais, J. C. 1992. *The demographic transition.* Oxford: Oxford University Press.

Coale, A. 1972. *The growth and structure of human populations: A mathematical investigation.* Princeton, N.J.: Princeton University Press.

Coale, A., and P. Demeny. 1983. *Regional model life tables and stable populations*, 2nd ed. New York: Academic Press.

Curran, S. R., S. McLanahan, and J. Knab. 2003. Does remarriage expand perceptions of kinship support among the elderly? *Social Science Research* 32:171–190.

Day, J. C. 1996. Population projections of the United States by age, sex, race, and hispanic origin: 1995 to 2050. *Current Population Reports, P25-1130* (U.S. Bureau of the Census). Washington, D.C.: U.S. Government Printing Office.

Disney, R. 2000. Crises in public pension programmes in OECD: What are the reform options? *The Economic Journal* 110:F1–F23.

Doty, P., M. E. Jackson, and W. Crown. 1998. The impact of female caregivers' employment status on patterns of formal and informal eldercare. *The Gerontologist* 38:331–141.

Downs, B. 2003. Fertility of American women: June 2002. *Current Population Reports.* P20–548:1–11.

Eberstadt, N. 1997. World population implosion. *The Public Interest* 129:3–22.

Edwards, S. 1998. The Chilean pension reform: A pioneering program. In *Privatizing social security.* Edited by M. Feldstein, 33–62. Chicago: University of Chicago Press.

Evandrou, M., and J. Falkingham. 2000. Looking back to look forward: Lessons from four birth cohorts for ageing in the 21st century. *Population Trends* 99:27–36.

Federal Interagency Forum on Aging Related Statistics. 2000. *Older Americans 2000: Key indicators of well-being.* Washington, DC: U.S. Government Printing Office.

Feldstein, M., and H. Siebert. 2002. *Social security pension reform in Europe.* Chicago: University of Chicago Press.

Freedman, V. A., and L. G. Martin. 1999. The role of education in explaining and forecasting trends in functional limitations among older Americans. *Demography* 36:461–473.

Freedman, V. A., H. Aykan, and L. G. Martin. 2001. Aggregate changes in severe cognitive impairment among older Americans: 1993 and 1998. *Journal of Gerontology: Social Sciences* 56:S100–S111.

Freedman, V. A., L. G. Martin, and R. F. Schoeni. 2002. Recent trends in disability and functioning among older adults in the United States: A systematic review. *Journal of the American Medical Association* 288:3137–3146.

Gee, E. M., and G. M. Gutman. 2000. *The overselling of population aging: Apocalyptic demography, intergenerational challenges, and social policy.* New York: Oxford University Press.

Grant, L. 2001. Replacement migration: The UN population division on European population decline. *Population and Environment* 22:391–399.

Jiang, L. 1995. Changing kinship structure and its implications for old-age support in urban and rural China. *Population Studies* 49:127–145.

Keyfitz, N. 1968. *Introduction to the mathematics of population.* Reading, Mass.: Addison-Wesley.

Keilman, N. 1997. Ex-post errors in official population forecasts in industrialized countries. *Journal of Official Statistics* 13:245–277.

Kingson, E. R., and J. B. Williamson. 2001. Economic security policies. In *Handbook of aging and the social sciences*, 5th ed. Edited by R. H. Binstock and L. K. George, 369–386. San Diego, Calif.: Academic Press.

Kinsella, K., and V. A. Velkoff. 2001. *An aging world: 2001*. U.S. Census Bureau, Series P95/01-1. Washington, D.C.: U.S. Government Printing Office.

Lutz, W., J. W. Vaupel, and D. A. Ahlburg, eds. 1998. *Frontiers of population forecasting*, Supplement to Vol. 24 of *Population and development review*. New York: Population Council.

Lye, D. N., D. H. Klepinger, P. D. Hyle, and A. Nelson. 1995. Childhood living arrangements and adult children's relations with their parents. *Demography* 32:261–280.

Manton, K. G., and X. Gu. 2001. Changes in the prevalence of chronic disability in the United States black and non-black population above age 65 from 1982 to 1999. *Proceedings of the National Academy of Sciences of the United States of America* 98:6354–6359.

Martin, L. G. 1990. Changing intergenerational family relations in East Asia. *Annals of the American Academy of Political and Social Sciences* 510:102–114.

Meyerson, F. A. B. 2001. Replacement migration: A questionable tactic for delaying the inevitable effects of fertility transition. *Population and Environment* 22:401–409.

National Academy on an Aging Society. 1999. *Demography is not destiny*. Washington, DC: National Academy on an Aging Society.

National Research Council. 2000. *Beyond six billion: Forecasting the world's population*. Edited by J. Bongaarts and R. A. Bulato. Washington, D.C.: National Academy Press.

National Research Council. 2001. *Preparing for an aging world: The case for cross-national research*. Washington, D.C.: National Academy Press.

Oeppen, J. , and Vaupel, J. W. 2002. Broken limits to life expectancy. *Science* 296:1029–1031.

Olshansky, S., and B. A. Carnes. 2001. *The quest for immortality: Science at the frontiers of aging*. New York: W. W. Norton.

O'Neill, B. C., and W. Lutz. 2003. Projections and forecasts, population. In *Encyclopedia of Population*. Edited by P. Demeny and G. McNicoll, 808–813. New York: Macmillan Reference USA.

Pavalko, E. K., and J. E. Artis. 1997. Women's caregiving and paid work: Causal relationships in late life. *Journal of Gerontology: Social Sciences* 52B:170–179.

Peterson, P. G. 1999. *Gray dawn: How the coming age wave will transform America—and the world*. New York: Times Books.

Pickard, L., R. Wittenberg, A. Comas-Herrera, B. Davies, and R. Darton. 2000. Relying on informal care in the new century? Informal care for elderly people in England to 2031. *Aging and Society* 20:745–772.

Preston, S. H., P. Heuveline, and M. Guillot. 2001. *Demography: Measuring and modeling population processes*. Malden, Mass.: Blackwell.

Rein, M., and H. Salzman. 1995. Social integration, participation and exchange in five industrialized countries. In *Older and active*. Edited by S. Bass, 238–263. New Haven, Conn.: Yale University Press.

Reinhardt, U. E. 2003. Does the aging of the population really drive the demand for health care? *Health Affairs* 22:27–39.

Reinhardt, U. E., P. S Hussey, G. F. Anderson, and F. Gerard. 2002. Cross-national comparison of health systems using OECD Data, 1999. *Health Affairs* 22:169–181.

Riley, J. C. 2001. *Rising life expectancy: A global history*. Cambridge: Cambridge University Press.

Schofield, H., and S. Bloch. 1998. Disability and chronic illness: The role of the family carer. *Medical Journal of Australia* 169:405–406.

Schulz, R., P. Visintainer, and G. M. Williamson. 1990. Psychiatric and physical morbidity effects of caregiving. *Journal of Gerontology: Psychological Sciences* 45:181–191.

Shirey, L., and L. Summer. 2000. Caregiving: Helping the elderly with activity limitations. *National Academy on Aging Society* 7:1–6.

Stone, R. I. 2000. *Long-term care for the elderly with disabilities: Current policy, emerging trends, and implications for the twenty-first century*. New York: Milbank Memorial Fund.

Tomassini, C., and D. A. Wolf. 2000. Shrinking kin networks in Italy due to sustained low fertility. *European Journal of Population* 16:353–372.

Traphagan, J. W., and J. Knight, eds. 2003. *Demographic change and the family in Japan's aging society*. Albany: State University of New York Press.

Uhlenberg, P. 1988. Population aging and the timing of old age benefits. In *Issues in contemporary retirement*. Edited by R. Ricardo-Campbell and E. P. Lazear, 353–377. Stanford, Calif.: Hoover Press.

Uhlenberg, P. 1993. Demographic change and kin relationships in later life. *Annual Review of Gerontology and Geriatrics* 13:219–238.

Uhlenberg, P. 1994. Implications of being divorced in later life. In *Ageing and the family*, 121–127. New York: United Nations.

Uhlenberg, P. 2005. Historical forces shaping grandparent-grandchild relationships: Demography and beyond. *Annual Review of Gerontology and Geriatrics* 24: 77–97.

Uhlenberg, P., and J. B. Kirby. 1998. Grandparenthood over time: Historical and demographic trends. In *Handbook of grandparenthood*. Edited by M. E. Szinovacz, 23–39. Westport, Conn.: Greenwood Press.

United Nations (Department of Economic and Social Affairs, Population Division). 2002. *World population ageing, 1950–2050*. New York: United Nations.

United Nations. 2000. *Replacement migration: Is it a solution to declining and aging populations?* New York: United Nations.

United States Bureau of the Census. 1976. *Historical statistics of the United States: Colonial times to 1970*. Washington, D.C.: U.S. Government Printing Office.

United States Bureau of the Census. 2001a. *Current population reports P20–538: Geographic mobility*. Washington, D.C.: U.S. Census Bureau.

United States Bureau of the Census. 2001b. The 65 years and over population: 2000. *Census 2000 Brief*, C2KBR/ 01–10. Washington, D.C.: U.S. Census Bureau.

Vallin, J. 2002. The end of the demographic transition: Relief or concern? *Population and Development Review* 28:105–120.

Wachter, K. W. 1997. Kinship resources for the elderly. *Philosophical Transactions of the Royal Society of London, Series B Biological Sciences* 352 (1363):1811–1817.

Walker, A. 1999. The future of pensions and retirement in Europe: Towards productive ageing. *The Geneva Papers on Risk and Insurance* 24:448–460.

Watkins, S. S., J. A. Menken, and J. Bongaarts. 1987. Demographic foundations of family change. *American Sociological Review* 52:346–358.

White, K. M. 2002. Longevity advances in high-income countries, 1955–96. *Population and Development Review* 28:59–76.

White, L. 1994. Stepfamilies over the lifecourse: Social support. In *Stepfamilies: Who benefits? Who does not?*. Edited by A. Booth and J. Dunn, 309–337. Hilldale, N.J.: Erlbaum Associates.

Williamson, J. B. 1997. A critique of the case for privatizing Social Security. *The Gerontologist* 37:561–571.

Wise, D. A. 1997. Retirement against the demographic trend: More older people living longer, working less, and saving less. *Demography* 34:83–95.

World Bank. 1994. *Averting the old age crisis: Policies to protect the old and promote growth*. Washington, D.C.

Zeng, Y., and L. George. 2001. Extremely rapid aging and the living arrangements of the elderly: The case of China. *Population Bulletin of the United Nations* 42/43:255–287.

CHAPTER 6

Demography of Race and Ethnicity

Rogelio Saenz and M. Cristina Morales

One of the most permanent features of many societies, especially the United States, is racial and ethnic stratification. Many immigrant groups have been integrated into the different dimensions of American life, while others have remained relatively marginalized. The road toward inclusion is particularly difficult for groups that initially gained entrance to the United States through involuntary means (e.g., warfare and conquest) and for those with more pronounced racial and cultural distinctions compared to the dominant group (McLemore and Romo 1998). Such patterns set apart the experiences of African Americans, American Indians, Mexican Americans, and Puerto Ricans, groups that have been labeled as "colonized groups" due to the aggression surrounding their initial incorporation into the United States, their racial and cultural distinctions, and their long-term location on the lower rungs of the American social and economic hierarchy.

The unique experience of these and other minority groups has major implications for the United States population. Race and ethnicity are important dimensions in understanding the demography of the United States, for racial and ethnic groups vary tremendously with respect to population composition, population processes, as well as their life chances and access to opportunity structures. Referring to the social world of African Americans, Weeks (2002:411) notes that "being of black-African origin in the United States is associated with higher probabilities of death, lower levels of education, lower levels of occupational status, lower incomes, and higher levels of marital disruption than for the non-Hispanic white population." The inequality of groups in American society along racial and ethnic lines has important implications for the future of the United States because of the major demographic transformations already underway in this country. Of the 75.8 million inhabitants that the United States is projected to add to its population between 2000 and 2030, non-Hispanic whites should account for less than one-fifth (18.9%) of the growth (U.S. Bureau of the Census 2000) and comprise less than half of the total population by 2060.

It is precisely these variations in population change that piqued the interest of demographers on racial and ethnic matters in the early part of the 20th century. Several prominent demographers of the time expressed alarm about the rapid growth of poor nonwhite populations and feared that the quality of the nation's population would diminish significantly (Zuberi 2001). However, most of the focus on the demography of racial and ethnic groups up to the middle of the 20th century was primarily relegated to the study of African Americans (e.g., Cox 1948; Drake and Cayton 1945; DuBois 1896, 1903, 1909; Frazier 1939, 1949, 1957). It is interesting to note that despite these many studies, Hauser and Duncan (1959) in *The Study of Population* devoted only four pages to race and ethnicity. And a recent inventory (Teachman, Paaselva, and Carvew 1993) of topics that demographers have addressed in articles published in *Demography* over the journal's first 30 years did not include a category on race and ethnicity.

In an examination we conducted of articles appearing in *Demography* between 1964 and 2003 (issues 1 to 3), of the 1,676 articles published, 187 were related to race and ethnicity (including immigration), accounting for approximately 11% of all the articles. Figure 6.1 shows, however, that most of the interest in the study of race and ethnicity occurred in the last two decades, with the peak taking place in the 1999 to 2003 period when about one-fifth of the articles dealt with this topic.

This chapter focuses on the demography of racial and ethnic groups and is broken down into four sections. First, it examines the conceptualization, substantive concerns, and relevance of race and ethnicity to demography. Second, it provides an overview of theoretical perspectives that have been used to understand racial and ethnic groups. Third, it discusses the methodological issues related to the study of race and ethnicity,

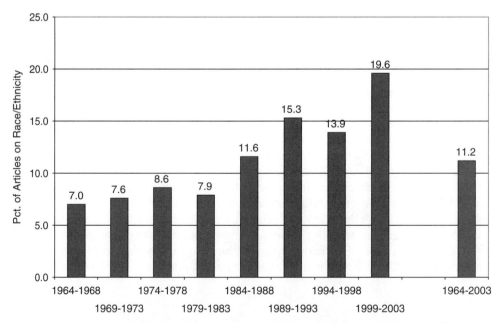

FIGURE 6.1. Percentage of articles in *Demography* focusing on race/ethnicity by period, 1964–2003.

along with key empirical findings. Finally, it focuses on directions for future research and a few research areas that merit attention. The chapter focuses almost exclusively on the demography of racial and ethnic groups in the United States.

SUBSTANTIVE CONCERNS

This section provides an overview of the concepts of race and ethnicity and demonstrates the importance of these concepts for demographic research. Specifically, the discussion focuses on the construction of race and ethnicity and the complexities associated with defining these concepts. Also illustrated are the distinct experiences of racial and ethnic groups associated with variations in population composition, population processes, and life chances.

The Construction of Race and Ethnicity

Race and ethnicity are important concepts for demographers. While they are often used interchangeably, they are distinct terms. The former is associated with physical characteristics, and the latter is related to behavioral or cultural attributes. Despite the supposed link between physical features and race, race is a social construct, which is defined by society rather than by genetics (Bonilla-Silva 2001; McFalls 1998).

Nonetheless, race and phenotype continue to be coupled. Historically, in the United States, the dominant white population identified skin color as the principal means for sorting people into varying locations on the social and economic hierarchy. At the outset, persons who resembled the dominant population were labeled as "us" while those who deviated from the ideal white image became the "other." In the process, white skin was associated with what was good, and black skin with what was bad. Even today, the English language serves as a reminder of this distinction. White is associated with purity and goodness (the "good guys" wear white hats), and black is associated with impurity and evil (the "bad guys" wear black hats).

In the United States, racism emerged as an ideology to justify the conquest of American Indians and the enslavement of Africans (Feagin 2001). Whites could live with themselves if they became convinced that American Indians and African slaves were subhumans who were mentally and biologically inferior creatures who could not rule themselves. Even after the hostilities against American Indians and the enslavement of Africans ended, institutional arrangements were established to maintain the second-class citizenship of these minorities. These institutional arrangements include the establishment of reservations and Jim Crow practices.

Although these are the most extreme cases, other groups (e.g., Irish, Southern and Eastern Europeans, Asians, and Latinos) have been racialized at different times in the historical past. In the process, these groups have been defined as "others" at one point or another and have been associated with inferior physical, mental, and moral attributes in relation to the dominant white population. Similar kinds of social construction have occurred in other societies (with regard to this phenomenon in China, see Borchigud 1995; Dikotter 1992; Gladney 1994; Khan 1995; with respect to Brazil, see Skidmore 1995; and with respect to Germany and Italy, see Teitelbaum and Winter 1998).

In its barest form, race and ethnicity can be viewed as ascribed characteristics. At birth, one is assigned a race and ethnicity based on the attributes of one's parents. Yet, racial classification systems associated with the social construction of race and ethnicity have inconsistencies and ambiguities (Obach 1999). Racial and ethnic categories are social constructs that vary across place, time, and situations (Eschbach and Gomez 1998; Saenz and Aguirre 1991; Waters 2002; for a discussion of the fluid and situational ethnic identity of indigenous populations in Mexico, see Tiedje 2002; for a discussion of the dynamic nature of the Hutu and Tutsi ethnic categories in Burundi, Congo, and Rwanda, see Longman 1999). As Waters (2002:25) emphasizes, racial and ethnic identities are "subject to a great deal of flux and change—both intergenerationally, over the life course, and situationally." For example, groups once considered neither "white" nor "black," such as the Irish, Lebanese, and Syrians in the United States as well as Chinese in Mississippi, have gained acceptance as "whites" over time (Gualtieri 2001; Ignatiev 1995; Warren and Twine 1997).

Immigrants who come to the United States from countries with different racial classification systems often experience significant alterations in the conception of their own race and ethnicity. For instance, race is more fluid and malleable in Latin America than in the United States (Cruz-Janzen 2002; Landale and Oropesa 2002; Rodriguez 2000). Brazil, for example, has more than 140 racial categories (Rodriguez 2000). Because "money whitens" in many Latin American societies (see de la Cadena 2001; Streicker 1998), ostensibly black individuals who are well off economically may refer to themselves, and be seen by others, as "white." When such individuals immigrate to the United States they are faced with the more dichotomous and static notion of racial classification of the United States (Landale and Oropesa 2002; Rodriguez 2000).

Finally, nationality represents yet another factor that complicates racial and ethnic identification and further illustrates the fluidity of identity (Waters 1999). For example, Waters (1999) observes that national identity for West Indian immigrants consists of multilayered identities including a national origin identity (Trinidadian), a subnational identity (black), and a supernational regional identity (West Indian). For a discussion of the construction of ethnicity among Latin American women in Australia, see the work of Zevallos (2003); for a similar discussion involving ethnic minorities in the borderlands of China, Burma, and Thailand, see the work of Toyota (2003).

White ethnic groups are much more likely to use ethnicity in a voluntary fashion, having the freedom to reveal or hide it at will. Sociologists (Gans 1979; Waters 1990) have illustrated the notions of "voluntary ethnicity" and "symbolic ethnicity" among whites, ethnic forms which represent temporal, ethereal emblems that white ethnics can don freely. In contrast, minority groups set apart from the mainstream population find it more difficult to shed their race and ethnicity at will (Nelson and Tienda 1985). In these instances, particular physical or cultural attributes make it difficult for minority group members to downplay their race or ethnicity. However, minority group members may alter their preference for racial or ethnic identities over time. For example, over the last several decades, the term *Negro* gave way to the term *black*, which has increasingly given way to the term *African American*. Similarly, persons of Mexican origin have used a variety of ethnic identities including *Mexican*, *Mexican American*, *Chicano*, *Latino*, and *Hispanic*, with preference for such terms being situational (Saenz and Aguirre 1991). Nonetheless, the complexities of racial and ethnic identification are especially apparent among people whose parents are from different racial or ethnic groups.

Multiracial Identities

The last few decades have seen an increase in the prevalence of intermarriage and a corresponding increase in multiracial persons (Riche 2000). A growing literature has developed about multiracial individuals and their construction of race and ethnicity (Chew, Eggebeen, and Uhlenberg 1989; Gatson 2003; Perlmann and Waters 2002; Root, 1992, 1996; Saenz et al. 1995; Spickard 1989; see, for an international perspective, Christian 2000). Multiracial individuals have numerous options for identifying themselves along racial and ethnic lines. They can select a single identity and discard part of their background, or they can decide to blend their cultural and racial allegiances to form a multiracial identity (Snipp 1997b). The numerous options of multiracial individuals are associated with a great degree of fluidity and instability in racial divisions (Snipp 1997b). Some of the difficulties with the racial classification of multiracial people include the lack of clarity and logic in distinguishing racial characteristics (Ferrante and Brown 1999; Glazer 2002; Spickard 1992), the absence of fixed racial boundaries pointing to the social construction of race (Allman 1996; Ferrante and Brown 1999; Outlaw 1990; Waters 2002; Zuberi 2001), and tremendous variation in the people identified as belonging to the same race (Ferrante and Brown 1999; Hummer 1996).

Prior to 2000, U.S. statistical agencies did not recognize multiracial respondents. Reflecting the increasing presence and voice of multiracial people, the 2000 U.S. census allowed individuals to select more than one racial group. Although there continues to be debate about the social and political implications of the identification and enumeration of multiracial people (Perlmann and Waters 2002) the construction of the multiracial category is seen by many as a positive move away from the dichotomous and rigid racial classification system of the United States.

Whiteness and Privilege

While much of the focus of research in race and ethnicity has dealt with minority groups, some recent work has focused on whites. The "whiteness" literature emphasizes the extent to which whites gain privileges because of structural arrangements benefiting them (Bonilla-Silva 2001, 2003; Doane and Bonilla-Silva 2003; Feagin 2001; Feagin and O'Brien 2003; Feagin and Vera 2000; Frankenberg 1993; Omi and Winant 1984; for a comparative base involving whiteness in the United States and South Africa, see Steyn 1999). For example, whites are less likely than minority group members to be denied access to the opportunity structure, to be singled out for suspicious behavior due to the color of their skin, or to bear psychological wounds resulting from membership in marginalized minority groups. Jensen (1998), a professor of journalism at the University of Texas at Austin, provides a personal introspective account of how he has benefited through white privilege:

> But no matter how much I "fix" myself, one thing never changes—I walk through the world with white privilege. What does that mean? Perhaps most importantly, when I seek admission to a university, apply for a job, or hunt for an apartment, I don't look threatening. Almost all of the people evaluating me for those things look like me—they are white. They see in me a reflection of themselves, and in a racist world that is an advantage. I smile. I am white. I am one of them. I am not dangerous. Even when I voice critical opinions, I am cut some slack. After all, I'm white....But, all said, I know I did not get where I am by merit

alone. I benefited from, among other things, white privilege. That doesn't mean that I don't deserve my job, or that if I weren't white I would never have gotten the job. It means simply that all through my life, I have soaked up benefits for being white. I grew up in fertile farm country taken by force from non-white indigenous people. I was educated in a well-funded, virtually all-white public school system in which I learned that white people like me made this country great. There I also was taught a variety of skills, including how to take standardized tests written by and for white people. All my life I have been hired for jobs by white people. I was accepted for graduate school by white people. And I was hired for a teaching position at the predominantly white University of Texas, which had a white president, in a college headed by a white dean and in a department with a white chairman that at the time had one non-white tenured professor....White privilege is not something I get to decide whether or not I want to keep. Every time I walk into a store at the same time as a black man and the security guard follows him and leaves me alone to shop, I am benefiting from white privilege. There is not space here to list all the ways in which white privilege plays out in our daily lives, but it is clear that I will carry this privilege with me until the day white supremacy is erased from this society (4C).

A growing literature has also demonstrated the stratification that exists within minority groups on the basis of skin color. Minority group members are not immune to the racist images favoring whiteness and often embrace such beliefs (Hall 1994, 1995; Hill 2002; for a U.S.–Latin American comparative base, see Uhlmann et al. 2002). As such, lighter-skinned minority group members have been shown to enjoy greater privileges within their groups as well as gain greater acceptance into the white world (Allen, Telles, and Hunter 2000; Espino and Franz 2002; Gomez 2000; Hill 2000; Hughes and Hertel 1990; Hunter 2002; Keith and Herring 1991; Murguia and Saenz 2002; Murguia and Telles 1996; Telles and Murguia 1990).

Racial and Ethnic Variations in Demographic and Socioeconomic Characteristics

It is clear that racial and ethnic groups have distinct life experiences. These unique experiences can be seen in their demographic and socioeconomic experiences, particularly their population composition, population processes, and socioeconomic status. These topics are also applicable for the minority groups of other societies. See, for instance, the work of Poston and Shu (1987) with regard to China and that of Anderson and Silver (1989) with regard to Soviet populations.

POPULATION COMPOSITION.   The distinct life experiences of racial and ethnic groups are associated with variations in their population compositions. Figure 6.2 shows age/ sex pyramids for 12 U.S. racial and ethnic groups: whites, African Americans, American Indians, six Asian groups (Asian Indians, Chinese, Filipinos, Japanese, Koreans, and Vietnamese), and three Latino groups (Mexicans, Puerto Ricans, and Cubans). The shapes of the pyramids clearly display the vastly different demographic and historical experiences of the 12 groups.

Here are some general patterns. First, Mexicans and Puerto Ricans have the youngest populations. Nearly one-third of Mexicans (31.8%) and almost three-tenths of Puerto Ricans (28.9%) are less than 15 years of age. These patterns reflect their relatively high fertility levels. Second, Japanese and Cubans are older populations. The elderly account for approximately one-fifth of their populations, a larger percentage

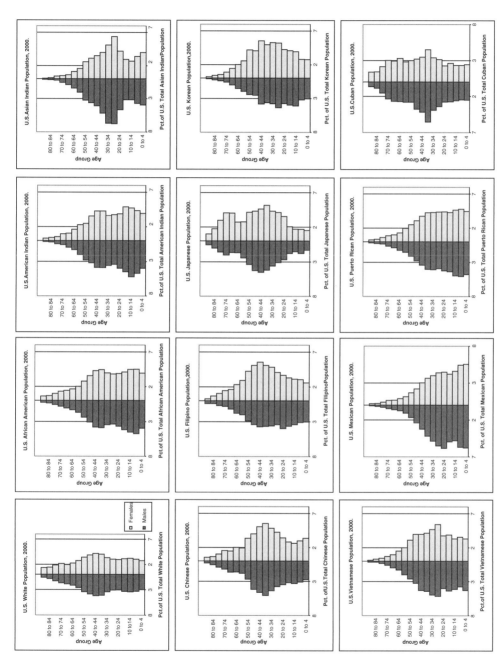

FIGURE 6.2. Age–sex pyramids for 12 selected racial/ethnic groups, 2000. Source: 2000 1% Public Use Microdata Sample (PUMS).

than that for persons less than 15 years of age (Japanese, 9.5%; Cubans, 14.6%). These patterns result from low fertility. Third, immigration has played a significant role in the shaping of the Asian and Latino groups. This is seen in the bulges associated with the primary working ages surrounding the 25 to 44 age categories. About two-fifths of Asian Indians (41.8%) and Vietnamese (37.2%) are 25 to 44 years of age. Fourth, the groups also vary in their sex ratios (number of males per 100 females). Males outnumber females among Asian Indians (115.0), Mexicans (111.1), Vietnamese (102.9), and Cubans (101.4). In contrast, females outnumber males in the other eight groups, with the sex ratios being especially low for Japanese (76.2), Koreans (79.9), Filipinos (82.2), and African Americans (89.9). The wide variability in sex ratios is primarily associated with sex selectivity in immigration. Immigration from Mexico and India, for example, is primarily male. Moreover, the formation of "war bride" marriages between Asian women and American men is reflected in the low sex ratios of the Japanese, Korean, and Filipino groups. The low sex ratio of African Americans reflects the high mortality rates of African American males (see below). Indeed, much of the racial and ethnic variation in age/sex composition reflects distinctions in population processes. See the more general discussion in this regard in chapter 1 in this *Handbook*.

FERTILITY.   Racial and ethnic groups differ in their fertility. Data from the National Center for Health Statistics (NCHS) (Hamilton, Martin, and Sutton 2003) may be used to examine these distinctions. Unfortunately, current data are not available for the fertility rates of specific Asian and Latino populations. NCHS presents data for the "Asian and Pacific Islander" and "Latino" aggregate groups. Figure 6.3 shows the total fertility rate (TFR) for five racial and ethnic groups in 2001. Latinas have the highest fertility rate, with a TFR of 2,737, and African American women have the second highest TFR (2,039); the TFRs are the lowest among American Indian (1,740), Asian and Pacific Islander (1,835), and non-Hispanic White (1,840) women. Research has also shown racial and

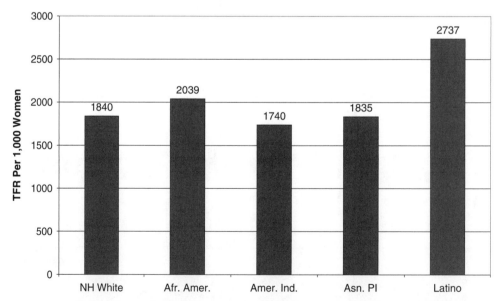

FIGURE 6.3. Total fertility rate by race/ethnic group, 2001. Source: Hamilton et al. 2003.

ethnic variations in fertility in other societies as well. For example, see research examining the fertility of aboriginal groups (Suwal and Trovato 1998) and Asians (Halli 1987) in Canada and ethnic groups in the former Soviet Union (Anderson and Silver 1989).

MORTALITY.   Racial and ethnic groups also have different mortality patterns. Data used here are from the NCHS (Arias et al. 2003) and are based on the same five racial and ethnic groups. Figure 6.4 presents the age-adjusted death rates (AADR) of males and females in each of the five racial and ethnic groups in 2001. The AADR, which adjusts for age differences across groups, indicates the number of deaths (per 100,000 persons) that members of a standard population (the United States) would have in a given year if they experienced the age-specific death rates of a given racial/ethnic group. A few patterns emerge. First, across all the groups, females consistently have lower death rates than males, with the rates of females being approximately two-thirds as high as those of their male counterparts. Second, African Americans have the highest death rates. The AADR of African American males is 38% higher than that of non-Hispanic white males, while the AADR of African American women is 30% higher than that of non-Hispanic white women. Third, the lowest death rates occur among Asian and Pacific Islanders (AADR of males, 597.4; AADR of females, 412.0), Latinos (802.5; 544.2), and American Indians (798.9; 594.0), each having lower death rates than those of non-Hispanic whites. For related discussions see chapter 10 in this *Handbook*.

The death rates of American Indians and Latinos are inconsistent with the relatively low socioeconomic positions of these groups. This is also the case with the relatively low fertility rates of American Indians. We suspect that the inconsistencies involving American Indians are related to their diversity and their high rates of intermarriage. Over the last few decades, a major reason for American Indian high growth is the greater prevalence of people identifying themselves as American Indian (Eschbach

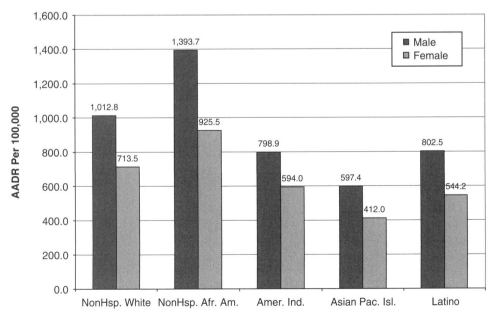

FIGURE 6.4. Age-adjusted death rates for race/ethnic groups by sex, 2001. Source: Arias et al. 2003.

1995; Passel 1997; Snipp 1992, 1997a). This occurs among American Indians living on reservations as well as those who are generations removed from these locales. The growth may also be due in part to problems of consistency, particularly among the offspring of the intermarried, in the identification of people in the census and in birth and death certificates, which could contribute to the unexpected levels of mortality and fertility described above. Similar reasons have been shown for the rapid growth of several of the minority nationalities of China (Poston 1993).

In the case of Latinos, there has been much debate and speculation about the cause of the "epidemiological paradox" involving the low death rates of Latinos (Abraido-Lanza et al. 1999; Echevarria and Frisbie 2001; Forbes et al. 2000; Hayes-Bautista 2003; Hummer et al. 2000; Landale, Oropesa, and Gorman 1999, 2000; Markides and Coreil 1986; Patel et al. 2004). Because the paradox is especially evident among Mexican immigrants, it has been suggested that the favorable mortality patterns are associated with strong levels of social support, the selective nature of immigration to the United States, and the return of immigrants to Mexico when they become seriously ill (the "salmon bias") (for a challenge to the paradox at the older ages, see Patel et al. 2004).

There are real difficulties associated with developing mortality rates for a mobile population such as Mexican immigrants. The low death rates of Latinos could well be a statistical artifact produced by immigrants who return to Mexico when they become seriously ill; this is especially the case if the death is not recorded in the United States. Hence, in the computation of the death rate, these individuals would be part of the denominator (population at risk of dying) but not the numerator (deaths). The problem is likely to be the most prevalent in the case of infant mortality since, especially along the U.S.-Mexico border, Mexican women may deliver babies in the United States and return to Mexico immediately thereafter. In such cases, infant deaths occurring in Mexico are not recorded in the United States, causing the infant mortality rate of Latinos to be artificially low. Data from the NCHS (Arias and Smith 2003) indicate that in 2000, Latinos (5.6) and whites (5.7) had similar infant mortality rates (number of deaths to babies less than one year of age per 1,000 live births) compared to a rate of 14.1 for African Americans. For mortality research in other societies, see the research of Ross and Taylor (2002) showing the high mortality rates of indigenous groups in Australia compared to nonindigenous groups in Australia and indigenous groups outside of Australia. See also the work of Trovato (2001) examining the mortality patterns of aboriginal groups in Canada, New Zealand, and the United States.

Internal and International Migration

Racial and ethnic groups also vary with respect to their propensity for migration within the United States and international migration to the U.S. Data from the 2000 One Percent PUMS (U.S. Census Bureau 2003) are used to measure the degree of interstate migration between 1995 and 2000 among persons five years of age and older who were living in the United States in 1995. The migration information is obtained through the use of the five-year migration query, which seeks information about where people were living in 1995 and 2000. Interstate migrants are those individuals who were living in a different state in 1995 and 2000. Because age is typically associated with migration, and because the different racial and ethnic groups differ substantially with respect to age structure, it is necessary to use age-adjusted interstate migration rates (AAIMR) that use the age-specific interstate migration rates of each racial and ethnic group and apply them to the population in the U.S. in 1995. The AAIMR refers to the number of interstate migrants in 1995 to 2000 per 1,000 persons five years and older living in the United States in 1995.

Figure 6.5 (dark bars) shows the AAIMRs for the 12 racial and ethnic groups in the U.S. Asian Indians (137.2) and Koreans (119.2) are the most geographically mobile groups with more than 1 in 10 persons five and older living in a different state in 1995 and 2000. Three other groups (Chinese, 99.3; American Indians, 97.9; and whites, 93.9) also show a considerable amount of geographical movement. On the other hand, Mexicans (56.1), Cubans (67.4), African Americans (71.1), and Filipinos (73.4) were the least likely to move across state boundaries between 1995 and 2000. These low AAIMRs of Mexicans and Cubans likely reflect their historical concentration in the Southwest and in Florida, respectively.

The 2000 PUMS data may also be used to estimate the number of persons from the different racial and ethnic groups who were living abroad in 1995 and in the United States in 2000. Abroad migration rates (AMR) indicate the number of persons who moved from abroad to the United States between 1995 and 2000 per 1,000 persons living in the United States in 1995. There is a significant amount of variation in the volume of international migration across the racial and ethnic groups (Figure 6.5, light bars). Asian Indians, again, have the greatest amount of movement, with 312.2 Asian Indians coming to the United States between 1995 and 2000 per 1,000 members of the group already living in the United States in 1995. Three other Asian groups (Japanese, 197.7; Koreans, 176.7; and Chinese, 170.1), along with Mexicans (112.6), have AMRs greater than 100. In contrast, three groups (American Indians, 10.5; whites, 11.4; and African Americans, 21.8) have extremely low levels of international movement between 1995 and 2000.

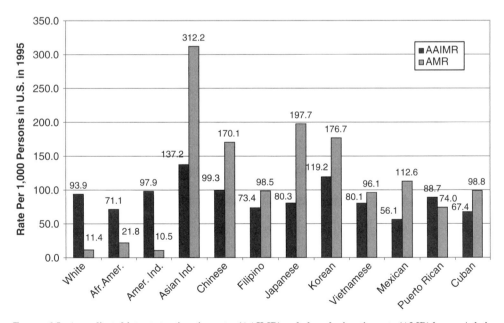

FIGURE 6.5. Age-adjusted interstate migration rates (AAIMR) and abroad migration rate (AMR) by race/ethnic group, 1995–2000. Source: 2000 1% Public Use Microdata Sample (PUMS).

Life Chances

The racial and ethnic groups also vary with respect to socioeconomic opportunities and life chances, specifically, educational attainment and poverty (for an international comparison base, see the work of Nattrass and Seekings [2001] on blacks and whites in South Africa). Educational attainment gauges the extent to which members of different racial and ethnic groups have access to human capital resources that are crucial for socioeconomic achievement. Poverty provides an indication of the degree to which people from different racial and ethnic groups lack the minimal economic resources required to sustain themselves. Because the groups differ significantly with respect to nativity, the analyses are conducted separately for native- and foreign-born groups. Note that due to relatively small numbers, foreign-born American Indians and Puerto Ricans are excluded from the analysis (here and in subsequent analyses below).

Figure 6.6 provides information on the percentage of persons 25 to 44 years of age in each racial and ethnic group and nativity group who have completed college (the equivalent of a bachelor's degree). There is a noticeable amount of variation across group on these percentages. Overall, with the exception of Vietnamese, Asians have the highest educational levels, with Asian Indians (native-born, 72.7%; foreign-born, 71.0%) positioned at the top alongside native-born Chinese (70.1%). Five other Asian groups have at least half of their members 25 to 44 years of age holding a college degree: native-born Koreans (63.6%), foreign-born Chinese (56.6%), foreign-born Japanese (56.6%), native-born Japanese (54.8%), and foreign-born Koreans (50.2%). Whites do not fare as well as many Asian groups and native-born Cubans with respect to college completion. In contrast, foreign-born Mexicans have by far the lowest level of education, with less than 1 in 20 having a college diploma. Furthermore, five other groups have fewer than one in five of their members 25 to 44 years of age who are college graduates: native-born American

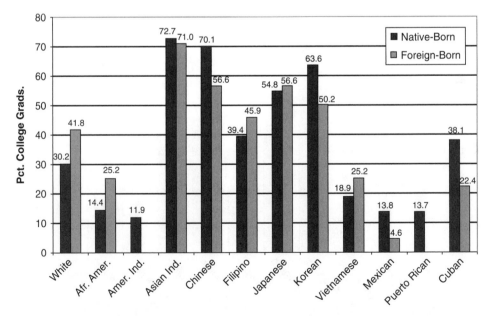

FIGURE 6.6. Percentage of persons 25 to 44 years of age who are college graduates by race/ethnic group and nativity, 2000. Source: 2000 1% Public Use Microdata Sample (PUMS).

Indians (11.9%), native-born Puerto Ricans (13.7%), native-born Mexicans (13.8%), native-born African Americans (14.4%), and native-born Vietnamese (18.9%). These groups have traditionally been associated with lower levels of socioeconomic status and are frequently referred to as minorities.

The poverty rates of the racial and ethnic groups may also be analyzed by nativity. The 2000 census asked individuals in households to report their incomes from all sources in the last complete calendar year (1999). The income of households and families was then compared to a poverty threshold based on household size, composition, and presence of children. Those in households or families with incomes below the poverty threshold were designated as being in poverty in 1999. Figure 6.7 presents the poverty rates for the 22 groups of interest. Selected Asian groups and whites have the lowest poverty rates. Fewer than one in a dozen native-born Japanese (4.6%), foreign-born Filipinos (5.5%), and native-born whites (7.9%) were living in poverty in 1999. Moreover, five other groups had fewer than one in nine of their members impoverished: native-born Filipinos (8.0%), native-born Asian Indians (8.5%), foreign-born Asian Indians (9.2%), native-born Chinese (10.2%), and foreign-born whites (10.4%). In contrast, the six groups with the lowest levels of education, and which are also viewed as minority groups, had the highest poverty rates: native-born American Indians (26.0%), foreign-born Mexicans (26.0%), native-born African Americans (25.0%), native-born Puerto Ricans (25.0%), native-born Mexicans (21.6%), and native-born Vietnamese (18.1%).

In this section the concepts of race and ethnicity have been discussed, and their importance for demographic analyses has been illustrated. It was shown that racial and ethnic groups differ significantly with respect to population composition, population processes, and life chances.

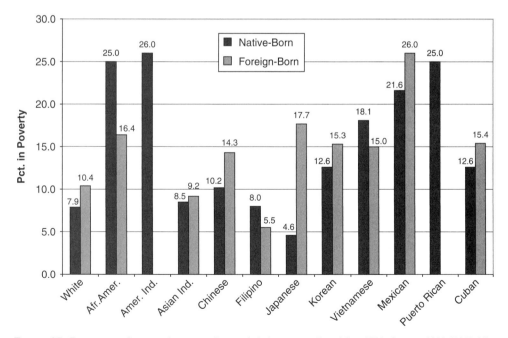

FIGURE 6.7. Percentage of persons in poverty by race/ethnic group and nativity, 1999. Source: 2000 1% Public Use Microdata Sample (PUMS).

THEORETICAL ISSUES

This section provides a general overview of the theoretical perspectives that have been used to explain racial and ethnic variations in demographic, social, and economic patterns. They may be grouped into two general categories—assimilation and structural.

Assimilation Perspective

The roots of the assimilationist perspective may be traced to the Chicago School of Sociology and the work of Robert Park (1950). Milton Gordon (1964), drawing on Park's ideas, developed the most popular exposition of the assimilationist perspective. He emphasized two key aspects of assimilation—cultural and structural. Gordon viewed assimilation as proceeding across eight subprocesses. The first subprocess is cultural assimilation (or acculturation), which involves minority group members learning the culture of the majority group. This phase is followed by structural assimilation, which Gordon distinguished into secondary structural assimilation and primary structural assimilation. Secondary structural assimilation involves members of the minority group coming into contact with majority group members in impersonal relationships in institutional and organizational settings. Primary structural assimilation involves the establishment of warm interpersonal relationships between minority and majority group members in the form of friendship groups.

For Gordon, primary structural assimilation represents the most crucial assimilation subprocess. Once this stage takes place, subsequent assimilation subprocesses are expected to ensue automatically (McLemore and Romo 1998). These subprocesses include marital assimilation (amalgamation), identificational assimilation (ethnic identification), attitudinal receptional assimilation (absence of prejudice), behavioral receptional assimilation (absence of discrimination), and civic assimilation (absence of value or power conflicts). Gordon's assimilationist perspective suggests that once minority group members achieve primary structural assimilation, they are likely to intermarry with members of the majority group, to shed their ethnic identities in favor of an American identity, to be less likely to experience prejudice and discrimination, and to hold universal—as opposed to particularistic—values and interests.

Because the assimilationist perspective is primarily based on the experiences of European immigrant groups, critics of this approach have questioned the extent to which the perspective applies to non-European groups. It generally took approximately three generations for European groups to be integrated into American society (McLemore and Romo 1998). However, some minority groups, such as African Americans, Mexican Americans, and Puerto Ricans, have been in this country for generations and have not been integrated. It has also been pointed out that ambiguity and controversy surrounding the concept of assimilation reinforces oppression (Yinger 1994). For instance, Alba (1999:9) argues that "today, assimilation is often depicted in terms of demands that minority individuals abandon their native cultures to accept the majority one, a demand that can be viewed as placing them in a position of inferiority and disadvantage." Therefore, the assimilationist perspective privileges the customs and values of some groups who emulate the majority group while devaluing the experiences of other groups that have not easily been integrated (Landsman and Katkin 1998).

MODIFICATION TO THE ASSIMILATION PERSPECTIVE. Despite critiques directed against it, the assimilationist perspective has not been abandoned, but has been modified (see Yinger 1994). For example, sociologists have recently paid an increasing amount of attention to the sons and daughters of immigrants—the second-generation—and have developed important insights that have helped better understand the assimilation process. In particular, Portes and his colleagues expanded the assimilation perspective in their development of the segmented assimilation perspective (Portes 1995; Portes and MacLeod 1996; Portes and Rumbaut 1996, 2001; Portes and Zhou 1993). This perspective suggests that immigrants today may be assimilated into one of three possible paths: (1) acculturation and subsequent assimilation into the white middle class, (2) assimilation into the underclass, which is marked by permanent poverty, and (3) the preservation of solidarity within the immigrant community, which promotes economic mobility. Portes and his associates (Portes and MacLeod 1996; Portes and Rumbaut 1996; Portes and Zhou 1993) argue that the route that immigrants take depends on their access to resources within their families and communities. It has also been suggested that the downward mobility path is associated with skin color, concentration in central cities, and the general lack of access to the opportunity structure in local labor markets (Landale, Oropesa, and Llanes 1998).

The assimilationist perspective has been used to examine racial and ethnic group differences in a variety of demographic patterns including fertility (Bean, Swicegood, and Berg 2000; Carter 2000; Pagnini 1997; Stephen and Bean 1992; Ford 1990), migration (Fang and Brown 1999), residential segregation (Alba and Logan 1993; Gross and Massey 1991; Logan, Alba, and Leung 1996; White and Omer 1997), marriage and divorce (Bean, Berg, and Van Hook 1996), and intermarriage (Hwang, Saenz, and Aguirre 1997; Kulczycki and Lobo 2002; Qian and Lichter 2001). It has also been shown to have utility for understanding the fertility of minorities in other societies. See, for instance, Chang's (2003) work dealing with the major minorities in China.

Structural Perspectives

Structural perspectives attribute the demographic, social, and economic standing of minority groups to macro-level or societal-level phenomena. In this respect, forces beyond the individual are shown to be primarily responsible for the observed demographic and socioeconomic patterns of minority groups. The structural perspectives that sociologists have developed to understand the stratification of minority groups are particularly useful. These include Blauner's internal colonialism model, Blalock's group size perspective, Blau's structural perspective, Wilson's structural perspective, Massey and Denton's structural perspective on segregation and poverty, and Bonilla-Silva's racialized social system perspective. These orientations generally seek to identify the forces and mechanisms that keep minority groups located at the bottom of the social and economic ladder of society.

The 1960s and 1970s represent a critical period in the United States for the development of scholarship related to the social and economic standing of minority groups. Blauner (1969, 1972) developed the internal colonialism model, which reflected the spirit of the era. Blauner applies ideas involving the colonization of Third-World people at the hands of European colonizers to the experiences of minority groups that have been colonized in the United States, i.e., groups that were originally incorporated through aggression. These groups include American Indians (conquest), African Americans (slavery), Mexican Americans (warfare), and Puerto Ricans (warfare). According to Blauner, these groups exist in internal colonies in the United States. Moreover, they are subjugated through the mechanisms of racism, cultural oppression, and lack of self-administration. Institutional forces are in place to keep colonized minorities within the confines of their colonies where they live as second-class citizens.

During the same period, Blalock (1967) developed the relative group size perspective. He reasoned that minority groups experience higher levels of discrimination and inequality in areas where they comprise a larger share of the population. In such instances, the minority group represents a threat to the existing power structure, with the majority group erecting barriers and obstacles to ensure that the minority group does not become upwardly mobile and gain access to power. The relative group size perspective has received a considerable amount of empirical support with respect to earnings (Frisbie and Neidert 1977; Tienda and Lii 1987), inequality (Fossett and Siebert 1997), poverty (Saenz 1997; Swanson et al. 1994), and interracial attitudes (Fossett and Kiecolt 1989).

Blau provided important insights for the study of the demography of racial and ethnic groups with his theoretical developments pertaining to the links between population structure and intergroup relations (Blau 1977, 1994). His structural contexts of opportunities perspective describe how macrostructural forces influence and constrain peoples' associations and choices (1994). Blau applied this macrosociological perspective to demonstrate that individual choices such as selecting a marriage mate and occupation are highly constrained and reflect the social structure. In the case of spouse selection, for example, even though people may prefer to marry an in-group member, structural constraints often prevent them from realizing their desires. One of the primary structural constraints is the size of one's group. Minority groups tend to have higher in-marriage rates in places where their own group is large and have higher out-marriage rates in areas where their group is small. A significant amount of research on intermarriage has provided support for Blau's perspective (Anderson and Saenz 1994; Blau and Schwartz 1997; Cready and Saenz 1997; Hwang, Saenz, and Aguirre 1997; Kalmijn 1998).

Wilson has also influenced the study of the demography of minorities. He set off considerable discussion and debate following the publication of his book *The Declining Significance of Race: Blacks and Changing American Institutions* (Wilson 1978), in which he argued that structural changes in the economy, along with civil rights legislation, led to a declining significance of race and an increasing significance of class. Wilson observed that the massive loss of manufacturing jobs between World War II and the late 1970s resulted in the loss of jobs that African Americans had relied on to achieve some degree of upward mobility. He also asserted that only a segment of the African American population was able to take advantage of opportunities that came about through the advent of civil rights legislation. Wilson observed that there was a bifurcation in the African American community with the increasing separation of the middle class and the "underclass." He noted that middle-class African Americans by and large moved to suburbs, leaving behind poor African Americans in central cities. Although Wilson did not deny that race was still a factor in the low socioeconomic standing of African Americans, he saw class as becoming a particularly important factor in explaining the condition of African Americans.

Wilson's (1978) thesis on the declining significance of race stirred a massive amount of debate and discussion (see also Wilson 1996). His ideas have found some support.

For example, Sakamoto and his colleagues (2000), using data from the Integrated Public Use Microdata Sample (IPUMS), observe that the relationship between race and earnings declined over time for all groups except Latinos. Other research has also found links between social class and occupational attainment (Hout 1984; Sakamoto and Tzeng 1999). However, others have challenged Wilson's assertion that the significance of race is declining (Herring 1989; Horton 1995; Morris 1996; Pattillo 1999; Willie 1978, 1989; Wilson 2000). For example, Feagin and Sikes (1994) observe that middle-class African Americans report a significant amount of racial discrimination even in corporate America. And Oliver and Shapiro (1995) clearly document the historical legacies of racism in their focus on wealth (accumulated assets and debts) as opposed to current income. Their study shows that slightly more than three-fifths of African American households do not have any wealth, twice the rate of their white counterparts. They show massive racial gaps in wealth across social classes as well.

Massey and Denton (1993) provide another structural perspective for explaining the social and economic plight of African Americans. Their primary focus is on the links between residential segregation and the elevated poverty rates among African Americans. Massey and Denton assert that the residential segregation of African Americans is part of a well-conceived plan, deeply embedded in the structure of American society, to keep African Americans away from whites, with federal policies, banking institutions, and the real estate industry helping to maintain this condition. The segregation of African Americans results in the absence of links to the opportunity structure. African Americans living in ghettoes lack access to most amenities that Americans take for granted. The following passage illustrates Massey and Denton's (1993:217) thoughts on the roots and consequences of the well-entrenched residential segregation of African Americans.

> After persisting for more than fifty years, the black ghetto will not be dismantled by passing a few amendments to existing laws or by implementing a smattering of bureaucratic reforms. The ghetto is part and parcel of modern American society; it was manufactured by whites earlier in the century to isolate and control growing urban black populations, and it is maintained today by a set of institutions, attitudes, and practices that are deeply embedded in the structure of American life. Indeed, as conditions in the ghetto have worsened and as poor blacks have adapted socially and culturally to this deteriorating environment, the ghetto has assumed even greater importance as an institutional tool for isolating the by-products of racial oppression: crime, drugs, violence, illiteracy, poverty, despair, and their growing economic costs.

There are theoretical developments emerging directly from the race and ethnicity literature that have important implications for the study of the demography of race and ethnicity. Of particular importance is Bonilla-Silva's (1997, 2001, 2003) racialized social system perspective. He challenges prevailing thinking that the continued inequality between minority and majority groups in the United States is due to prejudice and related phenomena centered at the individual level and that racial and ethnic relations have improved significantly over the last several decades. Bonilla-Silva emphasizes the structural interpretations of racism and the new racism that has emerged in the post-Civil Rights era. He asserts that racism is entrenched in the structure of American society and affects all segments of life. Whites benefit from their position in the stratification system and thus, consciously as well as unconsciously, exhibit behaviors and attitudes that support the existing stratification system. One important aspect of his work involves the use of a multimethod, triangulation approach, utilizing both traditional survey methods and in-depth interviews, to get at whites' "true, more innermost" feelings concerning race relations. Bonilla-Silva's research suggests that whites have developed a sophisticated and elusive language to mask their true feelings regarding African Americans in the post-Civil Rights era.

METHODS, MEASURES, AND EMPIRICAL FINDINGS

This section covers methods and measures related to racial and ethnic groups and brings in, where appropriate, empirical findings. In particular, it discusses the data, measures, and analytical procedures used to study racial and ethnic groups.

Data Issues

As noted earlier, race and ethnicity are social constructs that shift over time, space, the life course, and with altering situations. This conception of race and ethnicity stands in sharp contrast to how demographers use race and ethnicity in their research (Waters 2002). Their statistical models, for instance, examine variations in race/ethnicity across groups rather than within individuals. Furthermore, the lack of attention to the social construction of race and ethnicity affects population projections about the future racial and ethnic composition of any population. Indeed, population projections assume that racial and ethnic boundaries and patterns of identification remain static into the future (Bean et al. 1997; Hirschman 2002; Perlmann 2002; Waters 2002; for a discussion of population projections involving Jews and Arabs in Jerusalem, see DellaPergola 2001).

This conventional population projection approach also assumes that people belong to a single racial or ethnic group (Bean et al. 1997), that the current meaning of racial and ethnic categories will continue to be meaningful in the future (Alba 1999), and that the impact of intermarriage is not significant enough to have one generation change categories over time (Alba 1999; Edmonston, Lee, and Passel 2002; Hirschman 2002; Waters 2002). Although it is difficult to project the significance and stability of racial and ethnic groups into the future, it is well known that a segment of the population includes multiracial individuals and that some racial and ethnic groups have relatively high intermarriage rates (see below). These are issues that demographers will need to address in their presentation and interpretation of population projections.

There are other racial and ethnic classification issues worth mentioning. For example, in the collection of census data one individual usually provides information on all household members. While this practice is likely to produce fairly accurate data in many instances, there is the potential for inaccuracies in households composed of unrelated individuals. In addition, there may also be differences in how children from intermarried couples are classified racially and ethnically by their parents.

The accuracy in the racial and ethnic classification of individuals is a particular problem in mortality research. Death certificates, which represent the data base for much mortality research, may be filled out by people who did not know the deceased. Hospital personnel and funeral directors may inaccurately identify the deceased in terms of their race or ethnicity (Farley 1996). Similar problems emerge in the study of fertility when the father of the infant is not known or reported. Differences are also likely to exist in how infants from intermarried couples are designated with respect to their race and ethnicity.

There are other methodological problems related to the measurement of demographic phenomena. For example, in mortality research, death rates assume that the numerator (deaths) and the denominator (population at risk) refer to the same population. However, the numbers used to generate these rates usually come from different data sources: vital statistics records for deaths (the numerators) and census data or population estimates for the population at risk (the denominators). This conventional approach is problematic when race and ethnicity are fluid or when people from certain racial and ethnic groups are highly geographically mobile. Sullivan and her colleagues (1984) describe the problems associated with estimating mortality rates for the Mexican American population. Such problems may also be associated with the epidemiological paradox among Latinos. Although this problem has been discussed primarily with respect to the computation of infant mortality rates, it is likely that the problem also affects the computation of fertility rates when immigrant women come to the United States to deliver their babies and then return to Mexico. In such instances, the births are in the numerator, but the mothers are not in the denominator. This may result in the fertility rates of Mexican-origin women being artificially inflated.

Measures Associated with Race/Ethnicity and Inequality

There are a number of measures of race and ethnicity and inequality. Data from the 2000 One Percent PUMS and related sources are used to illustrate these measures. The approaches for identifying the racial and ethnic membership of individuals are first presented.

RACE AND ETHNIC GROUP IDENTIFICATION.   Most of the data associated with the classification of people along racial and ethnic lines are driven by governmental decisions (Office of Management and Budget [OMB]) about the appropriate categories to be used in generating the data. (For an excellent overview of the historical measurement of race in the U.S. census, see Snipp [2003] and Lee [1993].) Recently the Office of Management and Budget (1997; see also OMB 1977) issued a revision of the racial categories on which U.S. federal statistics are to be collected. This mandate established six categories: white; Black or African American; American Indian or Alaskan Native; Asian; Native Hawaiian or other Pacific Islander; and Hispanic or Latino. Hispanics/ Latinos are considered to be an ethnic group, with members belonging to any race. As such, two questions are used to obtain information on racial identification and Hispanic/Latino identification. The Office of Management and Budget (2000) also mandated that individuals be allowed to select two or more racial categories.

Table 6.1 (Panel A) shows the distribution of the U.S. population across the six OMB-designated categories as reported in the 2000 census (Grieco and Cassidy 2001). Of the 281.4 million counted in the 2000 census, non-Hispanic whites represent the largest group. Of those who reported only one race, approximately 69% are non-Hispanic whites. Latinos and non-Hispanic African Americans each accounted for about 12% of the national population, with non-Hispanic Asians making up slightly less than 4%. Multiracial individuals (persons who reported more than one race) accounted for 2.4% (for a total of 6.8 million people including 4.6 non-Hispanics and 2.2 Hispanics) of the overall U.S. population.

TABLE 6.1. **Population of the United States by Racial/Ethnic Group and Hispanic/Latino Population by Racial Classification, 2000.**

Panel A. U.S. Population

Racial/Ethnic Group	Population	% U.S. Pop.
Non-Hispanic/Latino		
White alone	194,552,774	69.1
Black or African American alone	33,947,837	12.1
American Indian and Alaskan Native alone	2,068,883	0.7
Asian alone	10,123,169	3.6
Native Hawaiian and other Pacific Islander alone	353,509	0.1
Some other race alone	467,770	0.2
Two or more races	4,602,146	1.6
Hispanic/Latino	35,305,818	12.5
Total	281,421,906	100.0

Panel B. U.S. Hispanic/Latino Population by Race

Race	Population	% Hsp. or Lat. Pop.
White alone	16,907,852	47.9
Black or African American alone	710,353	2.0
American Indian and Alaskan Native alone	407,073	1.2
Asian alone	119,829	0.3
Native Hawaiian and other Pacific Islander alone	45,326	0.1
Some other race alone	14,891,303	42.2
Two or more races	2,224,082	6.3
Total Hispanic/Latino population	35,305,818	100.0

Source: Grieco and Cassidy (2001).

Table 6.1 (Panel B) reports the distribution of Latinos by race. Close to half (47.9%) of Latinos classified themselves as white, and more than two-fifths (42.2%) classified themselves as "other." There is a significant amount of variation in the racial classification of Latino subgroups. Table 6.2 shows the racial distribution of Latinos in the three largest Latino subgroups (Mexicans, Puerto Ricans, and Cubans). Cubans stand out with respect to their preference for the white racial identity with nearly 85% identifying themselves as white compared to slightly less than half of Mexicans (47.3%) and Puerto Ricans (47.0%). Mexicans (45.4%) and Puerto Ricans (38.4%) are more likely than Cubans (7.2%) to choose the "other" racial category. Yet, a noticeable percentage of Puerto Ricans (5.8%) and Cubans (3.6%) identify themselves as black

TABLE 6.2. **Percentage Distribution of Latinos by Race for Selected Ethnic Groups, 2000.**

Race	Mexican	Puerto Rican	Cuban
White alone	47.3	47.0	84.5
Black or African American alone	0.7	5.8	3.6
American Indian and Alaskan Native alone	1.1	0.5	0.1
Asian alone	0.2	0.4	0.2
Native Hawaiian and other Pacific Islander alone	0.1	0.2	0.1
Some other race alone	45.4	38.4	7.2
Two or more races	5.2	7.8	4.3

Source: 2000 1% PUMS.

compared to a smaller percentage of Mexicans (0.7%). Finally, Puerto Ricans (7.8%) are more likely than Mexicans (5.2%) and Cubans (4.3%) to be multiracial.

Data from the 2000 One Percent PUMS are used to examine variation in the presence of multiracial people across racial and ethnic groups. To conduct this exercise, for the non-Hispanic racial groups, combined racial groups have been established which consist of individuals who chose a given race regardless of how many races they select. For example, the combined white group consists of individuals who report they were only white, as well as multiracial individuals whose race classification included white. Figure 6.8 shows the variation across groups regarding the prevalence of multiracial individuals. More than three-fourths of non-Hispanics who chose the "Other" racial category (77.0%) are multiracial, as are slightly more than half of Native Hawaiians and Other Pacific Islanders (51.3%) and American Indians and Alaskan Natives (43.3%). Asians (13.0%) represent the only other group with more than one-tenth of group members reporting multiple races. On the other hand, non-Hispanic whites (2.0%) and blacks (4.3%) have the lowest percentages of their members reporting two or more racial categories.

OTHER RACE AND ETHNICITY MEASURES: NATIVITY AND CITIZENSHIP STATUS.   There is another dimension of race and ethnicity, namely, nativity and naturalization citizenship status among the foreign-born. Data from the 2000 One Percent PUMS are used to develop actual measures for 12 groups—whites, African Americans, American Indians, six groups of Asians (Asian Indians, Chinese, Filipinos, Japanese, Koreans, and Vietnamese), and three groups of Latinos (Mexicans, Puerto Ricans, and Cubans). Note that the first nine groups are non-Hispanic (for the sake of simplicity, the non-Hispanic designator will not be used). These racial and ethnic groups are the focus of analyses in the remainder of the chapter, except where data are not available for specific groups.

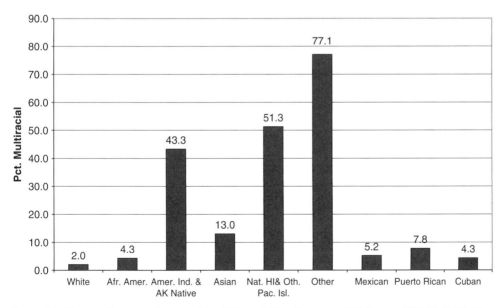

FIGURE 6.8. Percent of persons who are multiracial by racial/ethnic groups, 2000. Source: 2000 1% Public Use Microdata Sample (PUMS).

The 2000 census asked individuals to report their state and country of birth. Based on these data, persons may be classified into the native-born (including those born abroad to American citizens) and the foreign-born. Using these classifications, the percentages of members of each of the 12 groups who are foreign-born are computed (see Table 6.3). Six Asian and one Latino group have upward of two-thirds of their members who are foreign-born: Koreans (77.4%), Vietnamese (76.4%), Asian Indians (75.7%), Chinese (70.5%), Filipinos (69.0%), and Cubans (68.9%). Approximately two-fifths of Mexicans (41.3%) and Japanese (40.2%) were born outside of the United States. In contrast, relatively few African Americans (5.5%), whites (3.5%), Puerto Ricans (1.4%), and American Indians (1.0%) are foreign-born.

The 2000 One Percent PUMS data also permit the computation of naturalization rates for the foreign-born members of each of the 12 groups. The naturalization rate refers to the percentage of foreign-born individuals who have become U.S. naturalized citizens. Six groups have naturalization rates above 50%: Filipinos (62.2%), Cubans (60.6%), Vietnamese (58.9%), whites (54.8%), Chinese (52.5%), and Koreans (51.0%). On the other hand, Mexicans (22.1%) and Japanese (25.3%) have the lowest naturalization rates.

OTHER RACE AND ETHNICITY MEASURES: LANGUAGE AND INTERMARRIAGE. The final two dimensions of race and ethnicity to be examined are language (an indicator of acculturation) and intermarriage (an indicator of assimilation). The 2000 census asked individuals who were at least five years of age two questions related to language, namely, whether a language other than English was spoken at home and, for these individuals, their level of fluency in English. Using this information in the 2000 One Percent PUMS, respondents may be categorized into three categories: (1) monolingual English speakers (those speaking English at home); (2) bilingual (those speaking a language other than English at home and who speak English "well" or "very well"); and (3) monolingual non-English speakers (those speaking a language other than English at home and who speak English "not well" or "not at all"). This is not a perfect measure of language abilities. Indeed, individuals who are truly bilingual are classified as monolingual English speakers if they speak only English at home. In addition, respondents may inaccurately assess the language abilities of other household members.

Because language abilities are likely to be related to age and nativity, analyses are restricted to persons 25 to 44 years of age and conducted separately for the native- and foreign-born groups. Note that because of small numbers of foreign-born American Indians and Puerto Ricans, they are not included in subsequent analyses involving the foreign-born. Table 6.3 shows the percentage distribution of native- and foreign-born individuals in the 12 groups across the three language categories. Among the native-born groups, with the exception of Vietnamese and members of the three Latino groups, most people in the other groups are likely to be monolingual English speakers. Five groups have more than three-fourths of their members speaking English at home: African Americans (96.8%), whites (96.6%), Japanese (89.6%), Filipinos (75.5%), and American Indians (75.2%). However, the greatest portion of Puerto Ricans (71.0%), Cubans (68.1%), Mexicans (56.9%), and Vietnamese (48.7%) are bilingual speakers and also show the greatest tendency to be monolingual non-English speakers. Among foreign-born persons, except for Mexicans, most members are bilingual speakers with percentages ranging from 59.3% among whites to 84.8% among Filipinos. On the other hand, the majority (51.7%) of Mexicans are monolingual Spanish speakers.

TABLE 6.3. Selected Racial/Ethnic Indicators by Racial/Ethnic Group, 2000.

Indicators	White	African Amer.	Amer. Indian	Asian Indian	Chinese	Filipino	Japanese	Korean	Vietnamese	Mexican	Puerto Rican	Cuban
% Foreign-born	3.5	5.5	1	75.7	70.5	69	40.2	77.4	76.4	41.3	1.4	68.9
% of FB naturalized citizens	54.8	44.6	44.8	38.7	52.5	62.2	25.3	51	58.9	22.1	38.8	60.6
Language patterns (Pop. 25–44)												
% NB English	96.6	96.8	75.2	55	61.6	75.5	89.6	67.4	47.1	40	20.6	31
% NB bilingual	3.2	2.8	23.5	43.5	36.4	23.1	9.7	30.4	48.7	56.9	71	68.1
% NB native language	0.3	0.4	1.3	1.5	2	1.4	0.7	2.2	4.2	3.2	8.4	0.9
% FB English	31.9	51.4	53.6	12.8	6.2	12.5	9	11.4	4.5	5.3	11.5	5.2
% FB bilingual	59.3	43	34.3	82.5	71.4	84.8	66.9	63.7	66.2	43	58.2	66.1
% FB native language	8.8	5.6	12.1	4.8	22.4	2.8	24.1	24.9	29.3	51.7	30.3	28.7
Intermarriage with whites (<35)												
% NB male with white wife	N/A	8.8	47.2	*	*	*	*	*	*	23.4	20.2	41.2
% NB female with white husb.	N/A	3.1	45.1	*	*	*	*	*	*	23.9	20.3	36.7
% FB male with white wife	N/A	6.7	N/A	4.3	3.9	12.7	8.6	5.8	2.5	4.6	N/A	9.8
% FB female with white husb.	N/A	4.7	N/A	3.6	9.2	30.4	33	19.2	7.4	3.2	N/A	6.2

Source: 2000 1% PUMS.

Note: NB=native-born; FB=foreign-born.

*Because of small sample sizes, the percentages for the six NB groups have been aggregated into NB Asian: 25.2% of Asian NB males are married to white females; 39.5% of NB Asian females are married to white males.

The 2000 One Percent PUMS also allows the development of data to compare the racial and ethnic identity of spouses. Percentages of married persons in each of the 11 non-white groups who have a white spouse are obtained. Because the 2000 census data measure the incidence of marriage regardless of when the marriages were contracted, the analysis is limited to persons less than 35 years of age in order to capture more recent marriages as opposed to those that occurred in the more distant past. In addition, intermarriage percentages are computed separately for native- and foreign-born individuals. Moreover, because of the small size of native-born individuals in the six specific Asian groups, these are aggregated into a single native-born Asian group. Finally, the intermarriage percentages are broken down by gender.

Table 6.3 reports the intermarriage rates for the 11 groups broken down by nativity status and gender. Among native-born married individuals, American Indians (males, 47.2%; females, 45.1%), Cubans (males, 41.2%; females, 36.7%), and Asian females (39.5%) are the most likely to be married to whites. About one-fifth to one-fourth of Mexicans, Puerto Ricans, and Asian males have a white spouse. African Americans, particularly females, are the least likely to be married to whites, reflecting the rigid color line in American society. By and large, foreign-born individuals tend to be less likely to be intermarried with whites. Nonetheless, three groups of foreign-born Asian women— Japanese (33.0%), Filipinas (30.4%), and Koreans (19.2%)—are the most likely to have exchanged wedding vows with a white male. It is likely that some of these marriages consist of "war bride" unions involving U.S. servicemen and Asian women (see Saenz, Hwang, and Aguirre 1994). In addition, among foreign-born males, Filipinos (12.7%), Cubans (9.8%), and Japanese (8.6%) are the most likely to be married to white women. In contrast, seven foreign-born groups have intermarriage rates below 5%: Vietnamese men (2.5%), Mexican women (3.2%), Asian Indian women (3.6%), Chinese men (3.9%), Asian Indian men (4.3%), Mexican men (4.6%), and African American females (4.7%).

MEASURES OF INEQUALITY. A few measures of inequality that are commonly used to assess differences between racial and ethnic groups are now discussed. Readers interested in a wider array of measures of inequality should consult Iceland, Weinberg, and Steinmetz (2002), Lieberson (1975), Massey and Denton (1988), and Massey, White, and Phua (1996). Attention is focused here on two dimensions of inequality, namely, spatial inequality and earnings inequality.

MEASURES OF SPATIAL INEQUALITY. Two popular measures for assessing spatial inequality are the dissimilarity index and the isolation index. The dissimilarity index is the most common measure used for assessing distributional differences between two groups (Iceland et al. 2002). Although this index is commonly used to measure differences in residential patterns between groups, it is quite flexible and may be used to assess distributional differences in a wide variety of phenomena (e.g., income categories, educational categories, occupational categories, industrial categories, etc.). The dissimilarity index may be defined as:

$$\text{Dissimilarity Index} = [\Sigma \; |(pa_i - pb_i)|] / 2$$

where pa_i refers to the proportion of members of a given minority group in unit i, and pb_i refers to the proportion of members of the majority group in unit i. The absolute differences are summed across the units and divided by two. The dissimilarity index ranges from 0 to 1. It represents the proportional amount of one or the other group needing to change to certain other units in order to achieve the same distributions.

The isolation index is defined as:

$$\text{Isolation Index} = \Sigma[\,(x_i\,/\,X)\,(x_i\,/\,t_i)\,]$$

where x_i refers to the minority population size in a unit, X refers to the total minority population size across all units, and t_i is the total population in a given unit. The isolation index ranges from 0 to 1 and represents the probability that a given minority group member is likely to come into contact with a member of one's own group.

We use data from the analysis of Iceland and associates (2002) that is based on the construction of five indices, including the dissimilarity index and the isolation index, for Metropolitan Areas (MAs) in the United States, using census tract data from the 1980, 1990, and 2000 censuses. For an example of research using these two indexes in another country, China, see Poston and Micklin (1993). Iceland and his colleagues obtained weighted average indices based on all MAs, as well as others based on selected MAs that meet given population size criteria. For the sake of simplicity, weighted average indices based on all MAs are used. Figure 6.9 shows the weighted average dissimilarity and isolation indices for 2000. The results indicate that African Americans are the most segregated from whites. The dissimilarity index of 0.640 for African Americans indicates that, on average, in any given MA in the United States, nearly two-thirds (64%) of either African Americans or whites would need to move to certain other census tracts in order to bring about equal spatial patterns for the two groups. Latinos also tend to have a high level of spatial segregation, with approximately half of Latinos or whites having to shift to certain other census tracts to bring about the same geographical distributions for the two groups. The isolation indices for African Americans and Latinos indicate

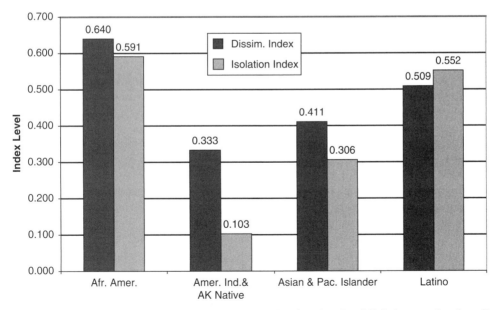

FIGURE 6.9. Weighted average dissimilarity and isolation indices for selected racial/ethnic groups based on all metropolitan areas, 2000. Source: Iceland et al. 2002.

that, on average, members of each group have a high likelihood of coming into contact with members of their own group, with African Americans having an average probability of 0.591, and Latinos a probability of 0.552. The results show that Asians and Pacific Islanders have a moderate level of spatial segregation, and American Indians and Alaskan Natives have the lowest degree of geographical separation. For an examination of research on residential segregation outside of the United States, see the work of Johnston, Forrest, and Poulsen (2002), Ladanyi (1993), Phillips (1998), Telles (1992), and Van Kempen and Van Weesep (1998).

MEASURE OF EARNINGS INEQUALITY.   Sociologists, demographers, and labor economists have observed a significant amount of variation in earnings across workers from different racial and ethnic backgrounds. Indeed, research has shown that certain groups, especially minority groups, forego a certain level of earnings due to their racial or ethnic group membership (Cotton 1985, 1988, 1989; Darity and Myers 2001; Dodoo and Takyi 2002; Durden and Gaynor 1998; Poston and Alvirez 1973; Poston, Alvirez, and Tienda 1976; Skinner 2002; Verdugo 1992; Verdugo and Verdugo 1984, 1988; Wong 1982. For a discussion of similar studies in Latin America, see Patrinos 2000; for research based on Israel, see Lewin-Epstein and Semyonov 1992; Semyonov 1997, Semyonov and Cohen 1990). These studies typically do not obtain direct measures of labor market discrimination based on race and ethnicity. However, they commonly treat differences in earnings between minority and majority workers that remain after making appropriate statistical adjustments as proxies of such discrimination. Data from the 2000 One Percent PUMS are now used to examine the earnings of a variety of racial and ethnic groups. The analysis is conducted separately on the basis of nativity and gender. For the analysis involving the native-born, the earnings of whites, African Americans, American Indians, Asians, Mexican Americans, Puerto Ricans, and Cubans are compared. For the analysis involving the foreign-born, the earnings of whites, African Americans, Asian Indians, Chinese, Filipinos, Japanese, Koreans, Vietnamese, Mexicans, and Cubans are compared. The samples consist of persons who worked for wages and for at least 1,040 hours in 1999. The criterion for amount of time worked during the year is imposed to ensure that the workers included in the analysis have fairly stable employment patterns. The minimum of 1,040 hours of work in 1999 translates to full-time employment for half a year or to half-time work over the entire year.

Hourly wages are obtained by dividing the wages of a given worker by the total number of hours he or she worked during 1999. For the multivariate part of the analysis, the natural logarithm of hourly wage is used to minimize the statistical influence of outliers in the distribution. Because the log of earnings is used, the regression coefficients may be interpreted as the proportion change in earnings given a unit change in a given independent variable. The major independent variable is race/ethnic membership measured with a series of dummy variables created for the nonwhite racial and ethnic groups noted above. Whites are the reference category. Many control variables that are commonly used in research examining earnings are included, such as age, language, educational level, occupation, experience (age-years of education-5), experience squared, marital status, disability, metropolitan/nonmetropolitan residence, and region of residence. In the foreign-born analysis, control variables based on period of entry into the United States and on naturalized citizenship status are also included; for the analysis involving women, a control variable based on the presence and age of children is also included in the analysis. Appendix A contains the list of variables in the analysis along with their operationalization. The analysis is carried out using ordinary least squares (OLS) regression.

Table 6.4 reports the results of the analysis. The left portion of the table shows the median hourly wages of the different groups in the analysis. Among the seven native-born groups, the highest hourly wages were earned by Asians, whites, and Cubans, with Mexicans and American Indians having the lowest earnings. Among the 10 foreign-born groups, Asian Indians, Japanese, Chinese, and whites clearly have the highest hourly wages, and Mexicans, Cubans, and Vietnamese have the lowest earnings. However, because the groups differ significantly on a variety of factors (e.g., education, age, occupation, and other variables), regression analyses should be conducted to control for the influence of these factors.

The right portion of Table 6.4 contains the regression coefficients reporting the relationship between racial and ethnic group membership and logged hourly wage, after controlling for a variety of other variables (see Appendix A). Among native-born workers, after taking into account the series of control variables, Asians and Cuban males have significantly higher wages than their white peers. For example, Cuban and Asian men have hourly earnings that are 7.4% higher and 2.6% higher, respectively, than those of white men. Asian women have hourly wages that are 9% higher than those of white women. In contrast, African American, American Indian, Mexican, and Puerto Rican workers have significantly lower hourly wages than their white counterparts. The

TABLE 6.4. **Median Hourly Wages and Ordinary Least Square Regression Coefficients Associated with the Relationship Between Racial/Ethnic Group Membership and the Logged Hourly Wages in 1999**

Race/Ethnic Group	Mdn. Hourly Wage ($)		OLS Regr. Coeff.			
	Male	Female	Male		Female	
Native-born						
White	16.15	12.36	RG		RG	
African American	12.50	11.22	−0.116	**	−0.022	**
American Indian	12.02	9.62	−0.120	**	−0.081	**
Asian	17.81	15.38	0.026	*	0.090	**
Mexican	11.80	10.35	−0.100	**	−0.045	**
Puerto Rican	12.79	11.06	−0.069	**	−0.015	*
Cuban	14.42	12.50	0.074	**	0.038	
Foreign-born						
White	18.91	13.26	RG		RG	
African American	13.84	12.50	−0.176	**	0.005	
Asian Indian	21.79	15.38	−0.011		0.034	**
Chinese	16.83	14.22	−0.158	**	−0.011	
Filipino	14.90	14.10	−0.161	**	0.016	
Japanese	23.69	13.46	0.219	**	−0.002	
Korean	15.63	12.00	−0.175	**	−0.038	*
Vietnamese	13.12	10.47	−0.127	**	0.030	*
Mexican	8.97	7.50	−0.199	**	−0.126	**
Cuban	12.28	10.83	−0.161	**	−0.056	**

Source: 2000 1% PUMS.

Note: RG = Reference group. The regression coefficients shown are from a model that includes a variety of control variables (see Appendix A).

*Significant at the 0.05 level.
**Significant at the 0.01 level.

gaps are greatest for American Indian men, African American men, Mexican men, and American Indian women.

Among foreign-born workers, only Japanese men, Asian Indian women, and Vietnamese women have significantly higher hourly wages compared to their respective white counterparts. In the case of men, workers in all other groups, except Asian Indians, have significantly lower earnings compared to white men. The greatest gaps occur among Mexicans, African Americans, Koreans, Filipinos, and Cubans. In the case of women, only Mexicans, Cubans, and Koreans have earnings that are significantly lower than those of white women, with the largest discrepancy taking place among Mexican women.

Analytical Procedures Issues

The final part of this section presents an overview of issues involving common analytical procedures that demographers use to study minority groups. One of the most debated issues deals with the measurement of discrimination. Specifically, a common methodological problem in the demography of race and ethnicity is measuring discrimination as a residual effect after controlling for differences in human capital and other attributes (Follett, Ward, and Welch 1993; Bonilla-Silva 2001; Hamilton 2000; Sakamoto, Wu, and Tzeng 2000). This procedure attributes to discrimination the portion of the behavior that is statistically unexplained or unmeasured.

One problem with this approach is that the controls may well mask the effect of minority status and thus underestimate the impact of discrimination (Killingsworth 1993; Sakamoto 2000; Bonilla-Silva 2001). This problem acknowledges that race/ethnicity is not a single factor that can be reduced to one variable, but one that is integrated in several other factors. For example, studies of labor market outcomes tend to overcontrol when including indicators such as occupational processes and educational status which are products of discrimination. Another problem involves the omission of relevant variables from the analysis (see Killingsworth 1993). These variables are hence subsumed in the error term, which is correlated with other variables in the model, resulting in biased estimates. Killingsworth (1993) notes two problems. First, the coefficients that already embody discriminatory aspects measure only "incremental" discrimination, or the effects that are not already embodied in the discrimination-induced differences in those variables. The second is a statistical problem in which the coefficients affected by discrimination suffer from statistical biases. Biased coefficients are then endogenous, and conventional regression estimates do not provide unbiased estimates on the extent of "increment" discrimination (see also the work of Shulman 1989; DeVaro and Lacker 1995; Hamilton 2000).

Zuberi (2001) also examines the intersection of race and methodology and provides a critical analysis of racial data. He asserts that in demography and the social sciences the definition of race has elements of eugenics, with statistical methods being mathematically rather than theoretically based. The major error in racial statistics deals with matters involving interpretation. He claims that researchers often mistakenly argue that race causes a certain dependent variable when in actuality the analysis only reveals an association between these variables. This interpretation of race as a causal factor has been used in theoretical arguments such as genetics, culture, or discrimination. This leads to erroneous conclusions about the significance and the implications of race.

Zuberi (2001) thus argues for the deracialization of statistical analysis by recognizing the importance of history and the goal of achieving racial justice.

Before leaving this topic, the critical demography paradigm of Horton (1999, 2002) is presented owing to the belief that this development has a significant amount of promise for the study of the demography of racial and ethnic groups. It permits the bridging of methodological and theoretical issues. Horton has critiqued traditional demography for paying relatively little substantive attention to the study of race and ethnicity. While demographers have used race and ethnicity in their work, much work in traditional demography has used race and ethnicity as controls. That is, many demographers tend to be interested in a given topic (e.g., health, fertility, or migration) and mechanically enter race and ethnicity into the model to control for racial and ethnic variation. They then report the relationships between race/ethnicity and the dependent variable without attempting to identify and understand the mechanism linking race and ethnicity to the outcome variable of interest. Horton (1999) calls on demographers to examine race and ethnicity with a more critical lens through greater attention to theoretical perspectives drawn from the race and ethnicity literature; to develop a more critical orientation toward the measures, indicators, and methods that demographers use; and to identify the mechanisms that produce and sustain racial and ethnic stratification. Specifically, he urges demographers to incorporate the concept of *racism* into their research to capture the mechanism underlying the relationship between race and ethnicity and inequality. Horton (2002:270) points out that:

> In the case of racial and ethnic demography, it is maintained here that one of the concepts that facilitates theoretical development is *racism*. Unlike the demographic transition, the baby boom and bust, the met-nonmetropolitan turnaround, or any of the major trends that we demographers have written about and debated, racism has consistently been an intrinsic element in the historical demography of the United States and the Western world. Moreover, there is ample evidence that it will play a major, if not pivotal, role in America's demographic future.

Some research that falls within the domain of critical demography includes the theoretical development of Hummer (1996) and the methodological critique of Zuberi (2001).

RESEARCH DIRECTIONS

This final section provides an overview of future directions for research in the demography of racial and ethnic groups. It first presents general discussion of the usefulness of the critical demography paradigm in guiding future research on the demography of race and ethnicity. In line with the critical demography paradigm, it argues that in order for demographers to uncover the essence of inequality involving minority groups, the use of race and ethnicity needs to move beyond the control variable approach to a more sophisticated understanding of these concepts. This will require that demographers historicize and contextualize the standing of racial and ethnic groups and how these factors are likely to affect the observed relationships uncovered through statistical analysis. Only with more substantive attention to race and ethnicity can demographers have any hope of uncovering the mechanisms that sustain the stratification of racial and ethnic groups. The training of the next generation of scholars to undertake research on minority groups needs to include theoretical developments in the area of race and ethnicity in sociology and related disciplines, the historical understanding of these groups, and the development of skills in both qualitative methods and quantitative methods.

Attention is now directed to specific areas that have the potential for important advancements related to the demography of race and ethnicity. These include research on multiracial individuals, the study of minority groups on the basis of nativity, and the intersection of race, class, gender, sexuality, and color. The 2000 U.S. census presents demographers with an excellent opportunity to advance beyond the traditional ways of viewing race and ethnicity. The multiracial category is a principal mechanism for moving beyond the static notion of race and ethnicity that has marked much of the existing work in the demography of racial and ethnic groups. Possible research projects based on multiracial individuals include the examination of the links between multiracial identity and social and economic outcomes, analysis of marriage patterns of the multiracial, study of the racial and ethnic identification of the children of multiracial individuals, and the development of population projections taking into account the presence of multiracial persons.

In addition, research based on groups with significant levels of immigration is needed, but the populations should not be treated as homogeneous. For example, existing research on Latinos and Asians is often based on the entire groups or on immigrant populations. Such research is likely to produce a slanted portrait of the experiences of these groups in the United States if the distinct social worlds of the native-born and foreign-born are not considered. The analyses shown in this chapter indicate that native-born Asians have experienced a significant amount of upward mobility, as have their foreign-born counterparts. Moreover, native-born Cubans have attained a significant amount of upward mobility compared to their Mexican and Puerto Rican counterparts. Foreign-born Mexicans are located at the bottom of the social and economic ladder on a wide variety of dimensions.

It will also be important to examine intragroup relations on the basis of nativity. In this respect, a research topic such as intragroup residential and marriage patterns holds promise for the better understanding of relationships between native- and foreign-born members of racial and ethnic groups. Moreover, given the changing demographic patterns based on race and ethnicity, it will also be important to examine shifting racial and ethnic boundaries and the establishment of panethnic groups, as well as interracial and interethnic coalitions.

Furthermore, it is clear that stratification and inequality are multidimensional and extend beyond simply race and ethnicity. Indeed, they exist also on the basis of other attributes, such as nativity, gender, class, sexuality, and skin color. To date, efforts to integrate these dimensions in a coherent fashion are limited. The development of integrative models requires that demographers use their sociological imaginations to develop theoretical models and creative research designs to enhance the understanding of how race and ethnicity interact with a variety of other attributes to produce and sustain stratification and inequality.

REFERENCES

Abraido-Lanza, A. F., B. P. Dohrenwend, D. S. Ng-Mak, and J. B. Turner. 1999. The Latino mortality paradox: A test of the "salmon bias" and health migrant hypotheses. *American Journal of Public Health* 89:1543–1548.

Alba, R. D. 1999. Immigration and the American realities of assimilation and multiculturalism. *Sociological Forum* 14:3–25.

Alba, R. D., and J. R. Logan. 1993. Minority proximity to whites in suburbs: An individual-level analysis of segregation. *American Journal of Sociology* 98:1388–1427.

Allen, W., E. Telles, and M. Hunter. 2000. Skin color, income and education: A comparison of African Americans and Mexican Americans. *National Journal of Sociology* 12:129–180.

Allman, K. M. 1996. (Un)Natural boundaries: Mixed race, gender, and sexuality. In *The multiracial experience: Racial borders as the new frontier*. Edited by M. P. P. Root, 277–290. Thousand Oaks, Calif: Sage Publications.

Anderson, R. N., and R. Saenz. 1994. Structural determinants of Mexican American intermarriages, 1975–1980. *Social Science Quarterly* 75:414–430.

Anderson, B. A., and B. D. Silver. 1989. Demographic sources of the changing ethnic composition of the Soviet Union. *Population and Development Review* 15:609–656.

Arias, E., and B. L. Smith. 2003. *Deaths: Preliminary data for 2001.* National Vital Statistics Reports, Vol. 51, No. 5. Hyattsville, Md.: National Center for Health Statistics.

Arias, E., R. N. Anderson, H., S. L. Murphy, and K. D. Kochanek. 2003. *Deaths: Final data for 2001.* National Vital Statistics Reports, Vol. 52, No. 3. Hyattsville, Md.: National Center for Health Statistics.

Bean, F. D., R. R. Berg, and J. V. W. Van Hook. 1996. Socioeconomic and cultural incorporation and marital disruption among Mexican Americans. *Social Forces* 75(2):593–617.

Bean, F. D., R. G. Cushing, C. W. Haynes, and J. V. W. Van Hook. 1997. Immigration and the social contract. *Social Science Quarterly* 78:249–268.

Bean, F. D., C. G. Swicegood, and R. Berg. 2000. Mexican-origin fertility: New patterns and interpretations. *Social Science Quarterly* 81:404–420.

Blalock, H. M. 1967. *Toward a theory of minority-group relations.* New York: Wiley.

Blau, P. M. 1977. *Inequality and heterogeneity: A primitive of social structure.* New York: Free Press.

Blau, P. M. 1994. *Structural contexts of opportunities.* Chicago: University of Chicago Press.

Blau, P. M., and J. E. Schwartz. 1997. *Crosscutting social circles: Testing a macrostructural theory of intergroup relations*, 2nd ed. Brunswick, N.J.: Transaction.

Blauner, R. A. 1969. Internal colonialism and ghetto revolt. *Social Problems* 16:393–408.

Blauner, R. A. 1972. *Racial oppression in America.* New York: Harper.

Bonilla-Silva, E. 1997. Rethinking racism: Toward a structural interpretation. *American Sociological Review* 62:465–480.

Bonilla-Silva, E. 2001. *White supremacy and racism in the post-civil rights era.* Boulder, Colo.: Lynne Rienner.

Bonilla-Silva, E. 2003. *Racism without racists: Color blind racism and the persistence of racial inequality in the United States.* Lanham, Md.: Rowman and Littlefield.

Borchigud, W. 1995. Transgressing ethnic and national boundaries: Contemporary "Inner Mongolian" identities in China. In *Negotiating ethnicities in China and Taiwan.* Edited by M. J. Brown, 160–181. Berkeley: Institute of East Asian Studies, University of California.

Carter, M. 2000. Fertility of Mexican immigrant women in the U.S.: A closer look. *Social Science Quarterly* 81:1073–1086.

Chang, C. 2003. *Fertility patterns among the minority populations of China: A multilevel analysis.* Unpublished Ph.D. dissertation. College Station: Texas A&M University.

Chew, K. S. Y., D. J. Eggebeen, and P. R. Uhlenberg. 1989. American children in multiracial households. *Sociological Perspectives* 32:65–85.

Christian, M. 2000. *Multiracial identity: An international perspective.* New York: Palgrave Macmillan.

Cotton, J. 1985. Decomposing income, earnings, and wage differentials: A reformulation of method. *Sociological Methods and Research* 14:201–216.

Cotton, J. 1988. Discrimination and favoritism in the U.S. labor market: The cost to a wage earner of being female and black and the benefit of being male and white. *The American Journal of Economics and Sociology* 47:15–28.

Cotton, J. 1989. Opening the gap: The decline in black economic indicators in the 1980s. *Social Science Quarterly* 70:803–819.

Cox, O. C. 1948. *Caste, class, and race.* New York: Monthly Review Press.

Cready, C. M., and R. Saenz. 1997. The nonmetero/metro context of racial/ethnic outmarriage: Some differences between African Americans and Mexican Americans. *Rural Sociology*, 62:355–362.

Cruz-Janzen, M. 2002. Ethnic identity and racial formations: Race and racism American-Style and *à lo latino*. In *Transnational Latina/o communities: politics, processes, and cultures*. Edited by C. G. Velez-Ibanez and A. Sampaio. Lanham, Md.: Rowman and Littlefield.

Darity, W. A., Jr., and S. L. Myers, Jr. 2001. Why did black relative earnings surge in the early 1990s? *Journal of Economic Issues* 35:533–542.

de la Cadena, M. 2001. Reconstructing race: Racism, culture and mestizaje in Latin America. *NACLA Report on the Americas* 34 (May–June):16–23.

DellaPergola, S. 2001. Jerusalem's population, 1995–2020: Demography, multiculturalism and urban policies. *European Journal of Population* 17:165–199.

DeVaro, J. L., and J. M. Lacker. 1995. Errors in variables and lending discrimination. *Federal Serve Bank of Richmond Economic Quarterly* 81:19–32.

Dikotter, F. 1992. *The discourse of race in modern China*. Palo Alton, Calif.: Stanford University Press.

Doane, A. W., and E. Bonilla-Silva, eds. 2003. *White out: The continuing significance of racism*. New York: Routledge.

Dodoo, F. N., and B. K. Takyi. 2002. Africans in the diaspora: Black-white earnings differences among America's Africans. *Ethnic and Racial Studies* 25:913–941.

Drake, S., and H. R. Cayton. 1945. *Black metropolis: A study of Negro Life in a northern city*. New York: Harper and Row.

Du Bois, W. E. B. 1896. *The suppression of the African slave-trade to the United States of America, 1638–1870*. New York: Schocken Books.

Du Bois, W. E. B. 1903. *The souls of black folk*. New York: Fawcett World Library.

Du Bois, W. E. B. 1909. *The Negro American family*. Cambridge, Mass.: MIT Press.

Durden, G. C., and P. E. Gaynor. 1998. More on the cost of being other than white and male: Measurement of race, ethnic, and gender effects on yearly earnings. *The American Journal of Economics and Sociology* 57:95–103.

Echevarria, S., and W. P. Frisbie. 2001. Race/ethnic-specific variation in adequacy of prenatal care utilization. *Social Forces* 80:633–654.

Edmonston, B., S. M. Lee, and J. S. Passel. 2002. Recent trends in intermarriage and immigration and their effects on the future racial composition of the U.S. population. In *The new race question: How the census counts multiracial individuals*. Edited by J. Perlmann and M. Waters, 227–258. New York: Russell Sage Foundation.

Eschbach, K. 1995. The enduring and vanishing American Indian: American Indian population growth and intermarriage in 1990. *Ethnic and Racial Studies* 18:89–108.

Eschbach, K., and C. Gomez. 1998. Choosing Hispanic identity: Ethnic identity switching among respondents to high school and beyond. *Social Science Quarterly* 79:74–90.

Espino, R., and M. M. Franz. 2002. Latino phenotypic discrimination revisited: The impact of skin color on occupational status. *Social Science Quarterly* 83:612–623.

Fang, D., and D. Brown. 1999. Geographic mobility of the foreign-born Chinese in large metropolises, 1985–1990. *International Migration Review* 33:137–155.

Farley, R. 1996. *The new American reality: Who we are, how we got there, where we are going*. New York: Russell Sage Foundation.

Feagin, J. R. 2001. *Racist America: Roots, current realities and future reparations*. New York: Routledge.

Feagin, J. R., and E. O'Brien. 2003. *White men on race*. Boston: Beacon Press.

Feagin, J. R., and M. P. Sikes. 1994. *Living with racism: The black middle-class experience*. Boston: Beacon Press.

Feagin, J. R., and H. Vera. 2000. *White racism: The basics*, 2nd ed. New York: Routledge.

Ferrante, J, and P. Brown, Jr. 1999. Classifying people by race. In *Race and ethnic conflict: Contending views on prejudice, discrimination, and ethnoviolence*. Edited by F. L. Pincus and H. J. Ehrlich, 14–23. Boulder, Colo.: Westview Press.

Follett, R. S., M. P. Ward, and F. Welch. 1993. Problems in assessing employment discrimination. *American Economic Review* 83:73–78.

Forbes, D., W. P. Frisbie, R. A. Hummer, S. G. Pullum, and S. Echevarria. 2000. A comparison of Hispanic and Anglo compromised birth outcomes and cause-specific infant mortality in the United States, 1989–1991. *Social Science Quarterly* 81:439–458.

Ford, K. 1990. Duration of residence in the United States and the fertility of U.S. immigrants. *International Migration Review* 24:34–68.

Fossett, M. A., and K. J. Kiecolt. 1989. The relative size of minority populations and white racial attitudes. *Social Science Quarterly* 70:820–835.

Fossett, M. A., and M. T. Siebert. 1997. *Long time coming: Racial inequality in the nonmetropolitan South, 1940–1990.* Boulder, Colo.: Westview Press.

Frankenberg, R. 1993. *White women, race matters: The social construction of whiteness.* Minneapolis: University of Minnesota Press.

Frazier, E. F. 1939. *The Negro family in the United States.* Chicago: University of Chicago Press.

Frazier, E. F. 1949. *The Negro in the United States.* New York: Macmillan.

Frazier, E. F. 1957. *Black bourgeoisie: The rise of a new middle class in the United States.* New York: The Free Press.

Frisbie, W. P., and L. Neidert. 1977. Inequality and the relative group size of minority populations: A comparative analysis. *American Journal of Sociology* 82:1007–1030.

Gans, H. 1979. Symbolic ethnicity: The future of ethnic groups and cultures in America. *Ethnic and Racial Studies* 2:1–20.

Gatson, S. N. 2003. On being amorphous: Autoethnography, genealogy, and a multiracial identity. *Qualitative Inquiry* 9:20–48.

Gladney, D. C. 1994. Representing nationality in China: refiguring majority/minority identities. *The Journal of Asian Studies* 53:92–123.

Glazer, N. 2002. Do we need the census race question? *The Public Interest* 149:21–31.

Gomez, C. 2000. The continual significance of skin color: An explanatory study of Latinos in the Northeast. *Hispanic Journal of Behavioral Sciences* 22:94 –103.

Gordon, M. 1964. *Assimilation in American life: The role of race, religion and national origins.* New York: Oxford University Press.

Grieco, E., and R. C. Cassidy. 2001. *Overview of race and Hispanic origin.* Census 2000 Brief C2KBR/01–1. Washington, D.C.: U.S. Census Bureau.

Gross, A. B., and D. S. Massey. 1991. Spatial assimilation models: A micro-macro comparison. *Social Science Quarterly* 72:347–360.

Gualtieri, S. 2001. Becoming "white": Race, religion and the foundations of Syrian/Lebanese ethnicity in the United States. *Journal of American Ethnic History* 20(4):29–58.

Hall, R. 1994. The "bleaching syndrome": Implications of light skin for Hispanic American assimilation. *Hispanic Journal of Behavioral Sciences* 16:307–314.

Hall, R. 1995. The bleaching syndrome: African Americans' response to cultural domination vis-à-vis skin color. *Journal of Black Studies* 26:172–184.

Halli, S. S. 1987. *How minority status affects fertility: Asian groups in Canada.* Westport, Conn.: Greenwood Press.

Hamilton, D. 2000. Issues concerning discrimination and measurement of discrimination in U.S. labor markets. *African American Research Perspectives* 6:98–111.

Hamilton, B. E., J. A. Martin, and P. D. Sutton. 2003. *Births: Preliminary data for 2002.* National Vital Statistics Reports, Vol. 51, No. 11. Hyattsville, Md.: National Center for Health Statistics.

Hauser, P. M., and O. D. Duncan. 1959. *The study of population: An inventory and appraisal.* Chicago: University of Chicago Press.

Hayes-Bautista, D. E. 2003. Research on culturally competent healthcare systems: Less sensitivity, more statistics. *American Journal of Preventive Medicine* 24(3S):8–9.

Herring, C. 1989. Convergence, polarization, or what?: Racially based changes in attitudes and outlooks, 1964–1984. *The Sociological Quarterly* 30:27–81.

Hill, M. E. 2000. Color differences in the socioeconomic status of African American men: Results of a longitudinal study. *Social Forces* 78:1437–1460.

Hill, M. E. 2002. Skin color and the perception of attractiveness among African Americans: Does gender make a difference? *Social Psychology Quarterly* 65:77–91.

Hirschman, C. 2002. Race and ethnic population projections: A critical evaluation of their content and meaning. In *American diversity: A demographic challenge for the twenty-first century.* Edited by N. A. Denton and S. E. Tolnay, 51–72. Albany: State University of New York Press.

Horton, H. D. 1995. Population change and the employment status of college educated blacks. *Research in Race and Ethnic Relations* 8:99–114.

Horton, H. D. 1999. Critical demography: The paradigm of the future? *Sociological Forum* 14:363–367.

Horton, H. D. 2002. Rethinking American diversity: Conceptual and theoretical challenges for racial and ethnic demography. In *American diversity: A demographic challenge for the twenty-first century.* Edited by N. A. Denton and S. E. Tolnay, 261–278. Albany: State University of New York Press.

Hout, M. 1984. Occupational mobility of black men: 1962 to 1973. *American Sociological Review* 49:308–322.

Hughes, M., and B. R. Hertel. 1990. The significance of color remains: A study of life chances, mate selection, and ethnic consciousness among black Americans. *Social Forces* 68:1105–1020.

Hummer, R. A. 1996. Black-white differences in health and morality: A review and conceptual model. *The Sociological Quarterly* 37:105–125.

Hummer, R. A., R. G. Rogers, S. H. Amir, D. Forbes, and W. P. Frisbie. 2000. Adult mortality differences among Hispanic subgroups and non-Hispanic whites. *Social Science Quarterly* 81:459–476.

Hunter, M. L. 2002. "If you're light you're alright": Light skin color as social capital for women of color. *Gender & Society* 16:175–193.

Hwang, S., R. Saenz, and B. E. Aguirre. 1997. Structural and assimilationist explanations of Asian American intermarriage. *Journal of Marriage and the Family* 59 (3):758–772.

Iceland, J., D. H. Weinberg, and E. Steinmetz. 2002. *Racial and ethnic residential segregation in the United States: 1980–2000.* Census 2000 Special Reports CENSR-3. Washington, D.C.: U.S. Government Printing Office.

Ignatiev, N. 1995. *How the Irish became white.* New York: Routledge.

Jensen, R. 1998. White privilege shapes the U.S. *Baltimore Sun* (July 19):1C, 4C.

Johnston, R., J. Forrest, and M. Poulsen. 2002. The ethnic geography of EthniCities: The 'American Model' and residential concentration in London. *Ethnicities* 2:209–235.

Kalmijn, M. 1998. Intermarriage and homogamy: Causes, patterns, trends. *Annual Review of Sociology* 24:395–421.

Keith, V. M., and C. Herring. 1991. Skin tone and stratification in the black community. *American Journal of Sociology* 97 (3):760–778.

Khan, A. 1995. Who are the Mongols? State, ethnicity, and the politics of representation in the PRC. In *Negotiating Ethnicities in China and Taiwan.* Edited by M. J. Brown, 125–159. Berkeley: Institute of East Asian Studies, University of California.

Killingsworth, M. R. 1993. Analyzing employment discrimination: From the seminar room to the courtroom. *American Economic Review* 83:67–72.

Kulczycki, A. and A. P. Lobo. 2002. Patterns, determinants, and implications of intermarriage among Arab Americans. *Journal of Marriage and the Family* 64:202–210.

Ladanyi, J. 1993. Patterns of residential segregation and the gypsy minority in Budapest. *International Journal of Urban and Regional Research* 17:30–41.

Landale, N. S., and R. S. Oropesa. 2002. White, black, or Puerto Rican? Racial Self-identification among mainland and island Puerto Ricans. *Social Forces* 81:231–254.

Landale, N. S., R. S. Oropesa, and B. Gorman. 1999. Immigration and infant health: Birth outcomes of immigrant and native women. In *Children of immigrants: Health, adjustments, and public assistance.* Edited by D. J. Hernandez, 244–285. Washington, D.C.: National Academy Press.

Landale, N. S., R. S. Oropesa, and B. Gorman. 2000. Migration and infant death: Assimilation or selective migration among Puerto Ricans? *American Sociological Review* 65:888–909.

Landale, N. S., R. S. Oropesa, and D. Llanes. 1998. Schooling, work, and idleness among Mexican and non-Latino white adolescents. *Social Science Research* 27:457–480.

Landsman, N., and W. Katkin. 1998. Introduction: The construction of American pluralism. In *Beyond pluralism: The conception of groups and group identities in America.* Edited by W. F. Katkin, N. Landsman, and A. Tyree, 1–10. Chicago: University of Illinois Press.

Lee, S. M. 1993. Racial classifications in the U.S. Census: 1890–1990. *Ethnic and Racial Studies* 16:75–94.

Lewin-Epstein, N., and M. Semyonov. 1992. Local labor markets, ethnic segregation, and income inequality. *Social Forces* 70:1101–1119.

Lieberson, S. 1975. Rank-sum comparisons between groups. In *Sociological methodology, 1976.* Edited by D. Heise, 276–291. San Francisco: Jossey-Bass.

Logan, J. R., R. D. Alba, and S. Leung. 1996. Minority access to white suburbs: A multiregional comparison. *Social Forces* 74:851–881.

Longman, T. 1999. Nation, race, or class?: Defining the Hutu and Tutsi of East Africa. *Research in Politics and Society* 6:103–130.

Markides, K. S., and J. Coreil. 1986. The health of Hispanics in the southwestern United States: An epidemiological paradox. *Public Health Reports* 101:253–265.

Massey, D. S., and N. A. Denton. 1988. The dimensions of residential segregation. *Social Forces* 67:281–315.

Massey, D. S., and N. A. Denton. 1993. *American apartheid: Segregation and the making of the underclass.* Cambridge, Mass.: Harvard University Press.

Massey, D. S., M. J. White, and V. Phua. 1996. The dimensions of segregation revisited. *Sociological Methods and Research* 25:172–206.

McFalls, J. A., Jr. 1998. *Population: A lively introduction*, 3rd ed. Population Bulletin 53 (3). Washington, D.C.: Population Reference Bureau.

McLemore, S. D., and H. D. Romo. 1998. *Racial and ethnic relations in America*, 5th ed. Boston: Allyn and Bacon.

Morris, A. 1996. What's race got to do with it? *Contemporary Sociology* 25:309–313.

Murguia, E., and R. Saenz. 2002. An analysis of the Latin Americanization of race in the United States: A reconnaissance of color stratification among Mexicans. *Race & Society* 5:85–101.

Murguia, E., and E. E. Telles. 1996. Phenotype and schooling among Mexican Americans. *Sociology of Education* 69:276–289.

Nattrass, N., and J. Seekings. 2001. "Two nations"? Race and economic inequality in South Africa today. *Daedalus* 130(1):45–70.

Nelson, C., and M. Tienda. 1985. The structuring of Hispanic ethnicity. *Ethnic and Racial Studies* 8:49–74.

Obach, B. K. 1999. Demonstrating the social construction of race. *Teaching Sociology* 27:252–257.

Office of Management and Budget. 1977. *Directive No. 15, Race and ethnic standards for federal statistics and administration reporting.* Washington, D.C.: Office of Management and Budget.

Office of Management and Budget. 1997. *Revisions to the standards for the classification of federal data on race and ethnicity.* Washington, D.C.: Office of Management and Budget.

Office of Management and Budget. 2000. *Provision guidance on the implementation of the 1997 standards for federal data on race and ethnicity.* Washington, D.C.: Office of Management and Budget.

Oliver, M. L., and T. M. Shapiro. 1995. *Black wealth, white wealth: A new perspective on racial inequality.* New York: Routledge.

Omi, M., and H. Winant. 1984. *Racial formation in the United States.* New York: Routledge.

Outlaw, L. 1990. Toward a critical theory of "race". In *Anatomy of racism.* Edited by D. T. Goldberg, 58–82. Minneapolis: University of Minnesota Press.

Pagnini, D. 1997. Immigration and fertility in New Jersey: A comparison of native and foreign-born women. In *Keys to successful immigration: Implications to the New Jersey experience.* Edited by T. J. Espenshade, 259–290. Washington, D.C.: Urban Institute Press.

Park, R. E. 1950. *Race and culture.* Glencoe, Ill.: The Free Press.

Passel, J. S. 1997. The growing American Indian population, 1960–1990: Beyond demography. *Population Research and Policy Review* 16:11–31.

Patel, K. V., K. Eschbach, L. A. Ray, and K. S. Markides. 2004. Evaluation of mortality data for older Mexican Americans: Implications for the Hispanic paradox. *American Journal of Epidemiology.* Forthcoming.

Patrinos, H. A. 2000. The cost of discrimination in Latin America. *Studies in Comparative International Development* 35(2):3–17.

Pattillo, M. 1999. *Black picket fences: Privilege and peril among the black middle class.* Chicago: University of Chicago Press.

Perlmann, J. 2002. Census Bureau long-term racial projections: Interpreting their results and seeking their rationale. In *The new race question: How the census counts multiracial individuals.* Edited by J. Perlmann and M. Waters, 215–226. New York: Russell Sage Foundation.

Perlmann, J., and M. Waters, eds. 2002. *The new race question: How the census counts multiracial individuals.* New York: Russell Sage Foundation.

Phillips, D. 1998. Black minority ethnic concentration, segregation and dispersal in Britain. *Urban Studies* 35:1681–1702.

Portes, A. 1995. Children of immigrants: Segmented assimilation and its determinants. In *The economic sociology of immigration: Essays on networks, ethnicity, and entrepreneurship.* Edited by A. Portes, 248–280. New York: Russell Sage Foundation.

Portes, A., and D. MacLeod. 1996. Educational progress of children of immigrants: The role of class, ethnicity, and school context. *Sociology of Education* 69:255–275.

Portes, A., and R. G. Rumbaut. 1996. *Immigrant America: A portrait*, 2nd ed. Berkeley: University of California Press.

Portes, A., and R. G. Rumbaut. 2001. *Legacies: The story of the immigrant second generation.* Berkeley: University of California Press and Russell Sage Foundation.

Portes, A., and M. Zhou. 1993. The new second generation: Segmented assimilation and its variants. *The Annals of the American Academy of Political and Social Science* 530 (Nov.):74–96.

Poston, D. L., Jr. 1993. The minority nationalities of China. In International Union for the Scientific Study of Population, *International Population Conference, Montreal 1993*, Volume 3, 483–495. Liege, Belgium: International Union for the Scientific Study of Population.

Poston, D. L., Jr., and D. Alvirez. 1973. On the cost of being a Mexican American worker. *Social Science Quarterly* 53:697–709.

Poston, D. L., Jr., D. Alvirez, and M. Tienda. 1976. Earnings differences between Anglo and Mexican American male workers in 1960 and 1970: Changes in the "cost" of being Mexican American. *Social Science Quarterly* 57:618–631.

Poston, D. L., Jr., and M. Micklin. 1993. Spatial segregation and social differentiation of the minority nationalities from the Han majority in the People's Republic of China. *Sociological Inquiry* 63:150–165.

Poston, D. L., Jr., and J. Shu. 1987. The demographic and socioeconomic composition of China's ethnic minorities. *Population and Development Review* 13:703–722.

Qian, Z., and D. T. Lichter. 2001. Measuring marital assimilation: Intermarriage among natives and immigrants. *Social Science Research* 30:289–312.

Riche, M. F. 2000. *America's diversity and growth: Signposts for the 21st century. Population Bulletin* 55(2). Washington D.C.: Population Reference Bureau.

Rodriguez, C. E. 2000. *Changing race: Latinos, the census, and the history of ethnicity in the United States*. New York: New York University Press.

Root, M. P. P., ed. 1992. *Racially mixed people in America*. Newbury Park, Calif.: Sage Publications.

Root, M. P. P., ed. 1996. *The multiracial experience: Racial borders as the new frontier*. Thousand Oaks, Calif.: Sage Publications.

Ross, K., and J. Taylor. 2002. Improving life expectancy and health status: A comparison of indigenous Australians and New Zealand Maori. In *Populations of New Zealand and Australia at the millennium: A joint special issue of the Journal of Population Research and the New Zealand Population Review*. Edited by G. A. Carmichael and A. Dharmalingam. Canberra, Australia, and Wellington, New Zealand: Australian Population Association.

Saenz, R. 1997. Ethnic concentration and Chicano poverty: A comparative approach. *Social Science Research* 26:205–228.

Saenz, R., and B. E. Aguirre. 1991. The dynamics of Mexican ethnic identity. *Ethnic Groups* 9:17–32.

Saenz, R., S. Hwang, and B. E. Aguirre. 1994. In search of Asian war brides. *Demography* 31(3):549–559.

Saenz, R., S. Hwang, B. E. Aguirre, and R. N. Anderson. 1995. Persistence and change in Asian identity among children of intermarried couples. *Sociological Perspectives* 38:175–194.

Sakamoto, A., H. Wu, and J. M. Tzeng. 2000. The declining significance of race among American men during the latter half of the 20th century. *Demography* 37:41–51.

Sakamoto, A., and J. M. Tzeng. 1999. A fifty-year perspective on the declining significance of race in the occupational attainment of white and black men. *Sociological Perspectives* 42:157–180.

Semyonov, M. 1997. On the cost of being an immigrant in Israel: The effects of tenure, origin and gender. *Research in Social Stratification and Mobility* 15:115–131.

Semyonov, M., and Y. Cohen. 1990. Ethnic discrimination and the income of majority-group workers. *American Sociological Review* 55:107–114.

Shulman, S. 1989. A critique of the declining discrimination hypothesis. In *The question of discrimination: Racial inequality in the U.S. labor market*. Edited by S. Shulman and W. Darity, Jr., 126–152. Middletown, Conn.: Wesleyan University Press.

Skidmore, T. E. 1995. Fact and myth: Discovering a racial problem in Brazil. In *Population, ethnicity, and nation-building*. Edited by C. Goldscheider, 91–118. Boulder, Colo.: Westview Press.

Skinner, C. 2002. High school graduate earnings in New York City: The effects of skill, gender, race and ethnicity. *Journal of Urban Affairs* 24:219–238.

Snipp, C. M. 1992. Sociological perspectives on American Indians. *Annual Review of Sociology* 18:351–371.

Snipp, C. M. 1997a. The size and distribution of the American Indian population: Fertility, mortality, migration, and residence. *Population Research and Policy Review* 16:61–93.

Snipp, C. M. 1997b. Some observations about racial boundaries and the experiences of American Indians. *Ethnic and Racial Studies* 20:667–689.

Snipp, C. M. 2003. Racial measurement in the American census: Past practices and implications for the future. *Annual Review of Sociology* 29:563–288.

Spickard, P. R. 1989. *Mixed blood: Intermarriage and ethnic identity in twentieth-century America*. Madison: University of Wisconsin Press.

Spickard, P. R. 1992. The illogic of American racial categories. In *Racially mixed people in America*. Edited by M. P. P. Root, 12–23. Newbury Park, Calif.: Sage Publications.

Stephen, E. H., and F. D. Bean. 1992. Assimilation, disruption and the fertility of Mexican-origin women in the United States. *International Migration Review* 26:67–88.

Steyn, M. 1999. White identity in context: A personal narrative. In *Whiteness: The communication of social identity*. Edited by T. K. Nakayama and J. N. Martin, 264–278. Thousand Oaks, Calif.: Sage Publications.

Streicker, J. 1998. Policing boundaries: Race, class, and gender in Cartegena, Colombia. In *Blackness in Latin America and the Caribbean: Social dynamics and cultural transformations*, Vol. I, Central America and Northern and Western South America. Edited by N. E. Whitten, Jr., and A. Torres, 278–308. Bloomington: Indiana University Press.

Sullivan, T. A., F. P. Gillespie, M. Hout, R. G. Spickard, and P. R. Rogers. 1984. Alternative estimates of Mexican American mortality in Texas, 1980. *Social Science Quarterly* 65:609–617.

Suwal, J., and F. Trovato. 1998. Canadian Aboriginal fertility. *Canadian Studies of Population* 25:69–86.

Swanson, L. E., R. P. Harris, J. R. Skees, and L. Williamson. 1994. African Americans in southern rural regions: The importance of legacy. *Review of Black Political Economy* 22:109–124.

Teachman, J. D., K. Paasch, and K. P. Carver. 1993. Thirty years of demography. *Demography* 30(4):523–532.

Teitelbaum, M. S., and J. Winter. 1998. *A question of numbers: High migration, low fertility, and the politics of national identity*. New York: Hill & Wang.

Telles, E. E. 1992. Residential segregation by skin color in Brazil. *American Sociological Review* 57:186–197.

Telles, E. E., and E. Murguia. 1990. Phenotypic discrimination and income differences among Mexican Americans. *Social Science Quarterly* 71:682–696.

Tiedje, K. 2002. Gender and ethnic identity in rural grassroots development: An outlook from the Huasteca Potosina, Mexico. *Urban Anthropology* 31:261–316.

Tienda, M., and D. T. Lii. 1987. Minority concentration and earnings inequality: Blacks, Hispanics, and Asians Compared. *American Journal of Sociology* 93:141–165.

Toyota, M. 2003. Contested Chinese identities among ethnic minorities in the China, Burma and Thai borderlands. *Ethnic and Racial Studies* 26:301–320.

Trovato, F. 2001. Aboriginal mortality in Canada, the United States and New Zealand. *Journal of Biosocial Science* 33:67–86.

Uhlmann, E., N. Dasgupta, A. Elguenta, A. G. Greenwald, and J. Swanson. 2002. Subgroup prejudice based on skin color among Hispanics in the United States and Latin America. *Social Cognition* 20:198–226.

U.S. Census Bureau. 2000. *Projections of the resident population by race, Hispanic origin, and nativity: Middle series, 1999 to 2100*. Washington, D.C.: Population Program, Population Division, U.S. Census Bureau. Internet release date: January 13, 2000. Last revised: August 2, 2002. Web page: *http://www.census.gov/population/www/projections/natsum-T5.html*.

U.S. Census Bureau. 2003. *United States Census 2000. 1-Percent Public Use Microdata Sample (PUMS) Files*. Washington, DC: U.S. Census Bureau.

Van Kempen, R., II and J. Van Weesep. 1998. Ethnic residential patterns in Dutch cities: Backgrounds, shifts and consequences. *Urban Studies* 35:1813–1833.

Verdugo, N. T., and R. R. Verdugo. 1984. Earnings differentials among Mexican American, black, and white male workers. *Social Science Quarterly* 65:417–425.

Verdugo, R. R. 1992. Earnings differentials between black, Mexican American, and non-Hispanic white male workers: On the cost of being a minority worker, 1972–1987. *Social Science Quarterly* 73:663–673.

Verdugo, R. R., and N. T. Verdugo. 1988. Overeducation and the earnings of black, Hispanic, and white male workers. *Sociological Perspectives* 31:190–212.

Warren, J. W., and F. W. Twine. 1997. White Americans, the new minority? Non-blacks and the ever-expanding boundaries of whiteness. *Journal of Black Studies* 28:200–218.

Waters, M. 1990. *Ethnic options*. Berkeley: University of California Press.

Waters, M. 1999. *Black identities: West Indian immigrant dreams and American realities*. Cambridge, Mass.: Harvard University Press.

Waters, M. 2002. The social construction of race and ethnicity: Some examples from demography. In *American diversity: A demographic challenge for the twenty-first century*. Edited by N. A. Denton and S. E. Tolnay, 25–49. Albany: State University of New York Press.

Weeks, J. R. 2002. *Population: An introduction to concepts and issues*, 8th ed. Belmont, Calif.: Wadsworth.

White, M. J., and A. Omer. 1997. Segregation by ethnicity and immigrant status in New Jersey. In *Keys to successful immigration: Implications to the New Jersey experience*. Edited by T. J. Espenshade, 375–394. Washington, D.C.: Urban Institute Press.

Willie, C. V. 1978. The inclining significance of race. *Society* 15 (July/Aug.):12–15.

Willie, C. V. 1989. *The caste and class controversy on race and poverty: Round two of the Willie/Wilson debate*, 2nd ed. Dix Hills, N.Y.: General Hall.

Wilson, G. 2000. Income in upper-tier occupations among males over the first decade of the work-career: Is race declining in its significance. *National Journal of Sociology* 12:105–127.

Wilson, W. J. 1978. *The declining significance of race: Blacks and changing American institutions*. Chicago: University of Chicago Press.

Wilson, W. J. 1996. *When work disappears: The world of the new urban poor*. New York: Knopf.

Wong, M. 1982. The cost of being Chinese, Japanese, and Filipino in the United States: 1960, 1970, 1976. *Pacific Sociological Review* 25:59–78.

Yinger, J. M. 1994. *Ethnicity: Source of strength? Source of conflict?* New York: State University Press.

Zevallos, Z. 2003. "That's my Australian side": The ethnicity, gender and sexuality of young Australian women of South and Central American origin. *Journal of Sociology* 39:81–98.

Zuberi, T. 2001. *Thicker than blood: How racial statistics lie*. Minneapolis: University of Minnesota Press.

Appendix A. List of Control Variables Included in the Ordinary Least Square (OLS) Regression of Logged Hourly Earnings

Age. 4 dummy variables: (1) Age 35–44; (2) age 45–54; (3) age 55–64; and (4) age 65 and older. Reference group = persons less than 35.

Language. 2 dummy variables: (1) Monolingual English speakers (speaks English at home) and (2) bilingual speakers (speaks a non-English language at home and speaks English "well" or "very well"). Reference group = monolingual non-English speakers (speaks a non-English language at home and speaks English "not well" or "not at all").

Education. 4 dummy variables: (1) Some high school education (completed 9 to 11 years of education or 12 years of education without high school diploma); (2) high school graduate; (3) some college (includes those with Associate degrees); and (4) college graduates (equivalent of Bachelor's degree or higher). Reference group = persons with 0 to 8 years of education completed.

Occupation. 5 dummy variables: (1) Management, professional, and related occupations; (2) service occupations; (3) sales and office occupations; (4) construction, extraction, and maintenance occupations; (5) production, transportation, and material-moving occupations. Reference group = persons working in farming, fishing, and forestry occupations.

Self-Employment. 1 dummy variable: (1) Persons who are self-employed in an incorporated or unincorporated business or company. Reference group = people who are not self-employed.

Experience. Age – Years of Education – 6

Experience squared. Experience * Experience

Marital status. 1 dummy variable: (1) Currently married. Reference group = persons not currently married.

Disability. 1 dummy variable: (1) Persons with a disability. Reference group = persons without a disability.

Metropolitan residence. 2 dummy variables: (1) Metropolitan residence; (2) mixed metropolitan and nonmetropolitan residence. Reference group = persons living in nonmetropolitan areas.

Region. 4 dummy variables: (1) Midwest; (2) South (excluding Texas); (3) West (excluding Arizona, California, Colorado, New Mexico); and (4) Southwest (Arizona, California, Colorado, New Mexico, Texas). Reference group = Northeast.

Presence/age of own children at home (female analysis only). 3 dummy variables: (1) Children less than 6 years of age; (2) children 6 to 17 years of age; and (3) children less than 6 and 6 to 17 years of age). Reference group = no children.

Period of immigration arrival in U.S. (foreign-born analysis only). 3 dummy variables: (1) Before 1970; (2) 1970–1979; and (3) 1980–1989. Reference group = persons that arrived in the U.S. from 1990 to 2000.

Naturalized citizenship status (foreign-born analysis only). 1 dummy variable: (1) naturalized U.S. citizen. Reference group = persons that are not naturalized U.S. citizens.

CHAPTER 7

Labor Force

Teresa A. Sullivan

The labor force refers to all members of the population above a minimum age who are either working or looking for work.[1] In terms of national economic accounts, the labor force can be thought of as the labor supply, the producers of the goods and services that are valued in the Gross National Product. In an early review, Jaffe (1959) notes that the significance of the labor force is that all members of a population consume goods and services, but only the members of the labor force produce those goods and services.

Because of its relationship to production and consumption, the labor force and its size, composition, and changes are significant to demographers, sociologists, and economists. Particularly in modern economies, where work is typically separated into times and places distinct from other life activities, the labor force is a useful subdivision of the adult population for further study.

This chapter first explores the relationship of the labor force to levels of economic development, which is a macrolevel approach to understanding the labor force. In the next section, the chapter distinguishes macrolevel from microlevel approaches to the labor force. Several theoretical approaches to the labor force are discussed, and a variety of methods and measurements relating to the labor force are presented. Several key empirical findings concerning the labor force are discussed, and the chapter concludes with directions for future research.

---

[1] The term *labor force* is used principally in the United States; in other countries, the more commonly used term is the *economically active population*. Both terms refer to the population that is working plus those actively seeking work.

SUBSTANTIVE CONCERNS

Labor Force and the Level of Development

One important issue in labor force research has been the differences in the labor force in advanced industrial countries versus developing nations. Typically, the concept has worked better in advanced developing countries, where there is usually a set of relationships between employers and employees that constitute more or less stable jobs, and where the distinction between the home and the workplace has been relatively sharp. In economies that are moving toward an industrial or postindustrial economy, however, the labor force participation rate for a demographic group or for an industry may be a powerful proxy variable for the development process.

The labor force concept assumes a monetized economy. As more types of work become incorporated into the money economy, the occupational structure of the labor force diversifies. Services that were previously performed at home enter the market economy, and previously unpaid workers (typically women) become labor force participants. Presser and Kishor (1991) document how labor force participation rates first declined and then increased for women as Puerto Rico experienced economic growth. Charles' (1992) work suggests that the incorporation of more women into the labor force may intensify occupational segregation because the new women workers are still doing traditionally women's work, only now for pay.

The self-employed, especially those in subsistence agriculture, have not always been adequately accounted for in labor force measurement. For this reason, the labor force has not always been an adequate measurement of the productive population in developing countries. Similarly, where many people are employed by other members of their own household, or where they may receive their pay as shares of produce or other in-kind provisions, the distinction between those in and not in the labor force becomes less obvious.

In addition, even in the advanced industrial countries labor force analysts typically ignore the nonmonetary contributions made by volunteers, housewives, and certain other adults, such as inmates of institutions whose work is typically not counted in the Gross National Product. The military are typically but not universally included in the labor force, although the reported labor force statistics may be limited to the civilian labor force. In advanced industrial countries, there are typically a fairly large number of retirees and students who do not work or who work only sporadically. Individuals who are sick or disabled may be unable to participate in the labor force.

The labor force is divided into two parts: the employed, those who are actively at work or who have a job from which they are temporarily absent, and the unemployed. Although the definition of unemployment varies from country to country, typically unemployment is defined as the active search for work by someone who does not currently hold a job. It is assumed that the unemployed person is legally of an age to work and is willing and able to work. Again, this is a concept that may better describe conditions in advanced industrial countries, especially those with transfer payments available for the unemployed. In countries with lower levels of living, the otherwise unemployed may pick up some casual labor or receive payment in kind rather than having a regular job. Whether they are truly employed or unemployed may be a matter of judgment.

Macrolevel versus Microlevel Approaches

One stream of demographic literature has viewed the labor force in macrolevel terms, analyzing its size, composition, and changes. These studies are typically undertaken with census or survey data that refer to an entire geographical area, such as a state or nation. The size of the labor force, especially relative to the entire population, is an indicator of considerable interest to demographers. For example, Bauer (1990) examined labor force growth and labor costs in Asian countries. A relatively large labor force indicates a large number of productive people to support the dependent population. A relatively small labor force may indicate high levels of dependency, either because the age structure is relatively young or old, or because many people in the usual working ages are unable or unwilling to work.

The composition of the labor force is also interesting. For example, a labor force that is principally made up of citizens of a country is likely to differ in important respects from a labor force with a high proportion of guest workers or immigrants. A receiving country's labor force may change in ways that reflect the presence of migrant workers (Shah 1995). Similarly, when a labor force is evenly divided between men and women, the population may have different norms about sex roles and lower fertility rates than a population whose labor force is predominantly male. Higher levels of economic development are typically associated with a larger share of women workers (Clark, Ramsbey, and Adler 1991).

Finally, there is great interest in the changes in the labor force, including accession rates of new workers, retirement rates of older workers, and movement in and out of the labor force by students, seasonal workers, temporary workers, or others.

Probably the most commonly used measure for comparative labor force studies is the labor force participation rate, which is defined as the number of eligible people in the labor force (employed or unemployed) divided by the number of people of working age eligible to be in the labor force, and evaluated for a specific time and place. Because it can be calculated for geographical subregions, the labor force participation rate is often used to evaluate local or regional labor markets (Odland 2001).

The female labor force participation rate is an indicator that has been of pervasive interest in understanding social change. The percent of the labor force engaged in agriculture can be a proxy variable for the level of economic development because nonagricultural employment typically grows as the economy develops (Nielsen and Alderson 1995; by contrast, Bollen and Appold 1993, use percent employed in industry as a proxy).

The unemployment rate, defined as the number of unemployed persons divided by the labor force, is a leading economic indicator and is closely watched in the advanced industrial countries. Unemployment rates are used to define recessions and to chart business cycles. The unemployment rate is often used as an indicator of hardship and is sometimes used in formulas for distributing block grants in aid to localities.

Another macrolevel indicator often used is the employment-population ratio, the ratio of employed persons to the total population. An indicator called the dependency rate is the ratio of people too young to work plus those older people who do not work, divided by the number of working age adults. Although the definition of working age varies among different countries, a conventional age grouping used in dependency ratios is ages 16 to 64. This ratio can be interpreted as the number of dependents supported, on average, by each worker.

Microlevel studies use data for individuals, typically from surveys or census micro-data samples. These studies can examine the reciprocal interactions of migration and fertility decisions with work behavior. Because labor force behavior typically differs among demographic groups, microlevel studies are often used to understand these differences. In the United States, for example, the labor force participation rate of black women has historically exceeded that for white women, but the unemployment rate for blacks has typically been twice that of whites. Labor force participation has been shown to be high for the well educated (Hill 1995), migrants (Borjas and Tienda 1993), and married men.

Such issues can be better understood with multivariate models that control other variables, such as education, that are known to affect labor force behavior. In such studies, labor force participation is typically the dependent variable. Bound, Schoen-baum, and Waldmann (1995), to take one example, discovered that health status differentials helped to clarify the differences in labor force participation among older black and white men. These differences explained most of the gap in participation attributed to education. In another study, the availability of cash and noncash transfers was related to declines in the labor force participation of young nonwhite males (Sanders 1990).

More frequently, labor force participation is an independent or control variable that is used to help understand other variables of interest. Fertility, for example, is lower for women who are labor force participants. Fertility studies commonly control for labor force participation. It is logical that labor force participation affects income, because most personal income comes from salaries and wages. Women's labor force participation, by increasing family income, affects inequality and income distribution (Maxwell 1990). But analysts have also found that women's labor force participation helps explain other phenomena, including the gender gap in U.S. presidential politics (Manza and Brooks 1998), grade retention of children (Guo, Brooks-Gunn, and Harris 1996), gender differences in child mortality (Kishor 1993), and even femicide (Avakame 1999).

Besides these uses of the labor force variables, there are also ecological studies that may use the local labor force participation rate or unemployment rate as control variables. Murthi, Guio, and Dreze (1995) used women's labor force participation among other district-level variables in India to explain differences in fertility, child mortality, and gender bias in child survival.

THEORETICAL CONSIDERATIONS

As the earlier section has suggested, labor force participation plays a role in macrolevel theories of economic development and social change. Although not always linked explicitly to the demographic transition, there is a close connection between the decline of fertility and the increase in women's participation, and there is likewise an association between the changed age structure of the early demographic transition and increased labor force participation (Avakame 1999). More commonly, however, labor force plays a role in the development of microlevel theory.

Human Capital Theory

Human capital theory is used to understand why some workers command high income while others do not. By extension, human capital theory also seeks to explain why some workers are more likely to be unemployed than others. Because labor force participation precedes earnings, the same variables used to predict income may also be used to predict labor force participation. Personal characteristics and endowments may increase or decrease a person's human capital. Education is the usual operational measurement, but levels of training, specialized licensure, and migration are also conceptually part of human capital theory.[2]

Enchautegai (1992) finds that geographical differences in the earnings of Puerto Rican women are due to their differing human capital characteristics. Wenk and Garrett (1992) find that human capital variables are significant in predicting employment exit after the birth of a baby. But Tienda and Wilson (1992) have found that the earnings return to migration are negligible, contrary to the expectation of human capital theory.

More recently, the concept of social capital has been introduced to account for the effect of social networks in helping to match workers with jobs. Workers with relatively extensive social networks through their extended families, churches, classmates, and other links may have an advantage in the labor market in terms of shorter search times for work and in terms of finding better jobs (see Lin 2001; Lin, Cook, and Burt 2001; Field 2003).

Labor Market Discrimination

Theories of labor market discrimination examine racial, ethnic, and gender differences in labor force participation, occupational attainment, or earnings. According to these theories, human capital variables alone are insufficient to explain the persistent differences in work experience. These differences are instead attributed to mechanisms within the labor market that steer certain workers to certain jobs, occupations, or industries. Such labor markets may be variously described as "split," "dual," or "segmented."

An important aspect of these studies is that ascriptive demographic characteristics, such as race or sex, are used to divide the labor supply into more preferred or less preferred workers. This is sometimes called statistical discrimination. The least preferred workers will not enter even the lowest-paid segments of the market, resulting in their higher levels of unemployment. Most such studies control for human capital variables such as education and attempt to identify the effect of discriminatory mechanisms that operate beyond the endowments of individual workers.

When it is impossible to examine discrimination directly, its presence may be inferred when differences persist even after many control variables have been applied. Stratton (1993), for example, finds that only 20% to 40% of the difference in unemployment rates between black and white men can be explained by variables such as education or local labor market conditions. Tienda, Donato, and Cordero-Guzman (1992) find that over a period of 20 years the labor market conditions of minority women worsened and that they received unequal returns to education. Evans and Kelley (1991), by contrast, found little evidence of discrimination against immigrants in Australia.

---

[2] For a concise assessment of human capital theory see Robinson and Browne 1994: 581–585.

Fertility and Women's Labor Force Participation

An important area of theorizing has been why some women and not others pursue paid work in the labor force. Structural characteristics of the economy help to shape the general demand for women's labor (Cotter et al. 1998). Women's family responsibilities, both as wives and as mothers, have often been seen as intervening variables between their human capital endowment and their eventual labor force participation. The relationships vary by generation, ethnicity and immigrant status (Stier and Tienda 1992), and religion. More recently, analysts have examined characteristics of jobs that facilitate or impede women's labor force participation. The availability of child care, or the ability of husbands and wives to work different shifts so that they can care for their children themselves, are currently important areas of research for understanding the circumstances under which mothers can participate in the labor force.

The Easterlin Effect is a theory that incidentally seeks to explain changes in women's labor force participation. The Easterlin Effect posits that the relative income of cohorts is inversely proportional to cohort size. Small cohorts are in high demand in the labor force. Large cohorts are in lower demand and may therefore have higher women's labor force participation, later marriage, and lower fertility (Pampel and Peters 1995). But both Pampel (1993, looking at Europe) and Carlson (1992, looking at Korea) suggest that institutional structures mediate the operation of the Easterlin Effect.

The empirical findings of this stream of research are reviewed below.

METHODS AND MEASURES

The fundamental concepts of labor force, employment and unemployment, and their corresponding rates, have already been introduced. These rates can be computed for different demographic groups and for different geographical areas. Labor force data are gathered from surveys or censuses because most administrative records of employment are incomplete. In particular, unemployment compensation records exclude a large number of the unemployed, including entrants to the labor force who have not yet found a job.

Combined with information concerning age structure, labor force participation rates form the basis for labor force projections, which are used by government agencies, employers, and insurers (Fullerton and Toossi 2001). The United States government makes labor force projections based on 136 age, sex, race, and Hispanic origin groups. The civilian labor force of the United States is projected to reach 158 million in 2010, with the share of women increasing slightly from 47% to 48%. The rates can also be combined into more complex measures.

Tables of Economically Active Life

Labor force participation rates can be used in multiple increment-decrement tables to model not only the effect of mortality but also the effect of entry and exit into the labor force on the expectation of economically active life (Willekens 1979). This measure can be interpreted as the expected length of working life if current age-specific labor force participation and mortality rates persist indefinitely. These measures are useful for predicting future labor supply and for making decisions concerning, for example, the investment of pension funds. Where labor force participation rates are changing rapidly, or whenever workers experience many exits and reentries into the labor force, these tables will be inaccurate. Recent developments have focused on successfully smoothing the transition probabilities to improve the tables (Land, Guralnik, and Blazer 1994).

In or Out of the Labor Force

In the United States and many other countries, the unemployed are a residual category identified only after all the employed have been counted. After the employed and the unemployed have been counted, the remainder of the adult population is counted as "not in the labor force," or NILF.

  To be employed, it is sufficient to have worked for just 1 hour a week for pay, or to work 15 hours unpaid in a family enterprise. It is also sufficient to have a job if one is only temporarily absent, such as a worker with a short-term illness, a vacation, or a holiday. Persons who are not employed are then counted as unemployed if they have actively sought work or are awaiting the results of a recent search. Norwood and Tanur (1994) describe the current measurement process in the United States.

  One criticism of this measurement technique is that the line between the not in the labor force adults and the unemployed is blurry. Gonul (1992) finds that these two states are distinct for young women but not for young men. Kreider (1999) finds that nonworkers in the Health and Retirement Survey overreport work limitations, suggesting that these people may have exaggerated their health conditions to justify their nonparticipation in the labor force. Retirement or disability are face-saving reasons for not seeking work.

  The concept of the *discouraged worker* refers to people who would accept work but who are no longer looking for work because they believe that no work is available (Buss and Redburn 1988). The National Commission on Employment and Unemployment Statistics (1979) recommended counting discouraged workers in the labor force, but government agencies do not yet include discouraged workers among the labor force.

  Another line of critique is directed at the very concept of "not in the labor force." Donahoe (1999) argues that the contemporary measurement methods underestimate women's productive activity, in particular. Bener'ia (1999) argues from feminist theory that the omission of women from labor force measurement renders women and their work invisible. Empirical data indicate that the simple participant/nonparticipant dichotomy is oversimplified for women who have recently experienced their first birth (Vandenheuvel 1997).

Underemployment: Refining the Employment Rate

Typically over 90% of the labor force is counted as employed. The employed status covers a wide range of job situations, from a person employed only one hour during a week at the minimum wage to the highest-paid corporate executive. A number of criticisms have been leveled at the great heterogeneity of the "employed" measure.

In developing countries, where the job market may have a large informal component, employment may also be informal and an unreliable source of income. Such employment is common in some developing countries, especially in urban areas (Cerrutti 2000).

In the advanced industrial countries as well, measured employment may disguise a fair amount of underemployment, a term that has been measured with the Hauser-Sullivan-Clogg labor utilization framework (Clogg and Sullivan 1983; Clogg 1979; Sullivan 1978). This framework identifies several types of employment that may nevertheless be considered normatively inadequate.

The first type of underemployment is involuntary part-time work. Although many workers are voluntarily part-time, others work only part-time because of partial layoff, slack work, or other economic reasons. Stratton (1996) finds that those classified as involuntarily part-time are 50% more likely than the voluntarily part-time to be full-time workers a year later, suggesting that the involuntary term is correctly applied. Involuntary part-time work varies with the business cycle. Many seasonal workers are also involuntarily part-year workers.

The second type of underemployment results from low pay rates. The underemployed under this criterion are full-time workers but earn less than some normative standard (such as the minimum wage or poverty rate). The third type of underemployment reflects a mismatch of skills and occupation and occurs when a worker's job requires significantly less education than the worker has. Using unemployment and these three types of underemployment, Clogg (1979) estimated that about 75% of the labor force was nonmarginal. These studies are reviewed in Sobel (1996).

Longitudinal Measures

A problem with all labor force indicators is that they are measured for a fairly short period of time and then presented in time series. These repeated cross-sections give a picture of changes in the labor force for the population, but they do not track changes in the behavior of individuals. Longitudinal studies or career studies permit the study of work histories for individuals, and the conclusions from these studies may often differ from those drawn from repeated cross-sections.

In the United States, the Current Population Survey provides a one-year retrospective supplement once a year. With this supplement, it is possible to answer questions such as, "How many people worked all year?" or alternatively, "How many people worked only seasonally?" (Mellor and Parks 1988). One finding from this study is that many more people are employed during the year, and many more people are unemployed at some time during the year, than the monthly surveys indicate.

Because the relationship between job market experiences and current job market behavior is strong and stable (Clogg, Eliason, and Wahl 1990), it is valuable to have information about the work background of workers. Moreover, workers who expect interruptions in their labor force participation tend to have lower earnings (Blau and Ferber 1991). Work histories are one tool for such studies (Rosenfeld 1996). Using the Panel Study of Income Dynamics, Harris (1993) found substantial work activity among single mothers on welfare, a conclusion that had not previously been drawn from studies using annual data.

EMPIRICAL FINDINGS

The Loss of the M-Curve

One of the most important changes in the labor force has been the shift in women's age-specific labor force participation rates (Bianchi 1995). In the middle of the 20th century, these rates when graphed against age formed the shape of the letter *M*. The rates rose through the young adult years, declined after marriage (or later, after first birth), rose after the children had left home, and finally declined again after retirement age. But with each succeeding year, the *M* shape changed. The graph rose higher each year as the overall labor force participation rates increased. In 1950, women represented less than 30% of the labor force, but by 1980 women were 42% of the labor force (Kutscher 1993). Along with this general rise, the center of the *M* shape slowly disappeared. Fertility began to decline after 1965. In addition, women were less likely to leave the labor force for any significant length of time following the birth of a child, thus removing the middle of the *M*. By 1990, the women's age-specific labor force participation rates looked like an inverted *U,* very much resembling the age-specific pattern traditionally found for men. An important set of empirical studies help to explain why the *M* shape disappeared.

An increase in the demand for female labor accompanied the development of advanced industrial economies, with greater numbers of service, sales, and clerical occupations (Charles 1992; Zsembik and Peek 1994). These are occupations that traditionally employ large numbers of women. Gender differences in labor force participation in many places and at many times appear to covary with the demand for female labor (Cotter et al. 2001).

In addition, the marital context for women still affects labor force participation, although wives' participation rates have risen relative to the 1950s (Gurak and Kritz 1996). Brinton, Lee, and Parish (1995), examining East Asian cases, found that where labor demand increases, married women joined the labor force, even where working wives had not been culturally accepted. Marital instability and divorce also lead to more continuous female employment (South 2001).

The increased number of single-parent households has fueled the continuous work participation of young mothers (Edin and Lein 1997a, 1997b). Although work may not be the only survival strategy that young mothers use, it is an important strategy both in the United States and in other countries (Parrado and Zenteno 2001). Several studies indicate that young women combine work and welfare to a greater extent than previously anticipated (Harris 1993, 1996). Lerman and Radcliffe (2001) find that single mothers find jobs without displacing other workers from jobs.

Married couples may also decide as a family investment strategy to have both partners work (Duleep and Sanders 1993). Immigrant families may have working wives even if that arrangement would have been stigmatized in the home country (Geschwender 1992; Gurak and Kritz 1996).

The most important reason for the change, however, has been the altered relationship of fertility to work (Carrasco 2001; Brewster and Rindfuss 2000). Fertility declines certainly play a role in the more continuous labor force participation of young women (Jacobsen, Pearce, and Rosenbloom 1999). Rindfuss, Brewster, and Kavee (1996) argue that the normative proscriptions on work for mothers of young children have also been reduced substantially.

For women who do bear children, one question has been whether the institutional arrangements friendly to working mothers have made a difference. Klerman and Leibowitz (1999) show that maternity leave provisions have relatively little impact on return to the labor force after delivery, but Glass and Riley (1998) find that employer policies such as leave reduced attrition. Gustafsson et al. (1996) find that social policy contributes to the return of women to work after childbirth.

The characteristics of a job also affect the likelihood that a woman with young children will work. Self-employment or work at home are possible arrangements for young mothers (Edwards and Hendry 2002). Desai and Waite (1991) find that occupations that raise the cost of labor force withdrawal (for example, occupations with a high education requirement) are associated with greater retention of young mothers. Women with better market skills are more likely than other new mothers to return to work (Klerman and Leibowitz 1994). But Stinebrickner (2002) finds that 67% of exiting female teachers leave the labor force entirely, most often to care for newborn children.

Child care costs form a major barrier to continuous labor force participation by young mothers (Baum 2002). Child care costs do lower women's labor force participation (Han and Waldfogel 2001). One-third of a sample of Detroit-area mothers of preschool-aged children reported that child care problems had reduced their employment (Mason and Kuhlthau 1992). Browne (1997) finds that the presence of children under the age of six, together with less than high school education and long-term welfare receipt, help to explain the black-white gap in labor force participation in women-headed households.

Some attention has been given to the women's labor force participation later in life. The likelihood of labor force reentry varies with education and marital status (Moen, Downey, and Bolger 1990). An interesting additional issue to consider is the withdrawal of women from the labor force to care for aging parents. One study has suggested that coresidence with a disabled parent leads to labor force withdrawal among women (Ettner 1995). With the baby boomers reaching the age at which their parents are becoming fragile, the care of elders might begin to affect the measured labor force participation of older women.

Marginalization of Workers

An issue that is closely associated with the topic of underemployment, discussed above, is the extent to which the labor force—the labor supply—is matched with labor demand in the labor market (Solow 1990). This issue is sometimes viewed in terms of the adequacy of the labor supplied, with examination of the numbers of available workers or of their human capital. More commonly, however, this issue is addressed in terms of the labor demand, especially the ways in which labor demand has been structured.

Many types of structure affect employment (DiPrete et al. 1997). The state, for example, may develop laws concerning the minimum working age, hours of work, minimum wage, and taxation of workers and of payrolls. The firm, or other employer, determines the number of workers hired, their job assignments, and changes therein. A firm may decide, for example, to close a plant in a relatively high-wage city and open a new plant in another country with lower prevailing wages, thereby affecting the labor force in both locations.

Workers also seek to gain some control over their employment through other structures, such as professions or unions. Both professions and unions seek to limit access, to prescribe minimum qualifications, to maintain some control over what work may be assigned to their members versus nonmembers, and to participate in disciplinary and job termination decisions.

The effect of state, firm, and worker decisionmaking is to limit the demand for workers, especially for workers with the best jobs—jobs that are the most skilled and the best paid. The labor supply nearly always exceeds labor demand, at least in recent decades, with the result that a larger or smaller fraction of the labor force must accept work that is poorly paid, unstable, boring, or in other ways undesirable. These are marginal jobs and the process of creating them is marginalization. The operation of these two sets of forces creates two tiers within the labor market: one that enjoys some job security and full-time employment, higher wages, and more interesting work, and a second tier with none of these benefits. Nonwork options, such as welfare or crime, may also compete with the labor force for the time of the lower tier of workers.

A number of studies have tried to define and analyze this dichotomizing process. In advanced industrial countries, the distinction can be expressed in terms of primary and secondary labor markets, or core and peripheral labor markets. In developing countries, the distinction is often made between formal and informal labor markets. In formal markets, jobs are contractual, comply with relevant laws, and are likely to be found in large, stable organizations. The informal labor markets involve casual labor for a short period of time, often are paid in cash or in kind, and are usually for a small firm or for an individual employer (Levin, Ruel, and Morris 1999). The secondary, peripheral, or informal market is also more likely to have temporary, part-time, or seasonal jobs (Hodson and Sullivan 2002: 352–375). Another conceptualization is that the two sectors represent the persistence of the traditional sector (the lower tier) with a modernizing sector (Nielsen 1994).

These dichotomizing trends are also associated with some division of the labor force into more preferred and less preferred groups of workers (Kerckhoff 1995). To some extent, the preferences are based on greater human capital, with more educated workers more likely to be in primary, core, or formal markets. In addition, there is often a demographic sorting, with urban males from dominant ethnic groups more likely to be preferred, and with women, minority group members, the very young and the very old, the disabled, and perhaps immigrants in the less preferred group (DeJong and Madamba 2001; DeAnda 2000). Hsueh and Tienda (1996) find that there is greater labor force instability for women and minority groups than for men and whites.

One interesting aspect of the research into two-tier labor markets is that there has been some effort to link real or imagined psychological outcomes, as well as economic and social outcomes, to the type of job one holds. The bottom-tier workers, who often have a work history of many short-term jobs, may then be thought of as unstable by future employers. By contrast, steady work is thought to produce psychological traits of responsibility and agency in workers (Roberts, Helson, and Klohnen 2002; but also see Kohn 1977 and Kohn et al. 1983 for a different argument about causation).

A key issue in this line of work is whether the bottom tier is growing or shrinking with respect to the top tier (Blank 1995). The development of temporary workers in many occupations is seen as a sign of marginalization. In addition, the growing use of nonstandard work arrangements is sometimes taken as a sign of greater instability and marginalization throughout the labor market (Kunda, Barley, and Evans 2002; Kalleberg 2000). Finally, globalization is seen as a means of decreasing job security for workers in several countries simultaneously because of the threat that jobs will flow to the areas with the lowest wages (Parrado and Zenteno 2001). An important and unresolved issue is how much the demographic and economic aspects of a two-tier system will overlap.

RESEARCH DIRECTIONS

Many of the most important labor force studies will continue the lines of research mentioned in the preceding section, but there are important additional research directions that are now receiving attention from researchers.

Age Structure and Retirement

In the advanced industrial societies, labor force participation rates have typically declined with advancing age. In many countries, there is a customary or even legally enforced retirement age. Programs such as Social Security must carefully model the number of retired dependents who will be eligible for transfer payments. Declining mortality rates have lengthened the number of years that elders will spend out of the labor force (Gendell 2002). In addition, declining fertility rates throughout the industrialized world have made it difficult to replace older workers with younger native-born workers. Thus, the rates of retirement are closely tied to issues of state spending and immigration policy (Coleman 1992).

In developing countries, older workers often continue to work almost until the time of death. In advanced industrial countries, the pattern is different (Clark, Ramsbey, and Adler 1999). American labor force participation rates at older ages dropped after the introduction of Social Security and private employer-sponsored pension plans (Wise 1997). Workers also have less available in savings upon retirement. Meanwhile the average length of expected time in retirement has increased (Lee 2001).

In the United States, where there is no longer mandatory retirement, the modeling of retirement is also important for projecting the future size of the labor force. Although this modeling is important, it has also become more difficult because retirement timing has become more irregular (Han and Moen 1999). Many researchers are looking for demographic regularities in retirement now that the institutional regularities are in abeyance (Guillemard and Rein 1993).

Some studies have shown that formerly married women plan much later retirements than formerly married men because they have had lower earnings and expect only small retirement payments (Hatch 1992). More generally, working and nonworking life expectancy vary according to occupation, class of worker, education, race, and marital status (Hayward and Grady 1990; Burr et al. 1996). Moreover, these economic and social characteristics, because they are related to income during working life, are also related to postretirement income (Pampel and Hardy 1994).

Given the economic and social significance of retirement and the growing share of the elderly in the population, it seems likely that labor force demographers will pay greater attention to retirement.

Youth Labor Force Attachment

Another issue of great interest to labor force demographers is how young people become attached to the labor force. It is known that youth do so over a period of time, often with multiple entries and reentries. The attachment process appears to differ for men and women. Attachment also seems to differ for blacks and whites (Deseran and Keithly 1994). Working during high school has a positive effect on many labor force behaviors, such as labor force participation and income, even 10 years later, but working during high school also appears to be negatively related to later finishing college (Carr, Wright, and Brady 1996).

Moreover, at least one study has found that time spent out of the labor force by youths is positively related to becoming engaged in crime (Crutchfield and Pitchford 1997). Thus, crime may be an alternative to work for some young men. Other studies have indicated that welfare may be an alternative to work for some young women, especially those who have had children.

Because young adulthood is a time for acquiring many roles simultaneously, there is great interest in how youths order family formation, schooling, and work, and the ways in which these statuses are entered and the overlap in statuses. Because of changes that occur in cohorts, it seems likely that the conclusions reached for previous generations may not hold for younger generations, leading to a continued need for additional research.

The Future of Work

A durable issue for labor force demographers is how the labor force will look when the demographic transition is complete and after the sectoral transition from agriculture to industry to services has been completed. By 2010, the median age of the U.S. labor force will be over 40, with a continuing shift toward knowledge work. One in five workers will be in a professional or related occupation (Francese 2002).

Demographers have become fairly sophisticated in projecting the labor supply, including the composition of potential workers who are available for work. Future progress in this area will rely more heavily on understanding labor demand and its intersection with the labor supply in the form of actual employment for specific workers. It is foreseeable that the effects of improved productivity, either because of technology or human capital improvements, will continue to affect the demand for labor. But a variety of institutional and organizational effects are more difficult to forecast and are likely to play a key role in shaping the future labor force.

REFERENCES

Avakame, E. F. 1999. Females' labor force participation and intimate femicide: An empirical assessment of the backlash hypothesis. *Violence and Victims* 14(3) (Fall):277–291.

Bauer, J. 1990. Demographic change and Asian labor markets in the 1990s. *Population and Development Review* 16(4) (December):615–645.

Baum, C. L. 2002. A dynamic analysis of the effect of child care costs on the work decisions of low-income mothers with infants. *Demography* 39(1) (February):139–164.

Bener'ia, L. 1999. The enduring debate over unpaid labour. *International Labour Review* 138(3):287–309.

Bianchi, S. 1995. Changing economic roles of women and men. In *State of the Union*, Vol. 1. Edited by R. Farley, 107–154. New York: Russell Sage.

Blank, R. M. 1995. Outlook for the U.S. labor market and prospects for low-wage entry jobs. In *The Work Alternative*. Edited by D. Smith Nightingale and R. H. Haverman, 36–69. Cambridge, Mass.: Harvard University Press.

Blau, F. D., and M. A. Ferber. 1991. Career plans and expectations of young women and men: the earnings gap and labor force participation. *The Journal of Human Resources* 26:581–607.

Bollen, K. A., and S. J. Appold. 1993. National industrial structure and the global system. *American Sociological Review* 58:283–301.

Borjas, G. J., and M. Tienda. 1993. The employment and wages of legalized immigrants. *International Migration Review* 27:712–747.

Bound, J., M. Schoenbaum, and T. Waldmann. 1995. Race and education differences in disability status and labor force attachment in the health and retirement survey. *Journal of Human Resources* 30:S227–S267.

Brewster, K. L., and R. R. Rindfuss. 2000. Fertility and women's employment in industrialized nations. *Annual Review of Sociology* 26:271–296.

Brinton, M. C., Y. Lee, and W. L. Parish. 1995. Married women's employment in rapidly industrializing societies: Examples from East Asia. *American Journal of Sociology* 100:1099–1130.

Browne, I. 1997. Explaining the black-white gap in labor force participation among women heading households. *American Sociological Review* 62:236–252.

Burr, J. A., M. P. Massagli, J. E. Mutchler, and A. M. Pienta. 1996. Labor force transitions among older African American and white men. *Social Forces* 74:963–982.

Buss, T. F., and F. S. Redburn. 1988. *Hidden unemployment: Discouraged workers and public policy.* New York: Praeger.

Carlson, E. 1992. Inverted Easterlin fertility cycles and Kornai's 'soft' budget constraint. *Population and Development Review* 18:669–688.

Carr, R. V., J. D. Wright, and C. J. Brody. 1996. Effects of high school work experience a decade later: Evidence from the National Longitudinal Survey. *Sociology of Education* 69:66–81.

Carrasco, R. 2001. Binary choice with binary endogenous regressors in panel data: Estimating the effect of fertility on female labor force participation. *Journal of Business and Economic Statistics*: 385–394.

Cerrutti, M. 2000. Intermittent employment among married women: A comparative study of Buenos Aires and Mexico City. *Journal of Comparative Family Studies* 31:19–43.

Charles, M. 1992. Cross-national variation in occupational sex segregation. *American Sociological Review* 57:483–502.

Clark, R., T. W. Ramsbey, and E. S. Adler. 1991. Culture, gender, and labor force participation: A cross-national study. *Gender & Society* 5:47–66.

Clogg, C. C. 1979. *Measuring underemployment.* New York: Academic Press.

Clogg, C. C., S. R. Eliason, and R. J. Wahl. 1990. Labor-market experiences and labor-force outcomes. *American Journal of Sociology* 95:1536–1576.

Clogg, C. C., and T. A. Sullivan. 1983. Labor force composition and unemployment trends, 1969–1980. *Social Indicators Research* 12:117–152.

Coleman, D. A. 1992. Does Europe need immigrants? Population and work force projections. *International Migration Review* 26:413–461.

Cotter, D. A., J. DeFiore, J. M. Hermsen, B. Marsteller Kowalewski, R. Vanneman. 1998. The demand for female labor. *American Journal of Sociology* 103:1673–1712.

Cotter, D. A., J. M. Hermsen, R. Vanneman. 2001. Women's Work and Working Women – the demand for female labor. *Gender & Society* 15:429–452.

Crutchfield, R. D., and S. R. Pitchford. 1997. Work and crime: The effects of labor stratification. *Social Forces* 76:93–118.

DeAnda, R. M. 2000. Mexican-origin women's employment instability. *Sociological Perspectives* 43:421–437.

DeJong, G. F., and A. B. Madamba. 2001. A double disadvantage? Minority group, status, and underemployment in the United States. *Social Science Quarterly* 82:117–130.

Desai, S., and L. J. Waite. 1991. Women's employment during pregnancy and after first birth: Occupational characteristics and work commitment. *American Sociological Review* 56(4) (August):551–566.

Deseran, F. A., and D. Keithly. 1994. Teenagers in the U.S. labor force: Local labor markets, race, and family. *Rural Sociology* 59(4) (Winter):668–692.

DiPrete, T. A., P. M. deGraaf, R. Luijkx, M. Tahlin, and H. Blossfeld. 1997. Collectivist versus individualist mobility regimes? Structural change and job mobility in four countries. *American Journal of Sociology* 103:318–358.

Donahoe, D. A. 1999. Measuring women's work in developing countries. *Population and Development Review* 25:543–576.

Duleep, H. O., and S. Sanders. 1993. The decision to work by married immigrant women. *Industrial and Labor Relations Review* 46:677–690.

Edin, K., and L. Lein. 1997a. *Making ends meet.* New York: Russell Sage.

Edin, K., and L. Lein. 1997b. Work, welfare, and single mothers' economic survival strategies. *American Sociological Review* 62:253–266.

Edwards, L. N., and E. F. Hendry. 2002. Home-based work and women's labor force decisions. *Journal of Labor Economics* 20:170–200.

Enchautegui, M. E. 1992. Geographical differentials in the socioeconomic status of Puerto Ricans : Human capital variations and labor market characteristics. *International Migration Review* 26:1267–1290.

Ettner, S. L. 1995. The impact of "parent care" on female labor supply decisions. *Demography* 32:63–80.

Evans, M. D. R. and J. Kelley. 1991. Prejudice, discrimination, and the labor market: Attainments of immigrants in Australia. *American Journal of Sociology* 97:721–759.

Field, J. 2003. *Social capital.* New York: Routledge.

Francese, P. 2002. The American work force. *American Demographics* February: 40–41.

Fullerton, H. N., Jr., and M. Toossi. 2001. Labor force projections to 2010: Steady growth and changing composition. *Monthly Labor Review* 124:21–38.

Gendell, M. 2002. Short work lives, long retirements make saving difficult. *Population Today* 30:5, 10.

Geschwender, J. A. 1992. Ethnicity and the social construction of gender in the Chinese diaspora. *Gender & Society* 6:480–507.

Glass, J. L., and L. Riley. 1998. Family responsive policies and employee retention following childbirth. *Social Forces* 76:1401–1435.

Gonul, F. 1992. New evidence on whether unemployment and out of the labor force are distinct states. *The Journal of Human Resources* 27:329–361.

Guillemard, A., and M. Rein. 1993. Comparative patterns of retirement : Recent trends in developed societies. *Annual Review of Sociology* 19:469–503.

Guo, G., J. Brooks-Gunn, and K. M. Harris. 1996. Parent's labor force attachment and grade retention among urban black children. *Sociology of Education* 69:217–236.

Gurak, D. T., and M. M. Kritz. 1996. Social context, household composition and employment among migrant and nonmigrant Dominican women. *International Migration Review* 30:399–422.

Gustaffson, S. S., C. M. M. P. Wetzels, J. D. Vlasblom, and S. Dex. 1996. Women's labor force transitions in connection with childbirth: A panel data comparison between Germany, Sweden, and Great Britain. *Journal of Population Economics* 9:223–246.

Han, S., and P. Moen. 1999. Clocking out: Temporal patterning of retirement. *American Journal of Sociology* 105:191–236.

Han, W. J., and J. Waldfogel. 2001. Child care costs and women's employment: A comparison of single and married mothers with pre-school-aged children. *Social Science Quarterly* 82:552–568.

Harris, K. M. 1993. Work and welfare among single mothers in poverty. *American Journal of Sociology* 99:317–352.

Harris, K. M. 1996. Life after welfare: Women, work, and repeat dependency. *American Sociological Review* 61:407–426.

Hatch, L. R. 1992. Gender differences in orientation toward retirement from paid labor. *Gender & Society* 6:66–85.

Hayward, M. D., and W. R. Grady. 1990. Work and retirement among a cohort of older men in the United States, 1966–1983. *Demography* 27:337–356.

Hill, E. T. 1995. Labor market effects of women's post-school-age training. *Industrial and Labor Relations Review* 49:138–149.

Hodson, R., and T. A. Sullivan. 2002. *The social organization of work.* Belmont, Calif.: Wadsworth.

Hsueh S., and M. Tienda. 1996. Gender, ethnicity, and labor force instability. *Social Science Research* 25: 73–94.

Jacobsen, J. P., J. W. Pearce III, and J. L. Rosenbloom. 1999. The effects of childbearing on married women's labor supply and earnings: Using twin births as a natural experiment. *The Journal of Human Resources* 34:449–474.

Jaffe, A. J. 1959. Working force. In *The study of population*. Edited by P. M. Hauser and O. D. Duncan, 604–619. Chicago: University of Chicago Press.

Kalleberg, A. 2000. Nonstandard employment relations: Part-time, temporary, and contract work. *Annual Review of Sociology* 26:341–365.

Kerckhoff, A. C. 1995. Institutional arrangements and stratification processes in industrial societies. *Annual Review of Sociology* 21:323–347.

Kishor, S. 1993. "May God give sons to all": Gender and child mortality in India. *American Sociological Review* 58:247–265.

Klerman, J. A., and A. Leibowitz. 1994. The work-employment distinction among new mothers. *The Journal of Human Resources* 29:277–303.

Klerman, J. A., and A. Leibowitz. 1999. Women's educational attainment, employment, and earnings: Job continuity among new mothers. *Demography* 36:145–155.

Kohn, M. L. 1977. *Class and conformity: A study in values, with a reassessment*. Chicago: University of Chicago Press.

Kohn, M. L., et al. 1983. *Work and personality: An inquiry into the impact of social stratification*. Norwood, N.J.: Ablex.

Kreider, B. 1999. Latent work disability and reporting bias. *The Journal of Human Resources* 34:734–769.

Kunda, G., S. R. Barley, and J. Evans. 2002. Why do contractors contract? The experience of highly skilled technical professionals in a contingent labor market. *Industrial and Labor Relations Review* 55:234–261.

Kutscher, R. E. 1993. Historical trends, 1950–92, and current uncertainties. *Monthly Labor Review* November: 3–10.

Land, K. C., J. M. Guralnik, and D. G. Blazer. 1994. Estimating increment-decrement life tables with multiple covariates from panel data: The case of active life expectancy. *Demography* 31:297–319.

Lee, C. 2001. The expected length of male retirement in the United States, 1850–1990. *Journal of Population Economics* 14:641–650.

Lerman, R. I., and C. Radcliffe. 2001. Are single mothers finding jobs without displacing other workers? *Monthly Labor Review* 124:3–12.

Levin, C. E., M. T. Ruel, and S. S. Morris. 1999. Working women in an urban setting: Traders, vendors, and food security in Accra. *World Development* 27:1977–1991.

Lin, N. 2001. *Social capital: A theory of social structure and action*. New York: Cambridge University Press.

Lin, N., K. Cook, and R. S. Burt, eds. 2001. *Social capital: Theory and research*. New York: Aldine de Gruyter.

Manza, J., and C. Brooks. 1998. The gender gap in U.S. presidential elections: When? Why? Implications? *American Journal of Sociology* 103:1235–1266.

Mason, K. O., and K. Kuhlthau. 1992. The perceived impact of child care costs on women's labor supply and fertility. *Demography* 29:523–543.

Maxwell, N. L. 1990. Changing female labor force participation: Influences on income inequality and distribution. *Social Forces* 68:1251–1266.

Mellor, E. F., and W. Parks, II. 1988. A year's work: Labor force activity from a different perspective. *Monthly Labor Review* September: 13–18.

Moen, P., G. Downey, and N. Bolger. 1990. Labor-force reentry among U.S. homemakers in midlife: A life-course analysis. *Gender & Society* 4:230–243.

Murthi, M., A. Guio, and J. Dreze. 1995. Mortality, fertility, and gender bias in India: A district-level analysis. *Population and Development Review* 21:745–782.

National Commission on Employment and Unemployment Statistics. 1979. *Counting the labor force*. Washington, D.C.: U. S. Government Printing Office.

Nielsen, F. 1994. Income inequality and industrial development: Dualism revisited. *American Sociological Review* 59:654–677.

Nielsen, F., and A. S. Alderson. 1995. Income inequality, development, and dualism: Results from an unbalanced cross-national panel. *American Sociological Review* 60:674–701.

Norwood, J. L., and J. M. Tanur. 1994. Measuring unemployment in the nineties. *Public Opinion Quarterly* 58:277–294.

Odland, J. 2001. Intermetropolitan variations in labour force participation rates of white and black men in the United States. *Urban Studies* 38:2327–2349.

Pampel, F. C. 1993. Relative cohort size and fertility: The socio-political context of the Easterlin Effect. *American Sociological Review* 58:496–514.

Pampel, F. C., and H. E. Peters. 1995. The Easterlin Effect. *Annual Review of Sociology* 21:163–194.

Pampel, F. C., and M. Hardy. 1994. Status maintenance and change during old age. *Social Forces* 73:289–314.

Parrado, E. A., and R. M. Zenteno. 2001. Economic restructuring, financial crises, and women's work in Mexico. *Social Problems* 48:456–477.

Presser, H. B., and S. Kishor. 1991. Economic development and occupational sex segregation in Puerto Rico: 1950–80. *Population and Development Review* 17:53–85.

Rindfuss, R. R., K. L. Brewster, and A. L. Kavee. 1996. Women, work, and children: Behavioral and attitudinal change in the United States. *Population and Development Review* 22:457–482.

Roberts, B. W., R. Helson, and E. C. Klohnen. 2002. Personality development and growth in women across 30 years: Three perspectives. *Journal of Personality* 70:79–102.

Rosenfeld, R. A. 1996. Women's work histories. *Population and Development Review* 22:199–222.

Robinson, R., and I. Browne. 1994. Education and the economy. In *The Handbook of Economic Sociology*. Edited by N. J. Smelser and R. Sweelberg, 581–599. Princeton, N.J.: Princeton University Press.

Sanders, J. M. 1990. Public transfers: Safety net or inducement into poverty? *Social Forces* 68:813–834.

Shah, N. M. 1995. Structural changes in the receiving country and future labor migration: The case of Kuwait. *International Migration Review* 29:1000–1022.

Sobel, M. E. 1996. Clifford Collier Clogg, 1949–1995: A tribute to his life and work. *Sociological Methodology* 26:1–38.

Solow, R. M. 1990. *The labor market as a social institution.* Cambridge, Mass.: Basil Blackwell.

South, S. J. 2001. Time-dependent effects of wives' employment on marital dissolution. *American Sociological Review* 66:226–245.

Stier, H., and M. Tienda. 1992. Family, work, and women: The labor supply of Hispanic immigrant wives. *International Migration Review* 26:1291–1313.

Stinebrickner, T. R. 2002. An analysis of occupational change and departure from the labor force—Evidence of the reasons that teachers leave. *Journal of Human Resources* 37:192–216.

Stratton, L. S. 1993. Racial differences in men's unemployment. *Industrial and Labor Relations Review* 46:451–463.

Stratton, L. S. 1996. Are 'involuntary' part-time workers indeed involuntary? *Industrial and Labor Relations Review* 49:522–536.

Sullivan, T. A. 1978. *Marginal workers, marginal jobs.* Austin: University of Texas Press.

Tienda, M., K. M. Donato, and H. Cordero-Guzman. 1992. Schooling, color, and the labor force activity of women. *Social Forces* 71:365–395.

Tienda, M., and F. D. Wilson. 1992. Migration and the earnings of Hispanic men. *American Sociological Review* 57:661–678.

Vanderheuvel, A. 1997. Women's roles after first birth: Variable or stable? *Gender & Society* 11:357–368.

Wenk, D., and P. Garrett. 1992. Having a baby: Some predictions of maternal employment around childbirth. *Gender & Society* 6:49–65.

Willekens, F. J. 1979. Tables of working life. *Population Index* 45:397–397.

Wise, D. A. 1997. Retirement against the demographic trend: More older people living longer, working less, and saving more. *Demography* 34:83–95.

Zsembik, B. A., and C. W. Peek. 1994. The effect of economic restructuring on Puerto Rican women's labor force participation in the formal sector. *Gender & Society* 8:525–540.

PART II

POPULATION PROCESSES

Part II of this Handbook continues discussion of the elements of the basic population model by focusing on population processes. While the notion of population structure portrays a static view of the organization of human populations, that is, a time-bound representation of a population's size, composition, and distribution, the concept of population processes encompasses the engines of change that account for differences in structural features over time. Most demographers recognize four population processes: fertility, mortality, migration, and social mobility (change of status at the individual level, compositional change at the population level) (Hauser and Duncan 1959; Ryder 1964a; Ryder 1964b; Ryder 1965).

The Study of Population contains four chapters devoted to population processes; they deal with fertility (Ryder 1959), mortality (Dorn 1959), internal migration (Bogue 1959), and international migration (Thomas 1959). This *Handbook* expands the coverage of population processes to six chapters, reflecting the increased knowledge of and attention to population processes over the past half century (see Preston, Heuveline, and Guillot 2001).

Morgan and Hagewen in chapter 8 review theoretical, methodological, and substantive developments in the study of fertility, a topic that continues to be a major concern of demographic inquiry. In chapters 9 and 10, Frisbie (chapter 9) and Rogers, Hummer and Krueger (chapter 10) turn their attention to the topics of infant and adult mortality, respectively. White and Lindstrom in chapters 11, and Brown and Bean in chapter 12 bring the field up to date in the sometimes neglected areas of internal and international migration. Their reviews are particularly important in light of several demographers' characterization of migration as the "step-child" of demography (Bouvier, Poston and Zhai 1997; Goldstein 1976; Kirk 1960, 1968). Finally, in chapter 13 Sakamoto and Powers emphasize another relatively neglected topic, changes in population composition through the process of social mobility. The editors of this *Handbook* believe these six chapters provide a fairly comprehensive treatment of the processes of demography.

REFERENCES

Bogue, D. J. 1959. "Internal Migration." pp. 486–509 in *The Study of Population: An Inventory and Appraisal*, edited by P. M. Hauser and O. D. Duncan. Chicago: University of Chicago Press.

Bouvier, L. F., D. L. Poston, Jr., and N. B. Zhai. 1997. "Population Growth Impacts of Zero Net International Migration." *International Migration Review* 31(2):294–311.

Dorn, H. F. 1959. "Mortality." pp. 437–471 in *The Study of Population: An Inventory and Appraisal*, edited by P. M. Hauser and O. D. Duncan. Chicago: University of Chicago Press.

Goldstein, S. 1976. "Facets of Redistribution: Research Challenges and Opportunities." *Demography* 13(4):423–434.

Hauser, P. M. and O. D. Duncan. 1959. "The Nature of Demography." pp. 29–44 in *The Study of Population: An Inventory and Appraisal*, edited by P. M. Hauser and O. D. Duncan. Chicago: University of Chicago Press.

Kirk, D. 1960. "Some Reflections on American Demography in the Nineteen Sixties." *Population Index* 26(4):305–310.

Kirk, D. 1968. "The Field of Demography." pp. 342–343 in *International Encyclopedia of the Social Sciences*, edited by D. L. Sills. New York: Macmillan.

Preston, S. H., P. Heuveline, and M. Guillot. 2001. *Demography: Measuring and Modeling Population Processes*. Oxford: Blackwell Publishers.

Ryder, N. B. 1959. "Fertility." pp. 400–436 in *The Study of Population: An Inventory and Appraisal*, edited by P. M. Hauser and O. D. Duncan. Chicago: University of Chicago Press.

Ryder, N. B. 1964a. "Notes on the Concept of a Population." *American Journal of Sociology* 69(5):447–463.

Ryder, N. B. 1964b. "The Process of Demographic Translation." *Demography* 1(1):74–82.

Ryder, N. B. 1965. "The Cohort as a Concept in the Study of Social Change." *American Sociological Review* 30(6):843–861.

Thomas, B. 1959. "International Migration." pp. 510–543 in *The Study of Population: An Inventory and Appraisal*, edited by P. M. Hauser and O. D. Duncan. Chicago: University of Chicago Press.

CHAPTER 8

Fertility

S. Philip Morgan and Kellie J. Hagewen

SUBSTANTIVE CONCERNS

Human fertility has attracted great attention over the past half-century.[1] In fact, the largest, coordinated social science research efforts in history (the World Fertility Surveys and Demographic Health Surveys) have had fertility as their focus. Motivation for this attention emanates from the important and wide-ranging consequences of fertility and fertility change. Fertility levels are key components of population change and have been, historically, the component most difficult to predict (Bongaarts and Bulatao 2000). Also, fertility levels alter cohort sizes that, in turn, impact a full set of age-graded institutions such as schools, the labor force, marriage, and social security. Finally, human fertility is strongly linked to "parenting" or social replacement, the process of socializing group members. Except perhaps for increasing longevity, no 20th-century change has impacted individual lives more than have fertility changes. Consider, for instance, the cascading consequences of declining fertility and the dramatic declines in the size of families, sibships and households, the number of close relatives, and the years spent as parents of small children.

Given the importance of fertility differences and trends and the effort devoted to their study, one should expect substantial scientific progress in this area of demography. Indeed, no social science subfield is more developed than fertility. Of course, not all

---

[1] Teachman and colleagues (1993) report in a 1993 article in *Demography*, the official journal of the Population Association of America, that of the 1,232 articles published in the journal between 1964 and 1991, by far the most common subject area was fertility and contraception, comprising 36% of all published articles.

answers are in hand and disputes exist. But highly useful analytic and theoretical frameworks have been developed, widely accepted methodologies for collecting and analyzing information have evolved, and significant knowledge has accumulated. We review this scientific progress in this chapter.

THEORETICAL ISSUES

We begin by distinguishing between analytic frameworks and causal/behavioral theories. Analytic frameworks are useful ways to organize data, and they capture structural aspects of the process. Fertility research has produced widely accepted and very useful analytic frameworks. However, these analytic frameworks are largely silent regarding the more distal social causes of fertility trends and group differences. There is much greater disagreement regarding the relative value of these more distal causal theories. We address analytic frameworks and causal theories in turn.

Analytic Frameworks

Two mutually informing analytic frameworks have been central to much recent fertility research: the *life course* and the *proximate determinants* frameworks. The biological nature of fertility determines the structure of each framework. In fact, both frameworks rest on very straightforward observations. The life course perspective adopts a sequential model because children tend to be born one at a time, not in lots (Namboodiri 1972: 198). Moreover, because women are biologically restricted to having children only between menarche and menopause, fertility may be considered as an irreversible, time-limited sequence.

This sequential structure can be used to decompose overall change into age and birth order (or parity) components (see Morgan 1996). Or it can be adopted to compare the fertility regimes of different groups. For instance, when do two groups behave differently and when do they behave similarly? This structure also makes explicit the fundamental life course principle that events and their circumstances at time t can influence behavior at time $t + 1$. Most researchers now view fertility outcomes as resulting from a series of sequential decisions. For instance, permanent childlessness results most often from a series of decisions to postpone childbearing and not from firm decisions made early in life to remain childless (see Rindfuss, Morgan, and Swicegood 1988).

The proximate determinants paradigm provides a second organizing framework. It rests on the observation that the sequential biological process is influenced through only a few mechanisms, specifically, variables that influence sexual activity, the likelihood of conception, and the likelihood that conceptions result in live births (see Davis and Blake 1956). Bongaarts and Potter's (1978) operationalization of the proximate determinants demonstrates that most fertility variability between populations and over time can be accounted for by the following four determinants: (1) marriage and marital disruption (as indicators of the segments of the life cycle when women are sexually active), (2) postpartum infecundability (the period after a birth without ovulation; its length is determined primarily by the duration and intensity of breastfeeding), (3) use and effectiveness of contraception, and (4) induced abortion. Three other determinants are occasionally or potentially important: (5) the onset of permanent sterility, (6) natural fecundability (frequency of intercourse), and (7) spontaneous intrauterine mortality. However, they do not vary as much among populations as the first four.

The life course and proximate determinant frameworks together provide a crucial foundation for understanding the mechanisms that influence individual and aggregate fertility. Descriptive work using these frameworks identifies precisely "what needs to be explained." As an example, the most dynamic fertility component in the U.S. baby boom and bust was the timing of the first birth (Ryder 1980). This observation begs the question: What accounts for this changing timing of family formation? Likewise, if an observed fertility decline can be attributed, within the proximate determinants framework, to changes in marriage, then a very different explanation is required other than that the change is due to increasing contraceptive use. Overall, then, theories of fertility change and variability are incomplete if they do not specify where in the life course and through which proximate determinants the social, economic, and cultural factors operate.

Causal/Behavioral Theories

Fertility transitions are complete in many developed countries and are in progress in much of the rest of the world. The transition model has three stages: relatively high and stable fertility, followed by a period of fertility decline, and then followed by relatively low and stable fertility. This fertility transition is part of the demographic transition model that includes similar changes/stages in mortality (see chapter 10 in this *Handbook*). The demographic transition theory, based heavily on observed, historical changes in the West, linked fertility and mortality changes to social, economic, and family changes caused by industrialization and urbanization (Notestein 1953). Given a very long time frame, all economic transitions (from rural/agrarian to urban/industrial) have been accompanied by fertility declines. But demographic transition theory has not performed as well in accounting for the timing of fertility decline. This poor fit of data to theory has led to a number of revisions, extensions, and elaborations of demographic transition theory.

Specifically, substantive behavioral explanations for fertility transition focus on at least one of three elements: the nature of fertility decisions, the information and knowledge available to decision makers, and the institutional context for decision making. We first consider high fertility in pre industrial settings. Widespread evidence indicates that the high fertility of many populations coincided with a "natural fertility" regime, one in which potential decision makers did not limit their number of births via changed behavior at higher parities (Henry 1961). There are three possible reasons: (1) decision makers were motivated to have as many children as possible, (2) decision makers did not know how to limit fertility, or (3) fertility control was not licit. Important behavioral theories focus on each alternative.

The first alternative is consistent with micro economic models of choice that stressed the economic value of children. Children provide substantial labor in preindustrial settings and have relatively low direct and opportunity costs. One version of the argument for the rationality of high fertility is found in Caldwell's (1982) work. Caldwell argued that preindustrial patriarchal family structure (an institutional context) allowed older individuals and males to appropriate wealth from younger and female family members. This positive "wealth flow" from children toward the senior generation motivated higher fertility. High fertility, in turn, produced greater wealth, power, and prestige for patriarchs. According to this and other arguments stressing the economic value of children, fertility was high in preindustrial contexts because children were net assets.

Empirical evidence regarding the economic value of children in preindustrial contexts is mixed. Children clearly performed substantial work, but their rearing and support also required substantial investment. The current consensus is that children were not universally perceived as net economic assets in preindustrial settings.[2] These mixed results on the economic cost of children shifted attention to children's roles as adults in supporting their parents. In many contexts older persons were dependent upon their children for support in old age. Prior to old age dependency, many relied upon children for support in case of crisis. A large literature has focused on the import of children in providing old age security and risk insurance (e.g., Cain 1983; Nugent 1985).

Finally, the cost-benefit analysis of high fertility focuses on noneconomic values of children. Across a range of institutional contexts, parents give reasons for having children, such as having a child to love and care for, having a sibling for a previously born child, having a son or a daughter, or bringing the family closer together (see Bulatao 1981).

Others have argued against individual cost-benefit calculations in many preindustrial contexts. van de Walle (1992), for instance, has claimed that many persons did not conceptualize family size as a key decision variable because factors determining it seemed beyond their ability or willingness to control. The vagaries of mortality or the social construction of morality pushed effective family size control beyond the reach of most.

Note that this argument does not mean that people had no knowledge of birth control. Rather it implies that they were not willing to use these mechanisms. In some settings knowledge of techniques may have been the limiting factor, while in others, limiting family size was beyond the "calculus of conscious choice." Proponents of these two positions have waged an intellectually engaging debate for over two decades. Evidence for both positions exists, and there is no reason to assume that a single answer is appropriate for all settings. For instance, evidence of infanticide in preindustrial China shows that under given institutional arrangements controlling family size and composition was of extreme importance. In addition, the extended family arranged marriage to control family size. Abstinence and abortion also have a long history in China (Lee and Feng 1999). In contrast, in Western Europe there was little evidence of family size control before the onset of fertility decline. Knodel and van de Walle (1979) have discussed the evidence in detail. For instance, they point out that nonmarital and marital childbearing declined in tandem. While one might argue that the desire to limit marital fertility was absent prior to the onset of decline, the European historical context included strong negative sanctions for nonmarital childbearing. Thus, incentives to avoid nonmarital childbearing clearly existed prior to the onset of fertility decline. Indeed, the nearly simultaneous decline of marital and nonmarital fertility suggests that knowledge of birth control means, not motivation, was the missing ingredient. As

---

[2] Evolutionary arguments point out that other mechanisms generally guaranteed a substantial supply of children (Potts 1997) and that exploitation of the younger generation is not a viable evolutionary strategy (Kaplan 1994).

further evidence, women in developing countries frequently report having more children than desired. This is prima facie evidence against the claim that families in preindustrial settings desired as many children as they could have (Shorter et al. 1971; Knodel and van de Walle 1979).

The fertility transition's second stage views family size declines as resulting from conscious actions by decision makers, specifically decisions to curtail childbearing at lower parities. Depending on their explanation for the preceding natural fertility regime, theorists point toward institutional change that transforms children from net assets to financial liabilities, or ones that provide new knowledge or changed norms that allow for family size control.

Caldwell (1982), for instance, points to schooling and nonfamilial employment opportunities that undermined the power and control of patriarchs and shifted the net flow of wealth toward children. Others have incorporated the importance of mortality decline. For instance, Easterlin and Crimmins's (1985) framework explicitly includes the possibility that declining infant and child mortality produced an increase in surviving children. For some decision makers, surviving children (the supply of children) now exceeded the desired number (the demand for children), producing a motivation for fertility control. In sum, a large body of work argues that rational decisions in changed contexts tended to lead to a new decision—to stop childbearing after a desired number was achieved.

For those arguments that stressed the lack of contraceptive knowledge or the presence of normative injunctions against using them, key factors in the decline were likely the spread of knowledge or new ideas legitimizing contraceptives or the small family size ideal. These ideas could have included broad, increasingly popular, anti-natalist ideologies of individualism and self-actualization. Such ideologies justified nonfamilial activities and aspirations (Lesthaeghe 1983). But the diffusing knowledge may have also included new information about techniques or the diffusion of the technologies themselves. The evidence suggesting a role for diffusion processes is powerful. For instance, the European Fertility Project (see Coale and Watkins 1986) characterized the geographical pattern of European fertility decline as a "contagion process." Geographical proximity and measures of interaction (e.g., shared language) were strong predictors of the timing of fertility decline. Likewise, reviews of evidence from developing country fertility surveys have shown patterns of change far too rapid to be attributed solely to decision-maker adjustment to changing objective, socioeconomic circumstances (Cleland and Wilson 1987).

Consistent with earlier adjudication between these positions, one need not choose one or the other as a universal answer (see Mason 1997). In an analysis that we believe best captures the contemporary demographic consensus, Bongaarts and Watkins' (1996) review of postwar fertility declines finds evidence that both structural change and diffusion processes are at work.

The third and final stage of the demographic transition is low fertility that approximates very low mortality. Such a balance is logically necessary; over the long run neither positive nor negative growth rates can continue. An emerging issue of both practical and intellectual import is the question of whether economically advanced societies will have fertility levels that even approximate replacement levels.

One position is nicely characterized by Bumpass (1990), who argues that the long-term factors that have reduced fertility "have not run their course." These factors include "structural" changes in the way we live and work that make children costly (in economic terms and in terms of foregone opportunities). Secular forces also include ideologies of self-actualization and individualism that could become even more powerful and pervasive antinatalist ideologies (see Lesthaeghe 1983; van de Kaa 2001).

As an example, many see increasing female labor force participation as a key structural, secular, antinatalist factor. The standard microlevel home economics approach posits that declining gender discrimination and greater access to the labor market increases the cost of having children. This increased cost results from women's exit from the labor force to bear and raise the children and the costs of labor force exit on career trajectories. This argument has led to the very widely held view that increased labor force participation by women would depress fertility rates. In the past, evidence for such an association was common at both the individual and aggregate levels.

More recent arguments, however, stress the importance of institutions in conditioning the effects of secular structural change (Rindfuss 1991, Rindfuss, Guzzo, and Morgan 2003). For instance, if one assumes that female labor force participation increases will continue, the question then becomes what societies using which institutions can make accommodations that allow women to more easily work and have children?

Perhaps the best evidence that societies vary on this dimension is the changing aggregate-level association between female labor force participation rates and the total fertility rate. Traditionally and according to most theories, this association should be negative; higher labor force participation is associated with lower fertility. But in low-fertility contexts, the opposite appears to be true (see Rindfuss and Brewster 1996; Rindfuss, Guzzo, and Morgan 2003). This cross-sectional association occurs because, in the past two decades, the association between labor force participation and fertility has varied dramatically by country. In the U.S., for instance, increases in labor force participation have not been accompanied by decreases in fertility. In Italy over the past two decades, for contrast, the association between labor force participation and fertility has been strongly negative (Rindfuss, Guzzo, and Morgan 2003). What aspects of context weaken the incompatibility of work and family obligations? Many point to available, high-quality day care, flexible work environments (flex time and parental leaves, for example), and more egalitarian gender roles that provide women with a domestic helpmate and a reduced "second shift." In sum, this second view holds that fertility levels are determined by adjustments in the institutions of family, economy, and public policy (for different conceptualizations of these adjustments see Esping-Anderson 1999; McDonald 2000). Thus, the future of fertility depends upon societal adjustments that ease work-family conflicts. Some countries will make or have made such adjustments, while others have not and may not (see Morgan and King 2001).

The above review underemphasizes several important issues. First, our review has largely ignored the larger social context in which the debate about fertility occurred. The politics of the Cold War period, concerns about a global "population explosion," and the feminist movement all provided an urgency and brought resources and attention to the study of fertility transitions. This political context helped define high fertility as a social problem of the highest order and thus motivated action at many levels (see Hodgson 1988; Hodgson and Watkins 1997). Two levels of action were by governments and by nongovernmental organizations, both of which organized and funded family planning programs. These programs clearly sped fertility declines in many countries. A second theme underemphasized here is linked to theories drawn from closely observed local experiences (e.g., Watkins 2000; Kertzer and Fricke 1997). Known as "thick description," these theories provide details of change specific to certain locales and resonate more closely with the experiences of the respondents. Such a focus is missed by the broad review just presented.

METHODS AND MEASURES

A mature science has reached agreement on definitions of key concepts, measurement strategies, and appropriate analysis procedures. Fertility research is clearly institutionalized in each of these domains. Fertility's success as a scientific area of study rests on fortuitous features of the phenomenon itself, the broader interest in fertility (for administrative and other reasons) that have encouraged data collections and standardization of measurement strategies, and an immense amount of research attention on a decadal time scale.

Fertility shares with the study of mortality fortuitous features of the study phenomenon. Births and deaths, the core events in demography, focus on observable events that are relatively easily measured, naturally quantifiable, highly structured, and can be easily incorporated into accounting frameworks or represented by descriptive demographic models (Morgan and Lynch 2001). In any science, conceptual clarity and intersubjective agreement across observers are essential for good measurement. Births are biologically based and are thus fixed in a universally accepted truth. Another important characteristic of births is that they are categorical by nature and thus inherently quantifiable, making measurement reliability attainable. The actual occurrence of a birth is universally recognized, although the actual meaning and consequences of a birth may be socially constructed. Therefore, valid cross-national and cross-temporal measurement of fertility is feasible. This is not to say that fertility measurement is easy or error free. But the inherent features of fertility provide a leverage for good measurement that is not found for many other concepts (Morgan and Lynch 2001).

The interest in fertility data for administrative purposes aids fertility measurement, increases data availability, and improves data quality. The importance of fertility data for administrative purposes has led to wide-scale collection. The usefulness of comparable fertility data across administrative units encourages the codification of definitions and standardization of measurement procedures.

While births are the event to be measured, the concept of an event/exposure rate is fundamental to all demographic measurement. The additional key concept needed for rate calculation is the *population at risk* or *person-years* of exposure. The essential measurement task is to estimate the risk of a specific event (e.g., a birth, a first birth, a nonmarital birth). The accepted strategy utilizes a ratio of a count of events (births to a specified group) to an estimate of the *person-years* exposed to the risk of an event in a given time period (Preston, Heuveline, and Guillot 2001). In the year 2000, for instance, a woman who survives the full year contributes a full year at risk of a birth and thus adds one to the denominator of a year 2000 birth rate. There is a range of strategies for estimating years at risk (Preston, Heuveline, and Guillot 2001).

Once rates have been estimated, how does one conceptualize social change? In general, birth rates can be examined by alternative dimensions of time: period or cohort. Period fertility measures look at fertility cross-sectionally, or births/exposure occurring at one period in time (usually across a set of age categories). Cohort analysis, conversely, follows a group longitudinally or over a women's reproductive history, again across age. Data for calculating period measures are more widely available, they have useful and interpretable meanings and, consequently, they are more frequently used (Newell 1988).

The two most commonly used period measures of fertility are age-specific fertility rates (ASFR) and the total fertility rate (TFR). When calculating age-specific fertility rates, the numerator is restricted to births occurring to women of a specified age interval, and the denominator is restricted to the number of person-years lived by women in the age interval (see Preston, Heuveline, and Guillot 2001). The teenage (age 15 to 19) birth rate is an age-specific birth rate, as is the rate for women aged 35 to 39.

The total fertility rate (TFR) is the most frequently used indicator of period fertility; it is the simple sum of the ASFRs across the childbearing years. Thus, the TFR is an age-standardized, single-value, summary measure of fertility. The TFR has a powerful yet easily understood interpretation. Specifically, the TFR is the number of children a woman would bear if she experienced, at each age, the current period age-specific fertility rates (and she survived to the end of her reproductive cycle). In the absence of mortality, a TFR of 2.0 would equal replacement level fertility. This means that the women are having enough births to replace themselves and their male partner. Other measures estimate replacement-level fertility in the presence of mortality (see Preston et al. 2001). Table 8.1 presents estimates of the highest and lowest TFRs for countries in 2002.

The TFR can be calculated from cohort data, that is, age-specific rates for an actual cohort. This measure (sometimes called children ever born) can be interpreted as the mean number of children produced by a birth cohort.

Data for fertility rate estimation come from several sources. Vital registration systems, if birth certificates are filed for all births, can provide an accurate count of births. One can then use various demographic procedures to estimate the denominator of desired rates, usually from census data projected forward or backward to correspond to the year in question. For instance, since birth certificates usually include the age of the mother, one can get a count of births to 20-year-old women. The census estimate of the midyear, 20-year-old, female population provides a commonly used estimate of years at risk, which is the denominator of the rate.

Frequently censuses contain data that can be used to measure fertility. Many censuses include the number of children ever born (a cohort measure of fertility). Also, since censuses generally include a household roster, one can count a woman's number of surviving children in the household. Strategies exist for estimating fertility from this count of *own children*. Specifically, one makes a set of adjustments to the count

TABLE 8.1. Selected High and Low TFRs from Around the World, 2002.

Country	TFR	Country	TFR
Niger	8.00	Spain	1.16
Somalia	7.25	Italy	1.20
Angola	7.20	Greece	1.30
Uganda	7.10	Germany	1.33
Yemen	7.10	Austria	1.36
Mali	7.00	Portugal	1.46

Source: United Nations Population Division, 2002.

of coresiding children (e.g., one estimates and includes the own children that did not survive to the census date and those not living with their mother at the time of the census (see Rindfuss and Sweet 1977). This clever strategy, known as *own children analysis*, can be used in some but not all settings.

Finally, surveys can ask about *retrospective fertility history*. That is, a respondent is asked to recall all her births and their dates. If her own age is reported correctly and if all birth dates are accurate, then accurate ASFR fertility rates for surviving women can be calculated. Specifically, one can for x years prior to the survey count births in year t-x and years of exposure in year t-x for women in the sample of a given age.

The survey strategy also allows for additional fertility-relevant information to be collected, resulting in estimates of fertility in the absence of high-quality vital registration and censuses. This methodology was used in the World Fertility Surveys and the Demographic Health Surveys carried out in many developing countries over the past three decades.

So far our discussion has been limited to measures of actual fertility, where measurement properties are strong. There are many other variables used in the study of fertility, each of which bring measurement challenges. These variables are fertility intentions or desires, measures of contraceptive use, coital frequency, marriage/union status, and breast-feeding. We only comment here on fertility intentions or desires. (See Chapter 3, "Marriage and Family," for a discussion of the measurement of marital/ union status.)

Virtually all contemporary populations, and presumably all future ones, will consist primarily of persons or couples that strategize about family size. Clearly, declining family size preferences constitute a primary cause of fertility transitions and will influence post transition fertility levels. In societies undergoing fertility transitions, observed fertility frequently exceeds stated preferences; in post transition countries of the 1990s the opposite was true (Bongaarts 2001). The study of emerging and changing family size preferences and their relation to behavior provides clues to the nature of fertility decision making and the causes of fertility trends and differentials.

Commonly used prospective questions are the following: Do you *intend* to have a (or another) child? And, if yes, How many more children do you intend to have? These questions raise two fundamental issues. The first is whether fertility intentions or, alternatively, fertility *expectations* or *desires*, should be of paramount, substantive interest. Intentions reflect the respondent's goals (what the respondent plans to do) and, as such, should be strongly linked to subsequent behavior in environments where fertility is controlled. In contrast, expectations invite (sometimes explicitly, but often implicitly) a consideration of impediments that might interfere with one's intentions (such as contraceptive failure or subfecundity) and produce an underestimate or overestimate (respectively) of future fertility. Fertility desires require an even more hypothetical exercise that is linked closely to the concept of *demand for children* (which is the number of children one would intend if there were no subjective or economic costs to fertility control).

Some empirical evidence indicates that many respondents do not detect the differences between these terms *or* are unable/unwilling to perform the implied conceptual tasks that distinguish them (Ryder and Westoff 1971). Further, the demographic literature frequently refers to these questions as family size preferences and ignores the distinctions noted above.

The second issue raised by this pair of questions is whether prospective intentions are best represented as a *fixed target* or as a *set of sequential decisions*. We have stressed earlier the importance of considering the inherent, sequential nature of fertility decisions. But prior to the 1960s, fertility intentions were mainly measured according to an alternative, the fixed-target model. This model posits that individuals or couples "formulate a desired completed family size and pursue this relative constant target throughout their reproductive life" (Lee 1980: 205). The fixed-target model, combined with reports of children already born, allowed the operationalization of *intended parity*. Specifically, intended parity is the sum of births to date and reported intended additional births. Mean intended parity for cohorts was frequently used to anticipate future fertility trends. The accuracy of forecasts based on intended parity depends on the predictive validity of reproductive intentions. This will be discussed in more detail later in this chapter.

Note that the first question above (Do you intend to have a/another child?) is a direct measure of sequential decisions that women or couples actually make and thus should be closely linked to fertility behavior. In fact, this indicator is highly predictive of subsequent fertility, especially if a time referent is included (explicitly asking do you intend to have a child in the next three years, three to five years, longer than five years, or intend no children). This variable is frequently used in analyses of factors influencing fertility decisions.

Respondents can also be asked about their intentions vis-à-vis births that they have had in the past. Demographers have developed a standard procedure and terminology for identifying *wanted* and *unwanted births*. Specifically, respondents are asked to recollect their fertility intention *at the time of each pregnancy*: 'At the time you became pregnant did you: (1) want to become pregnant at that time, (2) want to have children in the future, but not now, or (3) not want any additional children?' The first two responses are coded as *wanted* (although the second is termed a *timing failure*), and the third category as *unwanted*. For women who have completed childbearing, wanted fertility reflects their family size preferences and unwanted fertility a component that could have been avoided by effective birth control. Evidence clearly shows that the unwanted component of fertility declines as effective contraception and abortion become widely available.

EMPIRICAL FINDINGS

The fertility literature is huge. We will introduce it by identifying 10 major "social facts," i.e., empirical regularities from this literature.

1. Fertility in populations not using contraception and abortion varies substantially.
2. The timing of the onset of fertility transition (vis-à-vis objective socioeconomic conditions) is highly variable.
3. Existing institutions influence the fertility transition, thus the process of change varies from place to place and has historical continuity.
4. The fertility transition involves a collective evaluative assessment of social conditions and possible responses.
5. Once the fertility transition begins, it does not stop until fertility reaches levels of approximately two children or lower.

6. Fertility change is a period, not a cohort, phenomenon.
7. Fertility delay is fundamentally antinatalist.
8. Valid and reliable retrospective fertility histories can be collected from women in a broad range of settings. Reliable information on abortion cannot generally be obtained from respondents.
9. Long-range fertility intentions (individual or aggregate) have low predictive validity (at both the individual and aggregate level).
10. The fertility desires/intentions of men and women (and husbands and wives) are similar; and the impacts of their intentions/desires on subsequent fertility are similar.

We now discuss these in greater detail. These statements are not immutable "facts," but rather they reflect current, accepted wisdom.

1. In populations not using contraception and abortion, fertility varies substantially.

As noted earlier, *natural fertility* results if there are no attempts to control family size. In practice, however, natural fertility is frequently operationalized as involving no contraception or abortion (Henry 1961). Fertility is high in natural fertility populations—but how high? Females can have children as early as the midteens and can continue until the late 40s. Theoretically, women could have nearly one birth per year. Thus the theoretical maximum fertility, in the absence of all behavioral constraints, could be as high as 35 births!

In fact, no population has averaged anywhere close to this theoretical maximum level of fertility. Instead the classic example of a high-fertility population, the Hutterites, has fertility one-third this high. From 1880 to 1950, the U.S./–Canadian Hutterite population increased from 443 to 8,542 persons (Eaton and Mayer 1953). This is the world's fastest known natural growth rate (4.21% annually), with families averaging around 10 to 12 children (Ingoldsby 2001).

On the other end of the natural fertility spectrum lie the Dobe !Kung hunter-gathers, residents of the Kalahari Desert in Africa prior to 1975 (Howell 1979, 2000). The reported TFR for this natural fertility population was about 4.5 births per woman. Thus, the question, "How can natural fertility populations be so different from each other, and why are even the highest observed rates much lower than the theoretical maximum?"

The answer to both questions relies heavily on the *proximate determinants framework* described earlier. All known societies have encouraged practices that, through biological mechanisms, reduce fertility well below maximum levels. Key features are norms about union formation and dissolution (specifically, marriage) that impact coital frequency and the risk of pregnancy. Late marriage (indicating the postponement of sexual intercourse) reduces the years available for childbearing and thus the number of births.

The second important determinant of these differences in fertility is breast-feeding and postpartum amenorrhea (Bongaarts and Potter 1983). It is now well established that breast-feeding leads to a substantially longer postpartum period without ovulation than the typical 1.5- to 2-month interval that is experienced by women who do not breast-feed (Léridon 1977). Also, the intensity of breast-feeding affects the likelihood of ovulation. Women who exclusively breast-feed their children have a significantly lower chance of ovulating than do women who supplement breast-feeding with other food.

The !Kung typically breast-feed for three years and Hutterite women, for less than half this period.

In short, the Hutterite–Dobe !Kung natural fertility differential can be traced to greater time spent out of sexual unions (especially due to separation and union dissolution) and especially a much longer and more intense period of breast-feeding among the !Kung. In general, differences in natural fertility can be accounted for by these same two proximate determinants (see Bongaarts and Potter 1978, 1983).

2. The timing of the onset of the fertility transition (vis-à-vis objective socioeconomic conditions) is highly variable.

Demographic transition theory attributes fertility (and mortality) change to the process of economic development, especially the transition from a rural agrarian society to an urban industrial one. This leaves unanswered the question of what part of this process was most crucial for fertility decline. Was it changed occupations, urban living, or increased educational attainment that produced fertility decline? Further, what level of change in these aspects of economic development or its correlates was necessary to initiate a fertility decline?

The current consensus is that this view is overly mechanistic. There are no "threshold levels" of these macroeconomic indicators that consistently predict the onset of the transition. Likewise, there are no identifiable macrolevel changes that consistently predict the speed of the transition. Some argue that these findings must be interpreted cautiously, and one should not imply that economic development plays no causal role. Specifically, if multiple causes of decline are acknowledged, and if one views industrialization and urbanization as fundamental but distal causes (that need not produce synchronous change), then the role of economic development would receive greater support (Mason 1997).

3. Existing institutions influence the fertility transition, thus the process of change varies from place to place and has historical continuity.

Some of the reasons for the "loose" connections between socioeconomic change and fertility lie in preexisting differences in cultures and social institutions. For example, Greenhalgh (1988) argues that Chinese populations were among the first to experience fertility decline compared to others at similar levels of development. She attributes this to a historical and institutional context that made the number and sex composition of children a focal point of family strategy. In short, the Chinese populations began with a historical legacy that legitimated family size control and linked mobility strategies to number of children. Chinese groups quickly adopted modern contraception as a modern technology consistent with more costly traditional ones (including infanticide). In the Chinese context, the adoption of contraception was for limiting family size (specifically adopted by older women at higher parities).

In contrast, traditional African fertility regimes have been more concerned with a wide spacing of births as opposed to their number (Caldwell, Orubuloye, and Caldwell 1992). The link between limiting the number of children and upward social mobility was less apparent in these contexts. Institutions such as child fosterage may have played a role by spreading the costs of children across families, reducing the immediate impacts of rising child costs. Thus, the adoption of contraception was attractive as a substitute for postpartum abstinence and with the ideas that healthy children were produced by wide spacing (that could be aided by contraceptive use). As a result, the initial adoption of contraception in Africa tended to be simultaneous across ages and parities.

In short, Chinese and African family traditions influenced the speed and nature of their fertility transition. Chinese institutions hastened the transition (by its traditional emphasis on the size and composition of families and its use of postnatal control, explicitly, infanticide). African extended family and lineage institutions retarded change. The nature of the transition was also influenced. In Chinese populations fertility decline fell almost entirely due to contraceptive use after the desired number and composition of children were born. In Africa, fertility fell because of the wider spacing of births and birth limitation.

4. The fertility transition involves a collective evaluative assessment of social conditions and possible responses.

In a recent attempt to explain contemporary fertility transitions, Bongaarts and Watkins (1996) replicated the claim (discussed in 2, above) of a modest relationship between development indicators and changes in fertility. However, they argue that the diffusion of information about birth control techniques and ideas that legitimate small family size are important determinants of the timing of fertility change. This idea was central in the reports from the European Fertility Project (see Coale and Watkins 1986). Once a region of a country began a fertility transition, neighboring regions that shared a common language experienced a fertility decline shortly thereafter, regardless of the region's level of development. In this spirit, Bongaarts and Watkins (1996) conclude that social interaction in the form of exchanging information and ideas, evaluating their meaning in a given context, and social influences that encourage or discourage certain behaviors are significant factors in the transition from high to low fertility. Their measures of societal contact added significant explanatory power to their model of fertility transition. Watkins' work in contemporary African settings (e.g., Watkins 2000) describes at a microlevel how women's conversations helped to construct an understanding that fertility control was safe, appropriate, and advantageous.

5. Once the fertility transition begins, it does not stop until fertility reaches levels of approximately two children.

A well-known finding from the European Fertility Project is that once a 10% decline in fertility occurred (for any province), an irreversible transition was underway (Coale and Watkins 1986). Data in the Bongaats and Watkins study (1986) also show remarkably steady tendencies toward decline once the process is underway. Table 8.2 shows a cross-sectional, global view of the transition as of 2000. Of the 187 countries for which the UN provides data, only 19 have not yet shown evidence of fertility decline. These countries are primarily in Africa and include over 20% of the population of Africa. Thirty-two countries, again primarily in Africa, have recently begun a decline and another 73 are well into the transition. For practically all these countries, the lowest fertility observed is the most recent estimate, clearly indicating a steady march toward replacement level (or lower) fertility. Twenty-three countries, over half of the Asian countries, have TFRs that have fallen below 2.1 in the last decade or so. Coupled with the 39 countries that reached low fertility several decades ago (and experienced a post–World War II increase and then decline), these data indicate that by 2000 over 45% of the world's population lived in a country with replacement level fertility or below. Note that only two countries have experienced the transition to low fertility and have stabilized at levels above replacement (Argentina and Uruguay have levels that have remained close to 3.0 for the 1950 to 1980 period).

6. Fertility change is a period, not a cohort, phenomenon.

Earlier we noted that changing fertility rates can be described as occurring by cohort replacement or by pervasive period change. Ryder (1965) developed a paradigm of social change based on the concept of cohort replacement. The cohort perspective posits that trajectories of experience are frequently set by events early in life and are resistant to change subsequently. Cohort explanations stress the unique experience of a specified birth cohort (see Ryder 1965; Cherlin 1992). Change by cohort replacement comes slowly and steadily over time as new cohorts, in an orderly way, replace older ones.

Period explanations, on the other hand, emphasize the idea that shifts in fertility seem to affect all age groups at the same time. For example, shifts and changes in family attitudes and values may broadly impact nearly everyone's lives at once. Thus, the effects of these shifts are not unique to any one age group of people.

Twentieth-century U.S. fertility changes bear the unmistakable impact of period factors, including the Great Depression, wars, and economic cycles. Evidence from other developed countries is similar: changes in fertility are period driven, and cohort factors are weak or nonexistent (Ni Bhrolchain 1992).

7. Fertility delay is fundamentally antinatalist.

Although not invariant in magnitude, the timing of fertility is linked consistently to the number (or quantum) of births. This timing-number link can be seen for individual

TABLE 8.2. **Stages of the Transition to Low Fertility in the Major Areas of the World by 2000.**

Major Area and Region	NO Transition	Declining but TF>5	Declining with 5<TF<2.1	Declined to TF<=2.1	Early Transition 2.1<TF<3	Early Transition with "Baby Boom" TF<2.1	Total
			Number of countries				
Africa	15	21	16	1	0	0	53
Asia	1	10	25	12	0	0	50
Europe	0	0	1	3	0	35	39
Latin America/ Caribbean	0	0	24	7	2	0	33
North America	0	0	0	0	0	2	2
Oceania	0	1	7	0	0	2	10
World	16	32	73	23	2	39	187
		Percentage of People Living in Countries at Selected Stages of Transition					
Africa	20.7	43.2	36.0	0.1	0.0	0.0	100
Asia	0.5	6.3	49.6	39.9	0.0	3.6	100
Europe	0.0	0.0	0.4	0.9	0.0	98.7	100
Latin America/ Caribbean	0.0	0.0	88.8	3.4	7.8	0.0	100
North America	0.0	0.0	0.0	0.0	0.0	100.0	100
Oceania	0.0	1.5	21.9	0.0	0.0	76.5	100
World	3.0	9.5	39.0	24.6	0.7	19.6	100

Source: United Nations Population Division, 2002 (Table 1.1 World population Prospects: The 2000 Revision, Volume III) http://www.un.org/esa/population/ publications/wup2001/WUP2001report.htm.

women and cumulates in completed cohort fertility. A different dynamic operates between timing and quantum in period rates. We discuss each in turn.

Women who bear children early have larger numbers of children ever born (Morgan and Rindfuss 1999; Kohler, Billari, and Ortega 2002). There are several reasons for this association, and if all are operative in a particular setting, their cumulative effect can be substantial. To explain, as noted earlier, fertility is a nonreversible and time-bounded process. Given a relatively fixed mean age at menopause, a later start leaves less room for subsequent birth intervals (regardless of their mean length). This fact explains the powerful influence of marriage/union formation as a proximate determinant of natural fertility. But this mechanism can remain active in controlled settings because of the chance of contraceptive failure. Given a fixed number of children and fixed birth intervals, an earlier birth implies longer periods of exposure to an unintended pregnancy following the last intended birth. In addition, fecundity declines with age so that postponement can lead to couples being unable to have all of the children they intend. Finally, there are two potentially powerful social mechanisms. The first is a selective mechanism: those who desire more children and place a high priority on children may be less likely to postpone childbearing and thus start having them earlier. The second is more substantively interesting and follows from the sequential decision-making approach outlined earlier. Postponement can bring experience that competes with childbearing and increases the chance of additional postponement. Additional postponement can, in time, become a decision to have no (or no more) children.

Within a period framework, fertility postponement (in year t) is also associated with lower fertility (in year t). This is true even if the cohorts contributing to period fertility rates eventually have equivalent levels of completed fertility. For simplicity, assume a constant cohort level of childbearing. Fertility delay, a later age pattern of childbearing, can be viewed as postponing births into the subsequent year. This postponement lowers the number of births in year t by delaying them into year $t + 1$. Bongaarts and Feeney (1998) describe this process and show that the effects on period rates, including the widely used TFR, can be substantial and can operate for several decades. In fact, a major factor producing the very low contemporary TFR rates is a dramatic and continuing postponement of fertility.

8. *Valid and reliable retrospective fertility histories can be collected from women in a broad range of settings. Reliable information on abortion cannot generally be obtained from women.*

Women's fertility is revealed across a 30- to 35-year period of the life cycle. To collect information, one could collect data through an ongoing surveillance system. However, demographers have learned that in many settings retrospective fertility reports are of high quality and that trends constructed from these retrospective reports mirror those produced by vital registration systems or other data sources (e.g., Sirken and Sabagh 1968; Swicegood, Morgan, and Rindfuss 1984; Rindfuss, Morgan, and Offutt 1996: Figure 2). These retrospective histories have allowed for a wealth of cross-national data on fertility levels, trends, and differentials.

Fertility has many characteristics that make it an ideal event to be reported retrospectively: it is a discrete event that occurs at a clear point in time, births are usually positively sanctioned (increasing the respondent's willingness to report the event), recalling the exact date is often aided by celebrations (i.e., birthdays), and the event is recorded on administrative records (allowing verification).

Pregnancy histories, as opposed to birth histories, are much more problematic. First, in the case of an early-term spontaneous miscarriage, respondents may not recognize that they were pregnant. More problematic, in many contexts, pregnancies that end in abortions are underreported because of the stigma attached to abortions. In the U.S., for instance, only about one-half of abortions are reported in retrospective pregnancy histories (see Fu et al. 1998). In the U.S., more reliable data come from vital registration forms that doctors are required to fill out when performing an abortion and by surveys of abortion providers (see Henshaw 1998).

9. *Fertility intentions (individual or aggregate) are not reliable or valid indicators of future (individual or aggregate) fertility.*

As noted in an earlier discussion, a common question in fertility surveys asks women how many children they have now and how many more they intend to have. The sum of these is referred to as their *intended parity*. With longitudinal data one can ask how well these intentions predict subsequent fertility. Note that this question assumes a one-time decision model, instead of the sequential model favored in earlier discussions. Nevertheless, let us evaluate this model vis-à-vis accumulated evidence. One reason for such an exercise is to evaluate the one-time and sequential decision models.

Suppose that more distal social, economic, and psychological variables are linked to fertility only through fertility intentions. In other words, all relevant factors affect intentions directly, and intentions mediate these more distal effects. Indeed, numerous studies show that fertility intentions predict the subsequent behavior of individuals far better than do demographic and social indicators. However, evidence also clearly indicates a more complex process that produces a patterned inconsistency between intentions and behavior. Specifically, some groups (married women) are better than others (unmarried women) at predicting their future behavior. In other words, the link between intent and behavior can vary across groups (e.g., O'Connell and Rogers 1983; van de Giessen 1992). In addition, some subgroups and periods have higher fertility than others, net of intentions. That is to say, there is a direct effect of group membership and period that bypasses the proximate intention variable (Thomson 1997; Schoen et al. 1999). The fact that fertility differences or changes are not always foreshadowed by different or changed intentions challenges the usefulness of intention data for fertility forecasts (Campbell 1981). In explaining the failure of 1970 intended parity data to anticipate the fertility decline between 1970 and 1975, Westoff and Ryder (1977: 449) reasoned that "respondents failed to anticipate the extent to which the times would be unpropitious for childbearing, the same kind of forecasting error that demographers have often made." Thus, intentions and other preference measures can provide clues to future trends and differences, but they should not be expected to perform consistently as reliable and precise indicators of future individual or aggregate behavior. People can and do change their minds, as a sequential decision model suggests.

10. *The fertility desires/intentions of men and women (and husbands and wives) are similar; the impacts of their intentions/desires on subsequent fertility are similar.*

Social scientists have frequently speculated that the motivations for having children differed between men and women and that these differences made women (or men) more pronatalist. Mason and Taj (1987) have discussed these reasons, including the greater burden that women bear in pregnancy, birth, and childrearing (that might make women more willing to limit births than men) or the greater wealth and prestige that men might accrue through children (that might make men less willing to limit births than women). Mason and Taj's evidence shows, across a range of developing countries, that intended parity or desired family size varies little by gender. These results emphasize the social context that strongly and similarly influences the desires/intentions of both men and women. Results for couples show similar results in a number of Asian countries (see Mason and Smith 2000).

Results in developed countries are similar. Again the similarity could reflect the common conditions faced by husbands and wives. However, in the U.S. there is direct evidence that spouses know the fertility intentions and desires of their spouses and take them into account when stating their future intentions (Morgan 1985). Of course, not all spouses agree. Some evidence, again for U.S. couples, suggests that when spouses disagree, the wife's desire has somewhat greater predictive power than the husband's (Thomson, McDonald, and Bumpass 1990). But again, the primary findings are small gender differences in fertility intentions/desires and similar predictive validity of these intentions/desires.

RESEARCH DIRECTION

The scientific study of fertility is well advanced. We define an advanced science as one with agreed upon strategies of measurement and analysis, widely accepted frameworks for organization and interpretation of data, and widely accepted characterizations of phenomena that are "explained." In this chapter we have discussed each of these elements.

A logical way to conclude this discussion is to identify some important unanswered questions and to identify the ones most important to address in the next few decades.

For countries beginning or in the midst of the fertility transition, one is unsure whether to expect a more rapid or a slowed transition to low fertility. Studies of these transitions are key for refining our theories of fertility decline and because new phenomena could fundamentally alter the process. One argument holds that countries with currently high fertility are selected for their resistance to fertility decline. Perhaps they have pronatalist institutions that are especially resistant to change. Alternatively, reduced concern about population increase could reduce international aid, such as support for family planning programs, directed toward population concerns. This reduced aid could arrest ongoing fertility declines. Finally, new factors could alter the decision context making fertility control less acceptable (HIV/AIDS for instance). Or demographic differences could be politicized and linked to group identity and political disadvantage and thus perpetuated or exaggerated. Such a dynamic may account for Muslim–non-Muslim fertility differences in Asian countries with Muslim minority populations (see Morgan et al. 2002: 534). Such intergroup processes could emerge and operate at the international level, fueled by international events that foster pan-Islamic identity.

Other evidence suggests that recent declines have been more rapid than those begun in earlier decades, leading to the prediction that the pace of current and future declines will be the most rapid of all (Bongaarts and Bulatao 2000: 76–77). This expectation is linked to the importance of the diffusion of ideas and technology conducive to low fertility. The current globalization of trade, communication, and travel promotes these diffusion processes (Bongaarts and Watkins 1996).

Among low-fertility countries the key issue, as discussed earlier, is How low will fertility go? This question begs another (addressed by Morgan and King 2001): Why do couples have children in the 21st Century? Evidence that parenting is a powerful, life-defining event is widespread; most persons, men and women, desire and expect to have children. But substantial variation exists in intended family size, and we need to know more about the intensity of preference (Do persons strongly desire two or does a response of "two children intended" imply relative indifference in the one to three range?). The same question holds at the international level, where evidence suggests widespread mean desired family sizes of approximately two (Bongaarts 2001; 2002). More intensive study could reveal a general willingness in some countries to have fewer than this number. Such a finding may portend lower future fertility.

Nevertheless, the key contemporary question is: Can countries and will countries create environments where men and women can have the children they intend and also pursue careers and valued leisure activities? Or will competition among these valued life domains lead to decisions to postpone and forego childbearing? Covariation of institutional contexts with fertility levels shows that very low fertility is not inevitable (Morgan 2003). However, this claim leaves us a long way from precise answers to the question: What mix of societal institutions produces an environment conducive to replacement-level fertility? Answering this question tops the low fertility research agenda. The richness of future analyses will be aided by more (and more non-Western) societies to study as low fertility spreads (Morgan 2003).

Finally, future technology may alter the characteristics and experiences of pregnancy, childbirth, and parenting and thus contribute to making the future trends and differentials uncertain. For instance, postponed childbearing increases the risk of sub- or infecundity. But these risks can be partly offset by assisted reproductive technologies. Will new innovations and discoveries make this technology less intrusive, more effective, and more acceptable and thus virtually eliminate infecundity as an antinatalist factor? Also, genetic engineering, techniques that allow parents to choose the genetic makeup of their children, could have far reaching effects on reproduction, the family, and society (e.g., Silver 1998). But it remains unclear whether such technology will become available and whether it will be widely used. The debates over these new technologies will be among the most interesting and important of the coming decades.

REFERENCES

Bongaarts, J. 2001. Fertility and reproductive preferences in post-transitional societies. In *Global fertility transition*. Edited by R. A. Bulatao and J. B. Casterline, 260–281. New York: Population Council.

Bongaarts, J. 2002. The end of fertility transition in the developed world. *Population and Development Review* 28(3):419–444.

Bongaarts, J., and R. A. Bulatao, eds. 2000. *Beyond six billion: Forecasting the world's population*. Washington, D.C., National Academies Press.

Bongaarts, J., and G. Feeney. 1998. On the quantum and tempo of fertility. *Population and Development Review* 24:271–291.

Bongaarts, J., and R. G. Potter. 1978. Why are high birth rates so low. *Population and Development Review* 1:289–296.

Bongaarts, J., and R. G. Potter. 1983. *Fertility, biology and behavior*. New York: Academic Press.

Bongaarts, J., and S. C. Watkins. 1996. Social interactions and contemporary fertility transitions. *Population and Development Review* 22:639–682.

Bulatao, R. A. 1981. Values and disvalues of children in successive childbearing decisions. *Demography* 18:1–25.

Bumpass, L. 1990. What's happening to the family? Interactions between demographic and institutional change. *Demography* 27(4):483–498.

Cain, M. T. 1983. Fertility as an adjustment to risk. *Population and Development Review* 9:688–702.

Caldwell, J. 1982. *Theory of fertility decline.* New York: Academic Press.

Caldwell, J. C., I. O. Orubuloye, and P. Caldwell. 1992. Fertility decline in Africa: A new type of transition. *Population and Development Review* 18:211–242.

Campbell, A. A. 1981. Needed research on birth expectations. In *Predicting fertility.* Edited by G. E. Hendershot and P. J. Placek, 291–304. Lexington, Mass.: Lexington.

Cherlin, A. J. 1992. *Marriage, divorce, remarriage.* Cambridge, Mass.: Harvard University Press.

Cleland, J., and C. Wilson. 1987. Demand theories of the fertility transition: An iconoclastic view. *Population Studies* 41:5–30.

Coale, A. J., and S. C. Watkins. 1986. *The decline of fertility in europe.* Princeton, N.J.: Princeton University Press.

Davis, K., and J. Blake. 1956. Social structure and fertility: An analytic framework. *Economic Development and Cultural Change* 4:211–235.

Easterlin, R. A., and E. M. Crimmins. 1985. *The fertility revolution.* Chicago: University of Chicago Press.

Eaton, J., and A. Mayer. 1953. The social biology of very high fertility among the Hutterites. *Human Biology* 25:256–262.

Esping-Andersen, G. 1999. *Social foundations of post-industrial economies.* New York: Oxford University Press.

Fu, H., J. E. Darroch, S. K. Henshaw, and E. Kolb. 1998. Measuring the extent of abortion underreporting in the 1995 National Survey of Family Growth. *Family Planning Perspectives* 30:128–133, 138.

Greenhalgh, S. 1988. Fertility as mobility: Sinic transitions. *Population and Development Review* 14:629–674.

Henry, L. 1961. Some data on natural fertility. *Eugenics Quarterly* 8:81–91.

Henshaw, S. K. 1998. Abortion incidence and services in the United States, 1995–1996. *Family Planning Perspectives* 30:263–270.

Hodgson, D. 1988. Orthodoxy and revisionism in American demography. *Population and Development Review* 14:541–569.

Hodgson, D., and S. Cotts Watkins. 1997. Feminists and neo-Mathusians: Past and present alliances. *Population and Development Review* 23:469–523.

Howell, N. 1979. *Demography of the Dobe !Kung.* New York: Academic Press.

Howell, N. 2000. *Demography of the Dobe !Kung.* New York: Aldine de Gruyter.

Ingoldsby, B. B. 2001. The Hutterite family in transition. *Journal of Comparative Family Studies* 32:377–392.

Kaplan, H. 1994. Evolutionary and wealth flows theories: Empirical tests and new models. *Population and Development Review* 20:753–791.

Kertzer, D. I., and T. Fricke, eds. 1997. *Anthropological demography: Toward a new synthesis.* Chicago: University of Chicago Press.

Knodel, J., and E. van de Walle. 1979. Lessons from the past: Policy implications of historical fertility studies. *Population and Development Review* 5:217–245.

Kohler, H., F. C. Billari, and J. A. Ortega. 2002. The emergence of lowest-low fertility in Europe during the 1990s. *Population and Development Review* 28:641–680.

Lee, R. D. 1980. Aiming at a moving target: Period fertility and changing reproductive goals. *Population Studies* 34:205–226.

Léridon, H. 1977. H*uman fertility : The basic components.* Chicago: University of Chicago Press.

Lesthaeghe, R. 1983. A century of demographic and cultural change in Western Europe: An exploration of underlying dimensions. *Population and Development Review* 9:411–435.

Mason, K. O. 1997. Explaining fertility transitions. *Demography* 34:443–454.

Mason, K. O., and H. L. Smith. 2000. Husbands' versus wives fertility goals and use of contraception: The influence of gender context in five Asian countries. *Demography* 37(3):299–311.

Mason, K. O., and A. M. Taj. 1987. Differences between women's and men's reproductive goals in developing countries. *Population and Development Review* 13:611–638.

McDonald, P. 2000. Gender equity in theories of fertility transition. *Population and Development Review* 26:427–439.

Morgan, S. P. 1985. Individual and couple intentions for more children: A research note. *Demography* 22:125–132.

Morgan, S. P. 1996. Characteristic features of modern American fertility. *Population and Development Review* Suppl. Vol. 22:19–63.

Morgan, S. P. 2003. Presidential address: Is low fertility a 21st century demographic crisis? *Demography* 40: forthcoming.

Morgan, S. P., and R. B. King. 2001. Why have children in the 21st century? Biological predisposition, social coercion, rational choice. *European Journal of Population* 17:3–20.

Morgan, S. P., and S. M. Lynch. 2001. Demography's success and its future: The role of data and methods. In *Population health and aging: Strengthening the dialogue between epidemiology and demography*. Edited by M. Weinstein, A. I. Hermalin, and M. A. Stoto 35–51. Annals of New York Academy of Sciences, Vol. 954.

Morgan, S. P., and R. R. Rindfuss. 1999. Re-examining the link of early childbearing to marriage and to subsequent fertility. *Demography* 36:59–75.

Morgan, S. P., S. Stash, H. L. Smith, and K. O. Mason. 2002. Muslim and non-Muslim differences in female autonomy and fertility: Evidence from four Asian countries. *Population and Development Review* 28:515–538.

Namboodiri, N. K. 1972. Some observations on the economic framework for fertility analysis. *Population Studies* 26:185–206.

Newell, C. 1988. *Methods and models in demography*. New York: Guilford Press.

Ni Bhrolchain, M. 1992. Period paramount? A critique of the cohort approach to fertility. *Population and Development Review* 18:599–629.

Notestein, F. W. 1953. Economic problems of population change. In *Proceedings of the Eighth International Conference of Agricultural Economists*. New York: Oxford University Press.

Nugent, J. B. 1985. The old-age security motive for fertility. *Population and Development Review* 11:75–97.

O'Connell, M., and C. C. Rogers. 1983. Assessing cohort birth expectations data from the current population survey, 1971–1981. *Demography* 20:369–384.

Potts, M. 1997. Sex and the birth rate: Human biology, demographic change, and access to fertility-regulation methods. *Population and Development Review* 23:1–40.

Preston, S. H., P. Heuveline, and M. Guillot. 2001. *Demography: Measuring and modeling population processes*. Malden, Mass.: Blackwell.

Rindfuss, R. R. 1991. The young adult years: Diversity, structural change, and fertility. *Demography* 28:493–512.

Rindfuss, R. R., and K. L. Brewster. 1996. Childrearing and fertility. *Population and Development Review* 22:258–289.

Rindfuss, R. R., K. B. Guzzo, and S. P. Morgan. 2003. The changing institutional context of low fertility. *Population Research and Policy Review*. forthcoming.

Rindfuss, R. R., S. P. Morgan, and K. Offutt. 1996. Education and the changing age pattern of American fertility: 1963–89. *Demography* 33(3):277–290.

Rindfuss, R. R., S. P. Morgan, and C. G. Swicegood. 1988. *First births in America*. Berkeley: University of California Press.

Rindfuss, R. R., and J. A. Sweet. 1977. *Post-war fertility trends and differentials in the United States*. New York: Academic Press.

Ryder, N. B. 1965. The cohort as a concept in the study of social change. *American Sociological Review* 30:843–861.

Ryder, N. B. 1980. Components of temporal variations in American fertility. In *Demographic patterns in developed societies*. Edited by R. W. Hiorns, 15–54. London: Taylor and Francis.

Ryder, N. B., and C. F. Westoff. 1971. *Reproduction in the United States 1965*. Princeton, N.J.: Princeton University Press.

Schoen, R., N. M. Astone, Y. J. Kim, C. A. Nathanson, and J. M. Fields. 1999. Do fertility intentions affect fertility behavior? *Journal of Marriage and the Family* 61:790–799.

Shorter, E., J. Knodel, and E. van de Walle. 1971. The decline of nonmarital fertility in Europe, 1880–1940. *Population Studies* 25(3):375–393.

Silver, L. M. 1998. *Remaking Eden*. New York, Perennial, HarperCollins Publishers.

Sirken, M. G., and G. Sabagh 1968. Evaluation of birth statistics derived retrospectively from fertility histories reported in the National Population Survey: United States, 1945–64. *Demography* 5:485–503.

Swicegood, C. G., S. P. Morgan, and R. R. Rindfuss. 1984. Measurement and replication: Evaluating the consistency of eight U.S. fertility surveys. *Demography* 21:19–33.

Teachman, J. D., K. Paasch, and K. P. Carver. 1993. Thirty years of demography. *Demography* 30:523–532.

Thomson, E. 1997. Couple childbearing desires, intentions, and births. *Demography* 34:343–354.

Thomson, E., E. McDonald, and L. L. Bumpass. 1990. Fertility desires and fertility: His, hers and theirs. *Demography* 27:579–589.

van de Giessen, H. 1992. Using birth expectations information in National Population Forecasts. In *National population forecasting in industrialized countries*. Edited by N. Keilman and H. Cruijsen, 223–242. Amsterdam: Swets & Zeitlinger.

van de Kaa, D. J. 2001. Postmodern fertility preferences: From changing value orientations to new behavior. *Population and Development Review* 27:290–331.

van de Walle, E. 1992. Fertility transition, conscious choice and numeracy. *Demography* 29:487–502.

Watkins, S. C. 2000. Local and foreign models of reproduction in Nyanza Province, Kenya. *Population and Development Review* 26:725–759.

Westoff, C. F., and N. B. Ryder. 1977. The predictive validity of reproductive intentions. *Demography* 14:431–453.

CHAPTER 9

Infant Mortality

W. PARKER FRISBIE*

SUBSTANTIVE CONCERNS

Ultimately, the significance of research on infant mortality resides in the fact that few, if any, human experiences are more tragic or emotionally devastating as the death of an infant or child. At the societal level, the loss of human potential, economic or otherwise, occasioned by infant death is dramatic. Thus, the infant mortality rate (IMR) has been employed worldwide as a key social indicator (World Bank 1998), e.g., as a "critical test" for identifying countries as "superior health achievers," (Caldwell, 1986: 173), as an inverse proxy measure of development (Pattnayak and Shai 1995), and as "a synoptic indicator of the health and social condition of a population" (Gortmaker and Wise 1997: 147).

The general substantive issues motivating the study of infant mortality are the same as those in other areas of research—the documentation and explanation of variation in the outcome of interest. Demographers have documented variation in infant mortality along many dimensions—temporal, spatial (neighborhoods, communities, nations, etc.), and between groups within societies. There is also a growing interest in the development of conceptual frameworks that can adequately inform studies based on multilevel models (those which include both individual and contextual variables).

Among the most prominent, specific substantive issues are those having to do with inequalities in risk according to socioeconomic status (SES), race/ethnicity, nativity, and other socially relevant categories. The very substantial research efforts directed toward identifying and modeling the effects of factors that produce variation in infant mortality risk along these dimensions mirror the concerns and goals enunciated in such recent major public health policy statements as *Healthy People 2000* and *Healthy People 2010*.

* The author gratefully acknowledges the support for this analysis provided by the National Institute of Child Health and Human Development under Grant RO1 HD 41147.

It has proven advantageous for organizational and analytical purposes to group risk factors according to general substantive rubrics. Risk factor categories frequently employed include the demographic, socioeconomic, cultural, behavioral, and biomedical. A certain degree of theoretical utility accrues to such classifications, but it is limited by the seemingly inevitable overlap of categories. For example, there is strong consensus that the risk of infant death increases if the mother is a smoker. However, smoking can be classified as either a behavioral or a biomedical risk (or both), and some scholars view smoking behavior as representative of cultural differences (e.g., Scribner 1996).

Integral to demographic research on infant mortality are studies of three birth outcome dimensions: birth weight, gestational age, and maturity,[1] not only as risk factors typically viewed as having the most powerful and proximate impact on infant mortality, but also as pregnancy outcomes of interest in their own right (Cramer 1987, 1995; Frisbie, Fovbes, and Pullum 1996; Kiely and Susser 1992; Kline, Stein, and Susser 1989).[2] Among surviving infants, low birth weight, prematurity, and/or immaturity are associated with greater risk of congenital anomalies, neurodevelopmental and behavioral disorders, lower levels of educational achievement, and problems of family functioning (Hack, Klein, and Taylor 1995; McCormick 1985). Due to tremendous advances in neonatal technology and care in recent years, an increasing number and proportion of infants with highly adverse birth outcomes survive. Despite such progress, just as with infant mortality, the human costs of compromised birth outcomes for the child and its family are extremely high, as, of course, are the monetary costs of medical and social intervention designed to save such infants and maintain their health in subsequent months and years. Further, because infant mortality today is a relatively rare event in the U.S. and in many other societies, and since many of the variables believed to be crucial determinants are available only from surveys and/or small clinical data sets, it is often the case that inferences about the effects of risk factors must necessarily focus on birth outcomes which are very strongly correlated with infant mortality.

There is also an important literature on the consequences of infant mortality—consequences for demographic change in general and for reproductive behavior in particular (e.g., Palloni and Rafalimanana 1999; Preston 1978). This topic is not covered in this chapter because the focus of such research is typically on fertility differences and/or trends in population growth.

THEORETICAL ISSUES

General Conceptual Approaches

In general, two theoretical frameworks have been used by demographers to provide guidance and structure in research on pregnancy outcomes. The first has been termed the *social model*, and the second is often referred to as the *medical model* (e.g., Cramer

---

[1] *Lack* of maturity refers to infants who are small for gestational age (SGA) or intrauterine growth retarded (IUGR). These are terms that no doubt will (and should) continue to be employed. For the sake of clarity, I prefer the term *immature* to make clear that the focus is on the mortality risk of live-born infants, not the fetal growth curve (Frisbie et al. 1998b). As is conventional, I use *preterm* or *prematurity* synonymously with short gestation.

[2] Throughout, the term *pregnancy outcomes* will be employed to refer to both infant mortality and birth outcomes.

1995). "Social models stress the power of social variables to determine infant survival and the importance of structural change in overcoming disparate outcomes. Medical models stress pathways of frank pathophysiology and their potential interruption through clinical interventions" (Wise 1993: 9). Not surprisingly, most demographers and other social scientists have relied on the social model, while public health and medical researchers have primarily used the medical model. Until fairly recently, many researchers have proceeded as if the two approaches were competing. For example, Wise notes that, although "vast sociologic, anthropologic, and demographic literature exists on the causes of infant mortality," [this body of knowledge] "is rarely tapped in the exploration of clinical pathways to adverse birth outcomes." The reverse is also true, as "the social sciences continue to make little use of the clinical literature in refining the search for relevant social and behavioral factors" (1993: 9).

Today, the situation is changing. As evidenced in Wise's work, there is a growing interest in cross-disciplinary collaboration with social scientists on the part of public health and medical researchers. Further, I believe a consensus is emerging in support of the view expressed by Frank, who points out (citing Carey 1997) that, in demography, there is a growing recognition that "studies of biology of death, mortality, longevity, and life are all informed by biological processes that demographers cannot afford to ignore" (2001: 563).

The involvement of demographers in multidisciplinary research is facilitated by the fact that the social demography of infant mortality has drawn heavily on the proximate determinants approach advanced by Mosley and Chen (1984). Despite a keen interest in those factors, especially socioeconomic variables, that are more causally distant from the outcomes of interest, the heart of this approach "is the identification of proximate determinants that directly influence the risk of child morbidity and mortality" (Mosley and Chen 1984: 27). Although the Mosley-Chen typology includes maternal characteristics, it is heavily weighted in the direction of biomedical factors, including environmental influences, nutrition, injury, and personal illness control (preventive and remedial) as intervening factors, thereby helping to set the stage for integrating the social and medical approaches.

This conceptual scheme is most applicable in studies of child mortality and morbidity. However, in infant mortality research, this framework has been adapted and expanded so that race/ethnicity, nativity, and other factors have joined SES as the most distal variables. Birth weight, gestational age, and maturity of infant are viewed as the most vital proximate determinants.[3]

Specific Theoretical Issues

The number of specific hypotheses investigated in studies of infant mortality is probably as extensive as the number of researchers in the area. Simply listing the hypotheses that have been previously tested would be a formidable task, and providing even a very brief discussion of each is certainly not possible given any reasonable space limitations. Thus,

---

[3] This distinction is not exact. Sex and plurality are determined at the moment of conception but are often of slight theoretical importance, except as controls. Thus, these variables appear at different points in partially ordered models, depending on analytic aims.

this section focuses on broader theoretical concerns selected partly due to their prominence in the literature, but also because they represent conceptual issues in need of resolution.

CONCEPTUALIZING BIRTH OUTCOME EFFECTS.   It may be surprising to some that substantial differences of opinion exist over whether and how to assign causal importance to birth outcomes, which over many years have proven to be the most powerful predictors of infant mortality. Typically, the relationship between birth weight and infant mortality is stronger than that between gestational age and infant mortality, and, not uncommonly, length of gestation has been viewed as a determinant of birth weight, with the latter variable viewed as having the most proximate effect on infant survival chances (Gage 2000; Gage and Therriault 1998). Not all agree, however— witness Wilcox's contention (2001a, 2001b) that the relationship between birth weight and infant mortality is essentially noncausal. Further, it has been concluded that "[e]limination of LBW (low birth weight) is neither practical nor necessary in order to achieve the lowest possible rates of infant mortality" (Wilcox 2001a: 1238). The vast literature on low birth weight and its deleterious consequences for infant survival and subsequent child health is inconsistent with this conclusion, and challenges emerged immediately (David 2001; Hertz-Picciotto 2001).

     In any event, Wilcox's conclusion regarding the causal impact of birth weight (or lack thereof) remains to be fully tested at the microlevel, where rates do not apply. Limited modeling of the effects of both birth weight and gestational age (both main and interaction effects) on the odds of mortality for individual infants indicates that birth weight has the largest net effect (Solis, Pullum, and Frisbie 2000).

EXPLAINING RACE/ETHNIC VARIATION IN INFANT MORTALITY.   Discussion of the issue of how race/ethnicity should be conceptualized in infant mortality (or other) research can quickly become confusing or, worse, deteriorate into polarized and dogmatic exchanges. Fortunately, in recent years, the demographic literature on pregnancy outcomes has been relatively free of the latter. Nevertheless, current discourse in social science and public health ranges broadly from the recommendation of complete abandonment of race/ethnicity as a risk factor in health research (Bhopal and Donaldson 1998; Fullilove 1998) to the suggestion that genetic effects may explain some nonnegligible proportion of variation in pregnancy outcomes across races (especially between blacks and whites). For instance, Van Den Oord and Rowe (2000) have proposed that the greater likelihood of low birth weight (LBW) among black infants, as compared to white infants, may be partially attributable to race differences in maternal genes and that "racial groups should be regarded as both genetic and social categories" (Van Den Oord and Rowe 2000: 286). Critics of this notion have argued that, while human biological variation needs to be taken into account, "race as a way of organizing that variation is false" (Zuberi 2001: 569; see also Frank 2001).

     Most demographers, however, view race as a social category and probably would be comfortable with some variant of David's conclusion that race/ethnic differences in birth weight essentially "reflect the status at one point in time of a population defined by that combination of physical, historical, and cultural attributes commonly referred to as 'race.' The biological meaning of the term is questionable" (1990: 102; see also Gortmaker and Wise 1997). Given what appears to be the rather general acceptance of the notion that race and ethnicity are essentially (and essential) social constructs, there is every reason to continue to analyze health differentials (including disparities in infant mortality) between and within these categories.[4] The crucial relevance of biology for demographic studies of health outcomes in no way denotes support for any claim that one or another race/ethnic group is inherently superior or inferior. Specifically, "[t]he point here is not that a biological conceptualization of race should be avoided for fear of supporting a racist agenda. Rather, it should be recognized that "human biological variation is not racially patterned" (Frank 2001: 566). For demography, then, the basic substantive foci are (1) the specification of the demographic, social, economic, cultural, and biomedical covariates responsible for race/ethnic inequalities in pregnancy outcomes and (2) the interpretation of race/ethnic differences that persist in the face of numerous controls for potentially confounding covariates.

WHAT ARE THE BIOLOGICAL LINKS BETWEEN SOCIAL AND DEMOGRAPHIC FACTORS AND PREGNANCY OUTCOMES?. Inasmuch as death is a biological event, biomedical risk factors are of crucial importance for infant mortality research. Hence, the question that immediately and logically follows is, What are the *mechanisms* through which demographic and socioeconomic factors "get into the body" to influence the risk of adverse pregnancy outcomes? (Seeman and Crimmins 2001). In the medical and public health literature, it is possible to find reasonably clear notions of how biomedical factors are related to infant mortality and other pregnancy outcomes. For example, it has long been known that certain maternal morbid conditions such as abruptio placenta (premature separation of the placenta) or placenta previa (development of placenta low in the uterus, i.e., in the zone of dilation), are associated with premature birth and hypoxia, which in turn are known risk factors for infant mortality and morbidity (Shapiro, Schlesinger, and Nesbitt 1968).

Demographic theories dealing with the biological mechanisms through which socioeconomic and sociodemographic factors affect infant mortality risk are, by contrast, rather underdeveloped. The reasons for this are no doubt many and include the lack of data sets that facilitate the linking of sociodemographic and biomedical factors and the aforementioned scarcity of cross-disciplinary research agendas. Nevertheless, if the stance taken by Carey (1997) and Frank (2001) is any indication, demographers are now joining social epidemiologists (Wise 1993) at the forefront of efforts aimed at synthesizing conceptual and empirical models of demographers with those of public health and medical researchers.

METHODS AND MEASURES

Measuring Infant Mortality

Infant mortality refers to death within the first year of life to persons born alive. A live birth is defined as the "complete expulsion or extraction from its mother of a product of

---

[4] For a comprehensive discussion of the social origins and of the analytic importance of race and ethnicity as key dimensions in social science theory, see Bonilla-Silva (1999).

conception, irrespective of the duration of pregnancy, which after such separation breathes or shows any other evidence of life" and death as "the permanent disappearance of life any time after live birth has taken place" (United Nations 2001: 13). The *infant mortality rate* is conventionally measured as the number of deaths to infants under one year of age in a given year, per 1,000 live births in the same year. However, not all infant deaths occur in the calendar year of birth, so that the IMR as just defined is not a probability based on the population at risk. A true probability can be computed directly from birth cohort data of the sort routinely made available in the Linked Birth/ Infant Death Files by the US National Center for Vital Statistics (NCHS). Shryock and Siegel (1976) refer to the computation based on birth cohorts as the *infant death rate*. In the absence of substantial year-to-year fluctuations, the infant mortality rate and the infant death rate will be similar in magnitude. It is possible to apply separation factors that apportion vital events in a manner that moves calculations based on period data closer to what would be achieved with cohort data. Another frequently adopted alternative is the use of multiyear averages that "may serve adequately as adjusted measures" (Shryock and Siegel 1976: 237). Inasmuch as infant mortality is a rare event in many areas of the world, combining infant deaths occurring over a three-, five- or other multiple-year period and dividing by the corresponding grouped number of live births has often been employed as a way of ensuring that the number of cases is sufficiently large to yield stable estimates, as well as a means of adjustment. Throughout this chapter, the term *infant mortality rate* (*IMR*) is employed regardless of whether computations are based on period or cohort data.

Infant mortality is often subdivided into *neonatal mortality* (deaths to infants under 28 days) and *postneonatal mortality* (deaths during the remainder of the first year). By the last decade of the 20th century, about 65% of all infant deaths in the U.S. occurred during the first month of life, with the majority of the latter (about 80%) occurring during the first week (National Center for Health Statistics 1996: Table 23). While there is reason to be interested in the timing of infant death, per se, researchers have also used this dichotomy to proxy cause of death structure. Specifically, neonatal mortality has been used to approximate deaths due to *endogenous* causes, i.e., conditions that are related to genetic makeup or that are "a consequence of circumstances occurring during the prenatal period and/or the birth process" (Frisbie et al. 1992: 535). *Exogenous* infant mortality is due to environmental or external causes, such as infections, accidents, etc. (Bogue 1969). Although the absence of information on cause of death may force reliance on timing of death, there is evidence that, while the timing proxy may have been of acceptable validity in early research, such is no longer the case (Frisbie, Forbes, and Rogers 1992; Poston and Rogers 1985). For example, although for quite some time *exogenous* mortality represented more than half of all postneonatal deaths in the U.S., such is no longer the case. The reason that *endogenous* conditions are now the most prevalent cause of death in the postneonatal period "is that advances in perinatal care and extraordinary medical intervention...have resulted in the survival of nonviable infants past the first 27 days of life" (Frisbie, Forbes, and Rogers 1992: 544). In the more distant past, or in areas of the world today where modern perinatal care and technology are not widely available, the timing proxy may (unfortunately) retain a fair degree of validity. Finally, in the absence of cause-of-death data, the timing proxy may permit adequate *relative* comparisons if temporal trends for two or more groups are homogeneous as to direction of change (Frisbie, Forbes, and Rogers 1992).

Perinatal mortality combines late fetal deaths (often at 28 weeks or longer gestation) with deaths to infants less than one week of age.[5] The perinatal mortality *rate*
denotes late fetal and early infant death divided by the population at risk. In other
words, the denominator for the rate is the sum of live births plus fetal deaths. Use of
only live births in the denominator yields the perinatal mortality *ratio* (Shryock and
Siegel 1976: 246).

Fetal mortality, i.e., death prior to the complete expulsion or extraction of the fetus,
is excluded under the definition of infant mortality. Fetal death generally refers to both
stillbirth and abortion, whether spontaneous or induced (Shryock and Siegel 1976).
Although fetal death as an *outcome* is not considered further here (because infant
mortality can occur only in the case of a live-born infant), previous pregnancy loss
has been shown to be an important risk factor for infant mortality.

Measuring Birth Outcomes

A century ago, the concept of prematurity, operationalized as birth prior to 37 weeks
gestation, began to be widely recognized as a major threat to human survival (Kline,
Stein, and Susser 1989). Less than 2,500 grams birth weight as an alternative measure
emerged in 1919, but it was not until the mid-20th century that this datum "slowly became
a part of vital records in many countries" (Kline, Stein, and Susser 1989: 166–167), and
both gestational age and birth weight were recognized as distinct, but highly interrelated,
dimensions. The use of 37 weeks gestation to demarcate premature from term births and
2,500 grams to distinguish low weight from normal weight births has proven to be a useful
measurement strategy over many decades. Still, these venerable measures are problematic
in many respects. Since most infant deaths occur at very low birth weight ($< 1,500$ grams)
and during the neonatal period, finer-grained birth outcome typologies combining birth
weight and gestational age began to be constructed several decades ago (Yerushalmy
1967; see also Frisbie, Forbes, and Pullum 1996). Finally, categorical measurement of
birth outcomes, no matter how refined, inevitably sacrifices precision. For example, use
of the conventional 2,500 gram cut-point for birth weight means that an infant who
registers 2,499 grams at birth is viewed as conceptually quite different from one born
weighing 2,500 grams, while an infant born at, say, 1,600 grams, is treated as analytically
identical to the 2,499 gram birth. More fine-grained typologies provide a partial and, in
many instances, a sufficient, solution. Nevertheless, additional studies of infant mortality
that preserve the continuous metric of birth weight and gestational age are needed.

Immaturity of the newborn, often referred to as intrauterine-growth-retarded
(IUGR) or small-for-gestational-age (SGA) births, was added as a third dimension of
adverse outcomes around the middle of the 20th century (Kline, Stein, and Susser 1989;
Wilcox 2001a). Measurement of immaturity has proceeded along two general lines.[6] The
first relies on anthropometric indicators from clinical records, including crown-to-heel
length, a body mass index (ratio of height to length), skinfold thickness, and skull
circumference. Unfortunately, information of this sort is not routinely available to
demographers, and clinical data sets usually contain only a small number of cases

---

[5] Deaths occurring under 28 days are sometimes substituted for deaths in the first week.
[6] Both of these apply to live-born infants. Estimates of *in utero* development have for some time relied on
ultrasound evaluations (sonograms).

from one or a few local areas (Williams et al. 1982). Thus, many researchers have turned to indicators which can be obtained from survey data and from the largest and most representative data files available, viz., the vital statistics. Other measures of immaturity include identifying infants born at weights below the 10th percentile for gestational age such as SGA (Battaglia and Lubchenco 1967; Miller 1994) and the use of two standard deviations from the gestational age-specific birth weight mean (Gruenwald 1965; McCarton et al. 1996). A related approach involves the fetal growth ratio (FGR), introduced by Kramer and associates (1989), which identifies immature births, on a sex-specific basis, as those whose weight is less than 85% (or some other predetermined fraction) of mean weight at a given gestational age (Balcazar 1994; Kramer et al. 1989). Yet another alternative directly available from vital statistics classifies as immature those infants carried to term (37 weeks+), but who are born weighing less than 2,500 grams (Hummer et al. 1995; Kallan 1993).

Another important measurement issue emerges from the fact that the birth weight optimum for infant survival is not only much higher than the conventional 2,500 gram cut-point (Solis, Pullum, and Frisbie 2000) but also "is several hundred grams heavier than the mean of the birthweight distribution" (Wilcox and Russell 1983: 324). In addition, the gestational age associated with the lowest risk of infant death is in the neighborhood of 40 to 41 weeks, as contrasted with the 37-week cut-point that has been historically used to denote a full-term birth (Solis, Pullum, and Frisbie 2000). Again, the need for the use of alternative birth outcome measures, either in place of, or in conjunction with, conventional indicators is obvious.

Other Methodological Issues

Many of the methodological issues involved in the study of infant mortality are similar, if not identical, to those associated with research in other substantive areas and are more appropriately discussed in the demographic methods literature. However, certain methodological matters need to be addressed here because they are integral to the success of efforts to describe and/or account for variation in infant mortality.

DISTRIBUTIONAL ISSUES.   The birth weight distribution "is composed of at least two statistically identifiable subpopulations" (Gage 2000: 181). The first, sometimes denoted the predominant distribution (Wilcox and Russell 1986), is essentially normal (Gaussian) and consists of most infants born at normal weight and term gestation and among whom the infant mortality rate is low. The second is the "residual distribution of small births," among whom far and away the largest proportion of deaths in the first year occurs (Wilcox and Russell 1986).[7] A useful way of dealing with this heterogeneous distribution is through models of weight-specific perinatal mortality (Wilcox and Russell 1983). Wilcox and Russell have demonstrated that meaningful comparisons of the infant mortality *rate* across populations[8] can be achieved "by plotting each weight-specific mortality curve relative to its own birthweight distribution" (Wilcox and

---

[7] Actually, a third component of the distribution might be identified, namely, extremely heavy (macrosomic) births which are characterized by an upward inflection in mortality risk (Wilcox and Russell 1983).

[8] The Wilcox and Russell research also has implications for modeling the *individual risk* of infant death (Solis, Pullum, and Frisbie 2000). At this juncture, however, the focus is entirely on comparisons of rates across populations.

Russell 1986: 188). Failure to take these insights into account leads to a "low birth weight paradox," viz., puzzlement over the finding that "LBW babies in high-risk populations...usually have lower mortality than LBW babies in better-off populations" (Wilcox 2001a: 1234). A prime example occurs in what at first glance seems to be an enigmatic effect of smoking. While it early became clear that both low birth weight and infant mortality are more likely among babies of mothers who smoke, it was also discovered that "LBW babies born to mothers who smoked had lower infant mortality than the LBW babies of mothers who did *not* smoke" (Wilcox 2001a: 1234; emphasis in the original). The puzzle is solved when infant mortality is plotted by relative birth weight (adjusted to z-scores), in which case "[m]ortality with mother's smoking is higher across the whole range of weights" (Wilcox 2001a: 1237).

Another approach to analyzing the relationship between the primary (predominant) and secondary (residual) components of the birth weight distribution involves the use of "mixture models," as applied by Gage (2000) and Gage and Therriault (1998), in which the two components are taken as Gaussian, but with different means and standard deviations. One of the most important results emerging from mixture models is that both birth weight and gestational age distributions "vary significantly between the sexes and among ethnic groups" (Gage 2000: 181).

POPULATION-SPECIFIC STANDARDS.   Findings of heterogeneity in pregnancy outcome distributions by race/ethnicity and sex support the contention by Alexander and colleagues that "[g]iven that the general norms for preterm, postterm, and fetal growth measures may be largely derived from White populations, more information is needed to assess whether or not the ongoing use of these one-size-fits-all standards may result, for some ethnic groups, in invalid risk assessments and the misidentification of infants in need of intervention services" (1999a: 77). This argument is consonant with the conclusions by Kline and colleagues who note that "measures of development do not correspond with post-conception age in a way that is consistent (across populations)....Sex is one such criterion....Ethnicity or race is another" (1989: 188), as well as with the call by Wilcox and Russell (1990) for population-specific standards.

EMPIRICAL FINDINGS

It is unlikely that an entire volume on infant mortality, much less a single chapter, could adequately portray every empirical result that, even with strict selection criteria, could reasonably be viewed as worthy of discussion. Nevertheless, this chapter attempts to include sets of findings that are representative of major emphases in microlevel, macrolevel, and multilevel analyses. Most research covered in this section was conducted in the United States over the past few decades. Thus, to provide background and some modicum of balance, it will useful to begin with worldwide historical trends in, and current levels of, infant mortality.

Historical Trends: The Infant Mortality Transition

Historical research on infant mortality, and perhaps more frequently, child mortality, has long had a prominent place in the demographic literature (McKowen 1976; Preston

1976; Preston and Haines 1991). Demographers are well acquainted with the "epidemiological transition," which denotes the shift from acute and infectious diseases to chronic and degenerative conditions as leading causes of death (Omran 1971, 1977). An infant mortality transition parallels the epidemiological transition, both in regard to declining mortality and change in cause of death structure (though, obviously, degenerative conditions are not a cause of infant death).

While the infant mortality rate (IMR) has been substantially reduced in most of today's less developed countries, it remains high compared to that observed in more developed regions of the world. Further, the speed of decline in the IMR has varied across different societies and across different groups in the same society. Frenk and associates believe that in some world regions, "epidemiologic differentiation *within* each country is now producing internal polarization" (1989: 29; emphasis in original), with the implication that a simple dichotomy contrasting developed with less developed countries has come to provide less and less analytical leverage.

Vital statistics registration remains inadequate in most areas of the world today, and even modern-day international comparisons are difficult due to variability in definitions, completeness of registration, and data quality (United Nations 2001: 12–16). Nevertheless, it is possible to say with some confidence that "for most of human history, life expectancy probably fluctuated between 20 and 30 years" (Weeks 1999: 131). Life expectancies in this range imply that only 63% to 74% of infants survive the first year of life (Weeks 1999: Table 4.2). During the premodern period, IMRs were probably on the order of 260 to 370 per 1,000 live births.

Some time during the latter part of the 19th century, there was a major reduction in infant mortality in Western Europe. Scholars seem to agree that the transition to lower infant mortality, as well as to lower child and adult mortality and longer life expectancy during this early period, was largely due to a major reduction in deaths from infectious diseases and that, prior to 1935, the role played by physicians and drug therapy in the reduction of mortality was relatively slight (McKowen 1976). There is at least one point of major disagreement, however. McKowen (1976) has argued that most of the *early* decline in mortality may be attributed to greater food supplies and better nutrition. Others have expressed doubt that increases in material resources lie at the heart of the mortality transition, citing the high levels of child mortality that persisted in late 19th-century America, even though the U.S. was already the richest country in the world with a population that was "highly literate and exceptionally well-fed" (Preston and Haines 1991: 208). Even with such advantages, about 18% of U.S. children did not survive to age five. Preston and Haines believe that the continuation of high levels of child mortality resulted from the fact that neither physicians, nor public health personnel, nor the general public had yet achieved a good understanding of infectious disease processes (at least until the second decade of the 20th century) and that advances in health technology were slow to diffuse.

Current Levels of Infant Mortality

The association of infant mortality with economic development across world regions can be seen in Figure 9.1, which is based on recent information from the Population Reference Bureau (Haub and Cornelius 2001). Figure 9.1 juxtaposes infant mortality rates per 1,000 live births with Gross National Income *per capita adjusted for purchasing*

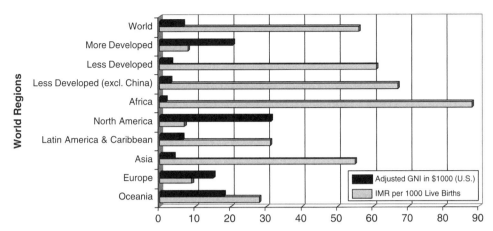

FIGURE 9.1. Infant mortality and Gross National Income (GNI) compared by world region. Source: Population Reference Bureau, *World Data Sheet 2001*.

power expressed in $1,000 U.S. The Population Reference Bureau (PRB) estimates put the average IMR in 2001 at 56 per 1,000 live births worldwide, 8 per 1,000 in the more developed countries, and 61 per 1,000 in the less developed countries. These data show a range across regions of from 88 for Africa (94 for sub-Saharan Africa [not shown]) to 7 for North America. At least two important conclusions emerge from Figure 9.1. First, societal variation in infant mortality continues to be very substantial and, second, there is a strong inverse relationship between level of societal development and infant mortality.

Over the past few decades, the IMR in many less developed countries has been substantially reduced in relatively brief periods of time, as basic sanitation improvements (potable water, hygienic disposal of waste) have occurred and relatively inexpensive perinatal care techniques (such as oral rehydration in the case of diarrheal disease) have been made available. Even so, tremendous inequalities remain. For example, the most recent data for world regions released by the United Nations (2001) indicate more than a half-century lag in the reduction of infant mortality. To illustrate, for today's developed regions, the IMR averaged 59.1 *for the period 1950 to 1955*. It was not *until 1995 to 2000* that the average for the world as a whole approximated this level.

Even within the same nation, the major point of downward inflection for one group or another may have lagged behind the general trend by several decades. One of the more striking illustrations of temporal disparity is seen in Bexar County (San Antonio), Texas, where during the mid-1930s, the mortality rate among white, Spanish-surnamed (largely Mexican American) infants exceeded 130 per 1,000 live births, about two and one-half times the white non-Spanish-surnamed ("Anglo") rate (Forbes and Frisbie 1991). That the infant mortality transition took place unevenly is evident in the cause of death distributions. At this early stage, the leading cause of Spanish-surname infant death was diarrhea/enteritis/colitis, which, together with pneumonia/influenza and infections (all conditions characteristic of pretransition mortality), accounted for 60% of total infant deaths (Blanchard 1996; Forbes and Frisbie 1991). By contrast, among Anglos, the leading cause of death in the mid-1930s was short gestation/low birth weight. That is, Spanish-surname infants remained at risk of death from acute, infectious conditions well after the prevalence of such causes had been sharply curtailed among Anglos. With the provision of modern sanitation facilities to Spanish-surname neighborhoods, the Spanish-surname IMR began a marked decline (Blanchard 1996). However, the lag in the transition was not overcome until the mid-1970s (Forbes and Frisbie 1991).

Factors Associated with Infant Mortality: Findings from MacroLevel, MicroLevel, and MultiLevel Research

Findings on infant mortality can be usefully organized according to the level of analysis at which the research was conducted. Although at its inception, public health research was "essentially ecological,"[9] over the past several decades, health research has been concentrated at the individual level (Diez-Roux 2001: 1783). Micro level findings will receive the most attention in this discussion because analyses at this level have dominated infant mortality research for quite some time and because efforts aimed at identifying the biological links between sociodemographic factors and risk of infant death must proceed largely with data on individuals. There is also a substantial and growing interest in multilevel, or contextual, analysis in which the effects of both area and individual predictors are modeled (Diez-Roux 1998; O'Campo et al. 1997; Robert 1998).

MACROLEVEL FINDINGS.   Geoffrey Rose has argued that, while the analysis of individual risk predominates and may be the best way to evaluate "aetiological force, . . . it is no measure at all of aetiological outcome or of public health importance" (1985: 32). Although it seems likely that few scholars in any discipline would subscribe to the view that individual-level analysis is of no importance for public health, there are numerous reasons to engage in research on socially meaningful aggregates, not the least of which is that "[to] find the determinants of prevalence and incidence *rates*, we need to study characteristics of populations" (Rose 1985: 34; emphasis added).

Higher infant mortality rates have been observed in lower socioeconomic status neighborhoods (Guest, Almgrew, and Hussey 1998), while at the societal level, unemployment is associated with elevated infant mortality rates in developed countries (Pampel and Pillai 1986). From his studies of metropolitan areas, Polednak (1991, 1996) concluded that racial residential segregation contributes to higher black infant mortality rates, net of the effects of black-white income inequality and the black poverty rate. Another study (Collins and David 1990) based on the Chicago census found that black LBW rates were twice as high as white rates and that residence in low-income areas was associated with higher LBW rates for infants among mothers of both races. However, racial *disparities* in birth weight were less pronounced in the poorest areas, perhaps because whites were able to preserve an advantage regardless of the level of income characterizing the areas. Further, high rates of violent crime are associated with elevated rates of both LBW and IUGR (Collins and David 1996). In the most recent installment

[9] The rubric *ecological* is often used to refer to analyses in which geographical areas (neighborhoods, communities, nations, etc.) are the units of analysis. Such analyses should be referred to as macrolevel or area-level so as to avoid confusion with sociological human ecology, as developed most fully in the work of Amos Hawley (1950, 1986), in which it is the *conceptual framework*, not the choice of analytical units, that distinguishes human ecology from other paradigms.

from this Chicago-based research agenda, Collins and colleagues (2001) have reported that, even in impoverished neighborhoods, the postneonatal mortality rate (attributed primarily to causes such as accidents, homicides, and infections) for infants of Mexican American mothers was twice as high as the rate for infants born to Mexico-born mothers—a finding speculated to be a result of loss of the protective influence of Mexican culture among U.S.-born women.

At the societal level, infant mortality tends to decline as income increases, at least until a threshold is reached at which basic health needs can be satisfied. Further, "income inequality rather than income level may be crucial," inasmuch as economic development that allows adequate health services does not ensure that the low-income portion of the population will have full access to services (Pampel and Pillai 1986: 527). Greater social, cultural, and ethnic heterogeneity may be linked to higher infant mortality rates to the extent that heterogeneity implies discrimination and inequities in the distribution of, and access to, societal resources. Government support for proper medical care should help to improve health in a society, including lowering rates of adverse pregnancy outcomes. Nonetheless, it may be that in developing countries neither overall prosperity, nor social and cultural heterogeneity, nor the presence of modern medical technology will be especially effective in lowering the infant mortality rate in the absence of political consensus regarding health goals, efficient provision of health services at the local level, and female autonomy sufficient to allow women to achieve the levels of education and freedom of action required to take advantages of economic growth and advances in health technology for themselves and their children (Caldwell 1986).

Pampel and Pillai's investigation of infant mortality in developed countries (1986) showed that all measures of infant mortality (total [IMR], neonatal [NMR], and postneonatal [PNMR]) varied inversely with per capita gross national product, percent urban, and percent of females with higher levels of education. Higher mortality was associated with ethnic/linguistic diversity and the unemployment rate. Total government expenditures for social welfare were not significantly associated with infant mortality after ethnic/linguistic diversity were controlled.

A recent societal-level analysis of infant mortality revisits the link between government health care spending per capita and the infant mortality rate for 19 countries (Conley and Springer 2001). Controlling for economic development and indicators that likely influence government welfare spending (e.g., fertility rates and proportion elderly), it was found that "public health spending does have a significant impact in lowering infant mortality rates, ... and that this effect is cumulative over a five-year time span" (Conley and Springer 2001: 768). Importantly, these results were obtained using country fixed-effects models to address the problem of unobserved heterogeneity bias and with adjustments for reciprocal causation and autocorrelation. The beneficial effects of health care for infant survival were theorized to be both direct through support for neonatal care and technology and indirect through a lowering of the LBW rate.

MICROLEVEL FINDINGS. Especially in light of the massive number of microlevel studies of infant mortality, it is useful to organize the discussion of this literature according to the hypothesized ordering of effects, beginning with background factors and proceeding through intervening variables to the most proximate determinants.

A delineation of risk factors according to this organizational strategy appears as Table 9.1 according to three categories: background factors, preparturition intervening factors, and postpartum proximate factors. However, as the earlier summary of the debate over the relevance of birth weight makes abundantly clear, there is less than full consensus regarding both the causal importance and causal ordering of risk factors for infant mortality.[10] It is not possible to include every variable that might be useful in accounting for variation in infant mortality. Based on a review of the literature, Table 9.1 presents a reasonable partial ordering and one which, at least in a general way, reflects demographic consensus regarding the nature of individual risk factor effects.

Among those effects are several background factors, including socioeconomic status, demographic factors, biological/biomedical variables, and race/ethnicity.

Socioeconomic Status. Infants born to low SES mothers are more likely to be of low birth weight and/or less likely to survive the first year of life (Fuentes-Afflick and Hessol 1997), possibly because these women are more apt to lack the resources necessary to acquire either prenatal or postnatal care (or both) and may have less knowledge of the need for, and/or access to, health services. *Maternal education* is the socioeconomic status (SES) indicator most frequently linked to birth outcomes and infant survival

TABLE 9.1. **Selected Microlevel Background and Proximate Factors Affecting the Risk of Infant Mortality.**

Background Factors	Prenatal Intervening Factors	Postpartum/ Proximate Factors
Race/Ethnicity	*Biomedical*	*Demographic*
	Prenatal care	Sex of infant
SES	Maternal weight gain	Plurality
Mother's education	Pregnancy complications	
Household/family income	Delivery complications	
Poverty	Maternal morbidity	
Health insurance		*Biomedical*
		Birth outcomes (birth weight, gestational age, maturity)
	Behavioral	Ambient smoke
Demographic	Smoking	Breast-feeding
Mother's age	Alcohol consumption	Infant morbidity
Parity	Drug use	Postnatal care
Marital status	Nutrition (weight gain)	
Mother's nativity		
	Psychosocial	
	Stress	
	Wantedness/intendedness of pregnancy	
Biological/Biomedical		
Maternal morbidity		
Pregnancy history (prior loss, prior adverse birth outcomes, etc.)		
Interpregnancy interval		
Parental birth weight		

[10] Recall also that specific variables can reasonably be included in different substantive categories.

chances because other measures that might be preferable, such as family income, are not usually available in the vital statistics records which constitute the basis for much demographic research in this area (Hummer, Eberstein, and Nam 1992: 1060). A positive effect of maternal education on infant survival chances has been shown to persist following adjustment for a wide range of other risk factors (Hummer et al. 1999). Part of the effect is likely mediated by birth outcomes. For example, Schoendorf et al. (1992) report that "black infants born to college-educated parents have higher mortality rates than similar white infants," but when only normal-weight infants were considered, the relationship vanished.

More than 20 years ago, Gortmaker noted that "significant direct relationships between income poverty and both neonatal and postneonatal mortality are indicated" (1979: 291). Much more recently, based on a data set that included health-related variables (e.g., health insurance, program participation), higher household income was associated with lower risk of both endogenous and exogenous infant mortality, even net of controls for birth weight and preterm birth (Moss and Carver 1998). In many instances, though, the effects of SES on birth outcomes and infant mortality have been reported to be inconsistent and/or small to nonexistent (Cramer 1995; Hummer et al. 1995; Scribner and Dwyer 1989). Cramer concludes, e.g., that while "women with higher income have larger babies . . . , the effects of income are small and not significant at conventional levels" (1995: 242).[11] These less than definitive findings do not mean that SES is of little or no consequence in accounting for variation in birth outcomes. Rather, SES is conceptualized as a background factor whose effect is primarily indirect through more proximate determinants.

The effects of *health insurance* are especially interesting from a policy standpoint. Having insurance to cover costs of pregnancy and delivery might be viewed as uniformly positive, were it not for negative selectivity bias. For example, in light of eligibility requirements, women who make use of Medicaid are more likely to exist under financial circumstances so severe as to diminish overall quality of life and to create psychological stress that may be detrimental to both mother and child. There is evidence that an increase in the odds of adverse birth outcomes is associated with reliance on government-provided health insurance, as compared to private insurance coverage (Frisbie et al. 1997) and that infants of Medicaid recipients are lighter than those born to mothers not part of the Medicaid program (Schwethelm et al. 1989). Moss and Carver (1998) found a consistently higher risk of *exogenous* infant mortality when Medicaid or other government insurance was used to pay for delivery. Odds of exogenous mortality were also elevated in the case of self-paid delivery, but the effect fell slightly below the level of significance ($p < .01$) in models where birth outcomes and other variables were controlled. Self-paid delivery was significantly related to higher risk of *endogenous* mortality in all models, while in the case of government-paid delivery, the higher risk from endogenous causes appears to be indirect through birth weight and gestational age. The ability to distinguish between the negative selectivity associated with eligibility for receipt of government assistance and the income effect of that

[11] Research on the effects of income, wealth, and poverty more often than not pertain to birth outcomes, rather than to infant mortality. This seems largely due to the fact that multivariate analysis of rare events, such as infant mortality, requires quite large data sets. The vital statistics provide files with huge numbers of cases, but they contain no information on income and no indication of poverty or wealth. There are, of course, exceptions, of which the Moss and Carver research (1998) is a prime example.

assistance may be crucial. For example, Cramer (1995: 243) demonstrated that women who receive public assistance "have much smaller babies than other people (the selectivity effect), but among women receiving assistance, those who obtain more assistance have larger babies (the income effect)."

Demographic Factors. Numerous analyses have found an association between *maternal age* and pregnancy outcomes that shows the risk of infant mortality to be higher for both teenage and older mothers (Singh and Yu 1996). Very young maternal age may be acting as a proxy for social disadvantage, and teenage childbearing has been associated with a life-long history of exposure to unhealthy conditions which may lead to "weathering," i.e., a diminution of a woman's health endowments (Geronimus 1987; Geronimus and Korenman 1993). Maternal age needs to analyzed jointly with *parity* (or birth order) because the chances of adverse pregnancy outcomes are greater for "primiparas 30 years of age and over and multiparas under 18 years of age" (Kleinman and Kessel 1987: 751). Others report that first births are more at risk of low birth weight, perhaps as a result of pregnancy complications (Kallan 1993). *Marital status* is an often included variable in studies of infant mortality. Infants born to unwed mothers are characterized by lower birth weight and higher mortality risk (Cramer 1987; Frisbie et al. 1997; Hummer et al. 1999; Kallan 1993). This relationship is often attributed to lifestyle differences and a greater likelihood of inadequate familial, social, and/or economic resources among unmarried mothers (Eberstein et al. 1990). Marital status effects may also vary by race and are strongest among groups for which childbirth outside formal marriage is nonnormative (Cramer 1987; Eberstein 1990).

Given the surge in growth of the immigrant population in the U.S., especially Hispanic and Asian immigrants (De Vita 1996), it is scarcely surprising that a large amount of attention has been given to *maternal nativity*. Over the years, lower mortality of adult immigrants, as compared to their native-born counterparts, has consistently been recorded (e.g., Marmot, Adelstein, and Bulusu 1984; Rogers, Nam, and Hummer 2000). Similar results have emerged regarding the survival chances of infants of foreign-born women. In fact, the social, economic, and cultural processes related to immigration have been offered as an explanation for the paradoxical coupling of relatively favorable pregnancy outcomes with a high-risk socioeconomic and demographic profile observed in the Mexican-origin population. This epidemiological paradox (which applies to adults, as well as infants, see Markides and Coreil 1986) is more fully described below.

Biological /Biomedical Variables. The health endowments characterizing women prior to conception may be crucial in determining pregnancy outcome. *Previous pregnancy loss* has been included in earlier research as a measure of reproductive efficiency, and women who previously have had a miscarriage or stillbirth are at greater risk of adverse birth outcomes and of infant mortality. The same is true of women who have experienced either *previous preterm* or *small-for-gestational-age births* (Eberstein, Nam, and Hummer 1990; Kallan 1993; Frisbie et al 1997; Hummer et al. 1999). As with other background risks, the effect of prior loss or previous small or preterm delivery is likely to be attenuated with controls for low birth weight (Hummer et al. 1999). A number of *maternal morbid conditions* increase the likelihood of adverse pregnancy outcomes. Hypertensive disorders (especially when preeclampsia is superimposed on chronic hypertension) are associated with increased risk of stillbirth, adverse birth outcomes, and neonatal mortality (Kallan 1993; National High Blood Pressure Education Program 2000). The likelihood of preterm and immature (IUGR) birth is increased for infants born to diabetic mothers, with the risk being greater in the case of chronic, as compared to gestational, diabetes (Kallan 1993). Diabetes is also implicated as a risk factor for excessively heavy (macrosomic) births, although only a small fraction of mothers of macrosomic infants are diabetic (Frank, Frisbie, and Pullum 2000).

Despite extensive preventive efforts that have involved nutritional supplementation, attempts to improve access to prenatal care, and "a greater use of pharmacologic agents to inhibit labor" (Goldenberg and Andrews 1996: 781), prematurity rates in the U.S. remain high. This has led to several investigations of the "urogenital infection hypothesis" (Fiscella 1996; Goldenberg and Rouse 1998; see also Kallan 1993 on the effect of pelvic inflammatory disease). Particular attention has been given to bacterial vaginosis, "defined as an overgrowth of various bacteria in the vagina," because this condition is associated with an odds ratio for spontaneous preterm birth of between 1.5 and 3.0" and because the first symptom of this condition is often spontaneous preterm labor itself (Goldenberg and Andrews 1996: 782).

Interpregnancy interval, i.e., the time between a live birth and next conception, may also be related to pregnancy outcomes. A short interval (less than 6 or 7 months) may result in physiological depletion of the mother and has been shown to increase the risk of adverse birth outcomes and infant mortality in samples of women in the U.S. and elsewhere in the world (Miller 1994; Moss and Carver 1998). Beneficial effects of longer birth intervals on the survivorship of infants and children have been observed in cross-national research, with impact apparently greatest in high mortality countries (Palloni and Millman 1986). The primary risk seems to arise from a combination of short intervals with higher parity births (Miller 1994).

Despite a growing interest in biological linkages between social factors and health, genetic explanations for adverse pregnancy outcomes are typically eschewed by social scientists. One notable exception is an analysis by Conley and Bennett (2000) that explores the relationship of *parental birth weight* and SES to infant birth weight. Based on the application of family-fixed-effects models (sibling comparisons) and intergenerational data, these authors find that "[a] mother or father having been low-birth-weight themselves is associated with a huge increase in the probability that their child will be born at a low birth weight—by roughly four-fold and six-fold, respectively" (Conley and Bennett 2000: 465).

Race/Ethnicity. Based on both volume of research and policy relevance, it can be argued that race/ethnic inequality in health outcomes constitutes the most significant and consistently troubling issue in empirical research where demography and public health research intersect. Race/ethnic variation in infant mortality, in particular, has been the topic of a vast amount of literature. The black-white differential has received most of the attention, but a very substantial amount of comparative research involving other minorities has emerged over the past decade or two.

Race/ethnic infant mortality trends in the U.S. for selected years from 1970 to 1998 are shown in Table 9.2. Hispanic ethnicity was not recorded on birth certificates until 1985. In 1985, fewer than half the states collected birth and death data on Hispanics, but these states (including California and Texas) were those where most Hispanics are

TABLE 9.2. U.S. Infant, Neonatal, and Postneonatal Mortality Rates[a] by Race and Hispanic Origin[b,c]

		1970	1985	1990	1998
All infants		20.0	10.6	9.2	7.2
	White	17.6	9.2	7.6	6.0
	Black	33.3	19.0	18.0	13.8
	Hispanic	NA	8.6	7.8	5.8
All neonatal		15.1	7.0	5.8	4.8
	White	13.7	6.0	4.8	4.0
	Black	23.2	12.6	11.6	9.4
	Hispanic	NA	5.4	5.0	3.9
All postneonatal		4.9	3.7	3.4	2.4
	White	4.0	3.2	2.8	2.0
	Black	10.1	6.4	6.4	4.4
	Hispanic	NA	3.2	2.8	1.9

Source: Abstracted from *Trends in the Well-Being of America's Children & Youth 2001*, Table HC3.1.A at http://aspe.os.dhhs.-gov/hsp/01trends/ack.htm.
[a] Per 1,000 live births.
[b] Race/ethnic identification according to race or national origin of mother.
[c] Estimates for separate race groups include Hispanics of those races. Persons of Hispanic origin may be of any race. Hispanic rates not available until 1985. NA = not available.

concentrated (Schick and Schick 1991).[12] Coverage was much more geographically extensive by 1990 and was nearly complete by 1995. The most striking patterns in Table 9.2 are the consistent reduction in the IMR, NMR, and PNMR over time, the fact that Hispanic rates are slightly lower than the rates for whites, and the roughly two-to-one excess of black over white infant deaths.

The IMRs for a larger number of specific race/ethnic groups for the period from the mid-1980s to 2000 appear as Table 9.3. The data in the final column of Table 9.3 are the latest available and, for that column only, non-Hispanic whites and non-Hispanic blacks are distinguished. Although the IMR fell over time for all groups, the trajectory of the decrease varied. American Indians have relatively high infant mortality, but the black IMR in 1998 was virtually identical to that recorded by American Indians more than a decade earlier. Table 9.3 also demonstrates substantial heterogeneity within the larger Hispanic and Asian populations and thereby emphasizes the importance of conducting separate analyses of subpopulations whenever data permit. The IMRs for most Hispanic groups are similar to, or slightly lower than, those of whites, but the Puerto Rican rate is elevated compared to all other Hispanic groups. Compared to other Asian and Pacific Islanders, Chinese and Japanese have modestly to substantially lower infant mortality—indeed, their IMRs are below the white rates for all years, while Hawaiian rates are considerably higher. Among certain of the smaller groups, stability of rates is less than optimal when calculations are based on single years.

However, it should be noted that a very recent report (Kochanek and Martin 2004) shows that there was an increase in the infant mortality rate in the U.S. between 2001 and 2002, which is a break in a more than four-decade-long set of annual declines. It

[12] Table 9.2 and Table 9.3 were derived from data sets in which race and Hispanic ethnicity overlap. While greater precision can be achieved by distinguishing non-Hispanic blacks, non-Hispanic whites, and non-black Hispanics—as is reflected in many of the studies cited herein—general race/ethnic differentials and trends are quite adequately represented in Tables 9.2 and 9.3.

TABLE 9.3. U.S. Infant Mortality Rates[a] by Race and Hispanic Origin[b,c]

Specific Subpopulations		1983–85	1989–91	1995	1998	2000[d]
Total		10.6	9.0	7.6	7.2	6.9
White		9.0	7.4	6.3	6.0	5.7
Black		18.7	17.1	14.6	13.8	13.6
American Ind./Alaska Native		13.9	12.6	9.0	9.3	8.3
Asian/ Pacific Islander		8.3	6.6	5.3	5.5	4.9
	Chinese	7.4	5.1	3.8	4.0	3.5
	Japanese	6.0	5.3	5.3	3.5	4.5
	Filipino	8.2	6.4	5.6	6.2	5.7
	Hawaiian	11.3	9.0	6.6	10.0	9.0
	Other API	8.6	7.0	5.5	5.7	NA
Hispanic		9.2	7.6	6.3	5.8	5.6
	Mexican American	8.8	7.2	6.0	5.6	5.4
	Puerto Rican	12.3	10.4	8.9	7.8	8.2
	Cuban	8.0	6.2	5.3	3.6	4.5
	Central/South Amer.	8.2	6.6	5.5	5.3	4.6
	Other/Unknown Hisp.	9.9	8.2	7.4	6.5	6.9

Source: 1983–85 through 1998 data abstracted from *Trends in the Well-Being of America's Children & Youth 2001*; Table HC3.1.B at http://aspe.os.dhhs.gov/hsp/01trends/ack.htm.
Data for 2000 abstracted from *Infant Mortality Statistics from the 2000 Period Linked Birth/Infant Death Data Set; Figure 1 and Tables 2 & 3 of National Vital Statistics Report, Vol. 50, No. 12, August 28, 2002.*
[a] Per 1,000 live births.
[b] Race/ethnic identification according to race or national origin of mother.
[c] Estimates for separate race groups include Hispanics of those races. Persons of Hispanic origin may be of any race. Hispanic rates not available until 1985.
[d] Data for 2000 are for non-Hispanic whites and non-Hispanic blacks. Persons of Hispanic origin may be of any race. NA = not available.

remains to be determined whether the recent upward inflection in the IMR marks the beginning of a set of increases or is only a short-lived deviation from the secular trend.

The race/ethnic differences in Table 9.3 are related to a wide range of demographic, SES, biomedical, and behavioral characteristics, but explanations of the differences are far from complete. Two of the most central questions remaining have to do with (1) the continuing disadvantage of blacks, among whom the risk of infant mortality has long been about twice that of whites—a relative gap which has recently shown an increase (Guyer et al. 1998), and (2) the epidemiological paradox—the term often applied to denote the finding that, despite a high-risk demographic and socioeconomic profile, Mexican American mortality rates and individual risk of infant mortality are typically similar to, and sometimes more favorable than, those of non-Hispanic whites (Anglos).

Blacks are disadvantaged relative to the white population in regard to most risk factors—most notably the fact that LBW has long been at least twice as common among blacks as whites (Guyer et al. 1998; Hummer et al. 1999; Schick and Schick 1991). Adjusting for birth weight tends to sharply reduce the disadvantage but begs the question of why LBW rates are so high among blacks.

Over the past decade or two, many analyses have attempted to account for the fact that the high-risk Mexican American population (adults, as well as infants) is characterized by relatively low mortality (Markides and Coreil 1986; Rogers, Nam, and Hummer 2000; Williams, Binkin, and Clingman 1986). The initial observation of the paradox among infants seems to have appeared about three decades ago in Teller and Clyburn's work (1974) based on Texas data. However, it was not until the mid-1980s that this enigma became the subject of a major research agenda. Even at this later point in time, along with surprise at the finding, came a certain element of disbelief—in particular, there was some tendency to view the finding as a data artifact. By the early 1990s, doubt about the validity of the finding was largely dispelled, and a major research agenda arose focused on both infant mortality and birth outcomes which demonstrated, at both national and local levels, that Hispanic infants, especially those of Mexican origin, were characterized by infant mortality risk similar to that of Anglo infants (e.g., Albrecht et al. 1996; Cervantes, Keith, and Wyshak 1999; Cobas et al. 1996; Cramer 1987, 1995; Forbes and Frisbie 1991; Frisbie, Forbes, and Pullum 1996; Frisbie, Forbes, and Hummer 1998a; Hummer et al. 1999; Rumbaut and Weeks 1991; 1996; Scribner 1996).

Two explanations for the paradox are prominent. The explanations are quite different in some ways, but both relate to the high proportion of immigrants in the Mexican-origin and other minority populations of the U.S. The first points to positive selection of migration according to health (Frisbie, Cho, and Hummer 2001; Marmot, Adelstein, and Bulusu 1984; Markides and Coreil 1986; Palloni and Morenoff 2001). The second is the *cultural hypothesis*, which proposes that Mexican-origin women, as well as those of Asian origin (see, e.g., Rumbaut and Weeks 1991), are the products of a more healthful cultural milieu and are therefore characterized by norms that make individuals less inclined to engage in risky behaviors. It has been demonstrated, for example, that women of Mexican origin, particularly first-generation immigrants from Mexico, are less likely to smoke cigarettes or consume alcohol and are more apt to have nutritious diets (Cobas et al. 1996; Guendelman and Abrams 1995; Rogers and Crank 1988). This, in turn, may be expected to impact positively on birth outcomes and infant survival (Cobas et al. 1996; Scribner and Dwyer 1989; Rumbaut and Weeks 1991, 1996; Singh and Yu 1996). Indeed, Scribner (1996) finds the evidence regarding the cultural hypothesis so persuasive that he suggests the phenomenon should be referred to, not as the epidemiological paradox, but rather as the epidemiological paradigm. It may be that the magnitude of the selectivity influence cannot be adequately determined without "pooled origin/destination data with comparable information for nonmigrants in the origin country and for migrants to the United States" (Landale, Oropesa, and Gorman 2000: 892). To my knowledge, other than Landale's study of Puerto Rican infant mortality, no other research has focused directly on that issue. Landale and colleagues find some evidence supporting both the selectivity and cultural hypotheses but are unable to account for "why the health advantage of infants of recent migrants erodes as duration of U.S. residence increases" (Landale, Oropesa, and Gorman 2000: 905).

My own evaluation is that it is more reasonable at this juncture to couch conceptual models in terms of behavioral, rather than cultural, differences. While useful proxies for cultural attachment exist (e.g., language use and nativity), we have no measures of cultural content (except, again, language). By contrast, we do have several indicators of behavior (including smoking), and it is the behavior involved in a more healthy life style that produces positive outcomes, regardless of whether the behavior has a cultural, or some other, basis.

Further, adults in virtually all immigrant groups, including immigrants from Africa, Asia, and Europe, have been found to have better health and/or lower mortality than their U.S. born counterparts (Cabral et al. 1990; Frisbie, Cho, and Hummer 2001; Marmot, Adelstein, and Bulusu 1984). Lower mortality risk also characterizes infants born to immigrant women from a number of different countries (Cervantes, Keith, and

Wyshak 1999; Hummer et al. 1999). Clearly, there are such substantial differences in the cultural milieus that characterize Hispanic, African, Asian, and European immigrants that there seems to be little reason to believe that these distinctive cultures all foster the same (or similar) healthy behaviors.[13] Thus, while findings exist in support of both the migration selectivity and cultural hypotheses, it would appear that the weight of the evidence favors the selectivity interpretation.

However, it should be noted that recent research has again begun to raise the data artifact issue in regard to the paradox. Patel and colleagues (2004) suggest that, due to "underascertainment" of ethnicity on some death records, the mortality rates of elderly Mexican Americans may be downwardly biased. Such a problem seems less likely in regard to infant mortality, especially in studies based on the NCHS-linked birth/infant death files because a match rate of better than 97% was achieved as early as 1989 (U.S. Department of Health and Human Services 1995). Further, while it is essential to explore possible distortions introduced by data problems, the consistent observation of health and survival advantages among immigrants to the U.S. from virtually all countries of origin suggests that the "paradox" cannot easily be dismissed as a data artifact.

Table 9.4 summarizes differential risks of infant mortality across a large number of race/ethnic groups, with additional attention given to whether the mother is an immigrant or U.S.-born, and with controls for a large number of demographic, SES, behavioral, and biomedical factors. The findings are based on logistic regression and presented in terms of odds ratios (i.e., the exponentiated coefficients). Anglos are the reference group for race/ethnic comparisons, and the U.S.-born serve as the referent for nativity. The control for birth outcome makes use of a six-category measure constructed from combinations of birth weight and gestational age (Frisbie, Forbes, and Pullum 1996). Model 1 of Table 9.4 shows that the bivariate odds ratio (OR) for infant mortality is twice as high for blacks (OR = 2.07) as for Anglos. All Asian groups experience a lower risk. Among Hispanics, the odds of infant death are significantly greater among Puerto Ricans (OR = 1.25) and slightly, but still significantly, higher among the Other Hispanic residual. Risk is lower for Cubans and Central/South Americans, and consistent with previous research, the risk for Mexican Americans is essentially the same as that for Anglos. Model 2 shows the bivariate effect of nativity. The odds ratio of .77 indicates the risk of an infant dying in the first year of life is reduced by 23% if the mother is foreign-born.

The findings from Model 3, which includes both race/ethnicity and nativity, emphasize the importance of immigration. When the beneficial impact of foreign birth is controlled, the survival advantage for all of the high-immigration groups (except Other Hispanics) is diminished and, in many cases, actually reversed.

All control variables, except the birth outcome measure, are included in Model 4, and the full model (Model 5) occupies the final column. With adjustment for demographic, SES, behavioral, and biomedical factors (Model 4), the odds for blacks are only 30% higher compared to whites, rather than more than 100% higher as seen in Models 1 and 3. Compared to Anglos, the odds of infant mortality among Puerto Rican infants become significantly *lower* in Model 4, thereby indicating that the initial Puerto Rican

---

[13] Further, it would seem that unqualified reliance on the cultural hypothesis is inescapably tied to the premise that American culture is "toxic" as compared to *all* others—a premise that is unwarranted based on any evidence with which I am familiar.

TABLE 9.4. Odds Ratios for Models of Race/Ethnic Differentials in Infant Mortality, United States

Race/Ethnicity[a]	Model 1	Model 2	Model 3	Model 4[c]	Model 5[c]
Black	2.07**		2.08**	1.30**	.96**
Chinese	.78**		0.95	1.00	1.01
Japanese	.64**		.70**	.76*	.74*
Filipino	.87*		1.06	0.96	.83**
Other Asian	0.94		1.16**	1.04	.91*
Mexican	1.00		1.14**	.82**	.82**
Puerto Rican	1.25**		1.37**	.93*	.80**
Cuban	.84*		1.00	1.03	0.91
Central/South American	.86*		1.07	.82**	.77**
Other Hispanic	1.06*		1.08**	.88**	.88**
Nativity[b]		.77*	.79**	.87**	.92**

Source: NCHS Linked Birth/Infant Death Files. 1989–91. Abstracted from Hummer et al. 1999.
[a] Reference group is non-Hispanic whites.
[b] Reference group is U.S.-born.
[b] Model 4 includes controls for maternal age, marital status, education, parity, previous loss, weight gain, medical risks, complications of labor and delivery, and smoking. In addition to these factors, Model 5 controls birth outcomes.
* = p < .05; ** = p < .01; all tests are two-tailed.

disadvantage can be fully accounted for by the controls. Further, Chinese, Filipinos, Other Asians, and Cubans are now statistically indistinguishable from Anglos. In the full model, which also incorporates the birth outcome measure, there are only a few notable changes as compared to Model 4. The most striking difference seen in Model 5, is that, net of the effect of birth outcome, blacks are at *lower* risk of infant mortality than whites. This is not especially surprising since LBW has long been about twice as common among blacks (Guyer et al. 1998; Hummer et al. 1999; Schick and Schick 1991). However, the question remains as to why LBW rates are so high among blacks in the first place. Another notable change seen in Model 5 is that every Asian group (except the Chinese) has a significant survival advantage compared to Anglos.

In addition to background factors, there are also a number of intervening factors that can affect infant mortality, including biomedical factors, behavioral factors, and psychosocial factors.

Biomedical Factors.   Until a decade or two ago, *prenatal care (PNC)*, as conventionally measured by trimester in which care began, was firmly "established as the key population-wide public health intervention for preventing low birthweight and preterm births," which in turn would reduce "infant morbidity and mortality and related neonatal intensive care costs...because fewer high risk infants would be delivered" (Alexander and Kotelchuck 2001: 116; see also Institute of Medicine 1988). Recent research, however, suggests that the positive and significant relationship often observed between adequate PNC and birth weight, and through birth weight on infant survival chances, is mainly the result of selectivity bias (see Alexander and Kotelchuck [2001]for a recent discussion). For example, it is reasonable to assume that women who seek PNC early and regularly during their pregnancy are in general also more apt to engage in healthy behaviors which in turn lead to more positive pregnancy outcomes. There may also be negative selection as when women experiencing problem pregnancies utilize PNC very intensively—i.e., women who record more PNC visits than the standard recommended by the American College of Obstetricians and Gynecologists (Kotelchuck 1994a, 1994b).

Essentially, the argument is that women who acquire adequate PNC are different in important, but often unmeasured, ways from those who do not acquire adequate care. Statistical approaches, such as two-stage least squares (Rosenzweig and Schultz 1983a, 1983b) are available to address this unobserved heterogeneity. Further, innovative measurement strategies have evolved to replace the conventional trimester approach. These newer measures include an "intensive" or "adequate plus" category that distinguishes women who have more than the recommended number of PNC visits. They also take length of gestation into account (Alexander and Kotelchuck 1996). Regardless of the effect on birth weight, adequate PNC continues to be regarded as a crucial intervention in that it provides "a package of necessary services" not related to birth weight (Shiono and Behrman 1995: 10), including education and referrals to other social services, such as smoking cessation and nutrition programs (Alexander, Kogan, and Himes 1999b; Shiono and Behrman 1995).

Complications of labor and delivery (such as moderate/heavy meconium, placenta previa, breech birth, and so on) and *maternal weight gain* during pregnancy are other examples of intervening biomedical factors. The threat posed by labor and delivery complications is obvious. There is a strong positive correlation between maternal weight gain and birth weight, an unsurprising finding in that much of the weight gain during pregnancy has to do with fetal growth (Chomitz, Cheung, and Lieberman 1995).

Behavioral Factors. The effects of maternal risky behavior, such as smoking, alcohol consumption, and drug abuse, are well known. Demographers often include measures of these behaviors, especially *smoking* (e.g., Frisbie et al. 1997; Hummer et al. 1999; Kallan 1993). Chomitz and associates have provided an extremely useful summary of such effects in which they noted that "[s]moking during pregnancy has been linked to 20% to 30% of low birth weight births and 10% of fetal and infant deaths" (Chomitz, Cheung, and Lieberman 1995: 124). In addition, heavy *consumption of alcohol* has been shown to be associated with congenital malformations, and *abuse of illicit drugs* is strongly implicated in delivery complications, adverse birth outcomes, and infant mortality.

Psychosocial Factors. A risk factor often cited, but rarely directly operationalized, in demographic research is *stress*, defined broadly as "perceived discrepancy between environmental demands and the individual's biological, psychological, or social resources" (Wadhwa et al. 2001: 120). Stress is believed to produce hormonal changes that negatively affect nueroendocrine, immune, and vascular processes (Wadhwa et al. 2001: 120). Cramer (1995) reports stress during pregnancy (as implied by conflicting occupational or educational demands) to be significantly associated with lower birth weight. A recent analysis of Puerto Ricans showed that a *subjective* measure of stress significantly increased the odds of infant mortality, even with birth weight controlled; on the other hand, reported *experience* of stressful life events had no significant effect (Landale et al. 1999).

It has been suggested that stress levels and actual behaviors will be different for women among whom a *pregnancy is wanted* as compared to those for whom it is not. A very modest tendency for an unplanned birth to be associated with late initiation of prenatal care has been observed in some research (Weller, Eberstein, and Bailey 1987). Another study reported that "unwantedness" was significantly related to increased risk of IUGR, and that some portion of the effect was indirect through smoking (Kallan

1993). Unfortunately, the retrospective nature of maternal reports (i.e., attitude toward the pregnancy was ascertained following the birth), which may well reflect either conscious or unconscious changes in attitude after parturition, make interpretation difficult or impossible (Hummer et al.1995).

Finally, in addition to background and intervening factors, a number of proximate factors also affect infant mortality.

Sex of infant is often included as a control variable, as it is well known that, although female babies have lower mean birth weight, their mortality risk is lower than that of males. At the same gestational age, females appear to be more fully developed than males (Kline, Stein, and Susser 1989). Thus, there is ample reason to control for sex of infant in multivariate analyses of pregnancy outcomes or to compute risk (and rates) on a sex-specific basis. *Plurality* needs to be taken into account because twins, triplets, and higher-order multiple births will typically be born lighter and earlier than single-tons—often for reasons unrelated to the substantive issue being addressed. Hence, many studies restrict analyses to singletons, while others control for plurality.

For healthy infants, regular *postnatal care* that involves checkups and a regular course of inoculations to prevent illness is consistently emphasized. Indeed, postnatal care for both well and sick infants significantly decreases the odds of infant death from exogenous causes, net of controls for a large number of other predictors, including birth weight and gestational age (Moss and Carver 1998). *Breast-feeding* is related to reductions in infant and child mortality and appears to be of particular benefit in high-mortality countries and "among groups which are socially and economically deprived" (Palloni and Millman 1986: 230). In addition, *ambient smoke* has been found to significantly add to the risk of death in the first year (Moss and Carver 1998).

Infant morbidity is obviously a cause of great concern. In recent years, the leading causes of infant death have been congenital anomalies, low-birth-weight/short gestation–related conditions, sudden infant death syndrome, and respiratory distress syndrome (U.S. Bureau of the Census 2001: Table 103). Of considerable interest currently is the impact of respiratory distress syndrome (RDS) and its implications for racial variation in neonatal mortality. Respiratory distress syndrome (hyaline membrane disease) "is generally considered to reflect the respiratory distress observed in premature infants as a result of a deficiency of pulmonary surfactant in the alveoli"[14] (Hulsey et al. 1993). It is a problem of preterm infants in that, prior to 26 weeks gestation, there is little or no natural secretion of surfactant. Interestingly, RDS "occurs less frequently, is less severe, and is accompanied by fewer complications in black preterm infants" (Hulsey et al. 1993: 572). The superiority of blacks in this regard is attributed to "the more rapid maturation of pulmonary surfactant in black fetuses" (Hamvas et al. 1996). Research based on clinical data from the St. Louis area indicated that pulmonary surfactant therapy was associated with substantial and statistically significant reductions in white neonatal mortality,[15] but not in black neonatal mortality (Hamvas et al. 1996). This differential may have led to an erosion of the advantage of very-low-weight black infants observed in much previous research (Wilcox and Russell 1986, 1990; Gortmaker and Wise 1997) and may help to explain the widening overall relative infant mortality gap between blacks and whites recorded in the 1990s (Guyer et al. 1998).

---

[14] The term *alveoli* refers to the air cells in the lungs.

[15] A relatively small fraction of RDS-related deaths occurs in the postneonatal period (Malloy and Freeman 2000).

Hamvas et al. (1996) attribute the greater improvement among white infants to a compositional effect (the fact that RDS is more prevalent among white, as compared to black, infants) and, perhaps, to differential access to intervention. Possible explanations offered by other scholars include racial differentials in efficacy of surfactant therapy and in timely access (Ranganathan et al. 2000). Another recent study also demonstrates a decline in the ratio of male-to-female risk of RDS-related infant deaths following wide-scale use of surfactant therapy (Malloy and Freeman 2000). Malloy and Freeman conclude that, while the narrowing of the male-female gap "may point to a biologically mediated difference," the shift in the black-white differential is viewed as the product of "behavioral, cultural, environmental, and economic conditions" (Malloy and Freeman 2000: 419).

Birth Outcomes. That birth weight and gestational age are the most powerful and proximate predictors of infant mortality is unquestionable. However, the question remains whether the debate over the causal importance of birth weight at the aggregate level of analysis should be extended to the microlevel.

Of direct relevance is the work by Solis, Pullam, and Frisbie (2000), which analyzed over 10 million cases from the 1989 to 1991 NCHS linked birth/infant death files in an effort to evaluate both the main and conjoint effects of birth weight and gestational age on the odds of infant mortality among Anglo females. These authors operationalized optimum birth weight for survival in terms of deviations from the mean transformed to z-scores (an adaptation of the macrolevel research of Wilcox and colleagues discussed earlier in this chapter). While not entirely precise, both 39 to 41 weeks gestation and +1 SD above the gestational-age-specific mean appeared to be close approximations of survival optimums.

Four different birth outcome dimensions were distinguished: (1) preterm or early births (E): (2) postterm or late births (L); (3) small births (S); and (4) heavy births (H). Early and late births were measured in their original metric as number of weeks before or after the 39- to 41-week interval, and small and heavy births were measured as relative deviations (i.e., in terms of z-scores) from the optimum described above. Net of the effects of gestational age and the interaction terms, birth weight was the strongest predictor of the risk of infant mortality. Specifically, the odds ratio representing the risk of infant mortality at the gestational-age-specific average was 114% higher (odds ratio = 2.137) than was the risk for an infant born +1 SD above that average. Consonant with previous research (Frank, Frisbie, and Pullam 2000; Wilcox and Russell 1983), heavy weight births also had an elevated mortality risk, but the impact was nowhere near as great as that for low-weight births. Risk was also significantly greater for early and late births, but the magnitudes of the net effects were a good deal smaller than those associated with birth weight.

Two significant interactions were uncovered by Solis and colleagues (2000). A combination of an early and small birth (the E*S term) significantly increased mortality risk. In addition, the E*H interaction had a beneficial effect. The odds ratio for that interaction is .961, indicating a modest, but statistically significant, reduction in risk, which was interpreted as evidence of the survival advantage of "heavy preemies" compared to their lower-weight counterparts observed in previous research (Brenner, Edelman, and Hendricks 1976; Frisbie, Forbes, and Pullum 1996). Extensions of this work to include males and other race/ethnic populations, with calculations based on race/ethnic- and sex-specific optimums (to avoid the need for "the one-size-fits-all" assumption), lend support to the conclusion that, at the individual level of analysis, both birth weight and gestational age (and some of their interactions) have independent, significant effects on infant mortality risk (Echevarria 2002; Frisbie and Echevarria 2002).

Multilevel Findings

Although the social, economic, and health contexts in which individuals reside are theorized to have potent consequences for individual health outcomes, multilevel studies of infant mortality are few. There seems to be considerably more interest in contextual effects on the health of adults, especially older adults (e.g., Seeman and Crimmins 2001) than is the case with infants. A greater focus on the adult population is reasonable in that many deleterious contextual effects emerge only after lengthy exposure—or at least at exposures greater than one year. Nevertheless, a few explorations of multilevel effects on infant mortality exist. In a study based on the NCHS 1995 to 1997 linked files, the effect on individual risk of infant death of residence in counties with varying concentrations of persons of Mexican origin was examined (Jenny, Schoendorf, and Parker 2001). Ethnic concentration was subdivided into high (66% to 100%), medium (33% to 65.9%) and low (< 33%) categories. Logistic regression results showed that infant mortality, net of individual controls, was significantly lower among infants of U.S.-born Mexican-origin women where concentration of the ethnic group was either medium or high. This result did *not* hold in the case of Mexico-born mothers or non-Hispanic white mothers, which led to the suggestion that residence in an area where exposure to Mexican culture is great "may reinforce healthy behaviors that Mexican-American women lose through acculturation" (Jenny, Schoendorf, and Parker 2001: 722). Other research (Landale et al. 1999) found either no significant effects, or ambiguous effects, of macro (tract-level) variables (e.g., neighborhood economic marginality and proportion of Latino residents) on infant mortality of mainland-born Puerto Rican infants.

One of the more elaborate and rigorous studies to date examined the relationship of a wide range of tract-level variables (unemployment rate, crime rate, average wealth, rate of violation of housing codes, per capita income) on the odds of infant mortality, allowing for both direct contextual effects and interactions between context and individual risk factors (O'Campo et al. 1997). Higher tract-level income had a positive influence on birth weight. More important for present purposes, "[a]ll individual risk factors showed an interaction with macro-level variables" (O'Campo et al. 1997: 1113). For the most part, it was observed that residence in higher-risk tracts reduced the protective influence of microlevel variables. "For example, women living in high-risk neighborhoods benefited less from prenatal care than did women living in lower-risk neighborhoods" (O'Campo 1997: 1113).

DIRECTIONS FOR FUTURE RESEARCH

Additional analyses exploring the interrelationships between birth outcomes and their main and conjoint effects on infant mortality would seem to hold considerable potential for generating insights into variation in perinatal health. More population-specific studies based on deviations from birth outcome survival optimums are needed, as alternatives to or in conjunction with, studies using conventional indicators of birth weight and gestational age.

We also need answers to the question of why the relative disparity between black and white infant mortality is increasing (Guyer et al. 1998). It would seem that part of the explanation likely resides in the erosion of the black survival advantage at short gestations and very low birth weights, which in turn may partially be due to the differential benefits of pulmonary surfactant therapy for neonates with RDS. Clinical study supports such an explanation. However, one recent study suggests that differential access to medical intervention is a likely explanation (Frisbie et al. 2004), One obstacle to large-scale studies is that, although infant deaths in which RDS is implicated can be identified from NCHS linked files, there is no record in these files of whether surfactant therapy was applied. Further, a comparison of the records of neonatal intensive care nursery systems in St. Louis with NCHS linked files indicated substantial underreporting of RDS (Hamvas et al. 1998).

Given the dearth of contextual research in this area, it seems eminently worthwhile to mount an effort to develop data sets designed especially for multilevel analyses. Moreover, using whatever relevant data are available, multilevel studies of pregnancy outcomes might profit from the application of random effects models. In the simplest case, the intercept is allowed to vary across areas (say, neighborhoods). Significant intercept variation "suggests either that neighborhood-level factors (or alternatively, omitted individual-level factors closely associated with neighborhoods) may be related to average outcomes for neighborhoods" (Diez-Roux 2000: 181). Random slope models would allow investigation of whether individual-level effects vary by area (Diez-Roux 2000: 182).

For the demography of health there is perhaps no more pressing need than to collaborate with social epidemiologists and medical researchers in the quest to identify biological mechanisms. In general, without such an effort, social scientists "are only able to infer physiologic pathways and therefore cannot rule out alternative explanations typically advocated by biomedical researchers" (Fremont and Bird 1999: 126). The need for interdisciplinary research of this sort is most palpable where the outcome of interest is a biological event, and no biological event should be of any greater interest to us than the survival and health of infants and children.

REFERENCES

Albrecht, S. L., L. L. Clarke, M. K. Miller, and F. L. Farmer. 1996. Predictors of differential birth outcomes among Hispanic subgroups in the United State: The role of maternal risk characteristics and medical care. *Social Science Quarterly* 77:407–433.

Alexander, G. R., M. E. Tompkins, M. C. Allen, and T. C. Hulsey. 1999a. Trends and racial differences in birth weight and related survival. *Maternal and Child Health Journal* 3:71–79.

Alexander, G. R., M. D. Kogan, and J. H. Himes. 1999b. 1994–1996 U.S. singleton birth weight percentiles for age by race, Hispanic origin, and gender. *Maternal and Child Health Journal* 3:225–232.

Alexander, G. R., and M. Kotelchuck. 1996. Quantifying the adequacy of prenatal care: A comparison of indices. *Public Health Reports* 111:408–418.

Alexander, G. R., and M. Kotelchuck. 2001. Assessing the role and effectiveness of prenatal care: History, challenges, and directions for future research. *Public Health Reports*. 116:306–316.

Balcazar, H. 1994. The prevalence of intrauterine growth retardation in Mexican Americans. *American Journal of Public Health* 84:462–465.

Battaglia, F. C., and L. O. Lubchenco. 1967. A practical classification of newborn infants by weight and gestational age. *Journal of Pediatrics* 71:159–163.

Bhopal, R., and L. Donaldson. 1998. White, European, Western, Caucasian, or What? Inappropriate labeling in research on race, ethnicity, and health. *American Journal of Public Health* 88 (September): 1303–1307.

Blanchard, K. S. 1996. *The decline in diarrhea-related infant mortality in San Antonio, Texas, 1935–1954: The role of sanitation*. Ph.D. dissertation. Austin: The University of Texas.

Bonilla-Silva, E. 1999. The essential social fact of race. *American Sociological Review* 64:899–906.

Bogue, D. J. 1969. *Principles of demography*. New York: Wiley.

Brenner, W., D. Edelman, and C. Hendricks. 1976. A standard of fetal growth for the United States of America. *American Journal of Obstetrics and Gynecology* 126:555–564.

Cabral, H., L. E. Fried, S. Levenson, H. Amaro, and B. Zuckerman. 1990. Foreign-born and US-born black women: Differences in health behaviors and birth outcomes. *American Journal of Public Health* 80:70–72.

Caldwell, J. C. 1986. Routes to low mortality in poor countries. *Population and Development Review* 12:171–220.

Carey, J. R. 1997. What demographers can learn from fruit fly actuarial models and biology. *Demography* 34:17–30.

Cervantes, A., L. Keith, and G. Wyshak. 1999. Adverse birth outcomes among native-born and immigrant women: Replicating national evidence regarding Mexicans at the local level. *Maternal and Child Health Journal*. 3:99–109.

Chomitz, V. R., L. W. Y. Cheung, and E. Lieberman. 1995. The role of lifestyle in preventing low birth weight. *The Future of Children* 5:121–138.

Cobas, J. A., H. Balcazar, M. Benin, V. M. Keith, and Y. Chong. 1996. Acculturation and low-birthweight infants among Latino women: A reanalysis of HHANES data with structural equation models. *American Journal of Public Health* 86:394–396.

Collins, J. W., and R. J. David. 1990. The differential effect of traditional risk factors on infant birthweight among blacks and whites in Chicago. *American Journal of Public Health* 80:679–681.

Collins, J. W., and R. J. David. 1996. Urban violence and African-American pregnancy outcome: An ecologic study. *Ethnicity and Disease* 7:184–190.

Collins, J. W., E. Papacek, N. F. Schulte, and A. Drolet. 2001. Differing postneonatal mortality rates of Mexican-American infants with United States-born and Mexico-born mothers in Chicago. *Ethnicity and Disease* 11:606–613.

Conley, D., and N. G. Bennett. 2000. Is biology destiny? Birth weight and life chances. *American Sociological Review*. 65:458–467.

Conley, D., and K. W. Springer. 2001. Welfare state and infant mortality. *American Journal of Sociology* 107:768–807.

Cramer, J. C. 1987. Social factors and infant mortality: Identifying high-risk groups and proximate causes. *Demography* 24:299–322.

Cramer, J. C. 1995. Racial and ethnic differences in birthweight: The role of income and financial assistance. *Demography* 32:231–247.

David, R. 1990. Race, birth weight, and mortality rates. *Journal of Pediatrics* 116:101–102.

David, R. 2001. Commentary: Birthweights and bell curves. *International Journal of Epidemiology* 30:1241–1243.

De Vita, C. J. 1996. The United States at mid-decade. *Population Bulletin* 50:1–48.

Diez-Roux, A. V. 1998. Bringing context back into epidemiology: Variables and fallacies in multilevel analysis. *American Journal of Public Health*. 88:216–222.

Diez-Roux, A. V. 2000. Multilevel analysis in public health research. *Annual Review of Public Health* 21:171–192.

Diez-Roux, A. V. 2001. Investigating neighborhood and area effects on health. *American Journal of Public Health*. 91:1783–1789.

Eberstein, I. W., C. Nam, and R. A. Hummer. 1990. Infant mortality by cause of death: Main and interaction effects. *Demography* 27:413–430.

Echevarria, S. 2002. *Race/ethnic- and sex-specific models of infant mortality among non-Hispanic whites, non-Hispanic blacks and Mexican Americans in the U.S.* Ph.D. dissertation. Austin: The University of Texas.

Fiscella, K. 1996. Racial disparities in preterm births: The role of urogenital infections. *Public Health Reports* 111:113.

Forbes, D., and W. P. Frisbie. 1991. Spanish surname and Anglo infant mortality: Timing and cause of death differentials over a half-century. *Demography* 28:639–660.

Frank, R. 2001. The misuse of biology in demographic research on racial/ethnic differences: A reply to Van Den Oord and Rowe. *Demography* 38 (November):563–567.

Frank, R., W. P. Frisbie, and S. G. Pullum. 2000. Race/ethnic differentials in heavy weight and cesarean births. *Population Research and Policy Review*. 19:459–475.

Fremont, A. M., and C. E. Bird. 1999. Integrating sociological and biological models: An editorial. *Journal of Health and Social Behavior*. 40:126–129.

Frenk, J., J. L. Bobadilla, J. Sepulveda, and M. L. Cervantes. 1989. Health transition in middle-income countries: New challenges for health care. *Health and Policy Planning*. 4:29–39.

Frisbie, W. P., D. Forbes, and R. G. Rogers. 1992. Neonatal and postneonatal mortality as proxies for cause of death: Evidence from ethnic and longitudinal comparisons. *Social Science Quarterly* 73:535–549.

Frisbie, W. P., D. Forbes, and S. G. Pullum. 1996. Compromised birth outcomes and infant mortality among racial and ethnic groups. *Demography* 33:469–481.

Frisbie, W. P., M. Biegler, P. B. de Turk, D. Forbes, and S. G. Pullum. 1997. Racial and ethnic differences in determinants of intrauterine growth retardation and other compromised birth outcomes. *American Journal of Public Health*. 87:1977–1983.

Frisbie, W. P., D. Forbes, and R. A. Hummer. 1998a. Hispanic pregnancy outcomes. *Social Science Quarterly*. 79:149–169.

Frisbie, W. P., D. Forbes, R. A. Hummer, and S. G. Pullum. 1998b. Birth outcome, not pregnancy process: Reply to Van Der Veen. *Demography* 35:518–527.

Frisbie, W. P., Y. Cho, and R. A. Hummer. 2001. Immigration and the health of Asian and Pacific Islander adults in the United States. *American Journal of Epidemiology*. 153:372–380.

Frisbie, W. P., and S. Echevarria. 2002. What's wrong with modeling infant mortality as a function of birth weight. Paper presented at the annual meeting of the Southern Demographic Association. Austin, Texas, October.

Frisbie, W. P., S. Song, D. A. Powers, and J. A. Street. 2004. The increasing racial disparity in infant mortality: Respiratory distress syndrome and other causes. *Demography* 41:773–800.

Fuentes-Afflick, A. T., and N. A. Hessol. 1997. Impact of Asian ethnicity and national origin on infant birth weight. *American Journal of Epidemiology* 45:148–155.

Fullilove, M. T. 1998. Comment: Abandoning "race" as variable in public health research—an idea whose time has come. *American Journal of Public Health* 88:1297–1298.

Gage, T. B. 2000. Variability of gestational age distributions by sex and ethnicity: An analysis using mixture models. *American Journal of Human Biology* 12:181–191.

Gage, T. B., and G. Therriault. 1998. Variability of birth-weight distributions by sex and ethnicity: Analysis using mixture models. *Human Biology* 70:517–534.

Geronimus, A. T. 1987. On teenage childbearing and neonatal mortality in the U.S. *Population and Development Review* 13:245–279.

Geronimus, A. T., and S. D. Korenman. 1993. Maternal youth or family background? On the health disadvantages of infants with teenage mothers. *American Journal of Epidemiology* 137:213–225.

Goldenberg, R. L., and W. W. Andrews. 1996. Editorial: Intrauterine infection and why preterm prevention programs have failed. *American Journal of Public Health* 86:781–783.

Goldenberg, R. L., and D. J. Rouse. 1998. Prevention of premature birth. *The New England Journal of Medicine*. 339:313–320.

Gortmaker, S. L. 1979. Poverty and infant mortality in the United States. *American Sociological Review* 44:280–297.

Gortmaker, S. L., and P. H. Wise. 1997. The first injustice: Socioeconomic disparities, health services technology, and infant mortality. *Annual Review of Sociology* 23:147–170.

Gruenwald, P. 1965. Terminology of infants of low birth weight. *Developmental Medicine and Child Neurology* 7:578.

Guendelman, S., and B. Abrams. 1995. Dietary intake among Mexican-American women: Generational differences and a comparison with white non-Hispanic women. *American Journal of Public Health*. 85:20–25.

Guest, A. M., G. Almgren, and J. M. Hussey. 1998. The ecology of race and socioeconomic distress: Infant and working age mortality in Chicago. *Demography* 35:23–34.

Guyer, B., M. F. MacDorman, J. A. Martin, K. D. Peters, and D. M. Strobino. 1998. Annual summary of vital statistics—1997. *Pediatrics* 102:1333–1349.

Hack, M., N. K. Klein, and H. G. Taylor. 1995. Long-term developmental outcomes of low birth weight infants. *The Future of Children* 5:176–196.

Hamvas, A., P. H. Wise, R. K. Yang, N. S. Wampler, A. Noguchi, M. M. Maurer, C. A. Walentik, W. F. Schramm, and F. S. Cole. 1996. The influence of the wider use of surfactant therapy on neonatal mortality among blacks and whites. *The New England Journal of Medicine*. 334:1635–1640.

Hamvas, A., P. Kwong, M. DeBaun, W. Schramm, and F. S. Cole. 1998. Hyaline membrane disease is underreported in linked birth-infant death certificate database. *American Journal of Public Health* 88:1387–1389.

Haub, C., and D. Cornelius. 2001. *World data sheet: 2001*. Washington, D.C.: Population Reference Bureau.

Hawley, A. H. 1950. *Human ecology: A theory of community structure*. New York: Ronald.

Hawley, A. H. 1986. *Human ecology: A theoretical essay*. Chicago: University of Chicago Press.

Hertz-Picciotto, I. 2001. Commentary: When brilliant insights lead astray. *International Journal of Epidemiology* 30:1243–1244.

Hulsey, T. C., G. R. Alexander, P. Y. Robillard, D. J. Annibale, and A. Keenan. 1993, Hyaline membrane disease: The role of ethnicity and maternal risk characteristics. *American Journal of Obstetrics and Gynecology*. 168:572–576.

Hummer, R. A., I. W. Eberstein, and C. B. Nam. 1992. Infant mortality differentials among Hispanic groups in Florida. *Social Forces* 70:1055–1075.

Hummer, R. A., C. P. Schmertmann, I. W. Eberstein, and S. Kelly. 1995. Retrospective reports of pregnancy wantedness and birth outcomes in the United States. *Social Science Quarterly* 76:402–418.

Hummer, R. A., M. Biegler, P. B. De Turk, D. Forbes, W. P. Frisbie, Y. Hong, and S. G. Pullum. 1999. Race/ethnicity, nativity, and infant mortality in the United States. *Social Forces* 77:1083–1118.

Institute of Medicine. 1988. *Reaching mothers, reaching infants*. Washington, D.C.: National Academy Press.

Jenny, A. M., K. C. Schoendorf, and J. D. Parker. 2001. The association between community context and mortality among Mexican-American infants. *Ethnicity & Disease* 11:722–731.

Kallan, J. E. 1993. Race, intervening variables, and two components of low birth weight. *Demography* 30:489–506.

Kiely, J., and M. Susser. 1992. Preterm birth, intrauterine growth retardation, and perinatal mortality. *American Journal of Public Health* 82:343–345.

Kline, J., Z. Stein, and M. Susser. 1989. *Conception to birth: Epidemiology of prenatal development*. New York: Oxford.

Kleinman, J. C., and S. S. Kessel. 1987. Racial differences in low birth weight: Trends and risk factors. *The New England Journal of Medicine* 317:749–753.

Kochanek, D. A., and J. A. Martin. 2004. Supplemental analysis of recent trends in infant mortality. National Center for Health Statistics: http://www.cdc.gov/nchs/products/pubs/pubd/hestats/infantmort/infant-mort.htm.

Kotelchuck, M. 1994a. An evaluation of the Kessner Adequacy of Prenatal Care Index and a proposed adequacy of prenatal care utilization index. *American Journal of Public Health* 84:1414–1420.

Kotelchuck, M. 1994b. The adequacy of the Prenatal Care Utilization Index: Its US distribution and association with low birthweight. *American Journal of Public Health*. 84:1486–1489.

Kramer, M. S., F. H. McLean, M. Olivier, D. M. Willis, and R. H. Usher. 1989. Body proportionality and head and length "sparing" in growth-retarded neonates: A critical reappraisal. *Pediatrics* 84:717–723.

Landale, N. S., R. S. Oropesa, D. Llanes, and B. K. Gorman. 1999. Does Americanization have adverse effects on health? Stress, health habits, and infant health outcomes among Puerto Ricans. *Social Forces* 78:613–641.

Landale, N. S., R. S. Oropesa, and B. K. Gorman. 2000. Migration and infant death: Assimilation or selective migration among Puerto Ricans. *American Sociological Review* 65:888–909.

Malloy, M. H., and D. H. Freeman. 2000. Respiratory distress syndrome mortality in the United States, 1987 to 1995. *Journal of Perinatology* 20:414–420.

Markides, K. S., and J. Coreil. 1986. The health of Hispanics in the Southwestern United States: An epidemiologic paradox. *Public Health Reports* 101:253–265.

Marmot, M. G., A. M. Adelstein, and L. Bulusu. 1984. Lessons from the study of immigrant mortality. *Lancet* 112:1455–1457.

McCarton, C., I. Wallace, M. Divon, and H. Vaughan. 1996. Cognitive and neurologic development of the premature, small for gestational age infant through age 6: Comparison by birth weight and gestational age. *Pediatrics* 98:1167–1178.

McCormick, M. C. 1985. The contribution of low birth weight to infant mortality and childhood mortality. *New England Journal of Medicine* 312:82–90.

McKowen, T. 1976. *The rise of modern population*. New York: Academic Press.

Miller, J. E. 1994. Birth order, interpregnancy interval, and birth outcomes among Filipino infants. *Journal of Biosocial Science* 26:243–259.

Mosley, W. H., and L. C. Chen. 1984. An analytical framework for the study of child survival in developing countries. *Population and Development Review* 10 (Suppl.): 25–45.

Moss, N. E., and K. Carver. 1998. The effect of WIC and Medicaid on infant mortality in the United States. *American Journal of Public Health* 88:1354–1361.

National Center for Health Statistics. 1996. *Health, United States, 1995*. Hyattsville, Md.: Public Health Service.

National High Blood Pressure Education Program. 2000 (revised). *Working group report on high blood pressure in pregnancy*. Bethesda, Md.: National Institutes of Health.

O'Campo, P., X. Xue, M. Wang, and M. O. Brien Caughy. 1997. Neighborhood risk factors for low birthweight in Baltimore: A multilevel analysis. *American Journal of Public Health* 87:1113–1118.

Omran, A. R. 1971. The epidemiologic transition: A theory of the epidemiology of population change. *Milbank Memorial Fund Quarterly* 49:509–538.

Omran, A. R. 1977. Epidemiologic transition in the U.S.: The health factor in population change. *Population Bulletin* 32:3–42.

Palloni, A., and S. Millman. 1986. Effects of inter-birth intervals and breastfeeding on infant mortality and early childhood mortality. *Population Studies* 40:215–236.

Palloni, A., and J. D. Morenoff. 2001. Interpreting the paradoxical in the Hispanic paradox. *Annals of the New York Academy of Sciences* 954:140–174.

Palloni, A., and H. Rafalimanana. 1999. The effects of infant mortality on fertility revisited: New evidence from Latin America. *Demography* 36:41–58.

Pampel, F. C., Jr., and V. K. Pillai. 1986. Patterns and determinants of infant mortality in developed nations, 1950–1975. *Demography* 23:525–541.

Patel, K. V., K. Eschbach, L. A. Ray, and K. S. Markides. 2004. Evaluation of mortality data for older Mexican Americans: Implications for the Hispanic paradox. *American Journal of Epidemiology* 159:707–715.

Pattnayak, S. R., and D. Shai. 1995. Mortality rates as indicators of cross-cultural development: Regional variations in the Third World. *Journal of Developing Societies* XI(2):252–262.

Polednak, A. P. 1991. Black-white segregation in infant mortality in 38 standard metropolitan statistical areas. *American Journal of Public Health* 81:1480–1482.

Polednak, A. P. 1996. Trends in US urban black infant mortality, by degree of residential segregation. *American Journal of Public Health* 86:723–726.

Poston, D. L., Jr., and R. G. Rogers. 1985. Toward a reformulation of the neonatal mortality rate. *Social Biology* 32:1–12.

Preston, S. H. 1976. *Mortality patterns in national populations*. New York: Academic Press.

Preston, S. H., ed. 1978. *The effects of infant and child mortality on fertility*. New York: Academic Press.

Preston, S. H., and M. R. Haines. 1991. *Fatal years: Child mortality in the late nineteenth century*. Princeton, N.J.: Princeton University Press.

Ranganathan, D., S. Wall, B. Khoshnood, J. K. Singh, and K. Lee. 2000. Racial differences in respiratory-related neonatal mortality among very low birth weight infants. *The Journal of Pediatrics* 136:454–459.

Robert, S. A. 1998. Community-level socioeconomic status effects on adult health. *Journal of Health & Social Behavior* 39:18–37.

Rogers, R. G. 1996. Assessing the accuracy of neonatal and postneonatal mortality: A comparison of cause- and period-specific infant mortality rates. *Social Science Journal* 23:411–418.

Rogers, R. G., and J. Crank. 1988. Ethnic differences in smoking patterns: Findings from NHIS. *Public Health Reports* 103:387–393.

Rogers, R. G., C. B. Nam, and R. A. Hummer. 2000. *Living and dying in the USA: Behavioral, health, and social differentials of adult mortality*. San Diego, Calif.: Academic Press.

Rose, G. 1985. Sick individuals and sick populations. *International Journal of Epidemiology* 14:32–38.

Rosenzweig, M. R., and T. P. Schultz. 1983a. Consumer demand and household production: The relationship between fertility and child mortality. *American Economic Review* 73:38–42.

Rosenzweig, M. R., and T. P. Schultz. 1983b. Estimating a household production function: Heterogeneity, and the demand for health inputs, and their effect on birth weight. *Journal of Political Economy* 91:723–746.

Rumbaut, R., and J. R. Weeks. 1991. *Perinatal risks and outcomes among low-income immigrants*. Final Report for the Maternal and Child Health Research Program. Rockville, Md.: Department of Health and Human Services.

Rumbaut, R. and J. R. Weeks. 1996. Unraveling a public health enigma: Why do immigrants experience superior perinatal health outcomes? *Research in the Sociology of Health Care* 138:337–391.

Schick, F. L., and R. Schick. 1991. *Statistical handbook on U.S. Hispanics*. Phoenix, Ariz.: Oryx.

Schoendorf, K., C. Carol, J. R. Hogue, J. C. Kleinman, and D. Rowley. 1992. Mortality among infants of black as compared with white college-educated parents. *The New England Journal of Medicine* 326:1522–1526.

Schwethelm, B., L. H. Margolis, C. Miller, and S. Smith. 1989. Risk status and pregnancy outcome among Medicaid recipients. *American Journal of Preventive Medicine* 5:157–163.

Scribner, R. 1996. Editorial: Paradox as paradigm—The health outcomes of Mexican Americans. *American Journal of Public Health* 86:303–305.

Scribner, R., and J. H. Dwyer. 1989. Acculturation and low birthweight among Latinos in the Hispanic HANES. *American Journal of Public Health* 79:1263–1267.

Seeman, T. A., E. Crimmins. 2001. Social environment effects on health and aging: Integrating epidemiologic and demographic approaches and perspectives. *Annals of the New York Academy of Sciences* 954:88–117.

Shapiro, S., E. R. Schlesinger, and R. E. L. Nesbitt, Jr. 1968. *Infant, perinatal, maternal, and childhood mortality in the United States.* Cambridge, Mass.: Harvard University Press.

Shiono, P. H., and R. E. Behrman. 1995. Low weight birth: Analysis and recommendations. *The Future of Children* 5:4–18.

Shryock, H. S., J. Siegel, and Associates. 1976. *The methods and materials of demography*, condensed ed. Edited by E. G. Stockwell. New York: Academic Press.

Singh, G. K., and S. M. Yu. 1996. Adverse pregnancy outcomes: Difference between US- and foreign-born women in major US racial and ethnic groups. *American Journal of Public Health* 86:837–43.

Solis, P., S. G. Pullum, and W. P. Frisbie. 2000. Demographic models of birth outcomes and infant mortality: An alternative measurement approach. *Demography* 37:489–498.

Teller, C. H., and S. Clyburn. 1974. Trends in infant mortality. *Texas Business Review* 29:97–108.

United Nations. 2001. *Demographic yearbook 1999.* New York: UN Publishing Division.

United Nations. 2001. *World population prospects 2001.* New York: United Nations Population Division.

U.S. Bureau of the Census. 2001. *Statistical abstract of the United States: 2001.* Washington, D.C.: U.S. Department of Commerce.

U.S. Department of Health and Human Services. 1995. Linked birth/infant death data set: 1989 cohort. *Public Use Data File Documentation.* Hyattsville, Md.: National Center for Health Statistics.

Van Den Oord, E. J. C. G., and D. C. Rowe. 2000. Racial differences in birth health risk: A quantitative genetic approach. *Demography* 37:285–298.

Wadhwa, P. D., J. F. Culhane, V. Rauh, and S. S. Barve. 2001. Stress and preterm birth: Neuroendocrine, immune/inflammatory, and vascular mechanisms. *Maternal and Child Health Journal* 5:119–125.

Weeks, J. R. 1999. *Population: An introduction to concepts and issues*, 7th ed. Belmont, Calif.: Wadsworth.

Weller, R. H., I. W. Eberstein, and M. Bailey. 1987. Pregnancy wantedness and maternal behavior during pregnancy. *Demography* 24:407–412.

Wilcox, A. J. 2001a. On the importance—and unimportance—of birthweight. *International Journal of Epidemiology* 30:1233–1241.

Wilcox, A. J. 2001b. Response: Where do we go from here? *International Journal of Epidemiology* 30:1245.

Wilcox, A. J., and I. T. Russell. 1983. Birthweight and perinatal mortality. II. On weight-specific mortality. *International Journal of Epidemiology* 12:319–325.

Wilcox, A. J., and I. T. Russell. 1986. Birthweight and perinatal mortality. III. Towards a new method of analysis. *International Journal of Epidemiology* 15:188–196.

Wilcox, A. J., and I. T. Russell. 1990. Why small black infants have a lower mortality rate than small white infants: The case for population-specific standards for birth weight. *Journal of Pediatrics* 116:7–10.

Williams, R. L., R. K. Creasey, G. C. Cunningham, W. E. Hawes, F. D. Norris, and M. Tashiro. 1982. Fetal growth and perinatal viability in California. *Obstetrics and Gynecology* 59Z: 624–632.

Williams, R. L., N. J. Binkin, and E. J. Clingman. 1986. Pregnancy outcomes among Spanish-surname women in California. *American Journal of Public Health* 76:387–391.

Wise, P. H. 1993. Confronting racial disparities in infant mortality: Reconciling science and politics. In D. *Racial differences in preterm delivery: Developing a new research paradigm.* Edited by D. Rowley and H. Tosteson, 7–16. Supplement to Vol. 9, *American Journal of Preventive Medicine.*

World Bank. 1998. *1998 World development indicators.* Washington, D.C.: World Bank.

Yerushalmy, J. 1967. The classification of newborn infants by birth weight and gestational age. *Journal of Pediatrics* 71:164–172.

Zuberi, T. 2001. One step back in understanding racial differences in birth weight. *Demography* 38:569–571.

CHAPTER 10

Adult Mortality

Richard G. Rogers, Robert A. Hummer
and Patrick M. Krueger

Demographic research on adult mortality is significant for understanding the health consequences of social inequality, human behavior, biological factors, and various other forces in human populations. In turn, mortality patterns may profoundly influence the size and composition of these populations. Thus, understanding adult mortality patterns is crucial to comprehending the dynamics of human society. This chapter begins by outlining the general substantive concerns that guide demographers who conduct research on adult mortality, especially by addressing the breadth of factors with which demographers are concerned by placing these factors in a general framework. Following this introduction is a discussion of the data and methods that are commonly used to conduct research in this area. The findings of specific influences on adult mortality are then summarized, revealing variations across a number of demographic, social, and behavioral factors. Most of the methodological and substantive issues could be applied to any geographical area, but this chapter uses data from the United States to illustrate most of our points. The chapter concludes with some ideas for ongoing research in this area.

SUBSTANTIVE CONCERNS

The study of mortality is a core area of demography. Indeed, some have argued that it antedates other core subjects, including fertility, migration, family, and population composition (Dorn 1959). Demographers typically examine the overall mortality patterns and trends among populations and are centrally concerned with mortality differentials across population subgroups. Because everyone eventually dies, demographers focus on when and how, rather than if, people experience death. Indeed, the chance of dying each year in the U.S. is higher for older individuals than for younger people, for males than for females, for individuals in the lower socioeconomic strata compared to those in the upper strata, and for individuals who are already in poor health. Table 10.1 presents a general framework for examining adult mortality and focuses on demographic characteristics, distal causes, proximate factors, and outcomes. Distal factors that indirectly influence mortality are differentiated from proximate factors, which have more direct impacts on mortality. Traditionally, population-based mortality research has focused on how demographic characteristics—age, sex, and race/ethnicity—relate to overall and cause-specific mortality. Indeed, demographers continue to place a great deal of focus on the demographic and social factors associated with adult mortality.

Proximate factors mediate the effects of demographic and distal factors on mortality and include health behaviors, health conditions, and psychosocial and physiological influences. These factors are acquired throughout a person's lifetime and, compared to demographic and social factors, have a more direct impact on the risk of mortality at particular ages. Many of these factors have been examined in the medical, public health, and epidemiological literatures because of their more direct biological links to mortality. Nevertheless, demographers have become increasingly interested in the behavioral, health, and genetic factors associated with adult mortality. This chapter highlights the traditional factors examined in a great deal of demographic research,

TABLE 10.1. **Framework Depicting Factors Related to Adult Mortality**

Demographic Characteristics	Distal Causes	Proximate Factors	Outcomes
Age	**Socioeconomic status**	**Health behaviors**	
	Education	Cigarette smoking	
Sex	Income	Alcohol drinking	
	Employment status	Diet	
Race/ethnicity	Occupational status	Exercise	
	Health insurance	Sleep	
	Wealth	Seat belt use	
		Use of violence	
	Social relations		
	Family relations	**Health conditions**	
	Marital status	Childhood health status	**Mortality**
	Family composition	Parent/sibling health status	Overall mortality
	Relatives	Self-reported health status	Underlying cause
	Friends	Functional limitations	Multiple cause
	Neighbors	Mental and addictive disorders	
	Community ties		
	Religion	**Physiological influences**	
		Height	
	Geographical factors	Weight	
	Region	Cholesterol	
	Urban/rural	Blood pressure	
	Migration	Stress	
	Neighborhood effects	Diabetes	
		Genetic markers	
	Human and environmental hazards		
	Natural disasters		
	Technological risks		
	Acts of terrorism and war		

Source: Expanded from Rogers, Hummer, and Nam (2000).

briefly reviews some research that examines the more proximate factors, and concludes by discussing new potential areas of demographic research on adult mortality. Outcomes examined in most mortality research include measures of overall mortality, measures of underlying causes of death, and multiple cause categorizations of mortality.

DATA AND METHODS

Conventional Methods and Techniques

Demographers rely on a number of techniques to understand mortality patterns and trends. Early demographic work employed straightforward approaches to understanding adult mortality, most often comparing overall, age-standardized, age-specific, and cause-specific mortality rates across population groups and geographical areas. Life tables have also been a staple of mortality researchers for many years; the earliest work using life tables goes back several centuries, but there are many current applications as well. More recently, hazard models, an extension of the life table model (Cox 1972), have enjoyed extensive use among researchers investigating adult mortality.

Demographers often examine mortality rates of specific populations and geographical areas, frequently comparing rates of one population group or geographical area with another. Most simply, the crude death rate divides the number of deaths in a population at a certain time interval to the number of person-years lived in the population during that interval (see Preston, Heuveline, and Guillot 2001). While informative, crude death rates fail to take age and sex structure differences between populations into account, which can seriously mislead comparisons. Thus, age-specific and age-standardized mortality rates are often used to compare population groups and geographical areas to one another. While age-specific rates have the same structure as the crude death rate, the age range for which the deaths and person-years used is restricted (usually in single- or five-year groupings) and thus provide much more specific and useful comparisons (Preston, Heuveline, and Guillot 2001). Age-standardized rates, in turn, compare overall mortality rates across populations by applying the age structure of one real or hypothetical population, i.e., a standard population, to the other populations, thereby controlling for the effects of differential age structures and allowing for more clear comparisons of mortality across population groups and geographical areas.

Life expectancy and life span are also critical measures used in mortality analyses. Life span refers to the maximum number of years a person can live (Nam 1994). Life span for humans is currently 122 years, based on the life of Jeanne Louise Calment, of Arles, France, who died in 1997 (National Research Council 1997). This life span could increase if a single individual outlived Madame Calment. Life expectancy is a summary measure of the average number of additional years a group of individuals can expect to live at a given exact age (Rogers, Hummer, and Krueger 2003b). U.S. life expectancy has increased remarkably over the last century, from just 47 years in 1900 to the present 77 years (Anderson and DeTurk 2002; Miniño et al. 2002).

Although the U.S. is now enjoying the highest life expectancy at birth ever achieved by individuals in this country, at least 20 other countries have higher overall life expectancies at birth. For instance, compared to a current U.S. life expectancy at birth of 77 years, Germany, Spain, Singapore, Greece, and Norway have life expectancies of 78 years; Italy, France, and Canada possess life expectancies of 79 years; Sweden and Switzerland have life expectancies of 80 years; and Japan currently enjoys the highest overall life expectancy at birth in the world, of 81 years (Population Reference Bureau 2001). Compared to some other industrialized countries, U.S. life expectancy is lower because of relatively high infant mortality, high rates of homicide, relatively high rates of smoking, and high levels of racial and social inequality. But U.S. mortality rates among the oldest old (aged 85 and above) population are the lowest in the world (Hill, Preston, and Rosenwaike 2000; Manton and Vaupel 1995).

The life table is one of the most fundamental and elegant demographic tools because in addition to providing life expectancies at birth, it also provides information on life expectancy estimates at any age, the proportion of the population that survives from one age to the next, mortality probabilities by age, and more. Life tables are constructed with data on the age-specific distribution of a population and the number of individuals who die in specific age groups during a particular year, and can be constructed to examine single decrements (e.g., survive versus die) or multiple decrements (e.g., competing causes of death) (Preston, Heuveline, and Guillot 2001).

Over the past three decades, life table methodology has been extended to simultaneously include the influence of various covariates on the risk of death across time periods (Cox 1972), an approach most often termed hazard modeling. Frequently employed in the current adult mortality literature, these models result in more complete mortality models that can encompass a number of formerly unobserved factors—most commonly referred to as unobserved heterogeneity in frailty—that influence the risk of mortality (Vaupel, Manton, and Stallard 1979). Further, hazard models are often described as the marriage of life tables and regression analysis, as they allow demographers to examine mortality risks over time, assess differential mortality risks among subpopulations (e.g., male/female mortality differentials), and control for any covariates of interest.

Common Data Sources

Myriad data sources can be used to study adult mortality patterns, just in the U.S. alone. Nevertheless, because death is a rare event, most data sources must exclusively focus on decedents or interview a very large number of individuals to capture mortality patterns during subsequent follow-up periods. Because space is limited, the following subsections present brief summaries of data sources that are widely used, that are nationally representative, that will likely include further updates or data collection into the future, and that possess notable strengths, although many others are also available for analysis.

Official U.S. mortality data—which are used to compare mortality rates across ages, sexes, race/ethnic groups, states, and more—are derived from two sources: death certificates and census data. Census data, which comprise the population denominator for the official U.S. mortality data, are collected decennially, with population estimates made between censuses and population projections utilized until new census figures are available. Death counts, which comprise the numerator for the official data, come from death certificates, which are first filed with state vital statistics agencies and then submitted to the National Center for Health Statistics (NCHS). The combined vital statistics and census data provide a large population base and rather stable estimates of mortality from year to year. Currently, there is a wealth of vital statistics information for the U.S. posted on the Internet (see www.cdc.gov/nchs). Additionally, there is similarly detailed mortality information available for many countries throughout the world, and for various time periods, on the internet (e.g., the Human Mortality Database www.mortality.org). The Human Life Table Database (www.lifetable.de) is a companion to the Human Mortality Database, providing two of the most comprehensive and useful data sets for understanding adult mortality variation throughout the world.

Disadvantages of using vital statistics information to calculate mortality rates include (1) actual census counts are only available once every decade; (2) some population groups are undercounted in the census; (3) there are a limited number of variables that are available in both the vital statistics and census data; and (4) there are some differences in the way that the information is collected in these two data systems that can bias mortality estimates. For example, data on age and race/ethnicity may not be consistently measured nor properly provided by individuals through the two data sources (see, for example, Hahn and Stroup 1994; Rogers, Carrigan, and Kovar 1997; Rosenberg et al. 1999). Official mortality data in a number of other countries—particularly in Japan and in Western Europe—are thought to be of higher quality than those of the United States.

In recent years, mortality researchers in the U.S. have made much greater use of linked files, where individuals identified in sample surveys are linked to follow-up death or survival information. In this case, the surveyed individuals most often provide the key information that is needed to analyze mortality risk, such as age, sex, race/ethnicity, education, and the like. But because linked files are sample-based, unstable mortality estimates for specific age and race/ethnic groups are an important limitation. Fortunately, a number of high-quality nationally based linked data sets now exist that are frequently used in the adult mortality literature. These data sets, in combination with the development of hazard modeling procedures, have enabled researchers to embark on broader analyses of demographic, social, and behavioral influences on adult mortality than has been previously possible.

The National Center for Health Statistics (NCHS) has linked the National Health Interview Survey (NHIS) to the Multiple Cause of Death Files (MCD) via the National Death Index (NDI) to create the NHIS-MCD files. The NHIS includes annual information from about 120,000 people (encompassing over 40,000 households yearly) regarding such items as age, race, sex, marital status, family size, income, education, and current occupation. It also includes supplemental questions that may vary from year to year, many of which are asked of the entire sample in a given year. These questions include items about religious attendance, income sources, social relations, health behaviors, and more. As this chapter was being written (2002), individuals aged 18 and over from the NHIS surveys of 1986 to 1994 have been successfully matched with the NDI through 1997 (NCHS 2000), with additional death matches expected in 2003. That is, although most of the adults surveyed in any given year live through the follow-up period, those who subsequently died have been identified.

Several federal agencies have collaborated to produce the National Longitudinal Mortality Study (NLMS), a data base that, when completed, will contain approximately three million survey records and over 250,000 identified deaths. The NLMS uses multiple Current Population Surveys and a cohort from the 1980 census as its population base and is designed to study the effects of socioeconomic influences on adult mortality risk (National Heart, Lung, and Blood Institute 1995; Singh and Siahpush 2002). Yet another key population data set of this type is the National Health and Nutrition Examination Survey (NHANES), which has also been linked to the NDI; an updated version of this linked data set is due out in late 2003.

The Health and Retirement Study (HRS) and Assets and Health Dynamics Among the Oldest Old (AHEAD) surveys are national longitudinal surveys that are particularly useful for examining how interrelations among health, socioeconomic factors, and family relationships that change over time predict future mortality. In 1992, the HRS initially interviewed over 12,600 individuals born between 1931 and 1941, whereas in 1993, the AHEAD initially interviewed nearly 7,500 individuals born in 1923 or earlier. Every two years these individuals were reinterviewed, until 1998 when several new cohorts were surveyed and the HRS and AHEAD samples were combined, thus making the 1998 data representative of all individuals aged 51 and over in the U.S. These data oversample blacks, Hispanics, and residents of Florida; allow researchers to examine changes in health, socioeconomic status, and family relationships over time; and are linked to several administrative data sources including the NDI, Social Security data, pension data, and Medicare files (Juster and Suzman 1995). Although both the HRS and AHEAD begin with a much smaller initial sample than the other data sources mentioned above, the rich array of covariates, the collection of data every two years into the indefinite future, and the inclusion of new cohorts every six years ensure that these data will be especially important for studying mortality in an aging population into the foreseeable future.

THEORETICAL ISSUES AND EMPIRICAL FINDINGS

This section presents recent empirical findings about the impacts of demographic, distal, and selected proximate factors on adult mortality. This section touches upon current debates that include: Will life expectancies keep increasing? Will we experience a reemergence of infectious diseases? Is there a black-white mortality crossover? How can we explain the epidemiological paradox, that is, the relatively favorable mortality patterns among Mexican Americans despite their high-risk socioeconomic profile?

Demographic Characteristics

AGE.   Age is the single most important factor affecting mortality. Indeed, as early as 1825, Benjamin Gompertz developed a mathematical formula depicting mortality by age. He found that age-specific mortality patterns were similar over different time periods and across different geographical areas and thus was daring enough to claim that he had revealed a law of mortality (see Olshansky and Carnes 2001). Ignoring age in an analysis of mortality would, therefore, introduce a major bias; demographers either control or standardize for age in their analyses of mortality, or they conduct their analyses separately by age categories.

The age-specific distribution of a population is often visually presented with a population pyramid, with males depicted on the left, females on the right, and age increasing from the youngest at the base of the pyramid to the oldest at the top. Just as we can represent the distribution of the population with a pyramid, so too can we depict the distribution of deaths by age and sex. Figure 10.1 is a death pyramid for the U.S. in 2000 and shows very few deaths at the youngest ages and increasingly more deaths at the older ages. This pattern is consistent with more developed countries; in contrast, deaths in less developed countries are much more concentrated in the youngest ages, with greater proportions of deaths in young and middle ages, and therefore relatively fewer deaths in

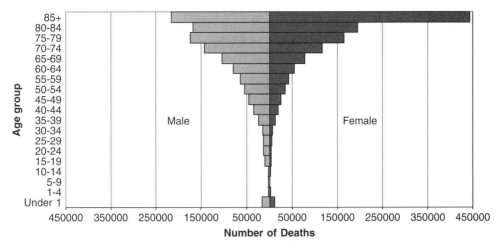

FIGURE 10.1. Death pyramid, U.S., 2000. Source: Derived from Meniño et al. (2002).

the oldest ages (see United Nations 1998). Compared to females, males in the U.S. experience more deaths at middle age and relatively fewer deaths at the oldest ages.

Mortality risk by age may be visually represented with survival curves that show the proportions of a synthetic birth cohort that survive to later ages. Figure 10.2 is a chart of survival curves that compares U.S. survival probabilities for selected years in the 20th century. Note that in the bottom curve, which depicts 1900, survival probabilities were relatively low, particularly at the young ages. In 1900, 20% of individuals died between birth and age 10; today, less than 1% of individuals face a similar fate. Thus, one distinguishing feature between survival rates of 1900 and today is substantial improvement among infants and children. In 1900, survival chances were also lower across the entire life span. Out of 100 newborns, only 77 were expected to reach age 20, fewer than half were expected to attain age 60, and just 32 were expected to reach age 70. In contrast, the curves based on 2000 survival rates indicate that almost 75% of U.S. newborns can expect to reach age 70, a historically unprecedented improvement over the course of just one century.

Between 1900 and 1920, survival drastically improved for infants and children, as well as for persons in other age groups. Between 1920 and 1940, and also between 1940 and 1960, survival improved substantially for middle-aged individuals, and between 1960 and 2000, mortality improvements were significant at older ages. In fact, individuals aged 85 and older in the U.S. have experienced remarkable declines in mortality over the last several decades. In 1920, out of 100 individuals born, just 3 could expect to live to age 90; by 1960, this number more than doubled, to over 7; and by 2000 it had increased by more than sixfold.

Further, from 1900 to the present, the survival curve has become more rectangular due to increased survival at all ages, but especially at young and middle ages. To describe the changing shape of the survival curve over time, Fries (1980) coined the concept the "rectangularization of mortality." Debate continues about future reductions in mortality and whether there is a limit to the human life span. Fries argued that while continued improvements will occur at the younger ages, we have witnessed most of the possible mortality improvements at the oldest ages. But current survival curves suggest that there is still ample room for improvement in the 50s, 60s, and 70s.

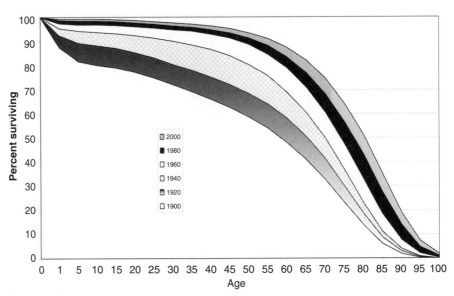

FIGURE 10.2. Percent surviving by age: United States, 1900–2000. Source: Derived from the Human Mortality Database (www.mortality.org) and Miniño et al. (2002).

Fries also suggested that greater proportions of individuals will survive to age 85, with fewer surviving beyond this age. Similarly, Olshansky, Carnes, and Cassel (1990) asserted that life expectancies will continue to increase but at a slow pace, noting that even though mortality has declined for those in the older age groups, neither the right tail of the age distribution nor the age of the verified longest-lived individual have substantially increased. Newer evidence, however, suggests that the survival tail may well continue to lengthen. There have been noticeable changes in the percentage of individuals in the U.S. and other countries surviving to the ages of 95, 100, and beyond (National Research Council 1997), and a number of researchers have raised the possibility of much higher future life expectancies (see Manton, Stallard, and Tolley 1991; National Research Council 1997). It seems reasonable to conclude that the life span is not fixed and can be extended through incremental social, economic, behavioral, and medical advances. For example, if the life span is currently 122 years and 165 days based on the documented length of life of Jeanne Calment (National Research Council 1997), then it seems logical for other individuals to be able to live the same length of time plus one day, and so on. In fact, at the oldest ages, mortality has declined and the distribution of ages of death has lengthened for more than a century. From 1870 through 1990 in Sweden, a country with excellent documentation of births and deaths, the oldest reported age has increased about 1 year for every 20 years of time (Wilmoth and Lundstrom 1996).

Figure 10.3 shows observed age-specific mortality rates for the U.S. population (the solid line). By using data from 1989 to 1991, based on the most recent census data currently available, it is possible to provide mortality rates by single years through age 109 on a logged scale. As the figure demonstrates, mortality is relatively high in infancy and early childhood, drops to its lowest levels at ages 10 to 11, increases in the late teens and early 20s, an age period particularly prone to accidental death, and steadily increases each year to the older ages. Compared to 10-year-olds, individuals aged 15

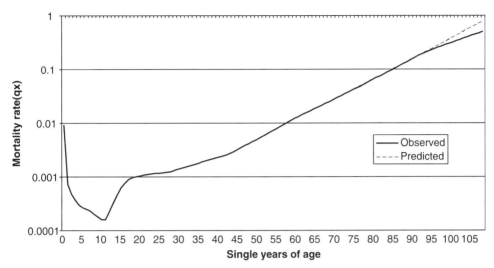

FIGURE 10.3. Age-specific mortality rates for the total population, 1989 to 1991, U.S. (logged scale). Source: Derived from Armstrong (1997).

are almost four times as likely to die, those aged 50 are over 30 times as likely to die, those aged 65 are over 100 times as likely to die, those aged 90 are almost 1,000 times as likely to die, and those aged 108 are almost 3,000 times as likely to die.

At the oldest ages, the pace of mortality increase may slow. Beyond childhood, each age increases the risk of death. Some demographers have assumed that at the oldest ages, mortality risks fit an exponential curve, with exponentially increasing mortality (Fries 1983). Yet observed data actually show a slight decline in the rate of mortality increase at the oldest ages, which Horiuchi and Wilmoth (1998) have termed the *deceleration of aging*. This deceleration can be seen in the right tail of the curve in Figure 10.3, with a fitted exponential curve (the dashed line) predicting higher mortality than the observed data (the solid line). Recent work has investigated this deceleration at the oldest ages among both human and nonhuman populations (National Research Council 1997).

SEX. Both sexes have enjoyed substantial improvements in life expectancy at birth over time. Table 10.2 reveals that U.S. females experienced life expectancy gains from 48.3 years in 1900 to 79.5 years in 2000; male life expectancy increased from 46.3 years to 74.1 years during the same period. The sex gap in life expectancy, which was 2 years in 1900, reached its lowest level of 1 year in 1920, gradually increased to its apex of 7.8 years in 1975, hovered around 7.8 years through 1979, and has been gradually narrowing to 5.4 years by 2000.

Sex differences in mortality are affected by a number of factors, including differences in health and risk behavior patterns, returns to marriage, and socioeconomic status. Females also have mortality advantages over males due to biological factors (including hormonal differences, especially differing levels of estrogen, and childbearing among women) that have been linked to lower risks of heart disease and cancer (Carey 1997; Waldron 1983). But the large variations in sex differences in mortality over time and by social status indicate that, although biology is important, it is not the sole, nor perhaps the central, determinant (Nathanson 1984; Rogers, Hummer, and Nam 2000; Waldron 1994).

TABLE 10.2. Life Expectancies at Birth by Sex, U.S. 1900–2000.

Year	Life Expectancies			Absolute Difference
	Total	Female	Male	
1900	47.3	48.3	46.3	2.0
1910	50.0	51.8	48.4	3.4
1920	54.1	54.6	53.6	1.0
1930	59.7	61.6	58.1	3.5
1940	62.9	65.2	60.8	4.4
1950	68.2	71.1	65.6	5.5
1960	69.7	73.1	66.6	6.5
1970	70.8	74.7	67.1	7.6
1980	73.7	77.4	70.0	7.4
1990	75.4	78.8	71.8	7.0
2000	76.9	79.5	74.1	5.4

Sources: Derived from Anderson and DeTurk (2002) and Miniño et al. (2002).

In the U.S., controlling for behavioral factors tends to close the sex gap in adult mortality, but accounting for social and economic differences widens the gap (Rogers, Hummer, and Nam 2000). That is, males are more likely than females to smoke, drink excessively, use drugs, and be overweight. This results in elevated male mortality risks, especially due to accidents and homicide, but also for cancer, circulatory disease, and respiratory diseases. Compared to males, females are more likely to be disadvantaged by earning less money, obtaining lower levels of education, working at lower-quality jobs, and living more years unmarried.

Some research examines whether increasing equity between the sexes would expand or close the sex gap in mortality (Jones and Goldblatt 1987). That is, women might receive a mortality advantage if their pay, education, and political power were the same as those of men. Conversely, as women began entering the labor force in greater proportions in the 1960s, some researchers speculated that labor force participation would lead to increased female mortality due to stress, risks associated with travel to and from work, and exposure to chemicals or physically deleterious labor in the workplace. Pampel (1998, 2001) directly examined this relationship and found that increasing equity between women and men first reduces the sex gap in suicide and accident mortality but then widens it as institutional adjustment occurs. Thus, following Durkheim (1897 [1951]), he found support for the notion that such social changes initially disrupt social norms and lead to relatively higher mortality for women, although over time, new norms develop and the sex gap returns to prior levels. Other research has further examined the reasons behind the more recent closure of the sex gap in mortality in the U.S. Much work emphasizes that this is due to a declining rate of mortality improvement for women, rather than an accelerating mortality improvement for men. Indeed, Pampel (2002) has demonstrated that increased rates of smoking among U.S. females in the 1960s through the 1980s may fully account for the recent narrowing of the sex gap in mortality.

RACE/ETHNICITY. With increased population heterogeneity, there is a growing amount of interest in the mortality of race/ethnic subpopulations in the U.S. Compared to whites, who had a life expectancy at birth of 77.3 in 1999, blacks had a considerably lower life expectancy, of 71.4 years (Anderson and DeTurk 2002). The life expectancy of Hispanics is thought to be similar to that of whites, while the life expectancy of Native Americans falls between the white and black life expectancy figures (Hummer, Reindl, and Rogers 2003; Kington and Nickens 2001). However, these estimates are based on data that are characterized by a number of known deficiencies (Rosenberg et al. 1999). Asian Americans appear to enjoy the highest life expectancy in the U.S., with recent careful demographic work verifying this notion (Lauderdale and Kestenbaum 2002). In 1992, U.S. life expectancy at birth was estimated to be 82.1 for Japanese Americans, 81.7 for Chinese Americans, and 80.6 for Filipino Americans (Hoyert and Kung 1997).

Race/ethnic estimates of overall adult mortality and life expectancy are characterized by a number of data quality issues that make further work necessary, particularly with the substantial growth of the Asian American, Hispanic, African American, Native American, and mixed race populations. Indeed, Rosenberg and his colleagues (1999: 9) found that for population groups other than non-Hispanic whites and blacks, "levels of mortality are seriously biased from mis-reporting in the numerator and under-coverage in the denominator of the death rates." Their findings suggest that officially reported death rates for Native Americans may be more than 20% too low, while those reported for Asian Americans and Hispanics may be about 11% and 2% too low, respectively. On the other hand, Rosenberg and associates (1999) found that officially reported rates for non-Hispanic whites and non-Hispanic blacks were most likely 1% and 5% too high, respectively. Their corrected estimates for age-adjusted death rates across the life course suggest that Asian and Pacific Islander and Hispanic death rates still remain the lowest (in that order), while Native American corrected rates are higher than those of non-Hispanic whites but lower than those of non-Hispanic blacks. Inconsistent reporting of race/ethnicity on different administrative records, small population sizes, small study sample sizes, immigration selectivity, and emigration selectivity can all bias race/ethnic differences in mortality. For example, immigrants might be enumerated in the U.S. Census but missed by the Vital Statistics System if they die after returning to their country of origin.

The closing black-white gap in life expectancy at birth is due to significant declines in African American mortality. This gap was estimated to be as high as 15.8 years from 1900 to 1902, declined to 6.9 years from 1989 to 1991, and has since declined to 5.9 years in 1999 (Anderson and DeTurk 2002). Compared to whites, blacks experience higher risk from most causes of death, save chronic obstructive pulmonary disease (COPD) and suicide. Rogers (1992) demonstrated that differences in age, sex, marital status, family size, and income virtually account for the entire race gap in overall mortality. The black-white gap in life expectancy is substantially influenced by black disadvantage across social categories: compared to whites, blacks are less likely to be employed, married, or wealthy, and more likely to live in poverty (Oliver and Shapiro 1995), and all of these factors have been shown to influence the adult mortality gap between the two populations (Bond Huie, Hummer and Rogers 2002; Hummer et al. 1999b; Rogers 1992; Rogers et al. 1996). This gap may also be sensitive to changes in social programs. Indeed, the race gap in life expectancy at birth narrowed substantially—from 7.5 to 5.4 years during the period 1965 to 1975—when Medicare and Medicaid were introduced (Sickles and Taubman 1997). Thus, social programs that lift individuals out of poverty and that provide health care may reduce adult mortality and help close the race gap in life expectancy.

Compared to whites, blacks do not experience higher mortality in all the adult years. Indeed, researchers consistently find a black-white mortality crossover among the oldest old (Nam 1995). That is, around age 90, blacks have lower age-specific mortality than their white counterparts. Although much research has been critical of these findings owing to concerns with poor quality data at the older ages, especially for blacks (Preston et al. 1996), this pattern persists even after careful corrections for data quality (Hill, Preston, and Rosenwaike 2000). Moreover, similar crossovers occur in other countries and between other majority and minority populations. The explanation for the crossover is that, compared to a more advantaged social group, a less advantaged social group may experience higher mortality in early ages, which could result in greater physical vitality and lower mortality at older ages (Johnson 2000).

Other recent work has focused on mortality differences between Hispanics and non-Hispanic whites. Compared to non-Hispanic Whites, most Hispanic groups (with the exception of Puerto Ricans) appear to have similar overall mortality rates, even though a much greater proportion of Hispanics live in poverty and lack health insurance (Elo and Preston 1997; Hummer et al. 2000; Sorlie et al. 1993). This incongruity between the overall socioeconomic status of Hispanics and mortality has been termed the *epidemiological paradox* (Markides and Coreil 1986). But this paradox is not inexplicable. The U.S. Hispanic population is composed of proportionally more immigrants than the non-Hispanic black or white populations. International migrants are often healthy and eager to succeed, compared to frail or unmotivated individuals who are less likely to migrate (Rosenwaike 1991). Further, immigrant and native Hispanics are less likely to smoke and drink than non-Hispanic blacks or whites (Hummer et al. 2000). These differences in composition and health behaviors between Hispanics and non-Hispanic whites are not only important in understanding the epidemiological paradox but might also explain differences in the most common causes of death despite similar overall life expectancies. Indeed, compared to non-Hispanic whites, Hispanics are more likely to die from diabetes, homicide, and chronic liver disease and cirrhosis, but have lower heart disease, cancer, suicide, Alzheimer's disease, and chronic lower respiratory disease rates of mortality (Miniño et al. 2002).

Distal Causes

SOCIOECONOMIC STATUS (SES).   SES has various dimensions, including not only education and income, but also community standing, power, and wealth (Moss and Krieger 1995). High levels of SES can reduce mortality risks through a number of mechanisms, in a variety of situations, and for numerous causes of death (Adler et al. 1994; Kitagawa and Hauser 1973; Link and Phelan 1995). First, high SES often reduces exposure to factors that lead to morbidity, disability, and eventually mortality. For example, individuals with higher incomes and occupational statuses often work in jobs that entail little exposure to physically demanding, emotionally stressful, or environmentally unsafe working conditions (Monson 1986; Moore and Hayward 1990), and can afford safer housing in less dangerous neighborhoods (Robert 1999). Second, high SES can attenuate the strength of health risks that individuals may face. Although all individuals face some risk from disease or accidents, those with higher incomes and higher levels of education are more likely to receive better medical care, comply with medicinal or therapeutic regimens, and more promptly seek medical attention. Finally, individuals with higher SES are more likely to undertake a number of behaviors that decrease their risks of mortality through access to health information, preferences for healthy lifestyles, or the economic means to put their preferences into action (Grossman 1972; Sickles and Taubman 1997). Indeed, higher SES individuals often exercise more, smoke less, eat better diets, use seat belts, and refrain from illicit drug use—factors that lower risks of mortality from diabetes, cardiovascular disease, various cancers, accidents, homicide, and many other causes of death (Mulatu and Schooler 2002; Preston and Taubman 1994; Rogers et al. 2000).

Some researchers have noted the potentially reciprocal relationship between SES and health outcomes. Better health may lead to higher earnings, more secure employment, and higher levels of education, whereas higher SES may also lead to better health well into the future. Most current research finds that both dimensions are important, although the most powerful relationship is between SES and health, and not the reverse (see Adler et al. 1994; Mulatu and Schooler 2002; Smith and Kington 1997). But much work remains, and future work that can track both health and SES over time will be better able to understand the health and socioeconomic experiences that unfold over the life course and lead to adult mortality outcomes.

Education has long been the most widely used indicator of SES in studies of adult mortality (e.g., Elo and Preston 1996; Kitagawa and Hauser 1973) because it is generally completed relatively early in life, is usually easy to ascertain for a large number of individuals, and has a substantial impact on other measures of SES, including income, occupational status, and wealth. Recent findings indicate that educational differences in U.S. adult mortality not only remain graded and very wide (Rogers, Hummer, and Nam 2000), but may also have increased in recent decades (Pappas et al. 1993; Preston and Elo 1995). Figure 10.4 shows that U.S. adults with less than 9 years of education were about twice as likely to die over a recent five-year period compared to persons with 17 or more years of education. Controlling for other dimensions of SES, including family income and employment status, reduces these educational differences in mortality, but they remain graded and substantial.

The multidimensional nature of SES is increasingly recognized in population research. Consequently, new measures include those that tap health insurance, credit card debt, food stamps and welfare receipt, childhood socioeconomic conditions, persistently low income and income insecurity, home ownership and other asset holdings, income inequality, and national-level economic swings (Becker and Hemley 1998; Bond Huie, Krueger, Rogers, and Hummer 2003; Drentea and Lavrakas 2000; Kawachi, Kennedy, and Wilkinson 1999; Krueger et al. 2003, 2004; McDonough et al. 1997; Robert and House 1996; Seccombe and Amey 1995; Smith and Kington 1997). Accounting for these various dimensions of SES can be especially important for understanding mortality in different race/ethnic groups, at various ages, across cultures, and within other subgroups of the overall population. Otherwise, researchers may understate the significance of SES in shaping overall mortality outcomes and in its impact on racial and ethnic differences (Kaufman, Cooper, and McGee 1997).

SOCIAL RELATIONS.   Social relations include ties to family, friends, neighbors, and the community at large. Family relations encompass marital status, family composition, social support, and social control. In general, married individuals have lower mortality risks than the unmarried because for the most part they exhibit more positive health

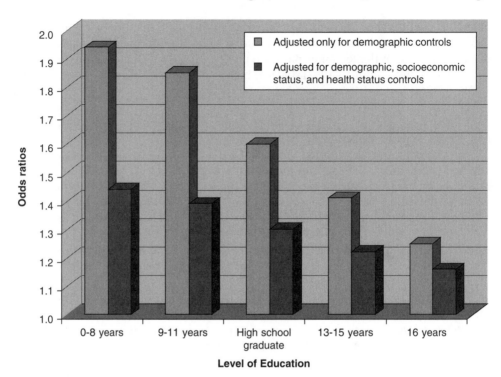

FIGURE 10.4. Risk of death by education level, U.S. adults, 1991 to 1995. Note: Referent is 17 years or more of education. Demographic controls include age, sex, race, and marital status. Socioeconomic and health status controls include income, employment status, and health status. Source: Rogers, Hummer, and Nam (2000).

behaviors, are wealthier, and are linked to tighter-knit social support networks (Lillard and Waite 1995; Rogers 1995; Waite and Gallagher 2000). Married individuals may have access to greater care and companionship, but it is not just marriage that works in this positive fashion. The specific characteristics of spouses are important in understanding the mortality of individuals. For example, the educational background, income generation, health behavior, and health status of one's spouse can influence the mortality of the other spouse (Smith and Zick 1994). Social support or stress also arises from other family members, other relatives and friends, and from participation in social activities—all factors that can affect adult mortality risks (Rogers 1996).

Religious involvement is a particular type of social activity that influences adult mortality, most notably through its social regulation and social integration functions (Durkheim 1897 [1951]). Measures of religion are rarely included in adult mortality studies, yet their effect—particularly that of public religious attendance—has been shown to be sizable in national level studies, even after controlling for socioeconomic and health characteristics, and substantively important for a number of causes of death and for males, females, blacks, and whites (Ellison et al. 2000; Hummer et al. 1999a; Musick, House, and Williams 2004). Some population-based work has also shown that individuals who belong to, and are active in, specific religious denominations, particularly those with strict proscriptions against risky health practices, tend to be characterized by lower mortality risks than the general population. For example, actively practicing Mormons and Seventh-Day Adventists have lower overall rates of mortality and higher life expectancies than other individuals living in the same geographical areas (Koenig, McCollough, and Larson 2001). Future work should examine how variations in religious involvement over time, interrelations between religion and health over the life course, and dimensions of religious involvement help to shape mortality outcomes by age, sex, race/ethnicity, and cause of death.

GEOGRAPHICAL FACTORS.   Life expectancy varies by state in the U.S. (see Figure 10.5). Several states enjoy exceptionally high life expectancy, exceeding 77 years at birth—Hawaii, Iowa, Minnesota, North Dakota, and Utah—although they are very much dispersed geographically. Other states display relatively low life expectancies at less than 73 years at birth, including Alabama, the District of Columbia, Georgia, Louisiana, Mississippi, and South Carolina. These states are clustered in the South and are characterized by lower average levels of education, and greater poverty, income inequality, and minority concentration. Note that the neighboring states of Nevada and Utah have similar physical environments but dissimilar social environments, which likely contributes to the 3.5 year difference in life expectancy. Nevada supports legalized gambling and exhibits high rates of smoking and drinking, whereas Utah is comprised of a large proportion of Mormons who tend to abstain from smoking and alcohol consumption (Fuchs 1974).

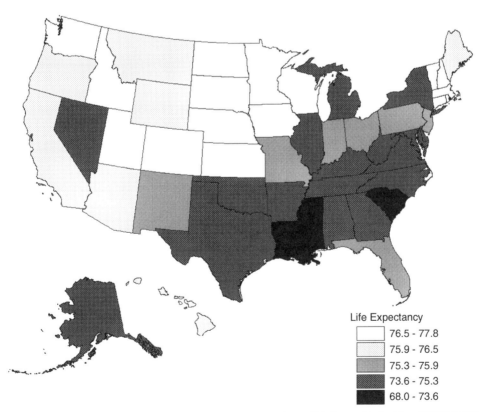

FIGURE 10.5.   U.S. life expectancies at birth, by state, both sexes, 1989 to 1991. Source: Derived from NCHS (1999).

Neighborhood or contextual effects—including social support and stress, social order and disorder, community-level poverty or inequality, and environmental amenities and insults—influence adult health and mortality (Bond Huie et al. 2002; LeClere, Rogers, and Peters 1997, 1998; Robert 1999). Areas with high rates of crime, poverty, drug and alcohol abuse, marital disruption, stress, substandard housing, overcrowding, illiteracy, unemployment, and air and water pollution may predispose residents to unusually high mortality due to heart disease, cancer, strokes, accidents, such infectious diseases as AIDS and tuberculosis, respiratory disease, cirrhosis of the liver, and homicides and suicides (Haan, Kaplan, and Camacho 1987; McCord and Freeman 1990). Conversely, stable social structure, low income inequality, and community support can lower mortality risks (Egolf et al. 1992).

HUMAN MADE AND ENVIRONMENTAL HAZARDS.   Human-made and environmental hazards—including technological risks, terrorist acts, and natural disasters—generally have demographically modest, but often very newsworthy, effects on adult mortality. Natural disasters include earthquakes, floods, landslides, droughts, volcanoes, and hurricanes, all of which may worsen health and increase mortality due to damaged housing and infrastructures, disruptions in local economies, and air or water pollution (Smith and McCarty 1996). Between 1975 and 1994, approximately 24,000 individuals died in the U.S. as a result of natural disasters (Mileti 1999). Generally, the risk of death due to environmental hazards can be much greater in less developed than in more developed countries due to lower-quality building materials, poorly developed emergency relief plans, and the inaccessibility of affected areas. Technological hazards may result from mining accidents, chemical spills and exposure, industrial mishaps, and transportation accidents. War and terrorist acts can also result in considerable levels of mortality that have dramatic effects on age and sex as well as family and household structures of a population (Heuveline 1998; Hirschman, Preston, and Loi 1995). Hirschman and his associates (1995) have provided estimates, for example, that approximately one million Vietnamese adults died in the Vietnamese-American War between 1965 and 1975. More recently, the September 11, 2001, terrorist attacks in the United States killed more than 2,600 individuals.

Proximate Factors

A number of proximate factors—which include health behaviors, health conditions, and physiological influences—have strong and more direct effects on adult mortality. Certainly, individuals can increase their longevity by shunning tobacco, avoiding excessive drinking, consistently engaging in exercise, maintaining regular sleep patterns, achieving positive mental health, avoiding drug and alcohol addictions, and regularly wearing seat belts while driving (Berkman and Breslow 1983; Rogers, Hummer, and Nam 2000). Functional status also influences overall health and mortality risks, especially but not exclusively among the elderly (for more detail, see the chapters 5 and 27 in this *Handbook*). Biodemography, an increasingly important field of demographic study, also focuses on a number of these characteristics and is reviewed in chapter 21 in this *Handbook*. Because proximate factors have been extensively studied within the public health, epidemiology, and medical literatures (e.g., Berkman and Breslow 1983) and have only recently been investigated by demographers, this section only briefly highlights recent work on cigarette consumption and body mass, two factors that profoundly influence adult mortality patterns in the U.S.

CIGARETTE SMOKING. Cigarette smoking is considered the single most important preventable determinant of mortality in developed nations. The adverse effects of smoking were identified relatively early, but it was not until the publication in 1964 of the Surgeon General's report that the public was sufficiently concerned about the ill effects of cigarette smoking to reduce consumption (U.S. Surgeon General's Advisory Committee on Smoking and Health 1964). Cigarette smokers experience a mortality gradient: as the number of cigarettes smoked increases, the risk of death increases (Rogers and Powell-Griner 1991). Cigarette smoking contributes to an increased risk of death through most major causes of death, including heart disease, stroke, cancer, respiratory diseases, and accidents. The immense mortal effects of cigarette smoking in U.S. society, which are estimated to account for nearly 400,000 U.S. deaths per year, will continue through much of the first half of the current century, with literally millions of lives prematurely lost because of cigarette smoking (Nam, Rogers, and Hummer 1996). Fortunately, much of the increased risk of death brought about by smoking can be reduced by quitting.

BODY MASS. Height and weight provide insight into a person's nutrition and patterns of exercise and can be assessed by the body mass index (BMI), calculated as weight in kilograms divided by height in meters squared (Elo and Preston 1992; Lee et al. 1993; Rogers, Hummer, and Krueger 2003a). Even though obesity is a major preventable cause of death, the prevalence of obesity in the general population has been increasing. In 1987, just 11.4% of the U.S. adult population was considered obese (BMI $\geq$ 30); today, that figure has jumped to 20.4% (Rogers et al. 2003a). Increasing obesity contributes to increased mortality due to such causes of death as diabetes, heart disease, stroke, hypertension, and cancer.

Some obesity is interrelated with cigarette smoking: compared to nonsmokers, some smokers lose weight or maintain lower weights. If increased rates of obesity result from individuals who have quit smoking and who are now gaining weight because they quit smoking, then their overall mortality risk should be lower, because cigarette smoking is a more pernicious risk factor for mortality than is obesity. If such a trend is occurring, then in time, as fewer individuals smoke, the prevalence of obesity should increase. But obesity—which is related to dietary patterns, exercise, and genetics—has continued to increase in the U.S. At some point, as the proportions of people who are obese increase, and as the proportions of individuals who smoke decline, we may see greater numbers of deaths attributed to obesity than to smoking.

Mortality Outcomes

Analyses of specific causes of death can inform social policies aimed at reducing mortality and can strengthen theories of adult mortality. Arising from demographic transition theory, the epidemiological transition theory states that as countries modernize, they increase their standards of living and improve their public health and medical technology, all of which result in declines in overall mortality and changes in causes of death. By far, the largest transition has been from infectious and parasitic diseases to chronic and degenerative diseases (Omran 1971).

In 1900 in the U.S., the majority of all deaths were infectious in origin—tuberculosis, bronchitis, smallpox, cholera, diphtheria, influenza, pneumonia, and malaria. Individuals in age extremes—infants, children, and the elderly—were most susceptible to deaths due to infectious diseases. Life expectancies were volatile. For example, between 1917 and 1918, life expectancy at birth in the U.S. plummeted 24%, from 48.4 to 36.6 years, due to the influenza epidemic.

Major reductions in infectious diseases and consequent gains in life expectancy were realized through improvements in health care, social programs, living conditions, medical advancements, and public health. Refrigeration protects food from spoilage, chlorination reduces the chance of infection through such water-borne diseases as cholera, pasteurization reduces the transmission of infectious diseases in milk, and improved sewage treatment reduces a whole host of infectious diseases, including cholera. Since the introduction of antibiotics in the 1930s, many infectious diseases have declined substantially, and some diseases, like smallpox, have been completely eradicated (Link and Phelan 1995). Further, better clothing and housing insulate individuals against temperature extremes. Thus, we have witnessed a major transition from deaths due to infectious and parasitic diseases to deaths due to chronic and degenerative diseases, especially cardiovascular diseases and cancer.

Debate continues over the etiology of diseases. Some diseases have persisted that are neither infectious nor chronic. Indeed, external causes—including suicides, homicides, and accidents—continue to plague Americans. Some diseases are defined as chronic and degenerative but originate in infections at earlier ages. For instance, rheumatic heart disease early in life contributes to heart disease mortality in later life. And some infectious diseases result from earlier chronic and degenerative diseases. For example, increased medical technology can now aggressively treat individuals with heart diseases, cancer, and diabetes, but invasive medical treatment through surgery, kidney dialysis, and other techniques can increase the chance of infections. This may be one reason for the increase in septicemia as a cause of death in the U.S. Furthermore, some health behaviors contribute to specific causes of death. For instance, overeating can contribute to diabetes, heart disease, and cancer; excessive drinking can contribute to cirrhosis of the liver, accidents, and cancer; and cigarette smoking can contribute to cancer, heart disease, and respiratory diseases.

Table 10.3 shows cause-specific mortality information for the top 15 causes of death in the U.S. in 2000. Heart disease, the major cause of death, accounted for almost 30% of all deaths. Cancer, the second major cause of death, was responsible for 23%. Over time, impressive declines in heart disease mortality have occurred, whereas the cancer mortality rate has declined much more slowly, leading to a convergence of these two rates. It is possible that in time, cancer will emerge as the number one cause of death in the U.S., as it has already in a number of other countries, including Japan. Other major causes of death include stroke (cerebrovascular diseases), contributing to 7% of all deaths; chronic lower respiratory diseases, contributing to 5% of all deaths; accidents, comprised of motor vehicle and other accidents; diabetes; pneumonia and influenza; Alzheimer's disease; renal disease; and septicemia.

Some causes of death are more important at younger than at older ages, and vice versa. For example, although HIV/AIDS was not one of the top 15 causes of death for the total population, it was the 10th leading cause of death among individuals aged 15 to

TABLE 10.3. Cause-Specific Mortality in the U.S., 2000.

Rank	Cause of Death	Percent of Total Deaths in 2000	Annual Percent Mortality Change 1990–2000
1	Heart disease	29.6	−1.8
2	Cancer	23.0	−0.7
3	Stroke	7.0	−0.7
4	Chronic lower respiratory diseases	5.1	1.9
5	Accidents	4.1	−0.9
6	Diabetes mellitus	2.9	1.8
7	Influenza and pneumonia	2.7	−3.1
8	Alzheimer's disease	2.1	16.2
9	Renal disease	1.5	4.3
10	Septicemia	1.3	3.1
11	Suicide	1.2	−1.6
12	Chronic liver disease and cirrhosis	1.1	−1.3
13	Essential (primary) hypertension and hypertensive renal disease	0.8	6.9
14	Homicide	0.7	−3.5
15	Pneumonitis due to solids and liquids	0.7	6.3
	All other causes	16.3	

Source: Derived from Miniño et al. (2002) and the NCHS website (www.cdc.gov/nchs/).
Note: Negative sign indicates mortality decline; positive sign, mortality increase. Annual percent mortality change based on age-adjusted rates.

24, the fifth cause of death among those aged 25 to 44, and the ninth cause of death among those aged 45 to 64 (see Table 10.4). Among individuals aged 15 to 24, the top three causes of death—accidents, homicide, and suicide, respectively—contributed to almost three-quarters of all deaths in this age group.

Among individuals aged 65 and above, chronic conditions are the central causes of death. Accidental mortality is the only external cause included among the major causes of death, and it is ninth. Alzheimer's disease is increasing as a major cause of death and is now the seventh leading cause among U.S. individuals 65 and older. The increase in Alzheimer's disease mortality relative to other causes of death is due in part to successful reductions in mortality due to other causes of death, in addition to improved diagnosis and reporting of the condition, greater knowledge of the disease within the medical community, and greater proportions of individuals dying at very old ages.

A central question is whether more developed countries, including the U.S., could witness a reemergence of infectious diseases. In addition to deaths due to HIV/AIDS, individuals are at risk of death due to tuberculosis, hepatitis C, influenza, and septicemia (Olshansky et al. 1997). There could be a resurgence of infectious diseases due to improper use of antibiotics that have resulted in drug-resistant diseases or due to increased travel around the world. However, it is unlikely that natural infectious outbreaks would affect anywhere near the number of individuals who, for example, died in the 1918 influenza epidemic. Over the course of about nine months, the 1918 influenza epidemic killed 500,000 people in the U.S. To place this in perspective, HIV/AIDS has accounted for a similar number of deaths in the U.S.—but over the course of about 20 years. The 1918 epidemic was unique in that it occurred at the end of World War I, it could interact with other infectious diseases like tuberculosis (Noymer and Garenne 2000), it happened during a period when standards of living were relatively low, and it took place before the development and widespread use of antibiotics. Thus,

TABLE 10.4. Top 10 Causes of Death by Age Group, Males and Females Combined, U.S., 2000.

Rank	Ages 15–24		Ages 25–44		Ages 45–64		Ages 65+	
	Cause of Death	% Deaths	Cause of Death	% Deaths	Cause of Death	% Deaths	Cause of Death	% Deaths
1	Accidents	45.1	Accidents	20.9	Cancer	34.2	Heart disease	33.0
2	Homicide	15.8	Cancer	15.7	Heart disease	24.6	Cancer	21.8
3	Suicide	12.8	Heart disease	12.4	Accidents	4.9	Stroke	8.2
4	Cancer	5.5	Suicide	8.7	Stroke	4.0	Lower respiratory diseases	5.9
5	Heart disease	3.3	HIV	6.4	Lower respiratory diseases	3.5	Pneumonia/flu	3.3
6	Congenital malformations	1.4	Homicide	5.7	Diabetes mellitus	3.5	Diabetes mellitus	2.9
7	Stroke	0.6	Chronic liver disease	2.9	Chronic liver disease	3.1	Alzheimer's disease	2.7
8	Lower respiratory diseases	0.6	Stroke	2.5	Suicide	2.1	Renal disease	1.7
9	Pneumonia/flu	0.6	Diabetes mellitus	2.0	HIV	1.3	Accidents	1.7
10	HIV	0.6	Pneumonia/flu	1.1	Renal disease	1.2	Septicemia	1.4

Source: Derived from Miniño et al. (2002).

with improved medical technology, the proper use of antibiotics and public heath efforts, and improved standards of living, it is unlikely that the U.S. will witness a natural outbreak of infectious diseases anywhere near 1918 levels.

Even though a particular disease may represent a large portion of all deaths, its elimination may not assure huge gains in life expectancy. On the contrary, it may result in relatively modest life expectancy increases, a phenomenon called *the Taeuber Paradox* (Keyfitz 1977). For example, even though cancer currently accounts for nearly one-quarter of all U.S. deaths, its elimination might add just 3.4 years to life expectancy at birth (Anderson 1999). This paradox results because most cancer deaths occur at older ages; thus, preventing or curing this one disease provides an opportunity for death to occur from other diseases.

Future research will extend our knowledge of variations in causes of death by exploring multiple-cause mortality, which refers to deaths in terms of all of the causes entered on the death certificate (see Nam 1990). Combinations of causes can be more lethal than single causes and can influence mortality differentials between subpopulations. Several demographic researchers have examined multiple causes of death (Nam, Hummer, and Rogers 1994).

CONCLUSIONS AND RESEARCH DIRECTIONS

A complex web of elements shapes adult mortality patterns, risks, and causes. As such, demography has arisen as an interdisciplinary field that derives insights from sociology, geography, economics, history, biology, epidemiology, and medicine to better understand the multidimensional forces that shape mortality in the contemporary world. Future work that seeks to better understand the causes and consequences of adult mortality in the U.S. and throughout the globe must capitalize on the interdisciplinary nature of demography if future gains in life expectancy are to be understood and maintained (Weinstein, Hermalin, and Soto 2001).

Although the U.S. population is generally healthy with good longevity prospects, several factors may hamper future gains. For instance, the increasing prevalence of obesity is an alarming trend and presages increasing mortality from diabetes, heart disease, and some forms of cancer. Further, in the four decades since the U.S. Surgeon General brought to public attention the hazards of cigarette smoking, nearly a quarter of the U.S. adult population continues to smoke, and surprisingly large proportions of individuals start smoking every year. These patterns threaten to offset improving longevity prospects that result from increasing levels of education and public health efforts and are especially pernicious as they disproportionately affect racial and ethnic minorities (U.S. Department of Health and Human Services 2000).

There is an opportunity to better understand the social and contextual influences on mortality. Although much work has focused on various social relationships, including marriage and family structure (Lillard and Waite 1995; Rogers 1995), less research has examined mortality patterns within couples or families. Because individuals live, work, and recreate in a larger social milieu, future work could capture part of these greater family and household environments. Some family members—through higher income, regular employment, or healthy behaviors—may buffer others in the household from additional mortality risk. On the other hand, some family members—through drug use, cigarette smoking, and other risky behaviors—may place other family members at increased risk of death—through passive smoking, increased chances of addiction, and family dysfunction. Similarly, neighborhood and regional risk factors, including social disorganization, unemployment, crime, risk of natural hazards, and environmental risks may influence mortality outcomes—a nascent research area (Robert 1999).

The interrelationships between migration and mortality should also be more thoroughly studied, particularly with the relatively high levels of immigration in countries such as the United States and increasing racial and ethnic diversity. In general, studies have identified the healthy immigrant effect: individuals who are healthy, who engage in healthy behaviors, with more social and human capital, and with ties to the country of destination are more likely to move and to exhibit low mortality risks. But epidemiological transition theory suggests that less developed countries will exhibit higher rates of infectious disease mortality, and other bodies of research suggest that diseases contracted in childhood and early adult periods can predispose individuals to early death (Elo and Preston 1992). Thus, immigrants from less developed countries could potentially experience higher mortality than the native born, due to infectious diseases and diseases that predominate in less developed countries. One's country of origin is rarely studied but could very well further elucidate the relationship between health, migration, and mortality. Further, immigrant status could be important: mortality may vary among legal immigrants, illegal immigrants, those who come for family reunification, refugees, and individuals seeking asylum. Thus, a more nuanced and theoretically driven analysis might uncover interesting relationships between migration and mortality.

Future research is necessary, not only for the sake of theoretical development, but also for shaping social and health policy and directly impacting longevity prospects. Social institutions, including the government, can have a profound effect on life expectancy. The government can fund research to help better understand health and mortality patterns and can fund disease prevention and health promotion programs. Further, government agencies can set priorities related to national health. The U.S. Department of Health and Human Services (2000) recently released *Healthy People 2010*, a set of health objectives for the country to meet in this decade. It highlights a number of objectives, including closing racial and ethnic disparities; limiting inactivity, smoking, and substance abuse; and increasing access to health care and public awareness of health-related information. The government provides public education, approval for food and drugs, and taxation and regulation on some products. Tax increases have lowered the incidence of new smokers among teens and even higher taxes might further inhibit smoking (Grossman and Chaloupka 1997). Moreover, the government distributes billions of dollars annually for health-related research through agencies including the National Institutes of Health, the National Science Foundation, and the Veterans Administration (Sickles and Taubman 1997). These funds will continue to be the major resource for understanding U.S. health and mortality patterns.

Previous reductions in mortality at younger and middle ages have dramatically increased the percentage of individuals surviving to older ages. Greater proportions of individuals living longer may increase the need for a variety of medical services, from organ transplants and joint replacements, to treatments for cancer and heart disease (Fogel and Costa 1997). Medicare is a health insurance program that targets individuals primarily aged 65 and above but also provides payments for individuals who are disabled, and it covers the costs associated with kidney dialysis, as well as cardiac transplantation for some medical centers (Sickles and Taubman, 1997). Some of the gains in U.S. life expectancy among the elderly may be attributed to the introduction of Medicare. But future advances are necessary to ensure that contemporary gains in life expectancy persist into the future, including more comprehensive health care coverage for individuals of all ages; further scientific research on the determinants of cancer, heart disease, diabetes, HIV/AIDS, and various other illnesses; and continued progress in implementing medical technologies and information about healthy behaviors.

Few demographic researchers would assert that no future mortality improvements will occur. Although there have been periodic setbacks in life expectancy increases over time, as with the influenza epidemic in the early 20th century and with the HIV/AIDS epidemic in Africa more recently, such setbacks are usually of short duration and are compensated for by later improvements in controlling and treating infectious diseases and by further improvements in other causes of death. Thus, the current question seems to be not whether mortality will improve in the future, but by how much it will improve, and what age, sex, race/ethnic, socioeconomic, and geographical groups will reap the greatest benefits. Overall, continued improvements in health behavior, medical technology, and overall quality of life bode for a generally bright future, most likely with steady but deliberate increases in average length of life accompanied by an increasingly healthy population.

REFERENCES

Adler, N. E., T. Boyce, M. A. Chesney, S. Cohen, S. Folkman, R. L. Kahn, and S. L. Syme. 1994. Socio-economic status and health: The challenge of the gradient. *American Psychologist* 49(1):15–24.

Anderson, R. N. 1999. *U.S. decennial life tables for 1989–91*. Vol. 1, No. 4, United States life tables eliminating certain causes of death. Hyattsville, Md.: National Center for Health Statistics.

Anderson, R. N., and P. B. DeTurk. 2002. United States life tables, 1999. *National Vital Statistics Reports* 50(6):1–40.

Armstrong, R. J. 1997. *U.S. decennial life tables for 1989–91*, Vol. 1, No 1. Hyattsville, Md.: National Center for Health Statistics.

Becker, C., and D. Hemley. 1998. Demographic change in the former Soviet Union during the transition period. *World Development* 26(11):1957–1977.

Berkman, L. F., and L. Breslow. 1983. *Health and ways of living*. New York: Oxford.

Bond Huie, S. A., R. A. Hummer, and R. G. Rogers. 2002. Individual and contextual risks of death among race and ethnic groups in the United States. *Journal of Health and Social Behavior* 43(3):359–381.

Bond Huie, S. A., P. M. Krueger, R. G. Rogers, and R. A. Hummer. 2003. Wealth, race, and mortality. *Social Science Quarterly* 84(3):667–684.

Carey, J. R. 1997. What demographers can learn from fruit fly actuarial models and biology. *Demography* 34(1):17–30.

Cox, D. R. 1972. Regression models and life tables. *Journal of the Royal Statistical Society, Series B*, 34:187–220.

Dorn, H. F. 1959. Mortality. In *The study of population: An inventory and appraisal*. Edited by P. M. Hauser and O. D. Duncan, 187–220. Chicago: The University of Chicago Press.

Drentea, P., and P. J. Lavrakas. 2000. Over the limit: The association among health, race and debt. *Social Science and Medicine* 50:517–529.

Durkheim, E. 1951/1897. *Suicide*. New York: Free Press.

Egolf, B., J. Lasker, S. Wolf, and L. Potvin. 1992. The Roseto Effect: A 50-year comparison of mortality rates. *American Journal of Public Health* 82(8):1089–1092.

Ellison, C. G., R. A. Hummer, S. Cormier, and R. G. Rogers. 2000. Religious involvement and mortality risk among African American adults. *Research on Aging* 22(6):630–667.

Elo, I. T., and S. H. Preston. 1992. Effects of early-life conditions on adult mortality: A review. *Population Index* 58(2):186–212.

Elo, I. T., and S. H. Preston. 1996. Educational differentials in mortality: United States, 1979–85. *Social Science and Medicine* 42(1):47–57.

Elo, I. T., and S. H. Preston. 1997. Racial and ethnic differences in mortality at older ages. In *Racial and ethnic differences in the health of older Americans*. Edited by L. G. Martin and B. J. Soldo, 10–42. Washington, D.C.: National Academy Press.

Fogel, R. W., and D. L. Costa. 1997. A theory of technophysio evolution, with some implications for forecasting population, health care costs, and pension costs. *Demography* 34(1):49–66.

Fries, J. F. 1980. Aging, natural death, and the compression of morbidity. *New England Journal of Medicine* 303:130–135.

Fries, J. F. 1983. The compression of morbidity. *Milbank Memorial Fund Quarterly* 61:397–419.

Fuchs, V. 1974. *Who shall live? Health, economics, and social choice*. New York: Basic Books.

Grossman, M. 1972. On the concept of health capital and the demand for health. *The Journal of Political Economy* 80(2):223–255.

Grossman, M., and F. H. Chaloupka. 1997. Cigarette taxes: The straw to break the camel's back. *Public Health Reports* 112 (July/Aug): 290–297.

Haan, M., G. A. Kaplan, and T. Camacho. 1987. Poverty and health: Prospective evidence from the Alameda County Study. *American Journal of Epidemiology* 125(6):989–998.

Hahn, R. A., and D. F. Stroup. 1994. Race and ethnicity in public health surveillance: Criteria for the scientific use of social categories. *Public Health Reports* 109:7–15.

Heuveline, P. 1998. Between one and three million: Towards the demographic reconstruction of a decade of Cambodian history (1970–79). *Population Studies* 25(1):49–65.

Hill, M. E., S. H. Preston, and I. Rosenwaike. 2000. Age reporting among white Americans aged 85+: Results of a record linkage study. *Demography* 37(2):175–186.

Hirschman, C., S. H. Preston, and V. M. Loi. 1995. Vietnamese casualties during the American war: A new estimate. *Population and Development Review* 21(4):783–812.

Horiuchi, S., and J. R. Wilmoth. 1998. Deceleration in the age pattern of mortality at older ages. *Demography* 35(4):391–412.

Hoyert, D. L., and Hsiang-Ching Kung. 1997. Asian or Pacific Islander mortality, selected states, 1992. *Monthly Vital Statistics Reports* 46(1):1–64.

Hummer, R. A., M. R. Benjamins, and R. G. Rogers. 2004. Racial and ethnic disparities in health and mortality among the U. S. elderly population. Chapter 3 (pp. 53–94) in *Critical perspectives on racial and ethnic differences in health in late life*. Edited by N. B. Anderson, R. A. Bulatao, and B. Cohen. National Research Council. Washington, D.C.: National Academies Press.

Hummer, R. A., R. G. Rogers, S. H. Amir, D. Forbes, and W. P. Frisbie. 2000. Adult mortality differentials between Hispanic subgroups and non-Hispanic whites. *Social Science Quarterly* 81:459–476.

Hummer, R. A., R. G. Rogers, C. B. Nam, and C. G. Ellison. 1999a. Religious participation and U. S. adult mortality. *Demography* 36(2):273–285.

Hummer, R. A., R. G. Rogers, C. B. Nam, and F. B. LeClere. 1999b. Race/ethnicity, nativity, and U. S. adult mortality. *Social Science Quarterly* 80(1):136–153.

Johnson, N. E. 2000. The racial crossover in comorbidity, disability, and mortality. *Demography* 37(3):267–283.

Jones, D. R., and P. O. Goldblatt. 1987. Cause of death in widow(er)s and spouses. *Journal of Biosocial Sciences* 19:107–121.

Juster, T. F., and R. Suzman. 1995. An overview of the health and retirement survey. *Journal of Human Resources* 30(5): S7–S56.

Kaufman, J. S., R. S. Cooper, and D. L. McGee. 1997. Socioeconomic status and health in blacks and whites: The problem of residual confounding and the resiliency of race. *Epidemiology* 8:621–628.

Kawachi, I., B. P. Kennedy, and R. G. Wilkinson. 1999. *The society and population health reader: Income inequality and health*. New York: The New Press.

Keyfitz, N. 1977. What difference would it make if cancer were eradicated? An examination of the Taeuber Paradox. *Demography* 14:411–418.

Kington, R. S., and H. W. Nickens. 2001. Racial and ethnic differences in health: Recent trends, current patterns, future directions. In *America becoming: Racial trends and their consequences, Vol. II*. Edited by N. J. Smelser, W. J. Wilson, and F. Mitchell, 253–310. Washington, D.C.: National Academy Press.

Kitagawa, E. M., and P. M. Hauser. 1973. *Differential mortality in the United States: A study in socioeconomic epidemiology*. Cambridge, Mass.: Harvard University Press.

Koenig, H. G., M. E. McCollough, and D. B. Larson. 2001. *Handbook of religion and health*. New York: Oxford University Press.

Krueger, P. M., R. G. Rogers, R. A. Hummer, F. LeClere, and S. A. Bond Huie. 2003. Socioeconomic status and age: The effect of income sources and portfolios on U.S. adult mortality. *Sociological Forum* 18(3):465–482.

Krueger, P. M., R. G. Rogers, C. Ridao-Cano, and R. A. Hummer. 2004. To help or to harm? Food stamp receipt and mortality risk prior to the 1996 Welfare Reform Act. *Social Forces* 82(4):1573–1599.

Lauderdale, D. S., and B. Kestenbaum. 2002. Mortality rates of elderly Asian American populations. *Demography* 39(3):529–540.

LeClere, F. B., R. G. Rogers, and K. D. Peters. 1997. Ethnicity and mortality in the United States: Individual and community correlates. *Social Forces* 76(1):169–198.

LeClere, F. B., R. G. Rogers, and K. D. Peters. 1998. Neighborhood social context and racial differences in women's heart disease mortality. *Journal of Health and Social Behavior* 39(2):91–107.

Lee, I-Min, J. E. Manson, C. H. Hennekens, R. S. Paffenburger, Jr. 1993. Body weight and mortality: a 27-year follow-up of middle-aged men. *Journal of the American Medical Association* 270(23):2823–2828.

Lillard, L. A., and L. Waite. 1995. Til death do us part: Marital disruption and mortality. *American Journal of Sociology* 100(Mar):1131–1156.

Link, B. G., and J. Phelan. 1995. Social conditions as fundamental causes of disease. *Journal of Health and Social Behavior* Extra Issue: 80–94.

Manton, K. G., E. Stallard, and H. D. Tolley. 1991. Demographic perspectives on human senescence. *Population and Development Review* 17:603–637.

Manton, K. G., and J. W. Vaupel. 1995. Survival after the age of 80 in the United States, Sweden, France, England, and Japan. *New England Journal of Medicine* 333:1232–1235.

Markides, K. S., and J. Coreil. 1986. The health of Hispanics in the Southwestern United States: An epidemiological paradox. *Public Health Reports* 101:253–265.

McCord, C., and H. P. Freeman. 1990. Excess mortality in Harlem. *The New England Journal of Medicine* 322(3):173–177.

McDonough, P., G. J. Duncan, D. R. Williams, and J. S. House. 1997. Income dynamics and adult health mortality in the United States, 1972 through 1989. *American Journal of Public Health* 87(9):1476–1483.

Mileti, D. S. 1999. *Disasters by design: A reassessment of natural hazards in the United States*. National Academy of Sciences. Washington, DC: Joseph Henry Press.

Miniño , A. M., E. Arias, K. D. Kochanek, S. L. Murphy, and B. L. Smith. 2002. Deaths: Final data for 2000. *National Vital Statistics Reports* 50(15):1–120.

Monson, R. R. 1986. Observations on the healthy worker effect. *Journal of Occupational Medicine* 28(6):425–433.

Moore, D. E., and M. D. Hayward. 1990. Occupational careers and mortality of elderly men. *Demography* 27(1):31–53.

Moss, N., and N. Krieger. 1995. Measuring social inequalities in health: Report on the Conference of the National Institutes of Heath. *Public Health Reports* 110:302–305.

Mulatu, M. S., and C. Schooler. 2002. Causal connections between SES and health: Reciprocal effects and mediating mechanisms. *Journal of Health and Social Behavior* 43(1):22–41.

Musick, M. A., J. S. House, and D. R. Williams. 2004. Attendance at religious services and mortality in a national sample. *Journal of Health and Social Behavior* 45(2):198–213.

Nam, C. B. 1990. Mortality differentials from a multiple cause-of-death perspective. In S. D'Souza, A. Palloni, and J. Vallin, eds., 328–342. *Measurement and analysis of mortality*. London: Oxford Press.

Nam, C. B. 1994. *Understanding population change*. Itasca, Ill.: FE Peacock Publishers.

Nam, C. B. 1995. Another look at mortality crossovers. *Social Biology* 42(1–2):133–42.

Nam, C. B., R. A. Hummer, and R. G. Rogers. 1994. Underlying and multiple causes of death related to smoking. *Population Research and Policy Review* 13:305–325.

Nam, C. B., R. G. Rogers, and R. A. Hummer. 1996. Impact of future cigarette smoking scenarios on mortality of the adult population in the U. S., 2000–2050. *Social Biology* 43:155–168.

Nathanson, C. A. 1984. Sex differences in mortality. *Annual Review of Sociology* 10:191–213.

National Center for Health Statistics. 1993. Advance report of final mortality statistics, 1990. *Monthly Vital Statistics Report* 41(7):1–52.

National Center for Health Statistics. 1999. *U. S. decennial life tables for 1989–91*. Vol. 1, No. 3. Some trends and comparisons of United States life table data: 1900–1991. Hyattsville, Md.

National Center for Health Statistics. 2000. *National health interview survey: Multiple cause of death public use data file, 1986–1994 survey years*. Computer file and documentation. Hyattsville, Md.: Public Health Service.

National Heart, Lung, and Blood Institute. 1995. *National longitudinal mortality study, 1979–89: Public use file documentation, Release 2*. Bethesda, Md.: Public Health Service.

National Research Council. 1997. *Between Zeus and the salmon: The biodemography of longevity*. Edited by K. Wachter and C. Finch. Washington, D.C.: National Academy Press.

Noymer, A., and M. Garenne. 2000. The 1918 influenza epidemic's effects on sex differentials in mortality in the United States. *Population and Development Review* 26(3):565–583.

Oliver, M. L., and T. M. Shapiro. 1995. *Black wealth / white wealth: A new perspective on racial inequality*. New York: Routledge.

Olshansky, S. J., and B. A. Carnes. 2001. *The quest for immortality: Science at the frontiers of aging*. New York: W. W. Norton.

Olshansky, S. J., B. A. Carnes, and C. Cassel. 1990. In search of Methuselah: Estimating the upper limits to human longevity. *Science* 250:634–640.

Olshansky, S. J., B. A. Carnes, R. G. Rogers, and L. Smith. 1997. New and ancient threats to world health. *Population Bulletin* 52(2):1–52.

Omran, A. R. 1971. The epidemiologic transition: A theory of the epidemiology of population change. *Milbank Memorial Fund Quarterly* 49:509–538.

Pampel, F. C. 1998. National context, social change, and sex differences in suicide rates. *American Sociological Review* 63(5):744–768.

Pampel, F. C. 2001. Gender equality and the sex differential in mortality from accidents in high income nations. *Population Research and Policy Review* 20(5):397–421.

Pampel, F. C. 2002. Cigarette use and the narrowing sex differential in mortality. *Population and Development Review* 28(1):77–104.

Pappas, G., S. Queen, W. Hadden, and G. Fisher. 1993. The increasing disparity in mortality between socioeconomic groups in the United States, 1960 and 1986. *New England Journal of Medicine* 329:103–109.

Population Reference Bureau. 2001. *2001 world population data sheet*. Washington, D.C.: PRB.

Preston, S. H., and I. T. Elo. 1995. Are educational differentials in adult mortality increasing in the United States? *Journal of Aging and Health* 7:476–496.

Preston, S. H., I. T. Elo, I. Rosenwaike, and M. Hill. 1996. African-American mortality at older ages: Results of a matching study. *Demography* 33(2):193–209.

Preston, S. H., P. Heuveline, and M. Guillot. 2001. *Demography: Measuring and modeling population processes*. Oxford: Blackwell Publishers.

Preston, S. H., and P. Taubman. 1994. Socioeconomic differences in adult mortality and health status. In *Demography of aging*. Edited by L. G. Martin and S. H. Preston, 279–318. Washington, D.C.: National Academy Press.

Robert, S. A. 1999. Socioeconomic position and health: The independent contributions of community socio-economic context. *Annual Review of Sociology* 25:489–516.

Robert, S. A., and J. S. House. 1996. SES differentials in health by age and alternative indicators of SES. *Journal of Aging and Health* 8(3):359–388.

Rogers, R. G. 1992. Living and dying in the USA: Sociodemographic determinants of death among blacks and whites. *Demography* 29(2):287–303.

Rogers, R. G. 1995. Marriage, sex, and mortality. *Journal of Marriage and the Family* 57(2):515–526.

Rogers, R. G. 1996. The effects of family composition, health, and social support linkages on mortality. *Journal of Health and Social Behavior* 37(4):326–338.

Rogers, R. G., J. A. Carrigan, and M. G. Kovar. 1997. Comparing mortality estimates based on different administrative records. *Population Research and Policy Review* 16(3):213–224.

Rogers, R. G., R. A. Hummer, and P. M. Krueger. 2003a. The effect of obesity on overall, circulatory-disease and diabetes specific mortality. *Journal of Biosocial Science* 35(1):107–129.

Rogers, R. G., R. A. Hummer, and P. M. Krueger. 2003b. Life expectancy, Vol. 3. In *Encyclopedia of aging*. Edited by D. J. Ekerdt, R. A. Applebaum, K. C. Holden, S. G. Post, K. Rockwood, R. Schulz, R. L. Sprott, and P. Uhlenberg, 789–790. New York: Macmillan Reference.

Rogers, R. G., R. A. Hummer, and C. B. Nam. 2000. *Living and dying in the USA: Social, behavioral, and health differentials in adult mortality*. New York: Academic Press.

Rogers, R. G., R. A. Hummer, C. B. Nam, and K. D. Peters. 1996. Demographic, socioeconomic, and behavioral factors affecting ethnic mortality by cause. *Social Forces* 74:1419–1438.

Rogers, R. G., and E. Powell-Griner. 1991. Life expectancies of cigarette smokers and non-smokers in the United States. *Social Science & Medicine* 32(10):1151–1159.

Rosenberg, H. M., J. D. Maurer, P. D. Sorlie, N. J. Johnson, M. F. MacDorman, D. L. Hoyert, J. F. Spitler, and C. Scott. 1999. Quality of death rates by race and Hispanic origin: A summary of current research. *Vital and Health Statistics* 2(128):1–13.

Rosenwaike, I. 1991. Mortality experience of Hispanic populations. In *Mortality of Hispanic populations.* Edited by I. Rosenwaike, 3–14. New York: Greenwood.

Seccombe, K., and C. Amey. 1995. Playing by the rules and losing: Health insurance and the working poor. *Journal of Health and Social Behavior* 36(2):168–181.

Sickles, R. C., and P. Taubman. 1997. Mortality and morbidity among adults and the elderly. In *Handbook of population and family economics: Vol. 1A.* Edited by M. R. Rosenzweig and O. Stark, 559–643. Amsterdam: Elsevier.

Singh, G. K., and M. Siahpush. 2002. Ethnic-immigrant differentials in health behaviors, morbidity, and cause-specific mortality in the United States: An analysis of two national data bases. *Human Biology* 74(1):83–109.

Smith, J. P., and R. Kington. 1997. Demographic and economic correlates of health in old age. *Demography* 34(1):159–170.

Smith, K. R., and C. D. Zick. 1994. Linked lives, dependent demise? Survival analysis of husbands and wives. *Demography* 31(Feb.):81–93.

Smith, S. K, and C. McCarty. 1996. Demographic effects of natural disasters: A case study of hurricane andrew. *Demography* 33(2):265–275.

Sorlie, P. D., E. Backlund, N. J. Johnson, and E. Rogot. 1993. Mortality by Hispanic status in the United States. *The Journal of the American Medical Association* 270(20):2464–2468.

United Nations. 1998. *Health and mortality: A concise report.* New York: United Nations Reproduction Section.

U.S. Department of Health and Human Services. 2000. *Healthy people 2010: Understanding and improving health*, 2nd ed. Washington, D.C.: U.S. Government Printing Office.

U.S. Surgeon General's Advisory Committee on Smoking and Health. 1964. *Smoking and health: Report of the advisory committee to the Surgeon General of the Public Health Service.* Washington, D.C.: U.S. Government Printing Office.

Vaupel, J. W., K. G. Manton, and E. Stallard. 1979. The impact of heterogeneity in individual frailty on the dynamics of mortality. *Demography* 16(3):439–454.

Waite, L. J., and M. Gallagher. 2000. *The case for marriage: Why married people are happier, healthier, and better off financially.* New York: Doubleday.

Waldron, I. 1983. Sex differentials in human mortality: The role of genetic factors. *Social Science and Medicine* 17(6):321–333.

Waldron, I. 1994. Contributions of biological and behavioral factors to changing sex differences in ischemic heart disease mortality. In *Premature adult mortality in developed countries.* Edited by A. Lopez, T. Valkonen, and G. Caselli. London: Oxford University Press.

Weinstein, M., A. I. Hermalin, and M. A. Soto, eds. 2001. *Population health and aging: Strengthening the dialogue between epidemiology and demography.* New York: Annals of the New York Academy of Sciences, Vol. 954.

Wilmoth, J. R., and H. Lundstrom. 1996. Extreme longevity in five countries: Presentation of trends with special attention to issues of data quality. *European Journal of Population* 12:63–93.

CHAPTER 11

Internal Migration

MICHAEL J. WHITE AND DAVID P. LINDSTROM

INTRODUCTION

Migration is usually combined with fertility and mortality in most introductory descriptions of the basic components of population change. The study of internal migration involves an examination of two questions: Who moves? and What places grow? At the level of the individual person or household, the answer to the question, Who moves?, is often found in a set of personal traits linked to economic activity, the life cycle, sociocultural context, and policies that vary over space. Likewise, the answer to the question, What places grow?, is usually found in the comparative economic advantages across regions, demographic dynamics that shift either population composition or the number of those likely to migrate, and again, policy—intended or not—that shifts the costs and benefits of location for persons and employers.

In this chapter, internal migration is examined as one event among several demographic phenomena that shift persons across space. Other chapters in this *Handbook* address related aspects of population distribution, including Chapter 2, "Population Distribution and Suburbanization"; Chapter 12, "International Migration"; Chapter 16, "Urban and Spatial Demography"; and Chapter 20, "Ecological Demography."

Much has changed in demography since Donald Bogue penned the "Internal Migration" entry in the 1959 collection, *The Study of Population*. Forms of data-gathering and analysis in population studies are sharply different than they were four or five decades ago. Yet some things have changed little. Migration is still "a major symptom of basic social change" (Bogue 1959: 486). As the least biologically determined of the three basic demographic processes, migration (and its companion, local mobility) is responsive to economic forces, attitudes and values, and shifts in population composition. Still, some of the major forces that stimulate migration and influence choice of destination operate as they did earlier, but our ability to analyze these forces and make inferences for social science and policy has improved.

This chapter begins with some general remarks on internal migration, discussing its definition and relationships with other kinds of mobility. Then, in keeping with the outline of most of the other chapters in this section, it turns to contemporary issues, data and methods, substantive findings, and then offers some remarks on the future. Since the study of internal migration is broad and interdisciplinary, and since mobility and migration behavior are closely linked to other demographic events, the extensive literature is not surveyed. Several good compendia, such as the *International Library of Studies on Migration* and several review articles (Becker and Morrison 1986, Greenwood et al. 1991b; Nam, Serow, and Sky 1990; Lucas 1997), offer a variety of disciplinary perspectives.

CONTEMPORARY SUBSTANTIVE CONCERNS

This section takes up some prevailing issues in the contemporary study of internal migration. While scholars have long been concerned with the determinants of population movement and the net redistribution of population across territory, contemporary discussions have raised new issues and focused on particular facets of internal migration. Some of the issues with respect to higher-income countries are first presented, followed by concerns manifest in the case of lower-income societies.

Internal Migration in More Developed Countries (MDCs)

Societies in North America, Europe, Japan, Australia, and other regions have generally passed through the demographic transition and its attendant shift from predominantly rural societies to overwhelmingly urban and metropolitan societies. To be sure, the transition was well on its way by the middle of the 20th century, and by the beginning of the 21st century all these populations had virtually completed the transition. Even in the wake of a completed transition, however, broad patterns of internal migration impinge on these contemporary societies. The themes to be described include:

- Population diffusion
- Urbanization and counterurbanization
- Intrametropolitan population distribution
- Structure of migration streams
- Policy concerns

POPULATION DIFFUSION. *Population diffusion* is the redistribution of population in ways that are less consistent with age-old paradigms, particularly those frameworks that see an overarching organizational structure to demographic redistribution. For example, while urbanization, with a concomitant internal urban structure, was once considered the master trend in population distribution, such a unidirectional and uniform pattern no longer holds in Europe and North America. Rather, the late 20th century and early 21st century have been characterized by alternate shifts in the relative growth and decline of core urban territory versus the fringe. Furthermore, the core metropolitan area itself has evolved to a point where it is far less beholden to long-standing models of urban ecological structure. While a number of forces are at work on these changes, internal migration is the predominant demographic factor that leads to the resulting population diffusion. Some of the migration trends described below illustrate these themes of population diffusion.

Several political and demographic developments accentuate the likely impact and relative importance of migration for regions in industrialized settings. First, political and regulatory obstacles to population movement have been removed in many places, the most sweeping of which is the increasing economic integration of the European Union. Although this movement is technically international, it is presumably responding to subnational relative advantages and disadvantages for economic opportunity. Indeed, European Union (EU) policy directs some of this. Second, the very low rates of natural increase in industrialized populations mean that migration (whether internal or international) composes a larger fraction of population change. For example, the range of rates of net migration for administrative units in the EU is about triple the range of rates of natural increase (Rees et al. 1996a).

Metropolitan extensification has contributed to population diffusion. Shifts in the technology of transportation—most notably the worldwide growth in automobile use over the 20th century—further eroded the old city-suburb (core periphery) model of urban organization. Especially in North America, suburban or other peripheral nodes of commerce and employment developed, competing as organizational structures for urban ecology.

URBANIZATION AND COUNTERURBANIZATION. For much of the 20th century, the predominant pattern of population distribution in industrializing societies was urbanization. This concentration of population in cities (and their surrounding suburban territory) was fed, of course, by migration. From 1900 through about 1970 almost all industrialized nations recorded increases in the proportion of their population residing in urban areas.

Counterurbanization, by contrast, is a decline in the share of population residing in cities and suburban territory. Counterurbanization began to appear first in the 1970s in the United States, and then in Europe and other industrialized countries (Champion 1992). Rees and his associates (1996b) went so far as to characterize counterurbanization as "dominant" or "significant" in several countries of the European Union. Poulain, for instance, finds that for much of the 1960s through the 1980s the core urban region of Brussels lost in migration flows to and from the more outlying Walloon and Flemish Brabants (Poulain 1996: Figure 6.6). Similarly, the core Copenhagen region lagged behind the national average in the 1970s and 1980s (Illeris 1996). In France, there is still selective population dispersion from the center to the periphery (Baccaini and Pumain 1996: 193). This broad characterization sweeps over some underlying temporal, geographical, and age-specific detail. Figure 11.1 (from Baccaini and Pumain 1996: Figure 11.3) indicates that in France throughout the 1968 to 1982 period, sparse population settlements there continued to lose population, while among urban settlements a modest negative relationship between size and net migration was observed.

This apparent resurgence of demographic growth in the hinterland, alternately termed the *nonmetropolitan turnaround* or *rural renaissance*, intrigued demographers even as it generated controversy about its cause and authenticity (Lichter and Fuguitt

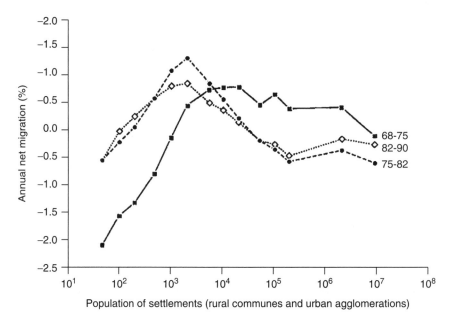

FIGURE 11.1. Net migration by settlement size, France 1968–1990. Source: Baccaini and Pumain (1996).

1982; Long and DeAre 1988). Scholars suggested reasons ranging from cultural redirection to technical issues in census geography to economic restructuring. All of these forces probably played a role. It is likely that economic restructuring was implicated in several of the explanations. Some views favored "back to the land" interpretations; others focused on the growth of retirement communities in amenity-rich nonmetropolitan locations. Still others saw a fundamental restructuring of economic geography, with technology of manufacturing, transport, and communication whittling away at urban advantage.

Demographic trends are documented most thoroughly for the United States, but research on Europe and other societies suggests that similar forces were driving the observed events, although the administrative categorizations may differ from country to country. In the U.S., some of the 1970s population deconcentration was exurban spillover, i.e., suburban growth outside of the existing boundaries of metropolitan areas, but a significant portion was due to growth in the hinterland. Many U.S. counties not adjacent to metropolitan areas experienced greater-than-average population growth.

Soon after this counterurbanization was identified, trends of *reurbanization* began to pick up again in the United States, with metropolitan growth outpacing nonmetropolitan growth (Richter 1985). The very same explanations—demographic accounting, migration back to urban cores, and underlying economic forces—were also named. And in the 1990s, evidence emerged again for another oscillation in the direction of increased nonmetropolitan growth (Long and Nucci 1997) in the United States. Since this time, the urban-rural balance seems to have exhibited few sharp trends in these societies.

INTRAMETROPOLITAN POPULATION DISTRIBUTION. Although "internal" migration in demography generally refers to the movement of persons across regions and between labor markets, it is useful to note the shift of persons within metropolitan areas. Again, the general trend in high-income societies during the last 50 years has been the growth of suburban territory at the expense of inner city areas. The inner sections of New York, London, Paris, and many other large and moderate-sized cities have seen this net shift.

Internal migrants contribute to the net redistribution of population within metropolitan areas to the extent that they exhibit specific origin and destination patterns. Evidence strongly suggests that in this period of metropolitan expansion and suburbanization, interregional labor migrants often choose suburban destination locations over central city locations. Such a phenomenon would reinforce the city-suburban movement within the metro area itself.

Inner city depopulation results partly from these dynamics: not only do urban residents move from the inner cities to suburbs, *new* arrivals to the metropolitan area may elect suburban residences. (This pattern may have been more pronounced in the United States than in other industrialized societies.) To the extent that these intermetropolitan migrants are selective for population traits (younger, higher socioeconomic status), they will accelerate (or in some cases retard) overall composition changes within the urban area.

THE STRUCTURE OF MIGRATION STREAMS.   Another contemporary set of substantive concerns involves the issue of the "structure" of migration streams. Just as some population scientists are concerned with the age structure of other demographic regularities, interest arises in the stability and change of flows between origin and destination communities. On the one hand these flows represent the aggregated migration decisions of many individuals and households; on the other hand, they may help tell about new patterns of population redistribution. For instance, there has been some discussion of the relative importance of regional restructuring versus decentralization perspectives in capturing the patterns of population redistribution in the United States and some other settings (Frey 1987; Wilson 1986). Analysis of the patterns and persistence of origin-destination migration often reveal economic and cultural connections between communities (Herting et al. 1997; Lin and Xie 1998; Plane and Mulligan 1997). In developing countries the concern may be for rural-urban or inland-coastal movement (NRC 2003).

POLICY CONCERNS.   The link to public policy permeates the study of internal migration. Most obviously, migration is linked to the spatial shift in the location of job opportunities. Some economic development programs have made population relocation a central feature, and studies of migration can help evaluate the consequences of such interventions (Baydar et al. 1990; Oberai 1988). There is a substantial literature on the spatial incentives and disincentives of government transfer policies in high-income societies. Some policies directly target population distribution. Others have an indirect impact, since migration allows people to "vote with their feet" and move toward or away from particular combinations of economic opportunities, public sector regulations, and amenities.

Internal Migration in Less Developed Countries (LDCs)

While the study of internal migration in less developed countries has many parallels to that in more developed countries, there are important distinctions in terms of the substantive focus of research and the theoretical approaches developed to explain migration behavior and migration flows. In this section we identify six substantive areas of research on internal migration in LDCs that are important either because they have received substantial attention from population experts or because they are new areas of research and concern. These areas are:

- Rural-urban migration and the growth of megacities
- Step migration and the growth of towns and secondary cities
- Rural-urban migrant adaptation
- Rural-rural migration and the extension of the agricultural frontier
- Circular migration
- The impact of migration on migrant places of origin

RURAL-URBAN MIGRATION AND THE GROWTH OF MEGACITIES.   Internal migration in LDCs has traditionally been studied by demographers in the context of urbanization. Migration from rural areas into towns and cities in some respects follows patterns observed earlier in MDCs. Economic and social changes occurring in urban areas made cities more attractive, and changes in rural areas that freed up agricultural labor precipitated the massive movement of people from rural areas into towns and cities. However, in several important respects the process in contemporary LDCs has differed from the historical experience.

The growth of urban centers, due in part to migration, has proceeded at a faster pace in LDCs than in MDCs, and in many cities has outpaced the rate of job growth in the modern sector and infrastructure development, producing squatter settlements, highly concentrated poverty, serious problems of congestion, and widespread deficiencies in vital services (McGee and Griffiths 1998). In some LDCs the high concentration of government employment, financial services, commerce, and industry in a single city, usually the capital, has created instances of high urban primacy, where urban growth and in-migration are concentrated in one location (Chen, Valente, and Zlotnik 1998). The growth of megacities is not restricted to LDCs, and many of the externalities associated with megacities, such as crime, congestion, and poor environmental quality, are also present in MDCs; however, concerns about the institutional capacity to address these externalities are greater in LDCs (United Nations 1998). Much of the interest in internal migration in LDCs has arisen out of concerns about rapid urban growth. Yet Chen, Valente, and Zlotnik (1998) estimate that of two principal components of urban population growth, natural increase has been the larger. For example, Table 11.1 indicates that during the 1960s and 1970s internal migration and the reclassification of rural places as urban places accounted for between 40% and 45% of annual urban

TABLE 11.1. Percent of Annual Urban Growth Rates Attributable to Internal Migration/ Reclassification. Selected Less Developed Regions.

	1960s	1970s	1980s
Africa	41.2	40.6	24.9
Latin America	40.1	40.5	33.9
Asia	40.4	46.7	63.6
Developing world	40.3	44.1	54.3

Source: Chen, Valente, and Zlotnik (1998: 82, Table 2–7).

growth in LDCs. During the 1980s the contribution of internal migration and reclassification to urban growth declined to 25% in Africa and 34% in Latin America, but rose to 64% in Asia. Excluding China, the figure for Asia was 48.9% (Chen, Valente, and Zlotnick 1998: 82). According to Chen, Valente, and Zlotnick (1998) this suggests that policies designed to reduce the rate of urban growth in LDCs should place more emphasis on reducing fertility than on focusing on migration.

Much of the research on rural-urban migration in LDCs has been concerned with understanding the relationship between migration and development and identifying the economic determinants of migration. Early studies viewed migration as a demographic response to geographical imbalances in the factors of production: land, labor, and capital. The division of the determinants of migration into forces of propulsion in places of origin and forces of attraction in places of destination was encapsulated in the "push-pull" framework. From a policy perspective, concerns about rapid urban growth produced an interest in identifying "push" factors that were amenable to policy interventions in places of origin and those "pull" factors in urban places that could be improved in rural places. The intention was to slow the pace of rural-urban migration or, in some instances, even to reverse it (Chen, Valente, and Zlotnik 1998; Obudho 1998; World Bank 1984). For example, in China, the government promoted rural industrialization and the development of small towns with urban amenities as a strategy to deter migration to cities (Zhu 1998: 158; Liang, Chen, and Gu 2002). Implicit in the equilibrium approaches to migration is the expectation that as LDCs achieve similar levels of economic development as those found in present-day MDCs, they will also achieve similar levels of urbanization. Hardoy and Satterthwaite (1989) find evidence of a positive correlation between the level of rural-urban migration in LDCs and the growth of GNP in recent decades, but it is far from clear whether there will be a global convergence in urbanization levels.

Changes in population distribution resulting from migration in LDCs are consistent with the idea that migration occurs in response to geographical differences in the distribution of economic resources and opportunities. However, at the aggregate level, equilibrium models fail to explain why migration streams begin when they do, why migration is directed to some destinations and not others that offer similar opportunities, and why there is not more migration given the persistence of significant regional disparities in resources and opportunities. Recent research on internal migration in LDCs devotes considerable attention to the social organization of migration. Migration decisions and migration behavior are seen as the outcome of social processes that influence everything from the decision to migrate, the type of migration, the choice of destination, and the process of adaptation and settlement.

STEP MIGRATION AND THE GROWTH OF TOWNS AND SECONDARY CITIES. Migration from the countryside to major urban centers in LDCs often involves a sequence of moves from smaller to larger places rather than a single leap from village to metropolis. The classic pattern is to move from a village to the nearest town, then from the town to the regional capital, and finally from the regional capital to the national capital. This sequential process is termed *step migration* and represents a response to factors which impede the flow of people from less developed to more developed regions. Step migration provides a way to moderate the financial and psychic costs of migration between dramatically different types of places by allowing for gradual adjustment and the collection of information about ultimate urban destinations. Two implications of step migration are (1) that the growth of some towns and secondary cities represents a transitional stage in the redistribution of population from rural areas to large urban agglomerations—although the growth of secondary cities in some instances is also fueled by counter-migration from megacities as a reaction to urban congestion (see Bilsborrow 1998b; Cunha 1998)—and (2) that urban-urban migration is an important component of the growth of major metropolitan areas in LDCs.

MIGRANT ADAPTATION.   Interest in internal migrants does not stop with the act of migration but continues with the process of adaptation to urban conditions. Major areas of interest are the economic adjustment of migrants, migrant fertility and, more recently, migrant health. Studies of urban economic activity and employment in LDCs identify a formal and an informal sector of the economy in which the organization and characteristics of work differ in terms of adherence to regulations, skill requirements, wages and benefits, opportunities for advancement, and job stability. The informal sector is a crucial source of employment for recently arrived migrants in LDC cities. Employment in this sector is often found in small family-run businesses in small-scale manufacturing or repair or in petty commerce and street vending. The absorption of migrants by the informal sector represents an important contrast to migration in MDCs, where the informal sector has historically been smaller. The addition of migrants to the urban labor force has fueled the growth of the informal sector in LDCs at a rate that has outstripped that of the formal sector of the economy. Whether the presence of a large and dynamic informal sector represents a transitional phase in economic development, and whether it has a positive or negative effect on long-run economic development, is a hotly debated subject in the development literature and will not be covered here. For many migrants, work in the informal sector represents a transitional phase. In the short-run, migrants may accept work conditions and wages that on the surface do not appear to represent a significant improvement over what they had before, but in the long-term they experience upward economic mobility as they move into more formal employment. Most studies of migrants in the urban areas of LDCs indicate that migrants tend to adapt well to their new environments and that differences between them and nonmigrants in labor force participation, occupational status, and income are due primarily to differences in age, gender, education, and time since migration (United Nations, ECLAC 1994).

Rural-urban fertility differentials in LDCs are often large, particularly in countries in the early stages of the fertility transition. The question of what happens to the fertility of rural women after they migrate to urban areas is of great interest for anticipating the rate of population growth at both urban and national levels. Continued high fertility after migration raises the rate of natural increase in cities and produces rates of urban growth greater than what would be predicted by the addition of migrants alone. On the other hand, the adoption of urban fertility levels by rural migrants will produce national fertility levels and rates of growth lower than what would be predicted by a gradual decline in rural fertility alone. Early studies of migration and fertility produced contradictory results with no clear pattern of findings across countries and historical periods. However, much of the confusion in the literature can be traced back to the use of data that did not provide sufficient detail or precision to measure the relative timing of migration and births. The largest body of evidence, nevertheless, places migrant fertility higher than urban native fertility, but lower than the fertility of rural nonmigrants. Recent studies, which utilize individual event histories with information on the timing of migration and births, are consistent with these findings (Brockerhoff and Yang 1994; Lindstrom 2003; White, Moreno, and Guo 1995). The rapid adjustment of migrant fertility to urban fertility patterns occurs in response to the higher real and opportunity costs of children in urban areas, greater acceptance of fertility control in urban areas, and increased access to contraceptive services and methods.

The gradual but steady decline in fertility in LDCs has alleviated many of the concerns about the contribution of migrant fertility to urban population growth. More attention is now being given to the health of migrants and their children in urban areas. Key questions that motivate this research include the impact of living conditions on migrant health, including access to potable water and human waste disposal, and access to medical services (Satterthwaite 1998).

RURAL-RURAL MIGRATION AND THE EXTENSION OF THE AGRICULTURAL FRONTIER. While certainly not as numerically large as rural-urban migration, rural-rural migration is nevertheless an important component of internal migration in LDCs. Migration to rural areas in many countries has been highly encouraged, openly orchestrated, and in some cases forcibly imposed by many national governments. The spontaneous migration of people from rural areas to other rural areas occurs in response to population growth and land scarcity in densely populated rural areas, the opening of more fertile lands to settlement, and as a response to soil exhaustion. Because tropical soils tend to be thin and rapidly exhausted, some settlers move again after several years into new unsettled forest areas and start afresh. Such patterns of successive rural-rural moves are documented in tropical forested areas of Central America and the Amazon, among other places, and are a major contributor to deforestation (Bilsborrow and DeLargy 1991; Fearnside 1986; United Nations 1994).

National governments have also sponsored colonization projects to relieve population pressure in more densely populated regions (see Cunha 1998; Jones 1990; Kay 1982; Oucho 1983; Wood 1982; United Nations 1997) or to establish sovereignty in sparsely populated border areas or in areas populated by ethnic minorities. Many colonization projects have failed when they have entailed the movement of peoples to ecological zones different from the ones in which they originated. Without proper technical assistance, farmers often fail to adapt to the new environment and eventually abandon the new locations to return to their places of origin or migrate to urban areas (Clay, Steingraber, and Niggli 1988).

Colonization projects have come under greater scrutiny from environmental groups and international development organizations because of their impact on fragile ecological systems and the destruction of tropical forest areas (Economic Commission for Latin America and the Caribbean 1994). In an interesting reversal from prior periods, economic development and employment growth in urban areas is favored as a way to attract rural migrants away from unsettled and fragile rural areas and into urban areas (United Nations Centre for Human Settlements 1994). However, for many LDCs, the expansion of the agricultural frontier and the settlement of sparsely populated forested areas are considered necessary steps in the process of economic development.

CIRCULAR MIGRATION.   Not all migration in LDCs is long-term or permanent. Many migrants remain in places of destination for relatively short periods either because the work itself is temporary, such as seasonal agricultural work, or the migrant has reached a particular savings target and then returns to his or her place of origin. Although the distinction between temporary and long-term or permanent migration is often blurred, there are several features that distinguish temporary migration, including short duration, the intention to return to the place of origin, and the maintenance of a residence and/or household in the place of origin. A pattern of repeated seasonal trips or regular movement back and forth between origin and destinations is termed circular migration. Circular migration is used by rural households to satisfy temporary income deficits or acquire savings for specific purchases without having to permanently abandon the community of origin. Internal circular migration generally involves rural-urban migration and rural-rural migration. In sub-Saharan Africa, circular migration is the dominant form of migration (Oucho 1998). Rural-urban circular migrants often are employed in the informal sector in work that is highly seasonal or irregular. There is some debate as to whether circular rural-urban migration represents a transitory phase in the process of urbanization and economic development or whether it constitutes a long-term feature of LDCs (Hugo 1982). While it is certainly true that for some rural-urban migrants, temporary migration is a prelude to permanent relocation and settlement in urban areas, for others it represents a long-term strategy to maximize the returns on low-wage urban employment by locating household consumption in rural places where the relative costs of living are substantially lower.

Temporary migration from rural to rural locations is another type of internal migration in LDCs with large commercial agricultural sectors. Producers of labor-intensive agricultural products depend on low-wage migrant workers to meet seasonal peaks in labor demand. The wages earned through temporary rural-rural migration are generally too low to provide any opportunities for economic mobility and are typically destined for household maintenance. Rural-rural circular migrants tend to have poorer human capital endowments than rural-urban migrants and therefore are less prepared for employment in urban areas.

IMPACT OF MIGRATION ON RURAL PLACES OF ORIGIN.   Long-term or settled rural-urban migrants often maintain close ties to their communities of origin through return visits, written and oral communication, and gifts of money and goods, and some eventually return to live in their communities of origin. When rural-urban migrants visit or return to their communities, they bring with them the experiences, behaviors, and attitudes that they acquired while living and working in urban areas, in addition to the money they have saved. While migrants' role in the spread of urban culture and lifestyles into rural areas is largely unmeasured, recent evidence from Guatemala, for instance, suggests that urban migrants may be diffusing information and positive attitudes about the adoption of innovative health behaviors, such as the use of prenatal care and modern contraceptives (Lindstrom and Muñoz-Franco 2003).

The gender composition of internal migration streams can influence those communities left behind. Circular migration streams vary by country according to levels of development and culturally specific norms regarding gender roles. In many countries, temporary migration streams are often dominated by men, but as streams become more stable and socially organized, women form an increasing fraction of the movers (Skeldon 1986; Donato 1993). In countries where temporary migration is predominantly a male activity, married women often become *de facto* heads of households while their husbands are away, exercising greater autonomy over decision making, which may lead to longer-term improvements in women's status (Palmer 1985). Internal migration from rural areas to towns and cities can also bring about greater autonomy for young women from highly traditional rural societies (Whiteford 1978; Tienda and Booth 1991).

The economic impact of internal migration on places of origin is mixed. Many studies view internal migration as a drain on human capital in rural areas. For instance, circular migration may create situations where origin households are forever dependent upon migrant wages (Simmons 1984). Other studies, however, have highlighted some of the positive benefits of remittance income for rural households (Oucho 1998). Studies confirm that remittances significantly improve the welfare of migrant households. Basic consumption and spending on housing are the two most common uses of remittance income. Investments in agricultural production and small businesses are more likely to occur in communities where the expected returns on such investments are positive.

THEORETICAL ISSUES

The study of migration is clearly an interdisciplinary exercise. Brettel, for instance, cites contributions from no fewer than seven disciplines contributing theoretical perspectives (Brettel 2000). These approaches range from the micro to the macro. After a short discussion of the reasons cited for different types of moves, attention is directed to a microlevel discussion of mobility models, which now permeate the several fields and are closely linked to the empirical modeling of geographical mobility. This is due in large part to the increasing availability of microlevel data for individuals and households.

Reasons for Migration

The reasons migrants cite for making a move are quite directly related to the type of move (migration or local mobility) and some of the traits of the migrants and their households. Simply stated, local moves tend to be tied to life-cycle changes and long-distance moves to job-related reasons, but this simple dichotomy may overstate the separability of the two types of geographical mobility.

Figure 11.2, taken from U.S. Current Population Survey data, illustrates broad consistency with this distinction. While housing and family reasons overwhelmingly dominate intracounty moves, a substantial fraction of intercounty movers (a common definition for U.S. migrants) cites these reasons. Similarly, one finds that in the U.K., moves of 10 miles or under are overwhelmingly linked to reasons regarding housing and life cycle, whereas nearly half of those citing work-related reasons involve moves of at least 50 miles (Owen and Green 1992). Often underappreciated, however, is the substantial fraction of job-related moves that involved job transfer without change of employer, with evidence on this point accumulated from the U.S., U.K., Japan, and Australia (Flowerdew 1992).

A Simple Micro-Decision making Model

The most logical and straightforward starting point in theory for the study of migration is a model of individual decision making. Scholars increasingly recognize that migration

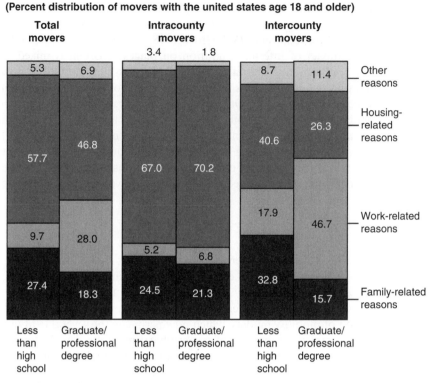

FIGURE 11.2. Reasons for moving by educational status and type of move: March 1990–2000. Source: U.S. Census Bureau Current Population Survey, March 2000.

is a social process in which the migrant's actions are embedded in a web of familial, friendship, and employment affiliations. Yet, casting the decision first at the individual level tracks the historical pattern of the development of theory, and it offers a basic building block on which more contemporary models stand. In this approach the individual labor migrant considers a decision in which a stream of annual income (discounted over time) at a potential alternative location j is compared to the corresponding stream at the existing location i. If the present value of the alternative stream exceeds the value of the current stream and the costs of moving over T years, the individual is predicted to migrate, to wit:

$$\sum_{t=1}^{T} \frac{Y_{jt} - Y_{it}}{(1+r)^t} - \sum_{t=1}^{T} \frac{C_{jt} - C_{it}}{(1+r)^t}$$

Of course this is the most rudimentary model, and it leaves much behavior unexplained.

Several straightforward elaborations of the model, still at the level of the individual migrant, make it more realistic. The costs of migration include more than the out-of-pocket expenses of moving one's self and one's possessions to a new location. They also include the *psychic costs* of leaving a community where one has local information and personal ties. A second element of an elaboration is the incorporation of *destination uncertainty,* especially regarding the income stream. Thus, in equation (1) above, the expected income stream at an alternative j might be discounted further by the uncertainty of realizing that stream in the future. It is likely that the potential migrant has more information about economic opportunities at the origin and hence a better estimate of the income stream from staying put. This uncertainty is especially relevant in developing country settings.

A further extension is seen in *job search models*. These models account for the fact that there is a cost to gathering information. In the migration case, this means that it is difficult for the worker (and prospective migrant) to be fully informed about wage opportunities for a large set of potential destinations (Molho 2001). The upshot of such elaborations—uncertainty and search costs—is that individuals may be less likely to move than wage rate difference alone would suggest.

Life Cycle and Internal Migration

In keeping with broad developments in the social sciences regarding life course approaches (both conceptual frameworks and data collection plans), some migration analysts have taken a life-cycle approach to mobility at all geographical scales. Movement through the life cycle impinges on the probability of moving in a variety of ways. Jumping off from the baseline microeconomic model above, one can see that the atomistic migrant may come to a different decision based upon his or her age. Simply stated, younger migrants will have a longer time over which to recoup the costs of moving, and they are therefore more likely to be responsive to differences in wages and employment opportunities.

A further elaboration is seen through the window of life-cycle stages. Union formation and dissolution, education, and entry and exit from the labor force all shift the parameters of the decision for individuals. These major events work over and above age to make certain points in the life cycle—most notably young adulthood and retirement—points at which the impetus for migration is increased.

Social Structure, Context, and Migration

Contemporary migration theory embeds the migrant in social context (De Jong 2000). It would be erroneous to claim the earlier theoretical approaches completely ignored such context. Psychic costs refer implicitly to social ties at the origin; life-cycle influences necessarily involve relationships with other people. Nevertheless, migration approaches have grown to more directly incorporate the social context in which people make decisions and, by extension, the social organization of migration. Empirically this is seen in the efforts to include various contextual variables in empirical analyses of migration and other demographic behaviors (Findley 1987; Bilsborrow et al. 1987; Brown and Goetz 1987).

There is a range of such contextual factors. At a minimum, the traits of other family or household members matter. Thus, the notion of a "tied" mover comes into play, especially in high-income societies where dual-earner couples make joint decisions about locations and labor markets. Other contextual factors include community effects. Thus the availability of a package of local public services and the opportunity to share amenities with persons of the same life-cycle stage could weigh into the decision. Thus in an equation predicting individual migration (e.g., equations 2 to 4 below), not only do the traits of the individual appear but traits of his or her household, neighborhood, and labor market may also appear. These may form part of the social capital upon which an individual may rely while developing a migration strategy.

Several theoretical and empirical developments examine the ways in which the composition of origin and/or destination region influences the flow of migrants. For instance, the labor market composition of the origin may influence the number of workers who are substitutes (persons with similar skills likely to drive down wages of the worker) or complements (persons with complementary skills that may actually improve wage and employment opportunities for the worker). Carrington, Detragiaeke, and Vishwanath (1996) argue that such mechanisms may operate by gathering momentum, hence reducing the relocation costs for succeeding waves of potential migrants. Such phenomena are also referred to in the migration literature as *cumulative causation* and may have contributed to the migration of African Americans within the United States (Carrington et al. 1996) and the continued arrival of immigrants to selected labor markets in high-income societies. At the other end of the spectrum, it has been argued that the increasing presence of immigrants (and other labor market competitors) spurs the internal migration of labor market substitute workers away from regions and metropolitan areas that have experienced heavy waves of new arrivals. For the 1990s, Frey observes that the concentration of foreign-born migrants in certain labor markets was accompanied by an apparent outmigration of less skilled U.S.-born individuals from such locales (Frey 1996). Correspondingly, the concentration of immigrants in the place of origin may influence the long-distance migration of the foreign-born (Kritz and Nogle 1994; White and Liang 1998).

Additional Theoretical Issues in LDCs

Theoretical approaches to the study of internal migration in LDCs have their origin in general theories of migration first developed to study migration in MDCs, but have been extensively modified and expanded to take into account structural differences in markets and differences in social organization at the household and community levels. Two important differences for which the theories adjust are (1) the absence of well-developed and smoothly functioning credit and insurance markets in many LDCs and (2) the presence of a large informal sector. These differences in economic structures have important implications for migration and the processes by which migrants become integrated into destination areas.

Neoclassical economic theory has been the dominant framework for explaining internal migration in LDCs. According to this theory, migration occurs as a response to regional differences in income opportunities generated by imbalances in the spatial distribution of the factors of production. Lewis (1954) and Ranis and Fei (1961) divided the economy into a rural subsistence sector and an urban industrial sector. Migration presumably continues until wage returns for labor become the same in urban and rural locations. This two-sector model, however, was not entirely appropriate for LDCs, where a large urban informal sector coexisted with the modern sector. To account for the continuation of rural-urban migration in the presence of significant urban underemployment, Todaro (1969) and Harris and Todaro (1970) changed the neoclassical focus on nominal wage rates to expected wage rates, where expected wages factored in the probability of eventually finding a job in the modern sector. According to the Todaro model, migrants are willing to experience what sometimes may even amount to a decline in real incomes resulting from a rural-urban move as long as they expect to eventually end up in higher-paying jobs. An important implication of this model is that the supply of urban labor may actually outstrip demand and that the growth of urban employment may increase levels of unemployment by spurring even more rural-urban migration in anticipation of acquiring urban jobs in the long run.

Cole and Sanders (1985) view the urban informal economy, or the urban subsistence sector, as they call it, as the expected end-point for many unskilled migrants from rural areas. In other words, not even the expectation of eventual employment in the modern urban sector is needed for rural-urban migration to occur. DeJong and Legazpi Blair's (1994) study of rural-urban migrant occupational mobility in the Philippines and Hugo's (1985) study of migration in Indonesia finds evidence consistent with this explanation: rural migrants in urban areas are often restricted by their social networks to low-status occupations in the informal sector of the urban economy.

Studies of internal migration flows and individual migration behavior provide evidence that is consistent with the neoclassical framework (Falaris 1979; Levy and Wadycki 1974; Schultz 1971). Migration tends to be directed from low-income places to high-income places. Studies that incorporate some measure of expected income also appear to have more explanatory power than models that include a measure of nominal wage rates or wage differentials (Bravo-Ureta, Quiroga and Brea 1996; Garrison 1982).

Both the individual decision maker and the income-maximization components of the neoclassical model have been put aside by subsequent theoretical developments in models of internal migration. First is the recognition that economic decisions and, in particular, decisions about the allocation of labor are made within the context of households (Banerjee 1981). Second is that satisfying current income needs and reducing economic vulnerability and risk are more important to households than income maximization (Collins 1985; Roberts 1985; Schaeffer 1987; Wood 1982). Households as income pooling units provide many benefits to individuals, including insurance against the risk of failed health, unemployment, and in the case of migration, failure to find work in an urban location (Schaeffer 1987; Katz and Stark 1986; Stark and Lucas 1988; Stark and Levhari 1982). According to Bilsborrow (1998a:17), "this approach adopts the common view that households in developing countries are 'closer' and more integrated than those in developed countries, with household members being more interdependent and having stronger affective ties."

The migration of one or more household members provides a means for rural households to insure themselves against crop failure or other unanticipated drops in household income by diversifying their sources of income across different locations and sectors of the economy. This implies that migration will occur even in the absence of nominal or expected wage differentials. Theoretical models of temporary or circular migration in LDCs also remove the assumption of income maximization. They depict migrants as target earners; once a particular savings target is reached, migrants return to their communities of origin (Berg 1961).

The neoclassical model also assumes that potential migrants possess information on employment opportunities in alternative destinations. Research, however, has shown that information is far from perfect and that potential migrants rely heavily on active migrants in places of destination and return migrants in places of origin for information about opportunities outside of the community of origin (Caces et al. 1985).

The different theoretical approaches to modeling internal migration are not mutually exclusive, of course. In combination, they highlight the importance of taking into account not only individual characteristics, but the characteristics of the household, community, and regional contexts within which decisions about migration are made. Geographical wage differences are often a necessary but not sufficient condition for migration. Where people migrate to, and how long they stay, are functions of the original motivations for migration, which are not restricted to income maximization, as well as the people to whom they are socially tied.

The role of gender is another important issue in migration research (de Lattes 1989; Pedraza 1991). Economic theories of migration assume that the process of migration decision making, whether it occurs at the individual or household level, is the same for men and women, and by extension the factors that influence migration decisions have the same effects for men and women. However, research shows that gender is an important factor in understanding migration patterns. This is so because first, labor markets are often stratified by gender due to the gender typing of occupations and employers' preferences for workers of a particular gender; second, women may not have the same influence on household decisions as men; and third, gender differences in household and familial roles and role relations factor into decisions about who migrates. De Jong (2000) finds in Thailand that men and women's decisions or intentions to move are differentially affected by origin and potential destination characteristics. Lauby and Stark (1988) find in the Philippines that daughters are more likely than sons to be sent by parents to urban locations to work temporarily because they are viewed as being more dependent on the family unit and thus are expected to be more reliable remitters.

METHODS AND MEASURES

This section reviews some key methods for collecting and analyzing internal migration. Because it is an event taking place in an identified population, it is important to properly define the population at risk and the "event" of internal migration. Despite the historical treatment of migration as a demographic phenomenon that is distinct from the vital events of fertility and mortality, methodologists conceptualize it well within the various population outcomes analyzed regularly by demographers. The major aspect of migration that separates it from conventional demographic methods is the intrinsic importance of geography. The measurement and analysis of migration also involves some specialized concerns in data collection and management.

Concept and Definition

Migration is best seen as a repeatable event (see Figure 11.3). The terminology of event history analysis is especially useful in this regard. The standard definition of migration is a relatively permanent change in usual place of residence. The identification of this transition event itself may have less precision than a birth or death, but probably no less than many other human transitions in residence, health, or labor force status. In this context, "relatively permanent" and "usual" are open to interpretation. There is no biological constraint governing migratory behavior (unlike, say conception through gestation to birth), and thus there is no obvious temporal unit or division for the event. Still, most data collection mechanisms sort out the temporal precision, and

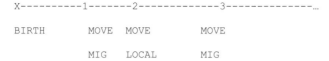

```
X----------1-------2-------------3------------...

BIRTH       MOVE  MOVE          MOVE

            MIG   LOCAL         MIG
```

FIGURE 11.3. Migration event history.

there are standard recording frameworks, which will be addressed later. Migration may thus be seen as a demographic process governed by transition probabilities for which a suitable population at risk needs to be defined (Rees et al. 2000).

The larger, and perhaps more pertinent, distinction involves geography, particularly the identification of the *migration-defining boundary* (or boundaries). The change of usual place of residence identifies general geographical mobility. The mover must cross a threshold to be considered to be a migrant. Thus, demographers generally distinguish between local mobility (the relocation within the migration-defining boundary) and internal migration (relocation across the migration-defining boundary).

International migrants are further defined as those who move across national borders, a phenomenon beyond our scope here (see chapter 12, "International Migration," in this *Handbook*). Hence in Figure 11.3, which records three residential moves in a span of time, move 1 and move 3 cross the migration-defining boundary and are classified as "migration." By contrast, move 2 remains within the boundary and is classified as "local mobility." This convention in terminology is quite common in American demographic usage but is less often observed in other settings. In other writings, often those for Europe, all moves are labeled "migration," and these are further distinguished as "intraregional" and "interregional" migration (see, e.g., Rees et al. 1996a).

Probably the most conceptually appealing distinction for the migration-defining boundary (MDB) is that which separates relocation *within* labor markets (and perhaps housing markets) and relocation *between* labor markets. Typical choices or operationalizations for this distinction are rural-urban territory and subnational political units. Each will be examined.

In a developing setting, the movement from rural to urban areas is seen as a fundamental shift of living environment. To invoke this MDB, it is necessary to dichotomize all places or territories as urban or rural. Sometimes subtypes are used. Only then can movers be classified as migrants.

However, states, provinces, and regions are widely used as migration-defining boundaries. Thus, movement between Sichuan and Hubei provinces in China or between California and Arizona in the United States would constitute migration. Interprovincial (or interstate) movement of this sort is a common feature of published material from national censuses. Subnational political units often fall short of the labor market concept described above. Provinces and states typically also vary widely in size, as a fraction of the national population, and in socioeconomic structure. Contiguous units have the feature that short distance moves might be regarded as migration, where the individual makes only a very modest social and economic change. Indeed it is possible in many parts of the world to make an interprovincial or interstate move and remain within the local labor market. Occasionally, analysts tabulate movement to noncontiguous states or provinces in an effort to be sure to examine migration that breaks a connection with the home territory.

Frequently a smaller administrative unit, a county or district, is used as the migration-defining boundary. In Malaysia, interdistrict movement is so regarded (Chattopadhyay 1998). Such lower-level units often work well, but they do run the risk of underbounding (and thus "overcounting") migration. Often, the choice of scale of unit rests on a compromise between the social scientist's preferred conceptualization and established practice (and data availability) in the statistical system. The choice of MDB has been shown to be consequential. Analysis of U.S. data shows differential selectivity of the population along socioeconomic characteristics when county, metropolitan, and state boundaries are used (White and Mueser 1988).

Metropolitan Territory and other Functional Units

Many statistical systems define a set of metropolitan areas as cities and their surrounding suburban territory. Although such functional units are themselves composed of lower-level administrative units, they have the virtue of coming closer to the analyst's conceptual preferences. In such a framework, movement from nonmetropolitan to metropolitan territory would be counted as migration, as would movement from one metropolitan area to another. Movement within a metropolitan area, even from one side of Cairo or Mexico City to the other, would generally be regarded as local mobility. This geographical structure has many advantages, but it does impose the burden of reclassification of territory.

Distance and Point-to-Point Measures of Migration

Distance figures prominently in migration discussions, yet direct measures of distance moved are harder to find. Some analysts measure distance moved by assigning a value from the point-to-point distance of the centroids of unit or residence (province, county) at origin and destination. Mueser, for instance, calculated interstate distance moved in a national U.S. sample (Mueser 1989b).

It is possible to identify "usual place of residence" as a point on the earth's surface, say by longitude and latitude. Therefore, in principle it is possible to measure all population mobility in terms of point-to-point movement. The analysis could further identify migration events as that subset of moves of minimum distance or (with use of appropriate GIS technology) crossing the MDB. Thus, one could work with continuous distance or reclassify the movement according to various geographical, administrative, or functional criteria. While such a high-resolution approach is theoretically and technologically feasible now (at least in some settings), applications are, suffice to say, not widespread.

Migration analysts frequently complain about the difficulty of establishing comparable migration statistics across national populations. The lack of comparable statistical geography has undoubtedly restrained the ability to provide cross-national analyses of internal migration. Some direct information about distance moved has been gathered for the United States, Sweden, and the United Kingdom by Long, Tucker, and Urton (1988). In the U.K., for instance, distance between the postal codes of current and previous residence can be used to calculate migration distance. Such calculations present the opportunity for comparisons across nations, even if somewhat rare, as illustrated in Table 11.2.

TABLE 11.2. Movers by Distance Moved.

	US 1976	UK 1981	Sweden 1974
Movers/1000 pop	171	90	NA
Moved < 50 km	125	75	NA
Moved >= 50 km	46	15	24
–Moved >= 300 km	*27*	*NA*	*7*

Source: Long, Tueker, and Urton (1988).

Nevertheless, several recent attempts have been made to improve our technical ability to generate comparable statistics. Some attempts directly address the lack of comparability; others concentrate on technical work to indirectly establish the population at risk and the count of events (Bell et al. 2002; Rees et al. 2000).

Analysts have often devoted their attention to streams of migration. In one of the earliest writings on the topic of migration, Ravenstein proposed a series of "laws" of migration (Ravenstein 1885). These include a number of regularities that are compelling today, particularly describing the negative association of distance with migration, the prevalence of "stages" of migration, the importance of economic motivation, and some demographic differentials. Ravenstein also introduced the concepts of *stream* and *counterstream*, arguing then that every stream produced a reverse flow. Lee built on these ideas in his classic article on migration theory (Lee 1966). Again, Lee emphasized the heterogeneity of population and geographical opportunity in generating migration, including migration streams.

The legacy of this early thinking is an orientation to gathering and analyzing migration for stream, i.e., place-to-place flows for a given migration interval. Not always has this been possible, but census data and some survey sources allow one to tabulate the origin-destination flow of persons in the last year or over a five-year interval. For many countries census data are made available in this form. At times the streams themselves become of interest, with applications of multistate methods and other techniques to describe and analyze the flows (Rogers 1984, 1985; Plane and Mulligan 1997) and other attempts to summarize the formal structure of the migration flow matrix, the implicit role of distance in the matrix (with this, the associated estimation of gravity models), and other population characteristics that influence the demographic structure of migration (Weidlich and Haag 1988; Stillwell and Congdon 1991). More substantively oriented approaches attempt to statistically explain the magnitude and direction of migration streams (including return migration streams) as a function of origin and destination place traits. A substantial empirical literature exists for this approach and it touches on a range of populations, although the degree of detail varies considerably across study and country (Nam, Serow, and Sly 1990). Recent applications can be found for a range of countries, including China (Poston and Mao 1998), Germany (Haag et al. 1988), Italy (Munz and Rabino 1988), and the United States (Plane and Mulligan 1997; Saenz and Davila 1992), with still others mentioned earlier in this chapter.

Data Sources

The sources of information for migration parallel those of other demographic behaviors. Censuses, surveys, and administrative data can all provide information on geographical mobility and, again, the role of time and space in the measurement of migration has important implications for the utility of any potential source of data.

CENSUS.   Censuses remain an important source of information in the migration field. Censuses are often one of the few data collection mechanisms that gather a sufficient number of events at a detailed geographical resolution to make the study of migration patterns possible. Of course, censuses give the complete picture of population distribution; they provide snapshots of who lives where at a particular point in time. By contrast, surveys are limited in how much they can cover, at least with suitable sample size, regarding place-to-place movement.

Typical census approaches to migration involve tabulation or analysis of place-to-place flows. Such flow matrices, often represented as a tabulation of current versus previous place of residence, are usually generated from responses to a simple question asking about residence one or five years ago. With sufficient numbers this can give a picture of the national migration system. The gain in geographical comprehensiveness with the census is usually accompanied by a loss of temporal detail.

ADMINISTRATIVE DATA.   Although administrative record sources are discussed widely throughout demography, they have conventionally played less of a role in geographical mobility, and their role will likely continue to decrease. This is both because of new data collection regimes and the decline in the availability and utility of administrative record data. There are, however, several interesting ways in which administrative data portray migration.

Population registers record individuals by place; thus, registers should give insight into net population movement, often by selected demographic traits such as age and sex. Registers are most common in parts of Europe and Asia, and they are relatively unknown throughout the Americas and Africa. Although registers offer, in principle, a continuous monitoring of the population, issues of data management and scant personal traits severely curtail their utility. Some have used population registers, however: Poulain (1996) reports the extensive coverage and updating of the Belgian population register and goes on to use it for analyzing trends and basic differentials in migration. In the United Kingdom, the National Health Service Central Register (NHSCR) has been used as an equivalent, but it faces obstacles with respect to geographical detail and other factors (Owen and Green 1992). Demographic surveillance systems for local areas in developing countries may offer selective insight into migration in some cases.

Population register information is of considerable ancillary value in certain settings. Most notably in China, individuals (households) hold an official registration in one location (*hukou*). Prior to market reforms, it was this registration that gave the household access to food allocations and social services. With the arrival of the market transition on the mainland, individuals often migrated to new locations beyond their official residence. Thus, they became known as the "floating population," akin to undocumented migrants in other contexts. The separation of *de jure* and *de facto* residence itself becomes an object of study, generating questions such as, Who is a floating migrant? How do those people integrate into the host economy and social structure? What is the pattern of future demographic behavior that we observe?, and the like (see Roberts 1997).

SURVEY DATA AND ASSOCIATED ANALYTICAL APPROACHES. To be sure, a major development in demographic analysis over the last generation has been the shift from aggregated, descriptive analysis to more micro and behavioral analysis. Such analyses are often supported by survey data or representative samples of a regional or national population for whom extensive information is collected. Many data are collected and released in a form that enables the statistical modeling of the timing of individual behavior. The availability of longitudinal information on "usual place of residence" immediately makes practical an event history approach to geographical mobility.

Thus, from a modeling point of view, irrespective of theoretical orientation, the study of internal migration has witnessed an increasing application of duration or hazard model, such as:

$$h(t) = f(X_1, X_2, X_3 \ldots)$$

where $h(t)$ is the hazard of migrating at time t. This hazard is seen to be influenced by a set of fixed and time-varying covariates, X. Typical are other core demographic traits including age and sex. Also key are human capital traits, such as education and occupation. More recently, concern has expanded to include traits that apply to other family members and wider communities of reference. Specifications for the hazard model use a variety of functional forms in continuous time. Alternatively, a large number of specifications make use of a discrete time model, for example, predicting the probability of a move, p:

$$\log[p_j/(1 - p_j)] = \beta_{oj} + \beta_{ij}X_{ij} + \beta_{2j}X_{2j} + \ldots e_j$$

The set of covariates is often the same in discrete and continuous models. While such longitudinal approaches have become widespread in demography, it is worth mentioning some of the key aspects of invoking them in the study of migration. Further variations in functional form allow the analyst to alter the predicted response of the outcome to the covariates or capture differently the influence of duration of residence in the existing locale.

Obtaining information on residential histories may be problematic, as has been the case in the Demographic and Health Surveys (DHS). While this round of internationally comparative surveys for developing countries has extensive information on fertility and child health histories, the collection of residence histories has lagged. In many versions of the DHS, only place of birth, residence at youth (typically age 15), and current residence are ascertained. Some surveys (often limited to populations with greater contraceptive prevalence) include a calendar, which includes residence information for the most recent five or six years.

As a pragmatic matter, the migration-defining interval is often defined by the data collection scheme. Census and national cross-sectional surveys typically include a one-year interval or five-year interval to capture geographical mobility. Usually, reports of prior residence in tandem with a geographical schema are used to classify migration. Thus, interprovincial or interstate migration is promulgated from many censuses. Dedicated event history data collection plans are more likely to collect residence information at a higher resolution. These fall into two types, namely, retrospective and prospective data collection.

Retrospective data collection requires the respondent to recall past demographic events, including residence spells. These have all the advantages and disadvantages of other retrospective data collection regimes. What is noteworthy from the viewpoint of internal migration is that the time interval is often determined by the overall data collection plan, which may or may not be consonant with the needs of other demographic or behavioral changes. Thus, the *life history calendar* approach has gained popularity in several quarters. Here the choice of monthly intervals or annual intervals determines the resolution of population mobility events. There seems to be little research on the optimal data collection intervals for the recovery of these dynamic processes.

Prospective data collection plans offer the advantage of multiple waves of interviews, where current status information is collected. However, sometimes intervening information since the last wave is ascertained. Such plans, while expensive, offer the advantage of reducing recall error. This may be particularly advantageous for improving the accuracy of reporting for residential histories, because current residence is accurately noted, and perception of a short migratory stay in a person's history does not cloud the information set.

Given that migratory behavior is so interwoven with other repeatable events, such as health episodes, fertility, and employment transitions, explicit timing information dramatically improves the (potential) quality of the analysis that can be conducted. Whereas analysts were once restricted to tabulations of migration differentials for a broad census-based or survey-based interval (with some of the traits of interest perhaps changing during that interval) contemporary analyses can begin to sort out the *temporal* ordering of events on the way to sorting out the *causal* ordering of events.

The discussion above has concentrated on the temporal dimension of migration, in keeping with the substantial growth of event-history models throughout the social sciences. A parallel methodological development has been the use of models that capture a variety of mobility outcomes or choices among a set of alternative destinations. Most of these approaches, now well established in the migration literature, rely on discrete choice models. Thus the analyst might use a multinomial logit model to predict interprovincial versus intraprovincial migration (Liang, Chen, and Gu 2002; Greenwood et al., 1991a). Along these same lines the "choice set" might include a number of metropolitan areas or states and in this way provide the microdata companion to the analysis of origin-destination streams discussed above. A further extension of this approach, building on some theoretical thinking about the migration decision itself (Speare, Goldstein, and Frey 1975), separates the departure decision from the destination choice. Outmigration is modeled as a dichotomous outcome, and destination choice is modeled as a multinomial set.

Contextual and Multilevel Models

We present here without much elaboration a discussion of the opportunities for contextual models in migration analyses. To some degree empirical analysis of internal migration has incorporated context for some time. Many studies have included characteristics of the region, metropolitan area, or other such information in the specification. For example, many analyses of internal migration have included among the regressors measures of climate or overall economic activity (industrial structure, unemployment rate, and the like). More recent studies add to the sophistication of the contextual approach. These have modeled the migratory behavior of the individual as a function of the characteristics of the household in the aggregate or of other specific household members. Such characteristics may include such examples as the employment status or income of a spouse or the number of young children in the household. Less well developed, but likely to increase, are approaches that are multilevel, where formal modeling of the community level effects is part of the focus.

Aggregate Data and Analysis

The above discussion has emphasized micro approaches. There still remains, however, a large array of instances in which aggregate data and the tools for their analysis come into play.

Tabulations of data by origin and destination produce a gross migration matrix. Such NxN matrices can, in turn, be analyzed by a variety of techniques based on regression models where the flow is taken to be a function of characteristics of the sending and receiving communities. Log-linear models, particularly suitable for cross-tables of this sort, have in some cases been used to capture, as discussed above, the structure of origin-destination relationships, often with the impact of having other regional characteristics measured as well (Herting et al. 1997; Lin and Xie 1998). Analysis of these tabulations can be extended to include a variety of origin and destination traits. Gravity models, where origin-destination distance figures prominently, constitute one major subset.

The parallel of such data structure with the approach to demographic analysis through multistate or multiregional models is clear (Schoen 1988; Rogers 1995). In such approaches one examines the structure of the transition matrix, fits parameters to predict the size of flows within, and conducts formal demographic analysis to understand the implications of transition probabilities. Moreover, the substantively oriented analyst can look at such transition processes, at the micro level or with aggregated data, and endeavor to discern the traits of individuals or places that govern population movement. Finally, transition probabilities arising from such models can be used to inform population projections in a manner superior to ad hoc adjustment for net migration.

There remains a place for net migration in demographic analysis. Improvements in theory, data, and method generally favor analysis of microdata and gross migration, wherever possible. In many cases, however, such detail is not available and net migration (NM), that is, the residual from a location's population change between two time points after removing the increments from births and deaths, will be the best available information. To be sure, net migration may be the only available information for smaller areas and locations in some settings where gross migration tabulations are not made. While often superseded, net migration calculations still provide a direct measure of the net population redistribution, often by age and sex, with telling insights into the forces of regional growth and decline.

EMPIRICAL FINDINGS

Descriptive empirical studies regularly turn up several regularities in the propensity for geographical mobility in the population. Certain regularities seem almost universal, while others seem to be true for most high-income settings, and others may vary with time and place. Perhaps the earliest and most complete compendium of the relationship of demographic traits to migration propensity was contained in the classic scholarly work of Dorothy Swaine Thomas, *Research Memorandum on Migration Differentials*, which included chapters on differentials by age, sex, family status, physical health, mental health, intelligence, occupation, and "motivation and assimilation" (Thomas et al. 1938). While the richness of data and sophistication of methods for contemporary scholars extend well beyond what Thomas could access, many of the same fundamental associations persist.

Age is the demographic trait that is probably most consistently related to migration. Theory insists it should be so. Age itself, of course, marks life-cycle stage and other behavioral characteristics. While the use of age profiles has been well established for decades in the literature on mortality, fertility, and nuptiality, the age regularity of geographical mobility has probably been less universally incorporated by demographers. (For more discussion, see chapter 1 in this *Handbook*.)

Tabulated data for geographical mobility in the past year (or five years) show a distinct age profile in almost any society. Figure 11.4 presents the one-year pattern identified by Long in survey data from six high-income countries (Long 1992). While it is true that New Zealand and the United States show relatively high levels of mobility at every age, it is also true that all of these profiles show a peak in the 20s and decline from there steadily to the elderly ages. The graph for the youngest ages also reveals a consistent pattern with rates of mobility highest in infancy and the first few years of life, declining to the teen years before rising to the peak in the 20s. The life-cycle behavior attached to these graphs is not hard to discern. Infants and young children move with their parents; teenage mobility is low, mirroring that of the parental

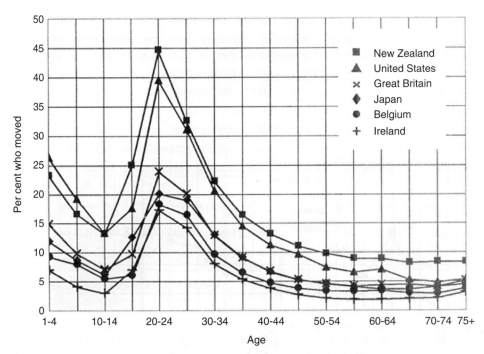

FIGURE 11.4. The age profile of mobility. Source: Long (1992).

generation; and young adulthood, a time of schooling, labor market entry and adjustment, and initial family formation, is a time of frequent moves.

International comparisons of moves across migration-defining boundaries that would separate local mobility from interregional migration are more difficult. The wide variation in national geography and administrative geography works against the uniformity that demographers covet. Nevertheless, the age profile persists (Rogers 1984), even as calculations of ratios across countries can identify likely differences in mobility regimes. Remarkably, too, this age profile has been fairly stable over time in many settings, shifting somewhat upward or downward to reflect broad societal forces. Poulain, for instance, finds that the 1970 and 1992 age-specific migration patterns (between *arrondissements*) are quite similar (Poulain 1996: Figure 6.4).

Stepping beyond these tabulations and graphs, it is possible to model the age pattern of mobility or migration. Rogers and colleagues have done this for a variety of populations and settings. Most age profiles fit reasonably well with a small set of parameters, built around a double-exponential model (Rogers 1984). The parameters describe the life-cycle pattern of declining mobility of children with age (reflecting parental mobility), increasing, then decreasing mobility in the labor force years, and then, in many societies, a "blip" linked to retirement migration.

Sex differentials in migration are less uniform. The best generalization that seems to be made is that internal migration to frontier areas of current LDCs is characterized by a relatively high sex ratio. As migration continues to the area, the sex ratio seems to come more into balance. Growth in labor market opportunities and the demographic diversification of the migrant stream, family formation and reunification all provide important incentives for female migration (Donato 1993). Moreover, as Pedraza argues, despite the persistent perception that migratory streams, especially LDC job-seeker streams, are overwhelmingly male, women do compose substantial fractions and even the majority of several major migration streams (Pedraza 1991).

In most societies migrants are identifiable as individuals seeking returns on their skills. This typically generates migrant streams that are differentiated by human capital. The more dispersed the geographical returns to human capital (educational and occupational status) the more visible the demographic differentiation. Such human capital differentials were identified in the earliest descriptive studies of migration, and they remain detectable in present data. These, of course, are differentials that are responsive to *relative* educational attainment; it is the more skilled who move, even as the average level of educational attainment increases. Generally, in high-income societies one finds a positive association between educational attainment (as a key indicator of human capital) and the probability of making a long-distance move. This certainly has been true of the United States for many decades of the 20th century (Long 1988: 173). In a recent study of the United States, Tolnay found that for about a century, black migrants out of the southern U.S. possessed higher educational attainment than the southern population they left behind and lower educational levels than the northern population they joined (Tolnay 1998). Such a study both confirms the continued relevance of migrant selectivity and indicates that "positive" selection from the origin may introduce a relatively disadvantaged migrant stream to a host community.

Has there been an overall increase in mobility and migration? And has there been a decline in the effect of distance in retarding migration? Much commentary would contest that contemporary industrial societies are highly mobile and becoming ever more so. At the same time, changes in transportation and communication technology should make long-distance moves easier by improving information about distant labor markets, reducing the outlay to relocate, and easing the psychic costs of leaving one's community of origin.

The characterization of ever-increasing mobility is not really borne out empirically, however, at least for the United States. While it is true that annual rates of overall mobility, intercounty migration, and interstate migration as a fraction of intercounty migration have all fluctuated over time, there is no strong, discernable trend in the pattern. Figure 11.5 shows various one-year mobility and migration rates for the United States from 1948 through 2000. One can observe that about 20% of the population moved in the preceding year; if anything, this fraction has declined slightly during the 50-year period. The share of all moves that are intercounty moves (a standard classification for migration) has increased modestly.

Even in advanced industrial societies, distance is a significant impediment to migration. Work with a gravity model for Belgium shows very little change in the effect of distance on migration from around 1980 to around 1990 (Poulain 1996). Detailed work on this issue across three 20th-century decades in the more geographically extensive United States found that a declining effect of distance came into play only at distances over 1,500 miles (Mueser 1989b).

Life cycle and family transitions also sharply differentiate mobility propensity. Moreover, they operate in distinguishable ways on local mobility and interregional migration. In any simple descriptive tabulation, rates of recent (overall) geographical mobility are higher for those who are young, unmarried, and have fewer children of school age. These simple differences point to a set of links between life course transitions and residential mobility and migration. The transition from adolescence through young adulthood and into established adulthood is "demographically dense" (Rindfuss 1991), meaning that a large number of life-cycle transitions are squeezed into a narrow age window. School completion, full-time labor force entry, marriage, and the onset of

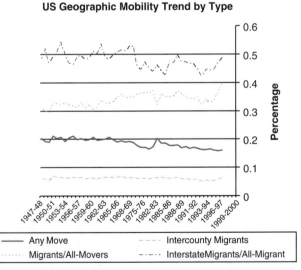

FIGURE 11.5. Trend in U.S. mobility and migration by type. Source: Tabulations from U.S. Census Bureau, Current Population Survey, March 2000.

parenthood all occur within the space of a few years in advanced industrial societies. These transitions are extraordinarily consequential for mobility. Virtually by definition, the household formation and reconstitution transitions generate local mobility while labor force transitions generate both local and, particularly, long-distance mobility, as described above. This combination gives rise, of course, to the sharp age profile of migration described earlier.

More focused multivariate empirical studies help tease out more information about the determinants of local mobility and migration. Housing and family structure transitions more clearly drive local mobility, something that has long been recognized and for which there is ample empirical support (Rossi 1980). One can even think of a set of moves across housing units as a life-cycle-linked "housing career," with the exact sequence predicted in part by income growth and family status (Clark, Deurloo, and Dieleman 2003). In almost every high-income society home ownership is associated with lower rates of mobility. Nevertheless, both age-profile indications and direct empirical measurement suggest that family life-cycle variables also influence migration. For example, in one nationally representative U.S. study, the hazard rate of intercounty and interstate mobility for married men is about half that of unmarried men, even after controlling for age (Sandefur and Scott 1981: 364). The presence of children or larger families further deters migration.

Just as human capital traits are strongly related to migration, so too are labor market conditions strongly related to migration in the adult years. It has long been found that economic opportunity at potential destinations attracts migrants. Empirical analyses of interregional migration almost universally find that measures of recent economic growth, economic base, and unemployment rates help predict the volume of migration. Specifications differ, with macromodels generally examining the flow of persons to and from provinces, counties, and states, and micromodels examining the determinants of migration at the level of the individual.

Interregional migration studies have long tried to incorporate the potential effects of fixed-place characteristics, also termed nontradable goods (Mueser and Graves 1995; Mueser 1989a). Sunshine, proximity to an ocean or mountains, and various other amenities can only be consumed via residential location. Desire to consume such amenities will generate a migratory flow to destinations that are amenity-rich. Although descriptive data clearly point to such amenity-influenced movements in many countries (U.S., France, and Germany, for example), statistically identifying their impact is nontrivial. The effects of amenities per se must be separated out from other factors which may be correlated, such as wage rates and the price of land and housing. Population redistribution to a lower-density location may indicate the appeal of lower wage rates (and land prices) for employers as well as any intrinsic appeal of the local landscape for potential migrants. Demographic traits of the current residential community and anthropogenic influences on the local environment are extensions of this line of thinking with respect to migration. Among anthropogenic effects, dis-amenities have also received some attention. The presumption here is that individuals will move away from, or be less likely to move to, locations where there is a significant amount of pollution or other environmental risk. Throughout all such studies a challenge exists to properly specify the relationship. Migrants undoubtedly care about the social and physical traits of current and potential communities, but they must weigh their value (and risks) against the other economic and social opportunities that these locations present.

Another class of characteristics that helps generate and guide migrant flows is that of human social networks. Social science writing has long recognized the importance of interpersonal connections in sustaining both internal and international movement. Boyd (1989) and Goldscheider (1987) write compellingly about the importance of family and other interpersonal networks in migration. But what is new is the availability of data and methods to capture the relative influence of such characteristics on movement. It is likely that both internal migration and international migration view the operation of networks in similar ways.

Networks, whether of family or friends, operate to influence the probability of migration and the choice of destination in several ways (Curran 2002). Networks carry information about potential destinations, including job opportunities. Even imperfect information may enhance the probability of movement to a particular locale where kin and friends already live. Migrant networks can aid adjustment and assimilation at the destination. Origin-destination connections, sustained by the circulation of individuals and the passage of remittances, help undergird the household risk management strategy discussed above. Recent research has uncovered clear evidence of the importance of family structure in determining the social organization of migration (Lauby and Stark 1988; Root and De Jong 1991; Smith and Thomas 1998). Work related to migration patterns diverse as Mexico-U.S. movement and internal migration in sub-Saharan Africa indicates that this social organization can become institutionalized and, to a degree, self-sustaining (Massey 1990; Guilmoto 1998). This phenomenon may be seen as a manifestation of the cumulative causation model of migration and is consistent with balancing risk.

Migrant adaptation is an issue as old as migration itself. The topic is suitable for more extensive review than is possible here, but a few key relationships merit discussion. It is a verity that the contemporary concern for the ability of rural-urban migrants to adapt to their host metropolitan communities in contemporary developing settings fairly parallels the concern during earlier times in present MDCs. Even more, the issues of adaptation by international migrants in their host societies offer yet another parallel. In fact, one could argue that the assimilation or adaptation process is really much the same in all such settings, with particular variations introduced by linguistic and cultural heterogeneity, by variations in the technology of communication and transport, and by crucial variation in the policies of the nation-state.

MIGRATION, URBANIZATION, AND ECONOMIC DEVELOPMENT.   Migration has long been linked to urbanization, especially during processes of economic development. For contemporary high-income countries, periods of industrialization were accompanied by urban growth. While some urban growth in any period is accounted for by natural increase, a substantial fraction and often the majority of urban growth was due to net rural-urban migration.

Empirical analyses and technical demographic work are more readily available for the current set of countries making the urbanization-development transition. For many of these middle and low-income countries, demographic analysis indicates that net migration (from rural areas) accounts for 40% to 60% of urban growth (Chen, Valente, and Zlotnick 1998; NRC 2003). A simulation analysis suggests that migration may account for a much larger fraction of urban growth in some developing settings with low fertility settings, such as contemporary China (NRC 2003). A couple of empirical patterns, almost natural experiments, provide simple examples of the link between migration and economic development. The case of China is particularly revelatory. As previously mentioned, China has regulated residence through the *hukou* system, in which local residents were registered at a particular location. In the times of state socialism these registrations gave access to certain state provisions and services. With market transformation, a huge flow of unregulated and conventional migrants sprung up. Analysis of the 1990 census points to nearly 11 million interprovincial moves in the preceding five years (Poston and Mao 1998). "Floating" or unauthorized migrants, persons living outside their place of permanent registration, have been estimated in the 1990s to be a large as 68 million (Liang 2001), and data from the 2000 census show that their number may be as large as 140 million (Liang and Ma 2002). The very size and persistence of these migration streams is testimony to the strong link between economic development and population redistribution.

Another example comes from Germany. After World War II partition, migration within East Germany, with its more stringent labor market and housing regulations, declined steadily to the point where, by the 1970s, migration rates were as low as one-third of those in West Germany (Bucher and Gatzweiler 1996).

While there is certainly an association between the occurrence of migration, urbanization, and economic development, the exact link between demographic processes and economic development is more difficult to discern. Concern has often been voiced in the literature with regard to whether certain regions or countries were "overurbanized" or "underurbanized" for their level of economic development. Of note, perhaps, is the fact that urbanization rates vary widely, and that, on average, contemporary urbanization rates (the change in the population fraction that is urban) are not out of line with the historical experience of contemporary industrialized countries (NRC 2003).

RESEARCH DIRECTIONS

In this final section we highlight some of the features of the demographic landscape that suggest new directions in the years to come.

Data

One of the most far-reaching changes for population investigators has been, as mentioned above, the tremendous growth of data, particularly microdata surveys. This pattern should continue, as both the interest in behavioral modeling and the techniques for such modeling spur efforts by scholars and government agencies to collect data for individuals.

Within the realm of microdata, one of the most promising developments is the movement toward longitudinal or event-history information about individuals, as already discussed. Despite concerns that many data collection efforts to date have been deficient in the collection of residential histories, there are optimistic signs. Many nationally representative life history surveys contain the needed detail for mobility studies. The Panel Study of Income Dynamics (U.S.) and the Indonesian and Malaysian Family Life Surveys are examples. The Mexican Migration Project and the Latin American Migration Project both contain a wealth of such information. The wide cross-national reach of the Demographic and Health Surveys has added value for migration studies in that some surveys do contain limited residential histories.

Geographical Information

In recent years there has been a virtual explosion in the technology of Geographic Information Systems (GIS). This new technology holds enormous promise for students of migration and population distribution. Quite obviously, GIS expedites and coordinates the systematic collection, organization, and merging of spatially identified data. Moreover, GIS has generally allowed both more refined geography *and* the "layering" of geographies. Where once the social scientist was bound by the set of administrative or statistical units contained in a census or some other geographical classification, it is now possible to identify origins, potential destinations, and additional features of the landscape that influence migration down to a point in a two-dimensional coordinate system. Moreover, the technology of GIS is allowing the analyst to nest households, employment sites, locational amenities, and the like into a set of hierarchically organized geographical units.

Such evolving technology can be invoked only with some burden, however. First, the user must master the new technology itself, although all developments point to a greater ease of using computer-assisted GIS for both descriptive and analytical purposes. Second, the availability of point-level information challenges the research community intellectually. Researchers will no longer be bound by given administrative and census categories, such as states, provinces, wards, and tracts. They must now think about what space means socially. Is it best for a particular analysis to proceed and to use the level of extreme resolution—the point? Or are those administrative units or catchment areas (metropolitan areas and provinces) of intrinsic value in the study of a migration behavior or pattern? Undoubtedly, state-of-the-art work in the coming years will address the issue of the relative merits (and most likely, the integration) of both point-level and aggregate information for understanding internal migration.

A third challenge lies in the management of this technology itself. The novice is readily swamped by an extraordinary amount of information, data that need to be coordinated and managed. As analysts move from using GIS software for simple description, as in maps, to more analytical application, as in multilevel statistical modeling with spatial autoregression, these challenges grow. Again it is likely that computer applications and the ability to work with these GIS sources will keep pace with the scale of the information itself. A greater challenge is that of data security and confidentiality. This problem permeates social science data collection, but it may be especially acute in the case of geographically augmented data sets. There are both administrative and technological ways to address this issue; secure data files and randomized, or "masked," data placed in the public domain are but two solutions. It is clear, however, that there will remain some tension between the need to preserve confidentiality and the desire to retain as much geographical and behavioral detail as possible.

Theory, Concept, and Empirical Frontiers

What are some of the new directions in the study of internal migration? New substantive concerns are probably most difficult to predict. To be sure, analysts will continue to be concerned directly with the adjustment of the labor force through migration. In both high-income and low-income societies a number of policy-oriented questions that link migration to the delivery of services (income security, health care provision, local schooling) will evolve as the issues themselves shift. There is likely to be growth in the study of the relationship between migration and other demographic events, a growth abetted by the improvement in data quality. Thus investigators will be able to gain increasing knowledge about the relationship—between family structure—for instance the number of children or spousal employment—and migration. Migrant adaptation has long been a concern of analysts. Future studies, exploiting the richness of longitudinal data, may be able to arrive at a better understanding of how well rural-urban migrants adapt in developing settings, parallel to an understanding of how well interregional migrants and immigrants adapt in high-income host countries.

Contextual models, themselves a growth area in the social sciences, will see further development in the field of migration and population distribution. As described above, research has for some time incorporated characteristics of place of origin or destination in models of interregional migration. Research at the frontier is likely to make more energetic use of contextual models: on the theoretical side, developing a more sophisticated notion of the way "place and space" influence behavior; and on the technical side, employing refined data management and statistical techniques for capturing the influence of distance, neighborhood, or province context on population redistribution. GIS and spatially augmented data are likely to stimulate more refined work on the relationship between migration and amenities, especially the role of environmental hazards and attractions to both local movers and interregional migrants (Hunter 2000).

It is also likely that future work will include efforts to integrate studies of internal migration with research on local mobility and international migration. These three subfields of geographical mobility have proceeded on somewhat independent tracks, partly due to understandable differences in the focal variables that drive the behavior and partly due to alternative sources of data. Clearly, however, space is continuous, determinants of movement are multiple, and the ability to stretch concepts may pay dividends to the analyst. In a related development there may be more efforts to integrate, especially theoretically, the study of migration for LDCs and MDCs. There are many points of intersection, with some clear points of separation, and historical parallels (see also Massey 1999). Other new developments—the role of networks, multilevel models, and concerns about heterogeneity and selection processes—are manifest simultaneously in both literatures.

Continued urbanization, changes in the technology of transport and communication, and the social science technology that allows researchers to understand population distribution all suggest changes in the categories of measurement, both at a point in time and across time (Hugo, Champion, and Lattes 2003; NRC 2003). Already this rethinking has begun on several fronts. These promising new developments in the study of population distribution are very likely to usher in another round of rethinking of the "settlement system" itself.

New technical tools, data, and conceptual frameworks will significantly impact the study of internal migration in the near future. These developments will provide insights into the behavioral determinants and consequences of migration.

REFERENCES

Baccaini, B., and D. Pumain. 1996. Migration in France between 1975 and 1990: A limited degree of decentralization. In *Population migration in the European Union*. Edited by P. H. Rees, J. Stillwell, A. Convey, and M. Kupiszewski, 191–206. New York: John Wiley.

Banerjee, B. 1981. Rural-urban migration and family ties: An analysis of family considerations in migration behavior in India. *Oxford Bulletin of Economics and Statistics* 43(4):321–355.

Baydar, N., M. J. White, C. Simkins, and O. Babakol. 1990. Effects of agricultural development policies on migration in peninsular Malaysia. *Demography* 27:97–109.

Becker, C. M., and A. R. Morrison. 1986. Urbanization in transforming economies. In *Handbook of regional and urban economics*. Edited by P. Cheshire and E. S. Mills. Amsterdam: Elsevier North-Holland.

Bell, M., M. Blake, P. Boyle, O. Duke-Williams, P. H. Rees, J. Stillwell, and G. Hugo. 2002. Cross-national comparison of internal migration: Issues and measures. *Journal of the Royal Statistical Society Series A-Statistics in Society* 165(Part 3):435–464.

Berg, E. J. 1961. Backward-sloping labor supply functions in dual economies—the Africa case. *Quarterly Journal of Economics* 75:468–492.

Bilsborrow, R. E. 1998a. The state of the art and overview of the chapters. In *Migration, urbanization, and development: New directions and issues*. Edited by R. E. Bilsborrow, 1–56. New York: United Nations Population Fund & Kluwer Academic Publishers.

Bilsborrow, R. E. 1998b. *Migration, urbanization, and development: New directions and issues*. New York: United Nations Population Fund & Kluwer Academic Publishers.

Bilsborrow, R. E., and P. F. DeLargy. 1991. Land use, migration, and natural resource deterioration: The experience of Guatemala and the Sudan. In *Resources, environment, and population: Present knowledge, future options*. Edited by K. Davis and M. S. Bernstam, 125–147. New York: The Population Council.

Bilsborrow, R. E., T. M. McDevitt, S. Kossoudji, and R. Fuller. 1987. The impact of origin community characteristics on rural-urban out-migration in a developing country. *Demography* 24(2):191–210.

Bogue, D. J. 1959. Internal migration. In *The study of population*. Edited by P. M. Hauser and O. D. Duncan. Chicago: University of Chicago Press.

Boyd, M. 1989. Family and personal networks in international migration. *International Migration Review* 23:638–670.

Bravo-Ureta, B. E., R. E. Quiroga, and J. A. Brea. 1996. Migration decisions, agrarian structure, and gender: The case of Ecuador. *The Journal of Developing Areas* 30:463–476.

Brettel, C. 2000. *Migration theory: Talking across disciplines*. New York: Routledge.

Brockerhoff, M., and X. Yang. 1994. Impact of migration on fertility in sub-Saharan Africa. *Social Biology* 41(1–2):19–43.

Brown, L. A., and A. R. Goetz. 1987. Development-related contextual effects and individual attributes in Third World migration processes: A Venezuelan example. *Demography* 24(4):497–516.

Bucher, H., and H.-P. Gatzweiler. 1996. Interregional migration patterns and processes in Germany. In *Population migration in the European Union*. Edited by P. H. Rees, J. Stillwell, A. Convey, and M. Kupiszewski, 123–144. New York: John Wiley.

Caces, F., F. Arnold, J. T. Fawcett, and R. W. Gardner. 1985. Shadow households and competing auspices. *Journal of Development Economics* 17:5–25.

Carrington, W., E. Detragiache, and T. Vishwanath. 1996. Migration with endogenous moving costs. *American Economic Review* 86(4):909–930.

Champion, A. G. 1992. *Migration processes and patterns*. London, New York: Belhaven Press.

Chattopadhyay, A. 1998. Gender, migration, and career trajectories in Malaysia. *Demography* 35(3):335–344.

Chen, N., P. Valente, and H. Zlotnik. 1998. What do we know about recent trends in urbanization? In *Migration, urbanization, and development: New directions and issues*. Edited by R. E. Bilsborrow, 59–88. New York: United Nations Population Fund & Kluwer Academic Publishers.

Clark, W., M. Deurloo, and F. Dieleman. 2003. Housing careers in the United States, 1968–93: Modeling the sequencing of housing states. *Urban Studies* 40(1):143–160.

Clay, J. W., S. Steingraber, and P. Niggli. 1988. *The spoils of famine: Ethiopian famine policy and peasant agriculture*. Cambridge, Mass.: Cultural Survival.

Cole, W. E., and R. D. Sanders. 1985. International migration and urban employment in the Third World. *American Economic Review* 75(3):481–494.

Collins, J. L. 1985. Migration and the life cycle of households in southern Peru. *Urban Anthropology* 14(4):279–299.

Cunha, J. M. P. D. 1998. New trends in urban settlement and the role of intraurban migration: The case of Sao Paulo/Brazil. In *Migration, urbanization, and development: New directions and issues.* Edited by R. E. Bilsborrow, 121–153. New York: United Nations Population Fund & Kluwer Academic Publishers.

Curran, S. 2002. Migration, social capital, and the environment: Considering migrant selectivity and networks in relation to coastal ecosystems. *Population and Development Review* 28:89–125.

De Jong, G. F. 2000. Expectations, gender, and norms in migration decision-making. *Population Studies* 54:307–319.

De Jong, G. F., and M. C. Legazpi Blair. 1994. Occupational status of rural outmigrants and return migrants. *Rural Sociology* 59(4):693–707.

de Lattes, Z. R. 1989. Women in internal and international migration, with special reference to Latin America. *Population Index* 55(4):95–107.

Donato, K. M. 1993. Current trends and patterns of female migration: Evidence from Mexico. *International Migration Review* 27(4):748–771.

Economic Commission for Latin America and the Caribbean. 1994. Latin America and the Caribbean: Notes on population, environment and development. In *Population, environment and development*, 235–239. New York: United Nations.

Falaris, E. 1979. The determinants of internal migration in Peru: An economic analysis. *Economic Development and Cultural Change* 27(2):327–341.

Fearnside, P. M. 1986. Spatial concentration of deforestation in the Brazilian Amazon. *Ambio* 15(2):74–81.

Findley, S. E. 1987. An interactive contextual model of migration in Ilocos Norte, the Philippines. *Demography* 24(2):196–190.

Flowerdew, R. 1992. Labour market operation and geographical mobility. In *Migration processes and patterns.* Edited by A. G. Champion and A. J. Fielding. London, New York: Belhaven Press.

Frey, W. H. 1987. Migration and depopulation of the metropolis: Regional restructuring or rural renaissance? *American Sociological Review* 52(2):240–257.

Frey, W. H. 1996. Immigration, domestic migration, and demographic balkanization in America: New evidence for the 1990s. *Population and Development Review* 22(4):741–763.

Garrison, H. 1982. Internal migration in Mexico: A test of the Todaro Model. *Food Research Institute Studies* 27:197–214.

Goldscheider, C. 1987. Migration and social structure: Analytic issues and comparative perspectives in developing nations. *Sociological Forum* 2(4):674–696.

Greenwood, M. J., G. L. Hunt, D. S. Rickman, and G. I. Treyz. 1991a. Migration, regional equilibrium, and the estimation of compensating differentials. *The American Economic Review* 81(5):1382–1390.

Greenwood, M. J., P. R. Mueser, D. Plane, and A. M. Schlottmann. 1991b. New directions in migration research: Perspectives from some North American regional science disciplines. *Annals of Regional Science* 25:237–270.

Guilmoto, C. Z. 1998. Institutions and migrations, short-term versus long-term moves in rural West Africa. *Population Studies* 52(1):85–103.

Haag, G., M. Munz, R. Reiner, and W. Weidlich. 1988. Federal Republic of Germany. In *Interregional migration.* Edited by W. Weidlich and G. Haag. Berlin: Springer.

Hardoy, J., and D. Satterthwaite. 1989. *Squatter citizens: Life in the urban Third World.* London: Earthscan Publications.

Harris, J. R., and M. P. Todaro. 1970. Migration, unemployment, and development: A two-sector analysis. *American Economic Review* 60:126–142.

Herting, J. R., D. B. Grusky, and S. E. Van Rompaey. 1997. The social geography of interstate mobility and persistence. *American Sociological Review* 62:267–287.

Hugo, G. 1982. Circular migration in Indonesia. *Population and Development Review* 8(1):59–83.

Hugo, G. 1985. Structural change and labour mobility in rural Java. In *Labour circulation and the labour process.* Edited by G. Standing, 46–88. London: Croom Helm.

Hugo, G., A. G. Champion, and A. Lattes. 2003. Toward a new conceptualization of settlements for demography. *Population and Development Review* 29(2):277–297.

Hunter, L. 2000. The spatial association between U.S. immigrant residential concentration and environmental hazards. *International Migration Review* 34:460–488.

Illeris, S. 1996. Changing patterns of net migration in Denmark: An explanatory analysis. In *Population migration in the European Union.* Edited by P. H. Rees, J. Stillwell, A. Convey, and M. Kupiszewski, 105–122. New York: John Wiley.

Jones, J. R. 1990. *Colonization and environment: Land settlement projects in Central America*. Tokyo: United Nations University Press.

Katz, E., and O. Stark. 1986. Labor migration and risk aversion in less developed countries. *Journal of Labor Economics* 4(1):134–149.

Kay, G. 1982. Population redistribution in Zimbabwe. In *Redistribution of population in Africa*. Edited by J. I. Clark and L. A. Kosinski, 85–94. London: Heinemann.

Kritz, M. M., and J. M. Nogle. 1994. Nativity concentration and internal migration among the foreign-born. *Demography* 31(3):509–524.

Lauby, J., and O. Stark. 1988. Individual migration as a family strategy: Young women in the Philippines. *Population Studies* 42(3):473–486.

Lee, E. S. 1966. A theory of migration. *Demography* 3(1):47–57.

Levy, M. B., and W. J. Wadycki. 1974. Education and the decision to migrate: An econometric analysis of migration in Venezuela. *Econometrica* 42:377–388.

Lewis, W. A. 1954. Economic development with unlimited supplies of labour. *Manchester School of Economic and Social Studies* 22:139–191.

Liang, Z. 2001. The age of migration in China. *Population and Development Review* 27(3):499–524.

Liang, Z., Y. P. Chen, and Y. Gu. 2002. Rural industrialisation and internal migration in China. *Urban Studies* 39(12):2175–2187.

Liang, Z. and Z. Ma. 2004. China's Floating Population: New Evidence from the 2000 Census. *Population and Development Review* 30(3):467–488.

Lichter, D. T., and G. Fuguitt. 1982. The transition to nonmetropolitan population deconcentration. *Demography* 19(2):211–221.

Lin, G., and Y. Xie. 1998. The loglinear modeling of interstate migration: Some additional considerations. *American Sociological Review* 63:900–907.

Lindstrom, D. P. 2003. Rural-Urban Migration and Reproductive Behavior in Guatemala. *Population Research and Policy Review* 22(4):351–372.

Lindstrom, D. P., and E. Muñoz-Franco. 2003. Migration networks and modern contraceptive knowledge and use in rural Guatemala. Minneapolis, Minn.: 2003 Annual Meeting of the Population Association of America.

Long, L. 1988. *Migration and residential mobility*. New York: Russell Sage.

Long, L. 1992. Changing residence: Comparative perspectives on its relationship to age, sex, and marital status. *Population Studies* 46:141–158.

Long, L., and F. DeAre. 1988. US population redistribution: A perspective on the nonometropolitan turnaround. *Population and Development Review* 14(3):433–450.

Long, L., and A. Nucci. 1997. The clean break revisited: Is US population again deconcentrating? *Environment and Planning A* 29(1):355–366.

Long, L., C. J. Tucker, and W. Urton. 1988. Migration distances: An international comparison. *Demography* 25(4):633–640.

Lucas, R. E. B. 1997. Internal migration in developing countries. In *Handbook of population and family economics*. Edited by M. R. Rosenzweig and O. Stark. New York: Elsevier.

Massey, D. 1990. Social structure, household strategies and the cumulative causation of migration. *Population Index* 56:3–26.

Massey, D. 1999. Why does immigration occur? A theoretical synthesis. In *The handbook on international migration*. Edited by C. Hirschman, P. Kasinitz, and J. DeWind, 34–52. New York: Russell Sage Foundation.

McGee, T. G., and C. J. Griffiths. 1998. Global urbanization: Towards the twenty-first century. In *Population distribution and migration*, 49–65. New York: United Nations.

Molho, I. 2001. Spatial search, migration and regional unemployment. *Economica* 68:269–283.

Mueser, P. R. 1989a. Measuring the impact of locational characteristics on migration: Interpreting cross-sectional analysis. *Demography* 26(3):499–513.

Mueser, P. R. 1989b. The spatial structure of migration: An analysis of flows between states in the USA over three decades. *Regional Studies* 23(3):185–200.

Mueser, P. R., and P. E. Graves. 1995. Examining the role of economic opportunity and amenities in explaining population redistribution. *Journal of Urban Economics* 37:176–200.

Munz, M., and G. Rabino. 1988. Italy. In *Interregional migration*. Edited by W. Weidlich and G. Haag. Berlin: Springer.

Nam, C. B., W. J. Serow, and D. Sly. 1990. *International handbook on internal migration.* New York: Greenwood Press.

National Research Council (NRC). 2003. Cities transformed: Demographic change and its implications in the developing world. Panel on Population on Urban Population Dynamics, M. R. Montgomery, R. Stren, B. Cohen, and H. E. Reed. Committee on Population, Davison of Behavioral and Social Sciences and Education. Washington, D.C.: The National Academies Press.

Oberai, A. S. 1988. *Land settlement policies and population redistribution in developing countries: Achievements, problems, & prospects.* New York: Praeger.

Obudho, R. A. 1998. Population distribution in Africa: Urbanization under weak economic conditions. In *Population distribution and migration.* New York: United Nations.

Oucho, J. O. 1983. The Kenyan land settlement programme: Its demographic and development implications. Nairobi, Kenya: A study specially prepared for the International Labour Organisation. Population Studies and Research Institute, University of Nairobi.

Oucho, J. O. 1998. Recent internal migration processes in sub-Saharan Africa: Determinants, consequences, and data adequacy issues. In *Migration, urbanization, and development: New directions and issues.* Edited by R. E. Bilsborrow, 89–120. New York: United Nations Population Fund & Kluwer Academic Publishers.

Owen, D., and A. Green. 1992. Migration patterns and trends. In *Migration processes & patterns.* Edited by A. G. Champion and A. J. Fielding. London, New York: Belhaven Press.

Palmer, I. 1985. *The impact of male out-migration on women in farming.* West Hartford, Conn.: Kumarian Press.

Pedraza, S. 1991. Women and migration: The social consequences of gender. *Annual Review of Sociology* 17:303–325.

Plane, D., and G. Mulligan. 1997. Measuring spatial focusing in a migration system. *Demography* 34:251–262.

Poston, D. L., Jr., and M. X. Mao. 1998. Interprovincial migration in China, 1985–1990. *Research in Rural Sociology and Development* 7:227–250.

Poulain, M. 1996. Migration in Belgium: Temporal trends and counterurbanization. In *Population migration in the European Union.* Edited by P. H. Rees, J. Stillwell, A. Convey, and M. Kupiszewski, 91–104. New York: John Wiley.

Ranis, G., and J. C. Fei. 1961. A theory of economic development. *American Economic Review* 51:533–565.

Ravenstein, E. G. 1885. The laws of migration. *Journal of the Royal Statistical Society* 48:167–227.

Rees, P. H., M. Bell, O. Duke-Williams, and M. Blake. 2000. Problems and solutions in the measurement of migration intensities: Australia and Britain compared. *Population Studies—A Journal of Demography* 54(2):207–222.

Rees, P. H., J. Stillwell, A. Convey, and M. Kupiszewski. 1996a. *Population migration in the European Union.* New York: John Wiley.

Rees, P. H., J. Stillwell, A. Convey, and M. Kupiszewski. 1996b. Introduction: Migration in an integrated Europe. In *Population migration in the European Union.* Edited by P. H. Rees, J. Stillwell, A. Convey, and M. Kupiszewski, 1–9. New York: John Wiley.

Richter, K. 1985. Nonmetropolitan growth in the late 1970s: The end of the turnaround? *Demography* 22(2):245–263.

Rindfuss, R. R. 1991. The young adult years: Diversity, structural change, and fertility. *Demography* 28:493–512.

Roberts, K. 1985. Household labour mobility in a modern agrarian economy: Mexico. In *Labour circulation and the labour process.* Edited by G. Standing, 358–381. London: Croom Helm.

Roberts K. D. 1997. China's "tidal wave" of migrant labor: What can we learn from Mexican undocumented migration to the United States? *International Migration Review* 31(2):249–293.

Rogers, A. 1984. *Migration, urbanization, and spatial population dynamics.* Boulder, Colo.: Westview Press.

Rogers, A. 1995. *Multiregional demography: Principles, methods and extensions.* New York: John Wiley.

Root, B. D., and G. F. De Jong. 1991. Family migration in a developing country. *Population Studies* 45:221–233.

Rossi, P. H. 1980. *Why families move.* Beverly Hills/London: Sage Publications.

Saenz, R., and A. Davila. 1992. Chicago return migration to the Southwest: An integrated human capital approach. *International Migration Review* 26(4):1248–1266.

Sandefur, G. D., and W. J. Scott. 1981. A dynamic analysis of migration: An assessment of the effects of age, family and career variables. *Demography* 18(3):355–368.

Satterthwaite, D. 1998. Health and environmental problems in the cities of developing countries. In *Population Distribution and Migration*, 150–177. New York: United Nations.

Schaeffer, P. V. 1987. A family model of migration. *Socio-Economic Planning Sciences* 21(4):263–269.

Schoen, R. 1988. *Modeling multigroup populations*. New York: Plenum Press.

Schultz, T. P. 1971. Rural urban migration in Colombia. *Review of Economics and Statistics* 53:157–163.

Simmons, A. B. 1984. Migration and rural development: Conceptual approaches, research findings and policy issues. Presented at International Conference on Population, 1984. Population Distribution, Migration and Development, 21–25 March, 1983, Hammamet, Tunisia.

Skeldon, R. 1986. On migration patterns in India during the 1970s. *Population and Development Review* 12(4):759–779.

Smith, J. P., and D. Thomas. 1998. On the road—Marriage and mobility in Malaysia. *Journal of Human Resources* 33(4):805–832.

Speare A., Jr., S. Goldstein, and W. H. Frey. 1975. *Residential mobility, migration, and metropolitan change*. Cambridge, Mass.: Ballinger.

Stark, O., and D. Levhari. 1982. On migration and risk in LDCs. *Economic Development and Cultural Change* 31(1):191–196.

Stark, O., and R. E. B. Lucas. 1988. Migration, remittances, and the family. *Economic Development and Cultural Change* 36(3):465–481.

Stillwell, J., and P. Congdon, eds. 1991. *Migration models*. London: Belhaven.

Thomas, D., R. Heberle, E. Hutchinson, E. Isbell, F. Meyer, and S. Riemer. 1938. *Research memorandum on migration differentials*. New York: Social Science Council.

Tienda, M., and K. Booth. 1991. Gender, migration and social change. *International Sociology* 6:51–72.

Todaro, M. P. 1969. A model for labor migration and urban unemployment in less developed countries. *American Economic Review* 59:138–148.

Tolnay, S. E. 1998. Educational selection in the migration of southern blacks, 1880–1990. *Social Forces* 77(3):487–514.

United Nations. 1994. Population dynamics in the large cities of Latin America and the Caribbean. Presented at International Conference on Population and Development, 1994, 18–22 January 1993, Santa Cruz, Bolivia.

United Nations. 1997. *Government views on the relationships between population and environment*. New York: United Nations.

United Nations. 1998. *Population distribution and migration*. New York: United Nations.

United Nations Centre for Human Settlements. 1994. Cities of the developing world. In *Population, environment and development*, 242–248. New York: United Nations.

U. S. Bureau of the Census. 2002. Current Population Survey. Annual Geographical Mobility Rates, By Type of Movement: 1947–2001. http://www.census.gov/population/socdemo/migration/tab-a-l.xls.

Weidlich W., and G. Haag, eds. 1988. *Interregional migration*. Berlin: Springer.

White, M. J., and Z. Liang. 1998. The effect of immigration on the internal migration of the native-born population, 1981–1990. *Population Research and Policy Review* 17(2):141–166.

White, M. J., L. Moreno, and G. Guo. 1995. The interrelation of fertility and geographic mobility in Peru: A hazards model analysis. *International Migration Review* 29:492–514.

White, M. J., and P. R. Mueser. 1988. Implications of boundary choice for the measurement of residential mobility. *Demography* 25(3):443–459.

Whiteford, M. B. 1978. Women, migration, and social change: A Columbian case study. *International Migration Review* 12(2):236–247.

Wilson, F. D. 1986. Temporal and subnational variations in the reversal of migration flows between metropolitan and nonmetropolitan areas: 1935–80. *Social Forces* 65(2):501–524.

Wood, A. P. 1982. Spontaneous agriculture resettlement in Ethiopia, 1950–1974. In *Redistribution of population in Africa*. Edited by J. I. Clarke and L. A. Kosinski, 157–164. London: Heinemann.

World Bank. 1984. *World development report 1984*. New York: Oxford University Press.

Zhu, J. 1998. Rural out-migration in China: A multilevel model. In *Migration, urbanization, and development: New directions and issues*. Edited by R. E. Bilsborrow. New York: United Nations Population Fund & Kluwer Academic Publishers.

CHAPTER 12

International Migration

Susan K. Brown and Frank D. Bean

INTERNATIONAL MIGRATION[1]

Births, deaths, migration: These form the triumvirate that determines the size of any population. Of the three, migration is the hardest to conceptualize and measure. Its very definition changes from country to country, as do the kinds and sources of data that provide possible gauges of its magnitude. According to the United Nations, international migrants in 2000 comprised slightly less than 3% of the world's population. However, international migration has been rapidly increasing. In the latter part of the 20th century, the global number of international migrants more than doubled (Martin and Widgren, 2002). For example, the United Nations Population Division estimates a rise from 75 million to 175 million international migrants between 1965 and 2000. And the increase occurring over the last 15 years of this period (1985 to 2000) represents a rate of growth of more than 4% per year, more than $2\frac{1}{2}$ times the 1.5% annual rate in overall population growth (see Table 12.1).

Countries vary substantially in their concentrations of international migrants. Some nations, like the United States, have always been known as immigration countries (that is, as countries whose policies allow for substantial immigration). Others, like Japan and Spain, have not. Still others, at least until recently, have not seen themselves or been known as immigration countries even though they in fact have been or have become countries of immigration. Germany is a good case in point. Like most developed countries in the world, Germany now receives migrants from elsewhere, either legally or "illegally," in one form or another. In this sense, most of the industrial countries of the world are now experiencing immigration, even if they have yet come

---

[1] Portions of this chapter are based on revised sections of chapter 2 from Bean and Stevens (2003).

TABLE 12.1. Estimated Foreign-Born Population, by Region, 1965–2000

| | Estimated foreign-born population (thousands) | | | | |
Area	1965	1975	1985	1990	2000
World total	75,214	84,494	105,194	119,761	174,781
Developed countries	30,401	38,317	47,991	54,231	104,119
Developing countries	44,813	46,177	57,233	65,530	70,829
	As percentage of total population of region				
Area	1965	1975	1985	1990	2000
World total	2.3	2.1	2.2	2.3	2.9
Developed countries	3.1	3.5	4.1	4.5	8.7
Developing countries	1.9	1.6	1.6	1.6	1.5
	Annual rate of change (percent)				
Area	1965–75	1975–85	1985–90	1990–2000	
World total	1.2	2.2	2.6	4.2	
Developed countries	2.3	2.3	2.4	4.4	
Developing countries	0.3	2.1	2.7	0.9	

Sources: Zlotnik 1999; UN 2002.

to view themselves as immigration countries. Certainly, the movement of peoples from country to country affects politics and economics both nationally and worldwide (see Chapter 23, "Political Demography," in this *Handbook* for more discussion).

This chapter examines definitions, data, trends, theories, and patterns of international migration—at the global level and in the United States. The first part of the chapter explores what migration is, who migrates, whence migrants come and go, and how many migrate. The second part examines theories about why people migrate. The third section focuses on methods and measures. Because the United States is the leading immigration country in the world, the fourth part presents empirical findings dealing with the nature and magnitude of U.S. migrant flows in recent years, together with the demographic and contextual factors that have shaped the reception migrants encounter after they arrive in the United States. The final section outlines some of the directions future research should take.

SUBSTANTIVE CONCERNS

What is Migration?

All migrants are movers, but not all movers are migrants. Migration involves both spatial and temporal dimensions. The temporal dimension of migration has been generally defined as a permanent or semipermanent move, generally of at least one year. Vacationers, seasonal farm workers, and nomads are not migrants, for their moves are not permanent. The spatial dimension generally involves moving a significant but unspecified distance and crossing a geopolitical border, such as a county line in the United States. As a result, migrants change their baseline population of reference and their local networks, whereas movers need not necessarily do so. *International* migration, obviously, involves crossing national borders and thus is distinguished from *internal* migration, which occurs within national boundaries. Internal migrants to and from an area are called in-migrants and out-migrants, while international migrants are known as immigrants when they are moving into a new country and emigrants when they are leaving an old one. The difference between in-migrants and out-migrants is net migration.

Who Migrates?

Migration can be described using several heuristic distinctions, but perhaps the most basic is the difference between voluntary and involuntary migrants. The great majority are voluntary migrants, those who choose to move, usually to join family and friends or to earn a better living. They may be or may not be authorized to move internationally. In a useful typology of migration, Petersen (1975) defines *free migrants* as those who move because of higher aspirations. These pioneering migrants are relatively few in number—first individuals, then groups banding together out of common beliefs or need for security. Despite relatively small numbers, free migrants have a big effect in that they set social patterns and lower the social and economic cost of migration. As these costs diminish, migration becomes a collective behavior, or what Petersen (1975) calls *mass migration*, which can involve millions of people. Such collective behavior characterized the vast European migration to the United States, Canada, Argentina, and Australia in the 19th and early 20th centuries. The second major type of migration is involuntary—those who move because they have to. Petersen distinguishes between *forced* migration, in which the migrants have no choice about whether to leave, from *impelled* migration, in which migrants retain some choice. Flight from wars is impelled; deportation or enslavement is forced. The numbers of such involuntary migrants fluctuate with political uprisings. Interestingly, Petersen does not consider flight from land because of natural elements like droughts or plagues to be a form of involuntary migration. Rather, he classifies it as a primitive form of migration more akin to hunting and gathering or nomadism.

Almost by definition, voluntary migrants are self-selected. Not everyone migrates. Overwhelmingly, migrants are healthy adults in their 20s. The unmarried are most likely to migrate, while families tend to move mainly when the children are young. Although migrants may be seeking better jobs, they tend not to come from the poorest, least educated members of the origin society, for such people have few resources and contacts to enable them to move. In many developing countries, the college-educated are far more likely to emigrate, because they have the most potential to benefit from the move. Even labor migrants are likely to come from families or communities that have already supported other migrants, so that their standard of living is above subsistence and their sense of relative deprivation is strengthened (Stark and Taylor 1989).

Worldwide, women and girls comprise almost half of the international migrant stream (Zlotnik 2003). The growth of the female migration stream has been small in the past 40 years. In the developed world, female migrants are in the slight majority, thanks to policies that promote family reunification and the desire of some women for more rights. In the developing world, men still predominate as labor migrants, although the number of women labor migrants has been rising for years. Even in countries that restrict women's roles, such as Saudi Arabia, women comprise a third of the migration flows. Many of them may be dependents of male laborers, but some work in jobs reserved for women.

How Many Move?

As of 2000, roughly 175 million people were international migrants. The number grew during the latter part of the 20th century at a rate more than double the rate of growth in world population. Although international migrants comprise roughly 3% of the world's population, their destination addresses are concentrated in the developed countries, where they make up almost 9% of the population overall. This proportion varies, from just over 1% in Japan to nearly 25% in Australia to more than 37% in Israel as of 2000 (Table 12.2). Among the OECD countries, many of which have birthrates below replacement, immigrants account for about 65% of population growth (UN 2002).

Over the last four decades, the overall levels and trends of migration have remained fairly stable, although with fluctuations caused by major events such as the breakup of the Soviet Union (Zlotnik 1999). The most notable trend has been toward a greater distribution of immigrants across countries as well as greater variation in the number of immigrants who have settled within countries. In particular, Western Europe, the United States, Canada, Australia, and New Zealand have admitted a disproportionate share of the world's migrants even as these countries' fertility rates have fallen. As a result, whereas in 1965 1 in 20 residents of these countries was a migrant, by the end of the century 1 in 13 had migrated internationally (Zlotnik 1999). However, these immigrants do not originate in the same areas. In the traditional Western receiving countries, the United States, Canada, and Australia, the proportion of migrants from developing countries has been high—up to 80% of all migrants—for several decades. By contrast, in Europe, migration from developing countries has risen, but not so much and not so consistently.

Among the recent events that have influenced migration flows, the breakup of the Eastern bloc has been crucial. Most notably, between 1988 and 1996, Germany repatriated 2.3 million *Aussiedler*, or ethnic Germans living in Eastern Europe, as well as 622,000 East Germans moving to West Germany between 1988 and 1990. But many other Eastern European countries have experienced rising migration with their neighbors, especially as many people returned to their ethnic homelands. In addition, emigration data from the newly independent states show that 1.6 million left between 1990 and 1994, mostly for Germany, Greece, Israel, and the United States. Some of this migration may be involuntary, since the UNHCR enumerated 700,000 refugees and 2.3 million internally displaced persons in the newly independent states in 1991. This level of displacement harks back to the partition of India in 1947, which resulted in one of the most massive "international" migrations in the historical record, with around 12 million people moving from or to India and Pakistan.

Labor migration has changed in the last four decades because of economic restructuring. Whereas many countries in Western Europe curtailed their recruitment of labor migrants after the price of oil rose in the early 1970s, the oil-producing countries of Western Asia began to seek workers. The sources of this labor have varied. In the early 1990s, Saudi Arabia repatriated Yemenis, Jordanians, and Palestinians and turned to workers from Bangladesh, India, Pakistan, and Egypt. In Western Europe, labor migration rose again in the 1980s and certainly in the boom years of the late 1990s, though many workers entered these countries as family members or refugees rather than as labor migrants. The development of the East Asian economy increased labor migration in countries along the Pacific Rim. Japan began to experience labor shortages in low-skilled occupations in the 1980s but had no legal provision to admit unskilled

TABLE 12.2. **Number of Migrants and Refugees and Net Migration in 2000, by Continents and Major Areas**

Region/country	Total population (thousands)	Migrant stock		Number of refugees (thousands)	Refugees as pct of migrant stock	Net migration (average annual, 1995–2000)	
		Number (thousands)	Percent of population			Number (thousands)	Rate per 1,000 pop.
Northern America[1]	314,113	40,844	13.0	635	1.6	1,394	4.6
Europe	727,304	56,100	7.7	2,310	4.1	769	1.1
Australia/New Zealand	22,916	5,555	24.2	63	1.1	103	4.6
Oceania[2]	7,604	150	2.0	37	24.6	−13	−1.7
Caribbean	37,941	1,071	2.8	2	0.1	−72	−2.0
South America	345,738	3,803	1.1	9	0.2	−75	−0.2
Mexico and Central America	135,129	1,070	0.8	28	2.6	−347	−2.7
Africa	793,627	16,277	2.1	3,627	22.3	−447	−0.6
Asia	3,672,342	49,781	1.4	9,121	18.3	−1,311	−0.4
Greatest net receiving countries							
USA	283,230	34,988	12.4	508	1.5	1,250	4.5
Rwanda	7,609	89	1.2	28	31.9	395	62.8
Russia	145,491	13,259	9.1	26	0.2	287	2.0
Germany	82,017	7,349	9.0	906	12.3	185	2.3
Canada	30,757	5,826	18.9	127	2.2	144	4.8
Italy	57,530	1,634	2.8	7	0.4	118	2.0
Bosnia[3]	3,977	96	2.4	38	39.7	100	27.0
Hong Kong	6,860	2,701	39.4	1	0.0	99	15.1
UK	59,415	4,029	6.8	121	3.0	95	1.6
Australia	19,138	4,705	24.6	58	1.2	95	5.1
Liberia	2,913	160	5.5	69	43.4	90	36.5
Saudi Arabia	20,346	5,255	25.8	5	0.1	80	4.3
Singapore	4,018	1,352	33.6	0	0.0	74	19.6
Japan	127,096	1,620	1.3	4	0.2	56	0.4
Israel	6,040	2,256	37.4	4	0.2	52	9.1
Greatest net sending countries							
Bangladesh	137,439	988	0.7	22	2.2	−60	−0.5
Tajikistan	6,087	330	5.4	15	4.7	−61	−10.3
Pakistan	141,256	4,243	3.0	2,001	47.2	−70	−0.5
Sudan	31,095	780	2.5	415	53.2	−77	−2.6
Egypt	67,884	169	0.2	7	4.0	−80	−1.2
Burundi	6,356	77	1.2	27	35.1	−80	−12.9
Iran	70,330	2,321	3.3	1,868	80.5	−91	−1.4
Ukraine	49,568	6,947	14.0	3	0.0	−100	−2.0
Indonesia	212,092	397	0.2	123	30.9	−180	−0.9
Philippines	75,653	160	0.2	0	0.1	−190	−2.6
Kazakhstan	16,172	3,028	18.7	21	0.7	−200	−12.2
India	1,008,937	6,271	0.6	171	2.7	−280	−0.3
Mexico	98,872	521	0.5	18	3.5	−310	−3.3
Congo	50,948	739	1.5	333	45.0	−340	−7.1
China[3,4]	1,275,133	513	0.0	294	57.4	−381	−0.3

Source: United Nations 2002

Note: For countries in italics, immigration data refer to noncitizens; for the others, data refer to those who are foreign-born.

[1] U.S., Canada, Bermuda, Greenland and Saint-Pierre-et-Miquelon.
[2] Micronesia, Polynesia, and Melanesia.
[3] Imputed data.
[4] Excludes Hong Kong and Macao.

immigrants. When it relaxed its immigration laws in 1990, Japan began to attract foreigners from other Asian countries as well as ethnic Japanese from Peru and Brazil. Developed countries also began to favor highly skilled migrants, particularly those trained in technology or other sectors facing labor shortages.

Warfare has led to vast refugee movements, from Cambodia, Laos, and Vietnam beginning after the Vietnam War ended and continuing until the mid-1990s. War in the 1980s, 1990s, and 2000s in Afghanistan and Iraq has led to large refugee populations in Pakistan and Iran. In Africa, refugee movements in the Horn of Africa have lasted 40 years or more. Ethnic conflict between Hutus and Tutsis in Rwanda and Burundi has led to repeated refugee movements. Many refugees are now in Western Africa, and the number of African countries involved in refugee movements has grown considerably. Conflicts in other parts of the world, such as Central America, also have led to refugee movements, although those who have fled have not always been given refugee status.

At the beginning of 2002, The United Nations High Commissioner for Refugees (UNHCR, 2002a) estimated a global refugee population of 12 million (see Figure 12.1), or roughly 9% of the total migrant stock. In addition, 3.7 million more Palestinians fall under the aegis of the U.N. Relief and Works Agency for Palestine Refugees in the Near East. The overall number of refugees remained about the same as in 2001, with half a million people uprooted and almost as many returning to their countries. One-third of the refugees came from Afghanistan. Africa accounts for about 3.3 million refugees, particularly from Burundi, Sudan, Angola, Somalia, and the Congo. Large numbers of refugees also come from Iraq, Bosnia and Herzegovina, and Vietnam. Most refugees tend to come from and go to less developed countries; more than 7 of every 10 refugees flee to a less developed country. Although the level of repatriation varies, only a small fraction of refugees resettle in industrialized countries: 1.2 million in all from 1992 to 2001. Nearly half of these resettled refugees originally came from Europe, particularly from Russia and from Bosnia and Herzegovina (UNHCR 2002a,b). Most of these refugees resettle in the United States.

Although asylum seekers are far fewer in number than refugees, they have accounted for considerable diversity in the migrant flows, particularly in Europe. In the first half of 2002, 28 countries, most of them industrialized, received almost 270,000 applications for asylum, according to provisional figures from the UNHCR (2002a,b). The United Kingdom received the most applications, more than 50,000, followed by Germany, the United States, and France. The top five origin countries of the asylum seekers were Iraq, Afghanistan, Turkey, Yugoslavia, and China. In 2001, industrialized countries accepted almost one-third of asylum applications (UNHCR 2002). Asylum applications in Europe peaked in 1992 in the wake of the breakup of the Soviet Union, instability in Romania, and fighting in the former Yugoslavia. Germany, which had been receiving the most applications for asylum, then changed its law to allow rejection of claims filed by asylum seekers entering Germany through a neighbor Germany considered safe (Zlotnik 1999).

THEORETICAL ISSUES

Why do people migrate internationally? Immigration is a phenomenon that by its definition comes about at least partly as a result of state policy (Zolberg 1999; Joppke 1999). Countries adopt rules about how many and what kinds of persons can enter for

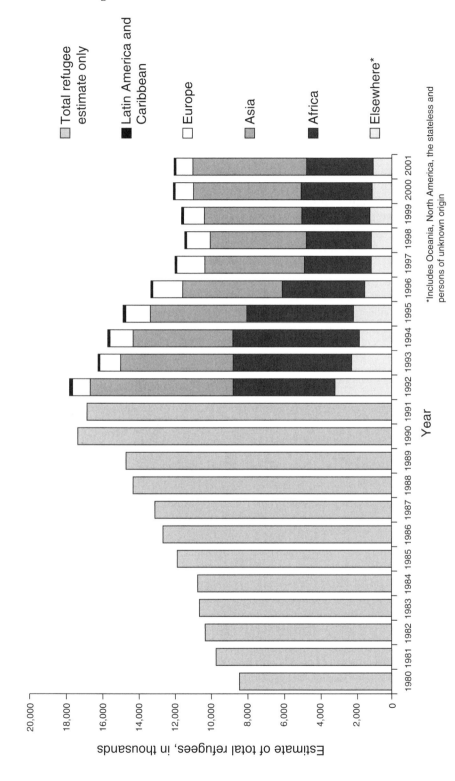

FIGURE 12.1. Estimated number of refugees, by area, 1980–2001. Source: UNHCR, 2001. 2002a,b.

the purpose of establishing long-term residence. But even the numbers and kinds of persons who enter countries illegally for the purpose of establishing long-term residence are affected by public policy because nations often implement border control practices that affect the ease or difficulty with which unauthorized border crossers can obtain entry (Andreas 2000; Bean et al. 1994). While it is clear that public policy shapes immigration processes, other forces also affect immigration. Although this would seem an obvious point, it often is lost in debates about immigration. Some observers speak of immigration as if it is *primarily* affected by policy, as if the reasons for permitting some kinds of people to enter a country can be largely separated from other sources of influence, such as family, personal, and political factors—as if only the rules concerning migration matter. Still other observers speak as if social and economic forces driving immigration operate independently of any rules about what kinds of people can obtain visas or of rules about whether borders can be crossed. While it is always difficult to ascertain whether policy or social and economic forces are more important in affecting immigration flows and patterns, it is crucial to recognize the fundamental importance of both kinds of influence. In this section, we examine a variety of theoretical perspectives that address the question of what forces drive international migration (see Massey et al., 1998; Massey 1999). These theories embody complementary but different views regarding the major reasons for migration, the predicted characteristics of migrants, and the nature of the societies that receive the migrants.

Neoclassical Economic Theory

Neoclassical economists envision migration as stemming from macrolevel imbalances between countries (or areas) in the supply of and demand for labor and the resultant wage differences these disequilibria generate (Harris and Todaro 1970). At the microlevel, this perspective assumes rational calculations on the part of individuals concerning the benefits (usually assumed to be economic) of a move relative to its costs (Todaro and Maruszko 1987). Migration is thus conceptualized to represent an investment strategy for individuals to maximize their returns to labor power. Migrants thus calculate their expected wages over their "time horizon," or expected lengths of stay at their destinations (Borjas 1990). Some migrants have short time horizons and therefore seek to maximize earnings within a framework of temporary, circular migration, while others have longer time horizons and are therefore more likely to settle permanently.

Costs of migrating may be incurred during the migration process or after settlement. For instance, Bean and his colleagues (1994) assessed the potential effectiveness of Operation Hold the Line, a U.S. Border Patrol operation in El Paso, Texas, in terms of increasing costs borne by unauthorized migrants. Eschbach, Hagan, and Bailey (1999) examined the deterrent effect of U.S.-Mexico border enforcement in terms of the ultimate cost: risk of death while crossing. Migrants also consider expected costs of living after they settle at their destination. Living costs include rents, food and clothing, and, especially in the United States, cost of automobile transportation (Grasmuck and Pessar 1991; Hagan 1994; Hondagneu-Sotelo 1994). There may also be psychological costs of adjustment or social benefits. For instance, women may find their social positions elevated, and men, their social positions weakened in the United States compared to their relative positions in their home countries (Hagan 1994; Hondagneu-Sotelo

1994). Expected wages and benefits must exceed expected costs of living after settlement to encourage migration, and social benefits must exceed psychic costs in order for migrants to stay in their new homes. These factors may affect the gender composition of immigrant populations in receiving countries. For instance, if men incur psychic costs because their social status has declined, they may be more likely to return home; at the same time, if women enjoy greater social benefits at their destinations than in their home communities, they may seek to become permanent residents (Grasmuck and Pessar 1991).

A variant of microeconomic theory—human capital theory—stresses the returns to investments in human capital. Workers are said to invest in their education based on expected returns over their time horizons (Becker 1964), in much the same way as migrants invest in moving to a new country and labor market. In addition, the concentration of larger, more prestigious educational institutions in developed countries may stimulate migration, and returns to education are often higher there than in developing countries. By moving to countries with better schools and more developed labor markets, migrants tend both to enhance their investment in human capital and to increase the likely return to that investment. Thus, human capital theory explains why countries like the United States attract so many well-educated migrants and cause a "brain drain" from other countries (Massey et al., 1998).

New Economic Theories of Migration

Some theorists (for example, Stark 1991; Taylor, Martin, and Fix 1997) have amended microeconomic theories by emphasizing the intersection of labor market factors and family/household variables in affecting migration decisions and by incorporating the notion of minimizing risk along with maximizing earnings. This perspective also predicts that social rank, relative income, and potential for social mobility will influence migration. For example, Taylor and associates (1997, 1994) have emphasized that not only lower average wages but also greater social and economic inequality in Mexico stimulate migration to the United States. Similarly, Roberts and Escobar Latapi (1997) have argued that urbanization generates emigration due to greater social inequality and atomization (i.e., fragmentation of families) in Mexico's largest cities.

Among the factors generating such inequalities are "market failures" (e.g., in the availability of investment capital or land allocation), which often impede social and economic mobility in sending countries. Households in these countries respond by sending one or more members to foreign labor markets to generate income and capital that can be used to minimize short- and long-term risk (i.e., household vulnerability to market failures) (Massey et al. 1998; Massey 1999). Members return income and capital to their home countries in the form of remittances, which are then either used for consumption or reinvested in household production, agriculture, or new small businesses (Lozano-Ascencio 1993; Taylor, Martin, and Fix 1997). In some communities in Mexico, the annual flow of remittances from the United States has been shown to be greater than the annual income earned locally (Massey and Parrado 1994). Moreover, once reinvested, remittances may raise household income by more than the value of the remittances themselves through migration-induced multiplier effects (Taylor 1992). Some Mexican households are "transnational" in the sense that they send members to the United States on a relatively permanent basis to earn supplemental income, while other members remain in the home community where the remittances are invested (Roberts, Bean, and Lozano-Ascencio 1999).

Because they emphasize household organizational factors operating in response to external economic conditions, new household economic theories better allow for the possibility that migration may often be temporary, especially when not all family members migrate. This contrasts with neoclassical theory, which essentially implies that migration will be permanent, or at least will last until macro imbalances giving rise to individual decisions to move shift appreciably. Otherwise, neoclassical theory can explain return migration only by making recourse to differences in "preferences" (i.e., differences in migration time horizons). But such preferences do not vary randomly. For example, using the theoretical concept of "social expected duration," Roberts (1995) showed how labor market conditions in both sending and receiving countries influence not only migrants' expected returns to their labor but the length of their time horizons as well. Thus, in the case of labor migration from Mexico, while neoclassical theory may provide an explanation for potential migrants' initial motivations to consider moving, new economic theories, because of their more adequate explanation of circular migration, better enhance our understanding of the dynamics of labor flows from Mexico, especially those involving unauthorized migrants.

Labor Market Segmentation Theory

In contrast to economic approaches, labor market segmentation theories emphasize how social stratification variables affect migration. Dual labor market theory envisions firms and their employees as stratified into primary and secondary sectors. The primary sector meets "basic demand" in the economy and consists of larger, better established firms that provide more capital-intensive, better-paying jobs. The secondary sector, by contrast, meets fluctuating or seasonal demand and relies primarily on lower-paid, labor-intensive jobs (Averitt 1968; Massey et al. 1998; Piore 1979; Tolbert, Horan, and Beck 1980). While human capital theorists argue that investments in education provide increasing returns for workers, segmentation theorists emphasize that barriers among segments and the nature of secondary sector employment and demand prevent upward mobility and limit returns to human capital in the secondary sector. These conditions often dissuade native-born workers from taking secondary sector jobs, especially when they are temporary or seasonal. Immigrants, however, are often willing to fill such jobs, especially if they expect to stay in the receiving country for only a short time (Piore 1979). Thus, labor market segmentation has implications both for the types of migrants who come to developed countries and for the structure of the labor market through which competition with native-born workers might occur.

Further segmentation may revolve around factors such as gender, ethnicity, and nativity. Waldinger (1996) and Bailey and Waldinger (1991), for example, have described New York City's labor markets as typified by a hierarchy or "queue" of hiring preferences. They argued that "ascriptive" characteristics (i.e., gender, skin color, ethnicity, and nativity) influence employers' hiring practices. Once an immigrant proves he or she is productive at a job, the employer then stereotypes the immigrant group positively and continues to hire from that group in the future and place other groups lower in the queue.

Similarly, labor market segmentation may derive from ethnic entrepreneurship: immigrants open businesses as "middleman minorities," providing goods and services in the least desirable industries or in areas where ethnic majority group members fear to go (Bonacich 1973; Bonacich and Modell 1980). Ethnic-owned businesses also serve co-ethnic communities or, in the case of the strictest segmentation, serve ethnic enclaves that are geographically and economically distinct from the larger economy (Light and Karageorgis 1980; Portes 1987; Portes and Bach 1985; Portes and Jenson 1989; Portes and Stepick 1993; Wilson and Portes 1980). Such developments, as we note below, can generate both economic opportunity as well as segregation by nativity. Further differentiation also derives from the structure of men's and women's labor market experiences. For example, immigrant men are often employed in construction (Stepick 1989) or migrant agriculture (Taylor, Martin, and Fix 1997), while many women work as domestics (Hagan 1994; Repak 1994, 1995), child care providers (Wrigley 1997), or garment industry sewing machine operators (Loucky et al. 1994; Morales and Ong 1991; Waldinger 1986). Labor market segmentation shapes migration when immigrant entrepreneurs seek to attract immigrant labor for their businesses or when other employers continue to hire or decide not to hire certain immigrant groups based on their ascriptive characteristics.

World Systems Theory

World systems analysts emphasize the influence on migration of the character of relationships among countries and among regions and cities within countries. World systems theory is heavily influenced by the dependency critique of capitalism, according to which capital accumulation depends on reserves of labor and materials, thus promoting development in some countries and underdevelopment in others. Core countries build capital by exploiting the labor power and materials of less developed, or peripheral, countries (Furtado 1964; Wallerstein 1983). Core cities such as New York, Los Angeles, and London are said to exercise control over the system through financial, labor, and commodity chains linking them to markets across the world. These links not only move labor-intensive production "offshore" to low-cost countries and regions of the world; they also concentrate capital in and attract migrants to the core cities. Thus, New York, Los Angeles, and London have great numbers of immigrants from countries all over the world, especially from those countries with the strongest specific financial and production links to these cities (Sassen 1988, 1991, 1994; Waldinger 1996).

The evolution of the global economy has not only stimulated international migration, it has also generated linkages between individual sending and receiving nations. The colonial and neocolonial history of capitalist expansion around the globe has resulted in ties between countries now in the semiperiphery, where industrialization is in its early stages, and core countries and their global cities in the more developed nations. For example, Mexico and the Philippines, which are sites for large numbers of U.S. multinational manufacturing plants, also send the most migrants to the United States (Yang 1995). Migration to the United Kingdom has been dominated by former colonies in India and the Caribbean, while migration to France has occurred mainly from Algeria and Morocco (Castles and Miller 1998).

The predictions of world systems theory, in contrast to those of other perspectives, are also useful in explaining why certain types of migrants fill certain types of jobs in global cities, for instance, the Asian garment entrepreneurs in Los Angeles. Loucky and his colleagues (1994) argued that growth in the garment industry in Los Angeles during the 1980s and 1990s was "inextricably linked" to large-scale immigration from Asia and Latin

America. That growth occurred alongside the evolution of a commodity chain linking garment production in Asia and Latin America to retailers and their markets in the United States. A large share of U.S. garment production moved overseas starting in the 1950s, generating a large share of the Asian economic miracle. Then, the arrival of large numbers of immigrants lowered labor costs, making domestic U.S. production competitive. In Los Angeles in the 1990s, the commodity chain included large numbers of small, Asian-immigrant-owned garment shops, employing mostly immigrant workers (Appelbaum and Gereffi 1994). Asian immigrants also created a new fashion market, and Asian entrepreneurs in California capitalized on their knowledge of this market, along with ties to producers in Asia, to open new garment-related businesses (Cheng and Gereffi 1994). The garment industry is but one example of how a global chain of production has both influenced and been influenced by large-scale international migration.

Network Theory

Network theory seeks to explain, at the microlevel, how connections among actors influence migration decisions, often by linking individual immigrants with their family members and with jobs, both before and after arrival. While labor markets in sending and receiving countries create push and pull factors stimulating migration, migration may continue after these push and pull factors have diminished. When large numbers of people have moved from one particular location to another, a process of "cumulative causation" is established whereby multiple ties to communities of origin facilitate on-going and at times increasing migration (Massey et al. 1993; Massey 1994). The exchange of information and the formation of relationships of trust are the building blocks of migration networks. Migrants often do not know the relative price of labor between their home country and their desired destination. Instead, they usually possess information about a particular job at a particular wage, and this information signals an opportunity in the destination labor market (Sassen 1995). Migrants also rely on informal trust rela-tionships to minimize the risks associated with moving to a foreign land (Granovetter 1985, 1995; Granovetter and Swedberg 1992). These networks—in the form of contacts with friends, families, and employers—provide an important means through which immigrants gain and accumulate social capital. By social capital, we mean the repertoire of resources such as information, material assistance, and social support that flow through ties to kin, to community, and to institutions (churches, for example). These ties constitute an important element in the migration process (Massey 1990; Massey and Espinosa 1997). Social capital is enhanced as the number and intensity of social ties between a focal individual (the migrant) and other persons increase (Hagan 1998).

Empirical studies have documented the influence of network variables. In a survey of two sending communities in Michoacán, Mexico, for example, Taylor (1987) found that having a close relative living in the United States strongly increased the likelihood of migration there, after controlling for age, sex, household income, prior migration, and the expected difference between earnings in Mexico and in the United States. Using survey data for 10 sending communities, Donato, Durand, and Massey (1992) found that social capital, in the form of family connections, raised Mexican immigrants' incomes, wages, and hours of work once they were in the United States. Thus, networks not only stimulate and channel migration, they also make it more lucrative. Studies documenting the presence and size of migration networks form an important basis for predicting future flows. Absent the imposition of significant checks on migration by state authorities, such networks can produce chain migration and thereby stimulate rapid increases in immigrant populations. Some authors have argued that this has been the case during the late 20th century in the United States with respect to the Asian and Latin American immigrant populations (e.g., Reimers 1985).

Political Economy Theories

While economic labor market and network factors drive migration, the immigration policies of receiving countries also play important roles in affecting flows. According to Hollifield's (1992) theory of "hegemonic stability," the world economic system rests on the political and military might of the dominant states. Following the Second World War, the victors established a global financial and trade system beginning with the international currency regime set up at Bretton Woods, followed by the General Agreement on Tariff and Trade (GATT) and the founding of the International Monetary Fund (IMF). The European Union and North American Free Trade Agreement (NAFTA) represent the most recent formal attempts by great powers to establish structures and institutions to influence and regulate the global economy. Such attempts have been guided by neoliberal economic principles, such as those governing the ownership of private property and the legal rights of individuals, as well as those protecting and enhancing the privileged position of capital.

Hegemonic states have employed the neoliberal economic order to regulate migration as well as global trade and finance, especially in times of labor shortages, when they have developed temporary direct labor importation programs. For example, by 1973, following decades of direct labor importation, between 10% and 12% of France and West Germany's labor forces consisted of temporary foreign workers, and Switzerland's labor force was 30% foreign-born (Salt 1981). Similarly, from 1946 to 1964 the United States imported 4.6 million temporary agricultural workers from Mexico under the *Bracero* program (Calavita 1992). The United States continues to import temporary agricultural workers—about 17,000 such workers entered with H-2A visas in 1995. During recent legislative sessions, the U.S. House of Representatives has considered proposals to admit up to 250,000 agricultural workers under an expanded temporary migrant program (Martin 1997: 102–103). As these examples show, receiving countries often attempt to control immigration by encouraging temporary work patterns rather than permanent settlement.

METHODS AND MEASURES

Measuring international migration is notoriously difficult. Many countries keep reasonably accurate data on the number of foreign migrants who enter a country with a valid passport or visa, and these data are often cited as the level of immigration. But even these data present some problems. For one thing, tourists or students who overstay temporary visas may wish to try to become authorized residents, but they have already migrated without being counted officially as migrants. Migrants who came without any authorization are unlikely to show up in records, because they avoid authorities. The result is that one cannot simply count visas to get an accurate record of migrants entering a country in any given year. Counting emigrants is even harder, since people often leave without being certain how long they will stay away. Few governments keep good records of those leaving, since governments are more interested in the people inside the country than those outside it. The United States stopped trying to count emigrants in 1957 and relies instead on estimates, often put at roughly 30% of the level of immigration to the United States (U.S. Immigration and Naturalization Service 2002a). Many times, governments estimate net migration over a given period as the difference between population change and natural increase.

Calculating migration rates can also be difficult, because the size of populations of origin is often unknown. With adequate emigration statistics, it is possible to obtain a rate of migration from a particular locale, since one can specify geopolitical boundaries and determine population size for an area that a resident might leave. But the calculation of in-migration rates with respect to the population at risk of moving to a given destination is difficult, since potential migrants might come from a multiplicity of origins, often unknown—in fact, from nearly anywhere *except* the destination. Thus, it is usually hard to specify a true denominator for a rate of in-migration. To circumvent this problem, demographers generally use the base population of the destination to calculate in-migration rates (Shryock and Siegel 1976: 376).

Using the same denominator for migration both in and out of an area allows demographers to calculate a crude net migration rate:

$$\frac{\text{Total in-migrants} - \text{total out-migrants in a time period}}{\text{Average total midyear population in that time period}} \times \frac{}{1000}$$

However, this rate assumes that adequate data on in-migrants and out-migrants exist for an area. Because this is often not the case, demographers often use vital statistics data to calculate net migration (e.g., in-migrants − out-migrants) as follows:

$$(\text{Total population}_{time2} - \text{total population}_{time\ 1}) - (\text{Births}_{t2,\ t1} - \text{Deaths}_{t2,\ t1})$$

This calculation is subject to error in the census enumeration and the vital statistics, but it provides an indicator of net migration. It does not allow the separation of in-migration from out-migration, however, so measurements with vital statistics make it impossible to compare net migration to total migration, or the sum of in-migration and out-migration. Still, it is possible to calculate a migration ratio as follows:

$$\frac{\text{Net number of migrants in a period}}{\text{Births} - \text{deaths in that period}} \times 1{,}000$$

This figure allows determination of the relative contributions of migration and natural increase to population growth.

Sources of Data

Although potential sources of data on international migration abound, the data are diverse, diffuse, and often difficult to obtain (United Nations 2002; Zlotnik 1987). Relevant data often are collected for administrative reasons unrelated to migration levels, so the data may come from various ministries or offices in formats that are hard to compile. In other cases, data may not be publicly available, or at least not in any timely way. The effectiveness of the offices collecting the data may vary widely. Furthermore, the data themselves may not exist, particularly data on emigration and unauthorized migration. Since administrative data, by definition, do not exist for unauthorized migration, the size of such flows must be estimated. In the United States, for instance, the 2000 census counted several million more people than the Bureau of the Census had initially expected. Some of the discrepancy stemmed from low estimates of unauthorized migration, currently thought to be about eight million (Bean et al. 2001).

Migration data may also vary according to how a country defines citizenship, since citizenship determines who is considered a "foreigner" versus "foreign-born." Most international migrants acquire citizenship by birth (*ius solis*) or by blood (*ius sanguinis*). In countries operating under *ius solis*, birth in the country confers citizenship. Immigrants born outside the country may naturalize under some circumstances and thereby acquire the rights of citizenship. In countries with *ius sanguinis*, citizenship is conferred through ancestry. Place of birth matters less than the ability to trace one's heritage to a country. Those lacking this ethnic heritage are considered foreigners, even if they are native-born or long-term residents. In Germany, *Aussiedler*, or the ethnic Germans born in Eastern Europe, have entered Germany nearly as citizens. Because of their ethnicity, they are considered returning nationals instead of immigrants, yet the data on inflows of migrants include them. As a result, migration data can reflect different definitions of citizenship and can obscure comparative studies on migrant flows.

For all these shortcomings, many types of data provide insight into different aspects of migration. In general, there are four sources of data about migration:

1. Administrative registers of populations or foreigners. These can be useful for determining migration. However, countries vary on their requirements for foreigners to register, so comparative analysis may be difficult.
2. Administrative records such as visas, work or residence permits, or deportations. In general, these are fairly weak proxies for migration, because they are collected for other purposes. But they can provide reasonable estimates for some subgroups of immigrants.
3. Entrances and departures at borders. These are direct measurements of migration flows, but the quality of the data often depends on geography. Countries that can control their points of entry and exit and have relatively few of them—island nations, for instance—are more likely to have accurate border data.
4. Censuses and household surveys. If censuses contain questions about nativity, they can yield estimates of immigrant stock at a country level and even local levels. Because censuses are taken infrequently, they cannot capture circulatory migration.

Used together, these data often provide useful and reasonably accurate indications of migration levels, but the limitations of the data need to be acknowledged.

Surprisingly, data on international refugees and asylum seekers tend to be better recorded (Hovy 2002). Most countries have agreed to a U.N. convention that defines a refugee as someone who is living outside his or her native country and who has a well-founded fear of persecution. The convention calls for governments to admit refugees and to collect data on them. On-site training in data collection comes from the Office of the United Nations High Commissioner for Refugees. Even so, political considerations often determine not only who is considered a refugee but also how many refugees are admitted to various countries. Estimates for people displaced within their own countries are much sketchier.

EMPIRICAL FINDINGS: IMMIGRATION TO THE UNITED STATES

Because more immigrants go to the United States than to any other country, it is particularly useful to examine some empirical evidence about the features of U.S. migrant flows and their significance for the country. In thinking about U.S. migration, it is worth reiterating what the term *immigration* means. The term has a legal connotation. That is to say, an immigrant is someone who has been granted a visa by a national government allowing that person to establish residence (and often to work) in the country. As noted above, the term immigrant thus does not necessarily denote the same thing as the term international migrant, because international migrants may move from one country to another without having been granted lawful permanent residency status. Thus, from a legal point of view, tourists, temporary students, and persons who illegally cross the border to live in the United States are not immigrants; they are international migrants. But what about people who have lived in the United States for two or three decades even though they entered the country illegally? Or people who enter legally and then stay beyond the time limit of their visas, often for years? Are such persons immigrants in a social science sense of the term, if not in a legal sense? Here we answer that question in the affirmative. That is, in addition to its legal connotation, we also adopt a settlement criterion when speaking of immigrants. Thus, we will define immigrants as persons who have established long-term residence in the United States, whether or not this has been done on a legal basis. Our consideration of immigrants thus focuses on a behavioral basis for residence; we consider an immigrant as someone who has settled in this country, either legally or illegally.

Immigration to the United States is important for three reasons. First, at the beginning of the 21st century, the United States occupies a new and historically unprecedented position: it is both the world's sole superpower and the locus of the new technologically driven information economy (Nye 2002). Immigration has been related to these developments in complex ways, sometimes operating as cause and sometimes as consequence of U.S. global military and economic power. Many envision immigration and globalization as essential to the future well-being of the country; others worry that these phenomena are threats to the vitality and security of the United States (Sassen 2000; Meissner 2001; Meissner and Martin 2001). Which of these views is more accurate and eventually comes to predominate will have important implications for the direction public policies are likely to take in the country over the next few decades. Formulating these policies requires taking stock empirically of the social, demographic, and economic effects of immigration in the recent past. The United States is not likely to be able to mold the various dimensions of immigration into phenomena that reinforce rather than contradict its major policy goals for the future if it does not better understand the nature and consequences of immigration in the recent past.

Second, immigration is also increasing in significance because of economic globalization, the forces of which draw the countries of the world even closer together (Gilpin 2000). Driven by technology and by the ascendance of the idea that freer international trade offers the prospect of more rapid economic growth, globalization has accelerated communications, capital flows, tourism, and trade among countries in many parts of the world. It has also exacerbated contradictions—antithetical themes and emphases that do not appear to fit well together, such as those encapsulated in the phrases "cosmopolitan-local," "universalism-particularism," "McDonaldization-jihad" and "globalism-tribalism." Globalization also exposes contradictions between immigration and the public policies that are both the causes and consequences of international migration. The major contradiction that many observers see emerging from this new international context is that many countries appear to support increased openness in flows of goods, capital, information, and technology but not increasingly free flows of people (Massey, Durand, and Malone, 2002). Globalization thus sets the context within which changes in migration and public policy must be interpreted.

Third, immigration is of increasing demographic importance to the United States. By the end of the 20th century, immigration had become the major component of population change in the United States (McDonald and Kippen 2001), especially since almost 20% of all births in the United States now occur to foreign-born mothers (Ventura, Curtin, and Mathews 2000: Table 13). Fertility rates peaked in the late 1950s and early 1960s and have since declined substantially. Soon after fertility peaked, immigration to the United States began to increase. As a result, immigration now directly (through the arrival of new residents) and indirectly (through the childbearing of immigrants) accounts for almost 60% of annual population growth in the country (Bean, Swicegood, and Berg 2000). This population growth has been accompanied by great racial/ethnic and cultural diversity in the U.S. population, thus complicating in the minds of some observers the question of national identity, a subject to which we return below.

Understanding immigration to the United States requires not only that we become knowledgeable about the shifting magnitude and nature of migration flows into the country occurring over the past few decades, but also that we consider the changes in the demographic and economic contexts that mark this period, shifts that usually affect the reception newcomers experience after arriving. In so doing we must not lose sight of the diversity in the kinds of flows that have occurred. If we lump all flows together under the same category and speak of immigration in blanket terms, we risk glossing over important differences in outcomes related to the various kinds of flows that channel newcomers into the country, the various migration policy auspices through which such flows occur, and the various contexts into which such flows take place. Newcomers to the United States have become more visible in recent years, in part because their numbers have increased, but also in part because they have increasingly been coming from different countries than previously. As we will see, there is considerable heterogeneity among newcomers, many of whom are not immigrants. Thus, we need to delve empirically into the various flows that contribute to migrant diversity and into the fluctuations in recent demographic and economic conditions that have confronted migrants after they have arrived in the United States.

Kinds of U.S. Migration Flows

The major migration flows to the United States in the post–World War II period have been (1) legal immigrants, (2) refugees and asylees, (3) unauthorized migrants, and

(4) persons admitted for short periods of time on so-called nonimmigrant visas. One of their most important features is that their numbers have generally been rising over this period. A second important feature, also in the case of each of the flows, is that the share of persons from Hispanic and Asian countries has been increasing and has come to constitute a majority of the flow. Both of these changes have occurred at the same time that economic growth has slowed, wages have stagnated, and earnings inequality has increased, with the notable exception of strong economic growth during the latter half of the 1990s that led to small countervailing trends at the end of the decade in wages and earnings inequality. Concerns about levels of immigration in the United States often reflect anxieties about potential changes in sociocultural identity and worries about economic conditions and job opportunities. Here we examine the recent changes in each of the major migration flows to the United States. Later we focus on the changes in the demographic and economic contexts in which they have occurred. The results help to set the stage for assessing what are the most important implications of U.S. immigration trends and policies for the country.

The Composition of Flows

A number of studies have examined changes in immigration trends and policies in the United States during the 20th century (e.g., Bean, Vernez, and Keely 1989; Borjas 1999; Reimers 1985, 1998; Suro 1998). All emphasize that the annual numbers of new entrants reached their highest totals during the first two decades of the century. The major pieces of legislation affecting immigrant flows are summarized in Table 12.3. Owing to the passage of the National Origins Quota Act in 1924, the Great Depression during the 1930s, and an unfavorable immigration climate during World War II, immigration numbers dropped tenfold from these record-setting levels during the next 25 years. Specifically, the number of entrants decreased from over 700,000 per year during the first 20 years of the century to less than 70,000 per year from 1925 through 1945 (U.S. Immigration and Naturalization Service, 1994). After this lull, and continuing for nearly 50 years now, legal immigration has again moved steadily upward, reaching by the late 1980s and into the 1990s levels approaching the all-time highs set in the early part of the 20th century (Figure 12.3). And if the legalizations resulting from the Immigration Reform and Control Act of 1986 (IRCA) are included in the totals, the levels in the early 1990s exceed all previous highs (U.S. Immigration and Naturalization Service 2002).

The results shown in Figure 12.2 reveal the dramatically changing national origins of U.S. immigrants. Prior to 1960, the vast majority came from European countries or Canada (often over 90% when examined on a decade-by-decade basis). Even as late as the 1950s, over two-thirds of all arrivals were from these countries. Things changed rapidly during the 1960s, when family reunification criteria, rather than national origins quotas, became the basis for granting entry visas (Bean, Vernez, and Keely 1989; Reimers 1983). That the vast majority of immigrants now enter on the basis of family criteria can be seen in Table 12.4, which shows admissions for the year 2000 by class of admission. Almost three-fourths were family-based admissions. By the 1980s, the influence of the new criteria on national origins was clear. In that decade, only 12.5% of legal immigrants came from Europe or Canada, whereas 84.4% were from Asian or Latin American countries (U.S. Immigration and Naturalization Service 1994).

TABLE 12.3. Selected Major Legislation Administered by the Immigration and Naturalization Service, 1920s–1990s

Title and date	Major provisions
Immigration Act of May 19, 1921 (first quota act)	Imposed national numerical limits according to the national origins of the white U.S. population in 1910
Immigration Act of May 26, 1924 (National Origins Quota Act)	Recalibrated national limits using 1890 census figures
Act of April 29, 1943	Provided for the importation of temporary agricultural laborers from South and Central America; served as the legal basis for the Bracero program, which lasted until 1964
Displaced Persons Act of June 25, 1948	Admitted émigrés fleeing war-ravaged areas; operated outside of limits imposed by immigration selection system
Immigration and Nationality Act of June 6, 1952 (McCarran-Walter Act)	Recodified national limits; also created separate preferences for skilled workers and relatives
Refugee Relief Act of August 7, 1953	Admitted European refugees from Communist countries
Immigration and Nationality Act Amendments of October 3, 1965	Eliminated national quotas; instituted a preference system employment-based skills and family reunification
Cuban Refugee Act of November 2, 1966	Admitted refugees from Cuba after the overthrow of the Cuban government
Refugee Act of March 17, 1980	Provided set procedures for the Attorney General to allow asylees to adjust to permanent resident status
Immigration Reform and Control Act of November 6, 1985	Banned employment of persons ineligible to work in the US; provided amnesty to former illegal aliens under certain conditions
Immigration Act of November 29, 1990	Instituted 3 preference categories: family-sponsored, employment-based, and "diversity" immigrants

These relatively recent changes in the national origin composition of immigrants have begun to convert the United States from a largely biracial society consisting of a sizable white majority and a small black minority, and a native American minority of less than 1%, into a multiracial, multiethnic society consisting of several racial/ethnic groups (Bean and Bell-Rose 1999; Passel and Edmonston 1994). This trend became discernible in the 1950s but began to accelerate in the 1960s (Table 12.5). In 2000, the U.S. census asked a question about Hispanic or Latino ancestry and another about race. In answer to the question on race, which for the first time allowed multiple responses, about 2.4% of all Americans chose two or more races, a percentage slated to grow as the increases in racial intermarriage produce more Americans with a complex racial heritage. About 12.3% chose Black or African American as their single response, 3.6% chose Asian, 0.9% chose American Indian or Alaska Native, and 5.5% chose some other nonwhite race (U.S. Bureau of the Census 2002a). In answer to the separate question on Hispanic or Latino ancestry, one in eight Americans (12.5%) identified themselves as Hispanic or Latino. The apparent growth in the multiracial population, and the clearly observed growth in the numbers of Americans of Hispanic and Asian

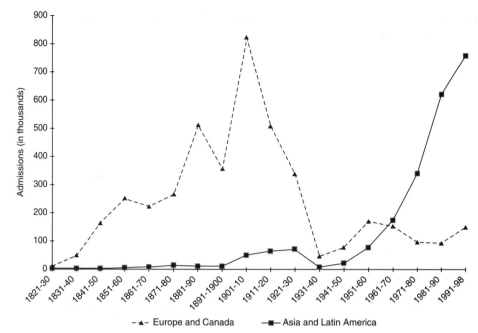

FIGURE 12.2. Average annual number of immigrants admitted to the United States by national origin, 1821–1998. Source: US INS 2002a.

TABLE 12.4. Immigrants Admitted by Type and Class of Admission, 2000

Type and class of admission	Number
Total, all immigrants	849,807
Total, subject to worldwide numerical limits[1]	393,304
A. Family-sponsored preferences	235,280
i. Unmarried sons/daughters of U.S. citizens	27,707
ii. Spouses/children of permanent residents	124,595
iii. Married sons/daughters of U.S. citizens, their spouses and children	22,833
iv. Siblings of U.S. citizens, their spouses and children	60,145
B. Employment-based preferences	107,024
C. Other (legalization dependents, diversity)	51,000
Total, not subject to worldwide numerical limits[2]	456,503
A. Immediate relatives of U.S. citizens	347,870
B. Refugee and asylee adjustments	65,941
C. Other	42,692

Source: U.S. Immigration and Naturalization Service 2002.
[1] Worldwide numerical limits include family-sponsored preferences, legalization dependents, employment-based preferences, and diversity programs.
[2] Immediate relatives of U.S. citizens in previous editions of the *Statistical Yearbook* are included with admissions not subject to a numerical cap. Immediate relatives may immigrate without limit, but the number affects the limit set for family-sponsored preference immigrants.

ancestries, means that the portion of the population that is white and non-Hispanic is shrinking and that Blacks no longer constitute a majority of the minority population (see chapter 6, "Demography of Race and Ethnicity," for more discussion).

TABLE 12.5. U.S. Population by Race/Ancestry, 1900–2000 (in thousands)

Year	Total	Non-Hispanic White	Black	Hispanic	Asian	American Indian
Population						
1900	76,195	66,225	8,834	656	243	237
1910	93,879	82,049	10,255	999	299	277
1920	110,747	96,969	11,512	1,632	389	244
1930	127,585	111,543	12,736	2,435	527	343
1940	136,928	119,425	13,767	2,814	577	345
1950	155,156	134,351	156,668	4,039	739	357
1960	182,055	154,969	19,071	6,346	1,146	524
1970	205,567	170,371	23,005	9,616	1,782	793
1980	226,625	180,392	26,482	14,604	3,726	1,420
1990	248,712	187,139	29,986	22,354	7,274	1,959
2000*	281,422	198,178	35,384	35,306	11,579	3,445
Percentage						
1900	100.0	86.9	11.6	0.9	0.3	0.3
1910	100.0	87.4	10.9	1.1	0.3	0.3
1920	100.0	87.6	10.4	1.5	0.4	0.2
1930	100.0	87.4	10.0	1.9	0.4	0.3
1940	100.0	87.2	10.1	2.1	0.4	0.3
1950	100.0	86.6	10.1	2.6	0.5	0.2
1960	100.0	85.1	10.5	3.5	0.6	0.3
1970	100.0	82.9	11.2	4.7	0.9	0.4
1980	100.0	79.6	11.7	6.4	1.6	0.6
1990	100.0	75.2	12.1	9.0	2.9	0.8
2000*	100.8	70.4	12.6	12.5	4.1	1.2

Source: Adapted from Table 2.3 in Passel and Edmonston 1994.
*For the various racial/ethnic groups (but not the total), the numbers include persons identifying with the group alone or in combination, and thus their sum exceeds the total, and their percentages exceed 100.0
Note: Populations include the 50 states and the District of Columbia for 1900–2000.

Refugees and Asylees

The United States, like most other Western democracies, did not admit refugees under the purview of immigration policy until after World War II, when it recognized the victims of political persecution as "a distinct category of international migrants to whom [it] owed special obligations" (Zolberg 1992: 55). In 1948, Congress passed the Displaced Persons Act, which was signed the month the Berlin blockade began in Germany, permitting the entry into the United States of 200,000 of the hundreds of thousands of displaced persons flooding into the American occupied zones in Europe. The drafters of the law tried to connect the refugee resettlement provisions in the legislation with U.S. immigration policy by stipulating that the number of refugees had to be charged against the immigration quotas of future years. In the ensuing years, the issue of what to do about refugees continued to arise but was viewed as conflicting with other features of U.S. immigration policy, particularly the national origins quotas, which severely restricted admissions from some countries. As a result of this dilemma and because it was largely driven by foreign policy considerations, U.S. refugee policy essentially had to be crafted and implemented on an *ad hoc* basis.

Whatever the vagaries of postwar refugee policy, the effects of the numerous *ad hoc* admissions programs introduced another source of new entrants into the United States.

Since the end of World War II, nearly three million refugees and asylees have been granted lawful permanent resident status by the United States (U.S. Immigration and Naturalization Service 2002a). During the 1940s and 1950s, the number of refugees and asylees averaged about 50,000 per year, a figure that declined to about 20,000 per year during the 1960s before moving to over 50,000 per year during the 1970s, to about 100,000 per year during the 1980s, and well over 100,000 per year in the 1990s (Figure 12.3). As with legal immigrants, the vast majority come from Asia, Latin America, and the Caribbean (49% overall since 1945 and 82% during the 1980s), although both the relative and absolute numbers coming from the former Soviet Union have increased substantially since 1990. In sum, as Figure 12.3 shows, the category of refugee and asylee admissions has constituted an increasing flow of persons into the country, predominantly Asian and Latino, over the past 50 years.

Unauthorized Immigrants

Persons who enter the United States illegally and persons who enter legally and then stay illegally constitute another major flow into the country. The former were called "EWIs" by the former U.S. Immigration and Naturalization Service (or simply un-documented migrants by other observers) because they "enter without inspection," whereas the latter are called "visa-overstays" because they consist of persons who stay beyond the expiration date of their visas. Almost all of the undocumented migrants

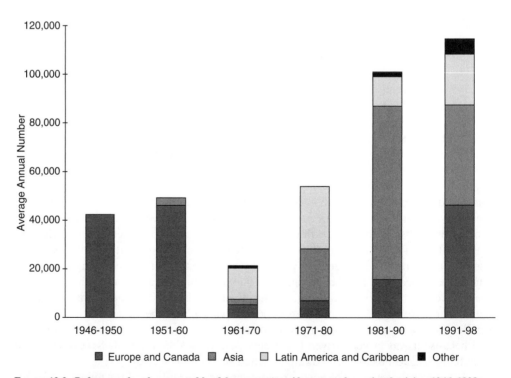

FIGURE 12.3. Refugees and asylees granted lawful permanent resident status by national origins, 1946–1998. Source: US INS 2002a.

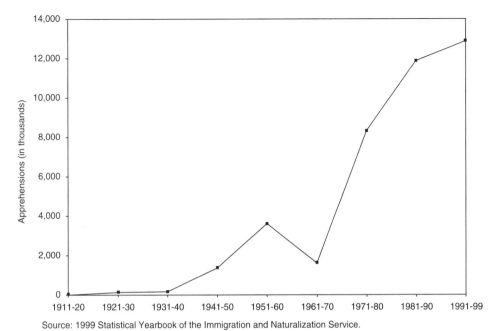

Source: 1999 Statistical Yearbook of the Immigration and Naturalization Service.

FIGURE 12.4. Average annual number of apprehensions by decade, 1911–1999 (US INS 2002a).

enter at the U.S.-Mexican border, with most originating in Mexico, although in recent years substantial numbers have also come from Central American countries (Bean, Passel, and Edmonston 1990) and a smaller yet significant number from Asia. The visa-overstays do not come predominantly from any one country, although in recent years such persons have represented approximately slightly less than half of the illegal population resident in the country at any one point in time (Warren 1990, 1992).

The Bracero program, which started in 1942 at the beginning of World War II, provided a means whereby temporary contract laborers from Mexico could enter and work in the country legally (Calavita 1992). After the Program ended in 1964, the flow of undocumented migrants from Mexico into the country began to increase. That the flows of such persons into the country has become substantial is reflected in Figure 12.4, which shows by decade the average annual number of apprehensions by the U.S. Border Patrol (mostly at the U.S.-Mexican border) of persons illegally resident in the United States (U.S. Immigration and Naturalization Service 1994). While it is well known that apprehension data do not directly indicate the number of *persons* who illegally reside in the country and that they better represent flows than stocks and refer to events, not people (Bean, Passel, and Edmonston 1990; Van Hook and Bean 1998), there is little doubt that the increasing numbers of apprehensions reflect increases in the number of undocumented migrants entering the country (Espenshade 1995).

Migration involves a social process consisting of transitions over time from temporary (and illegal) status to permanent (and often legal) migration status (Massey et al. 1987). Partly as a consequence, the stock of unauthorized migrants, together with the stock of persons illegally residing in the country because of visa-overstaying, began to grow in the 1960s and to increase substantially in the 1970s. The U.S. Bureau of the

Census included an annual net gain of 200,000 persons attributable to unauthorized immigration in its annual population estimates and projections (Campbell 1994). Other sources estimate the size of this net component currently in the range of 200,000 to 300,000 persons (Warren 1992).

It is more difficult to gauge the racial/ethnic composition of unauthorized migrants. However, the available evidence suggests that unauthorized migrants are also mainly Asian and Latin American in origin (Warren 1990, 1992; Warren and Passel 1987). This suggests that the implications of unauthorized immigration for changing racial/ethnic composition differ little from those of legal immigration, a conclusion corroborated by findings about the national origin composition of the persons who became legal immigrants under the provisions of the 1986 Immigration Reform and Control Act, nearly 70% of whom were of Mexican origin and over 90% of whom were either of Latin American or Asian origin (U.S. Department of Justice 1992).

Nonimmigrant Entrants

Nonimmigrants are persons admitted to the United States for a specified temporary period of time but not for permanent residence. Although the majority of nonimmigrants are tourists, large numbers of students and persons coming for various business and work-related reasons are also admitted. In fact, the numbers of persons coming for business-related reasons have increased substantially in the past two or three years, an outcome facilitated by the Immigration Act of 1990, which included compromise provisions allowing easier nonimmigrant business entry in lieu of the even higher levels of employment-related immigration that some proponents wanted to include in the legislation (Bean and Fix 1992). During fiscal year 1999, 31 million nonimmigrant admissions to the United States were recorded, the largest number ever, and an increase of over 9 million over fiscal year 1995 (U.S. Immigration and Naturalization Service 2002: 120).

Nonimmigrant admissions are an important source of flows into the country, and their implications for immigration issues go beyond their sheer magnitude. The dramatic increase in nonimmigrant admissions in recent years reflects the mounting demand both for tourism and for business and employment-related entry resulting from increased globalization of the economy. Nonimmigrant flows constitute the source from which visa-overstayers develop and currently have been estimated to make up slightly more than half of all illegal residents in the United States (Warren 1992). The picture that emerges from numerous ethnographic studies of migration implies that the nonimmigrant entrants who become illegal migrants through visa-overstaying may do so through a social process that in turn results in many eventually becoming legal immigrants. Hence, as the volume of nonimmigrant admissions continues to climb steeply, pressures on the legal immigration system are likely to increase, even if the rate of visa-overstaying remains constant.

While the number of nonimmigrant entrants has steadily risen over the past decade, the national origins of these flows have been somewhat more diverse than is the case for other kinds of flows (Figure 12.5). In 1998 about 56% of nonimmigrant entrants were from Asia, Latin America, and the Caribbean, up from about 41% in 1965. The number and racial/ethnic composition of persons in the United States on nonimmigrant visas are also likely to affect public perceptions about immigration to the country. The average citizen rarely seems able to distinguish among kinds of

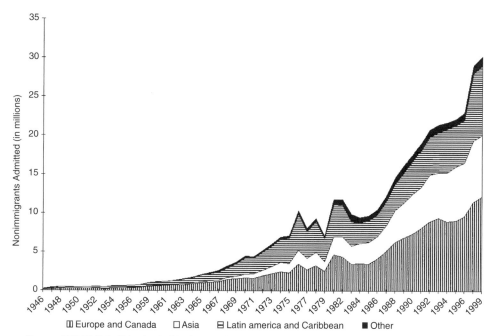

Source: 1999 Statistical Yearbook of the Immigration and Naturalization Service.

FIGURE 12.5. **Annual number of nonimmigrants admitted to the United States, fiscal years 1946–1999 (US INS 2002a).**

immigrants, let alone among kinds of nonimmigrants or between nonimmigrants and immigrants (Bean, Telles, and Lowell 1987). Thus, the rapidly rising numbers of nonimmigrants, over half of whom are from Hispanic and Asian countries, undoubtedly contribute to the impression that Latino and Asian immigration to the United States is higher than it actually is.

The Demographic and Economic Contexts of U.S. Migration

As the discussion above of migration trends indicates, the substantial rise in migration to the United States occurring since World War II has consisted of several kinds of flows occurring for a variety of reasons. What kinds of contextual factors in the United States might have influenced the flows and the ways these were received? The increases in each of the flows may be seen as rooted to some extent in conditions that emerged out of the postwar economic expansion. From the end of World War II to the early 1970s, the United States experienced rising economic prosperity and increasing affluence. Levels of productivity were high and wages and personal incomes rose (Landau 1988; Levy 1987). Not by coincidence, the country in 1965 eliminated the restrictive and discriminatory national origins criteria for the admission of immigrants that were embodied in the 1924 National Origins Quota Act and ratified in the 1952 McCarran-Walter Act. Adopted in their place were more inclusionary family reunification criteria reflecting the domestic policy emphases of the era on improving civil rights and the foreign policy emphases on establishing better relations with newly independent Third World countries (Cafferty et al. 1983). Partly as a result of such policies in general and the family reunification provisions in particular, legal immigration began to rise substantially (Reimers 1983, 1985). At about the same time, because of the termination of the Bracero program in 1964 and because of growing demand for inexpensive labor, undocumented (mostly Mexican) immigration began to increase (Massey 1981). And, as we noted above, compared to the so-called "old" immigrants, who were mostly European in origin, the so-called "new" immigrants (both legal and undocumented) came mostly from Third World Hispanic and Asian countries (Bean and Tienda 1987).

In the mid-1970s, growth in real wages began to level off, unemployment rose as the country experienced a recession (see Figure 12.6), and calls for immigration reform began to emerge (Bean, Telles, and Lowell 1987). Frequently these consisted of restrictionist outcries against the new immigration, often stated in the form of unsubstantiated claims about the pernicious nature of immigration and its harmful effects on the country. During the 1980s, a substantial body of social science research emerged that found little basis for the claims that immigration was generating strongly negative demographic, economic, or social effects. An important question is whether similar results would obtain during periods of continuing high immigration and during periods of continuing slow job and wage growth. These were the conditions characterizing the first half of the 1990s but not the second half. As of this writing, the strong economy of the latter half of the 1990s has collapsed into a significant recession during 2000–2002. Thus, the issue of the country's capacity (or willingness) to absorb immigration continues as a significant question.

Immigration issues have also frequently been addressed in terms of immigration's implications for population growth and, much less frequently, in terms of its implica-

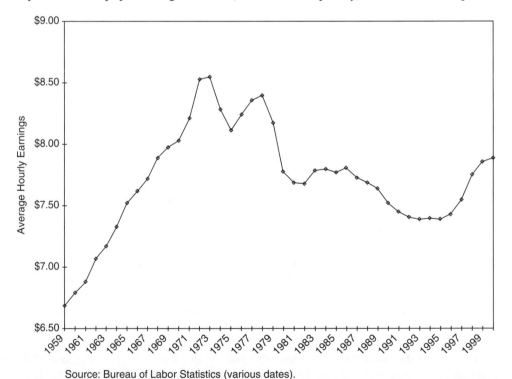

Source: Bureau of Labor Statistics (various dates).

FIGURE 12.6. **Hourly earnings in private nonagricultural industries, 1959–2000 (in 1982 dollars) (U.S. Bureau of Labor Statistics, 2001).**

tions for economic growth (Borjas and Tienda 1987; Easterlin 1982; Morris 1985). With respect to the former question, many observers have noted that the percentage of foreign-born persons in the population, even though rising during the 1970s and 1980s, has remained substantially below the percentage in the early part of the 20th century (Borjas 1990; Passel 1987; Portes and Rumbaut 1990; Simon 1987). In other words, although large in absolute terms relative to the size of the population, immigration during the 1970s and 1980s remained appreciably below the levels of the early 20th century (see Figure 12.7). But interestingly, because of higher fertility and because a larger share of the early 20th-century immigrants eventually returned to their countries of origin than appears now to be the case, immigration in the 1980s accounted for roughly similar fractions of population growth as it did at the turn of the century (about 35%) (Easterlin 1982; Passel and Edmonston 1994). But whether measured in terms of absolute numbers, in terms of the percentage foreign-born in the population, or in terms of the contribution of net immigration to population growth, the volume of immigration during the 1980s and 1990s has not exceeded the immigration to the United States that occurred during the first 20 years of the 20th century.

Efforts to assess immigration relative to the size of the economy have been much less frequent. Borjas and Tienda (1987) have examined immigration growth relative to the rate of growth in the civilian labor force. They noted that:

> Between 1951 and 1980, the U.S. labor force grew by 7.6 million, 12.3 million, and 22.5 million during each successive decade. On the basis of immigrant flows for each of these periods and assuming that all those admitted entered the labor force, recent immigrants could have accounted for at most 33 percent of this increase in employment during the 1950s, 27 percent during the 1960s, and 20 percent during the 1970s.

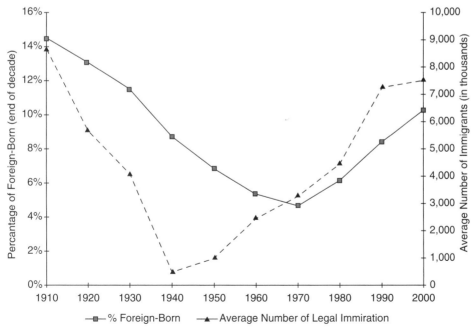

Source: U.S. Census Bureau (various dates) and U.S. Immigration and Naturalization Service. 2002b. "Immigration and Naturalization Legislation from the Statistical Yearbook." Vol.2.

FIGURE 12.7. **Average annual number of immigrants and percentage of foreign-born, 1910–2000.**

The rate of aggregate unemployment during this period varied from around 4.0% in 1950 to around 6.5% in 1980 (see Figure 12.8). Borjas and Tienda have also pointed out that only about half of all immigrants admitted to the country entered the labor force upon arrival during this period. Thus, however measured, the rate of labor force growth during this period exceeded the rate of growth in immigration.

The economic circumstances of the 1950s, 1960s, and 1970s thus seemed more than sufficiently healthy to absorb the numbers of immigrants arriving at the time. During the 1980s, however, several trends reversed. The rate of growth in immigration continued to increase while the rate of growth in the labor force began to decline. From 1970 through 1980, the growth rate in the U.S. labor force dropped to 20% from 27% during the 1960s. By contrast, the growth rate in the number of new immigrants jumped to 63% during the 1980s compared to 35% during the 1970s (see Figure 12.7). By the 1990s, the number of immigrants coming during the decade could have at most accounted for 54% of the growth in the labor force, assuming every immigrant who came held a job, a highly implausible assumption (see Table 12.6).

These changes in trends raise the interesting question of how the immigration experience of the late 1980s and 1990s compares both with other post–World War II years and with the early part of the 20th century; that is, how does the volume and growth of immigration compare to growth in the size of the economy? That this question so seldom seems to have been addressed is surprising. To our knowledge, the examination by Borjas and Tienda (1987) of growth in immigration relative to growth in the labor force is one of few attempts to address the issue. Easterlin (1982) has broadly discussed the

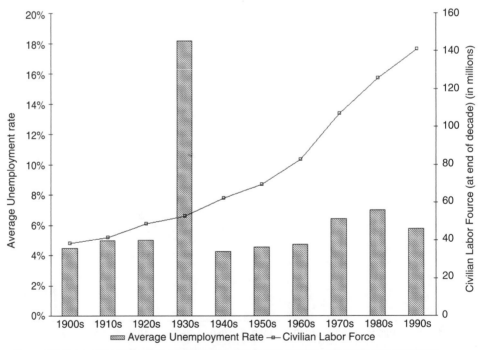

Source: U.S. Bureau of the census. 2001. Statistical Abstract of the United States, 2000, and Council of Economic Advisers, 2002. Economic Report of the President, 2001.

FIGURE 12.8. Average unemployment rate and the size of civilian labor force, 1900s to 1990s.

TABLE 12.6. Annual Percentage Change in Civilian Labor Force and the Percentage that Immigrants Make Up of Labor Force Change, by Decade, 1950–2000

Time period	Annual percentage change in civilian labor force	Number of immigrants as a percentage of labor force growth
1951–1960	1.8	33.0
1961–1970	1.9	27.0
1971–1980	2.6	20.0
1981–1990	1.6	36.0
1991–2000	1.2	53.5[1]

Sources: U.S. Bureau of Labor Statistics, various years, and US INS 2002a.
[1] Excludes IRCA-adjusted immigrants.

implications of immigration for growth in GNP, pointing out that at the simplest level of analysis, aggregate production clearly rises in some direct proportion to increases in immigration, but that the challenging problem is unraveling its effects on per capita output. To the extent that immigrants differ from the general population in characteristics that enhance production (higher proportions working, younger age structures, perhaps greater motivation), the effects would be favorable. To the extent that their characteristics lower production (lower education, less knowledge of English), the effect would be negative. In either case, the effects are not likely to be large because immigrants are still a relatively small fraction of the population, and the characteristics of many immigrants are not enormously different from those of natives (Fix and Passel 1994).

The coincidence of trends in economic growth and immigration growth, though *not* indicative of a causal relationship between the phenomena, is nonetheless likely to be informative concerning the emergence of conditions likely to influence the reaction of natives to immigration. Figure 12.9 shows average annual rates of growth in per capita GNP for decades of the 20th century. During the first 10 years of this century, when immigration reached the highest levels of any decade in the nation's history (and the population base was less than half the current base), the size of the economy grew faster than either population or inflation. For example, from 1900 to 1910, the average inflation- and population-adjusted growth rate was 2.8%. In other words, the economy expanded 2.8% faster than did population after adjusting for inflation. In the 1950s, this differential was 1.6%; in the 1960s, 2.5%; in the 1970s, 1.8%; and in the 1980s, 1.6%. During the 1990s, the average was 2.2%, although from 1991 through 1993, it was only 0.4%. More substantial economic growth began in 1992. After an initial year or two of continuing employment and wage stagnation, the economy in the latter half of the 1990s expanded at rates that were the strongest in many decades, rates that were stronger than at any time in the 20th century, and rates that also generated increases in real wages (see Figure 12.6). Rather than concerns about too much immigration, calls about labor shortages were increasingly heard. In 2001, the United States entered a recession, which as of this writing was continuing, at least insofar as job growth is concerned. A major question now is whether high rates of growth will resume during the ensuing few years.

RESEARCH DIRECTIONS

One of the most important questions for future research concerns the appropriate level and role for international migration in countries where low fertility and increasing

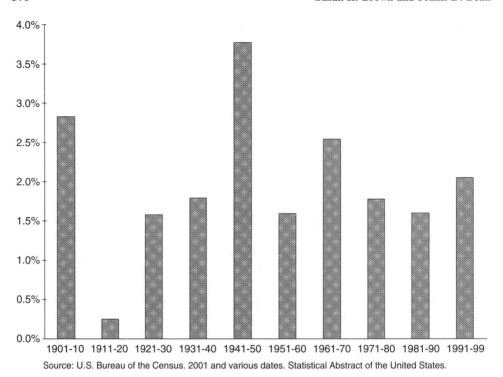

Source: U.S. Bureau of the Census. 2001 and various dates. Statistical Abstract of the United States.

FIGURE 12.9. **Average annual change in real GNP per capita by decade, 1901–1999 (in 1996 dollars).**

longevity have spurred a rapid aging of the population. The growth of the elderly population is more and more likely to tax these countries' capabilities of providing health care and pensions, as their ratios of "dependent" persons to the sizes of their workforces increase. The aging of populations has caused considerable anxiety, particularly in Europe, about national abilities to continue to provide for the elderly, or at least to provide the same quality of life as in the past. Such anxieties become all the more acute when private pension systems in advanced industrial economies have eroded and seem less likely to honor their commitments to future pensioners.

Despite resistance among many advanced countries toward more migrants, the international migration of working-aged adults may slow the onset of economic ills associated with an elderly age structure (Demeny 2003). Indeed, the United Nations (2002), in a widely disseminated report, suggested policy reliance on immigration as an antidote to population aging for advanced developed countries in the world. While the U.N. may be proven right in its recommendation of such measures, unemployment remains high in many countries for which the U.N. argues that immigration might provide demographic benefits. How immigration affects unemployment and other market outcomes in countries with relatively high unemployment remains a critical issue in need of more research. In other words, any long-term demographic balance regained through immigration must be considered in light of the short-term economic effects of such immigration. This is an important question with enormous significance for policy.

Another major set of questions for research involves the nature and extent of incorporation of immigrant groups in countries of destination. This is a critical issue driving much public debate about the need to reform immigration policy (Bean and Stevens 2003). Whether today's immigrant groups, particularly those from the less developed countries with low levels of education, will incorporate readily and join the economic mainstream holds considerable implications for the outcome of discussions about whether immigration policies should be changed. Many research projects on these kinds of issues are under way, but these projects often must focus on groups that are relatively recent arrivals. As a result, a definitive answer on incorporation is a long way off, even though policy decisions often cannot wait for final research answers and must be based on preliminary results based on incomplete evidence. In such circumstances, good theoretical models of incorporation will be vital for guiding research and interpreting preliminary results. Developing such models will thus itself constitute a major challenge for immigration scholars in the years ahead.

Another major research issue concerns how the more developed countries will respond to the ethnic diversity that immigration is bringing, especially if these countries adopt policies to increase immigration to cope with population declines and economic stagnation. Will diversity increase social tension or prove a new source of strength and resiliency and work to break down old ethnic barriers and divides? These are key questions for future research. Preliminary evidence suggests that in the United States, diversity stemming from immigration may be weakening historically rigid color lines and fostering greater ethnic tolerance (Lee and Bean 2004), but more research is needed on the pathways through which this takes place.

DISCUSSION AND CONCLUSION

Over the past 35 years or so the world has witnessed substantial increases in international migration. In the case of the United States, the country that receives more immigrants than any other, this period has also seen a remarkable rise in the size and diversity of in-flows to the country. These increases have occurred across all types of flows, from legal immigrants to refugees to unauthorized immigrants to nonimmigrants. The transition from flows originating mostly in European countries to those coming mostly from Asian and Hispanic countries has also generally been characteristic of the various types of flows. Because this diversity in national origins has spread to millions of nonimmigrants as well as immigrants, it reinforces the reality that the new immigration to the United States has substantially increased the country's national origin and racial/ethnic diversity. These patterns illustrate the applicability of various theories explaining the origins and magnitude of the flows. That is, migrants of all types tend to come more often from countries with which the United States has had prior and continuing relationships (whether primarily political or economic). Within those countries, migration tends to involve more often persons who have family and friends in the United States and persons whose own earnings and whose family's investments stand to gain the most from the migration.

The receptions immigrants receive when they arrive are affected by the strength of national economies at the time of arrival. Over the past four decades in the United States, for example, the economy has been reasonably strong and relatively easy to accommodate. But in periods of recession, when employment is stagnant or shrinking, new arrivals are harder to integrate into national workforces. Although such periods have not typically been of long duration in most developed countries in the post–World

War II era, they invariably heighten concerns about the social and economic repercussions of immigration. This potential volatility in public sentiment is a major factor for countries considering the adoption of more liberal immigration policies. In periods of rising employment, appreciation grows for the roles immigrants play in labor markets and the contributions they make to society and the economy, including the support of the elderly. But when jobs are scarce, resentment toward immigrants grows. Yet regardless of changes in public opinion toward newcomers, and despite temporal fluctuations in labor market conditions in many countries, international migration is likely to become an ever more important component of population dynamics in the more economically developed countries.

REFERENCES

Andreas, P. 2000. *Border games: Policing the U.S.-Mexico Divide*. Ithaca, N.Y.: Cornell University Press.

Appelbaum, R. P., and G. Gereffi. 1994. Power and profits in the apparel commodity chain. In *Global production: The apparel industry in the Pacific Rim*. Edited by E. Bonacich, L. Cheng, N. Chinchilla, N. Hamilton, and P. Ong. Philadelphia: Temple University Press.

Averitt, R. T. 1968. *The dual economy: The dynamics of American industry structure*. New York: W. W. Norton.

Bailey, T., and R. Waldinger. 1991. Primary, secondary, and enclave labor markets: A training systems approach. *American Sociological Review* 56:432–445.

Bean, F. D., and S. Bell-Rose, eds. 1999. *Immigration and opportunity: Race, ethnicity, and employment in the United States*. New York: Russell Sage Foundation.

Bean, F. D., R. Chanove, R. G. Cushing, R. de la Garza, G. P. Freeman, C. W. Haynes, and D. Spener. 1994. *Illegal Mexican migration and the United States–Mexico border: The effects of Operation Hold the Line on El Paso–Juarez*. Washington, D.C.: U.S. Commission on Immigration Reform.

Bean, F. D., R. Corona, R. Tuiran, K. A. Woodrow-Lafield, and J. Van Hook. 2001. Circular, invisible, and ambiguous migrants: Components of difference in estimates of the number of unauthorized Mexican migrants in the United States. *Demography* 38:411–422.

Bean, F. D., and M. Fix. 1992. The significance of recent immigration policy reforms in the United States. In *Nations of immigrants: Australia and the United States in a changing world*. Edited by G. P. Freeman and J. Jupp. New York and Sydney: Oxford University Press.

Bean, F. D., J. S. Passel, and B. Edmonston. 1990. *Undocumented migration to the United States: IRCA and the experience of the 1980s*. Washington, D.C.: Urban Institute Press.

Bean, F. D., C. G. Swicegood, and R. Berg. 2000. Mexican-origin fertility: New patterns and interpretations. *Social Science Quarterly* 81:404–420.

Bean, F. D., and G. Stevens. 2003. *America's newcomers and the dynamics of diversity*. New York: Russell Sage Foundation.

Bean, F. D., E. Telles, and L. Lowell. 1987. Undocumented migration to the United States: Perceptions and evidence. *Population and Development Review* 13:671–690.

Bean, F. D., and M. Tienda. 1987. *The Hispanic population of the United States*. New York: Russell Sage Foundation.

Bean, F. D., G. Vernez, and C. B. Keely. 1989. *Opening and closing the doors: Evaluating immigration reform and control*. Santa Monica, Calif.: Washington, D.C. and Lanham, Md.: Rand and Urban Institute Press.

Becker, G. S. 1964. *Human capital: A theoretical and empirical analysis, with special reference to education*. New York: Columbia University Press.

Bonacich, E. 1973. A theory of middleman minorities. *American Sociological Review* 38:583–594.

Bonacich, E., and J. Modell. 1980. *The economic basis of ethnic solidarity: Small business in the Japanese American community*. Berkeley: University of California.

Borjas, G. J. 1990. *Friends or strangers: The impact of immigrants on the U.S. economy*. New York: Basic Books.

Borjas, G. J. 1999. *Heaven's door: Immigration policy and the American economy*. Princeton, N.J.: Princeton University Press.

Borjas, G. J., and M. Tienda. 1987. The economic consequences of immigration. *Science* 235:645–651.

Cafferty, P., B. R. Chiswick, A. Greeley, and T. A. Sullivan. 1983. *The dilemma of American immigration*. New Brunswick, N.J.: Transaction.

Calavita, K. 1992. *Inside the state: The Bracero program, immigration, and the I.N.S.* New York: Routledge.

Campbell, P. R. 1994. *Population projections for states, by age, sex, race, and Hispanic origin: 1993–2020.* P25–1111. Washington, D.C.: U.S. Government Printing Office for U.S. Bureau of the Census.

Castles, S., and M. J. Miller. 1998. *The age of migration: International population movements in the modern world.* New York: Guilford.

Cheng, L., and G. Gereffi. 1994. U.S. retailers and Asian garment production. In *Global production: The apparel industry in the Pacific Rim.* Edited by E. Bonacich, L. Cheng, N. Chinchilla, N. Hamilton, and P. Ong. Philadelphia: Temple University Press.

Demeny, P. 2003. Population policy dilemmas in Europe at the dawn of the twenty-first century. *Population and Development Review* 29:1–28.

Donato, K. M., J. Durand, and D. S. Massey. 1992. Changing conditions in the U.S. labor market: Effects of the Immigration Reform and Control Act of 1986. *Population Research and Policy Review* 11:93–115.

Easterlin, R. 1982. Economic and social characteristics of the immigrants. In *Dimensions of ethnicity.* Edited by S. Thernstrom. Cambridge, Mass.: Belknap Press and Harvard University Press.

Eschbach, K., J. Hagan, and S. Bailey. 1999. Death at the border. *International Migration Review* 33:430–454.

Espenshade, T. J. 1995. Unauthorized immigration to the United States. *Annual Review of Sociology* 21:195–216.

Fix, M., and J. S. Passel. 1994. Setting the record straight: What are the costs to the public? *Public Welfare* 52:6–15.

Furtado, C. 1964. *Development and underdevelopment.* Translated by R. W. de Aguiar and E. C. Drysdale. Berkeley: University of California Press.

Gilpin, R. 2000. *The challenge of global capitalism: The world economy in the 21st century.* Princeton, N.J.: Princeton University Press.

Granovetter, M. 1985. Economic action and social structure: The problem of embeddedness. *American Journal of Sociology* 91:481–510.

Granovetter, M. 1995. The economic sociology of firms and entrepreneurs. In *The economic sociology of immigration.* Edited by A. Portes. New York: Russell Sage Foundation.

Granovetter, M. S., and R. Swedberg. 1992. *The sociology of economic life.* Boulder, Colo.: Westview Press.

Grasmuck, S., and P. R. Pessar. 1991. *Between two islands: Dominican international migration.* Berkeley: University of California Press.

Hagan, J. M. 1994. *Deciding to be legal: A Maya community in Houston.* Philadelphia: Temple University Press.

Hagan, J. M. 1998. Social networks, gender and immigrant incorporation: Resources and constraints. *American Sociological Review* 63:55–67.

Harris, J. R., and M. P. Todaro. 1970. Migration, unemployment and development: A two-sector analysis. *American Economic Review* 60:126–142.

Hollifield, J. F. 1992. *Immigrants, markets, and states: The political economy of postwar Europe.* Cambridge, Mass.: Harvard University Press.

Hondagneu-Sotelo, P. 1994. *Gendered transitions: Mexican experiences of immigration.* Berkeley: University of California Press.

Hovy, B. 2002. Statistics on forced migration. *Migration Information Source* (Sept. 1).

Joppke, C. 1999. *Immigration and the nation-state.* New York: Oxford University Press.

Landau, R. 1988. U.S. economic growth. *Scientific American* 258:44–52.

Lee, J., and F. D. Bean. 2004. America's changing color lines: Race/ethnicity, immigration and multiracial identity. *Annual Review of Sociology* 30:221–242.

Levy, F. 1987. *Dollars and dreams: The changing American income distribution.* New York: Russell Sage Foundation.

Light, I., and S. Karageorgis. 1980. Chinatown: The socioeconomic potential of an urban enclave. *Ethnic and Racial Studies* 16:742–743.

Loucky, J., M. Soldatenko, S. Gregory, and E. Bonacich. 1994. Immigrant enterprise and labor in the Los Angeles garment industry. In *Global production: The apparel industry in the Pacific Rim.* Edited by E. Bonacich, L. Cheng, N. Chinchilla, N. Hamilton, and P. Ong. Philadelphia: Temple University Press.

Lozano-Ascencio, F. 1993. Bringing it back home: Remittances to Mexico from migrant workers in the United States. Monograph Series, No. 37. San Diego: Center for U.S.-Mexican Studies, University of California, San Diego.

Martin, P. 1997. Do Mexican agricultural policies stimulate emigration. In *At the crossroads: Mexico and U.S. immigration policy*. Edited by F. D. Bean, R. O. de la Garza, B. R. Roberts, and S. Weintraub. New York: Rowman & Littlefield.

Martin, P., and J. Widgren. 2002. International migration: Facing the challenge. *Population Bulletin* 57:1–40.

Massey, D. S. 1981. Dimensions of the new immigration to the United States and the prospects for assimilation. *Annual Review of Sociology* 7:57–85.

Massey, D. S. 1990. The social and economic origins of immigration. *Annals of the American Academy of Political and Social Science* 510:60–72.

Massey, D. S. 1994. Immigrants and the American city. *American Journal of Sociology* 99:1346–1348.

Massey, D. S. 1999. International migration at the dawn of the twenty-first century: The role of the state. *Population and Development Review* 25:303–322.

Massey, D. S., R. Alarion, J. Durand, and H. Gonzalez. 1987. *Return to Aztlan: The social process of international migration From western Mexico*. Berkeley: University of California Press.

Massey, D., J. Arango, G. Hugo, A. Kouaouci, A. Pellegrino, and J. E. Taylor. 1993. Theories of international migration: A review and appraisal. *Population and Development Review* 19:431–466.

Massey, D., J. Arango, G. Hugo, A. Kouaouci, A. Pellegrino, and J. E. Taylor. 1998. *Worlds in motion: Understanding international migration at the end of the millennium*. Oxford and New York: Clarendon Press and Oxford University Press.

Massey, D. S., J. Durand, and N. J. Malone. 2002. *Beyond smoke and mirrors: Mexican immigration in an era of economic integration*. New York: Russell Sage Foundation.

Massey, D., and K. E. Espinosa. 1997. What's driving Mexico-U.S. migration? A theoretical, empirical, and policy analysis. *American Journal of Sociology* 102:939–999.

Massey, D., and E. Parrado. 1994. Migradollars: The remittances and savings of Mexican migrants to the USA. *Population Research and Policy Review* 13:3–30.

McDonald, P., and R. Kippen. 2001. Labor supply prospects in 16 developed countries, 2000–2050. *Population and Development Review* 27:1–32.

Meissner, D. 2001. After the attacks: Protecting borders and liberties. Washington, D.C.: Carnegie Endowment for International Peace.

Meissner, D., and D. Martin. 2001. Terrorism and immigration: Our borders, security, and liberties. Washington, D.C.: Carnegie Endowment for International Peace.

Morales, R., and P. Ong. 1991. Immigrant women in Los Angeles. *Economic and Industrial Democracy* 12:65–81.

Morris, M. 1985. *Immigration: The beleaguered bureaucracy*. Washington, D.C.: Brookings Institution Press.

Nye, J. S. 2002. *The paradox of American power: Why the world's only superpower can't go it alone*. New York: Oxford University Press.

Passel, J. S. 1987. Measurement of ethnic origin in the decennial census. Paper presented at the Annual Meeting of the American Association for the Advancement of Science, Chicago (Feb. 14–18).

Passel, J. S., and B. Edmonston. 1994. Immigration and race: Recent trends in immigration to the United States. In *Immigration and ethnicity: The integration of America's newest arrivals*. Edited by J. S. Passel and B. Edmonston. Washington, D.C.: Urban Institute Press.

Petersen, W. 1975. *Population*, 3rd ed. New York: Macmillan.

Piore, M. J. 1979. *Birds of passage: Migrant labor and industrial societies*. New York: Cambridge University Press.

Portes, A. 1987. The social origins of the Cuban enclave economy of Miami. *Sociological Perspectives* 30:340–372.

Portes, A., and R. L. Bach. 1985. *Latin journey: Cuban and Mexican immigrants in the United States*. Berkeley: University of California Press.

Portes, A., and L. Jensen. 1989. The enclave and the entrants: Patterns of ethnic enterprise in Miami before and after Mariel. *American Sociological Review* 54:929–949.

Portes, A., and R. G. Rumbaut. 1990. *Immigrant America: A portrait*. Berkeley: University of California Press.

Portes, A., and A. Stepick. 1993. *City on the edge: The transformation of Miami*. Berkeley: University of California Press.

Reimers, D. M. 1983. An unintended reform: The 1965 immigration act and Third World migration to the United States. *Journal of American Ethnic History* 3:9–28.

Reimers, D. M. 1985. *Still the golden door: The Third World comes to America*. New York: Columbia University Press.

Reimers, D. M. 1998. *Unwelcome strangers: American identity and the turn against immigration*. New York: Columbia University Press.

Repak, T. A. 1994. Labor market incorporation of Central American immigrants in Washington, D.C. *Social Problems* 41:114–128.

Repak, T. A. 1995. *Waiting on Washington: Central American workers in the nation's capital*. Philadelphia: Temple University Press.

Roberts, B. R. 1995. Socially expected durations and the economic adjustment of immigrants. In *The Economic Sociology of Immigration*. Edited by A. Portes. New York: Russell Sage Foundation.

Roberts, B. R., R. Bean, and F. Lozano-Ascencio. 1999. Transnational migrant communities and Mexican migration to the U.S. *Ethnic and Racial Studies* 22:238–266.

Roberts, B. R., and A. Escobar Latapi. 1997. Mexican social and economic policy and emigration. In *At the crossroads: Mexico and U.S. immigration policy*. Edited by F. D. Bean, R. O. de la Garza, B. R. Roberts, and S. Weintraub. New York: Rowman & Littlefield.

Salt, J. 1981. International labor migration in western Europe: A geographical review. In *Global trends in migration: Theory and research on international population movements*. Edited by M. M. Kritz, C. B. Keely, and S. M. Tomasi. New York: Center for Migration Studies.

Sassen, S. 1988. *The mobility of labor and capital: A study in international investment and labor flow*. New York: Cambridge University Press.

Sassen, S. 1991. *The global city: New York, London, and Tokyo*. Princeton, N.J.: Princeton University Press.

Sassen, S. 1994. *Cities in a world economy*. Thousand Oaks, Calif.: Pine Forge Press.

Sassen, S. 1995. Immigration and local labor markets. In *The economic sociology of immigration*. Edited by A. Portes. New York: Russell Sage Foundation.

Sassen, S. 2000. Urban economics and fading distances. Lecture presented to the Project "De Ondergang Van Nederland?" March 30.

Shryock, H. S., and J. S. Siegal. 1976. *The methods and materials of demography*. San Diego, Calif.: Academic Press.

Simon, J. L. 1987. *Effort, opportunity and wealth*. Oxford: Basil Backwell.

Stark, O. 1991. Migration incentives, migration types: The role of relative deprivation. *Economic Journal* 101:1163–1178.

Stark, O., and J. E. Taylor, 1989. Relative deprivation and international migration. *Demography* 26:1–14.

Stepick, A. 1989. Miami's two informal sectors. In *The informal economy: Studies in advanced and less developed countries*. Edited by A. Portes, M. Castells, and L. A. Benton. Baltimore, Md.: John Hopkins University.

Suro, R. 1998. *Strangers among us: How Latino immigration is transforming America*. New York: Alfred A. Knopf.

Taylor, J. E. 1987. Undocumented Mexico-U.S. migration and the returns to households in rural Mexico. *American Journal of Agricultural Economics* 69:616–638.

Taylor, J. E. 1992. Remittances and inequality reconsidered: Direct, indirect, and intertemporal effects. *Journal of Policy Modeling* 14:187–208.

Taylor, J. E. 1994. "Mexico-to-U.S., Migration in the Context of Economic Globalization: A Village CGE Perspective." Paper prepared for the annual meeting of the American Association for the Advancement of Science, San Francisco (Feb. 24).

Taylor, J. E., P. L. Martin, and M. Fix. 1997. *Poverty amid prosperity: Immigration and the changing face of rural California*. Washington, D.C.: Urban Institute Press.

Todaro, M. P., and L. Maruszko. 1987. Illegal migration and U.S. immigration reform: A conceptual framework. *Population and Development Review* 13:101–114.

Tolbert, C. M., P. M. Horan, and E. M. Beck. 1980. The structure of economic segmentation: A dual economy approach. *American Journal of Sociology* 85:1095–1116.

United Nations. 2002. *International migration report 2002*. New York: United Nations Press.

United Nations High Commissioner for Refugees. 2002a. *Statistical Yearbook, 2001*.

United Nations High Commissioner for Refugees. 2002b. *Refugees By Numbers, 2002*.

U.S. Bureau of the Census. 2002a. *Census 2000*. Demographic Profiles. Washington, D.C.

U.S. Bureau of the Census. 2002b. *Census 2000*. Supplementary Survey (C2SS) (computer file). Washington, D.C.

U.S. Bureau of Labor Statistics. 2001. "Employment Estimates." Available on-line at: *stats.bls.gov/bls/employment.htm*.

U.S. Department of Justice. 1992. Immigration Reform and Control Act: Report on the legalized alien population. Washington, D.C.: U.S. Government Printing Office.

U.S. Immigration and Naturalization Service. 1994. *1993 INS Yearbook*. Washington, D.C.: U.S. Government Printing Office.

U.S. Immigration and Naturalization Service. 2002. *2000 INS Yearbook*. Washington, D.C.: U.S. Government Printing Office.

Van Hook, J., and F. D. Bean. 1998. Estimating unauthorized Mexican migration to the United States: Issues and results. In *Migration between Mexico and the United States, binational study*, Vol. 2, 511–550. Mexico City and Washington, D.C.: Mexican Ministry of Foreign Affairs and U.S. Commission on Immigration Reform.

Ventura, S. J., S. C. Curtin, and T. J. Mathews. 2000. Variations in teenage birth rates, 1991–98: National and state trends. *National Vital Statistics Reports* 48:1–13.

Waldinger, R. 1986. *Through the eye of the needle: Immigrants and enterprise in New York's garment trades*. New York: New York University Press.

Waldinger, R. 1996. *Still the promised city? African-Americans and new immigrants in postindustrial New York*. Cambridge, Mass.: Harvard University.

Wallerstein, I. 1983. *Historical capitalism*. New York: Verso.

Warren, R. 1990. Annual estimates of nonimmigrant overstays in the United States: 1985–1988. In *Undocumented migration to the United States: IRCA and the experience of the 1980s*. Edited by F. D. Bean, B. Edmonston, and J. S. Passel. Washington, D.C.: Urban Institute Press.

Warren, R. 1992. Estimates of the unauthorized immigrant population residing in the United States, by country of origin and state of residence: October 1992. Report. Washington, D.C.: U.S. Immigration and Naturalization Service, Statistics Division.

Warren, R., and J. S. Passel. 1987. A count of the uncountable: Estimates of undocumented aliens counted in the 1980 United States census. *Demography* 24:375–394.

Wilson, K. L., and A. Portes. 1980. Immigrant enclaves: An analysis of the labor market experiences of Cubans in Miami. *American Journal of Sociology* 86:295–319.

Wrigley, J. 1997. Immigrant women as child care providers. In *Immigrant entrepreneurs and immigrant absorption in the United States and Israel*. Edited by I. H. Light and R. Isralowitz. Aldershot, U.K., and Brookfield, Vt.: Ashgate.

Yang, P. Q. 1995. *Post-1965 Immigration to the United States: Structural Determinants*. Westport, CT: Praeger.

Zlotnik, H. 1987. The concept of international migration as reflected in data collection systems. *International Migration Review* 20:925–946.

Zlotnik, H. 1999. Trends of international migration since 1965: What existing data reveal. *International Migration* 37:21–61.

Zlotnik, H. 2003. The global dimensions of female migration. *Migration Information Source*, March 1.

Zolberg, A. R. 1992. Response to crisis: Refugee policy in the United States and Canada. In *Immigration, language, and ethnicity: Canada and the United States*. Edited by B. R. Chiswick. Washington, D.C.: AEI Press.

Zolberg, A. R. 1999. Matters of state: Theorizing immigration policy. In *The handbook of international migration*. Edited by C. Hirschman, J. DeWind, and P. Kasinitz. New York: Russell Sage Foundation.

CHAPTER 13

Demography of Social Stratification

ARTHUR SAKAMOTO

AND

DANIEL A. POWERS

INTRODUCTION

Issues pertaining to social stratification are increasingly considered in demographic research. In recent studies of morbidity and mortality, for example, education, income, and occupation typically have substantially large net effects (e.g., Cambois, Robine, and Hayward 2001; Duleep 1989; Gortmaker and Wise 1997; Johnson, Sorlie, and Backlund 1999; Mare 1990; Rogers 1992; Ross and Mirowsky 1999; Ross and Wu 1995).[1] Similarly, studies of fertility frequently refer to education and other variables pertaining to social class (e.g., Li and Choe 1997; Kohler, Behrman, and Watkins 2001; Powers and Hsueh 1997)—or at least to socioeconomic considerations involved in labor force participation, child-care costs, and economic opportunity costs (e.g., Blau and Robins 1989; Borg 1989). Socioeconomic motives and consequences are also important issues in demographic research on immigration and migration (e.g., Boyle et al. 2001; Oropesa and Landale 2000; Reed 2001).

A recent presidential address to the Population Association of America focused provocatively on socioeconomic inequality and concomitant social problems (Massey 1996). The address was published in *Demography* along with the commentaries of noted experts in the demography of social stratification (Danziger 1996; Farley 1996; Hout,

---

[1] Needless to say, life expectancy and health tend to be better for persons with higher socioeconomic status. An unusual exception to this general pattern, however, is evident for the military deaths among the North Vietnamese during the American military involvement in Vietnam between 1965 and 1975 (Merli 2000).

Arum, and Voss 1996). A recent editor of *Demography* is a specialist in the study of social stratification, as was another recent editor.[2] Papers on social stratification topics are now commonly published in *Demography*, including studies on income inequality (e.g., Chevan and Stokes 2000; Deaton and Paxson 1997; Karoly and Burtless 1995), economic and social mobility (e.g., Duncan, Boisjoly, and Smeeding 1996; Duleep and Regets 1997; Gittleman and Joyce 1999), poverty (e.g., Bauman 1999; Guo and Harris 2000; Iceland 1997, 2003), educational attainment (e.g., Hannum 2002; Hirschman 2001; Pribesh and Downey 1999), occupational attainment (e.g., Grusky and DiPrete 1990; Hannum and Xie 1998), and occupational gender segregation (e.g., Weeden 1998; Grusky and Charles 1998).

Increasing attention to the demography of social stratification is evident in the articles published in *Demography*, *Population Studies*, and *International Migration Review* during the past few decades. In these journals from 1964 to 1978, only six articles were published that included in their titles "social mobility," "poverty," "stratification" or "inequality." In the subsequent 15 years, from 1979 to 1993, these journals published 26 articles that included those terms in their titles. In the seven years from 1994 through 2000, 36 such articles were published by these journals. Thus, these results show that during the last seven-year period, six times as many articles were published on the demography of social stratification as were published during the 15-year period from 1964 to 1978.

Given this increased interest, a review and assessment of the current state of the demography of social stratification is needed. In the following section we discuss the definition and scope of this field and consider its linkages with other areas. We then review major research strands in the demography of social stratification and highlight some notable contributions. We conclude by pointing out some topics for future research.

SUBSTANTIVE AND THEORETICAL ISSUES

Definition and Scope

Although topics relating to social stratification seem to have always been accepted as pertinent to modern demography, formal statements of its scope usually do not refer explicitly to socioeconomic inequalities as a specific aspect of population composition. Shryock and Siegel (1976: 1) define demography in its "broader sense" to include the study of the "social characteristics and economic characteristics" of populations but do not mention social inequality or stratification per se. Hauser and Duncan (1959: 31) do recognize "social mobility" as a fundamental population process, but they use that term very loosely to refer to the change in any status variable (e.g., "from 'single' to 'married' with respect to marital status"). While Hauser and Duncan's definition of the scope of demography is clearly meant to be broad enough to include the study of socioeconomic inequalities, the latter are nonetheless not explicitly referred to or identified.

In recent years, demographic research has shown greater overlap with related disciplines. More elaborate theoretical arguments have been developed, and increasingly

---

[2] We refer to Daniel T. Lichter and Robert D. Mare, respectively.

complex data and statistical models have been used (Crimmins 1993). As mentioned above, demographic research now routinely considers topics and variables that pertain to social stratification. At this stage, there is an obvious need to clearly define the scope of the demography of social stratification. Providing a definition of this field is expedient not only for theoretical clarity, but also because the vast number of studies on the subject of social inequality requires that we delineate our consideration of this literature.

The core of demography is the study of the size and territorial distribution of populations that depend on the components of the demographic equation: fertility, mortality, and migration. Associated with this core is the study of population composition, which refers to the characteristics of people that are related to fertility, mortality, and migration. Population composition is typically thought to include sex and age structure, racial and ethnic characteristics, patterns of health and morbidity, marital characteristics, family structure, the distributions of nativity and citizenship statuses, educational attainments, and labor force characteristics, but social inequalities can also be explicitly included as a relevant feature of population composition. Demography can thus be defined as the scientific study of the core demographic components (i.e., fertility, mortality, and migration) and of related aspects of population composition.

Social stratification can be defined as the study of socioeconomic inequality and mobility. As noted by Otis Dudley Duncan, one of the pioneers of the demography of social stratification, inequality can be defined as "the dispersion of the distribution over a population of any of the rewards and status distinctions conferred by a society on its members—such as income, wealth, level of living, leisure, prestige, recognition, power, authority, skill, information, civil liberties, welfare, or life chances" (Duncan 1969: 361). Understanding and investigating the sources of the dispersion of these scarce social and economic resources is an important task for the field of social stratification.

Although Duncan preferred the term *opportunity*, mobility can be defined as "the probability of finding one's self at a high, medium, or low position on any of the scales of status or reward just mentioned" (Duncan 1969: 361). As is commonly distinguished, *intragenerational mobility* refers to changes in one's status position during one's lifetime, while *intergenerational mobility* refers to differences in status positions between the generations of a family. With regard to the latter, the associations between parents' and offspring's statuses are the most highly investigated (e.g., Blau and Duncan 1967; Featherman and Hauser 1978; Hauser and Featherman 1977), although there have been a few interesting studies of relationships between offspring and grandparents' generations (Warren and Hauser 1997; Alba, Lutz, and Vesselinov 2001; Borjas 2001).[3] Whatever the reference points used, however, the study of mobility in terms of the attainments and changes in socioeconomic status is a central concern for the field of social stratification.[4]

The demography of social stratification may thus be defined as the study of how fertility, mortality, migration, and related aspects of population composition affect and

[3] As noted by Mare (2001: 479), "the association between the socioeconomic characteristics of parents and offspring is just one out of a large number of possible socioeconomic associations between pairs of kin, which include siblings, spouses, individuals and their parents-in-law, parents and parents-in-law, cousins, and grandparents and grandchildren."

[4] In contrast to Duncan (1969), we do not focus primarily on intergenerational mobility. Furthermore, we use the term stratification more broadly than he does. Duncan (1969: 361) defines it as referring to a low level of intergenerational mobility.

are affected by inequality and mobility. That is, this field can be defined as the study of both the causes and consequences of demographic variables in terms of the degree of dispersion in the distributions of socioeconomic rewards as well as the attainments and changes in the positions of individuals and their kin in these distributions. Not only do social stratification processes often help to explain or to predict the sorts of outcomes in which demographers have traditionally been interested, but demographic factors can also have major consequences for social stratification.

Methodological Orientation

While the foregoing provides a general definition of the demography of social stratification, perhaps equally important in delineating this field is its methodological orientation. First and foremost, demographic research typically places a high priority on objective measurement and empirical data analysis involving the scientific use of statistics or mathematics; the methodology for the demography of social stratification usually involves the quantitative analysis of empirical data. Many of the classic demographic studies of social stratification (e.g., Blau and Duncan 1967; Featherman and Hauser 1978) are noted for their methodological rigor, whereas other studies that are more theoretical in orientation (or less rigorous methodologically) are less likely to be considered demographic research, even though they may be concerned with similar substantive issues (e.g., Lipset and Bendix 1964).

The empirical and quantitative nature of demographic analysis represents an exceedingly important approach for the study of social stratification. Social inequality and mobility are topics that often elicit or relate to fundamental political beliefs, social values, moral principles, philosophical views, and even emotional responses. Demographic research is important for the study of social stratification because some disciplined, scientific empiricism is needed to help elucidate the relevant empirical facts that might otherwise become obscured by political passions and ideologies.[5]

The empiricism of demographic analysis also plays an important role in the study of social stratification because empiricism serves as a countervailing force against the tendencies of many explanations of inequality to emphasize unobserved variables. For example, in explaining various aspects of inequality, economists often refer to processes in which individuals are assumed to "maximize utility" and employers are said to pay hourly wages according to "marginal revenue products," although typically these concepts are not measured directly (e.g., Mansfield 1979). Marxist sociological discussions emphasize "exploitation" (e.g., Wright 2000), yet their data analyses are devoid of any actual empirical measure of it. In short, many theories of social stratification often involve unobservable variables, and the empiricism of demographic analysis plays an important countervailing role in clarifying what is known about the actual empirical facts pertaining to social stratification.

In addition to the priority placed on the study of empirical data, demographic analysis often investigates entry and exit processes or other mobility processes that may be time-dependent. This analytical perspective derives from the demographic equation

---

[5] Perhaps this point is indirectly evident in Duncan's (1969: 363) comment about the interpretation of regression coefficients in a status attainment model: "Analysts who are intolerant of ambiguity may join the ideologists, for whom questions have clear and decisive answers."

in which fertility, mortality, and migration depend on exposure time and age. The study of entry and exit processes is also central to the mechanics of the life table, which is perhaps the most classic of demographic tools. Although this characteristic is not an absolutely necessary feature of the demography of social stratification, analyses of entry, exit, or other mobility and transition processes are common in this field. Indeed, the study of social mobility per se is sometimes considered virtually synonymous with the demography of social stratification.

In sum, we define the demography of social stratification as the study of how fertility, mortality, migration, and related features of population composition affect and are affected by inequality and mobility. In terms of methodology, the demography of social stratification usually involves the quantitative analysis of empirical data and frequently investigates entry, exit, or other mobility processes. This field is concerned not only with how social stratification variables affect the core demographic components (i.e., fertility, mortality, and migration) but also how these processes and their associated aspects of population composition may in turn have consequences for social inequality and mobility.

Relation to Other Demographic Topics

Given this definition, portions of each of the chapters for Part I and Part II of this volume are relevant to the demography of social stratification. For example, as discussed by Parker Frisbie (chapter 9), socioeconomic variables have important effects on infant mortality. Rogelio Saenz reviews socioeconomic differentials between racial and ethnic groups (chapter 6). Teresa Sullivan's discusses underemployment and unemployment, which are inherently socioeconomic in nature, in chapter 7, "Labor Free." In addition, social stratification issues may also arise in the intersection between demography and other social sciences (i.e., Part III of this volume).

This chapter focuses primarily on studies that investigate the effects of demographic variables on stratification outcomes (i.e., inequality and mobility). The earlier chapters of this volume should be consulted for discussions of the effects of socioeconomic differentials, inequality, and mobility on the core demographic components of fertility, mortality, and migration.[6] In our review, we do not devote extensive consideration to gender, marriage and the family, or race and ethnicity because there are separate chapters on these aspects of population composition.

Demography and Mobility

An enduring concern in the study of mobility is the degree to which it is explained or dependent on demographic and ascriptive factors such as age, race, ethnicity, gender, social class, or other family background characteristics.[7] This interest in part derives from sociological theories that postulate an increase in universalism in modern societies

---

[6] See also Kasarda and Billy (1985) for an excellent summary of the literature on the relationship between social mobility and fertility.

[7] According to Ganzeboom, Treiman, and Ultee (1991: 283–284), the empirical analysis of this issue was promoted by the "second generation" of cross-national research on social stratification.

(e.g., Parsons 1970; Treiman 1970). The norm of universalism dictates that mobility and inequality should depend primarily on achieved factors (e.g., education, training, work experience, technical skills) rather than ascriptive characteristics per se. According to this modernization theory, basing social stratification on achieved factors promotes more rational and efficient social organizations and economic production.

Given this theoretical background, demographic studies of social mobility have frequently been concerned with monitoring temporal trends in social stratification. For example, although Herrnstein and Murray (1994) argue that the net effect of cognitive skills on socioeconomic outcomes has increased in recent decades, Hauser and Huang (1997) find no evidence for this trend in their analysis of a simple measure of verbal ability.[8] In studies of occupational mobility, a long-standing objective of researchers over the decades has been to assess the current trend in the level of intergenerational transmission of occupational status (Blau and Duncan 1967; Featherman and Hauser 1978; Hout 1988; DiPrete and Grusky 1990; Rytina 2000).

Monitoring trends in the net effects of achieved versus ascribed characteristics has also been of major interest in this literature. An illustration of this concern is provided by Sakamoto and associates (1998, 1999, 2000), who find increased net effects of education and decreased net effects of being a racial or ethnic minority on the income and occupational attainment of American men during the latter half of the 20th century. In a somewhat related study, when comparing the intergenerational occupational mobility of African American men before and after the civil rights legislation of the 1960s, Hout (1984) finds a substantial increase in the importance of class of origin during the latter period.

An additional research concern frequently observed in the literature is how much social mobility is structural versus circulation mobility. The basic idea is that structural mobility refers to that which is "forced" due to changes in the distribution of occupations (either intragenerationally or intergenerationally) as reflected by the differences in the marginal distributions of the mobility table. Structural mobility is generally assumed to reflect technological change and economic development. On the other hand, circulation (or "exchange") mobility refers to that which is said to more directly reflect the degree of openness or inherent social fluidity of a society. Circulation mobility is usually defined as that which is net of structural mobility.

Demography and Inequality

Empty places is a popular phrase used by Marxists to emphasize the institutional nature of socioeconomic inequality (Wright 1979: 20). Similarly, among non-Marxist sociologists, "the distinctive approach by sociology to the study of inequality is probably the idea that social structure is somehow relevant for the creation of inequality.... this idea is shared by most sociological stratification researchers" (Sørensen 1996: 1334). In short, a central concern of many sociological studies of inequality has been understanding its institutional nature.

---

[8] In a thorough analysis of data from the Wisconsin Longitudinal Survey, Hauser et al. (2000: 223–225) find that measured mental ability is only one variable among several that have at least equal or greater effects on the occupational attainment of adults in the early 1990s.

While we do not doubt the theoretical significance of the institutional perspective on inequality, an analysis of why some empty places (i.e., jobs) pay higher earnings than others cannot provide a complete accounting of the degree of inequality across units within a population. For example, some people may have two jobs while others may have none so that the degree of earnings inequality among individuals in the population would be much greater than the degree of earnings inequality among the empty places. Or, among families, if spouses' earnings are correlated, then the degree of inequality across families would be much greater than if persons tended to marry spouses whose earnings were uncorrelated with their own. Investigating inequality only among persons with jobs also ignores, as Mare (2001: 478) observes, "the stratification of the large non-working part of the population, including (1) children and teenagers; (2) 'working-age' persons who do not hold jobs because they are homekeepers, caregivers, students, disabled, incarcerated, independently affluent, or simply unable to find work; and (3) retired persons who are past the conventional working age." In sum, although organizations and social institutions certainly do influence the degree of inequality between jobs, the demography of inequality is still important because it analyzes the degree of inequality across units in a population.

Furthermore, the distribution of various population characteristics may influence the degree of inequality across jobs as well. Wages are not permanently fixed across all jobs but instead are often affected by the characteristics of the incumbents of the empty places. The distribution or supply of well-paid jobs may also be affected by population characteristics and processes. As Mare (2001: 485) describes, when a change in the distribution of personal characteristics in the labor force "affects the relative numbers of workers trained for various positions, the relative wages of these skill groups may change and, in turn, change employers' demands for workers of varying types and the resulting job and wage distributions."[9] Thus, demography affects the observed degree of inequality across workers.

METHODS AND MEASURES

Implicit in the study of attainment and mobility, just as in many areas of demographic research, is *change*. Fundamental demographic concepts and statistical methods have been instrumental in several major lines of inquiry relating to change as applied to social stratification. This section focuses on the demographic underpinnings of some aspects of the methodology for the study of social mobility and attainment.

At the individual level, socioeconomic attainment represents a process of change or a *transition* from one social status—or social origin—to another destination status such as current job.[10] At the aggregate level, interest often focuses on changes in the

---

[9] Mare (2001: 485) also argues that intragenerational mobility increases the "transitory" component of the variance in earnings so that "inequality in earnings at any time is greater in markets where workers make frequent moves than in markets with limited labor mobility."

[10] Of course, individuals may end up in the roughly the same social status they started out in. When considering a strictly quantitative dimension of social status, such as a socioeconomic index that varies over all occupations or earnings measured in constant units with infinite precision, the probability that an individual's destination status equals his or her origin status is infinitesimally small. With less detailed measures, such as broad occupational categories, such small changes may be undetectable, and individuals can be considered immobile.

occupational distribution induced by structural change in the past. Such change would include the growth and decline in certain types of jobs over time, the expansion and contraction of certain sectors of the economy, and gross flows of new labor force entrants as a result of differential fertility and migration. Additional sources of change in the occupational distribution include institutional changes in occupational barriers to entry, licensing practices, and educational institutions and policies that affect the supply of high-skilled labor. Also important is the alteration of normative patterns of labor market processes that may inhibit the movement of groups out of jobs in which they have been traditionally overrepresented into jobs in which they have been traditionally underrepresented.

Change Processes

Change processes can be formulated in many ways. In their now classic study of status attainment, Blau and Duncan (1967: 165) propose and estimate a path model using the OCG-I data set. This model was extended by Sewell, Haller, and Ohlendorf (1970) in their formulation of the so-called Wisconsin Model, which includes social-psychological variables. In these and later status attainment studies (e.g., Jencks, Crouse, and Mueser 1983), a central objective is to uncover the pathways to attainment and to estimate the relative impact of social origins on social destinations as mediated by intervening variables such as education, aspirations, and first job.

Other approaches (e.g., Spilerman 1976) focus more exclusively on the labor market career per se and take the first job as the starting point in an ongoing sequence of socioeconomic changes. Individual career lines, job trajectories, and yearly wage rates are indicators of the attainment process over the life course of individuals. In this sense, job mobility and changes in earnings can be viewed as natural extensions of the status attainment model of Blau and Duncan (1967). This approach focuses on the determinants of individual change over the life cycle (i.e., intragenerational mobility) and employs a methodology that is closely related to the demographic methods used in the study of vital rates.

The investigation of intergenerational processes typically considers intergenerational occupational mobility by examining the social origins of a current sample of workers. Such analyses hinge on the cross-classification of the occupational distribution of a current sample of sons by the occupations of their fathers when respondents were adolescents. The square contingency table formed by arraying father's and son's occupational categories in this manner provides the data for the statistical analysis of social mobility.

Methods for Individual Change

The process of attainment entails a temporal component in which individuals' values on quantitative dimensions of stratification change over time. When such change in a continuous variable results in a change in a qualitative dimension, then, in a nominalist sense, a *transition* occurs from one social status (or qualitative dimension) to another. The study of change can be viewed as a study of transitions. A fundamental concept in the statistical analysis of change is the transition probability, which has close ties with several demographic methods, including life tables and population projections. To study change at the individual level, it is necessary to first define the set of social statuses that can be occupied at any point in time, or the state space Y_t. The probability that an individual in state i changes to state $j (i, j \in Y_t)$ in the time interval of from t to $t + \Delta t$ (where $t > 0$ and $\Delta t > 0$) is the transition probability p_{ij}. The limit of this conditional probability as $\Delta t \to 0$ is the transition rate $r_{ij}(t)$ at time t. Other quantities of interest are derived from the transition rate. For example, the proportion "surviving" to time t, or remaining in the origin state until that time, is given by the survival function, $\exp\{ - \int_0^t r(u)du\}$, which can be derived from the usual life table methods by setting the radix $l(0) = 1$.[11] With data that have been aggregated by summing the individual transitions occurring over a set of time intervals, these rates can be defined empirically as the ratio of the number of i to j transitions divided by person-units of exposure to the risk of that transition in a particular time interval.[12]

Researchers typically focus on a subset of possible transitions such as upward moves, changes in earnings, or job shifts of various kinds. There are several notable examples of earlier empirical research along these lines. Lipset and Bendix (1952a, 1952b) examine employer change and occupational change and find variation in job change behavior by occupation and age. Palmer (1954) examines job change patterns in several mutually exclusive categories comprised of employer, industry, and occupation, and other shift types. Spilerman and Miller (1973) investigate variation in the quality of position left and position entered. Sørensen (1974) finds differential socioeconomic effects of voluntary versus involuntary job shifts. Tuma (1976) shows that the rate of job mobility decreases as job rewards increase, increases with levels of personal resources including education, social background, and place of origin, but decreases as duration in the job increases.

Recent work focuses on the linkages between states in Y_t. For example, Y_t^A may represent a fertility transition such as the birth of first child and Y_t^B may represent an employment transition (e.g., leaving or entering a job). Blossfeld (1986, 1994) outlines a strategy for analyzing interdependent processes such as these in which the researcher considers one focal process among the set of interdependent processes as the *dependent* one. Subsequent change in a dependent process is viewed as a function of current status, the past, as well as other exogenous variables in what is termed a *semi-Markov* process.[13] That is, transitions are independent of previous history but depend on the length of time spent in a previous state. Time dependence in transition rates can be specified parametrically by making assumptions about the profile of the rate over time and allowing the shape of the rate to be a function of one or more parameters that may themselves be functions of observed variables.[14]

---

[11] Namboodiri and Suchindran (1987) provide a concise treatment of the life table from a Markov perspective.

[12] In demography, this method is routinely applied to assess the impact of measured covariates on rates. For example, a common technique is to treat the counts as Poisson variates and fit a generalized linear model with the log of the exposure as an offset—a term whose slope coefficient is fixed at unity or some other constant (e.g., Holford 1980; Laird and Oliver 1981).

[13] A Markov process is one in which an individual's future status depends only on his present status, independent of the previous history leading up to present status.

[14] Time dependence may be specified semiparametrically, in which case transition rates are assumed to be constant within time intervals but can change in a stepwise fashion over time. Tuma's (1976) finding of the

In their work on social change processes, Tuma and Hannan (1984) state that time itself can be viewed as a proxy for time-varying causal factors which are difficult to observe. This idea has been used by Blossfeld (1986) to study job shifts by postulating that unobserved job-specific labor force experience Z_{LFX} assumes a value of 0 at the beginning of each new job and increases linearly over the a person's job spell t. The equation to describe this situation usually incorporates a set of explanatory variables X, and can be written as:

$$r(t) = \exp\{X\beta + \gamma Z_{LFX}(t)\}. \tag{1}$$

In this case, the observed job duration t is viewed as a proxy for job-specific labor force experience resulting in the following Gompertz model:

$$r(t) = \exp(X\beta + \gamma t) = \exp(X\beta)\exp(\gamma t) \tag{2}$$

Thus, $\gamma < 0$ would support the hypothesis that increasing the stock of job-specific labor-force experience leads to a monotonic decline in the job shift rate.[15] Other parametric forms would lead to alternative hypotheses about the rate of change in job shift rates. For example, using the logarithm of job-specific experience $Z_{LFX}(t) = \log t$ would imply that increasing employment duration leads to a relatively smaller stock of job-specific labor force experience than would be implied by the model above, resulting in a more gradual decline in the job shift rate as the duration of the employment spell increases.

Both of these models assume that job shift rates change monotonically over the length of the employment spell. It is more realistic—and consistent with existing theory and empirical research—to envision employment as the result of matching employees to jobs (Mincer and Jovanovic 1981), so that employment may involve an initial adjustment period in which mismatches are likely to be resolved. This results in increasing job shift rates early in an employment spell and declining job shift rates later on. As noted by Blossfeld and Rohwer (1995), this empirical relationship would be quite plausible on theoretical grounds and could result from the interplay of two contradictory forces—increasing job-specific investments on the one hand and decreasing need to resolve employment mismatches on the other. To accommodate both of these scenarios requires a more flexible model that allows for increasing initial rates of job shift followed by declining rates as employment durations increase.

Demographic Studies of Social Mobility

Cross-classification, or cross-tabulation, is one of the oldest and most widely used statistical tools available to social scientists. Prior to the upsurge in regression and regressionlike methods, cross-tabulation was *the* major analytical method used in sociology. Classic studies of social mobility rely on cross-classifications of occupational

---

existence of significant duration dependence in job mobility rates is taken as evidence against a stationary Markov process for job mobility and evidence in favor of a semi-Markov view that incorporates stationary person-specific characteristics on the one hand and time-dependence in job-shift rates on the other.

[15] The Gompertz model and its modification by Makeham are widely used in demography to describe the force of mortality at later ages.

categories (e.g., Glass 1954). Intergenerational mobility is typically studied using a cross-classification based on as few as 3 and as many as 17 categories of father's and son's occupation, corresponding to table rows and columns respectively. The resulting square contingency table forms the basis for a statistical analysis of social mobility in which the joint frequencies f_{ij} in the ith row and jth column are the observed outcomes of a mobility process and denote the number of sons in the jth occupational class category with social origin category (father's occupational class) i. Hauser (1978: 921) states that models for mobility are useful in informing "us where in the social structure opportunities for movement or barriers to movement are greater or less, and in so doing provide clues about stratification processes which are not less important, if different in kind, from those uncovered by multivariate causal models."

It is tempting to view the marginal distribution of fathers' occupations in a father-son mobility table as an occupational distribution at an earlier time. A great deal of early mobility research takes this approach. The basic techniques for analyzing changing occupational distributions are identical to those used for projecting population growth as a first-order Markov process. Using this perspective, some investigators equate differences in the marginal distribution of occupations of fathers and sons to trends or change in the occupational distribution of the workforce (Rogoff 1953; Kahl 1957). Kahl (1957) uses the marginal distributions of occupations in different historical periods approximately a generation apart, along with additional data on occupation-specific fertility and migration rates, to decompose total intergenerational social mobility into distinct components attributable to differential reproduction, immigration, and technological sources. Matras (1961) follows in this tradition but considers different assumptions about mobility and fertility rates in analyzing generation-to-generation change in occupational distributions as well as mobility patterns.

As Duncan (1966) points out, however, this approach is attractive in its elegance and innovativeness, but it ignores the fact that social surveys begin with a sample of sons and ask about the occupations of their fathers at the time when sons were age 16.[16] Fathers with no sons are not represented in the marginal distributions of mobility tables, whereas fathers with more than one son are overrepresented. Because major studies of social mobility (e.g., those based on the OCG-I and OCG-II data sets) are based on large-scale surveys that interview men ages 20 to 64 in the current year, it is possible that a father and his son are both represented in the same table. Moreover, sons in the sample have fathers of different ages and these fathers are likely to have started their careers at different times, under different structural conditions, and hence the information corresponds to different points in the careers of fathers. As Duncan (1966: 59) states "the transformations that occur via a *succession of cohorts* cannot, for basic demographic reasons, be equated to the product of a *procession of 'generations.'*" Therefore, the mobility table is probably best viewed as a distribution of the current occupations of a sample of men. As such, it should be viewed not as information about mobility, but as information about the dependence of sons' statuses on fathers' statuses (Duncan 1966; Mukherjee 1954).

---

[16] A notable exception to this is Rogoff's (1953) study in which data are obtained from marriage license applications eliciting men's current occupation as well as the current occupation of the respondent's father.

Social Mobility as a Probability Process

Despite the aforementioned limitations, early studies of social mobility consider as a basis for analysis the matrix of transition probabilities, or outflow percentages, implicit in the father-son occupational mobility table. This forms the starting point for a mathematical analysis of social mobility that has many close parallels with mathematical population models. Prais (1955a) and Glass (1954) carried out early work on social mobility in Great Britain using methods based on Markov chains. In a similar vein, studies by Matras (1961, 1967) provide insights into the interrelationships between differential fertility, intergenerational mobility, and change in the distribution of occupations using Markov chain theory.[17] In this tradition, transition probabilities, outflow proportions, or mobility rates, denoted by p_{ij}, represent the conditional probability of moving from origin state i to destination state j. The set of transition probabilities forms the transition matrix, or mobility rate matrix, $\mathbf{M} = p_{ij}$.[18] If $\mathbf{M}$ is stable over time, the theory of Markov chains can be applied to yield an occupational distribution at a later time, in the same spirit that a Leslie matrix is used for population projection in stable population theory (Leslie 1945; Keyfitz 1977). An important question is whether the marginal distribution of occupations of sons could have been generated from the occupational distribution of fathers, as $\mathbf{a}_0\mathbf{M} = \mathbf{a}_1$, or projected out to the tth generation as $\mathbf{a}_0\mathbf{M}^t = \mathbf{a}_t$, where $\mathbf{a}_0$ is the row vector of proportions in the respective occupational origin categories and $\mathbf{a}_t$ is the distribution in the tth generation.

Apart from the aforementioned limitations inherent in the Markov approach to social mobility, Hodge (1966), Prais (1955b), and others also argue that Markov models will seldom fit social mobility data due to the phenomenon of clustering on the main diagonal. That is, a son's broad occupational category will tend to be more similar to a father's broad occupational category owing to *status inheritance*. This phenomenon is also exhibited in intragenerational mobility matrices, which typically encompass several measurement points.[19] Although a first-order Markov chain cannot describe the tendency of clustering on the main diagonal, the data may obey some other stochastic process. In their research on intragenerational mobility, Blumen, Kogan, and McCarthy (1955) view this tendency as a particular form of unobserved heterogeneity and propose a "mover-stayer" model, in which a latent class of stayers never leave their origin status and a latent class of movers move according to a Markov chain.[20] White (1970) extends this idea to intergenerational mobility. Goodman (1965) considers a simplified version of the mover-stayer model that "blocks out" the diagonal entries and adjusts the marginal distributions accordingly.[21] Goodman's work can be viewed as the beginning of a contemporary literature on the statistical analysis of mobility tables.

---

[17] Recent work by Mare (1997) uses generalizations of these methods to examine the process by which a socioeconomically differentiated population reproduces itself.
[18] These are conceptually identical to the p_{ij}'s we defined earlier. By definition the transition probabilities sum to 1 over rows, $\Sigma_j p_{ij} = 1$. The empirical counterparts are outflow proportions (or row proportions) $p_{ij} = f_{ij}/f_{i.}$, where f_{ij} denotes the joint frequency in the ith row and jth column and $f_{i.} = \Sigma_j f_{ij}$ denotes marginal frequency in the ith row. By contrast, the cell proportions in the table are f_{ij}/N, where N is the sample size.
[19] In fact, it is rare to find intergenerational mobility tables that go back more than one generation, making application of these models problematic.
[20] Formally, for a continuous-time process this means that the distribution of t is defective, implying that a proportion of the population never experience a transition.
[21] This is equivalent to fitting a parameter to each diagonal entry in a table or for a subset of diagonal cells.

While space limitations prevent us from elaborating subsequent developments in the mathematical modeling of social mobility, suffice it to say that this earlier tradition spawned a great deal of later work on life-course and career mobility and dynamic models in general. It also gave rise to a new focus on structural or statistical models of social mobility. By the mid 1970s, researchers focused less on the study of mobility as a stochastic process and more on structural models of social mobility.

Statistical Models for Mobility Tables

Models for mobility tables express the expected frequencies in terms of the parameters describing the marginal and joint distributions. Letting R denote the row variable (father's occupation) with row indices $i, \ldots, K$ and C denote the column variable (son's occupation) with column indices $j, \ldots, K$, yields a model for the expected frequency in the ith column and jth row F_{ij} as:

$$F_{ij} = \tau \tau_i^R \tau_j^C \tau_{ij}^{RC} \tag{3}$$

As Hauser (1979) points out, each observed frequency in a father-son mobility table has two components—the effects of prevalence and the effects of interaction. Prevalence effects involve the tendency for the joint frequencies in certain diagonal cells to be large because the corresponding marginal frequencies are large. For example, using three occupational "class" categories corresponding to upper-, middle-, and lower-class jobs, we would expect to find many middle-class sons with middle-class fathers simply because there are more middle-class jobs. Interaction concerns the varying tendencies for categories to interact or occur jointly. For example, we would expect to find that relatively more men "inherit" the broad occupational position of their fathers than end up very far from their social origins. In Equation 3, prevalence effects are accounted for by the parameters governing the marginal distributions, or the τ_i^R and τ_j^C parameters. Interaction effects are captured by the τ_{ij}^{RC} parameters. Taking logs, we can write Equation 3 as a loglinear model:

$$\log F_{ij} = \mu + \mu_i^R + \mu_j^C + \mu_{ij}^{RC}. \tag{4}$$

We will describe several models that are constrained versions of this model.

When all $\tau_{ij}^{RC} = 1$ or $\mu_{ij}^{RC} = 0$ we have the *model of independence* or *perfect mobility*. This model constrains all row-specific and column-specific proportions to be equal to the respective marginal proportions—a property referred to as marginal homogeneity. If proportions are not homogeneous across rows or columns, then there is dependence between son's and father's occupational class. As outlined earlier, this model will rarely fit mobility data due to a failure to account for status inheritance. However, Goodman (1965) considers the situation where perfect mobility holds, except for those who are in the same occupational category as their fathers, resulting in a model for quasi-perfect mobility or quasi-independence.

The *model of quasi-independence* is obtained if R and C are independent of each other in the off-diagonal cells. That is, the expected frequencies in the ith row and jth column are given by $F_{ij} = f_i. f_{.j}/N$, where $f_i.$ and $f_{.j}$ denote the marginal frequencies for the row and column variables respectively. Independence also implies that the odds ratio for any 2×2 subtable is equal to 1. Because odds ratios are invariant under transformations of the marginal distributions, and are byproducts of the estimation of loglinear models, they are highly useful for studying comparative mobility. Goodman (1968) makes extensive use of odds ratios to gain information about the association in selected regions of a mobility table. Hauser (1979) uses the nonredundant odds ratios obtained from a saturated model to delineate areas in a social mobility table with similar levels of association.[22] The result is what is referred to as the *topological model*. The interaction parameters from the topological model can be used to quantify the association between any two occupational origins and any two occupational destinations.

The *model of symmetry* and the *model of quasi-symmetry* have also been widely used. Symmetric association patterns may also provide a good fit to the observed data in square tables. In terms of model parameters, we constrain interaction terms to be the same on both sides of the main diagonal $\tau_{ij}^{RC} = \tau_{ji}^{RC}$. This model can be decomposed into two components: marginal homogeneity and symmetric interactions. Fitting the diagonal cells as a special case, so that in addition to the constraint above we also allow additional τ_{ij}^{RC} parameters for $(i = j)$, results in a model of quasi-symmetry. Similar to the quasi-independence model, this model allows for marginal heterogeneity.

Sobel, Hout, and Duncan (1985) show that when quasi-symmetry holds, it is possible to obtain estimates that describe structural mobility derived from differences in father's and son's occupational distributions. As was mentioned above, estimating structural and circulation mobility has been a long-standing concern in the analysis of social mobility. Previous approaches were problematic due to the fact that the distribution of a son's social origins does not correspond directly to the occupational distribution in the past and due to an inadequate theoretical conceptualization of structural mobility based on the difference between total and exchange mobility. Sobel, Hout, and Duncan (1985) equate structural mobility with marginal heterogeneity and further assume that this effect operates uniformly on all social origin categories. They define exchange mobility as mobility resulting from equal flows between pairs of cells in a mobility table, implying symmetry.

Association models represent an alternative approach to modeling interaction effects in mobility tables. In this case, we incorporate information on the ordering of occupational categories to construct row and column scores. For a $K \times K$ table, the row and column scores can be constructed as $i = 1, \ldots, K$ and $j = 1, \ldots, K$, respectively.[23] This results in the uniform association model which can be written as:

$$\log F_{ij} = \mu + \mu_i^R + \mu_j^C + \beta_{ij}. \tag{5}$$

The odds ratios involving adjacent rows and columns are invariant and equal to $\exp(\beta)$. This result can be used to construct odds ratios for arbitrary pairs (i and i' for row and j and j' for column) as $\exp\{\beta(i - i')(j - j')\}$.

Goodman (1979, 1981) proposes two kinds of association models—the row-and-column-effects association Model I and the row-and-column-effects association Model II (referred to as the *RC* model). Model I estimates row and column scores from the data and is of the form

---

[22] A saturated model has a single parameter per cell and thus fits the data perfectly.

[23] Here we use integer scoring. The particular values used are inconsequential as long as they are uniformly spaced. Other scoring methods may be more reasonable, such as using midpoints or weighted means to linearize categories based on interval measures.

$$\log F_{ij} = \mu + \mu_i^R + \mu_j^C + j\phi_i + i\varphi_j. \tag{6}$$

This model specifies the association between father's and son's occupation as the sum of the two interaction terms involving a row score ϕ (or row effect) and a column score φ (or column effect). It is a generalization of the uniform association model insofar as the association parameters vary uniformly (linearly) by row and column. Whereas this model depends on a correct ordering of the occupational categories, Goodman's *RC* model makes no assumptions regarding the correct ordering of categories and can be written as a log-multiplicative model, in which the two-way interaction is characterized by a multiplicative term involving unknown row and column scores:

$$\log F_{ij} = \mu + \mu_i^R + \mu_j^C + \phi_i \varphi_j. \tag{7}$$

The estimated scores not only reveal the ordering of categories but also show the relative differences in occupational categories (e.g., Clogg 1982).

Association models are particularly attractive from the standpoint of parsimony and have advantages that carry over to the analysis of more complicated tables. Xie (1992) proposes a log-multiplicative layer effect model to handle the three-way interaction present in a three-country mobility table with country dimension or layer L. His proposed model is:

$$F_{ijk} = \tau \tau_i^R \tau_j^C \tau_k^L \tau_{ik}^{RL} \tau_{jk}^{CL} \exp(\psi_{ij}\phi_k) \tag{8}$$

where the parameters ψ_{ij} and ϕ_k can be viewed as latent scales for ordinal variables, with the ψ parameters describing origin-destination association and the ϕ parameters describing the country-specific deviations in the association.

Studies of Heterogeneous Populations

Although intergenerational occupational mobility has been a key topic in the demography of social stratification, other aspects of the study of mobility continue to attract increased attention. Among them are demographic studies of socioeconomic outcomes for populations characterized by heterogeneity. Demographers have had a long-standing interest in problems of unobserved heterogeneity, especially with regard to the study of mortality (e.g., Vaupal, Manton, and Stallard 1979; Vaupal and Yashin 1985). Unobserved heterogeneity denotes a collection of unknown factors that contribute—along with known factors—to an individual's risk of some outcome of interest.

Known risk factors are readily incorporated into the transition rate models that were discussed earlier. Suppose, however, that we now wish to account for unobserved heterogeneity. To consider this issue, the following proportional hazard model may be specified:

$$r(t) = r_0(t) \exp(X'\beta)v \tag{9}$$

where v is unobserved heterogeneity, or frailty, that acts multiplicatively to raise or lower an individual's risk (assuming an average frailty of 1). We commonly account for frailty by assuming a distribution for v and averaging (or integrating) it out of the expression for a likelihood conditional on v, and then maximizing the resulting marginal likelihood with respect to β and ancillary parameters describing the distribution of v.

There are, however, several limitations to this approach. As discussed by Heckman and Singer (1984), a misspecification arises in regard to the baseline hazard $r_0(t)$ or because the distribution of the unobserved heterogeneity could lead to serious biases. Heckman and Singer (1984) demonstrate how these problems arise in several models and propose a nonparametric approach for handling the distribution of v. The literature remains unclear about the extent to which it is possible to compare models that control for unobserved heterogeneity against alternative models without unobserved heterogeneity (Hoem 1990; Trussel and Rodríguez 1990). Trussel and Rodríguez (1990) show that an identification problem exists in the sense that a model specification with unobserved heterogeneity can be observationally equivalent to a model specified without unobserved heterogeneity even though the two models appear to be conceptually distinct.

Rather than viewing unobserved heterogeneity as a process that occurs at the individual level, a more fruitful approach may be to control for the shared unmeasured factors that are common to paired, clustered, or repeatedly measured observations. In this context, a generalization of the preceding model is a natural way to accommodate unobserved heterogeneity due to common unmeasured sources of variation. These sources may derive from observations sharing a common family, neighborhood, community, or other aggregation.

Sibling Studies

Sibling data have special relevance for research on social stratification and mobility because of the opportunity to control for sources of variability that cannot otherwise be captured. As noted by Griliches (1979), the correlation between sibling characteristics is likely the result of many factors, including shared genetic traits (i.e., heredity), shared home environments (i.e., cultural, physical, and financial resources), shared communities, friends, and schools. Some of these factors may be measurable. However, many are not or are measured imperfectly and would be represented as disturbances, residuals, or unobserved family-specific traits in models of socioeconomic outcomes.

Unobserved components of socioeconomic outcomes should be positively correlated across siblings. Of course, siblings differ on important dimensions and the extent of sibling differences will likely depend on the difference in age as a result of changes that may have occurred in the age interval that separates them. For example, changes in socioeconomic circumstances and family structure may have varying impacts on older and younger siblings which can lead to differences in outcomes. Outcomes can be influenced by the sibling-specific context of parent–child relationships and by the unique nature of peer group interactions. While there is a possibility of countervailing influences leading to differences in outcomes among siblings, most researchers in this tradition would argue that siblings share a set of generalized unmeasured traits that can be captured by a single variable. Accounting for this effect should help to eliminate potential biases in the effects of key variables such as education on socioeconomic outcomes.

The structural equation approach is ideal for analyses involving sibling pairs, though a more general approach that allows for family clusters of any size might be preferable in other contexts. One model that closely resembles the preceding multiplicative frailty model considers a socioeconomic outcome Y as a function of years of schooling E for the jth sibling in the ith family.

$$Y_{ij} = \alpha + \beta E_{ij} + v_i + \varepsilon_{ij}. \tag{10}$$

This is a multilevel regression model, where v is either a normally distributed random variable (random effect) or a fixed effect that varies over families. Our estimate of β will be unbiased as long as siblings have the same level of v. Griliches (1979: S40) refers to this as "the rationale, the promise, and the limitation of the siblings method." That is, if the components of v (the collection of unobserved family traits) are in fact "family-level" traits, then β will be unbiased. Otherwise, if v also represents some combination of individual- and family-level traits, it is not clear that the estimator of β is unbiased *in either the random-effects or fixed-effects model*. Other potential sources of bias include regressors correlated with v or u (i.e., endogeneity of E). In spite of these limitations, sibling data permit a richer set of analytical questions to be addressed, as evident from studies by Jencks et al. (1972, 1979), Olneck (1977), Hauser (1988), Hauser and Mossel (1985), Hauser and Sewell (1986), and Hauser and Wong (1989).

It is also worth noting that models such as that shown in Equation 10 can be cast as random coefficients models, which allow for family-specific effects of education. Such models provide estimates of additional components of variation, beyond the usual residual variance in the classic regression model. Although sibling data have the potential to shed light on estimates of covariates affecting socioeconomic outcomes, they are not a panacea for understanding family effects except in certain circumstances with specific kinds of models.[24] Nevertheless, sibling models have been instrumental in focusing attention on the role of families in the stratification process.[25]

Sibling models are especially relevant for the study of the effects of education. It is well known that investments in schooling have major and important direct effects on socioeconomic success. But socioeconomic outcomes are also affected by family background factors and personal characteristics. Therefore, the observed association between socioeconomic outcomes and schooling may not be entirely a causal effect. Models based on sibling data (specifically, sibling pairs) allow the researcher to decompose the cross-sibling variance into between-family and within-family components. As noted by Hauser (1988: 1402), "if fraternal differences in schooling lead to differences in adult success, we can be more confident that the association of schooling with success is not merely an artifact of school success running in families that are also economically successful."

In general, studies using sibling data do not find much upward bias in conventional estimates of the effects of schooling on socioeconomic outcomes (Hauser and Sewell 1986; Altonji and Dunn 1996; Ashenfelter and Zimmerman 1997). This conclusion is especially apparent after correcting for measurement error in the schooling data

---

[24] For example, when sibling data are used with a gamma distributed random effect in a proportional hazard model, the estimated variance in frailty has a *substantive* interpretation in terms of a relative risk (e.g., Guo and Rodríguez 1992; Guo 1993; Powers 2001.)

[25] This latter concern is underscored by Mare (2001, p. 480), who states "it is families rather than individuals that provide demographic continuity of social stratification from one generation to the next. . . . the stratification scholar should bear in mind that socioeconomic reproduction combines intergenerational social mobility with demographic reproduction, including differential fertility, fertility timing, mortality, assortative mating and family stability."

(Ashenfelter and Rouse 2000: 96). The basic finding that the direct effect of schooling is not appreciably reduced by an unobserved family factor is largely evident even in studies that are restricted to siblings who are identical or fraternal twins (Ashenfelter and Krueger 1994; Ashenfelter and Rouse 1998; Ashenfelter and Rouse 2000; Miller, Mulvey, and Martin 1995). Thus, the direct effect of schooling on socioeconomic outcomes is probably not a spurious artifact deriving from a common association with being from a family with higher socioeconomic standing.

ADDITIONAL DEMOGRAPHIC RESEARCH ON MOBILITY

Some Major Findings Regarding Social Mobility in the U.S.

In the extant literature, the common if not perennial fear among students of American social mobility is that it is on the decline.[26] For the most part, however, this conclusion has not been evident in the major modern studies of intergenerational occupational mobility for the U.S. Featherman and Hauser's (1978) meticulous study of the OCG-I and OCG-II data sets finds increased mobility and reduced ascription between 1962 and 1973 for a variety of models of various socioeconomic outcomes. Those authors state they have "detected two complementary trends: declining status ascription and increasing universalistic status allocation.... If anything, the weight of the evidence of change suggests that the acquisition of schooling, jobs, and earnings has become less constrained by social background" (Featherman and Hauser 1978: 481).

Another important study (Hout 1988) investigates intergenerational occupational mobility from 1972 to 1985. This analysis combines features of association models as well as an earlier model of (Sobel, Hout, and Duncan 1985) that incorporates parameters for structural mobility. An additional innovation is that Hout's (1988) model also includes occupation-specific measures of status, autonomy, and training. In doing so, he allows for various sources of heterogeneity within broad occupational categories. Especially relevant is the role of education and training, and Hout finds that origin-destination association varies by educational level. In particular, the origin-destination association is nil among the college educated.[27] Thus, as the proportion of college-educated workers increases, an increase in circulation mobility is evident. Although structural mobility decreased during this time period, circulation mobility increased. As Hout observes (1988: 1358), "the more college graduates in the work force, the weaker the association between origin status and destination status for the population as a whole. Overall mobility remains unchanged because a decline in structural mobility offsets the increased openness of the class structure."

DiPrete and Grusky (1990), using data for approximately the same period as Hout (1988), reach similar conclusions, although their methodology differs. They find little evidence of an increase in the effect of ascription on occupational attainment, although

[26] A decline in social mobility is also hypothesized by Herrnstein and Murray (1994), although in their view this decline is generated primarily as a consequence of the increasing stratification of cognitive skills.

[27] As Hout (1988) notes, the finding that college education erases the origin-destination association may help to explain the paradox of higher-than-average attainment (i.e., beyond what would be predicted by social origins) of certain ethnic minorities in the U.S. such as Asian Americans and Eastern Europeans, as these groups have a higher than average proportion of college graduates.

some of their results suggest a slowdown in the growth of universalistic practices. Overall, however, the findings of DiPrete and Grusky seem generally consistent with those of Hout, showing considerable social fluidity during the latter 1970s and the 1980s despite some slowdown in structural mobility. DiPrete and Grusky (1990) argue that part of the continued universalism during this period is political, deriving from the enforcement of equal-opportunity employment legislation.

Hauser et al. (2000) provide results for occupational attainment during the early 1990s using the Wisconsin Longitudinal Survey. This thorough and informative test of a status attainment model that includes a variety of social background variables indicates the continuing importance of schooling as key determinant of occupational attainment, even after controlling for a mental ability test score. The direct effects of social background variables (net of schooling) are small or negligible, yielding no obvious evidence of a direct increase in the role of ascription in occupational attainment during the early 1990s.

Some Major Findings From Cross-National Studies of Social Mobility

A great deal of the research on social mobility has been cross-national. Hout (2003) succinctly summarizes much of our current knowledge derived from this research. Several important empirical generalizations emerge from his review. Of particular significance is what has come to be known as the Treiman constant: "occupations are ranked in the same order in most nations and over time" (Hout 2003: 2). In other words, in terms of average levels of prestige and socioeconomic rewards, occupations tend to be ordered similarly across most nations and across time within nations. This result was first reported and analyzed in Treiman (1977) and was subsequently extended by Ganzeboom and Treiman (1996). The Treiman constant is important because it implies that occupation is a major dimension of social inequality that may be directly compared across nations and across time periods for the purpose of studying patterns of social mobility. This finding thus underlies comparative studies of social mobility.

The latter topic is sufficiently complex to have generated a variety of debates and viewpoints over the years. However, a general consensus seems to be emerging recently regarding several basic conclusions. The first is that there is a great deal of variation in levels and patterns of structural mobility across nations and and across time periods (Erikson and Goldthorpe 1992). These variations in structural mobility (which are also sometimes referred to as variations in absolute mobility rates) reflect the generally historical and idiosyncratic features of the economic development and class structures of different nations. As stated by Goldthorpe (2000: 232) "most mobility researchers came to accept the view, either implicitly if not explicitly, that variation in absolute rates cannot in fact usefully be regarded as systematic, and that explanations of such variation, whether over time or cross-nationally, will need to be provided far more in specific historical, than in general theoretical terms."

A second major conclusion from this literature is that relative mobility rates—which may be construed as indicative of circulation mobility—show a great deal of similarity across industrial nations, particularly in regard to the fundamental pattern of association between origins and destinations. In other words, industrial nations do not differ much in terms of their levels of inherent social fluidity or degrees of openness.

Although differences do exist between countries, they are small compared to the cross-national similarities. In fact, "such variations in pattern as do occur are not of any major quantitative importance" (Goldthorpe 2000: 234). Hout (2003: 7–8) states that this conclusion generally applies both to "vertical" and "class" models of mobility.

Although somewhat less well conceptualized and studied, another basic conclusion from comparative studies is that education plays a critical role in the status attainment process in industrialized nations. As stated by Hout (2003: 9) "education is the main factor in both upward mobility and the reproduction of status from generation to generation." For the U.S., this conclusion is evident in numerous studies such as Blau and Duncan (1967), Featherman and Hauser (1978), Jencks et al. (1979), and DiPrete and Grusky (1990). Studies of status attainment in other industrialized nations, however, also report similar findings (Hope 1985; Hout 1989; Ishida 1993; Treiman and Ganzeboom 1990). Because of the important role of education in determining occupational attainment, upward mobility is facilitated to the extent that persons from lower-status origins obtain high levels of education while status reproduction results when persons obtain levels of education that are consistent with their class origins (Bielby 1981: 6–10; Hout 2003: 9–12).

An additional important conclusion from comparative studies of social stratification is the persistence of class differentials in educational attainment in most industrialized nations. "Class differentials in educational attainment, considered net of all effects of expansion per se, have tended to display a high degree of stability: that is, while all children of all class backgrounds have alike participated in the process of expansion, the association between class origins and the relative chances of children staying on in education, taking more academic courses, or entering higher education has, in most societies, been rather little altered" (Goldthorpe 2000: 182). The main source of this finding is Shavit and Blossfeld (1993), who investigate educational attainment in 13 countries including Czechoslovakia, Germany, Hungary, Israel, Italy, Japan, Netherlands, Poland, Sweden, Switzerland, Taiwan, United Kingdom, and the U.S. Previous studies have also reported similar findings for France (Garnier and Raffalovitch 1984) and the Philippines (Smith and Cheung 1986). The stability in class differentials in educational attainments seems somewhat surprising given the considerable cross-national variation in educational systems and the general increase in average levels of educational attainment across cohorts in all industrialized nations. However, this finding is consistent with (if not implied by) the previous two general conclusions about the cross-national similarity in relative mobility rates and the important role of education in status attainment in industrialized nations.[28]

Other major conclusions from comparative studies of social stratification pertain to gender. The first in this regard is that, when measured in terms of years of schooling completed, gender differentials in educational attainment have notably declined throughout industrialized nations since World War II (Shavit and Blossfeld 1993; Breen and Goldthorpe 1997). Indeed, in some nations, recent cohorts of women actually attend schooling for more years than do men. As mentioned by Hout (2003: 12), this trend may derive from "rising returns to market work among women, the educational

---

[28] The two countries where class differentials in educational attainment do appear to be significantly attenuated are the Netherlands and Sweden (De Graaf and Ganzeboom 1993; Jonsson 1993), and these two countries are also characterized by somewhat higher levels of circulation mobility (Ganzeboom and De Graaf 1984; Erikson and Goldthorpe 1987).

and occupational aspirations of post-feminist women, the family resources of smaller families, and the interests of privileged parents who have daughters but not sons."

Another general result from comparative studies of social stratification is that "occupational distributions are gendered" (Hout 2003: 3). In other words, throughout industrialized nations there are significant gender differentials in occupational attainment. In particular, women are typically much more likely to be employed in lower-level white-collar occupations. The most systematic cross-national study of this phenomenon is Charles and Grusky (1995). Although this study finds notable gender segregation in the occupational distributions of each of the countries considered, nations nonetheless differ significantly in terms of their specific patterns and in the changes of these patterns over time. Future research on this topic may need to investigate more thoroughly the role of gender differentials in educational type and specialty that continue to persist in many nations (despite declines in gender differentials in total years of schooing completed).

In sum, comparative studies have yielded an impressive body of knowledge about cross-national commonalities in the basic facts and processes involved in social stratification. In our review, we have been careful to limit these generalizations to those pertaining to industrialized nations because almost all of these studies are based exclusively on data from such countries.[29] The extent to which these generalizations may also be applicable to developing nations thus remains a topic for future research. The main impediment to extending these studies to developing nations has been the availability of appropriate data.

DEMOGRAPHIC RESEARCH ON THE LEVEL OF INEQUALITY

Demographic Factors Affecting the Level of Poverty

One of the fundamental indicators of inequality in a population is its level of poverty, which is typically measured as the proportion of households whose income falls below some specified poverty threshold (i.e., the poverty rate).[30] Because poverty thresholds vary by household size (and, to a lesser extent, composition), Bumpass and Sweet (1981) note that processes of family formation and change can have direct effects on the incidence of poverty. These demographic factors may also have indirect effects via consequent reductions in labor supply or earnings capacities. Households may thus leave or enter poverty as the result of such demographic changes as marital dissolution, aging, retirement, death, childbirth, remarriage, the departure of children from the household, and the formation of new households.

The particular demographic issue that has been prominent in the poverty literature is the extent to which changes in family structure over the past few decades have contributed to the rate of poverty in the U.S. Earlier qualitative and ethnographic

---

[29] The one major exception here is Treiman (1977), who also uses data for developing nations. The Treiman constant is thus the one generalization that may be said to pertain to both developed and developing nations.

[30] Despite Sen's (1976) seminal contribution to the methodology of poverty indices, most empirical research seems to be based on the simple proportion of the poor in the total population (perhaps because Sen's [1976] index may be more unreliable than a proportion when the incomes of the poor are reported with significant error).

research by sociologists often interpreted family structure as being adaptive to poverty (e.g., Rainwater 1968; Schulz 1969; Stack 1974). According to this "situational view" of poverty, nonmarital fertility and increased proportions of female-headed households are seen as being in part a consequence of low wages, unemployment, and economic inequality rather than the primary causes of them (Valentine 1968). By contrast, the "culture of poverty" view maintains that poverty is substantially promoted and increased by the rejection of middle-class social values and normative behaviors (Banfield 1968). The resulting high rates of female-headed households and high school dropouts are predicted to be fundamental and important sources of increased poverty rates (Lewis 1966).

Bane's demographic study (1986) is one of the first to systematically investigate the effect of family structure on poverty rates. Her analysis is based on the U.S. Census Bureau definition of poverty, which is an absolute measure (i.e., it is invariant with respect to changes in average standards of living or household income in society). Using standardization methods and demographic data from 1960 to 1983, she finds that "the poverty rate in 1979 would have been about 16 percent lower than it was had family composition remained as it was in 1959" (Bane 1986: 214). For the black population separately, the corresponding figure is 22% (Bane 1986: 215). Bane interprets her results as lending some support to the "situational view" because "most poverty, even that of female-headed families, occurs because of income or job changes" (Bane 1986: 231). For African Americans, Bane (1986: 231) concludes that "although there has indeed been a dramatic and shocking increase in female-headed households among blacks and an equally dramatic feminization of black poverty, one cannot conclude that much of the poverty could have been avoided had families stayed together."

Another important study is Danziger and Gottschalk (1995), which also uses the U.S. Census Bureau definition of poverty. Unlike Bane (1986), however, Danziger and Gottschalk seek to evaluate simultaneously the effects of economic changes as well as demographic changes. To do this, they develop a decomposition that incorporates changes in mean household income, household income inequality, and race-specific family structure. Consistent with Bane's (1986) general conclusion, they find that changes in family structure (in particular, the increase in female-headed households) had a moderate effect on increasing poverty from 1973 to 1991. Danziger and Gottschalk's (1995: 102) results for this period also indicate, however, that economic factors had larger effects than did family structure, including the increase in mean household income (which reduced poverty) and the increase in household income inequality (which increased poverty). Economic factors, particularly the increase in mean household income, had the overwhelmingly largest impact on reducing poverty during the earlier period from 1949 to 1969 (during which time family structure did not change significantly).

An update and extension of Danziger and Gottschalk's (1995) analysis is provided by Iceland (2003), who uses both the U.S. Census Bureau definition as well as a relative measure of poverty for the period from 1949 to 1999. With regard to his results for the U.S. Census Bureau definition, Iceland also finds (as did Danziger and Gottschalk) that economic factors—particularly increases in mean household income—overwhelmingly had the dominant impact on reducing poverty from 1949 to 1969. However, in the subsequent period, from 1969 to 1990, Iceland's (2003: 512–513) results indicate that changes in family structure played a significant role, especially for African Americans. Even so, the total impact of economic factors was still larger than was the effect of family structure for this period. During the last period in their analysis, from 1990 to 1999, the poverty rate did not change much, and economic factors clearly had the greatest impact—while the distribution of family structure remained relatively constant.

An important contribution of Iceland (2003) is to extend the analysis to a relative definition, according to which the poverty threshold increases as the average standard of living increases in society.[31] Although absolute poverty (i.e., the U.S. Census Bureau definition) declined dramatically from 1949 to 1969, Iceland (2003: 507) finds that relative poverty was reduced only slightly. During the subsequent two periods, from 1969 to 1990 and 1990 to 1999, relative poverty actually increased—in marked contrast to the declines in absolute poverty. Whereas according to the official (i.e., absolute) definition, the poverty rate declined from 13.9% in 1969 to 11.8% in 1999, by Iceland's relative measure, the poverty rate substantially increased from 20.6% in 1969 to 26.1% in 1999.

Iceland's (2003: 509–512) decomposition results generally show that increases in mean household income have much less impact on reducing relative poverty than on reducing absolute poverty and that the former is more highly affected by changes in household income inequality. This result is not surprising given that the thresholds for relative poverty are defined as a percentage of the median household income. In addition, the decomposition results indicate that the impact of family structure for the period from 1969 to 1990 was slightly larger for relative poverty than for absolute poverty, especially in the case of African Americans.[32] From 1990 to 1999, however, family structure again had a negligible impact in the case of relative poverty.

In sum, the studies reviewed in this section used decomposition methods to analyze the impact of changes in family structure on the trend in the poverty rate in the U.S. All of these studies indicate that changes in family structure—and in particular, the increase in female-headed households—have increased poverty at least to some degree before 1990. This conclusion is probably somewhat more applicable to African Americans and to results that are based on a relative measure of poverty. Since 1990, however, changes in family structure have been minor and have not had a significant impact on the poverty rate.

At the same time, these studies seem to agree that although changes in family structure have sometimes played a significant role, economic factors have been the primary factors associated with the trend in poverty in the U.S. In the case of an absolute measure, the trend in poverty is more affected by changes in mean household income. In the case of a relative measure, the trend in poverty is more affected by changes in household income inequality. In reaching these general conclusions, however, we point out that these studies have not investigated whether changes in family structure may have had "indirect effects" on the poverty rate by affecting trends in mean household income and household income inequality. This may be a fruitful issue to explore in future research.

---

[31] In particular, Iceland (2003: 503) defines the poverty threshold as being one-half of the median household income after accounting for differences in household size.

[32] In a related study, Smith (1988) argues that the effect of family structure on poverty among blacks was slightly more substantial during this time period than had been concluded by Bane (1986). These somewhat different conclusions probably in part reflect their different measures of poverty because Smith (1988) uses a type of relative measure.

Before concluding this section, we point out that the social and economic disadvantages of female-headed families are also evident in other industrialized nations (Garfinkel and McLanahan 1994; Lichter 1997). Data for the early 1990s indicate significantly higher relative poverty rates for female-headed households in Canada, France, Germany, and the United Kingdom (Garfinkel and McLanahan 1994: 209). As discussed by McLanahan and Sandefur (1994), female-headed households tend to be inevitably disadvantaged (as compared to two-parent families) in terms of parenting, economic resources, and social ties to the community. Family structure therefore probably plays a significant role in influencing the level of poverty in other nations as well.

Nonetheless, comparative studies also indicate clearly that the impact of female-headed households on the level of poverty is highly variable and conditional on the role of government programs (Smeeding, Torrey, and Rein 1988). For example, the relative poverty rates of female-headed families in Sweden and the Netherlands are quite low, and these countries are notable for the effectiveness of their welfare programs (Garfinkel and McLanahan 1994). In other European countries as well, government benefits are far more effective (than is the case in the U.S.) in mitigating the adverse economic disadvantages faced by female-headed households (Garfinkel and McLanahan 1994; Rainwater 1995). To be sure, such programs are more costly but they do indicate that poverty among female-headed families can be reduced substantially without increasing appreciably the incidence of female-headed households (Bergmann 1996; Garfinkel and McLanahan 1994).

Inequality in the Distribution of Family Income

In addition to its relationship with the poverty rate, household income inequality is an important issue in itself. With regard to couple-headed families, Treas (1987: 265) notes that income inequality can be viewed as a function of income inequality among husbands plus income inequality among wives plus the covariance between the incomes of husbands and wives.[33] Thus, income inequality among couple-headed families would increase if wealthier men tended to be married to wealthier women but would decrease if wealthier men tended to be married to poorer women. The pattern of assortative mating can thus have a direct impact on the level of income inequality among couple-headed families.

Treas's (1987) review of the literature from the 1960s and 1970s finds that most studies report that the earnings of wives tend to reduce family income inequality. These results seem to derive primarily from (at least for whites) the higher labor force participation among the wives of husbands who have lower incomes. That is, the wives of wealthier white husbands were less likely to have an income through work in the paid labor force. In short, due to the reduced labor force participation and hence lower earnings of the wives of wealthier husbands, the correlation between the incomes of white spouses during this time period appears to be negative, which reduces the level of family income inequality (Cancian, Danziger, and Gottschalk 1993: 210).[34]

---

[33] The same basic function could also be applied to gay and lesbian couples.

[34] The negative correlation is evident only when nonworking wives' earnings are set equal to zero; the correlation between spouses' earnings among couples where both spouses work was actually slightly positive even during this time period (Cancian, Danziger, and Gottschalk 1993: 210).

During the late 1970s and the 1980s, the labor force participation of women continued to increase. Partly as a result of this increase, the correlation between the earnings of spouses became positive (Cancian, Danziger, and Gottschalk 1993: 210). Although this positive correlation should increase the level of family inequality, the effect was counterbalanced by a reduction in the inequality of earnings among women. That is, the variation in the earnings among women declined significantly as more women worked more hours in the paid labor force. The reduction in inequality in the earnings of women is greater than the effect of the increase in the correlation between the earnings of spouses. The overall result is that during the 1970s, 1980s, and early 1990s, women's earnings reduced family income inequality (Cancian and Reed 1999).

Perhaps the most thorough and informative analysis of this issue is provided by Cancian and Reed (1999). This study develops a decomposition approach that factors in the proportion of households consisting of single persons or single parents. In addition, Cancian and Reed clarify the importance of stipulating the "counterfactual" when assessing the impact of women's earnings on the level of family income inequality. For example, comparison of the observed level of family income inequality and the level that would be obtained if all wives had zero earnings yields a different result than comparison of the observed level of family income inequality and that which would be obtained if the earnings of wives were reduced only slightly. For 1994, the former comparison increases family income inequality while in the latter case inequality is reduced (Cancian and Reed 1999: 180). However, when comparing the level of family income inequality in 1967 with that in 1994, Cancian and Reed conclude that the increase in the latter period would have been substantially greater if wives' earnings in 1994 were the same as they had been in 1967 (i.e., if the mean and variance of the distribution of wives' earnings did not change over this time period). Thus, "the growth in family income inequality cannot be attributed primarily to changes in wives' earnings. Changes in husbands' earnings are substantially more important in explaining recent trends" (Cancian and Reed 1999: 184).

Although this conclusion is important, so is the caveat mentioned by Treas (1987: 275) that "working women trade off time for money. Women perform many valued services around the home (e.g., housekeeping, meal preparation, child care, entertaining, emotional support). When the wife goes to work, the family must either forego some of these services, find another family member to provide them, or spend money to purchase them in the marketplace." This loss in the value of home production is not reflected in the statistics on income distribution analyzed in the studies discussed above. On an hourly basis, however, working-class wives earn appreciably less than do upper middle-class wives, so the former group must work longer hours in order to obtain earnings that are equivalent to those of middle-class wives; working-class families may thus be forgoing more home production. For this reason, we agree with with Treas's (1987: 275) speculation that the equalizing effect of women's earnings on the distribution of full income among households may be overstated. Future research on this topic should address this issue.

An additional issue worth pursuing is the effect of women's earnings on men's earnings. This topic was mentioned by Dooley and Gottschalk (1985: 31) in their analysis of the increasing earnings inequality among men. In particular, the increased labor force participation of women may increase the level of market competition experienced by men and perhaps drive down the wages of less educated men through the sort of occupational queuing process described by Reder (1955).[35] The consequence is that, as more highly educated women work more and increase their labor market opportunities, the inequality in the earnings of men may increase. As we have seen, this inequality is an important source of the level of poverty and the recent increase in family income inequality. Thus, to the extent that such an effect is evident, the equalizing effect of women's earnings on the distribution of family income may be overstated.

Regarding international studies, we are aware of only two publications that have focused on the effects of wives' earnings on inequality in the distribution of family income. The United Kingdom was investigated by Layard and Zabalza (1979), and Gronau (1982) considered the case of Israel. Using data for the 1970s, when the labor force participation and earnings of married women were relatively low in these countries, both of these studies found that the earnings of wives significantly reduced inequality in the distribution of family income.[36] These results are consistent with the basic conclusion for the U.S. during this period (Treas 1987).

In addition to the issue of assortative mating, we also note some recent research on the effect of population growth on household income inequality. While the debate on the relationship between population growth and economic development is well known (e.g., Ahlburg 1998), the relationship between population growth and economic inequality has received little consideration.[37] It is worth noting, however, that Nielsen (1994) and Nielsen and Alderson (1995) consistently find large positive effects of the natural rate of population increase on household income inequality using data for 88 nations from 1952 to 1988. This result is evident in regression models that control for a variety of independent variables and use different specifications. It is thus a robust finding that merits further consideration.

RESEARCH DIRECTIONS

Much of the research on the demography of social stratification has involved highly detailed descriptive analysis. Although much has been learned from this work in the past few decades, we believe that, at this stage of its development, the field would benefit from increasing the scope and breadth of its analytical models. An important task in this regard is to integrate more varied elements of demography and stratification in order to develop richer (albeit increasingly more complex) models of the processes that generate patterns of mobility and inequality. Although valuable insights and results have been obtained from the usual approach, which predicts a dependent variable outcome as a function of a set of exogenous variables, the field would currently benefit from additional work that attempts to incorporate additional factors that may sometimes be

---

[35] This hypothesis is reminiscent of the so-called "Easterlin effect," according to which the average labor market outcomes for larger cohorts are worsened due to the greater level of competition. Pampel and Peters (1995) provide a review of studies that investigate the Easterlin effect.

[36] Winegarden's (1987) analysis of household income inequality during the early 1970s does not include data on the earnings of husbands and wives and does not consider the effect of assortative mating. However, his econometric model and results do suggest the possibility that, for developing countries with very low levels of female labor force participation (i.e., even lower than the levels for developed nations during the 1970's), small increases in the labor force participation of women may in itself increase household income inequality.

[37] In one relevant study, Boulier (1982) argues that there is no causal effect of income equality on fertility decline.

endogenous. This broader scope would yield results that are more realistic and hence more relevant to the concerns of both explanatory social science and informed public policy deliberations.

In this regard, an exemplary study is Mare's (1997) investigation of the impact of differential fertility (by race and education) on the level of educational attainment in the American population and on the racial differential in educational attainment. Mare (1997) develops a multigroup projection model which is then used in simulations based on a variety of possible assumptions about patterns of intergenerational social mobility, mortality, and the level and timing of fertility. Among his results, Mare finds that differential fertility by educational attainment has not been substantial enough to have had much impact on the overall level of educational attainment, particularly given the high level of intergenerational educational mobility that characterized much of the 20th century. Similarly, fertility differences both within and between the races have not been substantial enough to have had much of an effect on educational inequality between whites and African Americans. These important conclusions are evident in his simulations, which become feasible only after specifying a model that incorporates a variety of variables pertaining to demography and social stratification.

Another interesting study is Lerman's (1996) analysis of the effects of family structure on poverty and income inequality. The other studies on these topics reviewed above were based largely on decomposition methods that do not explicitly consider interaction or endogenous effects. By contrast, Lerman provides a richer analysis by incorporating the effects of changes in family structure on fertility, the composition of extended families, and the earnings of men and women (rather than treating the latter as being given by their observed values), which in turn have consequences for poverty and household income inequality.[38] After taking into account these endogenous effects, Lerman (1996) argues that the total impact of family structure on poverty and house-hold income inequality is significantly greater than that typically found in earlier studies based on decomposition methods. While we do not necessarily espouse this conclusion or agree with all of the details of his analysis, Lerman's (1996) more enriched approach nevertheless illustrates an important avenue for future research.

However, increasing the scope and breadth of the demography of social stratification should extend beyond simply applying more complex methods. An additional and complementary concern should be with understanding and developing cumulative knowledge about the commonalities in cross-national patterns of mobility and inequality. If increasing the complexity of analytical models means paying more attention to the details of a social process in a particular setting, the goal of understanding common patterns in cross-national research implies assessing the degree to which generic similarities may characterize the process under varied societal contexts. This latter objective of developing cumulative knowledge about generic processes is common to any scientific enterprise.

An important example of this type of research is that of Erikson and Goldthorpe (1992), who, as mentioned above, clarified the pattern underlying intergenerational class mobility throughout industrial societies. This pattern derives from particular features of the class structure, including its socioeconomic hierarchy, sectoral divisions,

---

[38] Earlier, we also raised the issue of how increases in female labor force participation may also affect men's earnings and thus generate an additional feedback mechanism affecting the level of household income inequality.

cleavages of inheritance, and social affinities (Erikson and Goldthorpe 1987: 64–69). The finding of their research—that these features of the class structure generate a similar pattern of circulation mobility throughout the industrialized world—"ranks as a major discovery" (Treiman and Ganzeboom 2002: 194). It also suggests important substantive and theoretical issues about the linkages between inequality and mobility that merit further investigation (Goldthorpe 2000: 232–258).

Prior to the publication of Erikson and Goldthorpe (1992), numerous influential studies of various substantive and methodological aspects of social mobility were available (some of which were reviewed above). In fact, in reaching their conclusions, Erikson and Goldthorpe build on dozens of prior studies and data collection projects that had been conducted by colleagues in various industrialized countries.[39] Thus, Erikson and Goldthorpe's conclusions were made possible only because of a general concern in the research community for developing cumulative knowledge about social mobility.

Shavit and Blossfeld (1993) provide another major achievement in building cumulative knowledge about cross-national commonalities in the demography of social stratification. As was discussed earlier, these investigators detail the differentials in educational attainment by class origins in 13 industrialized nations and find that they share a great deal of stability and commonality. Inspired by the seminal analysis of Mare (1981), Shavit and Blossfeld's conclusions are another example of a collective research endeavor, and they have already led to new theoretical work that has important implications for understanding cross-national commonalities in educational inequality (Breen and Goldthorpe 1997; Goldthorpe 2000).

In closing, we have suggested that the demography of social stratification should increasingly venture beyond conventional descriptive approaches and attempt to broaden the scope of its analytical methods. Previous work in the field has been highly informative, but it has reached a sufficiently mature stage of development that would benefit from developing more complex models that integrate related processes and explicitly include endogenous variables. At the same time, however, the field should continue to pursue cross-national research in order to promote the complementary objective of building cumulative knowledge about general commonalities in the demographic processes pertaining to mobility and inequality.

REFERENCES

Ahlburg, D. A. 1998. Julian Simon and the population growth debate. *Population and Development Review* 24: 317–327.

Alba, R., A. Lutz, and E. Vasselinov. 2001. How enduring were the inequalities among European immigrant groups in the United States? *Demography* 38: 349–356.

Altonji, J., and T. Dunn. 1996. The effects of family characteristics on the return to education. *Review of Economics and Statistics* 78: 692–704.

Ashenfelter, O., and A. Krueger. 1994. Estimating the returns to schooling using a new sample of twins. *American Economic Review* 84: 1157–1173.

Ashenfelter, O., and C. Rouse. 1998. Income, schooling, and ability: Evidence from a new sample of twins. *Quarterly Journal of Economics* 113: 253–284.

---

[39] Hout (2003: 8) affirms that "finding a common pattern of social fluidity has been a collective endeavor."

Ashenfelter, O., and C. Rouse. 2000. Schooling, intelligence, and income in America. In *Meritocracy and economic inequality*. Edited by K. Arrow, S. Bowles, and S. Durlauf, 89–117. Princeton, N.J.: Princeton University Press.

Ashenfelter, O., and D. Zimmerman. 1997. Estimates of the returns to schooling from sibling data: Fathers, sons, and brothers. *Review of Economics and Statistics* 79: 1–9.

Bane, M. J. 1986. Household composition and poverty. In *Fighting poverty: What works and what doesn't*. Edited by S. Danziger and D. H. Weinberg, 209–231. Cambridge, Mass.: Harvard University Press.

Banfield, E. 1968. *The unheavenly city*. Boston: Little and Brown.

Bauman, K. J. 1999. Shifting family definitions: The effect of cohabitation and other nonfamily household relationships on measures of poverty. *Demography* 36: 315–325.

Bergmann, B. R. 1996. *Saving our children from poverty: What the United States can learn from France*. New York: Russell Sage Foundation.

Bielby, W. T. 1981. Models of status attainment. *Research in Social Stratification and Mobility* 1: 3–26.

Blau, D. M., and P. K. Robins. 1989. Fertility, employment, and child-care costs. *Demography* 26: 287–299.

Blau, P., and O. D. Duncan. 1967. *The American occupational structure*. New York: Wiley.

Blossfeld, H.-P. 1986. Career opportunities in the Federal Republic of Germany: A dynamic approach to the study of life-course, cohort, and period effects. *European Sociological Review* 2: 208–225.

Blossfeld, H.-P. 1994. Causal modeling in event history analysis. Paper presented at the 1994 Meetings of the XIII World Congress of Sociology, Bielefeld, Germany. University of Bremen, Germany.

Blossfeld, H.-P., and G. Rohwer. 1995. *Techniques of event history modeling: New approaches to causal analysis*. Mahwah, N.J.: Lawrence Erlbaum Associates.

Blumen, I., M. Kogan, and P. J. McCarthy. 1955. *The industrial mobility of labor as a probability process*. Ithaca, N.Y.: Cornell University Press.

Borg, M. O. 1989. The income-fertility relationship: Effect of the net price of a child. *Demography* 26: 301–310.

Borjas, G. J. 2001. Long-run convergence of ethnic skill differentials, revisited. *Demography* 38: 357–361.

Boulier, B. L. 1982. Income redistribution and fertility decline: A skeptical view. *Population and Development Review* 8: 159–173.

Boyle, P., T. J. Cooke, K. Halfacree, and D. Smith. 2001. A cross-national comparison of the impact of family migration on women's employment status. *Demography* 38: 201–213.

Breen, R., and J. H. Goldthorpe. 1997. Explaining educational differentials: Towards a formal rational action theory. *Rationality and Society* 9: 275–305.

Bumpass, L. L., and J. Sweet. 1981. A demographic perspective on the poverty population. Institute for Research on Poverty Discussion Paper No. 669–81. Madison: University of Wisconsin.

Cambois, E., J.-M. Robine, and M. Hayward. 2001. Social inequalities in disability-free life expectancy in the French male population, 1980–1991. *Demography* 38: 513–524.

Cancian, M., S. Danziger, and P. Gottschalk. 1993. Working wives and the distribution of family income. In *Uneven tides: Rising inequality in America*. Edited by S. Danziger and P. Gottschalk, 195–221. New York: Russell Sage Foundation.

Cancian, M., and D. Reed. 1999. The impact of wives' earnings on income inequality: Issues and estimates. *Demography* 36: 173–184.

Charles, M., and D. B. Grusky. 1995. Models for describing the underlying structure of sex segregation. *American Journal of Sociology* 100: 931–971.

Chevan, A., and R. Stokes. 2000. Growth in family income inequality, 1970–1990: Industrial restructuring and demographic change. *Demography* 37: 365–380.

Clogg, C. C. 1982. Using association models in sociological research: Some examples. *American Journal of Sociology* 88: 114–134.

Crimmins, E. M. 1993. Demography: The past 30 years, the present, and the future. *Demography* 30: 579–591.

Danziger, S. 1996. Comment on "The age of extremes: Concentrated affluence and poverty in the twenty-first century." *Demography* 33: 413–416.

Danziger, S., and P. Gottschalk. 1995. *America unequal*. Cambridge, Mass.: Harvard University Press.

Deaton, A. S., and C. H. Paxson. 1997. The effects of economic and population growth on national saving and inequality. *Demography* 34: 97–114.

De Graaf, P. M., and H. B. Ganzeboom. 1993. Family background and educational attainment in the Netherlands for the 1891–1960 birth cohorts. In *Persistent inequality*. Edited by Y. Shavit and H.-P. Blossfeld, 75–100. Boulder, Colo.: Westview Press.

DiPrete, T. A., and D. B. Grusky. 1990. Structure and trend in the process of stratification for American men and women. *American Journal of Sociology* 96: 107–143.

Dooley, M., and P. Gottschalk. 1985. The increasing proportion of men with low earnings in the United States. *Demography* 22: 25–34.

Duleep, H. O. 1989. Measuring socioeconomic mortality differentials over time. *Demography* 26: 345–351.

Duleep, H. O., and M. C. Regets. 1997. Measuring immigrant wage growth using matched CPS files. *Demography* 34: 239–249.

Duncan, G. J., J. Boisjoly, and T. Smeeding. 1996. Economic mobility of young workers in the 1970s and 1980s. *Demography* 33: 497–509.

Duncan, O. D. 1966. Methodological issues in the study of social mobility. In *Social structure and social mobility*. Edited by N. Smelser and S. M. Lipset, 51–91. Chicago: Aldine.

Duncan, O. D. 1969. Inequality and opportunity. *Population Index* 35: 361–366.

Erikson, R., and J. H. Goldthorpe. 1987. Commonality and variation in social fluidity in industrial nations. II. The model of core social fluidity applied. *European Sociological Review* 3: 145–166.

Erikson, R., and J. H. Goldthorpe. 1992. *The constant flux: A study of class mobility in industrial societies*. New York: Clarendon Press.

Farley, R. 1996. The age of extremes: A revisionist perspective. *Demography* 33: 417–430.

Featherman, D. L., and R. M. Hauser. 1978. *Opportunity and change*. New York: Academic Press.

Ganzeboom, H. B., and P. De Graaf. 1984. Intergenerational occupational mobility in the Netherlands in 1954 and 1977: A loglinear analysis. In *Social stratification and mobility in the Netherlands*. Edited by B. F. Bakker, J. Dronkers, and H. B. Ganzeboom, 36–61. Amsterdam: SISWO Press.

Ganzeboom, H. B., and D. J. Treiman. 1996. Internationally comparable measures of occupational status for the 1988 International Standard Classification of Occupations. *Social Science Research* 25: 201–239.

Ganzeboom, H. B., D. J. Treiman, and W. C. Ultee. 1991. Comparative intergenerational stratification research: Three generations and beyond. *Annual Review of Sociology*. 17: 277–302.

Garfinkel, I., and S. McLanahan. 1994. Single-mother families, economic insecurity, and government policy. In *Confronting poverty: Prescriptions for change*. Edited by S. H. Danziger, G. D. Sandefur, and D. H. Weinberg, 205–225. Cambridge, Mass.: Harvard University Press.

Garnier, M. A., and L. E. Raffalovich. 1984. The evolution of equality of educational opportunities in France. *Sociology of Education* 57: 1–11.

Gittleman, M., and M. Joyce. 1999. Have family income mobility patterns changed? *Demography* 36: 299–314.

Glass, D. V. 1954. *Social mobility in Britain*. London: Routledge and Paul.

Goldthorpe, J. H. 2000. *On sociology: Numbers, narratives, and the integration of research and theory*. New York: Oxford University Press.

Goodman, L. A. 1965. On the statistical analysis of mobility tables. *American Journal of Sociology*. 70: 564–585.

Goodman, L. A. 1968. The analysis of cross-classified data: Independence, quasi-independence, and interaction in contingency tables with or without missing entries. *Journal of the American Statistical Association* 63: 1091–1131.

Goodman, L. A. 1979. Simple models for the analysis of association in cross-classifications having ordered categories. *Journal of the American Statistical Association* 74: 537–552.

Goodman, L. A. 1981. Three elementary views of log-linear models for the analysis of cross-classifications having ordered categories. In *Sociological methodology 1981*. Edited by S. Leinhardt, 193–239. San Francisco; Jossey-Bass.

Gortmaker, S. L., and P. H. Wise. 1997. The first injustice: Socioeconomic disparities, health services technology, and infant mortality. *Annual Review of Sociology* 23: 147–170.

Griliches, Z. 1979. Sibling models and data in economics: Beginnings of a survey. *Journal of Political Economy* 87: S37–S64.

Gronau, R. 1982. Inequality of family income: Do wives' earnings matter? *Population and Development Review* 8: S119–S136.

Grusky, D. B., and M. Charles. 1998. The past, present, and future of sex segregation methodology. *Demography* 35: 497–504.

Grusky, D. B., and T. A. DiPrete. 1990. Recent trends in the process of stratification. *Demography* 27: 617–637.

Guo, G. 1993. Use of sibling data to estimate family mortality effects in Guatemala. *Demography* 30: 15–32.

Guo, G., and K. M. Harris. 2000. The mechanisms mediating the effects of poverty on children's intellectual development. *Demography* 37: 431–447.

Guo, G., and G. Rodríguez. 1992. Estimating a multivariate proportional hazards model for clustered data using the EM algorithm, with an application to child survival in Guatemala. *Journal of the American Statistical Association* 87: 969–976.

Hannum, E. 2002. Educational stratification by ethnicity in China: Enrollment and attainment in the early reform years. *Demography* 39: 95–117.

Hannum, E., and Xie, Y. 1998. Ethnic stratification in Northwest China: Occupational differences between Han Chinese and national minorities in Xinjiang, 1982–1990. *Demography* 35: 323–333.

Hauser, P. M., and O. D. Duncan. 1959. The nature of demography. In *The study of population.* Edited by P. M. Hauser and O. D. Duncan, 29–44. Chicago: University of Chicago Press.

Hauser, R. M. 1978. A structural model of the mobility table. *Social Forces* 56: 919–953.

Hauser, R. M. 1979. Some exploratory methods for modeling mobility tables and other cross-classified data. In *Sociological methodology.* Edited by K. F. Schuessler, 413–458. San Francisco: Jossey-Bass.

Hauser, R. M. 1988. A note on two models of sibling resemblance. *American Journal of Sociology* 93: 1401–1423.

Hauser, R. M., and D. L. Featherman. 1977. *The process of stratification: Trends and analyses.* New York: Academic Press.

Hauser, R. M., and M.-H. Huang. 1997. Verbal ability and socioeconomic success: A trend analysis. *Social Science Research* 26: 331–376.

Hauser, R. M., and P. A. Mossel. 1985. Fraternal resemblance in educational attainment and occupational status. *American Journal of Sociology.* 91: 650–671.

Hauser, R. M., and W. H. Sewell. 1986. Family effects in simple models of education, occupational status, and earnings: Findings from the Wisconsin and Kalamazoo studies. *Journal of Labor Economics* 4: S83–S115.

Hauser, R. M., J. R. Warren, M.-H. Huang, and W. Y. Carter. 2000. Occupational status, education, and social mobility in the meritocracy. In *Meritocracy and economic inequality.* Edited by K. Arrow, S. Bowles, and S. Durlauf. Princeton, N.J. Princeton University Press.

Hauser, R. M., and R. S. Wong. 1989. Sibling resemblance and intersibling effects in educational attainment. *Sociology of Education* 62: 149–171.

Heckman, J. J., and B. Singer. 1984. A method for minimizing the impact of distributional assumptions in econometric models for duration data. *Econometrica* 52: 271–320.

Herrnstein, R. J., and C. Murray. 1994. *The bell curve.* New York: Free Press.

Hirschman, C. 2001. The educational enrollment of immigrant youth: A test of the segmented-assimilation hypothesis. *Demography* 38: 317–336.

Hodge, R. W. 1966. Occupational mobility as a probability process. *Demography* 3: 19–34.

Hoem, J. M. 1990. Limitations of a heterogeneity technique: Selectivity issues in conjugal union disruption at parity zero in contemporary Sweden. In *Convergent issues in genetics and demography.* Edited by J. Adams, 133–153. New York: Oxford University Press.

Holford, T. R. 1980. The analysis of rate of survivorship using log-linear models. *Biometrics* 36: 299–305.

Hope, K. 1985. *As others see us: Schooling and social mobility in Scotland and the United States.* Cambridge: Cambridge University Press.

Hout, M. 1984. Occupational mobility of black men: 1962 to 1973. *American Sociological Review* 49: 308–322.

Hout, M. 1988. More universalism, less structural mobility: The American occupational structure in the 1980s. *American Journal of Sociology* 93: 1358–1400.

Hout, M. 1989. *Following in father's footsteps: Social mobility in Ireland.* Cambridge, Mass.: Harvard University Press.

Hout, M. 2003. What we have learned: RC28's contributions to knowledge. Paper presented in March 2003 at the annual meeting of Research Committee #28 in Tokyo, Japan.

Hout, M., R. Arum, and K. Voss. 1996. The political economy of inequality in the "Age of Extremes." *Demography* 33: 421–425.

Iceland, J. 1997. Urban labor markets and individual transitions out of poverty. *Demography* 34: 429–441.

Iceland, J. 2003. Why poverty remains high: The role of income growth, economic inequality, and changes in family structure, 1949–1999. *Demography* 40: 499–519.

Ishida, H. 1993. *Social mobility in contemporary Japan.* Palo Alto, Calif.: Stanford University Press.

Jencks, C., et al. 1972. *Inequality: A reassessment of the effect of family and schooling in America.* New York: Harper & Row.

Jencks, C., et al. 1979. *Who gets ahead? The determinants of economic success in America.* New York: Basic Books.

Jencks, C., J. Crouse, and P. Mueser. 1983. The Wisconsin model of status attainment: A national replication of improved measures of ability and aspiration. *Sociology of Education* 56: 3–19.

Johnson, N. J., P. D. Sorlie, and E. Backlund. 1999. The impact of specific occupation on mortality in the U.S. National Longitudinal Mortality Survey. *Demography* 36: 355–367.

Jonsson, J. O. 1993. Persisting inequalities in Sweden. In *Persistent inequality*. Edited by Y. Shavit and H.-P. Blossfeld, 101–132. Boulder, Colo.: Westview Press.

Kahl, J. A. 1957. *The American class structure*. New York: Holt Rinehart and Winston.

Karoly, L. A., and G. Burtless. 1995. Demographic change, rising earnings inequality, and the distribution of personal well-being, 1959–1989. *Demography* 32: 379–405.

Kasarda, J. D., and J. O. G. Billy. 1985. Social mobility and fertility. *Annual Review of Sociology* 11: 305–328.

Keyfitz, N. 1977. *Applied mathematical demography*. New York: Wiley.

Kohler, H.-P., J. R. Behrman, and S. C. Watkins. 2001. The density of social networks and fertility decisions: Evidence from South Nyanza District, Kenya. *Demography* 38: 43–58.

Laird, N., and D. Oliver. 1981. Covariance analysis of censored survival data using log-linear analysis techniques. *Journal of the American Statistical Association* 76: 231–240.

Layard, R., and A. Zabalza. 1979. Family income distribution: Explanation and policy evaluation. *Journal of Political Economy* 87: S133–161.

Lerman, R. I. 1996. The impact of the changing U.S. family structure on child poverty and income inequality. *Economics* 63: S119–S139.

Leslie, P. H. 1945. On the use of matrices in certain population mathematics. *Biometrika* 33: 183–212.

Lewis, O. 1966. *La vida: A Puerto Rican family in the culture of poverty*. New York: Random House.

Li, L., and M. K. Choe. 1997. A mixture model for duration data: Analysis of second births in China. *Demography* 34: 189–197.

Lichter, D. T. 1997. Poverty and inequality among children. *Annual Review of Sociology* 23: 121–145.

Lipset, S., and R. Bendix. 1952a. Social mobility and occupational career patterns. I. Stability and job holding. *American Journal of Sociology* 57: 366–374.

Lipset, S., and R. Bendix. 1952b. Social mobility and occupational career patterns. II. Social mobility. *American Journal of Sociology* 57: 494–504.

Lipset, S., and R. Bendix. 1964. *Social mobility in industrial society*. Berkeley: University of California Press.

Mansfield, E. 1979. *Microeconomics: Theory and applications*. New York: W. W. Norton.

Mare, R. D. 1981. Change and stability in educational stratification. *American Sociological Review* 46: 72–87.

Mare, R. D. 1990. Socio-economic careers and differentials among older men in the United States. In *Measurement analysis of mortality: A new approach*. Edited by J. Vallin, S. D'Souza, and A. Palloni, 362–387. Oxford: Clarendon.

Mare, R. D. 1997. Differential fertility, intergenerational educational mobility, and racial inequality. *Social Science Research* 26: 263–291.

Mare, R. D. 2001. Observations on the study of social mobility and inequality. In *Social stratification: Class, race and gender in sociological perspective*, Edited by D. B. Grusky. Boulder, Colo.: Westview Press.

Massey, D. S. 1996. The age of extremes: Concentrated affluence and poverty in the twenty-first century. *Demography* 33: 395–412.

Matras, J. 1961. Differential fertility, intergenerational occupational mobility, and change in the occupational distribution: Some elementary interrelationships. *Population Studies* 15: 187–197.

Matras, J. 1967. Social mobility and social structure: Some insights from the linear model. *American Sociological Review* 32: 608–614.

McLanahan, S., and G. Sandefur. 1994. *Growing up with a single parent: What hurts, what helps*. Cambridge, Mass.: Harvard University Press.

Merli, M. G. 2000. Socioeconomic background and war mortality during vietnam's wars. *Demography* 37: 1–15.

Miller, P., C. Mulvey, and N. Martin. 1995. What do twins studies reveal about the economic returns to education? A comparison of Australian and U.S. findings. *American Economic Review* 85: 586–599.

Mincer, J., and B. Jovanovic. 1981. Labor mobility and wages. In *Studies in labor markets*. Edited by S. Rosen, 21–63. Chicago: University of Chicago Press.

Mukherjee, R. 1954. A further note on the analysis of data on social mobility. In *Social mobility in Britain*. Edited by D. V. Glass, 242–259. London: Routledge & Kegan Paul.

Namboodiri, K., and C. M. Suchindran. 1987. *Life table techniques and their applications*. New York: Academic Press.

Nielsen, F. 1994. Income inequality and industrial development: Dualism revisited. *American Sociological Review* 59: 654–677.

Nielsen, F., and A. S. Alderson. 1995. Income inequality, development, and dualism: Results from an unbalanced cross-national panel. *American Sociological Review* 60: 674–701.

Olneck, M. R. 1977. On the use of sibling data to estimate the effects of family background, cognitive skills, and schooling: Results from the Kalamazoo Brothers Study. In *Kinometrics: Determinants of socio-economic success within and between families*. Edited by P. Taubman, 125–162. Amsterdam: North-Holland.

Oropesa, R. S., and N. S. Landale. 2000. From austerity to prosperity? Migration and child poverty among mainland and island Puerto Ricans. *Demography* 37: 323–338.

Palmer, G. 1954. *Labor mobility in three cities*. New York: Social Science Research Council.

Pampel, F. C., and H. E. Peters. 1995. The Easterlin effect. *Annual Review of Sociology* 21: 163–194.

Parsons, T. 1970. Equality and inequality in modern society, or social stratification revisited. In *Social stratification: Research and theory for the 1970s*. Edited by E. O. Laumann, 13–72. Indianapolis: Bobbs-Merrill.

Powers, D. A. 2001. Unobserved family effects on the risk of a first premarital birth. *Social Science Research* 30: 1–24.

Powers, D. A. and J. C.-T. Hsueh. 1997. Sibling models of socioeconomic effects on the timing of first premarital birth. *Demography* 34: 493–511.

Prais, S. J. 1955a. Measuring social mobility. *Journal of the Royal Statistical Society. Series A*. 118: 56–66.

Prais, S. J. 1955b. The formal theory of social mobility. *Population Studies* 9: 72–81.

Pribesh, S. and D. B. Downey. 1999. Why are residential and school moves associated with poor school performance? *Demography* 36: 521–534.

Rainwater, L. 1968. *Behind ghetto walls: Black families in a federal slum*. Chicago: Aldine.

Rainwater, L. 1995. Poverty and the income packaging of working parents: the United States in comparative perspective. *Children and Youth Service Review*. 17: 11–41.

Reder, M. W. 1955. The theory of occupational wage differentials. *American Economic Review* 45: 833–852.

Reed, D. 2001. Immigration and males' earnings inequality in the regions of the United States. *Demography* 38: 363–373.

Rogers, R. 1992. Living and dying in the U.S.A.: Sociodemographic determinants of death among blacks and whites. *Demography* 29: 287–303.

Rogoff, N. R. 1953. *Recent trends in social mobility*. Glencoe, Ill.: The Free Press.

Ross, C. E. and J. Mirowsky. 1999. Refining the association between education and health: The effects of quantity, credential, and selectivity. *Demography* 36: 445–460.

Ross, C. E., and C.-L. Wu. 1995. The links between education and health. *American Sociological Review* 60: 719–745.

Rytina, S. 2000. Is occupational mobility declining in the U.S.? *Social Forces* 78: 1227–1276.

Sakamoto, A., J. Liu, and J. M. Tzeng. 1998. The declining significance of race among Chinese and Japanese American men. *Research in Social Stratification and Mobility* 16: 225–246.

Sakamoto, A., and J. M. Tzeng. 1999. A fifty-year perspective on the declining significance of race in the occupational attainment of white and black men. *Sociological Perspectives* 42: 157–179.

Sakamoto, A., H.-H. Wu, and J. M. Tzeng. 2000. The declining significance of race among American men during the latter half of the twentieth century. *Demography* 37: 41–51.

Schultz, D. A. 1969. *Coming up black*. New York: Prentice-Hall.

Sen, A. 1976. Poverty: An ordinal approach to measurement. *Econometrica* 44: 219–213.

Sewell, W., A. O. Haller, and G. W. Ohlendorf. 1970. The educational and early occupational status attainment process: A replication and revision. *American Sociological Review* 35: 1014–1027.

Shavit, Y., and H.-P. Blossfeld. 1993. *Persistent inequality: Changing educational attainment in thirteen countries*. Boulder, Colo.: Westview Press.

Shryock, H. S. and J. S. Siegel. 1976. *The methods and materials of demography, condensed ed.* New York: Academic Press.

Smeeding, T., B. B. Torrey, and M. Rein. 1988. Patterns of income and poverty: The economic status of children and the elderly in eight countries. In *The vulnerable*. Edited by J. L. Palmer, T. Smeeding, and B. B. Torrey, 89–119. Washington, D.C.: Urban Institute.

Smith, H. L. and P. P. Cheung. 1986. Trends in the effects of family background on educational attainment in the Philippines. *American Journal of Sociology* 91: 1387–1408.

Smith, J. P. 1988. Poverty and the family. In *Divided opportunities: Minorities, poverty, and social policy*. Edited by G. D. Sandefur and M. Tienda 141–172. New York: Plenum.

Sobel, M. E., M. Hout, and O. D. Duncan. 1985. Exchange, structure, and symmetry in occupational mobility. *American Journal of Sociology* 91: 359–372.

Sørensen, A. B. 1974. A model for occupational careers. *American Journal of Sociology* 80: 44–57.

Sørensen, A. B. 1996. The structural basis of social inequality. *American Journal of Sociology* 101: 1333–1365.

Spilerman, S. 1976. Careers, labor market structure and socioeconomic achievement. *American Journal of Sociology* 83: 551–594.

Spilerman, S., and R. E. Miller. 1973. The effect of negative tax payments on job turnover and job selection. In *The final report of the New Jersey graduated income tax experiment, Vol. 1.* Edited by H. W. Watts and A. Rees, 123–167. Madison, Wisc.: Institute for Research on Poverty.

Stack, C. 1974. *All our kin.* New York: Harper & Row.

Treas, J. 1987. The effect of women's labor force participation on the distribution of income in the United States. *Annual Review of Sociology* 13: 259–288.

Treiman, D. J. 1970. Industrialization and social stratification. In *Social stratification: Research and theory for the 1970s.* Edited by E. O. Laumann, 207–234. Indianapolis: Bobbs-Merrill.

Treiman, D. J. 1977. *Occupational prestige in comparative perspective.* New York: Academic Press.

Treiman, D. J. and H. B. Ganzeboom. 1990. Cross-national comparative status attainment research. *Research in Social Stratification and Mobility* 9: 105–127.

Treiman, D. J. and H. B. Ganzeboom. 2002. The fourth generation of comparative stratification research. In *International handbook of sociology.* Edited by S. R. Quah and A. Sales, 193–204. Thousand Oaks, Calif.: Sage Press.

Trussel, J., and G. Rodríguez. 1990. Heterogeneity in demographic research. In *Convergent issues in genetics and demography.* Edited by J. Adams, 111–134. New York: Oxford University Press.

Tuma, N. B. 1976. Rewards, resources, and the rate of mobility: A nonstationary multivariate stochastic model. *American Sociological Review* 41: 338–360.

Tuma, N. B. and M. T. Hannan. 1984. *Social dynamics: Models and methods.* New York: Academic Press.

Valentine, C. 1968. *Culture and poverty.* Chicago: University of Chicago Press.

Vaupel, J. A., and A. I. Yashin. 1985. The deviant dynamics of death in heterogeneous populations. In *Sociological methodology 1985.* Edited by N. B. Tuma, 179–211. San Francisco, Jossey-Bass.

Vaupel, J. A., K. G. Manton, and E. Stallard. 1979. The impact of heterogeneity in individual frailty on the dynamics of mortality. *Demography* 16: 439–454.

Warren, J. R. and R. M. Hauser. 1997. Social stratification across three generations: New evidence from the Wisconsin Longitudinal Survey. *American Sociological Review* 62: 561–572.

Weeden, K. A. 1998. Revisiting occupational sex segregation in the United States, 1910–1990: Results from a log-linear approach. *Demography* 35: 475–487.

White, H. C. 1970. Stayers and movers. *American Journal of Sociology* 76: 307–324.

Winegarden, C. R. 1987. Women's labour force participation and the distribution of household incomes: Evidence from cross-national data. *Economica* 54: 223–236.

Wright, E. O. 1979. *Class structure and income determination.* New York: Academic Press.

Wright, E. O. 2000. Class, exploitation, and economic rents: Reflections on Sorensen's "sounder basis." *American Journal of Sociology* 105: 1559–1571.

Xie, Y. 1992. The log-multiplicative layer effect model for comparing tables. *American Sociological Review* 57: 380–395.

PART III

POPULATION AND THE SOCIAL SCIENCES

Over the past 50 years the scope of demographic science has been expanded to the point that it may now be referred to as an "interdiscipline" (Stycos 1987). The implication is that while demography clearly qualifies as a discipline in its own right, its subject matter and methods show substantial overlap with those claimed by a number of other disciplines, including sociology, economics, anthropology, public health, epidemiology, geography, history, biology, and genetics. Further evidence of this expansion is seen in the list of contributors to a recently published population encyclopedia (Demeny and McNicoll 2003), representing the fields of anthropology, biology, demography, economics, geography, history, law, philosophy, political science, public health, and sociology. In short, demographic concepts, theories, methods, and research findings have been influenced by those developed in other disciplines and, in turn, have served to enrich inquiry in these other fields.

The Study of Population contains seven chapters relating demography to other disciplines, covering biological ecology (Frank 1959), human ecology (Duncan 1959), geography (Ackerman 1959), physical anthropology (Spuhler 1959), genetics (Kallman and Rainer 1959), economics (Spengler 1959), and sociology (Moore 1959). This *Handbook* offers 10 chapters highlighting connections and interrelations between demography and a variety of other, predominantly social science, disciplines. Six of the chapters reflect long-recognized branches of interdisciplinary demographic inquiry. Chapter 14 by Hirschman and Tolnay, chapter 16 by Fossett, chapter 17 by Kertzer, chapter 18 by Mason, chapter 20 by Poston and Frisbie, and chapter 23 by Teitelbaum deal, respectively, with sociology, urban structure, anthropology, economics, human ecology, and political science. The other four represent newer extensions of demographic principles, methods and subject matter across disciplinary boundaries. In chapter 15 Carroll and Khessina focus on the field of organizational and corporate demography, much of which involves the application of demographic ideas and methods to the study of populations of organizations. Chapter 19 by VandeWalle covers the intersection of demography and history. In Chapter 21 Carey and Vaupel review progress of the relatively new specialty of biodemography which draws on epidemiology, biology, and demography to examine a variety of interesting and important issues, e.g., human senescence, longevity, frailty, and genetic variation. Finally, chapter 22 by Land, Yang and Zeng is devoted to mathematical demography and covers efforts to increase the precision and power of demographic analysis through the incorporation of mathematical models and mathematical statistics.

As the chapters in this section show, or at least suggest, the future of demographic science can be expected to be increasingly interdisciplinary, with both partners in these joint ventures becoming stronger and more consequential sciences than if the collaboration had not been undertaken.

REFERENCES

Ackerman, E. A. 1959. "Geography and Demography." pp. 717–727 in *The Study of Population: An Inventory and Appraisal*, edited by P. M. Hauser and O. D. Duncan. Chicago: University of Chicago Press.

Demeny, P. and G. McNicoll. 2003. *Encyclopedia of Population*. New York: Macmillan Reference USA.

Duncan, O. D. 1959. "Human Ecology and Population Studies." pp. 678–716 in *The Study of Population: An Inventory and Appraisal*, edited by P. M. Hauser and O. D. Duncan. Chicago: University of Chicago Press.

Frank, P. W. 1959. "Ecology and Demography." pp. 652–677 in *The Study of Population: An Inventory and Appraisal*, edited by P. M. Hauser and O. D. Duncan. Chicago: University of Chicago Press.

Kallmann, F. J. and J. D. Rainer. 1959. "Genetics and Demography." pp. 759–790 in *The Study of Population: An Inventory and Appraisal*, edited by P. M. Hauser and O. D. Duncan. Chicago: University of Chicago Press.

Moore, W. E. 1959. "Sociology and Demography." pp. 832–851 in *The Study of Population: An Inventory and Appraisal*, edited by P. M. Hauser and O. D. Duncan. Chicago: University of Chicago Press.

Spengler, J. J. 1959. "Economics and Demography." pp. 791–851 in *The Study of Population: An Inventory and Appraisal*, edited by P. M. Hauser and O. D. Duncan. Chicago: University of Chicago Press.

Spuhler, J. N. 1959. "Physical Anthropology and Demography." pp. 728–758 in *The Study of Population: An Inventory and Appraisal*, edited by P. M. Hauser and O. D. Duncan. Chicago: University of Chicago Press.

Stycos, J. M. 1987. "Demography as an Interdiscipline." *Sociological Forum* 2 (4, Special Issue: Demography as an Interdiscipline): 616–618.

CHAPTER 14

Social Demography

CHARLES HIRSCHMAN

AND

STEWART E. TOLNAY

The history of demography in the United States is closely bound up with the discipline of sociology. In many countries, demography is a freestanding field or is considered to be part of a branch of applied statistics. This pattern is much less common in the United States, where demography (and demographic training) is often considered an area of specialization within one or more social and health science disciplines, including economics, geography, anthropology, and sociology. But sociology is the first among equals in its association with demography.

Close interactions between the breadth of the sociological vision and the rigor of demographic analysis create the potential of a symbiotic relationship (Davis 1959). Demography is given its widest exposure via sociology. One or more courses in population are considered part of the core undergraduate curriculum in most sociology departments. In addition, having a nucleus of demographers and a leading population research center appears to favorably impact the prestige and ranking of sociology departments in the United States. Prominent examples include the distinguished sociology departments and population centers at universities such as Brown, Chicago, Michigan, North Carolina, Pennsylvania, Pennsylvania State, Princeton, Texas, University of California—Los Angeles, Washington, and Wisconsin. This association is much less common in other social science and health science disciplines.

This close link between the evolution of demography and sociology in the United States is probably a conjuncture of several independent historical conditions. Lorimer (1959: 162–163) observes that several of the pioneers of American demography, including Walter Wilcox, William Ogburn, and Warren Thompson, received graduate degrees in sociology at Columbia University, where sociologist Franklin Giddings was an influential advocate of the application of statistical methods in empirical research. For several decades, Ogburn was a central figure in the "Chicago School" (along with Robert Park, Ernest Burgess, and Roderick McKenzie), which became the primary training ground for American sociology in the decades prior to World War II. The Chicago School of Sociology did not identify demography as a distinct branch of the discipline, but the Chicago School's emphasis on the empirical study of urban social and spatial structure (loosely organized under the theoretical rubric of human ecology) provided a congenial environment for the exploration of demographic data and topics (Namboodiri 1988).[1]

Unlike other social science disciplines, which have a primary institutional focus (e.g., economics, political science, etc.), sociology typically covers a variety of distinct areas of specialization. For example, the standard introductory sociology textbook will include chapters on marriage and the family, race and ethnic relations, crime and delinquency, rural and urban communities, formal organizations, religion, and other topics. The sociological study of population trends and patterns fits easily into this list of specialties as another topic in the undergraduate and graduate curriculum. Warren Thompson's *Population Problems* went through five editions from 1930 to the mid-1960s and was a standard undergraduate textbook in the sociology curriculum (Thompson 1930).

The status of demography in sociology was raised in the decades after World War II, when several sociologist-demographers published a series of important books and articles that helped to define modern sociology (Preston 1993). Kingsley Davis wrote an influential introductory sociology textbook in 1949 and also published a series of important theoretical and empirical books and articles on population, social stratification, the family, and other topics in sociology (Davis 1945, 1949, 1951, 1956; Davis and Moore 1945). At the University of Michigan, Amos Hawley and Ronald Freedman played pioneering roles in the development of human ecology and the sociological study of human fertility in the United States and in Asia (Hawley 1950; Freedman, Whelpton, and Campbell 1959; Freedman and Takeshita 1969). At the University of Chicago, Philip Hauser, Otis Dudley Duncan, and Donald Bogue formally brought demography into the Chicago School of Sociology and Human Ecology (Hauser and Duncan 1959; Duncan and Duncan 1957; Duncan et al. 1960). Duncan moved to Michigan in the early 1960s and in collaboration with colleagues and students, he founded the modern school of social stratification (Blau and Duncan 1967; Duncan, Featherman, and Duncan 1972). Another sociologist-demographer, Stanley Lieberson, has made a series of path-breaking contributions to the sociological study of American race and ethnic relations, research methodology, and cultural change (Lieberson 1980, 1985, 2000). These sociological demographers and their pioneering studies have established the centrality of demographic training and the demographic perspective as core elements of the modern discipline of sociology.

---

[1] The influential textbook, *Introduction to the Science of Sociology* by Park and Burgess, did not include a chapter on population, and neither "demography" nor "population" was listed in the subject index (Park and Burgess 1921).

In his assessment of the future of demography from a vantage point in the mid-1970s, Preston (1978) noted four schools of demography, which he identified as the Princeton tradition, the Chicago-Berkeley tradition, the Pennsylvania-Brown tradition, and the Michigan-Wisconsin tradition. The Princeton tradition emphasized formal mathematical demography; the Chicago-Berkeley was the most theoretical, with an emphasis on interrelations between populations and societies; and the Pennsylvania-Brown tradition focused on spatial distribution and labor force structure. The fourth tradition, the Michigan-Wisconsin tradition, which devoted more attention to socio-economic status and social mobility, presented the broadest scope of the emerging field of social demography. Preston suggested that the Michigan-Wisconsin tradition was becoming more prominent relative to the other schools. The influence of the Wisconsin and Michigan programs was due, in large part, to their productive faculty, both in terms of their published scholarship and in their training of successive generations of social demographers. The doctoral alumni of Michigan and Wisconsin have spread their vision of social demography to many other universities and colleges in the United States and abroad.

Although our claim is that demography has become more central to sociology in recent decades, the reverse is probably not true. In the late 1950s, Hauser and Duncan (1959: 107) reported that three-fifths of Population Association of America (PAA) members holding doctorates earned them in sociology. Of the more than 3,000 PAA members in March 2003, fewer than one-third identified sociology as their major professional field (Dudley 2003).[2] As demography has gained a more prominent niche within sociology, the field has also become a more attractive area of specialization in economics (economic demography), geography (population geography), anthropology (anthropological demography), and other social, statistical, and health sciences. The comparative success of demography may be due to the nature of the field (an empirical interdisciplinary science with porous boundaries), a reliance on well-measured and quantifiable concepts, a focus on real-world problems, and the relatively generous federal and foundation funding for training (predoctoral and postdoctoral) and research (Morgan and Lynch 2001). All of these factors have also been important for the development of the specialization of demography among sociologists.

The overlap between demography and sociology has come to be known as *social demography,* though this term has been widely used only since the 1970s. The term social demography does not appear in the index of the classic *The Study of Population*, edited by Philip Hauser and Otis Dudley Duncan (1959). Hauser and Duncan drew the distinction between "formal demography" and "population studies" to characterize the two major foci in the field (1959: 33–43). Formal demography includes the analysis of population change in terms of other demographic variables, fertility, mortality, migration, and the age-sex composition of the population. Research in formal demography is generally concerned with the development of mathematical or statistical models. In contrast, the subfield of population studies is typically much more broad ranging, with theories and hypotheses from other scientific disciplines combined with demographic data and variables. It is often difficult to draw a precise line between demographers conducting population studies research and disciplinary researchers who happen to use demographic data.

---

[2] The same ratio (one-third of PAA members claiming sociology as their major professional field) would hold if only regular (nonstudent) members were counted.

One of the earliest references to "social demography" was the title of a 1963 essay by Kingsley Davis (Davis 1963; only four years earlier Davis published an essay with the title, "The Sociology of Demographic Behavior, see Davis 1959). *Social Demography* was also the title of a textbook *cum* reader published in 1970 (Ford and DeJong 1970) and the title of a state-of-the-art collection of essays published in 1978 (Taeuber, Bumpass, and Sweet 1978). However, *sociological demography* was the term used to describe the field in an influential book by Calvin Goldscheider (1971: chapters 1 and 2), and one of the classic textbooks published in 1977 was titled, *Introduction to Population: A Sociological Approach* (Matras 1977). Our impression is that *social demography* has been popularly accepted by most sociologist demographers to describe their area of specialization as economists increasingly adopted the term *economic demography* (see chapter 18, "Economic Demography," in this *Handbook*).

Although the term *social demography* has been widely accepted, there may be less agreement on the primary content of the field and its boundaries. The difficulty is that the boundaries of the field have expanded as the marriage between sociology and demography has deepened, and more sociologists identify their work as social demography or they draw upon demographic logic and modes of inquiry. For example, the sociology of the family has a lineage that is largely independent of demography, represented by the seminal works of William Goode, Ruben Hill, and Marion Levy. In recent decades, however, the works of demographer-sociologists such as Larry Bumpass, Andrew Cherlin, Frances Goldscheider, S. Philip Morgan, Ronald Rindfuss, James Sweet, Arland Thornton, and Linda Waite have blurred the boundary between general sociological studies of the family and social demographic studies of the family. Other leading sociologists of the family, such as Frank Furstenberg and Glen Elder, frequently collaborate with demographers and have become mentors of many younger social demographers through their affiliations with university population research centers.

The field of social demography might be described as the analysis of sociological questions with demographic data, such as censuses and population surveys. But this definition would be far too narrow, since quite a few social demographers use qualitative methods. Almost every topic in sociology has drawn the interest of some social demographers. Nonetheless, there appear to be two broad sociological themes that encompass much of social demography—the family and the study of inequality (see chapter 3, "Marriage and Family," and chapter 13, "Demography of Social Stratification," in this *Handbook*).

More than any other social institution, the family is at the heart of sociology. Demographers are well positioned to contribute to empirical research on the family because census, vital statistics, and population surveys are the primary sources for contemporary studies of the family and often the only source for historical studies (Bumpass and Lu 2000; Sweeney 2002; Thornton and Lin 1994; Tolnay 1999). Among the important topics addressed by social demographers are trends in marriage and divorce, changes in age at marriage, childbearing patterns, living arrangements, employment trends of mothers of young children, and child welfare. New topics in demographic research, including population aging and intergenerational support, have direct implications for classic sociological questions about the structure and functions of the family. Two recent presidential addresses at the Population Association of America, Samuel Preston's "Children and the Elderly: Divergent Paths for America's Dependents" (Preston 1984) and Larry Bumpass's "What's Happening to the Family?" (Bumpass 1990) illustrate how demographic insights and analyses can inform the sociological study of the family.

Research on socioeconomic inequality and stratification has been another field-defining area of social demography. Hauser and Duncan's (1959) inclusion of social mobility in their definition of demography put studies of census and survey data on education, occupations, income, and other census measures of socioeconomic status at the core of the field. The ideas, data, and methods used to study inequality and social mobility by social demographers have been widely diffused throughout sociology and are applied to research on the status of immigrants, race and ethnic inequality, and residential segregation (see chapters 2, 6, 12, and 16 in this *Handbook*). New research directions have included comparisons of men and women in the labor force, race and ethnic identities of new immigrants, and health disparities. In addition to their familiarity with census and other national data sources, social demographers have been able to make important empirical contributions because they have developed innovative methods to study intercohort social change from cross-sectional data and to model the relationship between changes in social structure and social mobility.

Beyond substance, social demography is best described in terms of methodological genres or styles of research. Although these genres of research are not "owned" by social demography, they are common patterns that illustrate how and why social demography has had such an important impact on the discipline of sociology. In the following sections, we highlight three major themes of work that are identified with social demography, broadly defined as: Description of Social Patterns and Trends, Hypothesis Testing and Explanatory Sociology, and Contextual Analysis.

DESCRIPTION OF SOCIAL PATTERNS AND TRENDS

There is a great social and economic demand for objective information about population characteristics and trends. This need arises, in part, from popular curiosity of people wanting to know if others are like them and share common experiences. Businesses want to know about potential markets for goods and services and whether demand is likely to grow or shrink (see chapter 25, "Small Area and Business Demography," in this *Handbook*). Public authorities also seek information about current and future population size and composition to be able to plan where to locate schools and roads and how much revenue will be needed to provide for future pensions and health care needs. Although these "data needs" are sometimes met by generalizing from one's own (and acquaintances') experiences, it is widely recognized that broader and more representative data provide a more accurate portrait. Demographers, by virtue of their expertise in analyzing and interpreting census data and their scientific training, are generally thought to be objective reporters on the state of society as revealed through population data.

Many social demographers, along with social historians, statisticians, and other scholars have used census data to describe the fortunes and problems of the American people (and of other societies). For much of American history, the decennial population census has been the primary (and only) source of information about the size, distribution, and characteristics of the population. Moreover, census data can be analyzed to provide valuable insights on important social and economic issues (Anderson 1988). Demographic data, as with all evidence, can be manipulated by partisans to "speak" on one side or the other of contested issues. In spite of these tendencies, the tradition of the census as the nation's "fact finder" and as a source of public enlightenment has been an important backdrop for the development of contemporary demography.

This tradition of census-based societal description and accounting is exemplified by the title (and content) of Reynolds Farley's 1990 highly regarded census monograph, *The New American Reality: Who We Are, How We Got Here, and Where Are We Going* (Farley 1996) and the accompanying two volumes, *State of the Union: America in the 1990s* (Farley 1995, 1996), with chapters on income, labor force, education, housing, family, the older population, immigrants, and much more. Although Census Bureau publications occasionally go beyond basic tabulations to describe and analyze social phenomena, the book-length "census monographs" written by academic scholars were important milestones in the development of social demography, beginning with the 1920 census. Among the titles of the 1920 census monographs (published from 1922 to 1931) were *Farm Tenancy in the United States* (Goldenweiser and Truesdell 1924), *Women in Gainful Occupations* (Hill 1929), and *Immigrants and Their Children* (Carpenter 1927).

Although some of the census monographs (published following the 1920, 1950, 1960, 1970, and 1980 censuses) fit the caricature of "one damn statistic after another," quite a few of them have become minor classics and are well worth reading as models of social reporting and careful descriptive analysis. For example, the 1950 census monograph on *Social Characteristics of Urban and Rural Communities* (Duncan and Reiss 1956) illustrated how the rural-urban continuum varied across a number of dimensions. Herman Miller's 1950 and 1960 census monographs on income distribution in the United States became the basis of his popular book *Rich Man, Poor Man* (Miller 1955, 1966, 1971) and were the models for Frank Levy's *Dollars and Dreams*, based on the 1980 census, and the sequel *New Dollars and Dreams* (Levy 1987, 1998). One of the most important census monographs from the 1980 census, *From Many Strands: Ethnic and Racial Groups in Contemporary America* (Lieberson and Waters 1988) explored the implications of measuring "ancestry" as a parallel to standard measures of race, ethnicity, and nativity.

Other exemplars of social reporting were the two volumes on *Recent Social Trends in the United States* and 13 associated monographs, popularly known as the Hoover committee report on social trends (United States, President's Research Committee of Social Trends 1933). In response to a request from then President Herbert Hoover, a panel of distinguished social scientists, with support from the Rockefeller Foundation and the Social Science Research Council, produced detailed empirical overviews on the "physical, biological, and social heritage of the nation." William F. Ogborn, a social demographer at the University of Chicago, was the research director of the committee.

Among the 29 chapters in *Recent Social Trends* were "The Population of the Nation" by Warren S. Thompson and P. K. Whelpton, "Shifting Occupational Patterns" by Ralph G. Hurlin and Meredith B. Givens, "The Rise of Metropolitan Communities" by R. D. McKenzie, "The Status of Race and Ethnic Groups" by T. J. Woofter, and "The Family and its Functions" by William F. Ogburn. These reports were aimed to be "scrupulously empirical and factual" studies of social trends without policy prescriptions, but the latent intent was surely to provide knowledge on the state of American society to those who did make policy. It was rumored that the page proofs of *Recent Social Trends* were read by President-Elect Franklin Roosevelt before he took office, and that these studies had an influence on the formulation of New Deal social policy, including the social security program (Worcester 2001: 23).

Another important development in 20th-century social science was the "Social Indicators Movement" in the 1960s and 1970s (Land 2000). Although the development and publication of social indicators reached far beyond the field of social demography, there was a common perspective on the value and significance of social description and reporting. And just as William F. Ogburn had played a critical role as the research director of the President's Research Committee on Social Trends, sociologist-demographer Otis Dudley Duncan was one of the primary intellectual leaders of the development of the social indicators field (Duncan 1969a).

The high water mark of the social indicators field was the publication titled *Toward a Social Report*, which summarized the best social science evidence on the social health of the nation, including such topics as Health and Illness, Social Mobility, Our Physical Environment, and Public Order and Safety (U.S. Department of Health Education and Welfare 1969). As the title indicated, this preliminary government report, which drew on the work of academic researchers, was thought to be the beginning of a new federal initiative to monitor the social welfare of the nation's population. Among the ideas being considered was the creation of a Council of Social Advisors, whose role would complement that of the Council of Economic Advisors and would issue periodic reports on the social well-being of the nation. With the change in the political direction following the election of 1968, however, the initiative of a Council of Social Advisors and the mandate for future social reports were dropped (for a critical overview of the promise and limitations of the HEW report, see Karl Taeuber 1969).

Even with lukewarm support from the federal government, the social indicators movement continued for another decade. Several large volumes with multicolor charts of social indicators were published by the Census Bureau (U.S. Census Bureau 1980). The Social Science Research Council and the Russell Sage Foundation played a major role in sponsoring committees and projects related to social indicators (Worcester 2001:66–68). Conferences and edited volumes on the conceptual and methodological underpinnings of social indicators (Sheldon and Moore 1968; Land and Spilerman 1975) and glossy publications of social indicators on a variety of aspects of social welfare were among the most visible activities and products of social science in the 1960s and 1970s. These publications served a valuable purpose in informing university students (via their use in the classroom) and the general public on the state of American society.

In the early 1980s, the SSRC Committee on Social Indicators was disbanded, and the stream of social indicators publications ceased; even the term *social indicators* has receded to the margins of contemporary social science. One school of thought is that politics led to the demise of the social indicators movement. Social indicators were considered to be strictly scientific and neutral observations by their adherents, but the ascendant conservative politics of the 1980s considered all social sciences, especially those that pointed to the social problems in American society, as undeserving of governmental support or attention. Without interest and support from the government, there were simply insufficient funds from universities and private foundations to support the extensive infrastructure of social indicators programs and publications.

Another weakness of social indicators research was the lack of centrality to a particular school of social science. Although most social scientists considered social indicators to be a useful "public good," there was no single discipline or research community that was devoted to their collection and dissemination. Social science, as with all science, tends to hold in highest regard the development of new theories as well as the most complex and ambitious empirical analyses. Descriptive studies are often characterized as "mere description." This tendency means that reporting of social trends and societal patterns is less likely to be published in the leading disciplinary journals.

Social demography, however, retains a commitment to careful monitoring of the social pulse; with the decline of the social indicators movement, core demographic data collection, analyses, and publications provide an important window for the discipline of sociology. These works in descriptive social demography are published by the Census Bureau and in the publications of such organizations as the Population Reference Bureau and the Population Council, which have a long history in providing links between demographic science and public policy.

Perhaps the most illustrious publication of demographic research that attempts to reach beyond a completely academic audience is the journal *Population and Development Review* (PDR). Although the editorial direction of PDR is more in the direction of innovative demographic research than social description, the journal's discouragement of technical virtuosity for its own sake has created an opening for research that illuminates general societal trends and patterns. With its strong editorial vision, PDR has filled an important niche in the field and has a remarkable range of readership, from research scholars to students in undergraduate sociology classes.

Another valuable source of social demographic reporting is the quarterly *Population Bulletin*, published by the Population Reference Bureau. Each issue (around 40 pages) is an extended essay on a single topic with basic data (often summarized in charts and graphs) presented in an easy-to-digest style for the general reader. *American Demographics* began as an outlet for interesting accounts of demographic change in American society, but over the years, it has become more directed to the immediate information needs of business-oriented readers.

An extraordinarily valuable source of social demographic reporting on the United States is *Current Population Reports* (CPR), the periodic reports from the Census Bureau, based on the Current Population Survey (CPS). There are several series of CPR publications that describe the latest survey data on family and household living arrangements, school enrollment and attainment, fertility, migration, income and poverty, and other topics, usually presented in a time series with data from previous years. One of the great values of *Current Population Reports* is the methodological discussion of the details of data collection, processing, and adjustment. Reading these details, often in the appendices and footnotes of CPR publications, is encouraged by the character of graduate training in social demography, which emphasizes acquiring more than a casual knowledge of the methodological underpinnings of government statistics (Shyrock and Siegel 1976).

This knowledge gives social demographers an advantage in interpreting social trends relative to many sociologists (and other social scientists) who are oblivious to the problems in data collection and measurement in government surveys. For example, careful readers of CPR publications learn that about one-third of all 20- to 29-year-old black men in the United States are missed in the CPS (U.S. Census Bureau 2000: Chapter 16). This problem means that most measures of black-white inequality are underestimates of the true differences (assuming that underenumerated black men have lower socioeconomic status than those who are interviewed). The problem of undercoverage is probably evident in all other data sources, including primary data collected by sociologists.

Another important but rarely understood issue in the study of inequality and stratification is the problematic measurement of income. Individual and family income data are based on survey responses to questions on both earned income (wages and salary and self-employment) and unearned income (from wealth and transfer income). Income is the most sensitive question in any census or survey and always encounters a high level of nonresponse (about 10% in the CPS, see U.S. Bureau of the Census 1993: C-10). Even more consequential than nonresponse is selective underreporting of certain types of income. With imputation, the Census Bureau estimates that the CPS income questions capture 97% of all wage and salary income but only 51% of interest income and 33% of dividend income (U.S. Bureau of the Census 1993: C12-C13). Although income from wealth (interest and dividends) is less than 12% of the total estimated income in the United States, it is received almost exclusively by the richest fraction of the population. This "methodological detail" has important implications for the often-reported finding of increasing income inequality in the United States over the last two decades of the 20th century (DeNavas-Walt et al. 2001: 21).

Another part of the social demographic perspective is an appreciation of the significance of long-term population trends and differentials for understanding social change. The careful assembly of long-term trends in marriage, divorce, and remarriage (Cherlin 1992) and birth rates (Rindfuss and Sweet 1977) has provided important sociological insights about the economic and cultural changes in American society that produced the "return of tradition" in the 1950s and the tumultuous social changes of the 1960s and 1970s. The portrayal of cohort trends in educational attainment as the product of a series of continuation ratios from one grade level to the next is elegant and also a model that "explains" how the American educational system has changed over the 20th century (Duncan 1968: 640; Mare 1995). One of the most famous articles in social demography—Samuel Preston's (1984) comparison of diverging trends in the welfare of children and the elderly in the United States—was prescient in its conceptualization and interpretation, but analytically, it was straightforward social description.

The elementary logic of demographic analysis focuses attention on the parallels between the life histories of individuals and cohorts as well as the distinction between period and cohort measures (Ryder 1964). This demographic perspective helps social demographers appreciate the value of summary measurements that describe social reality in an intuitive way. For example, the standard period measures of fertility and mortality are constructed to resemble life-cycle experiences of cohorts, e.g., the total fertility rate and life expectancy.

The knowledge of methodological aspects of data sources, elementary demographic techniques, and the value of social description has permitted creative social demographers to "invent" new conceptual measures that illuminate the human condition. Unlike the social indicators noted earlier, these summary measures are often intermediate, but indispensable, steps in the founding of a school of sociological research.

For example, Larry Bumpass and Ronald Rindfuss (1979) created a summary measure of the probability that a child will experience a single-parent household because of a marital breakup by age 18 (or an earlier age). Although such data are not directly collected in any national survey, Bumpass and Rindfuss linked parental marriage history by age of children and created a child-centered life table of experiencing a parental divorce. Another example of creative social demographic description was the index of "excess mortality" by Kitagawa and Hauser (1968). Excess mortality refers to the number of deaths that could have been averted if the entire population had experienced the mortality rates of the top quartile of the education distribution.

In the 1940s and early 1950s, one of the major research foci of sociology was the study of the residential segregation of social classes and race and ethnic groups within cities. Empirical generalizations were rare, however, because of the confusion created by the variety of indexes used to summarize the distribution of different groups across small areas in cities (blocks, census tracts). The confusion was ended with a single paper: Duncan and Duncan's (1955a) systematic evaluation of all widely used measures of residential segregation (also see Taeuber and Taeuber 1965: Appendix A). In addition to showing the mathematical relationships among the measures, the Duncans provide a conceptual rationale for using one measure—the index of dissimilarity (delta). For the next generation, there was a cumulative sociological and demographic science of research on residential segregation because all scholars worked within the same analytic school.

Twenty-five years later, Lieberson (1980) brought back one of the "almost forgotten" measures of residential segregation, P^*, an index of exposure rather than evenness of distribution across neighborhoods in a city. Lieberson used P^* to answer an important empirical question about the different ways that native whites in northern cities responded to the growing presence of SEC (Southern, Eastern, and Central) European immigrants and African American migrants from the South. With careful attention to the differences in conceptualization and interpretation of both indexes of segregation, Lieberson was able to continue and broaden the cumulative science of research on residential segregation.

Another major contribution of social demographic research was the extension of a measure of occupational prestige to a standardized index of the socioeconomic status of all occupations. Job titles and descriptions of jobs of survey respondents are coded into a very detailed occupational classification, consisting of hundreds of occupational categories, by the U.S. Census Bureau and other national survey organizations. One of the major problems confronting cumulative sociological research was how to summarize occupational distributions in a way that captures the important underlying dimensions of occupational differentiation and stratification. Most sociologists have traditionally dealt with this problem on an ad hoc basis by collapsing categories (e.g., white collar, blue collar, farm).

Sociological research had shown that a measure of the "social standing" of occupations yielded an interval scale index of occupational prestige that was almost invariant over time and across different populations (Hodge, Siegel, and Rossi 1964; Treiman 1977). The only problem was that occupational prestige was measured by detailed survey questions and only a few dozen of the hundreds of occupations had ever been rated and ranked. Duncan (1961a, 1961b) "invented" a method that showed that prestige scores could be reliably predicted as a weighted average of the income and educational attainments of occupational incumbents. The product of this research, the "Socioeconomic Index of Occupations," has became a fundamental building block of modern social stratification research (Hauser and Warren 1997).

Although descriptive sociology is sometimes considered as a stepchild of the discipline, social demographers have invested considerable energy and ingenuity in social description and social accounting. This is not simply because social demographers attach greater value to social description than other sociologists, though this may be partially true. Social demographers would agree that mechanical social description is of marginal utility, but they also have a strong belief that cumulative science can develop only when important social science concepts are accurately and reliably measured.

SOCIAL DEMOGRAPHY AS EXPLANATORY SOCIOLOGY

Although good science begins with accurate and insightful description, this is only the first step. The ultimate goal of science is explanation of the natural and social world.

There are, of course, many meanings (and levels) of explanation. The forces that brought about a phenomenon may be quite different from the forces that account for its persistence, change, or demise. The explanation that accounts for how the properties or behaviors of elements of a system (e.g., people) contribute to the survival (or welfare) of the system as a whole may be quite different from the individual-level conscious motivations or the assessment of benefits/losses that are associated with the consequences of specific behaviors. Exploring the complexities of an adequate theory of scientific explanation and its application to the study of societies and human behavior is a task far beyond the bounds of this essay. Here, we simply review more generally the "practice of hypothesis testing" in social demography and sociology.

For most social science research, the standard method of explanatory science has been to attempt to account for variation in one variable (at one moment or over time) in terms of the variation in other variables. For example, can the variation in fertility across societies be "explained" by the level of socioeconomic development? At the individual level, how much of income inequality is a function of educational attainment? In most research, both the variable to be explained (the dependent variable) and the explanatory variables (the independent variables) are conceptualized and measured for comparable units of analysis. Units of analysis can be societies, individuals, cities, years, organizations, events, or person-years, but the standard presumption is that both the independent and dependent variables are measured for the same units. This assumption is not absolute, and it is possible to move across levels of analysis, but this usually requires some justification and appropriate analytical methods.

The most important assumption in deductive empirical research is that there is a testable hypothesis drawn from a general theory or, in other words, the assumption of a causal relationship between the independent variable and the dependent variable. As the popular saying goes, correlation does not equal causation. In fact, even the presumption of an assumption of causation and a high correlation do not necessarily "prove" causation. As will be discussed later in this section, assumptions about causation usually turn out to be more complicated than they seem initially. However, there is still a lot of useful and important research that can be done based on "weak" assumptions about causality.

Standardization and the Method of Expected Cases

Social demographers typically draw on general social science theories, the standard logic of the scientific method, and inferential statistical methods to test hypotheses, which are widely used in the broader sociological craft. However, sociologists with demographic training have a small comparative advantage in developing novel empirical tests with the "method of expected cases," which is akin to the demographic method of indirect standardization. Standardization is a widely used method in demography to compare mortality (or fertility) rates between two populations with differing age compositions (Preston, Heuveline, and Guillot 2001: chapter 2). For example, the unadjusted mortality rate in many developing countries may be lower than the mortality rate in many industrial countries because of a younger age structure, even though mortality is higher at each age in the less developed country. Even in the absence of age-specific mortality rates for both populations, the method of indirect standardization allows the analyst to estimate how much of the difference in overall mortality is due to population composition, assuming both countries have the same age-specific rates.

This logic of indirect standardization has been used by social demographers (and also by other sociologists) to test important hypotheses with relatively weak data. For example, Lieberson (1980: 354–357) used the method of expected cases or indirect standardization to estimate the degree of labor market discrimination experienced by white immigrants relative to native-born whites and blacks in 1940. He compared the actual occupational distribution of white immigrants to the occupational distribution they would have attained with their own education and the education-occupation relationship of (1) native whites and (2) blacks. Lieberson concludes that white immigrants were able to obtain much better occupations than blacks with the same levels of education (also, see Hirschman and Wong 1986: 19–22, for a comparable study of Asian American occupational patterns).

Another ingenious example of the power of the method of expected cases is Otis Dudley Duncan's (1965) estimate of the trend in social mobility in American society using only one cross-sectional measure of social mobility (the transition matrix of respondent's occupation by father's occupation) from the 1962 Occupational Changes in a Generation (OCG) survey. Duncan compared the observed occupational distribution for various birth cohorts for earlier times with their expected occupational distributions, assuming the earlier cohorts had the 1962 transition matrix (from father's occupation to respondent's occupation), but their own distribution of father's occupations. The 1962 OCG provided estimates of the distributions of fathers' occupations for earlier cohorts, which were represented by the successive age groups in the 1962 OCG. Hauser and Featherman (1973) used the same method to estimate the trend in social mobility from 1962 to 1972, in advance of their replication of the OCG survey in 1973.

Another innovative social demographic analysis using an extension of the same method was Lieberson and Fuguitt's (1967) analysis that addressed the question of how many generations it would take to eliminate racial inequality in occupational structures if discrimination were eliminated immediately. One of the elementary lessons of formal demography is that two population distributions (by age or any other characteristic) will converge if they experience the same processes of change. In this case, the process of change is not fertility and mortality, but the matrix of intergenerational occupational mobility transition rates. The impact of differential social origins (as represented by father's occupation) on black-white occupational inequality would largely disappear in two or three generations in the absence of discrimination (both blacks and whites experiencing the same intergenerational occupational transition matrix).

The application of direct standardization methods, or "holding other variables constant" in sociological parlance, laid the groundwork for what has become the standard method of social demography—and of nonexperimental social sciences more generally. One of the earliest examples of this genre of work was Siegel's (1965) "On the Cost of Being a Negro." Following the logic of direct standardization, Siegel asks how much of the black-white income gap observed in the 1960 census would persist if racial differences in geographical location and educational attainment could be eliminated. Although Siegel acknowledged that other factors affecting racial differences in income were not controlled, he concluded that the "unexplained gap" in income between black and white men was a proxy measure for racial discrimination.

Otis Dudley Duncan (1969b) extended Siegel's work in what he called a "statistical experiment" that asked how much of the black-white gap in earnings was due to the "inheritance of poverty" or the "inheritance of race." One of the most popular explanations for black-white inequality in the 1960s was the "cycle of poverty." This explanation posited that the primary handicap for black men was that they were born and reared in poor families or, simply put, poverty begets poverty. Using a regression approach that allowed for the inclusion of many more variables than are typically used in direct standardization, Duncan "statistically assigned" black men the values of white men on a variety of attributes, including socioeconomic status of the family of origin, the number of siblings, mental ability as measured by test scores, years of schooling completed, and current occupation. Even with all these sources of unequal background eliminated, black men would still earn about $1,200 less than white men in 1961 dollars, when the mean income of white men was only $7,100.

From Hypothesis Testing to Causal Modeling

The original logic of hypothesis testing in sociology (and in science more generally) focused on a single independent variable. The experimental method measures the impact of the experimental variable (or "the treatment") on the outcome variable, with random assignment to the experimental and control populations eliminating the effects of all other variables. In nonexperimental social science, however, the methodological problems are more complex because the effects of many variables are intertwined, and there is no statistical method to uniquely apportion their interdependence. With the development of multivariate statistical methods, the initial idea was to estimate partial correlations or the "net associations" between variables, holding constant the impact of other variables. This approach, however, is an unsatisfactory method to test hypotheses because partial correlations present somewhat arbitrary estimates of the causal impact of independent variables on a dependent variable. Distinguishing spurious from real causes and the specification of remote causes from proximate mechanisms are theoretical and logical problems that cannot be resolved by more powerful statistical techniques.

Social demographers had an important advantage in developing causal models because of their experience with the logic of temporal order in demographic analyses. Many demographic variables follow a sequence ordered by the life cycle or chronological time. Fertility is a sequence of events that begins with marriage (or union formation), first birth, second birth, and so on. The events can be broken down to even more refined steps, beginning with the age at first sexual intercourse, conception, pregnancy, and birth. The central method of demography, the life table, is a cross-sectional representation of a temporal process—the survival function by age of a cohort from birth until all members of the cohort have died. The life table model provides a number of important summary measures, such as life expectancy for any age (or period of duration after entry into the population) from birth to death. Extensions of life table methods have given rise to event-history analysis and other statistical methods in sociology and social science.

There is a long tradition in demography of developing conceptual and analytical approaches to the study of many sociological variables (statuses) through the lens of the life course and temporal order (Schnore 1961). One of the most important contributions of social demography was Duncan's concept of the *socioeconomic life cycle*, which applied demographic logic to a life course model, beginning with family background and, following in sequential order, schooling, job, income, and expenditures (Duncan 1967: 87). Duncan explained that these variables were indicators of larger social processes, ranging from life chances to their ultimate effects on satisfaction and morale. In related work, Duncan introduced statistical methods to sociologists, for example, path analysis (which originated in genetics), to show how to analyze and interpret causal models, and he also provided important research exemplars that popularized life-cycle causal models in sociology (Duncan 1966; Blau and Duncan 1967).

Not all developments in causal models in sociology (and in the social sciences) can be credited to the work of social demographers. Hubert Blalock (1964, 1971), Herbert Costner (1969), Judea Pearl (2000), and many other sociologists, statisticians, and social scientists have made fundamental contributions to the theory and methods of causal analysis. Nonetheless, the introduction of life-cycle sequential logic and temporal order into multivariate models by social demographers has helped to transform sociology from the study of partial associations to the specification and testing of causal models.

Although most of the examples presented here are drawn from the study of stratification, the impact of temporal order and life-cycle models on sociological analysis reaches across the discipline. For example, the concept of the life cycle has been adapted to studies of urban development with the notion that the construction of the physical structure of cities, including transportation systems and housing stock, bears the imprint of the period of initial construction and that the physical infrastructure will decline with age and become less attractive (Duncan, Sabagh, and Van Arsdol, Jr. 1962; Schnore 1963). In their study of the determinants of race riots, Lieberson and Silverman (1965) drew the distinction between underlying conditions (such as minority poverty and unemployment) and precipitating events (an altercation following a police arrest). Perhaps social demographers unconsciously draw upon their familiarity with temporal order in creating causal models of sociological phenomena.

Social Demography and Studies of Social and Spatial Assimilation

The debate over assimilation has been at the heart of sociology since the days of Robert Park and the origins of the Chicago School of Sociology (Park 1950; Park and Burgess 1921). In the early decades of the 20th century, primary attention was focused on the "new immigration" from Southern and Eastern Europe. In the middle decades of the century, following the Great Migration of African Americans to cities in the Northeast and Midwest and especially in the wake of the Civil Rights movement of the 1950s and 1960s, sociology was convulsed with attempts to explain the continuing legacy of racism after 300 years of settlement and 100 years after the Civil War. In the last third of the 20th century, with the renewal of mass immigration from Asia and Latin America, sociology was again asking questions about the absorptive character of American society.

The questions raised by Robert Park, and refined by Milton Gordon (1964), became part of the 20th-century sociological agenda, but for the most part it has been difficult to establish cumulative empirical generalizations that reach across the disparate findings of individual studies. The fundamental problem was the lack of common standards or a hegemonic research paradigm to test the assimilation hypothesis. Although social demographers have not "solved" the problem, there have been several important contributions, many of them arising from demographic familiarity with potential uses and limitations of census and survey data and with techniques of studying social change via inter- and intracohort models.

Karl Taeuber (1964: 375) offers a distinctive sociological definition of assimilation "as the process of dispersion of members of the group throughout the social structure." This definition is fairly similar to Milton Gordon's (1964) specification of "secondary group structural assimilation." Gordon defined the central element of structural assimilation as integration between minority and majority group members in associations where primary group affiliations prevail, such as kinship groups, friendship cliques, and neighborhoods. In addition, Gordon notes that integration may also occur in situations where secondary associations prevail, such as schools, places of employment, commercial establishments, and so on. Many social demographers have adapted Taeuber's and Gordon's ideas to the concept of *socioeconomic assimilation,* which is usually operationalized by measuring group differences in education, occupations, and income. Although socioeconomic assimilation does not necessarily imply integration—sharing of common institutions or even common spaces—the assumption is that the lessening of socioeconomic differences will minimize social barriers between groups. One of the advantages of having a well-defined dependent variable (and one that is widely available in many data sources) is the possibility of a cumulative research literature.

Social demographers have also contributed the concept of *spatial assimilation* as a basis for understanding racial and ethnic residential stratification. The idea that spatial patterns reflect socioeconomic inequality, and that some groups reside in more attractive and desirable neighborhoods than other groups, reflects the legacy of the Chicago School (Duncan and Duncan 1955b). Using a variety of measures of residential "segregation," but especially the index of dissimilarity and the index of exposure/isolation, social demographers have documented the uneven distribution of racial and ethnic groups within U.S. cities (Lieberson 1963, 1980; Massey and Denton 1993).

African Americans have been found to be especially disadvantaged in terms of their patterns of residential segregation and the quality of their neighborhoods. Faced with these descriptive patterns of residential distribution, social demographers turned to the search for explanations, drawing first from theoretical perspectives that had been used to account for other types of racial and ethnic inequality. According to the "spatial assimilation model," such group variation in neighborhood location and quality reflects corresponding group differences in the socioeconomic standing (e.g., education, occupational status, and income) or, for immigrant groups, the degree of cultural adaptation (e.g., language acquisition). The spatial assimilation model, therefore, suggests the research hypothesis that group differences in residential location should "disappear" once the appropriate root causes are controlled—or, put simply, when individuals are compared only to others with identical characteristics (Alba and Logan 1991; Guest 1980; Massey 1985). When that hypothesis is tested, however, residual group differences in residential location and quality often remain, with African Americans continuing to reside in more segregated and less desirable neighborhoods (Massey and Denton 1987; Massey and Mullen 1984).

Faced with the inability of the spatial assimilation model to fully account for racial and ethnic differences in residential patterns, social demographers have proposed the "place stratification" model, which describes institutional barriers that prevent some groups, primarily African Americans, from converting their higher socioeconomic status into preferred residential locations (Alba and Logan 1991, 1993; Logan and Alba 1993; Logan, Alba, and Leung 1996; Massey 1979; South and Crowder 1997, 1998). While not denying the importance of the causal mechanisms identified by the spatial assimilation model, the place stratification model suggests the additional hypothesis that groups will vary in their ability to translate a socioeconomic advantage into a residential one. Tests of this hypothesis have yielded mixed results, leading to the further specification of "weak" and "strong" versions of the place stratification model (Logan and Alba 1993). Although the literature on racial and ethnic patterns of segregation and locational attainment has yet to provide a complete accounting, it illustrates nicely how social demography approaches an explanation of social phenomena, employing both deductive and inductive strategies.

The focus on socioeconomic and spatial assimilation by social demographers has been developed in tandem with models (or at least multivariate analyses) that attempt to test hypotheses. One of the key variables in any analysis is time, often measured as a period of influence by comparing data from 1970, 1980, and 1990 (or data from 1920 compared to 1940). However, the majority and minority populations are not always comparable over time because of changes in immigration (or domestic migration patterns), generational succession, and age structure. For example, the current Japanese American population is largely a third- or even a fourth-generation population, the descendants of immigrants who arrived in the first two decades of the 20th century, while the majority of Chinese Americans are immigrants. Temporal comparisons of the average status (or residential segregation) of race and ethnic groups are apt to be very misleading because of the confounding effects of immigration generation and age structure (Taeuber and Taeuber 1967).

Because of the tradition of cohort analysis, social demographers have been very sensitive to generational differences when making temporal comparisons of the assimilation of race and ethnic groups. In his celebrated study, A *Piece of the Pie: Blacks and Immigrants Since 1880*, Stanley Lieberson (1980) compares the attainments of the children of SEC (Southern, Eastern, and Central European) immigrants and the children of black migrants from the South to northern cities. Immigrants, and black migrants to the North, were socialized and educated in "worlds" so different from their current place of residence that it is almost impossible to try to explain the reasons for their socioeconomic inequality with older-stock Americans. On the other hand, their children (the second generation) were born and reared in the United States (or, for blacks, in northern cities), and the temporal (intercohort) trend in their educational progress (which can often be inferred from successive age groups in a single census) can be a proxy for inferences about opportunities in American society. Much of the recent work on ethnic stratification in the United States by sociologists (not all of whom are social demographers) tries to control for generational differences by analyzing the second generation (Portes and Rumbaut 2001) or by creating proxies for the second generation (Hirschman 2001).

The Limits to Explanatory Social Demography

One of the general strategies in social demographic research, which has become part of mainstream sociology, is to identify an important social change (comparing the same population at two or more points in time) or a significant social difference between populations (race and ethnic groups, cities, social classes, etc.) and then attempt to explain these differences in terms of differences in other variables (the independent variables). For example:

- Can changes in birth rates (from baby boom to birth dearth) be explained in terms of changes in educational composition (or farm origins) of the population?
- Can race and ethnic differences in educational attainment be explained in terms of the socioeconomic status of their families of origin?
- Can the shift from extended to nuclear families in modern societies be explained by changing patterns of social and geographical mobility?

There are good sociological theories to motivate these hypotheses and there are reasonably good data to test them. Indeed, these are the sorts of interesting questions that have been addressed by social demographers and other sociologists in the scientific literature. However, these questions have been only partially resolved by research, since there are many anomalous findings that may be a function of data, research design, and the scope and measurement of covariates.

The fundamental problem is that not all social differences over time (or between populations) are a function of population composition. For example, Rindfuss and Sweet (1977) report that the upswing in fertility during the Baby Boom years affected all groups, and the subsequent downturn was also pervasive across all educational, age, race and ethnic, and other social categories. These dramatic period effects cannot be reduced to changes in characteristics of the population by standardization, regression, or any other statistical method that attempts to explain population differences in terms of the variance of other variables (Preston 1978: 301–302).

Sociologists and other astute social observers have no shortage of ideas on potential reasons for the fluctuations in the birth rate over time. The problem is there are an (almost) infinite number of such speculative propositions that are consistent with the observed trends, and it is very difficult to test one hypothesis relative to the others. Richard Easterlin (1962, 1978, 1987) has suggested an elegant and parsimonious interpretation of the reasons for long waves in fertility trends in American society based on the effects of age structure on age-specific rates of fertility (and other behaviors), but the empirical evidence is mixed and there are other competing hypotheses (or ad hoc speculation) that cannot be ruled out.

There are many unique (or relatively rare) historical, political, cultural, or environmental factors that could explain social trends, as well as specific momentous events such as wars, economic booms and busts, and electoral outcomes. Although historians and social observers often discuss social change in terms of historical turning points, it is difficult to specify the specific causes of societal transformations that condition the behaviors of peoples and social aggregates. For example, the discovery of gold in California in 1848 dramatically changed every aspect of subsequent 19th-century American society, but this event was completely exogenous to everything and everyone at the time. Although this is an example of an unusual incident, the basic principle holds—namely, that many important causes of human behavior cannot be derived from the variance of any contemporaneous variables.

In the years ahead, social demography is likely to broaden its scope and incorporate alternative approaches to the study of societal change and human behavior. One possible alternative perspective is evolutionary theory, which has been mentioned as an attractive theoretical paradigm by several social demographers (Knodel et al. 1997; Lieberson and Lynn 2002; Massey 2002) but has yet to become linked to a formal methodological orientation or analytical approach.

SOCIAL DEMOGRAPHY AND CONTEXTUAL ANALYSIS

The premise of sociology as a discipline is that social structure (e.g., societies, communities, organizations) is more than the sum of individual characteristics. In other words, there are emergent properties of social aggregates that affect macrolevel social change and also condition the lives of individuals (Hawley 1992). For example, the size and age distribution of a population (which are properties of the whole) influence the rate of social mobility. Societal attributes condition individual behavior and life chances through opportunities and constraints (Blau 1994). Although this logic is widely accepted by sociologists, it is striking how little contemporary sociological theory and research attempts to refine, develop, or test hypotheses about structural and systemic influences on human societies and social behavior. Most social demographic research uses microlevel variables to explain microlevel outcomes or macrolevel variables to understand variation in macrolevel characteristics. Increasingly, however, social demographers are combining information from different levels of observation in their conceptual and analytic models—especially to allow for the possible influences of macrolevel variables on microlevel outcomes. Fundamental to such mixed-level approaches is the recognition that individuals are embedded within different social contexts and that social contexts can have an important impact on the characteristics and behaviors of individuals. Indeed, the assumption of contextual influences is a hallmark of the sociological perspective

Human ecology, which developed as a theoretical branch of the Chicago School of Sociology and in tandem with social demography, is one of the relatively few sources for sociological hypotheses of macrosocietal influences on social change and individual behavior (Hawley 1950; Duncan and Schnore 1959; Micklin and Choldin 1984; Micklin and Poston 1998). Human ecological theory, which assumes the centrality of social structure, developed in an era when aggregate units such as cities, communities, and neighborhoods were the primary units of analysis for much of quantitative sociology. With the growing development of metropolitan areas and their influence on suburban growth, transportation systems, and economic organization, human ecology provided a coherent macrolevel theoretical framework to posit reciprocal influences of population, environmental, and technological forces on social organization (community structure) (Duncan 1959; Frisbie and Poston 1975). Most social demographers still find intellectual kinship with ecological theory (Namboodiri 1988), and it is even possible to draw close parallels between human ecology and the Marxist theory of social change (Hawley 1984).

Human ecology's star, however, has waned in recent decades. Part of the reason may be an ideological mindset that tends to be very skeptical of all structural approaches to explaining society and human behavior. Most people, including social scientists, have a very individualistic point of view. Success or failure generally appears to be a product of personal characteristics and motivations. Even hypothetical suggestions of social influences are often met with such responses as "not everyone from the wrong side of the tracks becomes a criminal." These "strawman" caricatures of structural influences are illogical, but they probably have resonance in the broader society.

But the deeper reason for the lack of a sociological commitment to structural analysis may be the revolution in the availability of microlevel data in recent decades. Social demographers have enjoyed access to a growing variety of individual-level, nationally representative, survey data sets that have enabled new directions in social science (and demographic) research. The Census Public Use Microdata Samples (PUMS) have become a "workhorse" of demographic research on both historical and contemporary topics (Watkins 1994). PUMS files are now available for virtually all U.S. Censuses from 1850 through 2000 (Ruggles and Sobek 2001). In addition, many of these data sets, such as the Panel Study of Income Dynamics and the National Longitudinal Surveys, have given social demographers added leverage for inferring causal processes by following the same respondents over relatively long periods of time. Interestingly, however, these same data sets may have contributed to the renaissance of structural analysis through their inclusion of geocodes that allow researchers to situate individuals and families within a variety of geographical/social contexts such as neighborhoods, cities, counties, and metropolitan areas. This capability has led to renewed interest in the question of how various contexts influence individual-level behaviors and characteristics. This line of inquiry, which extends far beyond social demography, goes by many different names, including multilevel modeling, contextual analysis, and hierarchical linear modeling.

At the heart of contextual analysis is the question of whether there are environmental factors that affect the behaviors of individuals—over and above the characteristics of the individuals themselves. One of the most celebrated examples of contextual-level analysis in social demography was the project to find community-level influences on fertility. As part of the World Fertility Survey (WFS) project, Ronald Freedman (1974) advocated the collection of community-level data (i.e., village) to supplement household survey data. Demographic transition theory, the leading social demographic model of fertility decline, provided strong arguments for the salience of social and institutional context (e.g., the economic value of children, the status of women, infant and child mortality, etc.) on reproductive intentions and behavior (Caldwell 1980; Freedman 1979; Smith 1989). The results of research on contextual effects on fertility have been mixed.

Most of the empirical research based on WFS data found only modest effects of community characteristics on variations in individual-level fertility (Casterline 1985). There are a number of methodological obstacles that confront analyses of contextual models, including selection into contexts, variations in length of exposure to community context, and heterogeneity of contexts (Blalock 1985). In his analysis of fertility in four Southeast Asian countries, Hirschman and his colleagues found only modest effects of context on cross-sectional variations in fertility but very substantial effects of contextual variables in explaining fertility decline over time (Hirschman and Guest 1990; Hirschman and Young 2000).

The expanding availability of multilevel data sources, and the development of new and more appropriate estimation techniques, has allowed social demographic researchers to include contextual variables in their investigations of a diverse set of outcome variables, including the sexual activity of youth (Baumer and South 2001), nonmarital sexual intercourse (Brewster 1994), nonmarital childbearing (Brooks-Gunn et al. 1993; Crane 1991), divorce (South, Trent, and Shen 2001), residential location and mobility (Crowder 2001; South and Crowder 1997, 1998; Tolnay, Crowder, and Adelman 2002), family structure (Tolnay and Crowder 1999), and adolescent schooling (Brooks-Gunn et al. 1993; Crane 1991). Although the literature is too extensive to summarize completely, the results from these analyses have revealed a number of significant impacts of social contexts on individual-level outcomes. What is less clear, in many cases, is the precise mechanisms through which these contextual influences on individual behavior are exerted. In one notable exception, however, Baumer and South (2001) showed that the supportive attitudes and behaviors of peers are largely responsible for the positive relationship between neighborhood disadvantage and the number of sex partners reported by adolescents.

There has also been an emerging interest in measuring the impact of context, conceptualized as opportunity structures, on processes of social and ethnic stratification, sometimes identified as part of the school of *new structuralism*. Although much of this work has been done by social demographers, it is impossible to draw clear boundaries from the work of other sociologists. The research findings are again very complex and do not point to a single conclusion or interpretation. There are city (or community area) differences in occupational and earnings structures (and other dimensions of inequality), and "places" appear to have significant, but relatively modest, impacts on race and ethnic inequality (Fossett and Swicegood 1982; Guest, Almgren, and Hussey 1998; Hirschman 1982; Hirschman and Kraly 1988, 1990; Parcel 1979; South and Xu 1990). Several studies have found that the percent of an ethnic minority in a city (or other geographical areas) has a significant impact on patterns of ethnic stratification (Cohen 1998; Frisbie and Neidert 1977; McCreary, England, and Farkas 1989; Tienda and Lii 1987; Tigges and Tootle 1993; Tolnay 2001).

Important conceptual, methodological, and analytical problems appear to have inhibited the development of cumulative research on contextual models of stratification processes. Perhaps the most fundamental problem has been the conceptualization of place on economic opportunities. In earlier times, cities (or labor markets) were very differentiated from one another, depending on the industrial structure of employment. Because of the limitations of local (and long distance) transportation, people worked where they lived. At the present time, national (and global) integration has lessened the differences between places, and it is possible for workers to travel substantial distances between home and work. Place and location may still be constraints on opportunities, but it is not clear how best to conceptualize and measure the flexibility that frequent geographical mobility and long distance commuting have created.

Researchers interested in conducting contextual analyses face a variety of conceptual and methodological challenges, including the appropriate definition of *context* for a given individual-level outcome, the process through which individuals are selected into contexts, the possibility that multiple contexts influence individual behavior, the heterogeneity of contexts, the clustering of similar individuals within the same contexts, and the need to consider more complex error structures when individual and contextual units are used to predict individual-level outcomes (Blalock 1985; Bryk and Raudenbush 1992; DiPrete and Forristal 1994; Mason, Wong, and Entwisle 1983; Teachman and Crowder 2002). In recent years significant progress has been made in designing statistical software that is capable of meeting many of these challenges (see Zhou, Perkins, and Hui [1999] for a review).

Regardless of the specific software that is used, however, the statistical methods that are appropriate for conducting contextual analyses are designed to answer two general kinds of questions. First, do aspects of the social context have an *additive effect* on individual-level outcomes, independent of appropriate individual-level covariates? That is, is the likelihood of a given outcome (or its intensity) increased or reduced by the characteristics of the setting within which individuals are located? Most contextual analyses of social demographic or stratification outcomes have restricted their attention to such additive effects. Second, do the effects of individual-level predictor variables vary across contexts? And, if so, is it possible to identify the specific contextual characteristics that account for such variation? Although less common in the literature, the latter effects (often referred to as *cross-level* interactions) have also been considered by social demographers.

For example, one element of the ethnic enclave debate has been whether immigrant workers are rewarded differentially for their human capital in mainstream firms compared to firms owned by coethnics (Portes and Jensen 1989; Zhou and Logan 1989). In other words, does the effect of immigrant status on earnings differ according to the employment context in which they are engaged? From the fertility literature, Entwisle and colleagues report that the microlevel effects of education and childhood residence on fertility and contraceptive use vary across countries depending on the level of economic development and the strength of family planning programs (Entwisle and Mason 1985; Entwisle, Mason, and Hermalin 1986). Moreover, the effects of context may not be linear. Crane (1991) finds that there are "tipping points" of ghetto neighborhoods on adolescent fertility and dropping out. The impact of context may be very important, but only for a small fraction of the population.

A major unresolved issue in contextual analysis is whether all differences between places and institutional settings should be assumed to be the product of structural influences. The alternative hypothesis is selectivity. People move to cities where their skills best match opportunities and parents move to neighborhoods to find better schools. In terms of research design, the question is whether structural effects should be assessed before or after individual-level variables have been included in explanatory models. Much of the research in the "school effects" literature has found that between-school variations in student achievement are relatively small (or smaller than expected) once individual-level differences are held constant. This was one of the principal findings of the Coleman report on equality of educational opportunity (Coleman et al. 1966). The basic findings of the Coleman report were confirmed in reanalyses of the data (Harvard Educational Review 1969; Mosteller and Moynihan 1972), and subsequent research has found few strong "school (or neighborhood) effects" on student achievement and aspirations (Sewell and Armer 1966; Hauser 1969; Hauser, Sewell, and Alwin 1976).

The theory that social structure matters is central to the sociological perspective and to social demography and human ecology in particular. However, it was easier to make claims about the salience of structural influences on social life in an era when aggregate-level analysis was the norm, and there were fewer microlevel data sources available to researchers. The fields of structural sociology and human ecology have become more muddled in recent years without a clear theoretical model and analytical approach. However, just as richer data sources and more powerful statistical methods have exposed some earlier assumptions about "structural determinism," they also make it possible to develop a more sophisticated theory of the influences of context on social change and social behavior.

Recall the earlier discussion on the limits of conventional hypothesis-testing models of social demography. Tests of whether the variance in the dependent variable can be fully explained by variance in independent variables is a much more successful strategy for disproving "false" hypotheses than in explaining the real causes of social change. Changes in population composition are important elements of how societies change, but more elusive are the reasons for social change when all groups (age groups, race and ethnic groups, social classes) change their behavior. The explanations for such patterns and changes are most likely to be found in changing contexts (economic, political, social, technological, environmental). The increasing use of contextual analysis by social demographers to study individual-level behavioral outcomes suggests that the discipline is well poised to be a major source of inspiration for future research on these and other important questions. And, as the role of context in shaping individual behaviors assumes a higher profile within social demographic research, the field necessarily becomes more "sociological," and perhaps moves closer to its intellectual roots in human ecology.

CONCLUSIONS

There are no clear boundaries for the field of social demography. Although the majority of social demographic research probably is located within the areas of family sociology and social stratification, broadly defined, there are sociological demographers whose work reaches every branch of sociology and beyond. For example, Reynolds Farley, Matthew Snipp, Josh Goldstein, Mary Waters, Charles Hirschman, Richard Alba, and other social demographers conduct research on changing racial identities (*Perlmann* and Waters 2002; Hirschman, Alba, and Farley 2000; Waters 2002); Richard Udry writes on biological influences on gendered behavior (Udry 1994, 2000); Scott South has outlined the intersections of social demography and criminology (South and Messner 2000); and Teresa Sullivan has become one of the leading specialists on debt and bankruptcy (Sullivan, Warren, and Westbrook 1989, 2000).

Nor can social demography be pigeonholed by data and methods. The majority of social demographers use statistical methods to analyze census or population survey data, but social demographers have also been among the pioneers and leading advocates of in-depth interviews and focus groups (Knodel 1997), the ethnosurvey (Massey 1987a; Massey and Zenteno 2000), simulation (Wachter, Knodel, and Vanlandingham 2002), and fieldwork methods (Waters 1999: 347–371). Increasingly, social demographers make important contributions by assessing the state of knowledge on specific topics in the social sciences with careful reviews of theoretical debates, the research design of prior work, and the quality of data and analyses (Cherlin 1999; Massey et al. 1998). Social demographers are sociologists and social scientists, whose research foci and methods of investigation are limited primarily by their imagination and creativity, not by artificial boundaries.

There are, however, certain features of a social demographic perspective or orientation that characterize much (but probably not all) of the research work by those trained in the field. Perhaps most common is an understanding of the interplay of cohorts and period in social change. Norman Ryder's (1965) essay on "The Cohort as a Concept in the Study of Social Change" is a canonical reading in social demographic training. The classic applications of the cohort perspective have been in studies of fertility trends (Ryder 1969; Rindfuss, Morgan, and Swicegood 1988), but there have also been illuminating cohort studies of life-cycle events, political attitudes, church attendance, and many other topics (Abramson 1975; Alba 1988; Uhlenberg 1969). To some extent, the application of the cohort perspective has been inhibited by methodological obstacles and the impossibility of obtaining independent estimates of age, period, and cohort effects (Mason and Feinberg 1985), but the logic of the cohort perspective remains a cornerstone of social demography. Armed with a cohort perspective of the short-term and long-term impacts of period influences, social demographers have a conceptual lens that allows for the study of social change via the changed experiences/behavior of young adults, persistence over the life cycle, and generational replacement (Mayer 1988; Winsborough 1978). Although the current balance of evidence appears to suggest that social change is driven more by period than cohort influences (Ni Bhrolchain 1992; Morgan 1996), these findings were reached within a cohort analytical framework.

Another central dimension of social demographic training is the logic of decomposition. The crude birth rate is understood as the weighted average of age-specific fertility rates. Urban growth is the sum of exits and entries (in and out migrants) to the city, but also of births and deaths in the city, and of the births and deaths of in-migrants (and of "lost" births and deaths of out-migrants). Each of these components may have quite different causes, and the construction of an overall model or theory must be sensitive to underlying mechanisms and their relative magnitudes.

For example, by careful specification of all the population flows between cities and suburbs within and between metropolitan areas, William Frey (1979, 1984) demonstrated that much of the widening racial balance between cities and suburbs in the United States is due to factors other than white flight. In another important contribution, Samuel Preston (1979) cast doubt on the popular view that rapid urban growth in developing countries was due to unprecedented levels of rural-to-urban migration drawn by the "bright lights" of cities. He showed that the major source of urban growth was a natural increase in cities, and the most important reason for rapidly growing cities in some countries was the national rate of population growth in those countries. Douglas Massey (1987b) changed the standard approach to the study of international migration by distinguishing the components of departure, repetition (multiple migrations), settlement, and return migration. Changes in the number of net migrants to the United States over time are a function of the relative volume of these four components, each of which has different individual and structural determinants. Most social phenomena that are studied by sociologists have an internal structure of interlocking components. The demographic logic of decomposition provides an analytical strategy to focus attention on each of these component processes.

Another dimension of the demographic style is the lack of concern with disciplinary boundaries. In traditional social scientific fields, neophytes (graduate students) are generally indoctrinated into thinking about the superiority of certain theories, methods, data sources, and the art of asking the right question. Anthropologists learn that fieldwork is the "preferred" method of inquiry, and economists learn that the proper method of expressing theory is in mathematical form. Sociologists learn that all good research questions must be related to some quotation from Marx, Weber, Durkheim, or other classic theorist. Considerable time and effort is spent in reinforcing disciplinary boundaries. Although many sociologists are interested in testing hypotheses derived from economics and biology, they are likely to incur scorn and derision for straying from the disciplinary heartland.

A fundamental problem with the adherence to traditional disciplinary boundaries is that neither the natural nor the social world is organized for the convenience of researchers who are embedded within the disciplinary organization of contemporary science. Individuals and groups have preferences (and interests) for certain styles of theory and modes of analysis, but nature does not. Unlike the transformation of many disciplines in the natural sciences in recent decades with the development of new knowledge and methods, most social sciences seem rooted in 19th-century thinking of status and turf protection. Should departments of government change their name to political science? Why was there an almost universal trend to divide departments of anthropology and sociology even though the only real difference was the populations they studied? Why is there such fear by noneconomists of economists who begin to study topics such as politics, the family, and other institutions far from their traditional concerns?

Social demographers tend to be socialized with less doctrinaire orientations about disciplinary boundaries. By claiming to be both demographers and sociologists, social demographers are often more likely to draw upon novel ideas and productive methods regardless of their origins. At most American population centers, graduate students and faculty members are exposed to research (and research styles) from other disciplines through research seminars and research projects. At meetings of the Population Association of America, in the pages of the leading journals of demography, and through conferences sponsored by funding agencies or foundations, interdisciplinary perspectives and communications are valued and rewarded.

As sociology, and the social sciences more generally, faces new challenges in the coming years to address problems of the environment, health and health care, aging, violence and war, and ethnic divisions, it will be difficult to maintain rigid disciplinary boundaries. One tack has been to create new academic units devoted to the policy sciences, ethnic studies, women's studies, and other specialized fields. Although these units often begin as interdisciplinary programs, the general tendency is to create autonomous units with a separate curriculum, hiring and promotion policies, and eventually to create wholly independent disciplines. Social demography offers an alternative model for the future of social science with interdisciplinary centers existing side by side with disciplinary departments.

To paraphrase Oscar Handlin's quip about the place of immigration in American history, we began this survey by looking for the place of social demography at the margins of sociology, but discovered that social demography is at the heart of sociology.

REFERENCES

Abrahamson, P. R. 1975. *Generational change in American politics.* Lexington, Mass.: D. C. Heath.

Alba, R. D. 1988. Cohorts and the dynamics of ethnic change. Social structures and Human Lives: Social change and the Life Course, Volume 1 (American Sociological Association Presidential Series) by Matilda White Riley, Bettina J. Hubes, Beth B. Hess, Newbury Park, CA: SAGE Publications.

Alba, R. D., and J. R. Logan. 1991. Variations on two themes: Racial and ethnic patterns in the attainment of suburban residence. *Demography* 28:431–453.

Alba, R. D., and J. R. Logan. 1993. Minority proximity to whites in suburbs: An individual-level analysis of segregation. *American Journal of Sociology* 98:1388–1427.

Anderson, M. J. 1988. *The American census: A social history.* New Haven, Conn.: Yale University Press.

Baumer, E. P., and S. J. South. 2001. Community effects on youth sexual activity. *Journal of Marriage and the Family* 63:540–554.

Blalock, H. M. 1964. *Causal inferences in nonexperimental research.* Chapel Hill: University of North Carolina Press.

Blalock, H. M., ed. 1971. *Causal models in the social sciences.* Chicago: Aldine.

Blalock, H. M. 1985. Contextual-effects models: Theoretical and methodological Issues. *Annual Review of Sociology* 10:353–372.

Blau, P. 1994. *Structural contexts of opportunities*. Chicago: University of Chicago Press.

Blau, P., and O. D. Duncan. 1967. *The American occupational structure*. New York: John Wiley.

Brewster, K. L. 1994. Race differences in sexual activity among adolescent women: The role of neighborhood characteristics. *American Sociological Review* 59:408–424.

Brooks-Gunn, J., G. J. Duncan, P. K. Klebanov, and N. Sealand. 1993. Do neighborhoods influence child and adolescent development. *American Journal of Sociology* 99:353–395.

Bryk, A. S., and S. W. Raudenbush. 1992. *Hierarchical linear models*. Newbury Park, CA: Sage.

Bumpass, L. 1990. What's happening to the family? Interactions between demographic and institutional change. *Demography* 27: 483–498.

Bumpass, L., and H. L. Lu. 2000. Trends in cohabitation and implications for children's family contexts in the United States. *Population Studies* 54: 29–42.

Bumpass, L., and R. R. Rindfuss. 1979. Children's Experience of Marital Disruption. *The American Journal of Sociology* 85: 49–65.

Caldwell, J. C. 1980. Mass education as a determinant of the timing of fertility decline. *Population and Development Review* 6: 225–256.

Carpenter, N. 1927. *Immigrants and their children, 1920. A study based on census statistics relative to the foreign born and the native white of foreign or mixed parentage*. Washington, D.C.: U. S. Government Printing Office.

Casterline, J., ed. 1985. *The collection and analysis of community data*. Voorborg, Netherlands: International Statistical Institute.

Cherlin, A. 1992. *Marriage, divorce, remarriage*, revised and enlarged edition. Cambridge, Mass.: Harvard University Press.

Cherlin A. 1999. Going to extremes: Family structure, children's well being and social science. *Demography* 36: 421–428.

Cohen, P. N. 1998. Black concentration effects on black-white and gender inequality: Multi-level analysis for U.S. metropolitan areas. *Social Forces* 77: 207–229.

Coleman, J., et al. 1966. *Equality of educational opportunity*. Washington, D.C.: Department of Health, Education, and Welfare, Office of Education.

Costner, H. 1969. Theory, deduction, and rules of correspondence. *American Journal of Sociology* 75: 245–263.

Crane, J. 1991. The epidemic theory of ghettos and neighborhood effects on dropping out and teenage childbearing. *American Journal of Sociology*. 96:1226–1259.

Crowder, K. D. 2001. Racial stratification in the actuation of mobility expectations: Micro-level impacts of racially restrictive housing markets. *Social Forces* 107: 1377–1396.

Davis, K. 1945. The world demographic transition. *The Annals of the American Academy of Political and Social Science* 237: 1–11.

Davis, K. 1949. *Human society*. New York: Macmillan.

Davis, K. 1951. *The population of India and Pakistan*. Princeton, N.J.: Princeton University Press.

Davis, K. 1956. The amazing decline of mortality in underdeveloped areas. *American Economic Review* 46: 305–318.

Davis, K. 1959. The sociology of demographic behavior. In *Sociology today: Problems and prospects*. Edited by R. K. Merton, L. Broom, and L. S. Cotrtrell, Jr., 309–333. New York: Basic Books.

Davis, K. 1963. Social demography. In *The behavioral sciences today*. Edited by B. Berelson, 204–221. New York: Harper & Row.

Davis, K., and W. E. Moore. 1945. Some principles of stratification. *American Sociological Review* 10:242–249.

DeNavas-Walt, Carmen, Robert. W. Cleveland, and Marc I. Roemer, 2001. Money income in the Unites States: 2000, current population reports, series p 60–213. Washington, D. C.: U.S. Government Printing Office.

DiPrete, T., and J. Forristal. 1994. Multilevel models: Methods and substance. *Annual Review of Sociology* 331–357.

Dudley, S. 2003. PAA members profile. Summary information based on memberships valid on 3/1/2003 faxed to C. Hirschman from PAA office on June 6, 2003.

Duncan, B. 1968. Trends in the output and distribution of schooling. In *Indicators of Social Change: Concepts and Social Change*. Edited by E. B. Sheldon, and W. E. Moore, 601–672. New York: Russell Sage.

Duncan, B., G. Sabagh, and M. D. Van Arsdol, Jr. 1962. Patterns of city growth. *The American Journal of Sociology* 67: 418–429.

Duncan, O. D. 1959. Human ecology and population studies. In *The study of population*. Edited by P. Hauser, and O. D. Duncan, 678–716. Chicago: University of Chicago Press.

Duncan, O. D. 1961a. A socioeconomic index for all occupations. In *Occupations and social status*. Edited by A. J. Reiss, Jr., 109–138. Glencoe, Ill.: The Free Press.

Duncan, O. D. 1961b. Properties and characteristics of the socioeconomic index. In *Occupations and social status*. Edited by A. J. Reiss, Jr., 139–161. Glencoe, Ill.: The Free Press.

Duncan, O. D. 1965. The trend in occupational mobility in the United States. *American Sociological Review* 30:491–498.

Duncan, O. D. 1966. Path analysis: Sociological examples. *American Journal of Sociology* 72:1–16.

Duncan, O. D. 1967. Discrimination against Negroes. *Annals of the American Academy of Political and Social Sciences* 371: 85–103.

Duncan, O. D. 1969a. *Toward social reporting: Next steps*. New York: Russell Sage.

Duncan, O. D. 1969b. Inheritance of poverty or inheritance of race. In *On understanding poverty: Perspectives from the social sciences*. Edited by D. P. Moynihan, 85–110. New York: Basic Books.

Duncan, O. D., and B. Duncan. 1955a. A methodological analysis of segregation indexes. *American Sociological Review* 20: 210–217.

Duncan, O. D., and B. Duncan. 1955b. Residential distribution and occupational stratification. *The American Journal of Sociology* 60: 493–503.

Duncan, O. D., and B. Duncan. 1957. *The Negro population of Chicago: A study of residential succession*. Chicago: University of Chicago Press.

Duncan, O. D., D. Featherman, and B. Duncan. 1972. *Socioeconomic background and achievement*. Chicago: University of Chicago Press.

Duncan, O. D., and A. J. Reiss, Jr. 1956. *Social characteristics of urban and rural communities, 1950*. New York: John Wiley.

Duncan, O. D., and L. Schnore. 1959. Cultural, behavioral, and ecological explantions of social organization. *American Journal of Sociology* 65:132–153.

Duncan, O. D., R. Scott, S. Lieberson, B. Duncan, and H. Winsborough. 1960. *Metropolis and region*. Baltimore: Johns Hopkins Press.

Easterlin, R. 1962. The American baby boom in historical perspective. Occasional Paper No. 79. New York: National Bureau of Economic Research.

Easterlin, R. 1978. What will 1984 be like? Socioeconomic implications of recent twists in the age structure. *Demography* 15:397–432.

Easterlin, R. 1987. *Birth and fortune: The impact of numbers on personal welfare*, 2nd ed. Chicago: University of Chicago Press.

Entwisle, B., and W. Mason. 1985. Multilevel effects of socioeconomic development and family planning programs on children-ever-born. *American Journal of Sociology* 91:616–649.

Entwisle, B., W. Mason, and A. I. Hermalin. 1986. The multilevel dependence of contraceptive use on socioeconomic development and family planning program strength. *Demography* 23:199–216.

Farley, R., 1995. *State of the Union: America in the 1990s*. 2 vol. New York: Russell Sage.

Farley, R., 1996. *The new American reality: Who we are, how we got here and where we are we going?* New York: Russell Sage.

Ford, T. R., and G. F. DeJong, eds. 1970. *Social demography*. Englewood Cliffs, N.J.: Prentice Hall.

Fossett, M., and G. Swicegood. 1982. Rediscovering city differences in racial occupational inequality. *American Sociological Review* 47: 681–689.

Freedman, R. 1974. *Community-level data in fertility surveys*. World Fertility Survey Occasional Paper No. 8. Voorborg, Netherlands: International Statistical Institute.

Freedman, R. 1979. Theories of fertility decline: A reappraisal. *Social Forces* 58: 1–17.

Freedman, R., and J. Y. Takeshita. 1969. *Family planning in Taiwan: An experiment in social change*. Princeton, N. J.: Princeton University Press.

Freedman, R., P. K. Whelpton, and A. Campbell. 1959. *Family planning, sterility, and population growth*. New York: McGraw Hill.

Frey, W. H. 1979. Central city white flight: Racial and nonracial causes. *American Sociological Review* 44: 425–448.

Frey, W. H. 1984. Lifecourse migration of metropolitan whites and blacks and the structure of demographic change in large central cities. *American Sociological Review* 49:803–827.

Frisbie, W. P., and L. Neidert. 1977. Inequality and the relative size of minority populations: A comparative analysis. *American Journal of Sociology* 82: 1007–1030.

Frisbie, W. P., and D. L. Poston. 1975. Components of sustenance organization and nonmetropolitan population change: A human ecological investigation. *American Sociological Review* 40:773–784.

Goldenweiser, E. A., and L. E. Truesdell. 1924. *Farm tenancy in the United States. An analysis of the results of the 1920 census relative to farms classified by tenure supplemented by pertinent data from other sources.* Washington, D.C.: U. S. Government Printing Office.

Goldscheider, C. 1971. *Populations, modernization and social structure.* Boston: Little, Brown, and Company.

Gordon, M. 1964. *Assimilation in American life.* New York: Oxford University Press.

Guest, A. M. 1980. The suburbanization of ethnic groups. *Sociology and Social Research* 64:497–513.

Guest, A. M., G. Almgren, and J. M. Hussey. 1998. The ecology of race and socioeconomic distress: Infant and working age mortality in Chicago. *Demography* 35: 23–34.

Harvard Educational Review. 1969. *Equal educational review.* An expansion of the Winter 1968 special issue of The Harvard Educational Review. Cambridge, Mass.: Harvard University Press.

Hauser, R. M., 1969. Schools and the stratification process. *American Journal of Sociology* 74:587–611.

Hauser, P., and O. D. Duncan, eds. 1959. *The study of population.* Chicago: University of Chicago Press.

Hauser, R. M., and D. L. Featherman. 1973. Trends in occupational mobility of U.S. men, 1962–1972. *American Sociological Review* 38:302–310.

Hauser, R. M., W. H. Sewell, and D. F. Alwin. 1976. High school effects on achievement. In *Schooling and Achievement in American Society.* Edited by W. F. Sewell, R. M. Hauser, and D. L. Featherman, 309–341. New York: Academic Press.

Hauser, R. M., and J. R. Warren. 1997. Socioeconomic indexes for occupations: A review, update, and critique. In *Sociological methodology 1997.* Edited by A. E. Raftery, 177–298. Cambridge: Basil Blackwell.

Hawley, A. 1950. *Human ecology: A theory of community structure.* New York: Ronald.

Hawley, A. 1984. Human ecological and Marxian theories. *American Journal of Sociology* 89:904–917.

Hawley, A. 1992. The logic of macrosociology. *Annual Review of Sociology* 18:1–14.

Hill, J. A. 1929. Women in gainful occupations, 1870 to 1920. *A study of the trend of recent changes in the numbers, occupational distribution, and family relationship of women reported in the census as following a gainful occupation.* Washington, D.C.: U. S. Government Printing Office.

Hirschman, C. 1982. Unemployment among urban youth in peninsular Malaysia, 1970: A multivariate analysis of individual and structural effects. *Economic Development and Cultural Change* 30 (January): 391–412.

Hirschman, C. 2001. The educational enrollment of immigrant youth: A test of the segmented-assimilation hypothesis. *Demography* 38: 317–336.

Hirschman, C., R. Alba, and R. Farley. 2000. The meaning and measurement of race in the U.S. census: Glimpses in the future. *Demography* 37: 381–393.

Hirschman, C., and P. Guest. 1990. Multilevel models of fertility determination in four Southeast Asian countries: 1970 and 1980. *Demography* 27:369–398.

Hirschman, C., and E. Kraly. 1988. Immigrants, minorities and earnings in the United States, 1950. *Ethnic and Racial Studies* 11 (July): 332–365.

Hirschman, C., and E. Kraly. 1990. Racial and ethnic inequality in the United States, 1940 and 1950: The impact of geographic location and human capital. *International Migration Review* 24 (Spring): 4–33.

Hirschman, C., and M. Wong. 1986. The extraordinary educational attainment of Asian Americans: A search for historical evidence and explanations. *Social Forces* 65: 1–27.

Hirschman, C., and Y. Young. 2000. Social context and fertility decline in Southeast Asia. In *Population and economic change in East Asia.* Edited by R. D. Lee and C. Y. Cyrus Chu, 11–39. A supplement to Vol. 26, *Population and Development Review.*

Hodge, R., P. Siegel, and P. Rossi. 1964. Occupational prestige in the United States: 1925–1963. *American Journal of Sociology* 70:286–302.

Kitagawa, E. M., and P. M. Hauser. 1968. Education differentials in mortality by cause of death: United States, 1960. *Demography* 5: 318–353.

Knodel, J. 1997. A case for nonanthropological qualitative methods for demographers. *Population and Development Review* 23: 847–853.

Knodel, J., B. Low, C. Saengtienchai, and R. Lucas. 1997. An evolutionary perspective on Thai sexual attitudes and behavior. *The Journal of Sex Research* 34: 292–303.

Land, K. 2000. Social indicators. In *Encyclopedia of sociology.* Edited by E. F. Borgatta and R. J. V. Montgomery, 2682–2690. New York: Macmillian Reference USA.

Land, K., and S. Spilerman. 1975. *Social indicator models.* New York: Russell Sage.

Levy, F. 1987. *Dollars and dreams: The changing American income distribution.* New York: Russell Sage.

Levy, F. 1998. *The new dollars and dreams: American incomes and economic change*. New York: Russell Sage.

Lieberson, S. 1963. *Ethnic patterns in American cities*. New York: The Free Press.

Lieberson, S. 1980. *A piece of the pie: Blacks and white immigrants since 1880*. Berkeley: University of California Press.

Lieberson, S. 1985. *Making it count: The improvement of social research and theory*. Berkeley: University of California Press.

Lieberson, S. 2000. *A matter of taste: How names, fashions, and culture change*. New Haven, Conn.: Yale University Press.

Lieberson, S., and G. Fuguitt. 1967. Negro-white occupational differences in the absence of discrimination. *American Journal of Sociology* 73: 188–200.

Lieberson, S., and F. B. Lynn. 2002. Barking up the wrong branch: Scientific alternatives to the current model of sociological science. *Annual Review of Sociology* 28: 1–19.

Lieberson, S., and A. Silverman. 1965. The precipitants and underlying conditions of race riots. *American Sociological Review* 30: 887–898.

Lieberson, S., and M. Waters. 1988. *From many strands: Ethnic and racial groups in contemporary America*. New York: Russell Sage.

Logan, J. R., and R. D. Alba. 1993. Locational returns to human capital: Minority access to suburban community resources. *Demography* 30: 243–68.

Logan, J. R., R. D. Alba, and S. Leung. 1996. Minority access to white suburbs: A multiregional comparison. *Social Forces* 74:851–881.

Lorimer, F. 1959. The development of demography. In *The study of population: An inventory and appraisal*. Edited by P. M. Hauser and O. D. Duncan, 124–179. Chicago: University of Chicago Press.

Mare, R. D. 1995. Changes in educational attainment and school enrollment. In *State of the union: America in the 1990s*. Vol. 1. Edited by R. Farley, 155–214. New York: Russell Sage.

Mason, W. M., and S. E . Fienberg, eds. 1985. *Cohort analysis in social research: Beyond the identification problem*. New York: Springer Verlag.

Mason, W. M., G. Y. Wong, and B. Entwisle. 1983. Contextual analysis through the multilevel linear model. In *Sociological methodology 1983–1984*. Edited by S. Leinhardt, 72–103. San Francisco: Jossey-Bass.

Massey, D. S. 1979. Effects of socioeconomic factors on the residential segregation of blacks and Spanish Americans in United States urbanized areas. *American Sociological Review* 44:1015–1022.

Massey, D. S. 1985. Ethnic residential segregation: A theoretical synthesis and empirical review. *Sociology and Social Research* 69:315–350.

Massey, D. S. 1987a. Ethnosurvey in theory and practice. *International Migration Review* 21: 1498–1522.

Massey, D. S. 1987b. Understanding Mexican migration to the United States. *American Journal of Sociology* 92: 1372–1403.

Massey, D. S. 2002. A brief history of human society: The origin and role of emotion in social life. *American Sociological Review* 67: 1–29.

Massey, D. S., et al. 1998. *Worlds in motion: Understanding migration at the end of the millennium*. Oxford: Claredon Press.

Massey, D. S., and N. A. Denton. 1987. Trends in the residential segregation of blacks, Hispanics, and Asians. *American Sociological Review* 50: 94–105.

Massey, D. S., and N. A. Denton. 1993. *American apartheid*. Cambridge, Mass.: Harvard University Press.

Massey, D. S., and B. Mullen. 1984. Processes of Hispanic and black spatial assimilation. *American Journal of Sociology* 89: 836–873.

Massey, D. S., and R. Zenteno. 2000. A validation of the ethnosurvey: The case of Mexico-U.S. Migration. *International Migration Review* 34: 766–793.

Matras, J. 1977. *Introduction to population: A sociological approach*. Englewood Cliffs, N.J.: Prentice Hall.

Mayer, K. U. 1988. German survivors of World War II: The impact of the life course on the collective experience of birth cohorts. In *Social structure and human lives. Vol. 1. Social change and the life course*. Edited by M. W. Riley, 229–246. Newbury Park, CA: Sage.

McCreary, L., P. England, and G. Farkas. 1989. The employment of central city male youth: Non-linear effects of racial composition. *Social Forces* 68:55–75.

Micklin, M., and H. M. Choldin. 1984. *Sociological human ecology: Contemporary issues and applications*. Boulder, Colo.: Westview Press.

Micklin, M., and D. L. Poston, Jr. 1998. *Continuities in sociological human ecology*. New York: Kluwer Academic/Plenum Publishers.

Miller, H. P. 1955. *Income of the American people*. New York: John Wiley.

Miller, H. P. 1966. *Income distribution in the United States*. Washington, D.C.: U.S. Government Printing Office.

Miller, H. P. 1971. *Rich man, poor man*. New York: Crowell.

Morgan, S. P. 1996. Fertility trends and differentials. In *Fertility in the United States: New patterns, new theories*. A Supplement to *Population and Development Review*, Vol. 22. Edited by J. B. Casterline, R. D. Lee, and K. A. Foote, 19–63. New York: The Population Council.

Morgan, S. P., and S. M. Lynch. 2001. Success and future of demography: The role of data and methods. *Annals of the New York Academy of Sciences* 954: 35–51.

Mosteller, F., and D. P. Moynihan, eds. 1972. *On equality of educational opportunity*. New York: Vintage Books.

Namboodiri, K. 1988. Ecological demography: Its place in sociology. *American Sociological Review* 53: 619–633.

Ni Bhrolchain, M. 1992. Period paramount?: A critique of the cohort approach to fertility. *Population and Development Review* 18: 599–629.

Parcel, T. L. 1979. Race, regional labor markets and earnings. *American Sociological Review* 44: 262–279.

Park, R. E. 1950. *Race and culture*. Glencoe, Ill.: The Free Press.

Park, R. E., and E. W. Burgess. 1921. *Introduction to the science of sociology*. Chicago: University of Chicago Press.

Pearl, J. 2000. *Causality: Models, reasoning, and inference*. Cambridge: Cambridge University Press.

Perlmann, J., and M. C. Waters. 2002. *The new race question: How the census counts multiracial individuals*. New York: Russell Sage.

Portes, A., and L. Jensen. 1989. The enclave and the entrants: Patterns of ethnic enterprise in Miami before and after Muriel. *American Sociological Review* 54: 929–949.

Portes, A., and R. Rumbaut. 2001. *Legacies: The story of the immigrant second generation*. Berkeley: University of California Press.

Preston, S. H. 1978. The next fifteen years in demographic analysis. In *Social demography*. Edited by K. Taeuber, L. Bumpass, and J. A. Sweet, 299–313. New York: Academic Press.

Preston, S. H. 1979. Urban growth in developing countries. *Population and Development Review* 5: 195–215.

Preston, S. H. 1984. Children and the elderly: Divergent paths for America's dependents. *Demography* 21: 435–457.

Preston, S. H. 1993. The contours of demography: Estimates and projections. *Demography* 30: 593–606.

Preston, S. H., P. Heuveline, and M. Guillot. 2001. *Demography: Measuring and modeling population processes*. Oxford: Blackwell.

Rindfuss, R. R., S. P. Morgan, and G. Swicegood. 1988. *First births in America: Changes in the timing of parenthood*. Berkeley: University of California Press.

Rindfuss, R. R., and J. A. Sweet. 1977. *Postwar fertility trends and differentials in the United States*. New York: Academic Press.

Ruggles, S., and M. Sobek. 2001. *User's guide: Integrated public use microdata series, Millennial ed.* Minneapolis: University of Minnesota, Minnesota Population Center.

Ryder, N. 1964. Notes on the concept of a population. *American Journal of Sociology* 69: 447–463.

Ryder, N. 1965. The cohort as a concept in the study of social change. *American Sociological Review* 30: 843–861.

Ryder, N. 1969. The emergence of a modern fertility pattern: United States, 1917–66. In *Fertility and family planning: A world view*. Edited by S. J Behrman, L. Corsa, Jr., and R. Freedman, 99–126. Ann Arbor: University of Michigan Press.

Schnore, L. 1961. Social mobility in demographic perspective. *American Sociological Review* 67: 406–417.

Schnore, L. 1963. The socioeconomic status of cities and suburbs. *American Sociological Review* 28: 76–85.

Sewell, W. H., and J. M. Armer. 1966. Neighborhood context and college plans. *American Sociological Review* 31: 159–168.

Sheldon, E. B., and W. E. Moore. 1968. *Indicators of social change: Concepts and social change*. New York: Russell Sage.

Shyrock, H. S., and J. S. Siegel and Associates. 1976. *The methods and materials of demography*, Condensed ed., E. G. Stockwell. New York: Academic Press.

Siegel, P. 1965. On the cost of being a Negro. *Sociological Inquiry* 35: 41–57.

Smith, H. L. 1989. Integrating theory and research on the institutional determinants of fertility. *Demography* 26: 171–184.

South, S. J., and K. D. Crowder. 1997. Escaping distressed neighborhoods: Individual, community, and metropolitan influences. *American Journal of Sociology* 102: 1040–1084.

South, S. J., and K. D. Crowder. 1998. Leaving the "hood": Residential mobility between black, white, and integrated neighborhoods. *American Sociological Review* 63:17–26.

South, S. J., and S. F. Messner. 2000. Crime and demography: Multiple linkages, reciprocal relations. *Annual Review of Sociology* 26: 83–106.

South, S. J., K. Trent, and Y. Shen. 2001. Changing partners: Toward a macrostructural-opportunity theory of marital dissolution. *Journal of Marriage and the Family* 63: 743–754.

South, S., and W. Xu. 1990. Local industrial dominance and earnings attainment. *American Sociological Review* 55: 591–599.

Sullivan, T., E. Warren, and J. L. Westbrook. 1989. *As we forgive our debtors: Bankruptcy and consumer credit in America*. New York: Oxford University Press.

Sullivan, T., E. Warren, and J. L. Westbrook. 2000. *The fragile middle class: Americans in debt*. New Haven, Conn.: Yale University Press.

Sweeney, M. 2002. Two decades of family change: The shifting economic foundations of marriage. *American Sociological Review* 67: 132–147.

Taeuber, K. 1964. The Negro as an immigrant group. *American Journal of Sociology* 69: 374–382.

Taeuber, K. 1969. Toward a social report: A review article. *Journal of Human Resources* 5: 354–360.

Taeuber, K., L. Bumpass, and J. A. Sweet, eds. 1978. *Social demography*. New York: Academic Press.

Taeuber, K., and A. Taeuber. 1965. *Negroes in cities: Residential segregation and neighborhood change*. Chicago: Aldine.

Taeuber, A., and K. Taeuber. 1967. Recent immigration and studies of ethnic assimilation. *Demography* 4: 798–808.

Teachman, J., and K. D. Crowder. 2002. Multilevel models in family research: Some conceptual and methodological issues. *Journal of Marriage and Family* 54:280–294.

Thompson, W. S. 1930. *Population problems*. New York: McGraw Hill.

Thornton, A., and H. Lin. 1994. *Social change and the family in Taiwan*. Chicago: University of Chicago Press.

Tienda, M., and D. T. Lii. 1987. Minority concentration and earnings inequality: A revised formulation. *American Journal of Sociology* 93: 141–165.

Tigges, L. M., and D. M. Tootle. 1993. Unemployment and racial competition in local labor markets. *Sociological Quarterly* 34: 279–298.

Tolnay, S. E. 1999. The *bottom rung: African American family life on southern farms*. Urbana, Ill.: University of Illinois Press.

Tolnay, S. E. 2001. African Americans and immigrants in northern cities: The effects of relative group size on occupational standing in 1920. *Social Forces* 80: 573–604.

Tolnay, S. E., and K. D. Crowder. 1999. Regional origin and family stability in northern cities: The role of context. *American Sociological Review* 64: 97–112.

Tolnay, S. E., K. D. Crowder, and R. M. Adelman. 2002. Race, regional origin, and residence in northern cities at the beginning of the great migration. *American Sociological Review* 67: 456–475.

Treiman, D. 1977. *Occupational prestige in comparative perspective*. New York: Academic Press.

Udry, J. R. 1994. The nature of gender. *Demography* 31: 561–573.

Udry, J. R. 2000. Biological limits of gender construction. *American Sociological Review* 65: 443–457.

Uhlenberg, P. 1969. A study of cohort life cycles: Cohorts of native born Massachusetts women, 1830–1920. *Population Studies* 23: 407–420.

United States, President's Research Committee on Social Trends. 1933. *Recent social trends in the United States*. 2 vol. New York: McGraw-Hill.

U.S. Census Bureau. 1980. *Social indicators III: Selected data on social conditions and trends in the United States*. Washington, D.C.: U.S. Government Printing Office.

U.S. Census Bureau. 1993. *Current population reports, Series P60–184, Money income of households, families and persons in the United States: 1992*. Washington, D.C.: U.S. Government Printing Office.

U.S. Census Bureau. 2000. *Current population survey design and methodology Technical Paper 63* (issued March 2000) Washington, D.C.: U. S. Census Bureau.

U.S. Department of Health, Education, and Welfare. 1969. *Toward a social report*. Washington, D.C.: U.S. Government Printing Office.

Wachter, K. W., J. E. Knodel, and M. Van Landingham. 2002. AIDS and the elderly of Thailand: Projecting family impacts. *Demography* 39: 25–41.

Watkins, S., ed. 1994. *After Ellis Island: Newcomers and natives in the 1910 census*. New York: Russell Sage.

Waters, M. 1999. *Black identities: West Indian dreams and American reality*. New York: Russell Sage.

Waters, M. 2002. The social construction of race and ethnicity: Some examples from demography. In *American diversity: A demographic challlenge for the twenty-first century*. Edited by N. Denton and S. Tolnay, 25–49. Albany: State University of New York Press.

Winsborough, H. H. 1978. Statistical histories of the life cycle of birth cohorts: The transition from school boy to adult male. In *Social demography*. Edited by K. Taeuber, L. Bumpass, and J. A. Sweet, 231–259. New York: Academic Press.

Worcester, K. W. 2001. *Social Science Research Council 1923–1998*. New York: Social Science Research Council.

Zhou, M., and J. R. Logan. 1989. Returns on human capital in New York City's Chinatown. *American Sociological Review* 54:809–820.

Zhou, X., A. Perkins, and S. Hui. 1999. Comparisons of software packages for generalized linear models. *The American Statistician* 53:282–290.

CHAPTER 15

Organizational and Corporate Demography

Glenn R. Carroll

AND

Olga M. Khessina

Although the importance of organizations in modern life has long been recognized by social scientists, only a few prescient demographers, such as Nathan Keyfitz (1977), sensed early on the potential power of demography for their analysis. Indeed, it was not until the last two decades that the new subspecialty of organizational demography began and in the last decade that it really developed. So, we imagine that for many this chapter will be an introduction to this now vibrant area of demographic theory and research.

Organizational studies in general display an abundance of theoretical approaches, including many that are qualitative, interpretive, and postmaterialistic. Doing demography within this theoretically diverse field sometimes makes one feel like Charles Darwin must have felt when he read Herman Melville's (1987:140) parody[1] of his early empirical research on the Galapagos Islands:

> If you now desire the population of Albermarle, I will give you, in round numbers, the statistics, according to the most reliable estimates made upon the spot:
> Men,... none.
> Ant-eaters,... unknown.
> Man-haters,.. unknown.

---

[1] For a detailed account of the contentious relationship between Melville and Darwin, see Larson (2001).

Lizards,.. 500,000.
Snakes, ... 500,000.
Spiders,.. 10,000,000.
Salamaders, ... unknown.
Devils,... do.
Making a clean total of.. 11,000,000.
exclusive of an incomputable host of fiends, ant-eaters, man-haters, and salamanders.

As Melville illustrates, Darwin's efforts to count phenomena and to draw inferences from the counts ran up against passionate arguments against the meaningfulness and appropriateness of systematic counting.[2]

Despite occasional similar misplaced complaints from organizational theorists about the "sterility" of counting, demographic analysis of organizations has flourished in recent years. Indeed, three distinct research traditions, each with its own conceptual framework, can be found in the contemporary organizations literature: workforce demography, internal organizational demography, and corporate demography. This chapter first briefly explains these various frameworks but then reviews only one of them in depth—that usually called corporate demography or organizational ecology.[3] The major theoretical models or "theory fragments" of organizational ecology are examined along with their associated research programs. The chapter points to methodological trends, research exemplars, and future prospects. (See chapter 20, "Ecological Demography," in this *Handbook* for another view.)

CONCEPTUAL FRAMEWORKS

The first conceptual framework, which Carroll and Hannan (2000) call workforce demography, examines the demography of organizational labor forces. This approach might be seen by demographers as an application of formal demography; it follows in the footsteps of Keyfitz (1973, 1977) in using models to analyze demographic flows and related processes within organizations. A second framework, which might be called "internal organizational demography," looks at the way demographic distributions affect important organizational outcomes. This approach can be viewed as a special type of population study in the sense of the term used by Hauser and Duncan (1959); it is concerned with the effects of demographic structure on behavioral outcomes. A third framework, which is the main focus of this chapter, is typically called corporate demography (Carroll and Hannan 2000) or organizational ecology (Hannan and Freeman 1989). It focuses on organizational populations and their evolution over time, especially as exhibited through vital rates—organizational founding, growth, transformation, and mortality. This framework, which encompasses most of the chapter, entails both formal demographic and population studies to examine the evolution of organizational populations. From a demographic perspective, the main difference among the three conceptual frameworks is that the third framework treats the demography of corporations and the first two deal with demographic processes within corporations.

---

[2] A milder form of resistance to the programmatic aspect of demographic research can be seen even among positivists such as Hedstrom (1992), who implicitly criticize work by referring to it as "normal science." Such comments only illustrate that in organizational studies normal science is not a normal activity.
[3] This line of work is distinct from that called "ecological demography," which is discussed in Chapter 1.

The Demography of the Workforce

Workforce demography concerns itself with the flows of individuals through positions in the workplace; it is especially interested in questions of individual turnover and mobility within organizational settings. Research conducted within this framework usually adopts an organization-level analysis; theories are developed from the perspective of a prototypical focal organization.

The theoretical arguments developed in this framework typically focus on the factors and conditions associated with movement between jobs within an organization (internal mobility); such arguments, however, also have implications for external mobility as well.[4] Research on mobility within an organization often adopts either an individualistic view, concentrating on the characteristics of individuals, or a structuralistic view, looking at the organizational conditions that create internal career paths.

The tradition that focuses on individual characteristics such as age and education is commonly known as human capital theory. As Barnett, Baron, and Stuart (2000: 92) explain:

> Human capital theorists attribute differences in promotions and wage attachment by sex, race, and jobs demography to variations in skills, training, ability, and labor force attachment among groups in the labor market.

The second, more structural, tradition is often linked to the study of established internal labor markets. Doeringer and Piore (1971: 1–2) define an internal labor market as:

> An administrative unit, such as a manufacturing plant, within which the pricing and allocation of labor is governed by a set of administrative rules and procedures. The internal labor market ... is to be distinguished from the external labor market of conventional economic theory where pricing, allocating, and training decisions are controlled by economic variables.

By this view, an internal labor market is buffered from the forces of the larger labor market, meaning that the "usual" effects of sex, ethnicity, social class, industrial sector, and the like on internal mobility are likely attenuated. Mobility within an organization with an internal labor market may differ from general mobility patterns in large part because it is rationalized according to some personnel plan, be it implicit or explicit and bureaucratic (Weber 1968). An individual's odds of movement, however, depend heavily upon his or her location within the organization's structure.

The early structuralist research went in two complementary directions, one concentrating on the workforce of the organization and its demographic makeup, the second examining dimensions of organizational structure directly. Research of the first kind usually involved longitudinal analysis of career-mobility patterns within a single organization. From empirical studies of this kind, we know that rates of mobility within and across organizations are driven by a variety of factors, including the rates of growth and decline of organizations, the distribution of employee cohorts, early career history, vacancy chains, and career lines. An active line of current research investigates the relationship between the demographic composition of occupations and jobs (usually in terms of race and sex composition) in an organization and career outcomes such as job shifts and compensation (Baron and Newman 1990; Petersen and Morgan 1995). These studies show that demographic compositions play an important, although

---

[4] This section is adapted from Carroll, Haveman, and Swaminathan (1990).

sometimes complex, role in affecting outcomes. For instance, in a study of the California civil service system, Barnett, Baron, and Stuart (2000: 88) find that:

> Although female- and minority-dominated occupations were disadvantaged in many respects, their incumbents moved among state agencies more frequently (and reaped greater economic benefit) than did employees in occupations dominated by white males. Intraorganizational promotions yielded roughly comparable salary gains for incumbents of male- and female-dominated occupations, but through distinct paths: male-dominated occupations had less frequent promotions with larger salary increases; female-dominated occupations experience more frequent job shifts with smaller pay changes.

Initial research of the second kind, on organizational structure and mobility, theorized linkages between organizational characteristics, such as the presence of departmental boundary-spanning units and average levels of wages and status. Research in this vein explores questions about the conditions creating internal labor markets, sex segregation in jobs, fragmentation of work, and the opportunity structure within an organization (for a review see Baron 1984). The demographic orientation of this work is typically neither explicit nor strong.

Internal Organizational Demography

A second line of demographic research on organizations also sometimes goes by the name of organizational demography, but it would be more appropriately labeled as "internal organizational demography."

A speculative essay by Pfeffer (1983) initiated the contemporary flurry of research on internal organizational demography. Pfeffer (1983: 303) defined demography as "the composition, in terms of basic attributes such as age, sex, educational level, length of service or residence, race and so forth of the social unit under study." He continued by explaining to organizational theorists that "the demography of any social entity is the composite aggregation of the characteristics of the individual members of that entity."[5]

The impact of Pfeffer's (1983) essay came from his novel arguments about the causes and consequences of demographic phenomena inside an organization. For the most part, these arguments focused on the properties of demographic distributions of persons within an organization, especially the tenure or length of service (LOS) distribution of members of the organization. The claims that initially generated the most new research specify that the LOS distribution affects a wide variety of organizational outcomes, including employee turnover (McCain, O'Reilly, and Pfeffer 1983; Wiersema and Bird 1993); organizational innovation (Flatt 1993); internal control structures, power distribution and interorganizational relations (Hambrick, Cho, and Chen 1996); and firm performance (Keck 1997).[6]

Although arguments vary depending on the particular outcome, most of them specify *unevenness or heterogeneity* in the LOS distribution as the demographic variable of primary interest.[7] In making these claims, theorists usually invoke some kind of

---

[5] This section draws from Carroll and Harrison (1998).

[6] Recent research has expanded beyond LOS distributions to look at the effects of numerous other demographic distributions in organizations, including sex, race, ethnicity, age, and citizenship. See Lawrence (1997) for a review.

[7] The most commonly used measure of unevenness is the coefficient of variation in tenure. See Sørensen (2002) for review and critique of this practice.

unobserved social process to motivate the expected association between heterogeneity in LOS and outcomes. For instance, Wagner, Pfeffer, and O'Reilly (1984:76) propose that there should be a relationship between variation in LOS and turnover because:

> Similarity in time of entry into the organization will positively affect the likelihood of persons communicating with others who entered at the same time ... the more frequent the communication, the more likely it is that those interacting will become similar in terms of their beliefs and perceptions of the organization and how it operates.

Other social processes often employed to motivate expected LOS-outcome associations include psychological processes of similarity and attraction (Glick, Miller, and Huber 1993), social psychological processes of homophily and group dynamics (O'Reilly, Caldwell, and Barnett 1989)—including especially communication patterns (Smith et al. 1994), and processes of norm formation and maintenance (Boone and van Olffen 1997).

In research on the effects of heterogeneity in LOS distributions, individual turnover is the most commonly studied outcome variable. LOS research, while initially about the distributions of whole organizations or complete subunits, now often looks only at the top management teams of firms, using readily available data on officers in public corporations (Finkelstein and Hambrick 1996).

In their review of 21 major empirical studies conducted on the effects of LOS heterogeneity, Carroll and Harrison (1998) show that most of the available evidence supports the theoretical arguments. By their assessment, 11 studies present solid supporting evidence, another 4 provide weak support, and 6 offer no support. Nonetheless, Carroll and Harrison (1998) pointed to a number of issues that deserve attention if the program on internal organizational demography is to continue to flourish. These include specification of a formal model, greater measurement precision, and controlling for the effects of unobserved heterogeneity, which creates a built-in relationship with turnover (see also Sørensen 2000). Because human demographers[8] have dealt with these and related issues at length in other contexts, it would be very beneficial to have greater participation from them in further development of internal organizational demography.

Corporate Demography or Organizational Ecology

Corporate demography focuses on the vital rates—founding, growth, structural transformation, and mortality—of organizational populations. The framework maintains that changes in vital rates alter the organizational composition of a population and, consequently, features of the social structures based on the population also change.

Figure 15.1, taken from Carroll and Hannan (2000), depicts the general logical structure underlying corporate demographic analysis. It shows four general conceptual components: (1) a social structural arrangement or pattern; (2) a set of organizations in the social system decomposed into specific organizational populations or subpopulations; (3) a set of population-specific vital rates; (4) the environmental conditions that move the rates up or down. In this figure, solid arrows indicate the typical direction of causal arguments. Researchers frequently analyze one or several of these arrows in isolation and treat the causes as exogenous; this has been especially the case for the analysis of population-specific vital rates. On other occasions, corporate demographers

---

[8] We use the term *human demographer* to refer to those who study the demography of human populations.

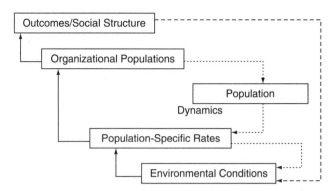

FIGURE 15.1. General structure of demographic explanations. Source: Carroll and Hannan (2000: 31).

focus on one or more of the feedback mechanisms in the system, shown by dotted lines; the resulting models possess endogenous causes. Finally, other longer-term feedback mechanisms thought to be operative in the system, shown by the dashed line, usually do not get modeled explicitly, mainly because available theory is deficient and many of the relevant events (e.g., revolution) are extremely rare.[9]

THEORETICAL MODELS

Corporate demography is characterized by a number of related but distinct theoretically driven research programs. The programs share a number of concepts and assumptions but differ in their orienting problems, theoretical arguments, specific models, and some assumptions. Corporate demographers now call these "theory fragments"; in general, the various theory fragments in organizational ecology complement rather than contradict or compete with each other. Both Pfeffer (1993) and Hargens (2000) have remarked on the high degree of coherence within the fragments and suggest that progress has been especially cumulative. We describe below the major demographically oriented theory fragments of organizational ecology.[10]

Structural Inertia and Change

Most theories about the behavior of organizations in the environment agree that when organizations are structurally aligned with their environment, they perform better. A common claim of this kind, for instance, holds that highly differentiated and decentralized organizational structures operate more effectively in heterogeneous environments. Theorists generally presume that as environments change, organizations do as

---

[9] A practical justification for this practice is that the rate of change among these structures is much slower than that of organizational populations.

[10] Other less demographically oriented fragments include evolution of organizational forms (McKendrick and Carroll 2001; Pólos, Hannan and Carroll 2002; Ruef 2000; Zuckerman 1999); niche width (Freeman and Hannan 1983; Péli 1997); social movement forms (Ingram and Simons 2000; Minkoff 1999; Olzak and Uhrig 2001; Swaminathan and Wade 2001).

well in attempting to maintain the alignment. So, by most theories, organizational change is considered to be adaptive, highly feasible, and beneficial.

In contrast, organizational ecology claims that organizational change is difficult because of various internal and external constraints (Hannan and Freeman 1977). If organizational structures are inertial, then the main mechanism driving change in the world of organizations cannot be the adaptation of its individual members. Instead, change proceeds via the selective replacement of "outdated" organizations (Hannan and Freeman 1977). It is important to recognize that the shift to a selection mechanism as the motor of change bumps the analysis up to the population level.

Organizational ecology does not claim that adaptation is impossible, only unlikely. The theory asserts that the general tendency in organizations is toward structural inertia, at least in their core structures. The *core* features of an organization are often defined as its general mission, its form of authority, its core technology, and its marketing strategy. Other more malleable features are considered *peripheral* (Hannan and Freeman 1984). Structural inertia is not absolute but relative: organizations can and do change, even occasionally in the core. But, in general, organizations cannot change fast enough to match the speed of environmental change and maintain alignment with shifting environmental demands (Hannan and Freeman 1984).

It strikes some as paradoxical that inertia can be a by-product of effective organizational operation. But reliability and accountability are important to customers and other external observers when judging organizational performance (Hannan and Freeman 1984). A precondition for reliability and accountability of organizational activity is reproducibility of organizational routines and structures, which runs hand in hand with inertia (Péli, Pólos, and Hannan 2000).

When environmental conditions shift dramatically, inertia can become a liability. Under these conditions, pressures to change may be so strong that inertia is overcome (Delacroix and Swaminathan 1991; Haveman 1992). However, changing such an entrenched and institutionalized system can be highly disruptive and hamper organizational survival chances. In particular, corporate demographers believe that changing the core features of an organization is more likely to generate detrimental consequences than does change in peripheral features (Baron, Hannan, and Burton 2001; Hannan and Freeman 1984).

A more complex view proposes that organizational change can have either beneficial or detrimental consequences for organizational operation, depending on certain boundary conditions. It has been proposed that a change of core organizational features can be beneficial in conditions of dramatic environmental shift. For example, for California savings and loan associations, changes of core features were largely beneficial for both organizational performance and survival if they were related to the previous activity and were undertaken in conditions of drastic environmental change (Haveman 1992). And, in the California wine industry, organizational changes undertaken under conditions of environmental shock tended to decrease probability of failure (Delacroix and Swaminathan 1991).

The distinction between content and process of organizational change helps to explain why organizational change can have both negative and positive outcomes (Barnett and Carroll 1995). *Content* of change refers to the difference in the structures before and after a successful transformation. *Process* of change refers to the path taken during the attempted change in content. The distinction is useful because an organization might be undertaking a potentially beneficial change of content, but its benefits might never be realized because the process of change creates so much disruption. So, process effects can prevent an organization from implementing what would be beneficial content changes. Much of the theory in organizational ecology about structural inertia (e.g., Hannan and Freeman 1984, 1989) concerns disruptive and detrimental process effects.

Empirical studies to date provide evidence supporting this speculation. The general model used in these studies specifies the organization-specific hazard of mortality as: $\mu_i(u, v) = \exp[\alpha \Delta_{iu} + \mathbf{BX}_{iu}] \cdot \varphi(u) \cdot \psi(v)$ where $\mu_i(u, v)$ is the instantaneous rate of mortality of organization i, u represents organizational age (or tenure), v gives the time elapsed since a major structural transformation (zero before the first), the X variables describe the organization, and Δ_{iu} is an indicator variable that takes the value of 1 after the transformation (it is 0 before). The usual tests of the structural inertia process arguments expect that estimates will show $\alpha > 0$ and $\psi(v) < 0$. For example, for a population of Finnish newspapers, Amburgey, Kelly, and Barnett (1993) found that, as a result of the process of change, the probability of organizational failure sharply increased right after a core change $[\alpha > 0]$ but then decreased with the elapsed time after the change $[\psi(v) < 0$ when $\psi(v)$ is specified as γv; that is, $\gamma < 0]$. This study pointed out that immediate and long-term effects of change can differ in their consequences: the former effects are usually disruptive, while the latter can be adaptive. Carroll and Hannan (2000) review a number of other similar studies using data from different populations. As they point out, the findings of these studies generally support the claims of structural inertia theory, but the research stream is not long and there are still some anomalous findings.[11]

A conceptual difficulty involves distinguishing core from peripheral organizational features. The list of features originally given by Hannan and Freeman (1984) is too malleable, and there is no strong conceptual basis for deciding if a feature belongs to the core or the periphery. To alleviate this problem, Hannan, Pólos, and Carroll (2003) propose a new model, one that focuses on the number of additional organizational changes induced from an initial change in an organization's architecture. They argue that an initial change exhibits "coreness" to the extent it prompts a long cascade of additional changes and requires more time to resolve any incompatibility generated in the various parts of the organization's architecture.

Age Dependence in Organizational Mortality Rates

As organizations age, they experience changes in their internal routines and structures and in their relations with the external environment. Some of these changes may increase an organization's chances of failure, whereas others may reduce them. Ecologists propose theories of age dependence aimed at explaining how and why organizational mortality rates depend on organizational age or tenure in the population.[12]

---

[11] Indeed, many empirical studies of effects of change on organizational outcomes have specification problems and should be interpreted with caution. The most common problem is a failure to separate effects of content and process of change. Another problem is incomplete modeling of the environment (Barnett and Carroll 1995).

[12] Some research is done on the effects of organizational age on organizational growth rates but it is rather slim due to the difficulty of getting growth data (but see Barron, West, and Hannan 1994).

Simple analyses of age dependence in organizational failure rates disagree about the direction of the age effect (Hannan 1998). One set of theoretical arguments and empirical studies finds that mortality rates decrease with organizational age; this is negative age dependence. Another set of arguments and findings establishes that mortality rates increase with organizational age: positive age dependence.

Predictions of negative age dependence are based on Stinchcombe's (1965) analysis of the "liability of newness." Contemporary applications of his ideas often can be boiled down to either one of two theoretical arguments. First, organizations are believed to have higher survival chances when they have well-developed capabilities—abilities to execute routines and solve problems (Hannan and Freeman 1984). Capabilities develop through experience, which comes with age (Nelson and Winter 1982). Because organizations with better capabilities are less likely to fail, organizational mortality rates decrease with age. Second, organizations are thought to have better survival chances when they hold positional advantages in the social structure. These include ties with important actors in the environment (Stinchcombe 1965), high status (Podolny 1993), bridges over structural holes (Burt 1992), market power (Barnett 1997), and political influence (Pfeffer and Salancik 1978). Positional advantages are acquired with age, and therefore, as organizations age, their risk of failure decreases.

A strict rendering of the "liability of newness" hypothesis predicts that mortality rates monotonically decline with age, as organizations develop capabilities and establish positional advantages (Carroll and Delacroix 1982; Carroll 1983; Freeman, Carroll, and Hannan 1983; Singh, Tucker, and House 1986). A looser version of negative age dependence takes into account the "liability of adolescence." It allows mortality rates first to increase momentarily during the first few months or years of operation and then to decrease with subsequent organizational age, yielding a negative pattern over most of the age dimension. The argument here is that organizations start by drawing down from an initial resource endowment, but then develop capabilities and positional advantages (Brüderl and Schüssler 1990; Fichman and Levinthal 1991).

Theories of positive age dependence in organizational mortality depend on three arguments. First, initial resource endowments become depleted and may even disappear as an organization ages. So, unless there is an offsetting inflow of resources, mortality rates are expected to increase with organizational age. Second, if an organization is perfectly aligned with the environment at founding but its structure is inertial, then its alignment will erode with the passage of time with environmental change (Carroll 1983). This is often referred to as the "liability of obsolescence." Because misalignment with the environment is likely to increase with age, mortality rates are thought to increase with organizational age as well. Third, capabilities may have a negative impact on survival chances if they code and preserve action-constraining features, such as political coalitions, precedents, and the like (Levitt and March 1988; March 1991). A "liability of senescence" results from dysfunctional organizational capabilities, the number of which increases with organizational age (Barron, West, and Hannan 1994; Hannan 1998).

The earliest empirical studies of age dependence sought to demonstrate the existence of age dependence (as compared to alternative explanations such as unobservable heterogeneity) and to establish its direction using stochastic survivor plots and hazard functions (e.g., Barron, West, and Hannan 1994; Brüderl and Schüssler 1990; Carroll 1983; Carroll and Delacroix 1982; Freeman, Carroll, and Hannan 1983). The hazard function models used include the Gompertz, the Weibull, Makeham's Law, and the log-logistic (for reviews, see Carroll and Hannan 2000; Tuma and Hannan 1984). Obviously, age dependence cannot simultaneously be both negative and positive, so the conflicting arguments and evidence led to attempts at reconciliation. One consequence of the effort is that mortality rate specifications of age or tenure now typically rely on piece-wise constant rate model (where the rate can vary across age, or tenure, segments but is constrained to be constant within a segment) rather than functional models that constrain the rate to behave in particular ways with respect to age. The typical piece-wise constant rate model for the organization-specific mortality μ_l rate as a function of tenure in the industry (u) and calendar time (t) has the form:

$$\ln \mu_l(u, t) = m_p + \mathbf{B}\mathbf{X}_{it}, u \geq 0, u \in I_p$$

where X_{it} represents measured covariates, m_p denotes a set of age or tenure-specific effects defined by the breakpoints $0 \leq \tau_1 \leq \tau_2 \leq \cdots \leq \tau_p$, and assuming that $\tau_{p+1} = \infty$, yielding P periods:

$$I_p = \{t|\tau_p \leq t \leq \tau_{p+1}\}, p = 1, \ldots, P$$

The estimated set of ordered constants m_p indicates whether age dependence follows any particular pattern.

One critical empirical consideration that was often missing in the earliest studies is size dependence. Organizational age and size are usually positively correlated, so to get good estimates of age dependence, one needs complete age-varying measures of size for all organizations in a population. This is a daunting data collection demand for large historical populations, but the more recent set of studies on age dependence do, in fact, collect and incorporate such information. (It is more readily available for regulated populations such as banks.) The bulk of these studies show evidence of positive age dependence when size is controlled, although the pattern is not fully conclusive (Hannan 1998). In perhaps the most complex attempt at reconciliation, Hannan et al. (1998a) estimated a piece-wise constant rate model where organizational age interacts nonproportionally with organizational size in analyzing historical populations of automobile producers in the U.S., France, Germany, and Great Britain. This model specifies the mortality μ_l rate as a function of tenure in the industry (u) and calendar time (t) as:

$$\ln \mu_l(u,t) = m_p + \gamma_p \ln S_{iu} + \mathbf{B}\mathbf{X}_{it}, u \geq 0, u \in I_p$$

where m_p denotes a set of age- or tenure-specific effects, S_{iu} measures organizational size, X_{it} represents other measured covariates, and I_p is defined as above. The estimates suggest that, in three countries, age dependence is negative for the largest organizations and generally positive for small ones (the exception is Britain, where large firms face increasing mortality with age). The pattern for the smaller organizations in these countries might be especially interesting for human demographers because of its similarity to the human mortality curve

> ...for relatively small firms in the German and French populations... the relationship of the rate of disbanding or exit has a bath-tub shape: the rate falls as tenure increases over the first three years and rises with increasing tenure beyond that point. Firms of sizes in the range of 50 to 1500 in the American population also show a bath-tub shape relationship: the rate declines over the first seven years and then rises (Hannan et al. 1998a: 297).

Hannan et al. (1998a) speculate that the pattern might simply represent a mixture of first newness and then obsolescence-senescence processes. But they also note that their reading of the historical data suggests that the initial decrease in mortality is the consequence of "selection driven by unobserved heterogeneity in the technical quality of products" (Hannan et al. 1998a: 298).

Future empirical research will need to find ways to disentangle these issues, a task for which human demographers may have important tools to offer. From the perspective of organizational theory, a promising approach might be to investigate the specific mechanisms thought to underlay different forms of age dependence. For example, in the semiconductor and biotechnology industries, Sørensen and Stuart (2000) claim that although older organizations develop better capabilities and acquire more positional advantages that allow them to patent innovations at a higher rate, their patents are more obsolete in relation to environmental demands than those made by younger companies. The inference about obsolescence comes from the finding that, in the patenting process, older firms disproportionately cite their own prior patents (self-citation) and cite the older prior art than younger firms. This study articulates a novel possible mechanism behind positive age dependence.

Important progress in understanding age dependence in organizational mortality is also evident at the theoretical level. Hannan (1998) develops several formalizations based on first-order logic to explain different forms of age dependence. His analysis uses different assumptions about endowment, capabilities, imprinting, inertia, and positional advantage to generate various types of age dependence. While the exercise does not lead to a grand unification of theoretical ideas, it does clarify "the mechanisms at work in each theoretical account and provides guidance for empirical research designed to discriminate among the competing theories" (Hannan 1998: 126).

A potentially path-breaking theoretical analysis by Pólos and Hannan (2001; 2002) takes these ideas further using tools of nonmonotonic logic. This framework offers a system of logic where knowledge about the world can be partial and knowledge statements need not be characterized by informational monotonicity, where "explanatory principles are not withdrawn, even when their first-order consequences get falsified" (Pólos and Hannan 2002: 140–141). The framework's basic assumptions fit remarkably well with much social science research—such as the program on age dependence—where there are seemingly contradictory arguments and evidence. How does the Pólos-Hannan nonmonotonic logic resolve such problems? For working theories, that is theories in progress, it uses a rule based on specificity. As Pólos and Hannan (2001: 436) explain:

> The basic methodological rule is that more specific knowledge (rules) override less specific knowledge. In making inferences, we want to use the most specific knowledge that applies. It is this feature of the strategy that gives the nonmonotonic character: adding new knowledge can overturn inferences that were valid without such knowledge.

Density Dependence in Vital Rates: Founding, Growth, and Mortality

The ecological theory of density-dependent legitimation and competition postulates that vital rates of organizations—founding, growth, and mortality rates—depend on population density, defined as the number of population members or organizations (Hannan 1986; Hannan and Carroll 1992). The legitimation construct is defined by a concept of constitutive legitimacy. According to this concept, an organizational form gains legitimation when it attains a "taken-for-granted" character in social interaction (Meyer and Rowan 1977)—that is, when relevant agents and gatekeepers see it as the "natural" way to perform some kind of collective action. A concept of diffuse competition is used to define the competition construct. According to this concept, organizations potentially compete with each other when they depend on the same pool of resources.

The theory proposes that legitimation enhances organizational founding rates and reduces mortality rates, while competition has mirror-image effects.[13] As a new population evolves and organizational density increases, the force of legitimation increases at a decreasing rate, whereas the force of competition increases at an increasing rate. So, legitimation is stronger at low levels of density while competition is stronger at high levels. Empirically, the combined operation of these forces implies curvilinear dependencies of organizational vital rates on density. At lower densities of population development, increasing density mainly increases the legitimation of a new organizational form; this, in its turn, decreases initially very high mortality rates and increases initially very low founding rates. At higher densities, increasing density mainly increases competition for diminishing supply of resources, which in its turn increases mortality rates and decreases founding rates. Thus, according to this theory, founding rates should show an inverted U-shape relationship with population density, whereas mortality rates should display a U-shape relationship with density. A common formulation used to specify these effects is a simple log-quadratic of the rate (either the population-specific founding rate or the organization-specific mortality rate): $\ln r(t) = \alpha_0 + \alpha_1 N_t + \alpha_2 N_t^2$ where N_t represents density at time t (see Hannan and Carroll (1992) for other model specifications used in the study of density dependence). Obviously, to get the relationships described above, the expected directions of the coefficients differ for founding and mortality.[14]

Another component of the theory concerns only organizational failure. It argues that organizations founded during periods of high density have higher age-specific failure rates because resources are scarcer and the only uncrowded spots available in the population are near the peripheries of the niche (Carroll and Hannan 1989). So, in addition to the curvilinear effects of contemporaneous density, the theory also expects a fixed positive effect of founding density on organizational mortality. With a log-quadratic specification of contemporaneous density, the complete density model for the organization-specific mortality rate : μ_i becomes: $\ln \mu_i(u) = \alpha_0 + \alpha_1 N_u + \alpha_2 N_u^2 + \alpha_4 N_{i0}$ where N_u represents density at age u and N_{i0} represents density at the time of organization i's founding ($u = 0$). The expectation is that $a_4 > 0$.

Figure 15.2 depicts the three basic expected relationships of density dependence theory, assuming a log-linear specification of rates.

Numerous empirical studies on a variety of population and industries overwhelmingly conclude that the curvilinear predictions of the density-dependence model hold generally (Carroll and Hannan 2000). Yet, differences in the timing and levels of turning points lead Carroll and Hannan (2000) to suggest that as with the demographic

---

[13] The density dependence theory has been criticized for using constructs of cognitive legitimacy and diffused competition as opposed to those of sociopolitical legitimacy and direct competition. These criticisms and responses to them are extensively discussed elsewhere (e.g., Carroll and Hannan 2000; Hannan and Carroll 1995).

[14] An odd criticism by Cole (2001) claims that the predictions of the model are obvious. This is undoubtedly news to the many organizational theorists who now use a different baseline specification for the study of organizational mortality than they did prior to the model's introduction.

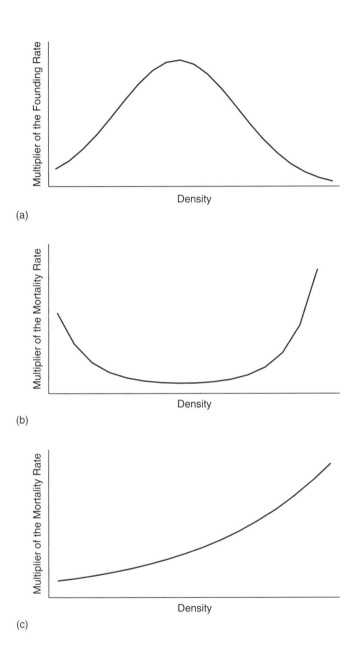

FIGURE 15.2. (A) Predicted relationship between density and founding rates. (B) Predicted relationship between density and mortality rates. (C) Predicted relationship between founding density and mortality rates.

transition in human demography, there is ample variation to support further theoretical development via meta-analysis. This exercise may lead to reformulation. For instance, some current evidence suggests that legitimation operates at a broader geographical scale than competition (Bigelow et al. 1997; Hannan et al. 1995).

The basic formulation of the density dependence theory (as laid out above) does not fully explain commonly observed late stages of population development, when the industry experiences decline or resurgence. Four explanations have been proposed for density decline and resurgence, observed at the late stages of population development. First, Hannan (1997) offers a population-level inertia model that suggests that legitimation and competition processes become increasingly sticky as the population evolves. Legitimation and competition strongly predict density only at earlier stages of population development. Hannan (1997) finds that the effects of density on entry rates of automobile producers vary systematically with population age in the five European countries studied. Density has powerful legitimating and competitive effects in young populations, but they diminish as populations age. However, density still matters in mature populations. The late effect of density echoes its earlier effect. Hannan et al. (1998b) find similar results in mortality analysis of automobile industries in four different countries.

Second, Barnett (1997) proposes a model of competitive intensity showing that as organizations age, large ones are more likely to survive, giving rise to industry concentration and decline. Paradoxically, large organizations tend to become weaker competitors, which opens a base for late density resurgence.

Third, Barron (1999) finds that industries have a tendency to become populated by large incumbents who outcompete small members when fierce competition at high densities occurs. This produces concentration as well.

Finally, resource-partitioning theory (Carroll 1985) explains density decline by the increase in market concentration over time caused by competition among large generalists (organizations operating in many ecological niches). At higher densities, when markets are highly concentrated, opportunities for specialists (organizations operating in one or very few ecological niches) increase, thus elevating founding rates and lowering mortality rates for specialists. The result of the growing number of specialists entering an industry is density resurgence, which is clearly observed in the automobile, brewing, and other industries (Carroll 1997; Carroll, Dobrev, and Swaminathan 2002). These explanations are not mutually exclusive or even necessarily contradictory, and future theory and research will undoubtedly need to parse out the unique aspects of each.

Resource Partitioning

Some mature organizational populations simultaneously display a trend toward increasing domination by a few large firms and a seemingly contradictory trend toward proliferation of small specialist firms. Resource-partitioning theory considers these two trends as potentially interdependent. It proposes that, under certain environmental and organizational conditions, increasing market concentration enhances the life chances of specialist firms (Carroll 1985; Carroll, Dobrev, and Swaminathan 2002).

Resource-partitioning theory assumes an environment consisting of unevenly distributed heterogeneous resources; it pays special attention to the locations of organizations within the resource space (Hannan, Carroll, and Pólos 2003). Organizations that aim for homogenous resource spots and therefore serve one or few market segments are *specialists*. Organizations that target heterogeneous resources and serve a broader spectrum of market segments are *generalists*.

The theory holds that, if the resource distribution is unimodal, competition among generalists involves strong advantages of scale, often economies of scale. The theory suggests that, at high densities, competition favors large generalists, who out-compete medium-sized generalists and small specialists (Dobrev and Carroll 2003). As large generalists force moderate-sized and weaker generalists out of the industry, market concentration increases and population density decreases. Eventually, only a few very large generalists—situated near the center of the resource space (on top of the unimodal peak)—populate the industry (Boone, Carroll, and van Witteloostuijn 2002). So, the generalist class of organizations becomes repositioned, from a wide range of space around the center (when many generalist organizations attempt to differentiate themselves) to a narrower space on the peak (dominated by fewer, very large generalist organizations). This repositioning leaves some previously occupied "peripheral" resource space free and unused. These free resources at the periphery of the market attract small entrepreneurial specialists, who are able to survive and prosper in the tiny resource niches (Carroll 1985; Péli and Nooteboom 1999). At the same time, generalists usually cannot take back this resource space because of one or more possibilities, including diseconomies of scope (Carroll 1985), anti-mass-production cultural sentiment (Carroll 1997; Carroll and Swaminathan 2000), customization needs of clients (Boone, Bröchler, and Carroll 2000; Jaffee 2000), size isomorphism with clients' firms (Boone, Bröchler, and Carroll 2000), or producer social status dynamics (Park and Podolny 2000).

In short, the empirical predictions of the theory are that when specific types of markets (e.g., heterogeneous resources with unimodal peak; scale advantages operative) are highly concentrated, opportunities for specialists increase, thus elevating their founding rates and lowering mortality rates for specialists (Dobrev, Kim, and Carroll 2002). The growing number of specialists entering the industry results in a resurgence of density. These predictions of resource-partitioning theory have been confirmed in a variety of industries (Carroll, Dobrev, and Swaminathan 2002).

Red Queen Competition

The Red Queen theory of organizational evolution proposes a reciprocal process of learning and competition (Barnett and Hansen 1996). According to this theory, when an organization faces direct competition, it undertakes a search for ways to improve performance. The search eventually results in some alterations of strategy, process, or structure, yielding a competitively strengthened organization. This increased competitive strength marginally increases the competition faced by the organization's rivals—it triggers in them a similar process of search and improvement. The rivals' responses in turn increase the competitive pressure faced by the focal organization, driving it to search again for improvements. According to the Red Queen theory, this self-reinforcing cyclical process of learning and competition is continuous (Barnett and Hansen 1996).

The theory holds that organizational improvement or learning is driven by exposure to direct competition. The Red Queen model has been interpreted to imply that organizations that experience intense competition acquire greater competitive strength. Furthermore, competitive strength increases (1) the longer the organization experiences direct competition, (2) the more recent the experience, and (3) the more homogenous the rivals. The theory receives some support from analysis of mortality rates (Barnett and Hansen 1996; Barnett and McKendrick 2001) and founding and growth rates (Barnett and Sorenson 2002).

The Red Queen evolution theory also implies two counterintuitive developments. First, it suggests that monopolists become weaker competitors over time because of their isolation (Barnett and Hansen 1996). Second, it implies that market leaders might have a greater chance of failing than market laggards because the former face more formidable competitors (Barnett and McKendrick 2001).

Localized Competition

Many predictions of ecological theory assume that organizations relying on the same mix of resources compete more intensely than organizations that rely on a different mix of resources (Carroll and Hannan 2000). The implications of the root idea can be seen clearly in the theory of size-localized competition. In the initial formulation, Hannan and Freeman (1977) proposed that organizations of different sizes employ different structures and strategies, implying reliance on a different mix of resources. If so, it follows that organizations compete most intensely with those of a similar size. Hannan and Freeman (1977) continued by suggesting that size-localized competition leads to population bifurcation. Because medium-sized organizations compete not only with those of similar size but also with both small- and large-sized organizations, their strategies are suboptimal and consequently lead to higher failure rates. As a result of this "liability of the middle," populations become dominated over time by organizations at the extremes of the size distribution—i.e., medium-sized organizations are selected out. Evidence suggests the operation of size-localized competition in populations of banks (Han 1998; Hannan, Ranger-Moore, and Banaszak-Holl 1990), credit unions (Amburgey, Dacin, and Kelly 1994), hotels (Baum and Mezias 1992) and insurance companies (Ranger-Moore, Breckenridge, and Jones 1995).

The modeling framework for size-localized competition can be readily generalized. Indeed, it is fairly simple to use dimensions other than size as the basis for localized competition. What is required is that organizations compete on the specified dimension and that this competition be intense and sustained enough to generate population segmentation (Carroll and Hannan 2000). For example, organizations sometimes compete along localized dimensions such as price (Baum and Mezias 1992), geographical proximity (Sorenson and Audia 2000; Sorenson and Stuart 2001), sociodemographic characteristics of their members (McPherson 1983) and customers (Baum and Singh 1994), status (Podolny, Stuart, and Hannan 1996), technological space (Barnett and McKendrick 2001), and so on. Of course, in each application of the model, analysts make sure to specify a metric along which distances between organizations can be meaningfully measured and assessed.

METHODOLOGICAL CHALLENGES

Corporate demography presents a variety of methodological challenges; some are well known to human demographers, and others appear not to be. Three general types of challenges recur regularly: those related to data collection; the lack of fully observed heterogeneity; and the simultaneity of different demographic processes.

Data Collection

As with much human demography, in organizational ecology systematic data on populations of interest are critical for scientific progress. Corporate demographers face three unique methodological challenges in compiling such data on organizational populations.

First, corporate demographers encounter multilayered organizational structures. Such structures make several different units of analysis possible, and analysts must choose among them. Choices include the establishment level, franchise, subsidiaries, strategic business units, divisions, firms, and complex, densely connected sets of firms known as business enterprise groups. As Carroll and Hannan (2000: 52) explain, the choice of unit has major implications for how events are defined and counted:

> For instance, bank branches open and close regularly in response to residential shifts in the human population. A study of the demography of banks cast at the establishment level might record considerable activity for this organizational form even though the larger banking firm remains basically stable as a corporation. Conversely, when two large banking firms merge and only one firm results, their underlying establishment structures might not change at all. In such a case, the combination (at the parent level) would be virtually invisible at the establishment level. Another likely possibility is that, following the merger, branches get consolidated—some closed and some merged—but at staggered dates. Then, an establishment-level study would record many corporate events, but none of them would coincide with the merger. What goes on in the bank holding companies that overarch the firms might involve a completely different story. Finally, when a banking company closes, all of its establishments close...

The most easily accessible data, from the government census bureaus or telephone book-like listings, typically list and count establishments. Accordingly, many analysts have constructed a corporate demography of establishments, often using the Census Bureau's Longitudinal Research Database.[15] Carroll and Hannan (2000) contend that such analysis is less sound than that based on higher-level units, especially strategic business units and firms (but not business enterprise groups). Why? They argue that two principles are important in choosing a level of analysis: (1) the resulting definition of corporate demographic events should conform to real-world conceptions of events and/ or meaningful theoretical concepts and (2) the underlying processes driving demographic activity must be stable enough to allow identification and systematic analysis.

The second challenge to collecting and compiling corporate demographic data is a common need to construct variables that require specific information on each and every member of the population. Models frequently used in theory fragments, such as structural inertia, density dependence, and localized competition, fall into this class, as do others, including even common control variable specifications. The significance of this requirement is that it usually precludes sampling as an effective data collection method; instead, data must be collected on the entire organizational population. This need might be partially mitigated for certain purposes (e.g., simple counts of density) if reliable aggregate data are available, but this is often not the case.

---

[15] The database also places severe limitations on establishment size for inclusion, resulting in a truncated observed size distribution.

Third, corporate demographers typically need to collect temporal data spanning a long time period. This is because many of the processes of interest—e.g., inertia, legitimation, concentration—take years, decades, or even centuries to unfold. While some panel studies have been conducted (see, for instance, Baron, Hannan, and Burton 2001; Freeman and Hannan 1983), researchers typically do not have the resources or patience to wait for enough corporate demographic events to occur. Panel studies also usually select for study a set of ongoing organizations, thus creating observation plans truncated on the left. As a result, the standard research design in corporate demography is backward-looking, using historical data culled from archival sources such as industry directories (for a detailed description, see Carroll and Hannan 2000). Identification and assembly of such data sets is usually a major undertaking.

Unobservable Heterogeneity

Corporate demographers routinely use hazard function methods to estimate vital rates of organizational population. Estimates of hazard models, of course, are known to be susceptible to bias introduced by unobservable heterogeneity, especially estimates of age or tenure effects (Tuma and Hannan 1984). In one respect, the problem is no different than that faced by human demographers, who often use the same methodological tools. However, organization theorists often assert that diversity is higher in the organizational world than it is within the human species (Carroll and Hannan 2000). If so, then it means that unobservable heterogeneity may be a potentially greater problem for corporate demography.

Corporate demographers' response to the challenge of unobservable heterogeneity sometimes takes the form of statistical control but more commonly relies on control by research design. Specifically, the diversity of organizations is narrowed down enormously by designs that focus on single types of interacting organizations (i.e., specific populations such as beer brewers, semiconductor manufacturers, and automobile producers) rather than diverse samples of many types of organizations. Indeed, the move from diverse to single-population designs is a dominant trend in all organizational studies.

Besides eliminating vast amounts of extrapopulation heterogeneity, the single-population design also facilitates measurement of intrapopulation heterogeneity. As researchers focus on single populations, they develop much institutional and historical knowledge about the population and its socioeconomic context. This knowledge allows researchers to pinpoint, among the many theoretical possibilities, the specific processes and mechanisms likely operating in the context. It also often allows them to locate and use population-specific data sources for particular features of organizations and their environments. Finally, institutional and historical knowledge about a population gives analysts the confidence to construct variables that periodize the population's history or classify organizations by some major feature when the available data cannot. Although such efforts do not completely eliminate the potential problems caused by unobservable heterogeneity, they surely reduce its impact.[16]

---

[16] While the single-population design might appear to hamper efforts to build general theory, this is not necessarily the case, as research in organizational ecology shows (Pfeffer 1993; Hargens 2000). What is critical for development of general theory is that the single-population studies focus on general issues and models and that the empirical findings are comparable (Carroll and Hannan 2000).

A type of heterogeneity that is particularly pronounced in corporate demography concerns the multiplicity of naturally occurring beginning and ending events that define an organization's lifetime. For example, organizations can die—cease to exist as independent entities—because of bankruptcy, voluntary disbanding, or merger. These differences may or may not be observable, but when they are, the analysis can potentially become very complicated because of the large number of possible transitions from beginning event to ending event. For instance, for European and American historical populations of automobile producers, Carroll and Hannan (2000) identify seven distinct types of life-beginning events (*de novo* founding, *de alio* entry, merger, acquisition, restart after bankruptcy, reentry, split, or spin-off) and seven types of life-ending events (disbanding, exit to another industry, merger, acquisition, takeover by creditors, nationalization, ended by war). If analyzed in its full elaboration, these data would yield 49 transitions for organizational lifetimes.

Simultaneity

Corporate demographers typically estimate each vital rate of a population in isolation from others. So, for instance, in investigating a population, an analyst might first study founding rates, then growth rates, and finally mortality rates. In any particular analysis, the prior events of other processes—or conditions that arise directly from them (e.g., density levels, which are functions of prior founding and mortality rates)—are taken as predetermined and treated as exogenous for future events.

Given precise measurement across time and weak interdependence across types of events, dealing with the various demographic processes in isolation from the other introduces no new problems. However, to the extent that data are clumped in time (temporal aggregation arising from sources such as annual industry directories) and event types are possibly interdependent, then simultaneity arises as a potential methodological challenge. For instance, theorists commonly believe that as a market grows, the carrying capacity of its associated organizational population increases. The market resources behind this increased carrying capacity might be absorbed by newly founded entrepreneurial organizations or by expansions of existing incumbent organizations. This implies that when a market expands, there is an interdependent trade-off between processes of organizational founding and organizational growth. What happens in one process directly affects the other. If the observation scheme is so precise that we can time exactly and order uniquely the events of the two processes relative to themselves and to each other, there is no problem treating prior events as predetermined (the ability to "see" and anticipate future events is also possible but related to a different issue). However, when both types of processes record events during the same (clumped or aggregated) observation period, the issue might be seen as a simultaneity problem. Unfortunately, corporate demographers have not yet widely recognized the issue and dealt with it in modeling demographic phenomena.[17] Doing so may be especially

---

[17] A similar type of simultaneity concerns institutional and political events in the broader environment, which are thought to be dependent on organizational population dynamics, as Figure 15.1 suggests. The problem here is often mitigated by the fact that events occur in the organizational population at a much higher rate than in the broader environment, thus justifying to some extent treating the latter as exogenous (Carroll and Hannan 2000).

challenging because the outcomes involved can be of different measurement types (e.g., discrete versus continuous measurement as with founding versus growth), and the processes involved might be cast at different levels of analysis (e.g., population versus organizational level as with founding versus growth). Of course, more precise measurement in the timings of events would eliminate the need to do so.

FUTURE PROSPECTS

Predicting the future of any human endeavor is always a precarious exercise, especially for an activity as intrinsically uncertain as research. Nevertheless, it is possible to look at current research trends in corporate demography and to extrapolate them into the future as what might be called default expectations. A good way to organize these future prospects is by their orientation to the theory fragments and the conceptual frameworks.

Within Theory Fragments

It can be stated with a great deal of certainty that the industrious level of research activity seen within the various theory fragments of organizational ecology will continue. The fragments have proven especially fertile in their ability to foster cumulative programmatic research and to spawn new theoretical ideas of broad interest. Seemingly simple issues, like the direction of age dependence in organizational mortality, often turn out to be much more challenging and interesting than expected, as reviewed above. Then, too, there is the demography of the researchers themselves: young talented doctoral graduates continually enter the field and make important contributions, ensuring a certain level of vitality and innovation. So it is more than reasonable to expect that corporate demography will continue to make considerable progress within the various theory fragments, as it has for the last 25 years or so.

Of the fragments reviewed above, density dependence has reached perhaps the most mature phase, meaning that its basic tenets have been accepted. This phase emerged only after a tremendous amount of research activity on the model, some heated controversy in interpretation, and considerable refinement and qualification in theory and models (see Carroll and Hannan 2000; Hannan and Carroll 1992). As a result, relevant aspects of the density model(s) are now included as controls in empirical analyses of many kinds of problems. The density dependence fragment has also generated an elaboration using weighted density variables that has proven extremely flexible for finer-grained analysis of particular organizational populations. From these developments, one might conclude that the fragment has run its course and will not spur much new research activity. However, as noted above, the fragment still faces the challenge of incorporating a generally accepted explanation of late-stage population declines and resurgences, despite some existing proposals for how to do so. On the more basic components of the theory, contemporaneous density dependence and the fixed effect of founding density, it would appear to be a rewarding time for a global assessment and comparison of findings: "enough evidence is piling up to allow soon an authoritative comparative meta-analysis of patterns of density dependence in a wide variety of organizational populations" (Carroll and Hannan 2000: 236). As with the human demographers' demographic transition, such an assessment might allow for explanation of variations in the timing and levels of density-dependent population evolution.

The structural inertia and resource-partitioning fragments are interesting contrasts to the density dependence fragment in that they show different and even unusual patterns of scientific activity. In both cases, the initial formulations of the research problem and theoretical ideas actually proceeded that of density dependence (the relevant studies are Hannan and Freeman [1984] for structural inertia, Carroll [1985] for resource partitioning, and Hannan [1986] for density dependence). However, both fragments were somewhat dormant for many years, only to be the subject of a great deal of research within the last 5 to 10 years (for a review of resource partitioning, see Carroll, Dobrev, and Swaminathan 2002; for a review of structural inertia, see Carroll and Hannan 2000: chapter 16). This new activity has strengthened the fragments' scientific bases considerably, but it also has raised many interesting questions and additional problems. For instance, whereas resource-partitioning theory originally relied only on notions of location in a crowded resource space, it now has three other mechanisms that plausibly operate, including customization, anti-mass production cultural sentiment, and conspicuous status consumption. Such developments suggest that these fragments may continue to flourish in the near future.

The future of the less developed fragments—Red Queen competition and localized competition—appears less clear. Certainly, the raw material is there for each to take off in the ways that structural inertia and resource partitioning did. But doing so may require a theoretical and empirical development not yet foreseen.

Across Theory Fragments

Perhaps the most ambitious efforts underway are those that attempt to achieve integration across the various theory fragments. Such efforts are of both an empirical and theoretical nature.

A casual or informal kind of empirical integration of findings across theory fragments often occurs as a natural matter of course. As analysts investigate specific organizational populations, they develop greater and deeper institutional understanding of the context and this leads naturally to the elaboration of models, especially when the data sets being used take years to assemble and compile. A concern in corporate demography that has arisen in the midst of such casual integration is about the cumulativity in model specifications, which is sometimes lacking (Carroll and Hannan 2000). It is likely that greater attention will be paid to this matter in the future.

More deliberate attempts at empirical integration also are of interest. These attempts occur when analysts aim to build models that explicitly take an insight from one area and confront it with that of another area using data. The following recent studies fall within this class of efforts: Barron's (1999) study of density dependence and concentration in the American credit union population; Dobrev, Kim, and Hannan's (2001) analysis of structural inertia and resource partitioning among European automobile producers; and Ruef's (2000) study of the density-dependent nature of institutional form emergence in the U.S. health care sector.

On the theoretical side, a major research program aimed at unification has also been initiated, using the tools of formal logic. As noted above, Hannan (1998) and Pólos and Hannan (2001, 2002) have already made headway using these methods to reconcile apparently contradictory evidence about age dependence. The theoretical analysis of organizational forms by Pólos, Hannan, and Carroll (2002) and of structural inertia by Hannan, Pólos, and Carroll (2003a, 2003b, 2004) attempts to build a common conceptual foundation across all the theory fragments of organizational ecology. This effort has been likened to the programs in sociology to build microfoundations to macromodels (e.g., Coleman 1990).

Across Conceptual Frameworks

In a remarkable development, several recent studies manage to bridge the broad conceptual frameworks of organizational demography sketched at the opening of the chapter. One set of studies links corporate demography and workforce demography, while the other brings together corporate demography and internal organizational demography. Given the high level of research interest in all three conceptual frameworks, it makes sense to expect that these and other cross-fertilization efforts are likely to increase in the future.

The bridge to workforce demography involves understanding how population-level vital events shape the demography of organizational labor forces. Because even a single population event might generate massive job turnover and mobility, the demography of corporations requires consideration in this research context (Carroll, Haveman, and Swaminathan 1992). A compelling empirical demonstration of the importance of population-level processes is provided by Haveman and Cohen (1994), who studied the full range of executive mobility within the California savings and loan industry from 1969 to 1988. They found that population events are "directly responsible for a large proportion of managerial job shift in the industry and affect directly a large fraction of the industry's managerial employees" (Haveman and Cohen 1994: 146).

During the period of Haveman and Cohen's (1994) study, the industry underwent deregulation, which perhaps caused a higher-than-usual number of population events. A similar study by Windzio (2001) looks at East Germany following reunification and also finds high associations of mobility with corporate demographic events. Although estimates in both studies might be heightened by their choice of observation periods, a strong association between labor mobility and population events likely exists, even in calmer times. This possibility is shown clearly by Phillips (2001) in a study of Silicon Valley law firms from 1946 to 1996. He focuses on a mechanism that he calls the "promotion paradox"—a negative relationship between the life chances of a law firm and the likelihood that an attorney will be promoted. He finds that "young, specialist and low-status firms are more likely to fail but are also contexts with the highest promotion likelihood. Moreover, except for those firms that are 'near death,' an associate's promotion likelihood increases with the law firm's probability of failure" (Philips 2001: 1058).

Two recent studies bring together internal organizational demography and corporate demography but achieve conceptual integration from the opposite ends. In the first, Haveman (1995) shows how population-level vital events can shape internal organizational demography. In the second, Sørensen (1999a, 1999b) explains how internal organizational demography can be consequential for events in the population.

Haveman (1995) proposes an ecological model of the antecedents of internal organizational demography that explains how vital events in organizational populations, such as foundings, mergers, and dissolutions, affect labor turnover and tenure distributions of executives in organizations. In the California savings and loan industry, she finds that organizational founding and failure significantly affect turnover of executives and, consequently, create shifts in firms' tenure distributions.

Sørensen (1999a, 1999b) advances a theory of recruitment-based competition that suggests that firms with similar organizational demography of top management teams, such as similar tenure distribution and managers hired from the same labor pool, experience more severe competition and, consequently, lower growth rates. The logic underlying this argument is that firms with a similar tenure distribution of top executives or with top executives hired from the same labor pool (e.g., from competitors) have employees with similar experiences and capabilities who are likely to pursue similar strategies and implement these strategies in similar ways. Homogeneity in strategic actions increases competition and decreases growth rates. Sørensen (1999a, 1999b) finds empirical confirmation to his theory on the analysis of organizational growth rates in the U.S. commercial television stations industry.

In conclusion, we return to our opening remarks, where we noted that organizational studies is a very diverse field within the social sciences and that demography is a relative newcomer to organizational studies. As our review here has shown, this observation should not be taken to imply that there is a shortage of important organizational problems and topics where demography might contribute—just the reverse. In fact, we expect that as organizational studies mature as a social science, some of its disparate approaches will disappear while others become more prominent because of their power and promise. And we have no doubt that organizational demography will be among the long-term survivors.

REFERENCES

Amburgey, T. L., T. Dacin, and D. Kelly. 1994. Disruptive selection and population segmentation: Interpopulation competition as a segregating process. In *Evolutionary dynamics of organizations*. Edited by J. Baum and J. Singh, 240–245. New York: Oxford University Press.

Amburgey, T. L., D. Kelly, and W. P. Barnett. 1993. Resetting the clock: The dynamics of organizational change and failure. *Administrative Science Quarterly* 38:51–73.

Barnett, W. P. 1997. The dynamics of competitive intensity. *Administrative Science Quarterly* 42:128–160.

Barnett, W. P., J. N. Baron, and T. E. Stuart. 2000. Avenues of attainment: Occupational demography and organizational careers in the California Civil Service. *American Journal of Sociology* 106:88–144.

Barnett, W. P., and G. R. Carroll. 1995. Modeling internal organizational change. *Annual Review of Sociology* 21:217–236.

Barnett, W. P., and M. T. Hansen. 1996. The Red Queen in organizational evolution. *Strategic Management Journal* 17:139–157.

Barnett, W. P., and D. G. McKendrick. 2001. The organizational evolution of global technological competition. Report 2001–02. San Diego: Information Storage Industry Center, University of California.

Barnett W. P., and O. Sorenson. 2002. The Red Queen in organizational creation and development. *Industrial and Corporate Change* 11:289–325.

Baron, J. N. 1984. Organizational perspectives on stratification. *Annual Review of Sociology* 10:37–69.

Baron, J. N., M. T. Hannan, and M. D. Burton. 2001. Labor pains: Change in organizational models and employee turnover in young, high-tech firms. *American Journal of Sociology* 106:960–1012.

Baron, J. N., and A. E. Newman. 1990. For what it's worth: Organizations, occupations, and the value of work done by women and nonwhites. *American Sociological Review* 55:155–175.

Barron, D. N. 1999. The structuring of organizational populations. *American Sociological Review* 64:421–445.

Barron, D. N., E. West, and M. T. Hannan. 1994. A time to grow and a time to die: Growth and mortality of credit unions in New York, 1914–1990. *American Journal of Sociology* 100:381–421.

Baum, J. A. C. and S. J. Mezias. 1992. Localized competition and organizational failure in the Manhattan hotel industry, 1898–1990. *Administrative Science Quarterly* 37:580–604.

Baum, J. A. C. and J. V. Singh. 1994. Organizational niches and the dynamics of organizational mortality. *American Journal of Sociology* 100:346–380.

Bigelow, L. S., G. R. Carroll, M-D. Seidel, and L. Tsai. 1997. Legitimation, geographical scale, and organizational density: Regional patterns of foundings of American automobile producers, 1885–1981. *Social Science Research* 26:377–398.

Boone, C., V. Bröchler, and G. R. Carroll. 2000. Custom service: Application and tests of resource-partitioning theory among dutch auditing firms from 1986 to 1992. *Organization Studies* 21:355–381.

Boone C., G. R. Carroll, and A. van Witteloostuijn. 2002. Resource distributions and market partioning: Dutch daily newspapers, 1968 to 1994. *American Sociological Review* 67:408–431.

Boone, C., and W. Van Olffen. 1997. The confusing state of the art in top management composition studies: A theoretical and empirical review. Research Memorandum No. 97–11. Netherlands Institute of Business Organization and Strategy, Maastricht.

Brüderl, J., and R. Schüssler. 1990. Organizational mortality: The liabilities of newness and adolescence. *Administrative Science Quarterly* 35:530–547.

Burt, R. S. 1992. *Structural holes: The social structure of competition.* Cambridge, Mass.: Harvard University Press.

Carroll, G. R. 1983. A stochastic model of organizational mortality: Review and reanalysis. *Social Science Research* 12:303–329.

Carroll, G. R. 1985. Concentration and specialization: Dynamics of niche width in populations of organizations. *American Journal of Sociology* 90:1262–1283.

Carroll, G. R. 1997. Long-term evolutionary change in organizational populations. *Industrial and Corporate Change* 6:119–143.

Carroll, G. R., and J. Delacroix. 1982. Organizational mortality in the newspaper industries of Argentina and Ireland: An ecological approach. *Administrative Science Quarterly* 27:169–198.

Carroll, G. R., S. Dobrev, and A. Swaminathan. 2002. Organizational processes of resource partitioning. *Research in Organizational Behavior* 24:1–40.

Carroll, G. R., and M. T. Hannan. 1989. Density delay in the evolution of organizational populations: A model and five empirical tests. *Administrative Science Quarterly* 34:411–430.

Carroll, G. N. R., and M. T. Hannan. 2000. *The demography of corporations and industries.* Princeton N.J.: Princeton University Press.

Carroll, G. R., and J. R. Harrison. 1998. Organizational demography and culture: Insights from a formal model and simulation. *Administrative Science Quarterly* 43:637–667.

Carroll, G. N. R., H. A. Haveman, and A. Swaminathan. 1990. Karrieren in Organizationen: Eine okologische Perspektive. *Kölner Zeitschrift für Soziologie und Sozialpsychologie* (Sonderheft) 31:146–178.

Carroll, G. R., H. A. Haveman, and A. Swaminathan. 1992. Careers in organizations: An ecological view. In *Life-span development and behavior*, Vol. 11. Edited by D. Featherman et al., 111–144. Hillsdale, N.J.: Earlbaum.

Carroll, G. R., and A. Swaminathan. 2000. Why the microbrewery movement? Organizational dynamics of resource partitioning in the American brewing industry after prohibition. *American Journal of Sociology* 106:715–1762.

Cole, S. 2001. What's wrong with sociology? In *What's wrong with Sociology?* Edited by S. Cole. New Brunswick, N.J.: Transaction.

Coleman, J. S. 1990. *Foundations of social theory.* Cambridge, Mass.: Harvard University Press.

Delacroix, J., and A. Swaminathan. 1991. Cosmetic, speculative, and adaptive organizational change in the wine industry: A longitudinal study. *Administrative Science Quarterly* 36:631–661.

Dobrev, S. D., and G. R. Carroll. 2003. Size (and competition) among organizations: Modeling scale-based selection among automobile producers in four major countries, 1885–1981. *Strategic Management Journal*, 24: 541–558.

Dobrev, S. D., T-Y. Kim, and G. R. Carroll. 2002. The evolution of organizational niches: U.S. Automobile Manufacturers, 1885–1981. *Administrative Science Quarterly* 47:233–264.

Dobrev, S. D., T-Y. Kim, M. T. Hannan. 2001. Dynamics of niche width and resource partitioning. *American Journal of Sociology* 106:1299–1337.

Doeringer, P. B., and M. J. Piore. 1971. *Internal labor markets and manpower analysis.* Lexington, Mass.: Heath.

Fichman, M., and D. A. Levinthal. 1991. Honeymoons and the liability of adolescence: A new perspective on duration dependence in social and organizational relationships. *Academy of Management Review* 16:442–468.

Finkelstein, S., and D. Hambrick. 1996. *Strategic leadership.* St. Paul, Minn.: West.

Flatt, S. 1993. The innovative edge: How top management team demography makes a difference. Unpublished doctoral thesis. Berkeley: University of California.

Freeman, J., G. R. Carroll, and M. T. Hannan. 1983. The liability of newness: Age dependence in organizational death rates. *American Sociological Review* 48:692–710.

Freeman, J., and M. T. Hannan. 1983. Niche width and the dynamics of organizational populations. *American Journal of Sociology* 88:1116–1145.

Glick, W. H., C. C. Miller, and G. P. Huber. 1993. The import of upper-echelon diversity on organizational performance. In *Organizational change and redesign.* Edited by G. P. Hubber and W. H. Glick, 176–214. New York: Oxford University Press.

Hambrick, D. C., T. S. Cho, and M-J. Chen. 1996. The influence of top management heterogeneity on firms' competitive moves. *Administrative Science Quarterly* 41:659–684.

Han, J. 1998. The evolution of the Japanese banking industry: An ecological analysis, 1873–1945. Ph.D. dissertation. Palo Alto, Calif.: Stanford University.

Hannan, M. T. 1986. Competitive and institutional processes in organizational ecology. Technical Report 86–13. Ithaea, N. O.: Cornell University, Department of Sociology.

Hannan, M. T. 1997. Inertia, density and the structure of organizational populations: Entries in European automobile industries, 1886–1981. *Organization Studies* 18:193–228.

Hannan, M. T. 1998. Rethinking age dependence in organizational mortality: Logical formalizations. *American Journal of Sociology* 104:85–123.

Hannan, M. T., and G. R. Carroll. 1992. *Dynamics of organizational populations: Density, legitimation, and competition.* New York Oxford: Oxford University Press.

Hannan, M. T., and G. R. Carroll. 1995. Theory building and cheap talk about legitimation: Reply to Baum and Powell. *American Sociological Review* 60:539–545.

Hannan, M. T., G. R. Carroll, S. D. Dobrev, and J. Han. 1998a. Organizational mortality in European and American automobile industries. Part I. Revisiting the effects of age and size. *European Sociological Review* 14:279–302.

Hannan, M. T., G. R. Carroll, S. D. Dobrev, J. Han, and J. C. Torres. 1998b. Organizational mortality in European and American automobile industries. Part II. Coupled clocks. *European Sociological Review* 14:303–313.

Hannan, M. T., G. R. Carroll, E. A. Dundon, and J. C. Torres. 1995. Organizational evolution in a multinational context: Entries of automobile manufacturers in Belgium, Britain, France, Germany, and Italy. *American Sociological Review* 60:509–528.

Hannan, M. T., G. R. Carroll, and L. Pólos. 2003. The organizational niche. *Sociological Theory*, forthcoming.

Hannan, M. T., and J. Freeman. 1977. The population ecology of organizations. *American Journal of Sociology* 82:929–964.

Hannan, M. T., and J. Freeman. 1984. Structural inertia and organizational change. *American Sociological Review* 49:149–164.

Hannan, M. T., and J. Freeman. 1989. *Organizational Ecology.* Cambridge, Mass.: Harvard University Press.

Hannan, M. T., L. Pólos, and G. R. Carroll. 2003a. Cascading organizational change. *Organization Science* 14:463–482.

Hannan, M. T., L. Pólos, and G. R. Carroll. 2003b. The fog of change: Opacity and asperity in organizations. *Administrative Science Quarterly* 48:399–432.

Hannan, M. T., L. Pólos and G. R. Carroll. 2004. The evolution of inertia. *Industrial and Corporate Change* 13:117–148.

Hannan, M. T., J. Ranger-Moore, and J. Banaszak-Holl. 1990. Competition and the evolution of organizational size distributions. In *Organizational evolution: New directions.* Edited by J. Singh, 246–268. Newbury Park, Calif.: Sage.

Hargens, L. L. 2000. Using the literature: Reference networks, reference contexts and the social structure of scholarship. *American Sociological Review* 65:846–865.

Hauser, P. M., and O. D. Duncan. 1959. *The study of population.* Chicago: University of Chicago Press.

Haveman, H. A. 1992. Between a rock and a hard place: Organizational change and performance under conditions of fundamental environmental transformation. *Administrative Science Quarterly* 37:48–75.

Haveman, H. A. 1995. The demographic metabolism of organizations: Industry dynamics, turnover, and tenure distributions. *Administrative Science Quarterly* 40:586–618.

Haveman, H. A., and L. E. Cohen. 1994. The ecological dynamics of careers: The impact of organizational founding, dissolution, and merger on job mobility. *American Journal of Sociology* 100:104–152.

Hedstrom, P. 1992. Is organizational ecology at an impasse? Review of *Dynamics of Organizational Populations* by M. T. Hannan and G. R. Carroll. *Contemporary Sociology* 21:751–753.

Ingram, P., and T. Simons. 2000. State formation, ideological competition, and the ecology of Israeli workers cooperatives, 1920–1992. *Administrative Science Quarterly* 45:25–53.

Jaffee, J. 2000. The resource partitioning of a corporate legal market: The proliferation of specialist law firms in Silicon Valley, 1966–1997. Presented at American Sociological Association Meetings, August, Washington, D.C.

Keck, S. L. 1997. Top management team structure: Differential effects by environmental context. *Organization Science* 8: 143–156.

Keyfitz, N. 1973. Individual mobility in a stationary population. *Population Studies* 27:335–352.

Keyfitz, N. 1977. *Applied mathematical demography*. New York: Wiley.

Larson, E. L. 2001. *Evolution's workshop: God and science on the Galapagos Islands*. New York: Basic Books.

Lawrence , B. S. 1997. The black box of organizational demography. *Organization Science* 8:1–22.

Levitt, B., and J. G. March 1988. Organizational learning. *Annual Review of Sociology* 14:319–340.

March, J. 1991. Exploration and exploitation in organizational learning. *Organization Science* 2:71–87.

McCain, B., C. A. O'Reilly, and J. Pfeffer. 1983. The effects of departmental demography on turnover. *Administrative Science Quarterly* 26:626–641.

McKendrick, D. G., and G. R. Carroll. 2001. On the genesis of organizational forms: Evidence from the market for dick drive arrays. *Organization Science* 12:661–682.

McPherson, M. 1983. An ecology of affiliation. *American Sociological Review* 48:519–532.

Melville H. 1987. The Encantadas, or Enchanted Islands. In *The piazza tales and other prose pieces 1839–1860*, 125–173. Evanston and Chicago: Northwestern University Press.

Meyer, J. W., and B. Rowan. 1977. Institutionalized organizations: Formal structure as myth and ceremony. *American Journal of Sociology* 83:340–363.

Minkoff, D. C. 1999. Bending with the wind: Change and adaptation for women's and racial minority organizations. *American Journal of Sociology* 104:1666–1703.

Nelson, R., and S. Winter. 1982. *An evolutionary theory of economic change*. Cambridge, Mass.: Harvard University Press.

Olzak, S., and S. C. N. Uhrig. 2001. The ecology of tactical overlap among new social movements in West Germany. *American Sociological Review* 66:694–718.

O'Reilly, C. A., D. Caldwell, and W. P. Barnett. 1989. Work group demography, social integration, and turnover. *Administrative Science Quarterly* 34:21–37.

Park, D., and J. M. Podolny. 2000. The competitive dynamics of status and niche width: U.S. investment banking, 1920–1950. *Industrial and Corporate Change* 9:377–414.

Péli, G. 1997. The niche hikers guide to population ecology: A reconstruction of niche theory using logic. In *Sociological methodology 1997*. Edited by A. Raftery, 1–46. Cambridge, Mass.: Blackwell.

Péli, G., L. Pólos, and M. T. Hannan. 2000. Back to inertia: Theoretical implications of alternative styles of logical formalization. *Sociological Theory* 18:193–213.

Péli, G., and B. Nooteboom. 1999. Market partitioning and the geometry of resource space. *American Journal of Sociology* 104:1132–1153.

Petersen, T., and L. A. Morgan. 1995. Separate and unequal: Occupation-establishment sex segregation and the gender wage gap. *American Journal of Sociology* 101:329–366.

Pfeffer, J. 1983. Organizational demography. In *Research in organizational behavior*, Vol. 5. Edited by L. Cummings and B. Staw, 299–357. Greenwich, Conn.: JAI.

Pfeffer, J. 1993. Barriers to the advance of organizational science: Paradigm development as a dependent variable. *Academy of Management Review* 18:599–620.

Pfeffer, J., and G. R. Salancik. 1978. *The external control of organizations*. New York: Harper & Row.

Phillips, D. J. 2001. The promotion paradox: Organizational mortality and employee promotion chances in Silicon Valley law firms, 1946–1996. *American Journal of Sociology* 106:1058–1098.

Podolny, J. M. 1993. A status-based model of market competition. *American Journal of Sociology* 98:829–872.

Podolny, J. M., T. E. Stuart, and M. T. Hannan. 1996. Networks, knowledge, and niches: Competition in the worldwide semiconductor industry, 1984–1991. *American Journal of Sociology* 102:659–689.

Pólos, L., and M. T. Hannan. 2001. Nonmonotonicity in theory building. In *Dynamics of organizations: Computational modeling and organization theory*. Edited by A. Lomi and E. Larsen, 405–438. Cambridge, Mass.: MIT Press.

Pólos, L., and M. T. Hannan. 2002. Reasoning with partial knowledge. In *Sociological methodology 2002*. Edited by R. M. Stolzenberg, 133–182. Cambridge: Blackwell.

Pólos, L., M. T. Hannan, and G. R. Carroll. 2002. Foundations of a theory of social forms. *Industrial and Corporate Change* 11:85–115.

Ranger-Moore J., R. S. Breckenridge, and D. L. Jones. 1995. Patterns of growth and size-localized competition in the New York State life insurance industry, 1860–1985. *Social Forces* 73:1027–1049.

Ruef, M. 2000. The emergence of organizational forms: A community ecology approach. *American Journal of Sociology* 106:658–714.

Singh, J. V., D. J. Tucker, and R. J. House. 1986. Organizational legitimacy and the liability of newness. *Administrative Science Quarterly* 31:171–93.

Smith, K. G., K. A. Smith, J. D. Olian, H. P. Sims, D. P. O'Bannon, and J. A. Scully. 1994. Top management team demography and process: The role of social integration and communication. *Administrative Science Quarterly* 39:412–438.

Sørensen, J. B. 1999a. Executive migration and interorganizational competition. *Social Science Research* 28:289–315.

Sørensen, J. B. 1999b. The ecology of organizational demography: Managerial tenure distributions and organizational competition. *Industrial and Corporate Change* 8:713–744.

Sørensen, J. B. 2000. The longitudinal effects of group tenure composition on turnover. *American Sociological Review* 65:298–310.

Sørensen, J. B. 2002. The use and misuse of the coefficient of variation in organizational demography research. *Sociological Methods and Research* 30:475–491.

Sørensen, J. B., and T. E. Stuart. 2000. Aging, obsolescence and organizational innovation. *Administrative Science Quarterly* 45:81–112.

Sorenson, O., and P. G. Audia. 2000. The social structure of entrepreneurial activity: Geographic concentration of footwear production in the U.S., 1940–1989. *American Journal of Sociology*, 106:424–469.

Sorenson, O., and T. E. Stuart. 2001. Syndication networks and the spatial distribution of venture capital investment. *American Journal of Sociology* 106:1546–1588.

Stinchcombe, A. L. 1965. Social structure and organizations. In *Handbook of organizations*. Edited by J. March, 142–193. Chicago: Rand McNally.

Swaminathan, A., and J. Wade, 2001. Social movement theory and the evolution of new organizational forms. In *The Entrepreneurship dynamic: Origins of entrepreneurship and the evolution of industries*. Edited by C. B. Schoonhoven and E. Romanelli, 286–313. Palo Alto, Calif.: Stanford University Press.

Tuma, N. B., and M. T. Hannan. 1984. *Social dynamics: Models and methods*. Orlando, Fla.: Academic Press.

Wagner, W. G., J. Pfeffer, and C. A. O'Reilly. 1984. Organizational demography and turnover in top-management groups. *Administrative Science Quarterly* 29:74–92.

Weber, M. 1968. *Economy and society: An outline of interpretive sociology*. 3 vols. New York: Bedmeister. [Originally published in 1924].

Wiersema, M., and A. Bird. 1993. Organizational demography in Japanese firms: Group heterogeneity, individual dissimilarity and top management turnover. *Academy of Management Journal* 36:996–1025.

Windzio, M. 2001. Organisationsökologie und Arbeitsmarktmobilität im sozialen Wandel. Eine empirische Analyse am Beispiel Ostdeutschlands. *Zeitschrift für Soziologie* 30:116–134.

Zuckerman, E. W. 1999. The categorical imperative: Securities analysts and the legitimacy discount. *American Journal of Sociology* 104:1398–1438.

CHAPTER 16

Urban and Spatial Demography

MARK FOSSETT

The spatial distribution of populations has long been a central focus of demographic inquiry. Structured patterns in spatial distribution are evident from the highest levels of macrospatial scale (e.g., global, national, and regional urban systems) to "fine-grained" patterns in metropolitan areas (e.g., central cities, suburbs, neighborhoods, and blocks) and nonmetropolitan hinterlands (e.g., towns, villages, and hamlets). The task of documenting and explaining these patterns has occupied the attention of sociologists, economists, and geographers, and their efforts have established a body of knowledge that is impressive for its cumulative nature, rigorous theoretical underpinnings, and extensive evidentiary base.

Without question, the dominant feature of spatial distribution in the United States and other developed countries is the concentration of population in densely settled urban areas. Not only do metropolitan centers contain the greatest share of the population in developed countries, these centers also exert influence over life in nonmetropolitan and rural areas. This occurs to such a degree that it is difficult to classify a significant portion of the population in a country such as the United States as nonurban in the sense that term would have evoked just a century ago. If nonurban is taken to mean populations living in low-density, small-scale communities that are largely self-sufficient in economic organization and substantially closed in terms of social organization, then nonurban populations are rare in developed countries. The daily rhythms of social and economic life of the vast majority of the population are fundamentally organized by, and integrated with, social and economic activity in metropolitan centers. Accordingly, this chapter focuses primarily on inter- and intrametropolitan spatial distribution. The chapter is also restricted to developed countries. It will not review the patterns and trends of urban and spatial distribution in developing countries, which easily could be the object of a separate paper.[1]

CONCEPTUAL FRAMEWORKS

Several theoretical frameworks guide the demographic understanding of urban and spatial patterns. Four major perspectives will be reviewed and comments will be offered on a fifth. The first three of these, namely, regional and urban economics, human and urban ecology, and urban geography, have long informed demographic perspectives on urban and spatial distribution and may be referred to as "traditional" or "conventional" demographic perspectives. A fourth perspective may be grouped under the heading of "critical and political-economic perspectives." Finally, there is a fifth approach representing sociocultural and postmodern views of the city. These last two perspectives are sometimes cast as standing in opposition to traditional demographic perspectives. In fact, however, insights emanating from them tend to supplement or complement insights from the traditional perspectives and do not force an "either-or-choice" between incompatible theoretical perspectives.

Urban Economics, Economic Geography, and Regional Science Perspectives

Urban economics, land economics, economic geography, and regional science apply the conceptual tools and theoretical methodology of economic analysis to derive implications for the spatial distribution of land use and population. Isard (1956, 1960) and Alonso (1964) provide statements on the spatial analysis of economic activity that integrate earlier influential work in the field (e.g., Hoover 1948; Zipf 1949; Weber 1929; and Christaller 1966). Cumulative theoretical advances continued through the 1960s and 1970s with important contributions by Muth (1969), Mills (1967, 1972), Henderson (1974), Thompson (1965), and Friedman and Alonso (1964). Recently, important work includes theoretical and empirical studies focusing on the spatial aspects of the economy (e.g., Krugman 1991; Fujita 1989; Fujita, Krugman, and Venables 1999; Black and Henderson 1999) and integrative reviews of the state of the field (e.g., Anas, Arnott, and Small 1998; Huriot and Thisse 2000; Fujita and Thisse 2002; Henderson and Thisse 2004).

Two important examples of the application of this perspective are central place theory and its implications for the spatial distribution of a population in an urban system and the theory of rents and its implications for the spatial distribution of economic actors within urban areas. The former builds on relatively simple assumptions about the costs associated with the movement of people, goods, and information in an idealized spatial domain to deduce patterns of population distribution into a cascading hierarchy of population centers arranged geometrically in space around central nodes. The latter also uses formal theoretical models to show that distinctive patterns of differentiated land use, economic activity, and population distribution emerge within urban areas based

---

[1] Recent reviews of urbanization in developing countries from different perspectives include Dogan and Kasarda (1988c), Kasarda and Crenshaw (1991), Roberts (1989), Knox (1995), Knox and Taylor (1995), Timberlake (1985), Sassen (1994), and Lo and Yeung (1998).

on the varying requirements of spatial actors and their differing ability to compete for spatial locations. Formulations such as the Alonso-Muth-Mills model of the monocentric city and the Krugman-Fujita-Thisse models of the new economic geography provide elegant descriptions of cities of the past. But more importantly, they provide a rigorous foundation for understanding ongoing transformations in the macrospatial arrangements in systems of cities and in the internal spatial organization of cities.

Human and Urban Ecological Perspectives

Human ecology and its subfield of urban ecology are the central perspectives informing the sociological understanding of population (Namboodiri 1988; Poston and Frisbie 1998), especially the dimension of spatial distribution (Berry and Kasarda 1977; Frisbie and Kasarda 1988). The "classic" form was set forth in the first half of the 20th century in the writings of Robert Park (1936a), Ernest Burgess (1925), and Roderick McKenzie (1924, 1926, 1933), along with other scholars who were inspired by, and drew on concepts from, evolutionary and ecological theory in biology. Subsequently, Otis Dudley Duncan (1959, 1964), and most especially Amos Hawley (1944a, 1950), recast the perspective in its present "neoclassical" form. It has been refined and carried forward by many influential figures. Without question, however, the dominant theoretical vision has been enunciated in the writings of Hawley (1968, 1971, 1984, 1986).

Hawley espouses a fundamentally materialistic view (1984, 1986) that focuses on macrolevel social organization rooted in and shaped by "human sustenance relations." The scope of human ecology is intentionally restricted (Hawley 1950: 73–74) and employs a small set of carefully chosen assumptions and concepts to pursue testable propositions about macrostructural processes such as functional differentiation in human populations, spatial differentiation within urban systems, metropolitan expansion, and the emergence of hierarchy and subordinate-dominant relations in urban systems. The strategy of limiting attention to a small number of organizing principles has served the ecological perspective well and has warded off problems of mysticism and teleology that plague some functionalist perspectives. At the same time, however, its narrow focus has inspired some critics to charge that it neglects important questions (Feagin 1998) and engages in technological reductionism and offers incomplete explanations of sociospatial patterns (Gottdeiner and Hutchinson 2000).

The ecological perspective is compatible with regional and urban economic perspectives, so much so in fact that proponents went to some lengths (e.g., Hawley 1944a, 1950) to point out that ecological principles involve more than the application of economic analysis (Gibbs and Martin 1959). One distinction is the ecological view that human communities adapt to their environment as a collectivity, and not as calculating individuals. As Hawley (1950) notes, humans not only have the capacity for social affiliation and nonrational attachments to other individuals and groups; this capacity is fundamental to their nature and is crucial to their survival. This impetus is expressed in social ties based on family, extended kinship, ethnicity, culture, and common interest. These rational and nonrational bases of sociality and affiliation give rise to group formation and social organization over and above what can be anticipated on the basis of narrowly circumscribed economic considerations. Thus, "the ecological viewpoint is that of individuals and groups seeking position in a developing system of relations" (Hawley 1950: 73). Signicantly, group-level adaptation can give rise to

group-based competition for "dominance" within ecological systems (Fossett and
Cready 1998: 169–174; Hawley 1950: 209–221; Noel 1968; Hannan 1979).

In short, human ecology draws heavily on insights from urban and regional
economics but directs theory and attention to a wider range of social phenomena.
Ecologists give attention to the potential spatial implications of diversity in ethnic
culture, social status, and the values, interests, preferences, and tastes associated with
social groupings. And ecologists invoke notions of competition that subsume not only
the dynamics of market processes but also intergroup competition and individual- and
group-based behavior that occur outside the framework of markets (e.g., conflict,
discrimination, protest, etc.). On this point, also see chapter 20, "Ecological Demography," in this *Handbook*.

Geography

The contributions of geographers to the understanding of spatial population distributions have changed considerably over time. In the 1960s and 1970s a cadre of geographers
heeded the call of Garrison (1959, 1960) and endeavored to extend economic and
ecological perspectives guiding geographical understandings of urban and regional population distributions. Yeates (2001) describes this as the emergence of a distinctive and
influential "Chicago School" of urban geography. Like the earlier "Chicago School" of
sociology, it was characterized by a coherent vision regarding theory, methodology, and
research agenda. Berry was visible in this movement and published prolifically on population distribution both within and between urban regions and urban areas. He collaborated with Horton (Berry and Horton 1970) and later with Kasarda (Berry and Kasarda
1977) on major integrative statements. Other influential contributions from this era (e.g.,
Haggett 1965; Chorley and Haggett 1967; Abler, Adams, and Gould 1971; Bourne 1971;
and Bourne and Simmons 1978) reflect the flowering of formal theoretical development
and quantitative research. While the impact of the this work was far reaching, the
discipline of geography, even more than sociology, fragmented in the 1970s and 1980s
as "critical" and "political economic" perspectives exemplified by Harvey's *Social Justice
and the City* (1973) deflected attention away from demographic perspectives on urban
systems and spatial patterns. Still, these interests continue to be pursued within the
specialty areas of urban geography and economic geography.

The more influential contributions coming from geography in recent decades are in
the areas of specialized techniques and methodologies such as techniques of quantitative
spatial analysis, the compilation of multidisciplinary geographical information system
data bases, advances in techniques for manipulating and visually representing spatial
data, and the analysis of data generated from aerial and satellite photography and
remote sensing. And, as noted earlier in the discussion of urban economics and regional
science, economic geographers are contributing to the refinement of theories of spatial
distribution.

Political Economic and Critical Perspectives

From the early decades of the 20th century through at least the 1960s the field of urban
sociology was dominated by the urban ecological perspective. This began to change

dramatically in the 1970s, and by the 1980s the work of scholars drawing on "political economic and critical perspectives" was receiving equal or greater attention in journals and in urban sociology textbooks. Loosely coalescing around such works as Logan and Molotch (1987), Gordon (1977, 1984), Hill (1977), Molotch (1976), Harvey (1973), Feagin (1985, 1988, 1998), Gottdeiner (1983, 1985), Gottdeiner and Feagin (1988), Castells (1977, 1985), Smith and Feagin (1987, 1995), Tabb and Sawyers (1984), Walton (1979, 1981, 1993), Scott (1988), and others, this new perspective is really many perspectives. Scholars seeking to stake out new ground apart from the traditional perspectives are doing so in different ways, often disagreeing among themselves on key issues. As yet, no dominant vision has integrated and consolidated the differing points of view, as has occurred in urban economics, regional science, and urban ecology.

Given the diversity of viewpoints it is instructive to note what is not embraced. Most eschew the models that undergird urban and regional economics and reject the functionalist orientations of ecology and economics and their reliance on notions of adaptation and equilibrium. They also tend to be skeptical of the emphasis traditional demographic perspectives place on technological change as the major factor providing the impetus for new equilibrium arrangements in the spatial distribution of population. Some are more open to traditional demographic perspectives than others. Smith (1995), for example, searches for common ground between traditional and new perspectives and suggests that "a reexamination of the old urban sociology may highlight some areas of theoretical overlap and continuity that are underappreciated and may provide real opportunities for the new urban sociologists to learn from urban ecology." In general, followers of the new "paradigm" studiously avoid drawing on the concepts and theoretical language of traditional demographic perspectives.

By way of a more positive identification, Jaret (1983: 499–503) notes the following rallying points in theory for those working in political economic and critical perspectives: an interpretation of urban structure and processes as "shaped by and rooted in the capital accumulation process," a focus on class conflict and social inequality, and the guiding hypothesis that urban and social problems reflect the "contradictions and limitations of capitalism." More broadly, he characterizes these scholars as seeing technological innovation, population redistribution, and urban transformations as driven by "capitalists' need for a large, cheap, easily controlled labor force and ever increased production" (1983:499). These perspectives also give more attention to the role of the state in urban patterns and the spatial distribution of population, although there is not complete agreement on the question of the degree to which the state is an autonomous actor or merely a reflection of capitalist interests.

There is another defining characteristic of critical perspectives which was alluded to earlier; they tend to address different questions and emphasize different issues than traditional economic and ecological perspectives. Specifically, there is a greater focus on issues of social inequality, concentration of power, uneven development, discrimination, and other contemporary social problems. In many ways, critics' objections to traditional perspectives may be traced as much to their dissatisfaction with the *questions* selected for attention as to the specific theories and empirical findings they develop in pursuing them. Feagin (1998: 185), for example, notes that some major statements in the field provide "no significant discussion of inequality, conflict, or poverty" and the field as a whole "has not dealt adequately with such critical factors in urban development as inequality, class conflict, vested capitalist interests operating in space, and government subsidy programs that are pro-real estate." On this point, there is a difference of approach and emphasis that would appear on the surface to be substantial. At a minimum, there does not seem to be much consensus regarding which problems should get attention. It may be fair to say that traditional and critical perspectives differ with regard to the balance between advancing general understanding by developing formal theory and abstract models and focusing attention on questions that bear more directly on contemporary social problems.

A major insight offered by political economic and critical theorists is that there is more to urban and spatial population distributions than the impersonal working of laissez-faire economics and the often (but not necessarily) decentralized population dynamics of human and urban ecology. The state, powerful institutional actors, and elites with vested interests of various kinds can and do play roles in shaping spatial population distributions. Traditional demographic perspectives are not well equipped to pursue that insight and tend to focus instead on what is likely to occur when law, regulation, and strategic interventions by powerful actors exert limited or moderate influence. A key difference, however, is that traditional perspectives set forth clear predictions regarding their theories' implications for spatial distribution. In contrast, new perspectives do not generate clear *a priori* expectations about spatial patterns. Their insight that the state and powerful actors have the *capacity* to shape spatial patterns is hardly controversial. What is less clear is whether the new perspectives offer compelling arguments that the actions of the state, institutional actors, and elites are likely to give rise to predictable, systematic spatial patterns that differ markedly from those predicted by traditional demographic perspectives.

In sum, critical and political economic perspectives address a void in the literature by investigating how powerful actors can exploit, manipulate, and distort spatial patterns predicted by traditional perspectives. They make the case that spatial distributions can be influenced by state decisions regarding the siting of military installations, universities, prisons, defense industries, dams, and other large-scale, public investments. Likewise, they make the case that institutions and elites can use political power and chicanery to influence spatial distributions by affecting the siting of airports, the development of harbors, the specific location of highway interchanges, tax subsidies to particular industries, incentives for downtown development projects, and so on. Critical and political economic perspectives are less successful when they suggest that insights from traditional economic and ecological perspectives are obsolete.

Sociocultural and Postmodern Perspectives

Before the rise of critical and political economic perspectives, there was an earlier sociocultural critique of economic and urban ecological theories. One of the most influential contributors to this view was Firey (1945, 1947), who showed that culture, symbolic meaning, and sentiment shaped spatial patterns in the center of the city of Boston, an area where conventional perspectives would predict that the intensity of land use would be at its maximum. The key insight of the sociocultural perspective is that even in secular, market-oriented capitalist societies, all land is not "in play" and subject to use determined solely by impersonal market forces. In societies where religion and tradition govern social relationships, the insight may be crucial. Understanding the cultural system may be fundamental for delineating land use and spatial patterns.

There are at least some parallels between the sociocultural perspective and the more recent literature examining the city from a postmodern vantage point (e.g., Dear and Flusty 1998; Dear 2000; Soja 1997, 2000). Both views stress that urban form and spatial distributions are guided by cultural values as well as by the factors identified in traditional spatial theories. However, where Firey's study points to the persistence of cultural values rooted in tradition and sentimental attachments to the past, postmodernist views point to a much wider range of cultural possibilities. This new view stresses that increasing wealth and technological advancement are freeing spatial arrangements from economic and material constraints and breaking down the importance of historically grounded sentiment and tradition. Consequently, an expanding array of "discretionary" cultural values may vie to influence land use and spatial distribution.

There is no denying the core insight of these perspectives; spatial arrangements can and are influenced by culture, symbolism, and sentiment. Guest (1984) is substantially correct, however, when he concludes that the sociocultural position (and, it may be added, postmodern views) can easily be overdrawn and do not seriously challenge the insights of traditional economic and ecological perspectives unless they are incorrectly construed as excluding other factors accounting for the spatial distribution of population. That is, while the impact of culture, tradition, and sentiment are evident, they are expressed in limited and highly selective ways and are not the dominant force in spatial patterns. At present it is too early to say that emerging spatial arrangements are divorced from the economic and ecological principles that served to organize them in the past.

Overview

In the remainder of this chapter, most of the attention will be directed to discussions of theory, methods, and research that fall squarely in the traditional demographic perspectives on urban and spatial distribution. Contrary to the views of some proponents of new perspectives, their best contributions tend to be supplementary and complementary, not substitutive. Traditional demographic perspectives remain vital and continue to stand as the central perspective for understanding urban and spatial population distributions.

THE SUCCESS OF CITIES: NODE AND HINTERLAND

Without question, the contemporary developed world is predominantly urban. Cities have proven to be enormously successful social inventions. They dominate spatial population patterns because they confer adaptive advantages to their populations by greatly facilitating communication, social interaction, trade, economic production, and administration. From their earliest inception, cities were imbedded in broader macrospatial systems. Fixed populations of any consequence must necessarily have extensive relationships with the outlying populations that sustain them with surplus food and resources. Thus, cities have never been isolated entities. They always are linked in a division of labor with hinterlands—that is to say that outlying regions socially, economically and, often but not necessarily, politically are integrated with urban centers. City and hinterland form a coherent unit of social organization. In the language of ecology they constitute a nodal-functional region that may be viewed as a relatively self-contained system.

When one views the burgeoning metropolitan areas of the present era, it is easy to lose sight of the fact that for most of human experience cities were hardly inevitable or enduring. Keyfitz (1965) points out that while the capacity to generate a stable agricultural surplus is a precondition for cities to emerge, the potential for urbanization often went unrealized for long periods of time. Thus, cities were possible but not inevitable forms of social organization. When cities did arise and prosper, history shows that their persistence was precarious. It is sobering to contemplate that most ancient cities thrived for a time and then disappeared, never to arise again. For this reason, demographic perspectives view the functional system of city and hinterland merely as an empirical possibility and do not take for granted the question of how organized populations adapt to their environment. This should dispel the charge that has been made that economic and ecological theory holds a mystical view of functional systems that obscures human agency (Gottdeinner and Hutchinson 2000). The social relations binding node and hinterland into a functional system are not inevitable. History has shown that they may not cohere and, when they do, may not necessarily endure.

Cities may grow through two primary processes. One is through expansion, that is, the process whereby the influence of the urban center is extended over an increasingly large hinterland. In the case of the most important cities, this often includes other urban centers. In expansion, new territory and population are drawn into the network of social interactions and interdependencies directly and indirectly coordinated by the dominant urban center. In one extreme exemplified in the imperial city, the incorporation of outlying populations is brought about by political compulsion and force. Alternatively, incorporation may emerge out of mutual benefit through exchange and trade. Either can give rise to a functionally integrated spatial system.[2] The latter obviously is more relevant for the U.S. urban system. As Hawley (1950) and Kasarda (1972) develop the idea, expansion generally proceeds until it reaches the limits of sustainable coordination, which can vary with a number of factors—including technologies of communication and transportation, the effectiveness and efficiency of social organization, and the nature of the relationships in the system. For example, systems expanding through mutually beneficial trade may be more easily sustained than systems expanding through imperial action. System expansion may be limited when the boundaries of other competing urban centers are reached.

The second way cities may grow is by adopting more efficient technologies and/or modes of social organization that increase the carrying capacity of the system. The notion of carrying capacity is not easy to operationalize, but one indication of its increase over time is the fact that the hinterland population needed to sustain an urban population of a given size has been reduced by multiple orders of magnitude. This permits the growth of the urban population through either migration from hinterland regions or natural increase or both. Over the long course of urbanization in world history, the steady increase in carrying capacity is the main factor allowing cities to reach enormous proportions, compared to their ancient counterparts, and to contain an ever larger fraction of regional, national, and global population.

---

[2] Note here that, as found in theoretical models of biological ecology, one should not equate the notion of functional relationship as implying mutual and symmetric benefit. The disparate elements that comprise the ongoing, functionally integrated empirical system do not necessary all benefit equally or influence each other symmetrically. Stable biological ecosystems include a wide array of relationships, including predator-prey relations, parasitism, as well as examples of direct and indirect mutual benefit.

MACROSPATIAL DISTRIBUTION

Cities do not arise in random locations nor do they all grow to the same size. Cities differ in their activities and in the nature and degree of their interrelations with other cities. Cities are embedded in regional, national, and global systems that are hierarchically structured. In systems, the relative positions of cities change over time. Some cities grow in relative size and influence, while others decline. These matters constitute the core concerns of economic and ecological theories explaining macrospatial population distribution.

Central place theory—a crucial building block in traditional demographic perspectives on the spatial distribution of population—is guided by the insight that spatial proximity reduces costs associated with communication, interaction, and exchange and thus provides a powerful impetus for the emergence of population nodes. Formal models building on this premise yield a number of important predictions about how populations will be distributed and organized in space. Under a fixed set of communication and transport technologies, (1) population will coalesce into nodes serving as focal points for trade, communication, and political and economic administration of a surrounding spatial domain, (2) nodes will vary in population size and region of influence, (3) the size distribution of nodes will be regular and strongly negative (i.e., smaller areas will be more common, and frequency will decline sharply with increasing size), (4) nodes will be functionally differentiated, with larger nodes having more coordinative functions and more extensive connections with other nodes in the system, (5) the spacing of nodes of a given size will be regular in relation to each other and in relation to nodes of other sizes, and (6) nodes will be hierarchically organized with the node at the center being the largest and most influential. The development of this perspective has taken place over many decades. Relatively recent reviews of central place theory (e.g., Berry and Horton 1970; Richardson 1969, 1980; Mulligan 1984; Fujita, Krugman, and Venables 1999) trace its intellectual foundations, identify the core assumptions of the perspective, and summarize the implications that flow from them.

Central place theory is an idealization, and economists and ecologists are well aware that the assumptions of the theory and hence some of its predictions are not fully approximated in real urban systems. While empirical patterns often depart in important ways from the predictions of the theory, the theory is nevertheless highly respected because the conceptual framework has been shown to be extensible, and supplementary theories have been developed to deal with spatial complications that arise when the model's core assumptions are not met. For example, special location theory deals with the fact that resources of different types are not distributed evenly in space (Ullman 1941). This provides a basis for predicting deviations from the geometric arrangements of centers and subcenters expected in the central place system. It also provides a basis for predicting more extensive functional specialization among cities (e.g., the concentration of petrochemical industries in regions where oil and gas deposits are found). Break-in-transportation theory (Cooley 1894) deals with the fact that the cost of movement in space is not uniform in all directions and leads to predictions that population nodes will arise where it is either necessary or cost-effective for goods and people to shift from one mode of transportation to another. Theories focusing on factors such as the bounding effects of national borders (especially for small countries) and uneven historical development of regional economies and transportation infrastructure help account for the occurrence of primate cities and other departures from the size distribution of cities predicted by central place theory (Walters 1985).

In sum, central place theory offers a powerful basis for understanding macrospatial population distributions. Scholars working within traditional demographic perspectives see it and associated theories as providing a rigorous foundation for understanding and interpreting macrospatial population distributions.

Borchert's (1967) review of changes in the U.S. urban system over a span of centuries provides a classic illustration of how abstract, ahistorical theories of location and spatial distribution can guide a historically informed account of how changes in technology influenced the evolution of the urban system. He traces how different cities in the urban system rose or fell in rank position in the urban system following major changes in technologies for transporting people and goods. For example, the steady increase in the size of ocean-going ships conferred advantages to ports with natural deep-water harbors such as New York and San Francisco and disadvantages to ports with shallow bays such as Charleston. Similarly, the emergence of rail and, later, trucking and air transport technologies substantially offset the advantages associated with proximity to a major navigable river or body of water. This made it possible for inland cities like Kansas City, Denver, and Dallas–Fort Worth to rise in rank position in the urban system. Correspondingly, it contributed to long-term declines in relative rank for cities like St. Louis, whose position in the urban system had been substantially predicated on inland water transport technologies. Significantly, the kinds of changes Borchert describes often spanned many decades. They would be instantaneous in an ahistorical formal model. But application of the models to empirical systems requires allowance for the significant inertia deriving from fixed capital investments and established social arrangements. These produce long lags in the restructuring of spatial distribution. Cities favored by new technologies may rise slowly and cities put at a disadvantage by new technologies may "drift" down the urban hierarchy slowly. This means that the macrospatial distribution of population at a particular point in time is rarely if ever in an equilibrium state. Nevertheless, the equilibrium arrangements predicted by the theory give a basis for understanding and anticipating patterns of change in population distribution.

FUNCTIONAL SPECIALIZATION, INTEGRATION, AND HIERARCHY IN URBAN SYSTEMS

Cities are embedded in regional, national, and global systems. These massive spatial systems are functionally integrated and hierarchically structured. Functional specialization is understood in terms of central place theory, special location theory, and break-in-transportation theory and is extensively documented in studies of industry and labor force profiles of metropolitan areas that provide a basis for identifying a city's "basic" function. These range from hand-crafted typologies developed from inspections of distributions of location-quotients for industries in different areas (e.g., Alexandersson 1956; Harris 1943; Mayer 1959; Harris and Ullman 1945; reviewed in Schwab 1992) to the use of the statistical technique of factor analysis to identify city "types" (e.g., Hadden and Borgatta 1965; Berry and Horton 1970; Kass 1973). Different approaches yield slightly different typologies (e.g., cities may be restricted to being single-function cities, or multiple-function cities may be permitted). All sustain the conclusion that cities specialize in economic activities and are implicated in an expansive macrospatial division of labor, sometimes termed the *horizontal dimension* of the urban system.

The other key dimension, the *vertical dimension*, reflects the fact that functions of influence, coordination, and control are not evenly distributed across cities in the system or within the nodal-functional system associated with a single city or metropolitan area (Wilson 1984). Taking the latter case first, cities compared to their hinterlands are more likely to be home to regional headquarters and the administrators and decision makers who work in them. They are located in urban centers so they can more easily coordinate with others in similar roles. This would be exceedingly difficult if they all were distributed evenly in space. This creates a powerful asymmetry in the functional relations between metropolis and hinterland. In the language of ecology, a relation of *dominance* holds (McKenzie 1933; Bogue 1949; Hawley 1950). In many matters, the metropolis exerts great influence over social and economic life in smaller cities, towns, and villages in the hinterland (e.g., regulating access to capital through regional financial institutions located in the metropolis). The subdominant areas in the hinterland often have little choice but to accept asymmetric "terms of trade" because the metropolis mediates their access to the broader urban system. This example shows that it is a mistake to conclude, as some critics have, that the ecological notion of a functionally integrated system implies that the relationships in the system reflect equality of influence and harmony of interest.[3]

Dominance attaches to key function, that is, the economic activity that is crucial to establishing the flow of sustenance (income) in the community (Hawley 1950, 1968; Meyer 1984, 1986). The key function is found in the specialized activity that marks the community's place on the horizontal dimension of the urban system, and it is in this area that a metropolis is most likely to be distinguished from other metropolitan areas. Galle (1963) shows that industries have higher concentrations of executive, administrative, and technical staff in metropolitan areas where they represent the key function (sometimes called "basic" or "city-building" industries) than the same industries have in metropolitan areas where they do not represent the area's key function. In contrast, metropolitan areas tend to be relatively similar in the occupational profiles of their "nonbasic" industries. Central place theory predicts that key functions follow the size of a city, with higher-order cities having a greater degree of specialization in "metropolitan" functions involving administration, coordination and control, and the flow and distribution of information, capital, and goods. Special location theory and break-in-transportation theory are also used to explain why lower-order cities specialize in particular key functions.

Dominance is a matter of degree, and there are many levels of hierarchy. All metropolitan areas perform "metropolitan" functions for their hinterlands, but the degree of specialization in these functions varies greatly. A subregional metropolis that exerts influence over a small hinterland may be "nested" under a regional metropolis that exerts influence over the subregional metropolis and, through it, indirect influence over its hinterland. The regional metropolis will itself be nested under a national metropolis and so on. The key prediction emerging from central place theory

---

[3] As Smith (1995) notes, the distinction between ecological perspectives and critical and political economic perspectives in this area is not great. The difference often boils down to the fact that ecological theory, reflecting its intellectual roots in bioecology, uses relatively neutral terms such as *dominant* and *subdominant* when describing actors with varying degrees of influence and power.

is that functions of coordination and control are found in greatest concentration in cities at the apex of the urban hierarchy, and so they exert tremendous direct influence over the entire urban system (Berry and Horton 1970; Berry and Kasarda 1977). The dominance relations predicted by the theory have been extensively documented in ecological research. Early studies by McKenzie (1933) and Bogue (1949) and Vance and Sutker (1954) used relatively simple data and somewhat imprecise methods for assessing dominance and position within the urban hierarchy. Duncan and his colleagues (1960) drew on more extensive data and more exacting methods of measurement to establish the outline of a national urban hierarchy for the United States. Wanner (1977) drew on the data reduction capabilities of factor analysis to simultaneously place cities on the horizontal and vertical dimensions of the urban system. Eberstein and Frisbie (1982) and Eberstein and Galle (1984) established the relations of functional interdependence between metropolitan areas in regional and national systems based on commodity flow data documenting patterns of trade. And many different analyses drawing on various methodological approaches have documented patterns of persistence and change in national and regional metropolitan hierarchies (e.g., Duncan and Lieberson 1970; South and Poston 1980, 1982; Galle and Stern 1981).

In recent decades the study of urban systems has increasingly focused on global systems and regional systems at the world level. Studies informed by ecological theory and traditional demographic perspectives are prominent (e.g., Dogan and Kasarda 1988a, 1988b; Lo and Yeung 1998; Meyer 1986; Kasarda and Crenshaw 1991; Bollen and Appold 1993; Kim and Shin 2002; London 1987; London and Smith 1988), but studies guided by critical and political economic perspectives are equally numerous (e.g., Chase-Dunn 1984; Chase-Dunn and Hall 1993; Chase-Dunn, Kawano, and Brewer 2000; Chase-Dunn and Grimes 1995; Rossem 1996; Wallerstein 1974; 1980; Walton 1976; Timberlake 1985; King 1990; Smith and White 1992; Smith and Nemath 1988). A smaller number of studies draw on both orientations (London 1987; London and Smith 1988; Hudson 1987; Smith 1995) and seek common ground. This burgeoning literature is not reviewed here. Suffice it to note that many of the patterns documented in it have close parallels in research on national urban systems.

One area of controversy is the question of how interdependency and the macrospatial division of labor are related to uneven development, economic restructuring and economic dislocation, dominance relations, and the spatial structuring of inequality. Ecologists take it for granted that when populations are drawn into broader functional systems that are characterized by a macrospatial division of labor, there are many consequences. The population gains access to the productive efficiencies and possibilities for economic growth that are associated with specialization, a refined division of labor, and greater access to markets. At the same time, however, the population loses autonomy and independence and is exposed to direct and indirect competition with other urban areas. This makes the population vulnerable to significant social and economic dislocations.

Certain kinds of changes are presumed to be especially likely owing to the standard ecological assumption that many processes operate to bring about a balance or equilibrium between population and opportunities for living. Chief among these processes is migration. It is presumed that, *unless impeded*, population in low-wage regions will flow toward high-wage regions. This underlies much rural-to-urban migration and migration between regions and nations. Of course, the latter is much more highly restricted by institutional barriers such as national borders. Another process outlined in the economic literature is "filtering," in which industries commanding higher wages at a given time and place are likely to be redistributed from the initial spatial locations where they were "spawned" to new spatial locations. The classic example is the high-wage, high-skill manufacturing industry that undergoes incremental "refinements" such as routinization and mechanization that permit the use of less skilled labor. This leads production and employment in this sector of the economy to be redistributed from high-skill, high-wage areas to low-skill, low-wage areas, resulting in job loss and wage declines in the origin region and new jobs and wage increases in the destination regions (Vernon 1966; Thompson 1965). One of the dynamics of globalization is that many barriers that have historically impeded movement toward equilibrium adjustments of the sort just described are falling at the same time that cities and nations are becoming more tightly integrated into a single global system. Consequently, both negative and positive consequences flowing from participation in the global system of cities (and nations) occur more often, and their impacts reach dramatic proportions in ever shorter time frames.

Not surprisingly, traditional demographic perspectives emphasize the role of transportation and communication technologies. For example, the rise of the Internet and cheap, high-speed telecommunications have made the business services sector in high-wage regions vulnerable to macrospatial competition for the first time in history. Thus, for example, high-tech jobs in computer programming and computing support are "filtering" down the global urban hierarchy from high-wage "incubator" areas in the United States (e.g., the Silicon Valley region in California) to lower-wage, high-tech centers in India. Dramatic positive economic growth in high-tech cities in India is the flip side of economic dislocation and restructuring in U.S. counterparts. The general phenomenon has been seen throughout history, but the scale and pace of contemporary transitions are unprecedented. In the present high-tech example, the birth of a high-wage industry in core areas of the global system is filtering to the developing world within the span of a few decades and is bypassing the traditional "intermediate stops" in the spatial economy. For example, to a substantial degree job movement is "leap-frogging" over low-wage metropolitan areas in the U.S.

The combination of interdependency and the increasing ease of movement of goods, information, capital, and labor have the capacity to produce major social and economic disruption and thus are frequently linked to important social problems. In the ecological view, this is an unsurprising consequence associated with economic growth and development. At the same time it highlights both the need to better predict negative consequences so they can be managed and regulated more effectively and the importance of recognizing that negative consequences in one spatial location are usually associated with positive consequences elsewhere. Kasarda and Crenshaw (1991) note that while uneven development can be seen to have undesirable as well as desirable consequences, no accepted models point the way to "even development." Traditional demographic perspectives assume that living standards tend to expand unevenly. Innovations that set off new waves of economic growth invariably confer initial advantages to the urban centers that "incubated" and "spawned" them. Economic growth and wealth creation associated with the rise of new, high-wage sectors create disparities between old and new sectors of the economy and give rise to increasing inequality in the short run (Kuznets 1955)—inequality that is likely to be spatially structured. This view obviously carries different implications for policy and regulation than the view that uneven development is an "aberration" or that it primarily reflects predation and "exploitation."

Urban hierarchy theory predicts that these innovations and the rise of new high-wage sectors are most likely to originate, and/or be exploited to their maximum, in cities at the top of the urban hierarchy. This introduces an expected spatial dimension to inequality, with average wages declining with movement from global to national to regional to subregional metropolises and eventually down to the lowest wages in the hinterlands of cities at the bottom of the urban hierarchy. Significantly, however, the same theory predicts that high-wage areas must continually innovate. In the long-run, cultural diffusion, population movement, routinization and deskilling, or other processes make these advantages available more broadly; this simultaneously reduces inequality while raising overall income and carrying capacity within the urban system. Evidence for this is seen in the fact that areas of relative high wages can, and historically do, lose their relative advantage and fall back toward the average, while cultural diffusion and economic restructuring can lift incomes in lower-wage areas toward the average.

INTRAURBAN SPATIAL DISTRIBUTION: LAND USE AND POPULATION DENSITY

A century ago, the intensity of land use in the typical American city followed a fairly basic pattern. The density of the combined residential and work-day population was greatest in and around a central core (usually termed the Central Business District or CBD); "peak density" and "central density" were usually the same. Intensity of land use fell with increasing distance from the CBD, declining with such rapidity that satisfactory mathematical descriptions necessarily drew on nonlinear, namely, negative exponential, functions that fall dramatically at first but then level out. Today this pattern is not uncommon, but other significant patterns have emerged. Larger metropolitan areas and newer metropolitan areas today are typically characterized by multiple centers and subcenters, and density of land use is highly variegated. Density gradients are "flatter," and thus the disparity between central density and densities elsewhere is less pronounced. Density is "patchier," with peaks and valleys found throughout the metropolitan region. The changes are definitely real, but they can be exaggerated. Density of land use in real cities never conformed exactly to the mathematical ideal of a monocentric field in which density declined with distance from the center at a uniform rate in all directions. To the contrary, intensity of land use has always been marked by subcenters and patchiness, and these patterns are noted in the earliest efforts to account for spatial patterns of population distribution (e.g., Burgess 1925).

In contemporary cities, spatial distribution may coalesce around single centers of extreme density, multiple centers of varying density in the fashion of center and subcenter, or multiple diffuse centers that create broad population "domes." Theoretical models of increasing sophistication (Anas, Arnott, and Small 1998; Fujita and Ogawa 1982; Henderson and Thisse 2004; Huriot and Thisse 2000) set forth these possibilities. Cost of communication and transportation play a key role in these models. Monocentric cities with dense urban cores are expected when the time costs of moving goods and people in space are high. In such circumstances, accessibility to the center of the city becomes an overriding factor in location decisions and promotes intense land use and high population densities at the center of the city. In the late 19th century, reliance on inflexible hub-and-spoke transportation systems (i.e., water and fixed rail) for moving people and goods over significant distances helped produce the typical spatial pattern in American cities. The state of construction technologies also figures in shaping population density by determining whether it is feasible to "stack" population and economic activity vertically in space as well as "pack it in" horizontally. A progression of innovations in this area over the late 19th and early 20th century played a prominent role in promoting increases in peak densities in American cities.

When considering the monocentric city, it is useful to distinguish between central or core density, the maximum density observed at the center of the urban region, and the density gradient, the rate at which density declines with distance from the center of the city. As noted by Winsborough (1963) (who uses the terms *congestion* and *concentration*), they are separate and distinct aspects of urban spatial distribution; they may vary independently and can be affected by different factors. So long as the costs associated with transportation and communication are nontrivial, competition for access causes centrally located land to be more valuable and thus to be developed more intensively. As Frisbie and Kasarda (1988) observe, the prediction from economic and ecological theory that intensity of land use will decline with distance from the city center is confirmed by a massive base of empirical studies documenting that density declines exponentially with distance from the city center for cities in a wide range of historical and cultural settings.[4] The slope of the density gradient is predicted to vary with the costs of communication and transportation; the higher the costs, the steeper the density gradient. This prediction also receives strong support in studies showing that density gradients in cities have been declining over the past 150 years and even longer as communication and transportation costs have been steadily declining (Clark 1951; Rees 1968; Winsborough 1961, 1963; Berry and Horton 1970). Holding the density gradient constant, the central density will be a positive function of overall city size.

The primary value of monocentric models is *not* that they yield an exact description of spatial patterns in contemporary urban areas (although they can serve as a passable first approximation for many purposes).[5] It is that they provide a framework from which to develop a rigorous understanding of the structuring principles of spatial distribution. Monocentric models rest on a variety of assumptions that are clearly simplistic: actors have location needs that are qualitatively identical (i.e., they seek only centrality), space is uniform and undifferentiated, it is possible to move with equal ease in all directions, and the city has no history. Still, these models are a useful point of departure because they can be elaborated to accommodate a wide range of complexities found in contemporary urban form.

As reviewed in Berry and Horton (1970), the Mills-Muth model of land use implies that specialized actors who have the greatest need for centrality and the greatest ability to pay for it will occupy the most intensely developed central portions of the city. Progressively distant "rings" will be used by actors with less demand for centrality. This leads to the familiar zonal progression from business district, to

---

[4] They cite the work of Colin Clark (1951), who found that an exponential equation of the form $d_x = d_0 e^{bx}$ (where d_x is density at distance x, d_0 is the central density, e is base of the natural logarithms, and b is the rate at which density changes with distance) provides a good fit in most applications and that b is estimated as negative in a wide range of historical and cultural settings.

[5] For example, I conducted an analysis of spatial population distribution for the quintessential sprawling metropolis of Houston, presumably a prototype of "new" urban form, and found that the simple negative exponential relationship between distance and population density accounts for more than half of the areal variation in population density.

residential zones, to agricultural areas. Harris and Ullman (1945) noted that different actors have different location needs and that some are complementary while others are at odds. This leads to expectations of multinucleation in which density distributions emanate not from a single point but from multiple points and which cause further spatial differentiation in the composition of population at various points in the city. Fujita and Ogawa (1982) extend the Muth-Mills framework to show how, depending on assumptions, it can explain a wide range of urban spatial forms, including monocentrism, polycentrism, diffuse centers. Long ago Hurd (1903) and Burgess (1925) noted that ease of movement in space is not even but is distorted by axial and radial transportation arteries. Accordingly, Frisbie and Kasarda (1988) note that distance should be seen as a proxy for the time-costs of travel, which obviously will vary with the spatial organization of the transportation system. This insight leads to several obvious predictions: high-density corridors will arise around highways and commuter rail lines, subcenters of varying magnitude will arise at major intersections, and "hollow spaces" of less intense development will be found in between major transportation arteries (see White 1987: 247–249).

Finally, not to exhaust the possibilities but to end this brief list, it is readily apparent that allowing for history and inertia also variegates the spatial pattern of population distribution in important ways. When transportation and communication technologies improve, the development of outlying areas, suddenly made more feasible, will occur under the new set of conditions. In contrast, interior areas will change little in the short run, since fixed capital investments in infrastructure, buildings, and housing stock cannot be easily rearranged. As a result, the spatial development of the city over time can be highly irregular. Discontinuities in spatial patterns do not imply that the logic of the underlying spatial processes is changing but reflect that these processes are playing out under changing historical conditions.

The above paragraphs show that simple models of an idealized monocentric city can be readily extended to handle the complexity of modern cities with multinucleated urban fields, irregular density surfaces, and sprawling patchworks of suburban and exurban development. Significantly, all of the ideas introduced here are part and parcel of conventional demographic perspectives set forth in classic works (Burgess 1925; Harris and Ullman 1945; Hawley 1950, 1971, 1981; Hoyt 1939, 1971; Hurd 1903; Ullman and Harris 1970) and summarized repeatedly in authoritative reviews (Berry and Horton 1970; Berry and Kasarda 1977; Frisbie 1980a, 1980b; Frisbie and Kasarda 1988). Thus, conventional demographic perspectives provide a highly serviceable framework for understanding intraurban spatial distributions for both contemporary and past cities in America.

Frisbie and Kasarda (1988: 634) offered a similar conclusion more than a decade and a half ago, noting that traditional demographic perspectives have endured criticism and stand as "the dominant (and, arguably, the only) general theory of urban form and process that has been generative of systematic, empirically verifiable models." Frisbie and Kasarda also argue that critics of conventional models largely miss the point. The value of these models is found less in the specific patterns they predict (e.g., concentric zones, sectors, etc.), but rather in their articulation of basic principles of spatial process that readily apply to new realities and thus remain relevant to understanding spatial distributions of land use and population even today (1988: 633; see also Clark 2000).

Critical and political economic theorists have sometimes characterized traditional demographic perspectives as examples of "technological reductionism" (Gottdeinner and Hutchinson 2000) for giving inappropriate weight to the impact that changes in communication and transportation technology have on spatial patterns of land use and population density. By its nature, science engages in reductionism, so that is not a point of concern to population specialists. The specific charge of technological reductionism would be telling if technological change were a minor factor in long-term trends in spatial patterns, but that is hardly the case. In the past century the rise of auto and truck transport and modern telecommunications has had dramatic effects: reducing transport costs, increasing the possible distance between employment and residence, and under-mining the scale economies of older transport technologies (Brueckner 2000; Brueckner and Fansler 1983; Glaeser and Kahn 2004).

The transition to decentralized transport systems organized around autos and trucks has been largely irresistible and is the dominant trend globally, not only in U.S. metropolitan areas. Focusing on the U.S., the transition to auto transport has generally reduced *total* commute and trip times and increased flexibility in trip sched-uling and in the selection of origin and destination points (Gordon, Kumar, and Richardson 1991; Glaeser and Kahn 2004).[6] Economies associated with outlying devel-opment often reduce housing costs (per square foot) substantially (Glaeser and Kahn 2004) and thus provide powerful economic incentives for population decentralization ("sprawl"). The economics of transporting goods via trucking versus fixed rail and water transport systems are equally if not more important in their impact on urban structure. Glaeser and Kohlhase (2003) estimate that the costs of transporting goods declined by approximately 90% over the past century.[7] They argue that this played a dominant role in cost calculations for business location decisions and helped fuel the decentralization of manufacturing, wholesaling, and retailing industries.

The consequences for cities have been far reaching. Schwirian, Hankins, and Ventresea and colleagues (1990: 1160) articulate the view advanced by many ecological researchers (Kasarda 1985; Berry and Cohen 1973; Frey and Speare 1988) that cities in the United States are continuing to undergo a dramatic transformation in which central cities "are shifting from being centers of production and distribution of goods to being centers of information exchange, service provision, and corporate and government administration." With this trend the value residential actors attach to central loca-tion—already declining with steady reductions in the time-cost of travel—has dimin-ished further, since it derived primarily from access to jobs and shopping.

Theory and evidence supporting this view continues to grow (Schwirian, Hankins, and Ventresca 1990; Edmonston and Guterbock 1984), and recent statements in the field assert the position with increasing vigor (Glaeser and Kahn 2004; Glaeser and Kohlhase 2003). What is needed to substantially refute it? Analyses emphasizing factors other than technological change (e.g., economic interests of suburban developers, real estate interests, growth machine boosters, postwar state subsidization of home owner-ship, racial dynamics, etc.) will have to overcome at least two hurdles to gain wider acceptance in demographic circles. First, they would have to provide a compelling

---

[6] Glaeser and Kahn (2004) report that in 2000, median total trip time nationwide was 24 minutes by car and 47 minutes by public transport. Much of total trip time for public transport involves getting to and from access points and waiting.

[7] These declining costs reflect multiple, technical changes and changes in business practices: improvements in transportation technology, reduction in the size and weight of goods, changes in the mix of goods; improve-ments in efficiency of shipping based on evolving business practices (e.g., just-in-time distribution, electronic monitoring of goods in transit, etc.).

alternative to the conventional interpretation of the long established association between declining time-costs of travel and declining density gradients in urban areas. Second, they would have to make the case that developers, boosters, and others who profited from trends in urban spatial distribution did so, not by "cashing in on" a powerful demographic trend, but by generating a massive spatial redistribution that *otherwise would not have occurred*.

In short, alternative views are faced with the task of establishing baseline models of spatial redistribution that *should* have been expected based on economic and ecological principles operating in the absence of political-economic factors and then identifying how spatial redistribution deviated from these expectations, specifically in conjunction with changes in political-economic factors. So far, critics of traditional demographic perspectives rarely pursue this kind of analysis, and when they do the results are mixed. A case in point is the body of research on "white flight" and suburbanization. In this literature the hypothesis that suburbanization was substantially accelerated by racial dynamics initially received some support but ultimately was not found to be the important factor that critics of traditional demographic perspectives suggested (Frisbie and Kasarda 1988). Frey (1979) provides quantitative evidence supporting the hypothesis but also shows that conventional ecological variables are very powerful factors. Later research (Farley, Richards, and Wurdock 1980; Smock and Wilson 1991) indicates that analyses focusing on the 1970s tended to exaggerate racial effects by picking up short-term effects that were stronger than long-term consequences. As additional research has accumulated, it is increasingly clear that, while racial dynamics should not be dismissed as trivial, they have not been the driving force in long-run trends in population deconcentration.

A number of problems are obvious: decentralization and deconcentration are extremely broad based and are not limited to metropolitan areas with relatively large nonwhite minority populations; the most highly decentralized cities are found in the fast-growing areas of the South and Southwest, which are characterized by the lowest overall levels of white-minority residential segregation; long-term decentralization is observed for all status groups (Frey 1985); and minority populations have been suburbanizing at high rates over several decades (Stahura 1986; Massey and Denton 1987; Schneider and Phelan 1993; Frey and Fielding 1995). It is interesting to note that while the white-flight hypothesis was not implausible, critical and political-economic scholars did not lead the way in rigorously assessing the hypothesis empirically. This helps explain why scholars guided by traditional demographic perspectives tend to view political economic arguments discounting the role of technological change in population decentralization and deconcentration as premature at best.

INTRAURBAN SPATIAL DISTRIBUTION:
SEGREGATION OF SOCIAL GROUPS

Sociologists writing in the early decades of the 20th century advanced some of the earliest comprehensive theories of the segregation of population groups in urban areas (Burgess 1928; Cressey 1938; McKenzie 1926; Park 1936b). Their efforts gave rise to one of the richest literatures in all of sociology. It remains vital today and is notable for its continuity and cumulative character. Briefly, the descriptive literature evolved from tabulations and impressionist maps, common in the earliest years, to sophisticated quantitative assessments of segregation patterns based on increasingly refined indices and the multidimensional scaling of factorial ecology. The literature exploring process began with case studies of neighborhoods and expanded to include processual studies of succession and neighborhood change, comparative analyses of variation and change in segregation at the city level, and most recently, investigations of the microlevel processes underlying aggregate segregation patterns.

While racial and ethnic segregation received the greatest amount of attention from early ecologists, they studied segregation among all manner of social groupings. As outlined in the writings of Park, Burgess, and McKenzie (1925), Burgess (1925, 1928), Park (1926, 1936a, 1936b); McKenzie (1924, 1926, 1933) and Cressey (1938), their theories emphasized processes of mutual attraction among members of the same group and processes of spatial competition between social groups. One key insight advanced was that differences in social characteristics (e.g., ethnicity, socioeconomic position, age, stage in the life cycle, etc.) give rise to "social distance" between population groups, which can influence their differential distribution in residential space. Another idea introduced was that differential means associated with intra- and intergroup inequality in socioeconomic status played a major role in competition for higher-quality housing in spatially structured housing markets and served to relegate lower economic classes and ethnic minority groups to older, centrally located neighborhoods with lower-quality housing and less desirable living conditions marked by disproportionate exposure to crime and other social problems.

They also observed that population growth and the arrival of new groups served to initiate cycles of "invasion" and "succession." New groups with limited resources usually settled in poor inner city areas, and their entry would set off a chain reaction in which existing groups would expand out and "invade" adjacent areas. As the process continued, the affected areas were likely to undergo succession; that is, the replacement of one population group with another. But full invasion-succession sequences were not inevitable; succession sometimes terminated in intermediate stages, producing integrated neighborhoods. This outcome typically marked the final stage of a process of spatial assimilation in which, over a period of time and successive generations, an immigrant group first acculturated, then assimilated on socioeconomic characteristics, and then moved on to higher-status areas and residential proximity with majority ethnic populations.

The core theoretical concepts from this early era of research, such as *social distance*, *congregation*, *centralization*, *competition*, *invasion*, *succession*, *segregation*, and *spatial assimilation*, remain central to sociological efforts to describe and explain residential segregation and neighborhood change. Urban ecological theory identifies a wide variety of mechanisms that can give rise to segregation between social groups. These include socioeconomic inequality and economic competition, "variation in need or requirements," social distance (affinity/aversion) dynamics, cultural differentiation, and informal and institutional exclusion and discrimination. Significantly, *these various mechanisms are not mutually exclusive; any one can be a sufficient cause of segregation; and they may operate in any combination.* For analytic purposes it is useful to group them into demand side and supply side dynamics. The former produces segregation when systemic differences in preferences and/or differences in means lead groups to cluster in different areas of the city as they select and attain residential locations in urban housing markets. The latter produces segregation when the spatial choices available to lower-status groups and ethnic minorities are restricted by discrimination and institutional barriers.

The strains of ecological theory that emphasize demand-side dynamics hypothesize that households of similar social position, based on ethnicity, status position, and stage of the life cycle, will have low "social distance" from each other based on one or more of the following: shared interests, similar "tastes," common ethnic culture, sense of mutual acceptance, and in-group solidarity. At one level, similar households are likely to select similar residential locations and will thus tend to congregate in the same areas, and dissimilar households will tend to select different residential locations and live in different areas. At another level, low social distance may give rise to attraction to in-group contact, and high social distance may give rise to aversion to out-group contact. For example, higher-status households and households from majority ethnic groups often have an aversion to coresiding with lower-status households and minority ethnic groups and seek to maintain spatial separation from them. They do so to minimize association with perceived social inferiors and to demonstrate and consolidate their position in the status hierarchy. Demand-side effects of attraction and aversion between different types of households can be amplified by status inequality and economic competition. Higher-status households seek to live together *and are able to do so* because they are advantaged in economic competition for high-quality housing and desirable neighborhoods (Duncan and Duncan 1955b; Jargowsky 1996, 1997; White 1987). Lower-status households and ethnic minorities are disadvantaged in this competition and are disproportionately relegated to lower-quality housing in less desirable neighborhoods over and above any specific desire to reside with coethnics or other households of similar social characteristics (Jargowsky 1996; 1997; Simkus 1978; Farley 1977).

Demand-side dynamics operating in decentralized housing markets have the capacity to produce "natural areas," that is, areas that are relatively homogeneous with respect to the social characteristics of their residents and that tend to maintain their character over time even as individual households in the neighborhood come and go. Since population homogeneity in neighborhoods necessarily gives rise to city-wide residential segregation, this establishes a model by which segregation can arise out of uncoordinated, microlevel interactions without any *necessary* assistance from law or formal institutional practices.[8]

If no other structuring principles are operating, the result would be a hodgepodge of different areas. But Burgess' concentric zone model (1925) posited that area stratification would emerge along a distance gradient resulting in concentric zones by socioeconomic status. Hoyt's (1939) insights about the housing market joined with Burgess' insights about the dynamics of urban growth to establish the idealized Burgess-Hoyt sectored-zone model. As the city grows, high-status groups tend to locate in newer, low-density, expensive housing added at the perimeter of the city; older, depreciating housing stock in the interior of the city tends to be occupied by lower-status groups who use it more intensively (i.e., by subdividing it or sharing it). Within status zones, population separates into ethnic sectors based on social distance. Processes of succession accompanying growth lead ethnic sectors to align across zones to yield the ethnic "wedges" described by Hoyt. Massey (1985) outlines how these dynamics overlay with

---

[8] In recent decades, analytic and simulation models by nonecologists (Schelling 1972; Epstein and Axtel 1996; Krugman 1996; Young 1998) lend formal theoretical support to the basic ecological insight that uncoordinated and unconstrained location decisions based on affinity for households of similar social characteristics (or aversion to others) can create stable segregation patterns in space that are featureless save for the characteristics of the households that reside in different locations.

theories of ethnic assimilation to yield a model of spatial assimilation. Minority groups initially are dissimilar in culture and social status and locate in the poorer areas of the central city. As they acculturate and assimilate on socioeconomic characteristics, they are better able to secure housing in higher-status areas, both because they have the means to do so and because they are more accepted based on lower social distance. Eventually, they gain acceptance into such primary relationships as coresidence, friendship, and marriage with the majority population and are fully spatially assimilated.

Reviews by Hawley (1950), Schnore (1965), Berry and Horton (1970), Guest (1984), Berry and Kasarda (1977), and Frisbie and Kasarda (1988) all stress that the significance of the Burgess-Hoyt model is found not in its descriptive utility but rather in the fact that it provides an idealized model of urban spatial segregation that is anchored in clear assumptions and theoretical principles. Despite being simple in many ways, the model has been found to provide reasonable descriptions of many U.S. urban areas (Berry, Horton, and Abiodun 1970; Rees 1968), at least in a certain historical era.

Critics have raised concerns that the model applies only to industrial cities of a certain era in western societies. But this does not gainsay the crucial insight of the model, which is that social distance and market dynamics operating in a particular urban form yield systematic patterns of residential segregation. One may investigate or even presume that the location decisions of high-status households (which along with growth drive the model) may differ across cultures or urban form (e.g., the location of high-status areas or the nature of urban transportation systems), but this only changes the specific expression of segregation; it does not negate the expectation of systematic segregation.[9] Because critics often miss this last point and, more importantly, because they have not offered any well-specified alternative model of segregation that generates testable predictions, the Burgess-Hoyt model continues to exert considerable influence on contemporary research on segregation.

One area where this is evident is the urban-ecological understanding of several well-known empirical regularities in minority segregation patterns. Massey and Denton (1988a) brought conceptual clarity to the theory of segregation measurement by identifying five dimensions of segregation: uneven distribution, isolation, clustering, centralization, and concentration. These dimensions resonate with ecological theory and the Burgess-Hoyt model and provide a framework for predicting when minority groups will be subject to what Massey and Denton (1989) term *hypersegregation,* that is, the condition where a minority population simultaneously experiences high levels of segregation on several dimensions of segregation. Park's notion of social distance based on ethnic culture generates the expectation of uneven distribution between minority and majority and the isolation of minority groups in ghettos. Economic disadvantage and market processes relegate minorities to the poorer, higher-density areas of the central city, promoting high levels of minority concentration and centralization. The process of ethnic succession under conditions of city growth similar to those outlined by Hoyt (1939) promotes clustering, that is, the formation of larger regions of ethnic homogeneity spanning many adjacent neighborhoods. Based on this framework, hypersegregation is to be expected in situations where minority-majority social distance is pronounced, where minority-majority economic disparity is high, and where urban spatial structure follows the Burgess-Hoyt pattern.

---

[9] Thus, if high-status groups consistently locate in the center of the city, for whatever reason, this change in assumption produces an inverted zonal pattern.

It is not surprising then, that Massey and Denton (1989) report that hypersegrega-tion of African Americans is especially common in the older, industrial metropolitan areas of the Midwest and Northeast, where the Burgess-Hoyt model is most apt. Hypersegregation is not as common for Hispanic and Asian minority populations, but this is consistent with ecological theory based on two important and closely related factors: social distance between non-Hispanic whites and Hispanic and Asian minorities is lower than social distance between non-Hispanic whites and African Americans (Zubrinsky and Bobo 1996; Charles 2000a, 2000b), and social and spatial assimilation dynamics, which undercut hypersegregation patterns, are stronger for Hispanics and Asians than for African Americans (Massey and Mullan 1984). Even holding these two factors constant, hypersegregation might still be predicted for Hispanics and Asians in cities with large recent settlements of homogeneously poor immigrants. This is not observed, however, because Asian immigrants are socioeconomically diverse and be-cause Hispanic immigrants tend to settle in largest numbers in cities where Hispanic population presence and spatial assimilation are already established.

The Burgess-Hoyt framework also provides a basis for understanding the fact that minority suburban settlement is disproportionately concentrated in older, "inner-ring" suburbs (Massey and Denton 1988b). The prediction that minorities will lag behind whites in suburbanization (and in neighborhood resources associated with suburban-ization) flows directly from spatial assimilation theory and the Burgess-Hoyt model. The economically advantaged majority population will disproportionately reside in the newest "outer-ring" suburbs. Following the progression originally documented for European ethnic groups in studies by Cressey (1938) and Ford (1950), minorities undergoing spatial assimilation tend to move from central cities to older "inner-ring" suburbs during the intermediate stages before full spatial assimilation is achieved. Since inner-ring suburbs are lower on housing quality, area status, and exposure to social problems, suburbanizing minorities lag behind on these outcomes. The lag is greater for African Americans since the spatial assimilation process for them is weaker than that seen decades ago for European immigrant groups and presently for Hispanic and Asian groups.

Two important changes in recent decades suggest that the spatial assimilation dynamic for African Americans is strengthening. One is that the slow rise of a signifi-cant black middle class fulfills a necessary precondition for spatial assimilation. The other is the onset of significant movement of middle-class African Americans out of inner-city neighborhoods and into inner-ring suburban neighborhoods. These neigh-borhoods, while still substantially segregated and lower in overall status, provide significantly higher residential attainment outcomes and higher levels of contact with majority households.

These trends represent a striking departure from earlier patterns and carry import-ant implications for the spatial distribution of urban poverty. Massey and Denton (1993) and Jargowsky (1996, 1997) differ in their assessment of the relative importance of the two dynamics, but both agree that the combination of strong racial and class segregation dynamics visits extreme residential disadvantage to the poorest segments of minority populations. Again, the Burgess-Hoyt framework provides a lens for inter-preting the well-documented emergence of highly concentrated inner-city poverty for poor African Americans (Massey and Eggers 1990; Massey 1990; Massey and Denton 1993; Jargowsky 1996, 1997). The emergence of a black middle class that is suburban-izing at a very rapid rate has produced a spatial separation between working-class and middle-class African Americans that previously was less pronounced (Jargowsky 1997). In a Burgess-Hoyt city, poor minorities will be centralized, concentrated, and socially isolated in devastatingly poor inner city ghettos devoid of social resources. Their conditions will worsen with any of the following: increases in the severity of racial segregation, increases in the severity of class segregation, and increases in class segregation within the minority population. The first catagory is declining, but the latter two are increasing (Jargowsky 1996; 1997). If the overall poverty rate by group is constant, then one would expect that the number of "underclass" neighborhoods will increase, that they will house an increasing fraction of the minority poor, and that they will be subject to especially pronounced social problems.

Before turning to supply-side factors in segregation patterns it is important to briefly mention the literatures associated with social area analysis and factorial ecology. Influential studies of residential patterns by Shevky and Williams (1949), Bell (1953, 1955), Shevky (1955), and Shevky and Bell (1955) popularized the concept of the "social area," which is very similar to the notion of "natural area" in classic ecology. Social area studies stress that socioeconomic status and ethnicity/race do not exhaust the important bases of segregation. In particular, they call attention to segregation associated with family and life-cycle status and demonstrate its importance empirically.[10] The effort to assess the primary "axes" of spatial differentiation in urban areas spawned the literature on factorial ecology, which uses factor analysis (or closely related statistical methods) to identify empirically distinct dimensions of residential clustering in urban areas. Reviews of this literature (e.g., Berry and Horton 1970; Berry, and Kasarda 1977; Hunter 1971, 1972) note that three primary dimensions of spatial differentiation are identified in American cities: ethnicity/race, socioeconomic position, and family/life cycle. Additional dimensions are sometimes found, but not consistently, and they rarely rival the first three in importance.

The literatures on social area analysis and factorial ecology document that spatial differentiation in American cities can be linked to a number of social characteristics and thus lend firm empirical support to the widely accepted but previously "fuzzy" notion that cities are complex spatial "mosaics." In recent decades, this empirical literature has diminished as empirical analysis of spatial differentiation within cities has focused on ethnic and socioeconomic segregation. Studies of segregation associated with age and stage in the family life cycle are still found in the literature (Guest 1972, 1977; Cowgill 1978; Chevan 1982; Pampel and Choldin 1978; White 1987) but are much less common. The basic insight driving social area analysis and factorial ecology, that many social characteristics are implicated in spatial patterns in urban areas, lives on. But nowadays empirical investigations of other, more nuanced dimensions of the urban mosaic, such as gentrification of neighborhoods, gay and lesbian enclaves, and bohemian districts, are most commonly pursued via ethnographies and historical case studies (Nyden et al. 1998; Abrahamson 1996; Anderson 1990; Eschbach et al. 1998).

Critics sometimes suggest that ecological theory does not acknowledge supply-side aspects of residential segregation, including factors such as exclusion, discrimination, conflict, and violence (e.g., Feagin 1998; Gottdeiner and Hutchinson 2000; Logan and Stearns 1981; Stearns and Logan 1986a). At one level the charge is unwarranted.

---

[10] Social area analysis also attempts to provide a broader societal-level theory for why certain social characteristics would become salient in segregation dynamics, but this is not well integrated into the ecological framework and is not vigorously pursued today.

Ecological theory has always recognized that social distance and prejudice can lead to formal and informal dynamics of exclusion and discrimination on the part of high-status groups and ethnic majority populations who seek to separate themselves from lower-status populations and ethnic minority groups (Hawley 1944b, 1950; Hawley and Rock 1973; Berry 1979; Berry and Kasarda 1977; Fossett and Cready 1998). This view is on clear display in Cressey's (1938: 62–63) classic study of ethnic succession in Chicago, which states that "[c]onflict may accompany invasion, varying in intensity with the cultural differences and prejudice of the groups involved. ... But where marked prejudices exist and there is fear that the invading group will cause a serious loss in real estate values, violent opposition may develop." McKee (1993) and Fossett and Cready (1998) provide more recent examples of how ecological theory gives attention to ethnic competition, discrimination, conflict, and violence.

Important studies rooted in ecological theory attempt to understand and predict the conditions under which interethnic contact and competition will result in discrimination and inequality (Blalock 1956, 1957, 1967; Barth and Noel 1972; Frisbie and Niedert 1977; Lieberson 1961a; Nagel and Olzak 1982; Noel 1968; Olzak and Nagel 1986; Fossett and Siebert 1997; Fossett and Kiecolt 1989; Hannan 1979; Heer 1959; Wilcox and Roof 1978). Conversely, a closely related literature seeks to understand and predict when conditions will moderate discrimination, facilitate assimilation, and promote movement toward minority incorporation and the dissolution of group boundaries (Blalock 1959; Lieberson 1961b, 1963, 1980; Duncan and Lieberson 1959; Duncan and Duncan 1957; Burr, Fossett, and Galle 1991). Studies in this tradition routinely explore questions of inequality and subordination as well as assimilation; many explicitly pursue ecological theories of ethnic competition, protest, and violence, including lethal violence (Olzak and Nagel 1986; Beck and Tolnay 1990; Tolnay and Beck 1992; Tolnay, Beck, and Massey 1989; Corzine, Creech, and Corzine 1983; Creech, Corzine, and Huff-Corzine 1989; Reed 1972). A number of ecological studies explicitly focus on urban areas and offer hypotheses regarding how race discrimination in housing and segregation outcomes may vary in relation to intergroup competition, city growth, and socioeconomic inequality (Hawley 1944b; Bahr and Gibbs 1967; Jiobu and Marshall 1971; Marshall and Jiobu 1975; Roof 1972) and thereby in relation to patterns of spatial assimilation (Duncan and Lieberson 1959; Lieberson 1980; Farley and Frey 1994; Massey and Denton 1987).

While critics err if they say ecological theory does not recognize dynamics relating to exclusion, discrimination, and conflict, they are correct to say that many ecological studies direct attention to social dynamics other than discrimination. Indeed Massey (1985) notes that the studies of the experiences of European immigrant groups to industrial cities of the late 19th and early 20th century have tended to disproportionately stress spatial assimilation dynamics. This is unfortunate because no minority population's history is devoid of significant discrimination. Thus, even when spatial assimilation dynamics are documented, as they have been for European ethnic groups of past eras and Hispanic and Asian immigrant populations in contemporary eras, it is important to recognize that spatial assimilation invariably entails overcoming discrimination. In this context, it is useful to stress again that demand-side and supply-side theories are not incompatible and do not necessitate an "either-or" choice between mutually exclusive processes.

The above leads to several points. One, it is a fallacy to interpret evidence of the operation of one process as having negative implications for the empirical relevance of other processes. Two, a full explanation of segregation patterns will need to draw on all viable perspectives and ignore none. And three, the relative merits of the various viable perspectives cannot be established by theory or by extrapolation from a few well-chosen studies. Precise estimates of relative contributions require rigorous quantitative analyses that are beyond the reach of current data and research designs.

METHODOLOGICAL CHALLENGES

Many important questions about urban and spatial distributions present difficult methodological challenges to researchers. Since new questions come to the fore when previous challenges are met, this is a perpetual condition. In the area of interurban spatial patterns, several long-standing challenges can be readily identified. To begin, the measurement and analysis of functional specialization, functional interdependence, and dominance, which are crucial concepts in theories of urban system and hierarchy, have always been difficult. Key advances in the analysis of functional specialization have included drawing on factor analysis or similar methods to identify dimensionality and continuous variation in functional specification, rather than assigning cities to discrete categories based on cut points for location quotients. The continuing problem with these methods is that complex factor structures are often sensitive to model specifications, such as the choice of orthogonal or oblique rotations, and may not be robust when applied to multiple time periods or differing samples. Consequently, they are serviceable for static descriptions at a given point in time but are less so in longitudinal research focusing on the causes and consequences of functional specialization.

The closely linked notions of interdependence and dominance present even more difficult challenges, since they involve measurements of communication, exchange, and coordination among multiple actors. Eberstein and Frisbie's (1982) analyses of commodity flow data provide an example of how to establish interdependence empirically rather than simply assuming it exists based on observing functional specialization. The task of measuring dominance is even more complicated, since it rests not only on establishing the magnitude of linkages of communication, coordination, capital flow, and decision making, but also their directionality. The concept of dominance itself is multidimensional and could be explored more carefully. It is an empirical question whether dominance is highly generalized and holds across many functions and broadly throughout the urban system (as might be implied by central place theory) or whether it is "uneven" and varies by sector of the economy. Answering such questions requires more detailed analysis of data on directional exchange on an industry-by-industry, area-by-area basis.

These are long-standing problems, and theoretical advance has been blunted because of difficulties of assembling the requisite data. The limitations of the data necessitate creativity in "making due" with available data, tempered with realism regarding what questions can be addressed in an adequate way and what questions currently defy empirically grounded answers. These problems are worsening with the rising coherence of the global system. Studies of national and regional urban systems will continue, but clearly the new game in town is the global urban system. All national urban systems are becoming less autonomous and increasingly must be understood in terms of their integration into the global system. True before, but now more than ever, the functions, scope of interdependencies, and dominance relations associated with cities such as New York, Los Angeles, Miami, and Houston cannot be fully understood without considering each area's involvement in global and regional systems extending beyond the U.S. economy. This not only increases the scale of analysis in terms of the geographical scope and the number of cities, but it also brings with it complexities of reconciling data on urban systems drawn from many different sources. Furthermore, where researchers studying a national urban system have the luxury of assuming a relatively homogeneous political and regulatory environment, this can hardly be assumed for the global system or even for subglobal systems.

Analyses of intermetropolitan growth and decline, long a staple of demographic studies of macrospatial distribution, have become increasingly refined. Perhaps the greatest challenge for future work in this area is to develop measures and analytic strategies that permit empirically rigorous assessments of the relative importance of factors emphasized in traditional demographic perspectives and those emphasized in new perspectives. Champions of new perspectives have shown varying degrees of willingness to pursue the implications of their ideas with systematic empirical analysis beyond questionable extrapolations from case studies and broad-brush historical analyses. Markusen (1985) provides an example of how new ideas can be pursued with greater attention to analytic rigor, careful measurement, and quantitative assessments of relationships and effects. But such work is rare. Researchers grounded in traditional demographic perspectives would do well to draw on the best examples of research motivated by new perspectives to explore opportunities for theoretical refinement and to expand the understanding of spatial patterns.

Kasarda and Crenshaw (1991) and Smith (1995) note that the marriage of differing perspectives is certain to be uneasy. But Kasarda's (1995) overview of the restructuring of the U.S. metropolitan system in recent decades shows that selective consideration of ideas emphasized in new perspectives can be fruitful. It would be naive to suppose that efforts along these lines will be appreciated everywhere. Nevertheless, efforts to promote greater engagement between traditional and new perspectives may invigorate traditional research and demonstrate its value to a growing number of researchers who are unfamiliar with the best that it has to offer. Failure to pursue engagement between perspectives will ensure further balkanization in the field.

This admonition can also be offered in the area of intraurban spatial patterns. In the interperspective debate over the causes of population decentralization, there are particular opportunities to advance the field by drawing on the analytic rigor of traditional perspectives to explore patterns more carefully. The field has long been burdened by the problems of measuring the boundaries of metropolitan regions and the patterns of spatial distribution within these boundaries. Measurements of density and other features of urban areas based on central city and metro area boundaries are based more on convenience than the close correspondence with nodal-functional notions of urban system. Conventional approaches to city-suburb comparisons (used by researchers from all perspectives) have always been problematic, and the limitations of this approach have increased decade by decade. Data on population and employment for small-scale geographies are growing in availability and dropping in cost, and the same is true of the computational power needed to exploit these data. As a result, it is increasingly feasible to examine suburbanization and decentralization dynamics using more appropriate approaches than census-based city-suburb comparisons. Such a move would likely spark a reexamination of the conceptual foundations of the notions of city and suburb and the relative importance assigned to factors such as the absolute and relative densities for population and employment, the mix of land use and economic activity, and the relative spatial position in an expanding urban field.

More easily than ever before, spatial density distributions can be modeled directly and population deconcentration can be examined based on systematic, comparative measurements of density gradients, central or peak density, critical density, and other staples of the analytic framework advanced by traditional demographic perspectives on intraurban spatial distribution. Hypotheses regarding polycentrism, declining density differentials between centers, subcenters, and the broader urban field can be explored using more systematic comparisons of how these vary over time and across areas. The literature is rife with inexact claims of "new" urban forms and "new" principles of spatial organization. These claims will gain credence with demographic audiences only after rigorous analysis establishes whether emerging spatial patterns truly reflect new spatial principles, reexpressions of established spatial principles at new spatial scales permitted by advances in communication and transportation technologies, or some mixture of both.

Spectacular advancements in the capabilities, ease of use, and cost-effectiveness of geographical information systems (GIS) permit easier analysis of such complex variations in density patterns that traditional demographic perspectives predict, such as density corridors around transportation arteries and subcenters around interchanges. Accordingly, analyses of population and employment deconcentration need not be limited to a consideration of the several parameters of Colins' negative exponential density-distance function, even though the benefits of drawing on that relatively simple descriptive tool have hardly been exhausted. GIS technology and methods make it possible to conceive of integrating political economic and traditional demographic perspectives in systematic empirical analyses that allow for direct assessments of relative explanatory power. For example, now more than ever it is possible to integrate spatial data on political boundaries of various types and obtain direct measurements of factors that are linked with them, such as tax rates, ethnic composition of school districts, and political fragmentation, and to explore their linkages with patterns and trends in population density and composition.

On another front, researchers interested in testing the implications of traditional spatial perspectives may find that special opportunities are being presented in non-U.S. settings. In particular, a "natural" experiment is unfolding in China, an urban and spatial system that was for many, many decades governed by the strict, centralized regulation of population movement. China is now moving in the direction of greater decentralization of employment and population. This new macro-spatial "laboratory," already the object of preliminary explorations by Mao (1998) and Poston and Frisbie (1998), may yield insights into the underpinnings of inter- and intraurban spatial distribution. Since there is no *necessary* requirement that planning and central decision making be in conflict with ecological principles (a point worth stressing generally), it is an open question as to whether or not the urban system in China will change in dramatic ways. Similarly, patterns of density distribution and social segregation within urban areas may or may not evolve in new directions. Of course, China is hardly the only setting where these opportunities may be found. But its population size and geographical scale combine with the relative paucity of prior research to make it a prime candidate for closer study.

In the area of social differentiation in American urban areas, important methodological challenges need to be met on several fronts. Fortunately, recent advances in conceptualization, methodology, and the creative exploitation of available data are likely to continue in the immediate future.

I believe that this field is about to enter a new era. Research on residential segregation and spatial differentiation in the future will be distinguished from the past by a more detailed understanding and documentation of the linkages between individual-level processes and aggregate residential distributions. While the need for improvements in this area is great, both in research focusing on the demand-side and supply-side theories of segregation, the likelihood of significant breakthroughs is probably greater in research exploring demand-side dynamics because factors involved in individual choice dynamics are easier to measure and study than the microdynamics of discrimination.

Survey data provide ample evidence that residential preferences, tastes, and priorities vary systematically with individual- and household-level characteristics such as age, family-life-cycle, gender, social class, and ethnicity and race (McCauley and Nutty 1982; Shlay 1986; Shlay and DiGregorio 1985; Emerson, Yancey, and Chai 2001; Farley et al. 1978; Bobo and Charles 1996; Charles 2000a, 200b; Clark 1992). Accordingly, demand-side elements of ecological theory predict that variation in preferences should, all else equal, contribute to the formation of natural and social areas—the "urban mosaic." Social area analysis and other approaches to documenting social differentiation in urban space produce a certain kind of evidence consistent with these predictions. However, research of this type has always faced a major problem: data for small geographical areas have historically provided limited opportunities for examining the distribution and movement of social groups defined on the basis of multiple social characteristics. Thus, studies examining the spatial distribution of groups delimited by a single characteristic such as race have been much more common than studies examining the spatial distributions of groups delimited by two or more social characteristics such as race *and* socioeconomic status *and* stage in the family life cycle. The literature has been reaching the limits of what can be learned from studying city-level summary measures of segregation on one or two characteristics for some time.

Two recent innovations may be noted. One is the adaptation of large-scale surveys, such as the Panel Survey of Income Dynamics and the Annual Housing Survey, to the investigation of residential outcomes at low levels of geography (South and Crowder 1997, 1998; Crowder 2000) and the use of special individual-level census files with certain kinds of neighborhood data attached to individual records (Massey and Denton 1985). Much has been gained from these approaches, but they are limited in their ability to sustain the in-depth analysis of individual metropolitan areas or the comparative analysis of many metropolitan areas. The second innovation is the methodology of Alba and Logan (1992, 1993), which creatively combines aggregate-level and microdata to permit the individual-level analysis of locational attainments. This has spawned an important literature. The full exploitation of the methodology has not yet run its course, but two problems loom. One is that limitations of the aggregate-level tabulations for census microgeography restrict the options for subgroup analysis and model specification in significant ways.

Another is that clear connections between individual-level location attainment processes and aggregate-level segregation patterns have yet to be fleshed out in a way that might extend the appeal of the method. This may yet occur, and the effort should be given high priority. Success in this regard would elevate the methodology of Alba and Logan to the forefront in segregation research and make the literature based on city-level segregation scores alone obsolete. Unfortunately, it is an open question as to whether the goal of connecting individual-level location attainment processes to aggregate-level segregation patterns can be realized. The problem is long standing; Duncan and Duncan (1955a: 216) noted more than 50 years ago that nowhere in "the literature on segregation indices measures is there a suggestion about how to use them to study the *process* of segregation or change in segregation pattern" (emphasis in original). This remains largely true today.

One possible approach is to shift the focus from measures based on the segregation curve, i.e., the dissimilarity index and the related and conceptually superior Gini index, toward Bell's (1954) revised index of isolation and related "exposure" or "contact" measures. The revised index of isolation is attractive for modeling purposes because it can be conceptualized as an individual attainment outcome, namely, the probability of in-group contact, expressed in relation to the expected value of this outcome in the absence of segregation. Thus, it can be used to link aggregate-level segregation directly to the effects in individual-level, spatial attainment models. James and Taeuber (1985) note that this measure is not without flaws. But it is well known that the ubiquitous index of dissimilarity is flawed in serious ways, and it cannot be linked to spatial attainment models. So Bell's measure and other variations of measures comparing actual-to-expected group contact should be explored.

A new option is now available that can overcome at least some of the limitations of past research. This is the use of restricted-access census files to gain the possibility of accessing individual-level data with full geographical detail. Bayer and colleagues (2003) conduct analyses based on this approach and explore the question of whether or not the effects of individual characteristics on spatial location outcomes may combine with group differences in distribution on these characteristics to produce systematic group differences in residential distribution. Their detailed analysis of the San Francisco–Oakland region suggests that individual characteristics account for 80% of Hispanic isolation, approximately 50% of Asian isolation, and 30% of black isolation. The results are preliminary, but the method is promising; it permits detailed decompositions of the sources of segregation and is extensible to cross-area comparisons. Unfortunately, the phrase "restricted access" should not be taken lightly. The census files in question are not available to the public and can only be accessed by special arrangement with the U.S. Census Bureau at a limited number of physical sites.

The overriding problem facing supply-side theories of segregation parallels that facing demand-side theories: it is the chasm between the identification of microlevel processes of discrimination and constraint on housing choice and establishing their impact on city-level segregation measures. The documentation of ongoing discrimination in the current era is widely accepted. Large-scale audit studies (Yinger 1995), while not without serious methodological problems (Heckman and Siegleman 1993), are by and large accepted as convincing (Yinger 1998). Unfortunately, they are not suited for estimating the quantitative effects of discrimination on minority location attainments or aggregate residential distributions. Observers who conclude that the quantitative impact is large and accounts for observed segregation to the extent that other factors can be dismissed must rest their conclusions on a chain of assumptions and indirect inferences that are speculative and difficult to evaluate or verify. The problem is not that the hypothesis is implausible; the problem is that defensible quantitative assessments are unavailable. At one end of the spectrum, Butters (1993), Thernstrom and Thernstrom (1997), and Patterson (1997) argue that in many, perhaps most, cities, minority families with sufficient means experience few constraints on their location choices and can settle where they wish with little realistic concern of being subject to physical intimidation or violence. Whether they would be welcomed and accepted into the social life of the local community is another question, but that is a separate phenomenon. The controversy in this area is likely to endure until better linkages between measures of the incidence of discrimination and aggregate-level segregation patterns can be developed.

One methodology that may help in this regard is computer simulation. While not used extensively, isolated examples of simulation methodology have explored segregation dynamics (e.g., Schelling 1971, 1972; Young 1998; Krugman 1996; Epstein and Axtell 1996; Freeman and Sunshine 1970; Fossett 1999, 2001, 2004a, 2004b). At present the potential value is primarily in the area of conducting theoretical analysis of the causal potential of hypothesized microlevel social processes. Given the present gap between studies of microlevel process and macrolevel segregation patterns, this is not without value. But simulation models would have to advance considerably before they could be used to anchor the quantitative assessments of the impact of discrimination or other factors on segregation outcomes. One possible strategy to pursue in this regard is to examine results from simulation analyses to try and identify "signature" patterns that mark the effects of particular microlevel processes and then see if these can be found in data for "real" cities. The limitation of this approach is that exploratory research along these lines suggests that most familiar aggregate-level segregation patterns can be produced by multiple microlevel processes and thus no particular microlevel process may be ruled out (Fossett 2004a).

RESEARCH EXEMPLARS: INTRAURBAN SPATIAL DISTRIBUTION

Recent research in the area of urban and spatial patterns provides many candidates for exemplars. Regarding macrospatial distributions, this chapter now reviews a compilation of points developed in several recent analyses by Frey (1995), Glaeser and Shapiro (2003), Glaeser and Kohlhase (2003), and Kasarda (1995), all of whom draw on traditional demographic perspectives leavened with selected insights from new perspectives to explain and interpret trends in regional and intermetropolitan population shifts in recent decades. Kasarda (1995) and Frey (1995) draw on urban ecological theory; Glaeser and colleagues draw on the new economic geography (Anas, Arnott, and Small 1998; Fujita and Thisse 2002). These theoretical perspectives are highly compatible, so it is not surprising that they advance similar findings and interpretations. The impact of long-term changes in communication and transportation technologies receives the greatest attention, with secondary emphasis going to factors such as climate and amenities, government (although not always for the reasons suggested by critical theorists), and the implications of globalization.

While all four stress the impact of technological change, Glaeser and Kohlhase (2003) are especially forceful. "A revolution in transportation technologies unfolded in the twentieth century; it would have been surprising had a revolution in urban form and location not occurred as well" (2003: 31). They argue that at the beginning of the 20th century transportation costs were high and created powerful economic incentives for cities to be located near natural resources and natural transport hubs. Transportation costs declined dramatically over the century and became less hub-centered. At the same time, cities shifted from being centers of goods production to centers of service production. This made it increasingly possible for population to redistribute, spatially guided by business and consumer preferences regarding climate, amenities, and the business environment. Cities still continued to be centers of economic activity because they brought people together in close proximity, creating significant agglomeration economies especially for educated and higher-skilled workers. But urban economies became more "footloose" in space, and cities were less tied to resources and break-in-transportation locations. Consequently, population followed business and consumer preferences and shifted from the interior of the country and toward coastal regions, toward warmer and dryer regions, and "favorable" business environments. In addition, the population increasingly concentrated in cities which, due to the consequences of reduced transportation costs within cities, shifted from being organized around an urban core to being organized around sprawling urban regions. As dramatic as these trends are, Glaeser and colleagues speculate that they would have been even stronger if not for the massive inertia in the urban system associated with sunk costs in infrastructure and housing.

Glaeser and Shapiro (2003) and Glaeser and Kohlhase (2003) document the long-term declines in specific transportation costs and in the declining fraction that transportation costs represent in the total economy, both key factors in their overall arguments. They also find support for the hypotheses they advance by drawing on a variety of data sets to perform relevant empirical analyses. Analysis of urban growth patterns in recent decades shows, as they predict, that certain kinds of cities gained relative to others and certain kinds lost: cities with resource-based economies, such as extraction and agriculture, lost; cities with warm, dry climates gained; cities organized around auto and truck transport gained; cities with higher skill mixes gained; and cities specializing in goods production lost. Their arguments also generate predictions about urban form that figure into their overall analysis. Declining transport costs for goods freed manufacturing from rail and water transport hubs. With the reduction in economic incentives to locate near resources, customers, and suppliers, manufacturing moved from the center of the city to the fringe, and from larger to smaller metropolitan areas. Service industries requiring significant amounts of nonroutine face-to-face interaction continued to promote high densities in central cities, since time-costs of bringing people together over very long distances tend still to be high. However, service industries did not sustain the urban core in the same way as hub-and-spoke rail and water transport and mass transit systems. Thus, density was falling generally but was varying positively with services and level of education and negatively with manufacturing.

Finally, they present evidence on long-term population shifts consistent with the prediction that population is shifting toward large, sprawling urban regions. Specifically, they show that the fraction of national population found in counties in the bottom decile of density and in counties in the top 1% of density *both* declined substantially between 1920 and 2000, and the share of population found in the top decile (excluding the top 1%) increased substantially.[11]

Essentially these regions are large population and employment "domes," which may or may not have single, multiple, or no dominant centers. Even when dominant centers are present, the majority of employment is spread diffusely, since the primary transport consideration is moving people and, in cities with car-oriented transport systems, movement within the suburban ring (now the most common kind of commute) has lower time-costs than movement from periphery to center due to congestion effects. The emergence of these large, sprawling urban regions is leading to important shifts in the national urban hierarchy. This is consistent with central place theory because the

---

[11] Between 1920 and 2000 the population share for the bottom decile of counties by density fell from 19% to 9% and the share for the top 1% fell from 20% to 11%. The share for the top decile (excluding the top 1%) increased from 30% to 49%.

decline of cities at the lower tiers is expected under conditions of declining transportation costs for goods and information.[12] Interestingly, Ogburn (1946) more than half a
century ago forecast that this would occur based on his analysis of how maturation of
auto and air transit would lead to consolidation of city-based trading areas into
progressively smaller numbers of large regions.

Kasarda (1995) or Frey (1995) would take issue with little in this capsule summary.
Both endorse the notion that cities that made the transition from producing goods to
providing services fared better in intermetropolitan restructuring over recent decades.
They also note the resumption of the long-term decline of nonmetro areas despite the
"blip" of the 1970s; population movement toward the West and the South; population
movement from the interior to coastal areas (also see Rappaport and Sachs 2003), and
the vitality of population growth in metro areas with high education and skill mixes
(especially after controlling for immigration). Kasarda gives greater attention to globalization and how it is implicated in some of the macrospatial changes observed in
recent decades. One interpretation of the positive education-growth relationship and the
negative manufacturing-growth relationship is that in a global economy, cities specializing in most forms of manufacturing are vulnerable to global competition due to the
dynamics identified in the product-cycle theory of Vernon (1966) and the neo-Marxian
profit cycle theory of Markusen (1985). Both predict that high-wage regions must
continually innovate to maintain their relative standing in a spatially integrated economy, especially one in which transportation costs are declining, political barriers to
trade are falling, and centers of high-skill labor are emerging in the developing world.
Thus, Kasarda reports that cities specializing in new "leading" industries fare better
than those specializing in "lagging" industries, which are vulnerable to "filtering."

While all these studies emphasize the growing importance of consumer preferences
in location decisions, Kasarda (1995) gives more attention to business "climate" and
quasipolitical economic concerns. His point is that in an economy where declining
transport costs increasingly free businesses from specific locations, areas within the
United States must increasingly compete with each other and with extranational locations on considerations such as tax incentives, regulatory burdens, and related factors to
capture and retain business and industry. Labor costs and unionization factor into both
this and product cycle theory. Closely related is the question of local government
policies regarding growth and the provision of government-based services such as public
education, crime, and low pollution. These considerations do not always line up nicely,
but Kasarda notes that the match between local government policies and the class
ideology of affluent business leaders and elite workers is likely to play an increasing
role in location decisions. Ironically, this political-economic consideration is elevated in
importance because conventional ecological dynamics give affluent decision makers
greater discretion in location decisions. Finally, Kasarda notes that some have hypothesized that federal fiscal policies have influenced interregional restructuring, but the
impact of this relative to other factors is not well established.[13] In sum, the four studies
highlighted here (plus the larger literature they draw on) document important long-term
trends in interurban and intraurban population distribution and link them to changes in

---

[12] The spacing between nodes in central place theory is an inverse function of the cost of communication and
transportation. Along these lines Cottrell's (1951) study "Death by Dieselization" documented how a small
layer of the central place system in rural areas disappeared as advances in rail transport technologies obviated
the need for closely spaced stops.

[13] For a discussion, see Markusen (1987).

factors that have long been central to traditional demographic perspectives on urban and spatial distribution of population.

FUTURE PROSPECTS

The discussion in this chapter has been guided primarily by traditional demographic perspectives regarding urban and spatial distributions. This is likely to resonate with many readers of this *Handbook*. But the fact is that undergraduate texts on urban sociology and an increasing number of journals focusing on urban issues give less attention to these perspectives now than in the past. Many urban sociologists, including some who proclaim particular interests in spatial patterns, express skepticism about the relevance and value of these traditional perspectives. Indeed, some have written that the traditional demographic-ecological paradigm has been supplanted (Feagin 1998; Gottdeiner and Hutchinson 2000). Without question, the field has bifurcated. In the area of population, traditional perspectives generally hold sway. Elsewhere, traditional population perspectives are receiving less attention. This is certainly true in sociology and appears to be the case in geography (Yeates 2001; Berry 2001). Population specialists may see little impact in the field of demography directly, and it will surprise no one that critical and political economic perspectives have made lesser inroads in economics and regional science.[14] But the general trends in sociology and geography are that insights from traditional population perspectives are being compartmentalized and are having less of an impact in these disciplines, even in areas where population perspectives would seem highly relevant.

Two questions arise. What are the points of departure between traditional and new perspectives on urban and spatial patterns? Are there any opportunities for a meeting of the minds? To anticipate the conclusion, I hold that the answer to the second question is probably yes, but that opportunities for constructive dialog are unlikely to be seized in the near term. In short there is little reason to be optimistic about the chances for any serious reconciliation of the perspectives in the near term, although efforts along the lines of Smith's (1995) search for common ground are to be commended and could pave the way for constructive engagement and mutual benefit. One reason for this view is that there is relatively little engagement between adherents of traditional perspectives and proponents of new perspectives, even in areas where outsiders might see considerable overlap in views. There are several points of fundamental difference between the traditional and new perspectives that contribute to this situation.

Problem Selection and Research Agenda

Scholars who are proponents of critical and political economic perspectives address different questions and emphasize different issues than those subscribing to traditional economic and ecological perspectives. Specifically, there is a greater focus among the former on issues of social inequality, concentration of power, uneven development, discrimination, and other social problems. In many ways, critics' objections to traditional

---

[14] To the contrary, in urban economics and the subfield of economic geography traditional economic and ecological perspectives seem to be enjoying a renaissance of sorts.

perspectives trace as much to their dissatisfaction with the *questions* selected for theoretical and empirical attention as to the development of specific theories and empirical findings. While there is never complete consensus in any field regarding which problems should receive attention, it is fair to say that traditional and critical perspectives differ more than is usual. This is especially true regarding views about the appropriate balance to strike between pursuing "basic" science questions versus questions that are more immediately related to contemporary social problems.

Differences in Research Practices

There is considerable heterogeneity in research design and method of analysis in both perspectives and a significant overlap across perspectives. That said, there also are clear aggregate differences in methodological practice between the traditional and new perspectives. Demographic researchers are more likely to perform quantitative analyses using census and survey data and large samples. Critical and political economic researchers are more likely to draw in-depth studies of a small number of cases. Even when researchers from the two perspectives use similar methods, differences are evident. Researchers drawing on traditional perspectives tend to see case studies as valuable for making exploratory inquiries to identify new patterns and dynamics. The guiding presumption, however, is that hypotheses emerging from qualitative studies will be taken as exploratory and tentative until they are assessed with quantitative studies using large, representative samples and sophisticated techniques of multivariate analysis. In contrast, scholars working within "critical" or "political economic" frameworks are more willing to draw strong causal inferences and broad conclusions from case studies; some rarely use any other methodology. Reciprocal skepticism greets research generated by both perspectives.

Approaches to Conceptualization and Measurement

Proponents of traditional perspectives are more likely to place stock in abstract conceptualization, technical measurement strategies, and formal approaches to theory development and construction. "Critical" and "political economic" urban researchers are more inclined to draw on concepts that are "naturalistic" and less technical.

Appreciation of Formal Models

Researchers drawing on traditional demographic perspectives generally hold formal theory and abstract models in higher regard than proponents of other perspectives. Economists, regional scientists, and urban ecologists subscribe to the view that causal effects should be assessed in the context of well-understood "baseline" models. They believe that it is difficult to develop rigorous conclusions in the absence of such models. This leads them to be skeptical of strong conclusions developed from discursive theory, which they are likely to view as a precursor to "serious" theory development that entails formalization. In contrast, many researchers working within the "critical" and "political economic" perspectives subscribe to a decidedly different view of theory. They often do not embrace the development of formal models. Many are openly suspicious of the value of such models and may view them as simplistic and ahistorical. Consequently, while proponents of new perspectives are not shy about criticizing the "simplistic models" of traditional perspectives, they rarely engage in systematic efforts to formalize their own theories and expose them to similar critique.

Approaches to Standards of Evidence and the Philosophy of Science

Traditional researchers subscribe to goals of developing nomothetic explanations and evaluating theories against evidence along the lines of practices in the natural sciences. New perspective researchers are a heterogeneous group, but most tend to be ambivalent at best toward traditional science approaches and the goal of nomothetic explanation. This ambivalence underlies the skepticism many have of formal theory and models. It also leads many to place a lower priority on the task of developing specific empirical predictions from their theories and pursuing a sustained program of assessing these predictions with rigorous quantitative studies.

Orientation to Social Policy

Ironically, while critical theorists often criticize traditional perspectives for giving inadequate attention to inequality and other social problems, some argue that, because they seek to develop rigorous, predictive science grounded in basic models of urban and spatial dynamics, traditional perspectives are more likely to create the possibility for developing effective social policy to address normative concerns. Yeates (2001) for example, suggests that one of the legacies of the Chicago School of urban geography is that planners and regulators often pursue normative goals such as preserving historic downtowns, maintaining traditional neighborhoods, moderating residential segregation, stemming inner-city decline, and managing sprawl by using tools and strategies that derive in part from the theories and models of traditional spatial perspectives. Significantly, these policies can be pursued regardless of whether the originators of the models and theories endorse them or not. Some critical theorists respond that planners and regulators have limited options for at best reformist intervention. But more dramatic (radical) social interventions are especially unlikely to be entertained if they are not grounded in a model-based, predictive science that can provide a sound basis for anticipating the full range of consequences that might flow from the interventions.[15] Recent studies by Logan and Zhou (1989, 1990) advance a similar view from a grounding in political-economy perspectives.

The Future Directions of Traditional and New Perspectives

The future direction of traditional perspectives on urban and spatial population distribution is relatively easy to forecast. It will be given direction by questions that have long

---

[15] It goes without saying that for regulation and intervention to be predictable in their consequences, they must be grounded in a basic understanding of what would take place in their absence.

motivated the literature. They include the following: Why do cities exist and provide a home to an ever increasing fraction of the worlds' population? Why are cities found in particular locations? Why do they vary in size? How do they come to be functionally differentiated and linked together in a complex system of ever changing interdependencies? What are the patterns of their internal form, and how and why do these change over time? In pursuing these questions, traditional perspectives will likely follow the trajectory established now for more than eight decades; they will refine general models of urban areas and urban systems and will assess these models by pursuing systematic programs of cumulative empirical research.

Proponents of new perspectives have called attention to the limitations of traditional perspectives. The defenders of established views accept that this criticism can and has stimulated the consideration of interesting new questions (e.g., Yeates 2001; Clark 2001; Markusen 2003). But the criticism is often overdrawn and unnecessarily antagonistic. Traditional perspectives are *intentionally* restricted in scope and goals. This is a hallmark of scientific "reductionism." On the one hand, this helps explain why criticism grounded in new perspectives has sparked little change in the direction or orientation of traditional perspectives. On the other hand, it is clear that the restricted focus of traditional perspectives provides an opening for new perspectives to contribute to expanded understandings of urban and spatial distributions.

It is difficult to forecast whether the new perspectives will fully exploit this opportunity. To date the impact of new perspectives outside of their own circles has been severely blunted by the fact that no clear consensus has been built behind a single, theoretically coherent, alternative vision. The "call to arms" for the new perspectives is clear: there is more to urban and spatial patterns than traditional demographic perspectives can fully explain. But this is hardly an adequate basis for establishing that new theoretical perspectives on spatial distribution must be *substituted* for old. New perspectives cannot simply provide alternative conceptual frameworks for interpreting *established* empirical patterns in different ways. They must make significant positive contributions by accounting for patterns of spatial distribution that proponents of *all* perspectives agree are both important and difficult to explain with traditional perspectives alone. Overviews of the field by scholars sympathetic to political-economic efforts implicitly recognize this need when they express concern that the initial blush of success the perspective enjoys has promoted a degree of "overconfidence" and a lack of "a sense of genuine puzzlement" (Walton 1993:318). Some worry that this may slow the impetus to refine concepts and establish empirical linkages more carefully (Pahl 1989).[16]

There are many reasons why new perspectives have not had great impact in demographic circles. Sociocultural, postmodern, and related perspectives establish that culture "matters" in spatial distributions but do not capitalize on this insight to explain spatial patterns in any general way. Scholars working with critical and political economic perspectives have often tried to change the focus of the field rather than seriously pursue new and compelling answers to the long-standing questions motivating the research of demographers, economists, and urban ecologists who study urban and spatial patterns. Those who have addressed these questions often adopt antagonistic stances toward traditional theory and research practices that are unproductive and guarantee that their impact in demographic circles will be limited.

---

[16] It would be wrong to interpret these misgivings as an endorsement for traditional perspectives since they are intended as a rallying call for adherents of another view.

For their part, adherents of traditional perspectives have shown little inclination to see past differences and examine new perspectives for useful insights (Kasarda and Crenshaw 1991; Markusen 2003; Adams 2001; Clark 2001; Yeates 2001; for exceptions see London 1987 and Smith 1995). As the situation presently stands, the traditional and new perspectives are barely engaged. Smith (1995) is probably correct in arguing that opportunities are being missed all around. In sum, the situation is ripe for efforts that can bridge the conceptual and philosophical divide between traditional and new perspectives and yield a more comprehensive understanding of urban and spatial patterns.

REFERENCES

Abler, R. F., J. S. Adams, and P. R. Gould. 1971. *Spatial organization: The geographer's view of the world.* Englewood Cliffs, N.J.: Prentice-Hall.

Abrahamson, M. 1996. *Urban enclaves: Identity and place in America.* New York: St. Martin's Press.

Adams, J. S. 2001. The quantitative revolution in urban geography. *Urban Geography* 22: 530–539.

Alba, R. D., and J. R. Logan. 1992. Assimilation and stratification in the homeownership patterns of racial and ethnic groups. *International Migration Review* 26: 1314–1341.

Alba, R. D., and J. R. Logan. 1993. Minority proximity to whites in suburbs: An individual-level analysis of segregation. *American Journal of Sociology* 98: 1388–1427.

Alexandersson, G. 1956. *The industrial structure of American cities: A geographic study of urban economics in the U. S.* Lincoln: University of Nebraska Press.

Alonso, W. 1964. *Location and land use: Toward a general theory of land rent.* Cambridge, Mass.: Harvard University Press.

Anas, A., R. Arnott, and K. A. Small. 1998. Urban spatial structure. *Journal of Economic Literature* 36: 1426–1464.

Anderson, E. 1990. *Streetwise: race, class, and change in an urban community.* Chicago: University of Chicago Press.

Bahr, H. M., and J. P. Gibbs. 1967. Racial differentiation in American metropolitan areas. *Social Forces* 45: 521–532.

Barth, E. A. T., and D. L. Noel. 1972. Conceptual frameworks for the analysis of race relations: An evaluation. *Social Forces* 50: 333–348.

Bayer, Patrick, Robert McMillan, Kim Rueben. 2003. "What Drives Racial Segregation? New Evidence Using Census Microdata." Discussion Paper No. 859. Public Policy Institute of California.

Beck, E. M., and S. E. Tolnay. 1990. The killing fields of the deep South and the market for cotton and the lynchings of blacks 1882–1930. *American Sociological Review* 55: 526–539.

Bell, W. 1953. The social areas of the San Francisco Bay region. *American Sociological Review* 18: 39–47.

Bell, W. 1954. A probability model for the measurement of ecological segregation. *Social Forces* 32: 357–364.

Bell, W. 1955. Economic, family, and ethnic status: An empirical test. *American Sociological Review* 20:45–52.

Berry, B. J. L. 1979. *The open housing question: Race and housing in Chicago, 1966–1976.* Cambridge, Mass.: Ballinger.

Berry, B. J. L. 2001. The Chicago School in retrospect and prospect. *Urban Geography* 22: 559–561.

Berry, B. J. L., and Y. Cohen. 1973. Decentralization of commerce and industry: The restructuring of metropolitan America. In *The urbanization of suburbs.* Edited by L. H. Masotti and J. K. Hadden, 431–455. Beverly Hills, Calif.: Sage Publications.

Berry, B. J. L., F. E. Horton, and J. O. Abiodun. 1970. *Geographic perspectives on urban systems.* Englewood Cliffs, N.J.: Prentice-Hall.

Berry, B. J. L., and J. D. Kasarda. 1977. *Contemporary urban ecology.* New York: Macmillan.

Black, D., and V. Henderson. 1999. A theory of urban growth. *Journal of Political Economy* 107: 252–284.

Blalock, H. M., Jr. 1956. Economic discrimination and Negro increase. *American Sociological Review* 21: 584–588.

Blalock, H. M., Jr. 1957. Percent nonwhite and discrimination in the South. *American Sociological Review* 22:677–682.

Blalock, H. M., Jr. 1959. Urbanization and discrimination in the South. *Social Problems* 7:146–152.

Blalock, H. M., Jr. 1967. *Toward a theory of minority-group relations.* New York: Wiley.

Bogue, D. J. 1949. *The structure of the metropolitan community: A study of dominance and subdominance.* Ann Arbor: University of Michigan Press.

Bollen, K. A., and S. J. Appold. 1993. National industrial structure and the global system. *American Sociological Review* 58:283–301.

Borchert, J. R. 1967. American metropolitan evolution. *Geographical Review* 57:301–332.

Bourne, L. S. 1971. *Internal structure of the city: Readings on space and environment.* New York: Oxford University Press.

Bourne, L. S., and J. W. Simmons. 1978. *Systems of cities: Readings on structure, growth, and policy.* New York: Oxford University Press.

Brueckner, J. K. 2000. Urban sprawl: Diagnosis and remedies. *International Regional Science Review* 23:160–171.

Brueckner, J. K., and D. A. Fansler. 1983. The economics of urban sprawl: Theory and evidence on the spatial sizes of cities. *Review of Economics & Statistics* 65: 479–482.

Burgess, E. W. 1925. The growth of the city. In *The city.* Edited by R. E. Park, E. W. Burgess, and R. D. McKenzie, 47–62. Chicago: University of Chicago Press.

Burgess, E. W. 1927. The determination of gradients in the growth of the city. *American Sociological Society* 21: 178–184.

Burgess, E. W. 1928. Residential segregation in American cities. *Annals of the American Academy of Political and Social Science* 140: 105–115.

Burr, J. A., O. R. Galle, and M. Fossett. 1991. Racial occupational inequality in southern metropolitan areas, 1940–1980: Revisting the visibility-discrimination hypothesis. *Social Forces* 69: 831–850.

Butters, R. D. 1993. The real estate industry's view of audit results: Comments. In *Clear and convincing evidence: Measurement of discrimination in America.* Edited by M. Fix and R. J. Struyk, 153–163. Washington, D.C.: Urban Institute Press.

Castells, M. 1977. *The urban question.* Cambridge, Mass.: MIT Press.

Castells, M. 1985. *High technology, space, and society.* Beverly Hills, Calif.: Sage Publications.

Charles, C. Z. 2000a. Neighborhood racial composition preferences: Evidence from a multiethnic metropolis. *Social Problems* 47:379–407.

Charles, C. Z. 2000b. Residential segregation in Los Angeles. In *Prismatic metropolis: Inequality in Los Angeles.* Edited by L. D. Bobo, M. L. Oliver, J. H. Johnson, Jr., and A. Valenzuela, Jr., Chapter 4. New York: Russell Sage.

Chase-Dunn, C. K. 1984. Urbanization in the world-system: New directions for research. In *Urban affairs annual review,* Vol. 26. Cities in transformation. Edited by M. P. Smith. Thousand Oaks, Calif.: Sage Publications.

Chase-Dunn, C. K., and P. Grimes. 1995. World-system analysis. *Annual Review of Sociology* 21:387–417.

Chase-Dunn, C. K., and T. D. Hall. 1993. Comparing world-systems: Concepts and working hypotheses. *Social Forces* 71:851–886.

Chase-Dunn, C., Y. Kawano, and B. Brewer. 2000. Trade globalization since 1795: Waves of integration in the world-system. *American Sociological Review* 65:77–95.

Chevan, A. 1982. Age, housing choice, and neighborhood age structure. *American Journal of Sociology* 87:1133–1149.

Chorley, R. J., and P. Haggett, eds. 1967. *Models in geography.* London: Methuen.

Christaller, W. 1966. *Central places in southern Germany.* Translated from *Die zentralen Orte in Süddeutschland,* by C. W. Baskin [1933]. Englewood Cliffs, N.J.: Prentice-Hall.

Clark, C. 1951. Urban population densities. *Journal of the Royal Statistical Society* 114:490–496.

Clark, W. A. V. 1992. Residential preferences and residential choices in a multiethnic context. *Demography* 29:451–466.

Clark, W. A. V. 2000. Monocentric to polycentric: New urban forms and old paradigms. In *A companion to the city.* Edited by G. Bridge and S. Watson. Oxford: Blackwell.

Clark, W. A. V. 2001. Pacific views of urban geography in the 1960s. *Urban Geography* 22:540–548.

Cooley, C. H. 1894. The theory of transportation. *Publications of the American Economic Association* 9:312–322.

Corzine, J., J. C. Creech, and L. Corzine. 1983. Black concentration and lynching in the South: Testing Blalock's power threat hypothesis. *Social Forces* 61:774–796.

Cottrell, W. F. 1951. Death by dieselization: Study in the reaction to technological change. *American Sociological Review* 16:358–365.

Cowgill, D. O. 1978. Residential segregation by age in American metropolitan areas. *Journal of Gerontology* 33:446–453.

Creech, J. C., J. Corzine, and L. Huff-Corzine. 1989. Theory testing and lynching: Another look at the power threat hypothesis. *Social Forces* 67:626–630.

Cressey, P. F. 1938. Population succession in Chicago: 1898–1930. *American Journal of Sociology* 44: 59–69.

Crowder, K. 2000. The racial context of white mobility: An individual-level assessment of the white flight hypothesis. *Social Science Research* 29:223–257.

Dear, M. J. 2000. *The postmodern urban condition*. Oxford: Blackwell.

Dear, M. J., and S. Flusty. 1998. Postmodern urbanism. *Annals of the Association of American Geographers* 88:50–72.

Dogan, M., and J. D. Kasarda, eds. 1988a. *The metropolis era, Vol. I. A world of giant cities*. Newbury Park, Calif.: Sage Publications.

Dogan, M., and J. D. Kasarda, eds. 1988b. *The metropolis era, Vol. II. Mega-cities*. Newbury Park, Calif.: Sage Publications.

Dogan, M., and J. D. Kasarda. 1988c. How giant cities will multiply and grow. In *The metropolitan era, Vol. I. A world of giant cities*. Edited by M. Dogan and J. D. Kasarda, 12–29. Newbury Park, Calif.: Sage Publications.

Duncan, B., and S. Lieberson. 1970. *Metropolis and region in transition*. Beverly Hills, Calif.: Sage Publications.

Duncan, O. D. 1959. Human ecology and population studies. In *The study of population*. Edited by P. M. Hauser and O. D. Duncan, 678–716. Chicago: University of Chicago Press.

Duncan, O. D. 1964. Social organization and the ecosystem. In *Handbook of modern sociology*. Edited by R. E. L. Faris, 37–82. Chicago: Rand McNally.

Duncan, O. D., and B. Duncan. 1955a. A methodological analysis of segregation indices. *American Sociological Review* 20:210–217.

Duncan, O. D., and B. Duncan. 1955b. Residential distribution and occupational stratification. *American Journal of Sociology* 60:493–503.

Duncan, O. D., and B. Duncan. 1957. *The Negro population of Chicago*. Chicago: University of Chicago Press.

Duncan, O. D., and S. Lieberson. 1959. Ethnic segregation and assimilation. *American Journal of Sociology* 64:364–374.

Duncan, O. D., R. W. Scott, S. Lieberson, B. Duncan, and H. H. Winsborough. 1960. *Metropolis and region*. Baltimore, Md.: Johns Hopkin University Press.

Eberstein, I. W., and W. P. Frisbie. 1982. Metropolitan function and interdependence in the US urban system. *Social Forces* 60:676–700.

Eberstein, I. W., and O. R. Galle. 1984. The metropolitan system in the South: Functional differentiation and trade patterns. *Social Forces* 62:926–940.

Edmonston, B., and T. M. Guterbock. 1984. Is suburbanization slowing down? Recent trends in population deconcentration in U.S. metropolitan areas. *Social Forces* 62: 905–925.

Emerson, M., G. Yancey, and K. J. Chai. 2001. Does race matter in residential segregation? Exploring the preferences of white Americans. *American Sociological Review* 66:922–935.

Epstein, J. M., and R. Axtell. 1996. *Growing artificial societies: Social science from the bottom up*. Cambridge, Mass.: MIT Press.

Eschback, K., J. M. Hagan, N. P. Rodriguez, and A. Zakos. 1998. Houston Heights. *Cityscapes* 4:245–259.

Farley, R. 1977. Residential segregation in urbanized areas of the United States in 1970: An analysis social class and racial differentials. *Demography* 14:497–518.

Farley, R., and W. H. Frey. 1994. Changes in the segregation of whites from blacks during the 1980s: Small steps toward a more integrated society. *American Sociological Review* 59:23–45.

Farley, R., T. Richards, and C. Wurdock. 1980. School desegregation and white flight: An investigation of competing models and their discrepant findings. *Sociology of Education* 53:123–139.

Farley, R., H. Schuman, S. Bianchi, D. Colasanto, and S. Hatchett. 1978. Chocolate city, vanilla suburbs: Will the trend toward racially separate communities continue? *Social Science Research* 7:319–344.

Feagin, J. R. 1985. The global context of metropolitan growth: Houston and the oil industry. *American Journal of Sociology* 90:1204–1230

Feagin, J. R. 1988. *Free enterprise city: Houston in political-economic perspective*. New Brunswick, N.J.: Rutgers University Press.

Feagin, J. R. 1998. *The new urban paradigm: Critical perspectives on the city*. Lanham, Md.: Rowman and Littlefield.

Firey, W. 1945. Sentiment and Symbolism as Ecological Variables. *American Sociological Review* 10: 140–148.

Firey, W. 1947. *Land use in central Boston.* Cambridge, Mass.: Harvard University Press.

Fix, M., and R. J. Struyk, eds. 1993. *Clear and convincing evidence: Measurement of discrimination in America.* Washington, D.C.: The Urban Institute Press.

Ford, R. G. 1950. Population succession in Chicago. *American Journal of Sociology* 56:156–160.

Fossett, M. A. 1999. Ethnic preferences, social distance dynamics, and residential segregation: Results from simulation analyses. Paper Presented at the Annual Meetings of the American Sociological Association, Chicago.

Fossett, M. A. 2001. Ethnic preferences and residential segregation: What goes up does not necessarily come down (at least not rapidly). Paper Presented at the Annual Meetings of the American Sociological Association, Anaheim, Calif.:

Fossett, M. A. 2004a. Simulation analysis of residential segregation: Advantages and disadvantages. Paper Presented at the Annual Meetings of the Southwestern Sociological Society, Corpus Christi, Tex.

Fossett, M. A. 2004b. Racial preferences and racial residential segregation: Findings from analyses using minimum segregation models. Paper Presented at the Annual Meetings of the Population Association of America, Boston.

Fossett, M. A., and C. Cready. 1998. Ecological approaches to the study of racial and ethnic differentiation and inequality. In *Continuities in sociological human ecology.* Edited by M. Micklin and D. L. Poston, Jr., 157–194. New York: Plenum.

Fossett, M. A., and K. J. Kiecolt. 1989. The relative size of minority populations and white racial attitudes. *Social Science Quarterly* 70:820–835.

Fossett, M. A., and T. M. Siebert. 1997. *Long time coming: Trends in racial inequality in the nonmetropolitan South since 1940.* Boulder, Colo.: Westview.

Freeman, L. C., and M. H. Sunshine. 1970. *Patterns of residential segregation.* Cambridge, Mass.: Schenkman.

Frey, W. 1979. Central city white flight: Racial and nonracial causes. *American Sociological Review* 44:425–448.

Frey, William H. 1985. Mover destination selectivity and the changing suburbanization of meteropolitan Whites and Blacks. *Demography* 22:223–243.

Frey, W. 1995. The new geography of population shifts. In *State of the Union: America in the 1990s, Vol. 2. Social trends.* Edited by R. Farley, 271–337. New York: Russell Sage.

Frey, W., and E. L. Fielding. 1995. Changing urban populations: Regional restructuring, racial polarization, and poverty concentration. *Cityscapes* 1:1–66.

Frey, W., and A. Speare. 1988. *Regional and metropolitan growth and decline in the United States.* New York: Russell Sage.

Friedmann, J., and W. Alonso, eds. 1964. *Regional development and planning: A reader.* Cambridge, Mass.: MIT Press.

Frisbie, W. P. 1980a. Urban sociology in the U. S.: The past 20 years. *American Behavioral Scientist* 24:177–214.

Frisbie, W. P. 1980b. Theory and research in urban ecology: Persistent problems and current progress. In *Sociological theory and research: A critical appraisal.* Edited by H. M. Blalock, Jr., 203–219. New York: Free Press.

Frisbie, W. P., and J. D. Kasarda. 1988. Spatial processes. In *Handbook of sociology.* Edited by N. J. Smelser, 629–666. Newbury Park, Calif.: Sage Publications.

Frisbie, W. P., and L. Niedert. 1977. Inequality and the relative size of minority populations: A comparative analysis. *American Journal of Sociology* 82:1007–1030.

Fujita, M. 1989. *Urban economic theory: Land use and city size.* Cambridge, U.K.: Cambridge University Press.

Fujita, M., P. Krugman, and A. J. Venables. 1999. *The spatial economy: Cities, regions, and international trade.* Cambridge, Mass.: MIT Press.

Fujita, M., and H. Ogawa. 1982. Multiple equilibria and structural transition of nonmonocentric urban configurations. *Regional Science and Urban Economics* 12: 161–196.

Fujita, M., and J. Thisse. 2002. *Economics of agglomeration Cities, industrial location, and regional growth.* Cambridge, U.K.: Cambridge University Press.

Galle, O. R. 1963. Occupational composition and the metropolitan hierarchy: The inter- and intra-metropolitan division of labor. *American Journal of Sociology* 69: 260–269.

Galle, O. R., and R. Stern. 1981. The metropolitan system in the South: Continuity and change. In *The population of the South*. Edited by D. L. Poston, Jr., and R. H. Weller, 155–174. Austin: University of Texas Press.

Garrison, W. L. 1959. Spatial structure of the economy. *Annals of the Association of American Geographers* 49:232–239, 471–482.

Garrison, W. L. 1960. Spatial structure of the economy. *Annals of the Association of American Geographers* 50:357–373.

Gibbs, J. P., and W. T. Martin. 1959. Toward a theoretical system of human ecology. *Pacific Sociological Review* 2:29–36.

Glaeser, E. L., and M. E. Kahn. 2004. Sprawl and urban growth. In *The Handbook of Urban and Regional Economics, Vol. 4*. Edited by J. V. Henderson and J. Thisse. Amsterdam: North Holland Press.

Glaeser, E. L., and J. Kohlhase. 2003. Cities, regions, and the decline of transportation costs. Working Paper 9886. National Bureau of Economic Research.

Glaeser, E. L., and J. M. Shapiro. 2003. City growth: Which places grew and why? In *Redefining urban and suburban America: Evidence from census 2000*. Edited by B. Katz and R. E. Lang, 13–32. Washington, D.C.: Brookings Institute.

Glazer, N. 1999. Impediments to integration. In *The African American predicament*. Edited by C. H. Foreman, Jr., 97–115. Washington, D.C.: Brookings Institute.

Gordon, D. 1977. Class struggle and the stages of urban development. In *The rise of the sunbelt cities*. Edited by D. Perry and A. Watkins, 55–82. Beverly Hills, Calif.: Sage Publications.

Gordon, D. 1984. Capitalist development and the history of American cities. In *Marxism and the metropolis*. Edited by W. Tabb and L. Sawyers, 21–53. New York: Oxford University Press.

Gordon, P., A. Kumar, and H. Richardson. 1991. The influence of metropolitan spatial structure on commuting time. *Journal of Urban Economics* 26: 138–151.

Gottdeinner, M. 1983. Understanding metropolitan deconcentration: A clash of paradigms. *Social Science Quarterly* 64:227–246.

Gottdeinner, M. 1985. *The social production of urban space*. Austin: University of Texas Press.

Gottdeinner, M., and J. R. Feagin. 1988. The paradigm shift in urban sociology. *Urban Affairs Quarterly* 24:163–187.

Gottdeinner, M., and R. Hutchinson. 2000. *The new urban sociology*. Boston: McGraw-Hill.

Guest, A. M. 1972. Patterns of family location *Demography* 9:159–171.

Guest, A. M. 1977. Residential segregation in urban areas. In *Contemporary topics in urban sociology*. Edited by K. P. Schwirian, 268–336. Morristown, N.J.: General Learning Press.

Guest, A. M. 1984. The city. In *Sociological human ecology: Contemporary issues and applications*. Edited by M. Micklin and H. M. Choldin, 277–322. Boulder, Colo.: Westview Press.

Hadden, J. K., and E. F. Borgatta. 1965. *American cities: Their social characteristics*. Chicago: Rand McNally.

Haggett, P. 1965. *Locational analysis in human geography*. New York: St. Martin's Press.

Hannan, M. T. 1979. The dynamics of ethnic boundaries in modern states. In *National development and the world system: Educational, economic, and political change, 1950–1970*. Edited by J. W. Meyer and M. T. Hannan, 253–275. Chicago: University of Chicago Press.

Harris, C. 1943. A functional classification of cities in the United States. *Geographical Review* 33:86–99.

Harris, C., and E. Ullman. 1945. The nature of cities. *Annals of the American Academy of Political and Social Science* 242:7–17.

Harvey, D. 1969. *Explanation in geography*. London: Edward Arnold.

Harvey, D. 1973. *Social justice and the city*. Baltimore: Johns Hopkins University Press.

Hawley, A. H. 1944a. Ecology and human ecology. *Social Forces* 22:398–405.

Hawley, A. H. 1944b. Dispersion versus segregation: Apropos of a solution of race problems. *Papers of the Michigan Academy of Sciences, Arts, and Letters* 30:667–674. Ann Arbor: University of Michigan.

Hawley, A. H. 1950. *Human ecology: A theory of community structure*. New York: Ronald Press.

Hawley, A. H. 1968. Human ecology. In *International encyclopedia of the social sciences*. Edited by D. L. Sills, 323–332. New York: Crowell, Collier, and Macmillan.

Hawley, A. H. 1971. *Urban society: An ecological approach*. New York: Ronald Press.

Hawley, A. H. 1972. Population density and the city. *Demography* 9:521–529.

Hawley, A. H. 1981. *Urban society: An ecological approach*. New York: Wiley.

Hawley, A. H. 1984. Human ecology and Marxian theories. *American Journal of Sociology* 89:904–917.

Hawley, A. H. 1986. *Human ecology: A theoretical essay*. Chicago: University of Chicago Press.

Hawley, A. H., and V. P. Rock. 1973. *Residential segregation in urban areas: Papers on racial and socio-economic factors on choice of housing*. Washington, D.C.: National Academy Press.

Hawley, A. H., and B. G. Zimmer. 1970. *The metropolitan community: Its people and government*. Beverly Hills, Calif.: Sage Publications.

Heckman, J. J., and P. Siegelman. 1993. The Urban Institute audit studies: Their methods and findings. In *Clear and convincing evidence: Measurement of discrimination in America*. Edited by M. Fix and R. J. Struyk, 187–258, 271–276. Washington, D.C.: Urban Institute Press.

Heer, D. M. 1959. The sentiment of white supremecy: An ecological study. *American Journal of Sociology* 64:592–598.

Henderson, J. V. 1974. Size and nature of cities. *American Economic Review* 64: 640–656.

Henderson, J. V., and J. Thisse, eds. 2004. *Handbook of Urban and Regional Economics, Vol. 4*. Urban Economics. Amsterdam: North Holland Press.

Hill, R. C. 1977. Capital acumulation and urbanization in the United States. *Comparative Urban Research* 4:39–60.

Hoover, E. M. 1948. *Location of economic activity*. New York: McGraw-Hill.

Hoover, E. M., and F. Giarratani. 1984. *An introduction to regional economics*. New York: Knopf.

Hoyt, H. 1939. *The structure and growth of residential neighborhoods in American cities*. Washington, D.C.: U. S. Government Printing Office.

Hoyt, H. 1971. Recent distortions of the classical models of urban structure. In *Internal structure of the city: Readings on space and environment*. Edited by L. S. Bourne, 84–96. New York: Oxford University Press.

Hunter, A. A. 1971. The ecology of Chicago: Persistence and change, 1930–1960. *American Journal of Sociology* 77:421–444.

Hunter, A. A. 1972. Factorial ecology: A critique and some suggestions. *Demography* 9:107–117.

Hurd, R. M. 1903. *Principles of city land values*. New York: The Record and Guide.

Huriot, J., and J. Thisse, eds. 2000. *Economics of cities: Theoretical perspectives*. Cambridge, U.K.: Cambridge University Press.

Isard, W. 1956. *Location and space economy: A general theory relating to industrial location, market areas, land use, trade, and urban structure*. Cambridge, Mass.: MIT Press.

Isard, W. 1960. *Methods of regional analysis*. Cambridge, Mass.: MIT Press.

James, D. R., and K. E. Taeuber. 1985. Measures of segregation. *Sociological Methodology* 15:1–32.

Jaret, C. 1983. Recent neo-Marxist urban analysis. *Annual Review of Sociology* 9:499–525.

Jargowsky, P. A. 1996. Take the money and run: Economic segregation in U. S. metropolitan areas. *American Sociological Review* 61:984–998.

Jargowsky, P. A. 1997. *Poverty and place: Ghettos, barrios, and the American city*. New York: Russell Sage.

Jiobu, R. M., and H. H. Marshall, Jr. 1971. Urban structure and the differentiation between blacks and whites. *American Sociological Review* 36:638–649.

Kasarda, J. D. 1972. The theory of ecological expansion: An empirical test. *Social Forces* 51:165–175.

Kasarda, J. D. 1985. Urban change and minority opportunities. In *The new urban reality*. Edited by P. E. Peterson, 33–67. Washington, D.C.: Brookings Institute.

Kasarda, J. D. 1995. Industrial restructuring and the changing location of jobs. In *State of the Union, Vol. 1.: Economic trends*. Edited by R. Farley, 215–267. New York: Russell Sage.

Kasarda, J. D., and E. M. Crenshaw. 1991. Third World urbanization: Dimensions, theories and determinants. *Annual Review of Sociology* 17:467–501.

Kass, R. 1973. A functional classification of metropolitan communities. *Demography* 10:427–445.

Keyfitz, N. 1965. Urbanization in South and Southeast Asia. In *The study of urbanization*. Edited by P. M. Hauser and L. F. Schnore, 265–310. New York: Wiley.

Kim, S., and E. Shin. 2002. A longitudinal analysis of globalization and regionalization in international trade: A social network approach. *Social Forces* 81:445–468.

King, D. 1990. Economic activity and the challenge to local government. In *Challenges to local government*. Edited by D. King and J. Pierre, 265–287. New York: Russell Sage.

Knox, P. 1995. World cities and the organization of global space. In *Geographies of global change*. Edited by R. J. Johnston, P. Taylor, and M. Watts. Oxford: Blackwell.

Knox, P., and P. Taylor, eds. 1995. *World cities in a world-system*. Cambridge, U.K.: Cambridge University Press.

Krugman, P. 1991. *Geography and trade*. Cambridge, Mass.: MIT Press.

Krugman, P. 1996. *The self-organizing economy*. Oxford: Blackwell.

Kuznets, S. 1955. Economic growth and income inequality. *American Economic Review* 65:1–28.

Lieberson, S. 1961a. A societal theory of race relations. *American Sociological Review* 26:902–908.

Lieberson, S. 1961b. The impact of residential segregation on ethnic assimilation. *Social Forces* 40:52–57.

Lieberson, S. 1963. *Ethnic patterns in American cities*. New York: Free Press.

Lieberson, S. 1980. *A piece of the pie: Blacks and white immigrants since 1880*. Berkeley, Calif.: University of California Press.

Lo, F., and Y. Yeung, eds. 1998. *Globalization and the world of large cities*. Tokyo: United Nations University Press.

Logan, J. R., and H. L. Molotch. 1987. *Urban fortunes: The political economy of place*. Berkeley: University of California Press.

Logan, J. R., and L. B. Stearns. 1981. Suburban racial segregation as a nonecological process. *Social Forces* 60:61–73.

Logan, J. R., and M. Zhou. 1989. Do suburban growth controls control growth? *American Sociological Review* 54:461–471.

Logan, J. R., and M. Zhou. 1990. Adoption of growth control measures. *Social Science Quarterly* 70: 118–129.

London, B. 1987. The structural determinants of Third World urban change: An ecological and political economic analysis. *American Sociological Review* 52:28–43.

London, B., and D. A. Smith. 1988. Urban bias, dependence, and economic stagnation in noncore nations. *American Sociological Review* 53:454–463.

Mao, M. X. 1998. Determinants of the division of labor in China. In *Continuities in sociological human ecology*. Edited by M. Micklin and D. L. Poston, Jr., 241–250. New York: Plenum.

Markusen, A. R. 1985. *Profit cycles, oligopoly, and regional development*. Cambridge, Mass.: MIT Press.

Markusen, A. R. 1987. *Regions: The economics and politics of territory*. Totowa, N.J.: Roman & Littlefield.

Markusen, A. R. 2003. Fuzzy concepts, scanty evidence, policy distance: The case for rigour and policy relevance in critical regional studies. *Regional Studies* 33:869–884.

Marshall, H., and R. Jiobu. 1975. Residential segregation in United States cities: A causal analysis. *Social Forces* 53:449–460.

Massey, D. S., and Brendan P. Mullen. 1984. Processes of Hispanic and Black Spatial Assimilation. *American Journal of Sociology* 89:836–873.

Massey, D. S. 1985. Ethnic residential segregation: A theoretical synthesis and empirical review. *Sociology and Social Research* 69:315–350.

Massey, D. S. 1990. American apartheid: Segregation and the making of the underclass. *American Journal of Sociology* 96:329–357.

Massey, D. S., and N. A. Denton. 1985. Spatial assimilation as a socioeconomic process. *American Sociological Review* 50:94–106.

Massey, D. S., and N. A. Denton. 1987. Trends in the residential segregation of blacks, Hispanics, and Asians. *American Sociological Review* 52:802–825.

Massey, D. S., and N. A. Denton. 1988a. The dimensions of residential segregation. *Social Forces* 67: 281–309.

Massey, D. S., and N. A. Denton. 1988b. Suburbanization and segregation in U.S. metropolitan areas. *American Journal of Sociology* 94:592–626.

Massey, D. S., and N. A. Denton. 1989. Hypersegregation in U.S. metropolitan areas: Black and Hispanic segregation along five dimensions. *Demography* 26:373–391.

Massey, D. S., and N. A. Denton. 1993. *American apartheid: Segregation and the making of the underclass*. Cambridge, Mass.: Harvard University Press.

Massey, D. S., and M. L. Eggars. 1990. The ecology of inequality: Minorities and the concentration of povery, 1970–1980. *American Journal of Sociology* 95:1153–1188.

Mayer, H. M. 1959. The economic base of cities. In *Readings in urban geography*. Edited by H. M. Mayer and C. F. Kohn, 85–126. Chicago:University of Chicago Press.

McCauley, W. J., and C. L. Nutty. 1982. Residential preferences and moving: A life-cycle analysis. *Journal of Marriage and the Family* 44: 301–309.

McKee, J. B. 1993. *Sociology and the race problem: The failure of a perspective*. Urbana: University of Illinois Press.

McKenzie, R. D. 1924. The ecological approach to the study of human community. *American Journal of Sociology* 30:287–301.

McKenzie, R. D. 1925. The ecological approach to the study of the human community. In *The city*. Edited by R. E. Park, E. W. Burgess, and R. D. McKenzie, 63–79. Chicago: University of Chicago Press. (Reprint of AJS 1924.)

McKenzie, R. D. 1926. The scope of human ecology. Publications of the American Sociological Society 20:141–154. Reprinted in *Roderick D. McKenzie on human ecology: Selected writings*. Edited by A. H. Hawley (1968). Chicago: University of Chicago Press.

McKenzie, R. D. 1927. The concept of dominance and world organization. *American Journal of Sociology* 33:28–42.

McKenzie, R. D. 1933. *The metropolitan community*. New York: McGraw-Hill.

Meyer, D. R. 1984. Control and coordination links in the metropolitan system of cities: The South as a case study. *Social Forces* 64:553–581.

Meyer, D. R. 1986. The world system of cities: Relations between international financial metropolises and South American cities. *Social Forces* 64:553–581.

Mills, E. S. 1967. An aggregative model of resource allocation in a metropolitan area. *American Economic Review* 57: 197–210.

Mills, E. S. 1972. *Studies in the structure of the urban economy*. Baltimore, M.D.: Johns Hopkins Press.

Molotch, H. L. 1976. The city as a growth machine: Toward a political economy of place. *American Journal of Sociology* 82:309–333.

Mulligan, G. F. 1984. Agglomeration and central place theory: A review of the literature. *International Regional Science Review* 9:1–42.

Muth, R. 1969. *Cities and housing*. Chicago: University of Chicago Press.

Nagel, J., and S. Olzak. 1982. Ethnic mobilization in new and old states: An extension of the competition model. *Social Problems* 30:127–143.

Namboodiri, K. 1988. Ecological demography: Its place in sociology. *American Sociological Review* 53:619–633.

Noel, D. L. 1968. A theory of the origin of ethnic stratification. *Social Problems* 16:157–172.

Nyden, P., J. Lukehart, M. T. Maly, and W. Peterman. 1998. Overview of the 14 neighborhoods studied. *Cityscape* 4:19–27.

Ogburn, W. F. 1946. Inventions of local transportation and the patterns of cities. *Social Forces* 24:373–379.

Olzak, S., and J. Nagel. 1986. Introduction, competitive ethnic relations: An overview. In *Competitive ethnic relations*. Edited by S. Olzak and J. Nagel, 1–16. Orlando, Fla.: Academic Press.

Pahl, R. E. 1989. Is the emperor naked? Some questions on the adequacy of sociological theory in urban and regional research. *International Journal of Urban and Regional Research* 13:709–720.

Pampel, F. C., and H. Choldin. 1978. Urban location and segregation of the aged: A block-level analysis. *Social Forces* 56:1121–1139.

Park, R. E. 1926. The urban community as a spatial pattern and a moral order. In *The urban community*. Edited by E. W. Burgess, 3–20. Chicago: University of Chicago Press.

Park, R. E. 1936a. Human ecology. *American Journal of Sociology* 42:1–15.

Park, R. E. 1936b. Succession: An ecological concept. *American Sociological Review* 1:171–179.

Park, R. E., and E. W. Burgess. 1921. *Introduction to the science of sociology*. Chicago: University of Chicago Press.

Park, R. E., E. W. Burgess, and R. D. McKenzie. 1925. *The city*. Chicago: University of Chicago Press.

Patterson, O. 1997. *The ordeal of integration: Progress and resentment in America's "racial" crisis*. Washington, D.C.: Civitas/Counterpoint.

Poston, D. L., Jr., and W. P. Frisbie. 1998. Human ecology, sociology, and demography. In *Continuities in sociological human ecology*. Edited by M. Micklin and D. L. Poston, 27–50. New York: Plenum.

Rappaport, J., and J. D. Sachs. 2003. The United States as a coastal nation. *Journal of Economic Growth* 8:5–46.

Reed, J. S. 1972. Percent black and lynching: A test of Blalock's hypothesis. *Social Problems* 50:356–360.

Rees, P. H. 1968. *The factorial ecology of metropolitan Chicago*. Masters thesis. Chicago: University of Chicago

Richardson, H. W. 1969. *Regional economics: Location theory, urban structure, and regional change*. New York: Praeger.

Richardson, H. W. 1977. *The new urban economics, and alternatives*. London: Pion.

Richardson, H. W. 1980. *The new urban economics*. New York: Routledge.

Roberts, B. R. 1989. Urbanization, migration and development. *Sociological Forum* 4:665–691.

Roof, W. C. 1972. Residential segregation and social differentiation in American metropolitan areas. *Social Forces* 51:87–91.

Rossem, R. V. 1996. "The World-System Paradigm as General Theory of Development: A Cross-National Test." *American Sociological Review* 61:508–527.

Sassen, S. 1994. *Cities in a world economy*. Thousand Oaks, Calif.: Pine Forge.

Schelling, T. C. 1971. Dynamic models of segregation. *Journal of Mathematical Sociology* 1:143–186.

Schelling, T. C. 1972. The process of residential segregation: Neighborhood tipping. In *Racial discrimination in economic life.* Edited by A. Pascal, 157–184. Lexington, Mass.: D.C. Heath.

Schneider, M., and T. Phelan. 1993. Black suburbanization in the 1980s. *Demography* 30:269–279.

Schnore, L. 1965. On the spatial structure of cities in the two Americas. In *The study of urbanization.* Edited by P. M. Hauser and L. F. Schnore, 347–398. New York: Wiley.

Schwab, W. A. 1992. *Sociology of cities.* Englewood Cliffs, N.J.: Prentice-Hall.

Schwirian, K. P., M. Hankins, and C. A. Ventresca. 1990. Residential decentralization of social status groups in American metropolitan communities, 1950–1980. *Social Forces* 68:1143–1163.

Scott, A. 1988. *Metropolis: From the division of labor to urban form.* Berkeley: University of California Press.

Shevky, E., and W. Bell. 1955. *Social area analysis: Theory illustrative application and computational procedures.* Palo Alto, Calif.: Stanford University Press.

Shevky, E., and M. Williams. 1949. *The social areas of Los Angeles: Analysis and typology.* Berkeley: University of California Press.

Shlay, A. B. 1986. Taking apart the American dream: The influence of income and family composition on residential evaluations. *Urban Studies* 23: 253–270.

Shlay, A. B., and D. A. DiGregorio. 1985. Same city, different worlds: Examining gender- and work-based differences in perceptions of neighborhood desirability. *Urban Affairs Quarterly* 21:66–86.

Simkus, A. A. 1978. Residential segregation by occupation and race in ten urbanized areas, 1950–1970. *American Sociological Review* 43:81–93.

Smith, D. A. 1995. The new urban sociology meets the old: Re-reading some classical human ecology. *Urban Affairs Review* 30:432–457.

Smith, M., and J. R. Feagin. 1987. *The capitalist city: Global restructuring and community politics.* Oxford: Blackwell.

Smith, M., and J. R. Feagin, eds. 1995. *The bubbling cauldron: Race, ethnicity, and the urban crisis.* Minneapolis: University of Minnesota Press.

Smith, D. A., and R. J. Nemeth. 1988. An empirical analysis of commodity exchange in the international economy: 1964–80. *International Studies Quarterly* 32:227–40.

Smith, D. A., and D. R. White. 1992. Structure and dynamics of the global economy: Network analysis of international trade, 1965–1980. *Social Forces* 70:857–893.

Smock, P. J., and F. D. Wilson. 1991. Desegregation and the stability of white enrollments: A school-level analysis 1968–1984. *Sociology of Education* 64:278–292.

Soja, E. W. 1997. *Postmodern geographies: The reassertion of space in critical social theory.* London: Verso Books.

Soja, E. W. 2000. *Postmetropolis: Critical studies of cities and regions.* Oxford: Blackwell.

South, S. J., and G. D. Deane. 1993. Race and residential mobility: Individual determinants and structural constraints. *Social Forces* 72:147–167.

South, S. J., and D. L. Poston, Jr. 1980. A note on the stability of the US metropolitan system: 1950–1970. *Demography* 17:445–450.

South, S. J., and D. L. Poston, Jr. 1982. The US metropolitan South: Regional change, 1950–1970. *Urban Affairs Quarterly* 18:187–206.

South, S. J., and Kyle Crowder. 1997. Residential mobility between cities and suburbs: Race, suburbanization, and back to the city moves. *Demography* 34:525–538.

South, S. J., and Kyle Crowder. 1998. Leaving the 'Hood: Residential mobility between Black, White, and integrated neighborhoods. *American Sociological Review* 63:17–26.

Stahura, J. M. 1986. Suburban development, black suburbanization, and the Civil Rights Movement since World War II. *American Sociological Review* 51:131–144.

Stearns, L. B., and J. R. Logan. 1986a. The racial structuring of the housing market and segregation in suburban areas. *Social Forces* 65:28–42.

Stearns, L. B., and J. R. Logan. 1986b. Measuring segregation: Three dimensions, three measures. *Urban Affairs Quarterly* 22:124–150.

Tabb, W. K., and L. Sawyers, eds. 1984. *Marxism and the metropolis.* New York: Oxford University Press.

Taeuber, K. E., and A. F. Taeuber. 1965. *Negroes in cities.* Chicago: Aldine.

Thernstrom, S., and A. Thernstrom. 1997. *America in black and white: One nation, indivisible.* New York: Simon and Schuster.

Thompson, W. 1965. *A preface to urban economics.* New York: Wiley.

Timberlake, M., ed. 1985. *Urbanization in the world economy.* Orlando, Fla.: Academic Press.

Tolnay, S. E., and E. M. Beck. 1992. Racial violence and black migration in the American South, 1910 to 1930. *American Sociological Review* 57:103–116.

Tolnay, S. E., E. M. Beck, and J. L. Massey. 1989. Black lynchings: The power threat hypothesis revisited. *Social Forces* 67:605–623.

Turner, M. A., S. L. Ross, G. C. Galster, and J. Yinger. 2002. *Discrimination in metropolitan housing markets: National results from Phase I HDS 2000*. Washington, D.C.: US Department of Housing and Urban Development.

Ullman, E. L. 1941. A theory of location for cities. *American Journal of Sociology* 46:853–864.

Ullman, E. L., and C. Harris. 1970. The nature of cities. In *Urban man and society: A reader in urban ecology*. Edited by A. N. Cousins and H. Nagpaul, 91–100. New York: Knopf.

Van Valey, T. L., and W. C. Roof. 1976. Measuring segregation in American cities: Problems of intercity comparisons. *Urban Affairs Quarterly* 11:453–468.

Vance, R. B., and S. S. Sutker. 1954. Metropolitan dominance and integration in the urban South. In *The Urban South*. Edited by R. B. Vance and N. J. Demerath. Chapel Hill: University of North Carolina Press.

Vernon, R. 1966. International trade and international investment in the product cycle. *Quarterly Journal of Economics* 80: 190–207.

Wallerstein, I. 1974. *The modern world system: Capitalist agriculture and the origins of the European world-economy in the sixteenth century*. Orlando, Fla.: Academic Press.

Wallerstein, I. 1980. *The modern world system II: Mercantilism and the consolidation of the European world-economy, 1600–1750*. Orlando, Fla.: Academic Press.

Walters, P. B. 1985. Systems of cities and urban primacy: Problems of definition and measurement. In *Urbanization in the world economy*. Edited by M. Timberlake, 63–85. Orlando, Fla.: Academic Press.

Walton, J. 1976. Urban hierarchies and patterns of dependence in Latin America: Theoretical bases for a new research agenda. In *Current perspectives in Latin American urban research*. Edited by A. Portes and H. L. Browning, 43–70. Austin: Institute for Latin American Studies, University of Texas.

Walton, J. 1979. Urban political economy. A new paradigm. *Comparative Urban Research* 7:5–17.

Walton, J. 1981. The new urban sociology. *International Social Science Journal* 33:374–390.

Walton, J. 1993. Urban sociology: The contributions and limits of political economy. *Annual Review of Sociology* 19:301–320.

Wanner, R. A. 1977. The dimensionality of the US urban functional system. *Demography* 14:519–537.

Weber, A. 1929. *Theory of the location of industries*. Chicago: University of Chicago Press.

Wheeler, J. O. 2001. Assessing the role of spatial analysis in urban geography in the 1960s. *Urban Geography* 22:549–558.

White, M. J. 1987. *American neighborhoods and residential differentiation*. New York: Russell Sage.

Wilcox, J., and W. C. Roof. 1978. Percent black and black-white status inequality: Southern versus non-southern patterns. *Social Science Quarterly* 59:421–434.

Wilson, F. 1984. Urban ecology: Urbanization and systems of cities. *American Review of Sociology* 10:283–307.

Winsborough, H. H. 1961. *A comparative study of urban population densities*. Doctoral dissertation. Chicago: University of Chicago.

Winsborough, H. H. 1963. An ecological approach to the theory of suburbanization. *American Journal of Sociology* 68:565–570.

Yeates, M. 2001. Yesterday as tomorrow's song: The contributions of the 1960s "Chicago School" to urban geography. *Urban Geography* 22:514–529.

Yinger, J. 1995. *Closed doors, opportunities lost: The continuing costs of housing discrimination*. New York: Russell Sage.

Yinger, J. 1998. Housing discrimination is still worth worrying about. *Housing Policy Debate* 9:893–927.

Young, H. P. 1998. *Individual strategy and social structure: An evolutionary theory of institutions*. Princeton, N.J.: Princeton University Press.

Zipf, G. 1949. *Human behavior and the principle of least effort*. Cambridge, Mass.: Addison-Wesley.

Zubrinsky, C. L., and L. Bobo. 1996. Prismatic metropolis: Race and residential segregation in the City of the Angels. *Social Science Research* 25:335–374.

CHAPTER 17

Anthropological Demography

DAVID I. KERTZER

In the last dozen years of the 20th century anthropological demography as both a specialty within anthropology and as a recognized part of demography began to come into its own. Special graduate programs sprang up, a regular committee of the International Union for the Scientific Study of Population devoted to the field, begun somewhat earlier, attracted an increasing number of anthropologists, and meetings of the Population Association of American began to feature sessions focusing on anthropological work. Yet obstacles remained. Anthropologists working in demography often found themselves caught between those anthropologists for whom *positivist* was the worst epithet imaginable and those demographers suspicious of ethnographic research and uncomfortable at the relentless deconstruction of analytical categories that characterizes anthropology.

The development of anthropological interests in demography has a much longer history, going back well into the 19th century. In this longer view, the renascence of the field in the late 20th century was simply a move to return demographic research to a prominent place it had earlier occupied in anthropology. This chapter briefly sets out the nature of this history and also discusses the forces within demography that have led in recent years to an ever greater interest in anthropology. While anthropology's methodological emphasis on ethnography has received much of the attention when demographers have referred to the potential contributions of anthropological demography, this chapter emphasizes the theoretical contributions that anthropological demography can make, partially by exploring contemporary cultural theory within anthropology insofar as it relates to the explanation of demographic behavior. In this respect, the chapter addresses various kinds of anthropological research, ranging in focus from work on fertility to studies of marriage and household, as well as migration.

In this manner, the chapter covers examples of innovative demographic research done recently by anthropologists.

CONCEPTUAL FRAMEWORK

Anthropology's intersections with demography are many, although often anthropologists working on issues of demographic interest are unaware of the connections. American anthropology consists of three principal subdivisions (four if anthropological linguistics is considered): sociocultural anthropology, archaeology, and biological anthropology. The largest of these, and the one that has thus far drawn the greatest attention in the demographic world, is sociocultural anthropology, the comparative study of cultures and societies. It is to the demographically relevant works in this subfield that this chapter is dedicated, and "anthropology" is here used as shorthand for sociocultural anthropology. For an introduction to work in archaeological demography, see Hassan (1979) and Paine (1997). For an overview of the different ways in which biological anthropologists have been engaging in demographic study, see Wood (1990), Ellison (1994), Gage (1998), Voland (1998), and Meindl and Russell (1998).

History

Demographers and, indeed, many anthropologists themselves are unaware of how important demographic topics were to many of the pioneers of modern anthropology. The kind of anthropology that developed in Britain beginning in the late 19th century, focusing on documenting the diversity of human societies, turned its attention to issues of social organization and kinship at a time when American anthropology was developing its distinctive focus on culture. The British focus, along with the developing emphasis on prolonged, intensive fieldwork, led to a concern for documenting family processes that lie at the heart of demography. In the late 19th century, the classic British manual of anthropological investigation, *Notes and Queries in Anthropology*, called on field workers to conduct censuses to provide the framework for their investigations. Many of the most influential British anthropologists of the first decades of the 20th century attempted population surveys or estimates of one kind or another, Radcliffe-Brown's (1922) Andaman Island work notable among them.

By the 1930s, anthropologists such as Meyer Fortes and Raymond Firth, sharing a strong interest in kinship systems, began to work on population issues. Firth (1936) devoted a whole chapter of his classic study of the Polynesian island of Tikopia to "A Modern Population Problem," while Fortes (1943) examined fertility among the West African Tallensi, concluding that due to the lack of reliable demographic data, "anthropologists have had to be their own demographers, in however a rough-and-ready fashion." British social anthropology continued for decades to show great interest in the study of marriage, divorce, household dynamics, and fertility.[1]

For a variety of reasons, American anthropology took a different path, one in which demographic issues were not as central. Partly this had to do with the heavy emphasis that American Indian studies had in the first decades of the 20th century.

---

[1] For a fuller account of this history, see Kertzer and Fricke (1997).

Studying people on reservations whose lives were radically different from that of their grandparents, anthropologists placed greater emphasis on oral history, mythology, and ritual and showed less interest in the actual population processes at work in the present. However, some strands of American anthropology did lend themselves to demographic topics, including work in cultural ecology (Steward 1936) and the study of foraging (hunting and gathering) peoples (Lee and Devore 1968). Cultural materialism, pioneered by Marvin Harris (1966), similarly highlighted demographic questions (Harris and Ross 1987) and the use of scientific paradigms, although this approach has remained controversial in American anthropology.

The growth in interest in anthropological demography among demographers over the past two decades has sprung from various sources and has found its center in the United States. Partly the interest derived from social organizational issues once largely identified with British social anthropology: questions of domestic group dynamics and marriage in particular (Hammel 1972; Kertzer 1989). Partly they have come from some feminist concerns that have strongly influenced anthropology in this period (Greenhalgh 1995b). Here studies of fertility and of women's positions in their households have been prominent. Likewise, the influence of cultural ecological and materialist concern—renewed by John Bennett (1976)—can be seen in the work of a number of anthropologists involved in demographic study (Fricke 1994). But, in addition, a huge amount of demographically related work is being done by anthropologists under the general rubric of medical anthropology. This, the largest subfield within sociocultural anthropology, has a long tradition of studies of childbirth, menstruation, morbidity and mortality, yet has had remarkably little contact with demographers.

Interest in anthropology among demographers similarly goes back quite a way. Emblematic, and influential, was the work of the International Union for the Scientific Study of Population (IUSSP) Committee on Population Problems of Countries in Process of Industrialization, founded in 1951, which counted Raymond Firth among its most active members. The influential literature synthesis which the Committee commissioned Frank Lorimer (1954) to do on the "social and cultural conditions affecting fertility in nonindustrial societies" turned out to be very largely a survey of the existing anthropological literature.

More recent interest in what anthropology could contribute to demography has been triggered by two developments within demography, one theoretical and the other methodological. Theoretically, demography came by mid-20th century to be dominated by modernization theory in general and demographic transition theory in particular. It was within this paradigm that the ambitious and influential Princeton European fertility history project was launched by Ansley Coale in 1963. In their attempts to test the paradigm by using historical provincial-level European data, Coale and his colleagues came to the surprising conclusion that demography's reigning paradigm did not hold. The course of fertility decline in Europe did not follow the path suggested by such standard predictor variables as urbanization, literacy, infant and child mortality, or industrialization. As two of the core members of the project put it: "Cultural setting influenced the onset and spread of fertility decline independently of socioeconomic conditions" (Knodel and van de Walle 1986: 412).

Likewise, based on the Princeton findings and also work coming out of the World Fertility Survey, demographers John Cleland and Christopher Wilson (1987: 20) concluded that "the most striking feature of the onset of transition is its relationship to broad cultural groupings." A series of critiques of the reigning theoretical paradigm resulted (e.g., McNicoll 1980). All of a sudden, that hoary concept of culture had placed itself at the center of demographic discussion, and with it the need for anthropological work and for an infusion of anthropological theory came increasingly to be recognized.

The methodological impetus for paying attention to anthropology came from a different quarter, although around the same time. By the 1970s the sample survey had become the dominant methodology in demography. But while it offered the prospect of gaining nationally representative data, and furnishing straightforward means for cross-national comparison, the limitations of the approach soon became apparent. The most influential voice within demography proved to be John Caldwell, whose critique of survey methods was based initially on his exposure to village studies and his reading of the anthropological ethnographic literature on West Africa. He pointed out in 1982 that "Most demographers work on large data sets, often with little contact with the people whom the statistics describe."

Believing that such first-hand understanding was essential, Caldwell undertook a series of projects involving, as he wrote, "borrowing methodology from the anthropologists (and reading them) and becoming intimately acquainted with each village and its families in turn" (Caldwell 1982: 4). Not only were surveys limited in the kind of data they could collect, the responses they generated were of questionable validity, for, as Caldwell later wrote with Allan Hill (1988: 2), "the tendency is to obtain normative responses or reflections on the rules, particularly on sensitive topics." To remedy this problem they called for greater adoption of what they termed, more or less without distinction, *microlevel*, or *anthropological*, approaches.

In somewhat parallel fashion, studying migration rather than fertility and mortality, Douglas Massey and colleagues (Massey et al. 1990; Massey and Zenteno 2000; Kandel and Massey 2002) criticize the tendency of demographers to rely solely on survey methods and argue vigorously for the adoption of qualitative and ethnographic methods to complement quantitative approaches. An influential product of this movement, as promoted by Caldwell in particular, was the establishment by the IUSSP of a Committee on Anthropological Demography. Yet, until an anthropologist (Anthony Carter) took over the chair of this committee in the late 1990s and turned it in more cultural and theoretical directions, anthropological demography was in effect defined in terms of methodology—referring to all qualitative, microlevel, nonsurvey demographic research.

The Problem of Culture

Put crudely, there are two ways in which anthropologists and nonanthropological demographers can collaborate. One is to employ anthropologists to assist mainstream demographic research. This follows from an emphasis on anthropology's methodological contribution. In this context, anthropologists can be employed to do fieldwork which will allow survey researchers to design better questions or feed ethnographic information that can be used to contextualize the results of demographic studies. Ethnographic work can, along similar lines, be used to generate variables at an ethnic group level which can be entered into statistical models in which populations are compared.

While this use of anthropology in demography can lead to significant improvements in mainstream demographic research, it is understandably not a model that has great appeal to anthropologists. Anthropologists in general have a different way of viewing the world than do most demographers. The implicit assumptions behind survey research—rooted in a focus on the individual—conflict with anthropological emphasis on social organization and on culture. And while not all mainstream demographers embrace a rational choice model, something quite similar to an assumption of economic rationality is widely found (e.g., Sigle-Rushton and McLanahan 2002; Oppenheimer 2003) and conflicts with most anthropologists' understanding of how culture works.

Anthropologists tend to view culture not as a set of norms or a laundry list of customs. Gene Hammel (1990) makes the distinction in this regard between "culture for the people" and "culture by the people." The former, a more traditional view now rejected by many anthropologists, sees people as the products of their culture, simply following the norms that have been handed down to them. The latter approach, by contrast, focuses on individual agency, with culture seen as offering a stock of symbols that are invested with moral weight, but which people are able to manipulate for their own ends. Through this continuous process of manipulation culture itself changes. Bledsoe (1990) has employed this approach in her work on the Mende of Sierra Leone. She argues, for example, that "cultural labels such as kinship and fosterage are best viewed not as relationships that compel future support, but as idioms for making demands or asserting claims with respect to children" (1990: 82). For Kreager (1985: 136), at the heart of culture is "the application of criteria of right and wrong." Cultures, however, do not dictate a particular code of conduct, but instead involve "an endless process of negotiation."

Yet this negotiation itself involves the individual in a larger social, economic, and political context. A number of anthropologists working on demographic topics have called attention to the importance of this context. This has, on the one hand, put them in conflict with the more extreme cultural determinist wing of anthropology, those who stress human behavior as the product of the symbolic construction of reality. However, a focus on this larger institutional level also moves anthropology away from survey approaches to understanding demographic behavior. Greenhalgh (1995b: 20, 17), calling for a "culture and political economy perspective," argues that "the real challenge is to construct whole demographies that illuminate mutually constitutive relations between culture and political economy, and the implication of these relations for reproductive actors."

An example of this approach is found in Kertzer's (1993) study of large-scale infant abandonment in 19th-century Italy. Kertzer tries to explain a variety of demographic outcomes (abandonment, infant and child mortality) in terms of the action of the Roman Catholic Church and the civil authorities, while considering the impact of cultural beliefs about illegitimacy and the effects of a particular kinship system. He argues that while people's interests are defined for them by their culture, and their menu of choices is heavily constrained by their culture, their behavior must also be viewed as constrained by a variety of political economic and institutional forces (Kertzer 1997).

THEORETICAL MODELS

Fertility

Not unlike demographic research more generally, the bulk of anthropological demography to date has concentrated on fertility and related issues. This can be roughly divided between those studies that directly engage the larger demographic literature and those that deal with fertility and reproduction without great familiarity with or interest in the work of nonanthropological demographers. The latter tends to fall into two categories: work stemming from a medical anthropology tradition and that arising from feminist anthropology.

Anthropologists have typically been critical of notions of "natural fertility," and a good deal of their work in predemographic transition populations has been devoted to showing that fertility is the result of a series of culturally influenced behaviors and decisions. More generally, anthropologists have tried to explicate the links between various kin systems and fertility. A classic argument here regards the impact of polygyny on fertility (Borgerhoff-Mulder 1989), an issue that continues to generate disagreement. In a remarkable study, Skinner (1997) examines the various ways in which family systems shape demographic processes, with evidence ranging from Europe to China. He views causation operating in both directions, with the demographic regime constraining and shaping family systems. Using historical demographic data, Skinner adduces evidence in support of his argument that "family system norms imply, if not specify, the relative desirability of differently configured offspring sets and that, in many if not most populations, families did what they could (and do what they can) to shape the size and configuration of their progeny accordingly" (1997: 66).

Rather than respect the classic compartmentalization in mainstream demography between fertility and mortality, Skinner insists that the key phenomenon for study is reproduction, not fertility, and hence neonatal and early childhood mortality must be examined together with fertility in the context of family strategizing behavior. A similar argument is made by Scrimshaw (1983), who objects to traditional demographic theory, which sees high infant and child mortality rates as supporting high fertility rather than vice versa. As Carter (1998: 257–258) points out, there is considerable evidence that the sex composition of the offspring set affected the timing of the decision to stop having children in such "traditional" populations as the 18th-century Japanese (Smith 1977). All these studies call into question the concept of natural fertility.

The importance of the larger kinship system is also highlighted in Caroline Bledsoe's work on child fosterage in West Africa. As the title of one of her pieces (Bledsoe 1990) suggests—"The Politics of Children: Fosterage and the Social Management of Fertility Among the Mende of Sierra Leone"—she argues that fertility in many Western African societies can only be understood in light of the widespread practice of child fosterage. Women can regulate the number of their dependent children without necessarily regulating their fertility. Bledsoe's more recent work in The Gambia, which will be discussed later, in parallel fashion shows how women use contraceptive methods in order to facilitate fertility, as they see it, rather than as a means to limit births.

Another strand of anthropological work on fertility flows from basic ethnographic research on folk systems of belief regarding reproduction, women's bodies, and related matters. From the time that Malinowski argued that Trobriand Islanders recognized no role for men in reproduction, there has been interest in these issues. Much of the recent literature here comes from a medical anthropology tradition (e.g., MacCormack 1994; Davis-Lloyd and Sargent 1997). Here there is little direct engagement with the larger demographic literature on fertility. Typical of this tradition is a recent collection on *The Anthropology of Pregnancy Loss* (Cecil 1996), which in reviewing fields that have something to contribute to the anthropological study of this topic focuses on literary studies and does not mention demography.

Yet even in the field of reproductive ethnography there have been collaborations between anthropologists and demographers. A good example is provided by anthropologist Elisha Renne and demographer Etienne van de Walle (2001), who co-edited a collection on menstrual regulation. The rich historical and ethnographic studies in the volume provide a glimpse into a phenomenon that has great implications for fertility. Nevertheless, it had been little considered by demographers and had been examined by anthropologists mainly in symbolic terms, as part of that complex of rites associated with a belief in female pollution.

Anthropologists have also tended to show more interest than most demographers in problems of infertility in high-fertility societies. While from a traditional demographic transition theory perspective, this issue is of only marginal interest, in an anthropological perspective it sheds light on the central importance of childbearing to people's lives (Inhorn 1994, 1996; Becker 1994).

Among the most recent directions in anthropological research on fertility has been a focus on men (Bledsoe, Guyer, and Lerner 2000). This work builds on classic anthropological research on kinship systems, which places considerable emphasis on theories of paternity, on which parent children are thought to belong to, and on distinctions between biological and social paternity (Guyer 2000). While much of the literature on the implications of unilineal (especially patrilineal) kinship systems for fertility behavior concerns Africa, such studies as that by Setel (2000) on fertility and the male life course in Papua New Guinea show just how widely we find the strong male belief in the need to produce children to have a proper claim to rights in one's kinship group.

But not all of this literature, even in Africa, emphasizes corporate kin groups. In a series of publications, Townsend (1997, 2000) looks at male responsibility for children in the United States and in Botswana. In the latter case, he shows the importance, in understanding fertility, of viewing not only the father's role but also that of the woman's brother, who may often be the most reliable male source of support. Townsend also shows that a man's age at marriage and his desirability as a partner may be closely linked both to his own father's situation and to that of his sisters and brothers. Townsend (1997: 108–109) concludes, more generally, that an individual's fertility, rather than being viewed in individual terms, should be seen as "a description of a place in a web of relationships with offspring, with other kin, and with a range of social groups and institutions."

Interest in the male role in fertility decisions has also sprung from the medical anthropology tradition, itself influenced by feminist anthropology. In a comparative study of various Hispanic populations, for example, Carole Browner (2000) tries to disentangle the interaction of structural and cultural factors that affect a man's ability to influence his partner's reproductive decision making. She places special emphasis on the importance of changing gender ideologies.

Feminist influence can be seen in a variety of studies of reproduction that focus on how fertilization itself is conceived. In two influential publications, Emily Martin (1987, 1991) used methods of cultural analysis to probe how contemporary Americans' views of ova and sperm, and of male and female reproductive biology, are influenced by the metaphors that guide modern Western medicine. Part of the science studies movement, this work challenges naïve views of medical science and reveals how important it is to investigate the ways in which science and medicine create their own symbolic systems that influence people's perceptions and behavior.

But people's symbolic understandings of procreation involve much that goes beyond science or medicine, extending to religious and other cultural influences. In a study of a Turkish village, Carol Delaney (1991) focuses on the key symbolism of seed and soil. Although her study is set in Turkey, she sees this symbolism as of much broader and deeper significance. The image of the man as planting the seed and the woman furnishing the nurturing soil in which it can grow has biblical antecedents and is widespread in the West. Delaney, following a now well-developed line of work in feminist anthropology, examines how this central reproductive metaphor has much broader and more socially consequential ramifications. Men are the creators and thus are linked to God. Women, providing material sustenance to support life, are reduced to what God created, the earth.

Feminist anthropologists who have turned their attention to reproduction have often cast their work in terms of the study of sexual politics. In an influential volume, *Conceiving the New World Order: The Global Politics of Reproduction*, editors Ginsburg and Rapp (1995a) draw not on demography but on feminist studies in order, as they put it, "to transform traditional anthropological analyses of reproduction and to clarify the importance of making reproduction central to social theory" (1995b: 1). They fault traditional ethnographic approaches to the study of fertility, infanticide, and child care for ignoring larger, nonlocal, and even global forces that affect reproductive behavior. Focusing on what they term "stratified reproduction," they look at the power relations that help empower some people to make their own reproductive decisions and disempower others. They are especially interested in how cultural images related to reproduction are produced and become broadly accepted in a society. Influenced by Foucault, they examine the influence that the dominant culture's categories have, even for those who seek to rebel against them.[2] Like feminist anthropology more generally, their scholarly agenda is combined with explicitly political aims, using research to help map a path of political activism.

Feminist inspiration can also be found in the research of anthropologists working on fertility who are more closely tied in to the demographic research world. Candace Bradley (1995), for example, has examined the relationship between the empowerment of women as a result of recent social and economic changes in Kenya and the beginnings of fertility decline. Here she examines the context in which women are able to exercise greater influence over social, political, and economic decision making, both within their own households and beyond them. Based on ethnographic research conducted in the hills of western Kenya, as well as census and survey data, Bradley examines the onset of fertility decline. However, she provides a nuance lacking in most survey-based studies in showing the complexities of the female life course and exactly how it is that a woman reaches a point in her reproductive, family, and socioeconomic career in which she can exercise greater influence over reproductive decisions.

Among those anthropologists who have directly taken part in the larger interdisciplinary demographic research community, perhaps the most influential theoretical perspective on fertility to emerge has been one that combines political economic and cultural analysis. Greenhalgh brought attention to this approach in a 1990 article in *Population and Development Review*, calling for a "political economy of fertility."

---

[2] Kertzer and Arel (2002) employ an anthropological perspective to examine the power of state-backed demographic categories and bottom-up resistance to them in the context of the use of ethnic, racial, and language categories in national censuses.

However, by this she did not mean political economy in the most commonly used sense. She referred to "a new analytic perspective ... with a new research agenda that has the potential for appreciably enhancing our understanding of the sources of fertility decline". Such an approach, she writes, "directs attention to the embeddedness of community institutions in structures and processes, especially political and economic ones, operating at regional, national, and global levels, and to the historical roots of those macro-micro linkages" (1990: 87). Following this approach, rather than seeking to identify a single set of factors to explain fertility decline, the researcher tries to shed light on the combination of institutional, political, economic, and cultural forces that bring it about. She draws attention to the failure of demographers to pay sufficient attention to political factors and calls for an emphasis on the political-economic dimensions of social and cultural organization (1990: 95).

Renne's work on the impact of government land tenure policy on fertility among the Yoruba in Nigeria offers an example of this approach. She finds that, paradoxically, while the government has been engaged in attempts to encourage smaller families, its rural land tenure policies have the opposite effect. By generating uncertainty regarding land tenure, Renne finds, the Nigerian Land Use Act has led many people to seek alternative means of security through having many children. Moreover, among the rural population, "ideas about the reproduction of family houses and names, like ideas about land tenure and children, are intimately linked, thus underscoring the inappropriateness of analyzing fertility levels in abstraction from this broader social context" (1995: 123).

The political implications of fertility have been cast in a somewhat different way by Handwerker, who begins his introduction to a volume of anthropological studies of fertility by writing "The birth of a child is a political event. So is its absence, for any part of all of the events that comprise human reproduction may be part of a strategy to acquire or extend power, may create new ties of dependence or may provide a means to break ties of dependence" (1990: 1). Here Handwerker draws on a definition of the political in terms of the distribution of power among people. Anthropologists following this perspective show special interest in how people's fertility reflects strategizing behavior that seeks to maximize resources. However, rather than see this in narrowly economic terms, they try to contextualize behavior in terms of culture, social organization, and political power structures.

Anthropological attempts to combine political economic and cultural analysis in understanding fertility behavior have often turned to historical rather than ethnographic sources of evidence. Part of the reason for this is that the kinds of theories of change they champion are best examined by use of data that cover a relatively long period. Jane and Peter Schneider's (1996) historical demographic research in Sicily focuses on a community they had previously studied ethnographically, and their interpretation of the historical evidence is informed, in part, by that intensive involvement with the population. In showing that the decline in fertility that occurred there took place at different historical moments for the three broad social classes under study—the elite, the artisans, and the peasantry—they examine not only larger political and economic changes that affected these classes differently, but also how people's cultural understandings and social relations changed.

Kertzer (1995) explores these issues theoretically in examining the relationship of political-economic and cultural explanations of demographic behavior. Focusing on an urbanizing, sharecropping town outside Bologna, Italy, in the period 1861 to 1921, he finds that there is no simple relationship between economic change and change in demographic behavior. In the case of fertility, he found a pattern similar to that described by the Schneiders in Sicily. Different economic segments of the population reduced their fertility at different times, in reaction to changes in their own family economic situations. Hence sharecroppers kept up high fertility throughout the period, despite the falls taking place in fertility of the rest of the population, because pressures on sharecroppers to have numerous sons continued and even increased, while the cost to them of raising children in households that remained large and complex remained modest (Kertzer and Hogan 1989). On the other hand, despite massive economic changes, very little change was observed in age at marriage, suggesting that here cultural norms proved resilient, a finding of other historical European studies of marriage age as well.

There is some irony here, for it seems that while an increasing number of demographers are expressing dismay about the possibility of explaining fertility decline based on economic factors, and pointing instead to culture, most of the anthropologists with the greatest involvement in demography continue to stress the importance of economic forces. This is certainly true of one of the most influential anthropologists to work in demography, Gene Hammel. Putting the matter boldly, in a piece titled "Economics 1, Culture 0," Hammel (1995) urges demographers not to reject economic factors in explanations of historical fertility decline in Europe. Examining data from the northwest Balkans over two centuries—1700 to 1900—he finds that neither religious lines of difference nor linguistic borders (often used by demographers as proxies for lines of cultural difference) correspond to fertility differentials. By contrast, he concludes that "variables apparently more closely related to the activities of extracting a living from the land and the exchange system, such as female labor-force participation, the strength of the primary sector, and the kind of agriculture, seem strongly predictive of fertility differences" (1995: 247).

Anthropologists' growing interest in state-level politics—a relatively new development—has produced other recent work related to reproduction. Most notable is Kligman's (1998) study of the politics of reproduction in Romania under Ceausescu's regime (1965 to 1989). It turns an ethnographic gaze on state policy, examining the rhetorical and institutional practices of the state in the public sphere and their integration into local life. It is a work that builds as well on the concept of reproduction in terms of politicization. As Kligman (1998: 5) puts it, "the politics of reproduction center attention on the intersection beween politics and the life cycle, whether in terms of abortion, new reproductive technologies, international family planning programs, eugenics, or welfare." The study examines the extreme pronatalist policies of the Romanian government, their rhetorical symbolism, and the effects all these had on individuals.

Marriage and Households

Although not for the most part viewing the issue in demographic terms, anthropologists have long been interested in marriage and domestic groups. Moreover, having developed this expertise in important part through the study of marriage in societies having corporate kin groups, especially those following unilineal descent rules, anthropologists have often theorized relationships between marriage systems and broader kinship systems.

Probably no aspect of nonwestern marriage systems has so struck western observers as polygamy, which anthropologists divide into two types. Polygyny, by far the more common, involves men having multiple wives and continues to be widespread today in sub-Saharan Africa. Polyandry, which entails a woman having two or more husbands, finds its *locus classicus* in the Himalayas but can be found in parts of sub-Saharan Africa. While the nature and dynamics of these systems have long fascinated anthropologists, demographers' interest in these systems has tended to focus on two issues: (1) the impact that plural marriage has on fertility and (2) the implications of plural marriage for concepts of household. The latter question derives its demographic interest not simply from the desire to better understand household relations but, at least as importantly, from its implications for survey research methods.

Polyandry has received considerable anthropological attention for the theoretical questions it raises. A recent spike of interest can be traced to its relevance to sociobiological theory (Levine and Silk 1997), for it seems, at least at first glance, to contradict the basic tenets of sociobiology. By contrast, polyandry has been largely ignored by demographers because of the small numbers of peoples who practice it.

Given the ever greater prominence that sub-Saharan Africa has achieved within demography, anthropological theorizing on marriage relations—including but not limited to plural marriage and the relationship of marriage to formalized kin systems—takes on ever more relevance. Guyer (1994), for example, notes that Nigeria alone has 250 different ethnic groups and two world religions—each with various distinct subgroups—and each of these has its own norms regarding marriage. In such a context, how can one define marriage? Nigerian law largely leaves such questions to local "customary law," resulting in marriage statistics that violate basic demographic principles of comparability and standardization.

What is most worrisome to demographers about all this is that marriage may be a much less clear-cut status in these societies. There is often no single event one could call a wedding, no single date at which one changes marital status, either in marrying or in divorcing. Marriage is often described in Africa as a process, and the fact of widespread polygyny makes the situation all the more complex (Bledsoe and Pison 1994: 2). In her study of the Yoruba in Nigeria, Guyer (1994: 247) finds that informality of first marriage has a long history and that such informality has been the prevalent form of higher-order marriages throughout Yoruba recorded history. She concludes that the formality of first marriage was partially an imposition of colonial powers, which tried to formalize bride-wealth payments and place them into a European understanding of marriage.

Although marriage has not been a major focus of anthropologists working in western societies, no discussion of anthropological theory and marriage in the context of demographic study can fail to mention the work of Jack Goody. Like many of the anthropologists with demographic interests who have worked on Europe, Goody takes a broad historical perspective, although in his case the history has unusual depth. In his influential *The Development of the Family and Marriage in Europe*, Goody (1983) looks at European marriage systems from the perspective of an anthropologist who has specialized in West Africa. He seeks to explain the broad and deep differences he observes, many of which he attributes to the impact and development of Christianity in Europe. Among the features of the European family system Goody tackles are bilineality; strength of the conjugal pair bond; lack of lineages among the bulk of the population; lack of rigid separation of the sexes; monogamy; absence of adoption (until recently); absence of provision for divorce and remarriage; the banning of marriage with kin. His explanation for these distinctive patterns rests on his argument that they all served the purposes of the Church, partly by undermining alternative institutions (e.g., the lineage) and partly by funneling property over the generations into Church coffers.

Mortality

Anthropological theorizing on mortality remains poorly developed—in contrast with the robust anthropological interest in funerary rites. Aside from recent work in anthropology on HIV-AIDS, most of which has little articulation with demographic research (Herdt 1997), most anthropological theorizing on mortality has involved work on infant and child mortality. The literature that most closely engages the larger demographic literature in this regard is that which examines the impact of various kinship and marriage systems on infant and child mortality in general and on sex-selective survivorship in particular (Skinner 1993). We will look at one example of this, the work of Monica Das Gupta, in a later section of this chapter.

Within anthropology in general the most influential recent theoretical work in this area has been Scheper-Hughes' (1992) *Death Without Weeping*, based on ethnographic work done in a northeastern Brazilian town. Seeking to position herself between what she calls the "mindlessly automatic 'maternal bonding' theorists," on the one hand, and those like Edward Shorter, who write historically of maternal indifference, on the other, Scheper-Hughes (1992: 356) takes the unpopular position that in the area of extreme poverty she studied, "mortal selective neglect and intense maternal attachment coexist." She finds that women in this environment regard those small children who are weak and fragile as doomed and so do little to try to keep them alive.

Branding theorists such as Nancy Chodorow and Carol Gilligan, who speak of a universal female ethos as suffering from a culture- and history-bound perspective, Scheper-Hughes argues that the "invention of mother love corresponds not only with the rise of modern, bourgeois, nuclear family . . . but also with the demographic transition." It was only with the sharp decline in infant and child mortality, she argues, that a new reproductive strategy arose, one involving bearing few children but investing heavily in each of them. Where high mortality and high fertility are found, as in northeastern Brazil, "a different, or a pre-demographic transition, reproductive strategy obtains." This entails giving birth to many children but investing emotionally and materially in only those who are seen as the best bets for survival (1992: 401–402). This thesis has produced a heated debate within anthropology, primarily in the confines of medical anthropology, with Scheper-Hughes accused of blaming impoverished mothers—at least in part—for the death of their children (Nations 1988).

Migration

Although its initial focus on isolated island communities can be exaggerated, anthropology did long have what Malkki (1995: 508) has called a "sedentarist analytical bias." The prototypical anthropological study was based on participant observation in a single locality; the main kind of movement envisioned was that of pastoralists who moved seasonally in repetitive fashion. Since the 1960s, however, anthropological interest in migration has mushroomed, although until recently little of it articulated directly with mainstream demographic research.

Brettell (2000) has recently provided an excellent overview of anthropological migration studies. Anthropologists have come to the study of migration via different routes. Some, seeking to undertake more traditional forms of rural community study, have found that local life has been dramatically affected by out-migration and by return migration, necessitating the study of population movement that was not originally envisioned. Others, part of the now 40-year-old tradition of anthropological studies of urban life in nonwestern societies, found that the lives of the urban dwellers they studied were lived not only in the cities but in rural areas of origin as well. Moreover, the lives of many of these people in the city appeared to be organized by social networks involving ties to such home areas.

Early migration study in anthropology was influenced by Redfield's (1941) rural-urban continuum, which portrays rural life as traditional and urban life as modern. Among the early concerns of migration study in anthropology was the likelihood of return and its social and cultural implications both for the migrant and for the home community. In more recent years, there has been considerable emphasis on the question of how migrants see themselves and whether they envision themselves as having given up their former residence and taken on a new identity in their new home. While paying attention to economic factors of push and pull, anthropologists typically place greater emphasis on understanding the social and cultural context in which decisions to migrate and decisions to return are made. These tend to involve a focus on household decision making and on kinship bonds and obligations, as well as analysis of the cultural norms and social arrangements surrounding property transfer, including inheritance.

Today anthropologists study migrants in the receiving community, those who have returned to their original homeland, and those in the sending area who themselves may never have migrated but who are affected by migrant kin and neighbors. Some anthropologists follow migrants, generally between a home area and a single other destination. It is not uncommon for an anthropologist to begin her or his career working in a nonwestern society and then subsequently studying migrants from that society closer to (the anthropologist's) home. While some anthropologists engaged in these studies do surveys and examine quantitative data, most rely largely if not entirely on qualitiative methods. Typical of the latter is George Gmelch's (1992) study of the lives of migrants from the Caribbean island of Barbados. His book is based largely on oral histories collected from just 13 return migrants who had lived portions of their lives in Britain or North America. There is not a single table in the book.

While a good deal of the most recent anthropological work on migration has focused on migrants in the West, an older anthropological research tradition continues to focus on the role of migration in nonwestern countries. Here Africa has received the greatest attention. Anthropologists working in this area are apt to criticize various aspects of reigning social science theory on urbanization and migration. Cliggett (2000), for example, shows the inadequacies of an exclusive focus on economic factors in explaining who moves in Zambia and when and why they do so. By examining the nature of control over farming resources and its link to social support networks, she shows the importance of understanding the dynamics of local power relations. She concludes that "social organization and social conflicts over access to resources play as great a role in migration decisions as do economic and ecological factors" (2000: 125). This also leads her to emphasize the diversity of situations found among migrants, some of whom in fact did not want to return to their home communities, nor did they send remittances there.

In a different kind of study in the same country, James Ferguson—whose intellectual links are closer to postmodernism and postcolonial studies than Cliggett's, which lie closer to the traditions of British social anthropology and demographic anthropology—looks at urban life on the Zambian Copperbelt. Showing the cruel delusions suffered by Zambians who bought into the myth of "modernization," Ferguson identifies two different cultural patterns in the city that reflect people's migration strategies. He found that discussions of the urban dwellers' decision of whether to retire back in "home" rural communities "centered less on such straightforward social and economic matters than on what we might call the cultural characteristics necessary for successful rural retirement." In considering what life would be like for them in rural retirement, people "turned quickly from questions of remittances or visits to matters of dress, styles of speech, attitudes, habits, even body carriage" (1999: 83). Curiously, while Ferguson himself rejects modernization theory, his informants all embraced it, lamenting the fact that their lives are suspended between two worlds, one modern, industrial, urban and western, the other traditional, rural, and African. In coping with this divide, people in the city adopted either what Ferguson terms a "localist" cultural style, more in harmony with rural norms and signaling a commitment to continued attachments to rural communities, or a "cosmopolitan" style, including characteristic modes of dress, speech, and behavior, signaling a rejection of such ties.

The large and rapidly growing body of anthropological studies of immigrants in the United States and other western countries has focused on a variety of issues, including the importance of immigrant networks in social, economic, and cultural adaptation, the changing nature of gender norms, and the role of religion and religious institutions. Among the most active researchers in this area is Leo Chavez (1991), whose studies of Mexican migrants to the United States have given special emphasis to the plight of illegal (or "undocumented") migrants. Here he shows the importance of studying the reception that migrants receive in the host community as a means of understanding the nature of their adaptation.

Taking this approach a step further, Cole, in his study of immigrants in Sicily, focuses attention on what he calls "everyday European responses to immigrants" (1997: 130). He finds that the Sicilians, contrary to some expectations, did not exhibit marked racist views. Based on participant observation and related qualitative methods, he unearths a much more subtle dynamic in the tensions that beset relationships between the immigrants and the "natives." Such anthropological studies have increasingly come to focus on questions of changing conceptions of national identity in the receiving societies, as in the case of the reception that the large population of Turkish immigrants has experienced in Germany (White 1997).

New York City is the site of an especially large number of anthropological studies of migrant adjustment, with research on Dominicans and assorted other Caribbeans, Russians, Chinese, Koreans, West Africans, Indians, Mexicans, southeast Asians and others (Foner 2000, 2001). A good example is offered by Margolis's study of Brazilians in New York. Motivated in part by the fact that Brazilians were a largely invisible minority in New York, lost amidst the sea of "Hispanics," Margolis combined a survey based on snowball sampling with informal interviewing and participant observation to produce an ethnography of "Little Brazil." She was particularly interested in examining the permanency of the migration. While people mainly viewed themselves as "sojourners," in the U.S. only temporarily to make money before returning to Brazil (a status reinforced by the fact that many lacked legal migrant status), she found that, as in so many other similar migrant cases, many of these sojourners became permanent migrants. Moreover, she also identified a pattern she termed "yo-yo migration" (1994: 263), the remigration to the U.S. of people who had said they were returning to Brazil "for good."

Of special interest to a number of anthropologists working in this area is the question of women's lives and the relation of gender norms in the sending and receiving societies. Typically a contrast is found between more patriarchal norms prevailing in many nonwestern or poorer sending societies and norms favoring greater gender equality in the major western receiving societies. Rather than viewing women as more traditional than men—a classic view in western social science—this line of work has viewed women as less eager to return to the home community insofar as such a move would mean giving up a degree of autonomy only available in the destination society (Gmelch and Gmelch 1995). Hirsch (1999), in order to get a better handle on these issues, studied Mexicans both in their home community in western Mexico and in the receiving community of Atlanta, comparing pairs of sisters or sisters-in-law living on either side of the border. She found that the women in Atlanta were better able to achieve their goal of a companionate marital relationship.

In recent years, a growing number of anthropologists have called for a reconceptualization of migration study—away from a dichotomous notion of sending and receiving communities and toward a transnational model of life lived across national boundaries (Kearney 1995). "Transmigrants," as such people who maintain multiple familial, social, religious, and political relationships across borders are called, "take actions, make decisions, and feel concerns, and develop identities within social networks that connect them to two or more societies simultaneously" (Glick-Schiller, Baseh, and Blanc-Szanton 1992: 1–2; Glick-Schiller, Basch, and Blanc-Szanton 1995). Whether this phenomenon is as new as some of its students suggest may be questionable. However, it is clear that recent developments in communication and transportation, as well as increased levels of wealth, have greatly facilitated it. The emphasis of transnationalism studies is on the network of relations tying people across national borders, viewing migrants not as situated in a geographical community (even an ethnic enclave), but rather as situated in transnational space.

The recent demographic interest in refugees has links to this transnational perspective, for the anthropologists who have turned their attention to refugee studies have emphasized the importance of examining just such transnational social networks and called for revision of common images of society as a territorially based entity (Marx 1990). Rather than view people in refugee camps as having their entire social lives circumscribed by their location, anthropologists have argued that people maintain important links with kin and others in a variety of locations, including their areas of origin. Without analyzing these links and these networks, studies of refugees will continue to produce unsatisfactory results. Lubkemann (2000), examining Mozambican refugees produced by the civil war, found that their lives and decisions could not be understood apart from an understanding of preexisting patterns of migration and gender relations. Moreover, their decisions as to whether and where to move following the ending of the war could similarly be understood only in terms of this larger understanding of cultural norms, social organization, and the meaning of geographical mobility.

METHODOLOGICAL CHALLENGES

Anthropologists have had mixed feelings about the way in which the larger demographic community has viewed anthropological methodology. The fact that demographers, in discussing what anthropology might contribute to demographic research, often seem to have in mind only methods, and not theory, has been a sore point. However, the loose use of the term "anthropological methods," when qualitative methods in general are intended, similarly provokes dismay among anthropologists. Furthermore, anthropologists, in their recognition of the cultural construction of analytical categories, see an important potential contribution to be made in critiquing and improving survey and other quantitative methods of research.

The cornerstone of anthropological methodology has long been participant observation. Since the time of Malinowski, the goal has been total immersion in a culture and in people's daily lives so that their understanding of the world and the nature of their social relations can be understood in holistic context. A corollary of this is a focus on the difference between what people say they do and believe on the one hand and what they actually do and (more problematically) what they actually believe on the other. The implications of this emphasis for a field like demography, which is heavily dependent on survey research methods, are enormous. A survey researcher can ask a respondent how often she goes to church but rarely checks this against actual church attendance. For an anthropologist, it is just this disjunction that is of particular interest. Nonanthropological demographers have sometimes turned to focus group methods to deal with some of these issues, but while a kind of informal focus group approach is often used by anthropologists in their research, much greater weight is placed on observing behavior in normal social contexts.

In historical demographic studies, as well, differences are evident between the work done by anthropologists and nonanthropological demographers. In the latter (the Princeton European fertility study being a good example), heavy emphasis is placed on machine-readable data and statistical analysis. Anthropologists working on historical demographic topics, while typically employing such data and statistical methods, also tend to place heavy emphasis on qualitative archival sources aimed at explicating the political economic and cultural context (Kertzer 1993, 1997).

Anthropologists have challenged the use of standardized terms for cross-cultural or cross-national research. Typically, such concepts are based on western folk terms and then given the status of scientific instruments. What is meant by a household may be (relatively) straightforward in a western context (though becoming less so with children of divorced parents moving between two residences), but it is much more problematic in polygynous societies and where great population flux is endemic (Hollos 1990). Van der Geest (1998: 41) points out that even such a seemingly simple question as "Are you married?" may entail a series of assumptions that mean that the answer given is based on considerations that the survey researcher never had in mind. Such concerns have led some survey researchers to call on anthropologists to do preliminary research on cultural and social context and meanings that would allow them to construct better survey questions. However, this skirts the more fundamental problem of a lack of cross-cultural comparability in survey data.

Many anthropologists have been influenced in recent years by an interpretivist approach. This focuses on local knowledge and the cultural construction of reality and generates deep skepticism regarding the use of standard social categories for comparative purposes. Some of its practitioners marry this approach to a concern for power relations, in which case the standard categories of social scientific analysis are of interest principally as objects of study in their own right, part of the dominant ideology that serves certain vested interests. Such a perspective tends to reject quantitative research, and, as is the case of Nancy Scheper-Hughes (1997), results in a call for "a demography without numbers." Castigating those anthropologists who would work as "hand-maidens" to statistical demographic science, she argues that "the piling up of quantitative data that relies on biomedical and Western categories will not generate fresh insights" (1997: 219).[3]

Yet on closer inspection one finds that even the most arch antipositivists in anthropology cannot escape from an interest in such standardized and quantifiable data as those documenting the spread of AIDS or rates of infant mortality. Just as anthropologists would argue that demographers must submit their categories of analysis to a deconstruction that is sensitive to local cultural understandings and social practices, so too demographers can point to important realms of human experience that require the use of cross-culturally applicable categories of analysis. Those anthropologists who have over the past two decades been working self-consciously at the intersection with demography remain committed both to the need for fundamental rethinking of demographic categories and methods and to the search for methods that will allow cross-cultural analysis, generalization, and theory.

RESEARCH EXEMPLARS

The range of recent work in anthropological demography can be illustrated by the example of three anthropologists who have been working in close contact with the larger demographic research community. These studies show some of the contributions that anthropology can make and, especially, the role of anthropological theory in demographic research.

Monica Das Gupta, working in a British social anthropological tradition, focuses on the relationship linking kinship and inheritance systems, gender ideology, and demographic outcomes. While her work concentrates primarily on northern India, she is interested in much larger comparative issues as well. In a series of publications (Das Gupta 1987, 1995, 1997), she has explored links between kinship systems and demographic regimes, with a special focus on mortality. Demographers have paid considerable attention in recent years to the link between women's status and fertility. What Das Gupta does is to put the question of women's status in the larger context of kinship systems and to relate these not only to fertility behavior, but also to a range of other demographic variables. Employing a broader anthropological perspective and adopting a life course view, she also demonstrates the importance of not viewing women's status as a simple variable with a single value characterizing a particular society. Rather, depending on the kinship system and the coresidential arrangements that are linked to it, women may have greater or lesser autonomy and influence at different stages of their lives. Hence, in northern India, while young married women have very low status and

---

[3] Expressions of doubt regarding the ability of anthropologists working on demographic questions and more traditional demographers to combine their forces in a single interdisciplinary field of demography are also raised by Hill (1997) and Greenhalgh (1997).

little autonomy, once women become mothers-in-law themselves, they typically gain considerable domestic power. These patterns in turn are shown to have demographic consequences; young mothers are unable to get the resources they need to nurture their newborns (especially daughters) and hence face high likelihood of infant mortality. In addition, in their young adult years women face higher death rates than men of the same age. Yet, later in their lives, as their power increases, women are able to marshal greater resources and in fact show greater survivorship rates than men.

Susan Greenhalgh's (1995a) attempts to develop a political economy of fertility that incorporates both feminist and cultural perspectives has been noted earlier. In her own work examining the nature and effects of China's one-child policy, she further develops these theoretical ideas while placing demographic behavior in China in a perspective different from that commonly found in the demographic literature. The fact that the state plays a major role in shaping fertility behavior is certainly no surprise in the Chinese context. What Greenhalgh sheds light on, though, through her anthropological approach, is how state-level policy comes to be contested at the local level and how contestation by peasant women and men affects local-level implementation of the state policy. She refers to her approach as "negotiational," focusing on three aspects of "reproductive micropolitics." These include "resistance to the birth control program; negotiation over family size and contraceptive practice; and the consequences, both beneficial and deleterious, for women, their bodies, and reproductive outcomes" (1994: 6). She does not romanticize women's resistance. Quite the contrary, she points out its paradoxical effect, which enables women to raise more sons than daughters. She also recognizes that peasant culture is itself changing as a result of its exposure to the state's antinatalist campaign.

Partially influenced by feminist theory, anthropologists have in recent years paid increasing attention to the body, to the ways in which it is conceptualized and its metaphoric use in symbolizing the social world. Caroline Bledsoe (2002), drawing on this tradition and linking it to the demographic study of fertility, aging, and mortality, calls for a new way of thinking about demographic issues. Rooted in a collaborative study with demographers and assorted other scientists in The Gambia (Bledsoe, Banja, and Hill 1998), Bledsoe's work was influenced by her surprising finding that contraceptive methods were often used in this West African society to increase rather than to limit the number of births. She shows the importance of gaining an understanding of how local people themselves conceptualize reproduction and relate it to understandings of body, health, and social support. Here Bledsoe stresses the fact that western notions of linear time do not capture how the women under study think of their bodies and their reproductive lives. Understanding their reproductive behavior entails an understanding of Gambian ideas relating to the wearing out of the body occasioned by reproductive episodes. These include not only childbirth but also miscarriage and other events as well.

FUTURE PROSPECTS

Had it not been for a strong feeling within mainstream demography that anthropological methods and theory could help enrich the field, it is possible that anthropologists investigating demographic topics would have continued working in almost total independence of demographers studying the same topics. It is still the case today that much of the anthropological work on such topics as fertility and migration takes place without reference to the demographic literature (and, one could add, vice versa). There are various reasons for this, including a certain degree of disciplinary insularity among anthropologists, as well as a strong antipositivist and antistatistical bias among many (but far from all) sociocultural anthropologists.

What has been so exciting about recent developments in anthropological demography, however, is that they have not simply come from the more behaviorist, or postivist, wing of anthropology, which is linked to studies of social organization. Rather, this new work has been enriched by anthropological theory on culture and the role of symbolism. The three research exemplars mentioned above all illustrate this in various ways, as political economic, social organizational, feminist, and symbolic theoretical strands from within anthropology are all brought into play.

Those demographers who, in calling for anthropological involvement in their field, simply sought advisors who would help them do better what they were already doing (e.g., in designing survey questions) may be either pleasantly or unpleasantly surprised that what they are getting is something quite different. Anthropological demography, as it is now developing, is poised to enrich demography as an interdisciplinary field by forcing it to confront some very basic epistemological and ontological questions. While this may produce some discomfort, the potential payoffs for both demography and anthropology are great.

REFERENCES

Becker, G. 1994. Metaphors in disrupted lives: infertility and cultural constructions of continuity. *Medical Anthropology Quarterly* 8: 383–410.

Bennett, J. W. 1976. *The ecological transition.* New York: Pergamon.

Bledsoe, C. 1990. The politics of children: Fosterage and the social management of fertility among the Mende of Sierra Leone. In *Births and power: The politics of reproduction.* Edited by W. P. Handwerker, 81–100. Boulder, Colo.: Westview.

Bledsoe, C. 2002. *Contingent lives: Reproduction, time and aging in West Africa.* Chicago: University of Chicago Press.

Bledsoe, C., F. Banja, and A. Hill. 1998. Reproductive mishaps and western contraception: An African challenge to fertility theory. *Population and Development Review* 20:81–113.

Bledsoe, C., J. Guyer, and S. Lerner, eds. 2000. *Fertility and the male life cycle in the era of fertility decline.* Oxford: Oxford University Press.

Bledsoe, C., and G. Pison. 1994. Introduction. In *Nuptiality in sub-Saharan Africa: Contemporary Anthropological and Demographic Perspectives.* Edited by C. Bledsoe and G. Pison, 1–22. Oxford: Clarendon.

Borgerhoff-Mulder, M. 1989. Marital status and reproductive performance in Kipsigis women: Re-evaluating the polygyny-fertility hypothesis. *Population Studies* 43:2:285–304.

Bradley, C. 1995. Women's empowerment and fertility decline in Western Kenya. In *Situating fertility.* Edited by S. Greenhalgh, 157–178. Cambridge: Cambridge University Press.

Brettell, C. 2000. Theorizing migration in anthropology. In *Migration theory.* Edited by C. Brettell and J. Hollifield, 97–135. New York: Routledge.

Browner, C. 2000. Situating women's reproductive activities. *American Anthropologist* 102:773–788.

Caldwell, J. C. 1982. *Theory of fertility decline.* New York: Academic Press.

Caldwell, J. C., and A. Hill. 1988. Recent developments using micro-approaches to demographic research. In *Micro-approaches to demographic research.* Edited by J. C. Caldwell, A. Hill, and V. Hull. London: Kegan Paul.

Carter, A. T. 1998. Cultural models and demographic behaviour. In *The methods and uses of anthropological demography.* Edited by A. Basu and P. Aaby, 246–267. Oxford: Clarendon.

Cecil, R., ed. 1996. *The anthropology of pregnancy loss.* Oxford: Berg.

Chavez, L. R. 1991. Outside the imagined community: Undocumented settlers and experiences of incorporation. *American Ethnologist* 18:257–278.

Cleland, J., and C. Wilson. 1987. Demand theories of the fertility transition: An iconoclastic view. *Population Studies* 41:5–30.

Cliggett, L. 2000. Social components of migration: Experiences from Southern Province, Zambia. *Human Organization* 59:125–135.

Cole, J. 1997. *The new racism in Europe: A Sicilian ethnography*. Cambridge: Cambridge University Press.

Das Gupta, M. 1987. Selective discrimination against female children in rural Punjab, India. *Population and Development Review* 13:77–100.

Das Gupta, M. 1995. Lifecourse perspectives on women's autonomy and health outcomes. *American Anthropologist* 97:481–491.

Das Gupta, M. 1997. Kinship systems and demographic regimes. In *Anthropological demography*. Edited by David I. Kertzer and Tom Fricke, 36–52. Chicago: University of Chicago Press.

Davis-Lloyd, R., and C. F. Sargent, eds. 1997. *Childbirth and authoritative knowledge: Cross-cultural perspectives*. Berkeley: University of California Press.

Delaney, C. 1991. *The seed and the soil*. Berkeley: University of California Press.

Ellison, P. T. 1994. Advances in human reproductive ecology. *Annual Review of Anthropology* 23:255–275.

Ferguson, J. 1999. *Expectations of modernity: Myths and meanings of urban life on the Zambian Copperbelt*. Berkeley: University of California Press.

Firth, R. 1968. (orig. 1936). *We, the Tikopia*. Boston: Beacon.

Foner, N. 2000. *From Ellis Island to New York*. New Haven, Conn.: Yale University Press.

Foner, N., ed. 2001. *New immigrants in New York*, rev. ed. New York: Columbia University Press.

Fortes, M. 1943. A note on fertility among the Tallensi of the Gold Coast. *Sociological Review* 35:4–5:99–113.

Fricke, T. 1994. *Himalayan households: Tamang demography and domestic processes*. Enlarged ed. New York: Columbia University Press.

Gage, T. B. 1998. The comparative demography of primates. *Annual Review of Anthropology* 27:197–221.

Ginsburg, F., and R. Rapp. 1995a. *Conceiving the New World Order: The global politics of reproduction*. Berkeley: University of California Press.

Ginsburg, F., and R. Rapp. 1995b. Introduction. In *Conceiving the New World Order: The global politics of reproduction*. Edited by F. Ginsburg and R. Rapp, 1–17. Berkeley: University of California Press.

Glick-Schiller, N., L. Basch, and C. Blanc-Szanton. 1992. Transnationalism: A new analytic framework for understanding migration. In *Towards a transnational perspective on migration*. Edited by N. Glick-Schiller, L. Basch, and C. Blanc-Szanton, 1–24. New York: Annals of the New York Academy of Science.

Glick-Schiller, N., L. Basch, and C. Blanc-Szanton. 1995. From immigrant to transmigrant: Theorizing transnational migration. *Anthropological Quarterly* 68:48–63.

Gmelch, G. 1992. *Double passage: The lives of Caribbean migrants abroad and back home*. Ann Arbor: University of Michigan Press.

Gmelch, G., and S. Gmelch. 1995. Gender and migration: The readjustment of women migrants in Barbados, Ireland, and Newfoundland. *Human Organization* 54:470–473.

Goody, J. 1983. *The development of the family and marriage in Europe*. Cambridge: Cambridge University Press.

Greenhalgh, S. 1990. Toward a political economy of fertility: Anthropological contributions. *Population and Development Review* 16:85–106.

Greenhalgh, S. 1994. Controlling births and bodies in village China. *American Ethnologist* 21:3–30.

Greenhalgh, S., ed. 1995a. *Situating fertility: Anthropology and demographic inquiry*. Cambridge: Cambridge University Press.

Greenhalgh, S. 1995b. Anthropology theorizes reproduction: Integrating practice, political economic, and feminist perspectives. In *Situating fertility*. Edited by S. Greenhalgh, 3–28. Cambridge: Cambridge University Press.

Greenhalgh, S. 1997. Methods and meanings: Reflections on disciplinary difference. *Population and Development Review* 23:819–824.

Guyer, J. I. 1994. Lineal identities and lateral networks: The logic of polyandrous motherhood. In *Nuptiality in sub-Saharan Africa: Contemporary anthropological and demographic perspectives*. Edited by C. Bledsoe and G. Pison, 231–252. Oxford: Clarendon.

Guyer, J. I. 2000. Traditions of studying paternity in social anthropology. In *Fertility and the male life cycle in the era of fertility decline*. Edited by C. Bledsoe, S. Lerner, and J. Guyer, 61–90. Oxford: Oxford University Press.

Hammel, E. A. 1972. The Zadruga as process. In *Household and family in past time*. Edited by P. Laslett and R. Wall, 335–373. Cambridge: Cambridge University Press.

Hammel, E. A. 1990. A theory of culture for demography. *Population and Development Review* 16:455–485.

Hammel, E. A. 1995. Economics 1, Culture 0: Fertility change and differences in the Northwest Balkans, 1700–1900. In *Situating fertility*. Edited by S. Greenhalgh, 225–258. Cambridge: Cambridge University Press.

Handwerker, W. P. 1990. Politics and reproduction: A window on social change. In *Births and power: Social change and the politics of reproduction*. Edited by W. P. Handwerker, 1–38. Boulder, Colo.: Westview.

Harris, M. 1966. The cultural ecology of India's sacred cattle. *Current Anthropology* 7:51–59.

Harris, M., and E. B. Ross. 1987. *Death, sex and fertility*. New York: Columbia University Press.

Hassan, F. A. 1979. Demography and archaeology. *Annual Review of Anthropology* 8:137–160.

Herdt, G., ed. 1997. *Sexual cultures and migration in the era of AIDS*. New York: Clarendon.

Hill, A. G. 1997. "Truth lies in the eye of the beholder": The nature of evidence in demography and anthropology. In *Anthropological demography*. Edited by D. I. Kertzer and T. Fricke, 223–247. Chicago: University of Chicago Press.

Hirsch, J. S. 1999. En el norte la mujer manda: Gender, generation, and geography in a Mexican transnational community. *American Behavioral Scientist* 42:1332–1349.

Hollos, M. 1990. Why is it difficult to take a census in Nigeria? The problem of indigenous conceptions of households. *Historical Methods* 25:12–19.

Inhorn, M. C. 1994. *The quest for conception: Gender, infertility, and Egyptian medical tradition*. Philadelphia: University of Pennsylvania Press.

Inhorn, M. C. 1996. *Infertility and patriarchy: The cultural politics of gender and family life in Egypt*. Philadelphia: University of Pennsylvania Press.

Kandel, W., and D. S. Massey. 2002. The culture of Mexican migration: A theoretical and empirical analysis. *Social Forces* 80:981–1004.

Kearney, M. 1995. The local and the global: The anthropology of globalization and transnationalism. *Annual Review of Anthropology* 24:547–565.

Kertzer, D. I. 1989. The joint family revisited: Demographic constraints and complex family households in the European past. *Journal of Family History* 14:1–15.

Kertzer, D. I. 1993. *Sacrificed for honor: Italian infant abandonment and the politics of reproductive control*. Boston: Beacon Press.

Kertzer, D. I. 1995. Political-economic and cultural explanations of demographic behavior. In *Situating fertility*. Edited by S. Greenhalgh, 29–52. Cambridge: Cambridge University Press.

Kertzer, D. I. 1997. The proper role of culture in demographic explanation. In *The continuing demographic transition*. Edited by G. W. Jones et al., 137–157. Oxford: Clarendon.

Kertzer, D. I., and D. Arel. 2002. Censuses, identity formation, and the struggle for political power. In *Census and identity*. Edited by D. I. Kertzer and D. Arel, 1–42. Cambridge: Cambridge University Press.

Kertzer, D. I., and T. Fricke. 1997. Toward an anthropological demography. In *Anthropological demography*. Edited by D. I. Kertzer and T. Fricke, 1–35. Chicago: University of Chicago Press.

Kertzer, D. I., and D. P. Hogan. 1989. *Family, political economy, and demographic change*. Madison: University of Wisconsin Press.

Kligman, G. 1998. *The politics of duplicity: Controlling reproduction in Ceausescu's Romania*. Berkeley: University of California Press.

Knodel, J., and E. van de Walle. 1986. Lessons from the past: Policy implications of historical fertility studies. In *The decline of fertility in Europe*. Edited by A. Coale and S. Watkins, 420–429. Princeton, N.J.: Princeton University Press.

Kreager, P. 1985. Demographic regimes as cultural systems. In *The state of population theory*. Edited by D. Coleman and R. Schofield, 131–155. Oxford: Blackwell.

Lee, R. B., and I. DeVore, eds. 1968. *Man the hunter*. Chicago: Aldine.

Levine, N., and J. Silk. 1997. Why polyandry fails. *Current Anthropology* 38:3:375–398.

Lorimer, F., et al. 1954. *Culture and human fertility*. Paris: UNESCO.

Lubkemann, S. 2000. The transformation of transnationality among Mozambican migrants in South Africa. *Canadian Journal of African Studies* 34:41–63.

MacCormick, C. P., ed. 1994. *Ethnography of fertility and birth*, 2nd ed. Prospect Heights, Ill.: Waveland.

Malkki, L. H. 1995. Refugees and exile: From "refugee studies" to the national order of things. *Annual Review of Anthropology* 24:495–523.

Margolis, M. L. 1994. *Little Brazil: An ethnography of Brazilian immigrants in New York City*. Princeton, N. J.: Princeton University Press.

Martin, E. 1987. *The woman in the body: A cultural analysis of reproduction*. Boston: Beacon.

Martin, E. 1991. The egg and the sperm. *Signs* 16:485–501.

Marx, E. 1990. The social world of refugees: A conceptual framework. *Journal of Refugee Studies* 3:189–203.

Massey, D. S. 2000. When surveys fail: An alternative for data collection. In *The science of self-report*. Edited by A. A. Stone, et al., 145–160. Mahwah, N.J.: Erlbaum.

Massey, D. S., R. Alarcón, J. Durand, and H. González. 1990. *Return to Aztlan: The social process of international migration from western Mexico*. Berkeley: University of California Press.

Massey, D. S., and R. Zenteno. 2000. A validation of the ethnosurvey: The case of Mexico-U.S. migration. *International Migration Review* 34:766–793.

McNicoll, G. 1980. Institutional determinants of fertility change. *Population and Development Review* 6:441–462.

Meindl, R. S., and K. F. Russell. 1998. Recent advances in method and theory in paleodemography. *Annual Review of Anthropology* 27:375–399.

Nations, M. 1988. Angels with wet wings won't fly: Maternal sentiment in Brazil and the image of neglect. *Culture, Medicine and Psychiatry* 12:141–200.

Oppenheimer, V. K. 2003. Cohabiting and marriage during young men's career-development process. *Demography* 40:127–149.

Paine, R., ed. 1997. *Integrating archaeological demography: Multidisciplinary approaches to prehistoric population*. Carbondale: Center for Archaeological Investigations, Southern Illinois University.

Radcliffe-Brown, A. R. 1964 (orig. 1922). *The Andaman Islanders*. Glencoe, Ill.: Free Press.

Redfield, R. 1941. *The folk culture of Yucatan*. Chicago: University of Chicago Press.

Renne, E. P. 1995. Houses, fertility, and the Nigerian Land Use Act. *Population and Development Review* 21(1): 113–126.

Renne, E. P., and E. van de Walle, eds. 2001. *Regulating menstruation*. Chicago: University of Chicago Press.

Scheper-Hughes, N. 1992. *Death without weeping: The violence of everyday life in Brazil*. Berkeley: University of California Press.

Scheper-Hughes, N. 1997. Demography without numbers. In *Anthropological demography*. Edited by D. I. Kertzer and T. Fricke, 201–222. Chicago: University of Chicago Press.

Schneider, J., and P. Schneider. 1996. *Festival of the poor: Fertility decline and the ideology of class in Sicily, 1860–1980*. Tucson: University of Arizona Press.

Scrimshaw, S. 1983. Infanticide as deliberate fertility regulation. In *Determinants of fertility in developing countries, II*. Edited by R. Bulatao and R. Lee, 245–266. New York: Academic Press.

Setel, P. 2000. "Someone to take my place": Fertility and the male life-course among coastal Boiken, East Sepik Province, Papua New Guinea. In *Fertility and the male life cycle in the era of fertility decline*. Edited by C. Bledsoe, S. Lerner, and J. Guyer, 61–90. Oxford: Oxford University Press.

Skinner, G. W. 1993. Conjugal power in Tokugawa Japanese families: A matter of life or death. In *Sex and gender hierarchies*. Edited by B. Miller, 236–270. Cambridge: Cambridge University Press.

Skinner, G. W. 1997. Family systems and demographic processes. In *Anthropological demography*. Edited by D. I. Kertzer and T. Fricke, 53–95. Chicago: University of Chicago Press.

Sigle-Rushton, W., and S. McLanahan. 2002. The living arrangements of new unmarried mothers. *Demography* 39:415–433.

Smith, T. C. 1977. *Nakahara: Family farming and population in a Japanese village, 1717–1830*. Palo Alto, Calif.: Stanford University Press.

Steward, J. H. 1936. The economic and social basis of primitive bands. In *Essays in honor of A. L. Kroeber*. Edited by R. L. Lowie, 331–345. Berkeley: University of California Press.

Townsend, N. 1997. Reproduction in anthropology and demography. In *Anthropological demography*. Edited by D. I. Kertzer and T. Fricke, 96–114. Chicago: University of Chicago Press.

Townsend, N. 2000. Male fertility as a lifetime of relationships: Contextualizing men's biological reproduction in Botswana. In *Fertility and the male life cycle in the era of fertility decline*. Edited by C. Bledsoe, S. Lerner, and J. Guyer, 343–364. Oxford: Oxford University Press.

van der Geest, S. 1998. Participant observation in demographic research: Fieldwork experiences in a Ghanaian community. In *The methods and uses of anthropological demography*. Edited by A. Basu and P. Aaby, 39–56. Oxford: Clarendon.

Voland, E. 1998. Evolutionary ecology of human reproduction. *Annual Review of Anthropology* 27:347–374.

White, J. 1997. Turks in the new Germany. *American Anthropologist* 99:754–769.

Willey, G. 1992. Precolumbian population history in the Maya lowlands. *Journal of Field Archaeology* 19:527–530.

Williams, B. F. 1994. What determines where transnational labor migrants go? Modifications in migration theories. *Human Organization* 53:269–278.

Wolf, A. P. 1984. Family life and the life cycle in rural China. In *Households: Comparative and historical studies of the domestic group*. Edited by R. Netting, R. Wilk, and E. Arnould, 279–298. Berkeley: University of California Press.

Wolf, A. P., and C. Huang. 1980. *Marriage and adoption in China, 1845–1945*. Palo Alto, Calif.: Stanford University Press.

Wood, J. W. 1990. Fertility in anthropological populations. *Annual Review of Anthropology* 19:211–242.

CHAPTER 18

Economic Demography

Andrew Mason[1]

There is a long tradition of research on population and economics. The work of Thomas Malthus is well known, but other early economists, including William Petty and William Godwin, were also concerned about the economic effects of population growth. Interest in the links between population and economics was rekindled during the Great Depression and was featured prominently in the writing of John Maynard Keynes. Rapid population growth during the second half of the 20th century led to renewed interest in the development effects of population growth. The consequences of population aging have emerged as an active research area as countries have entered the later stages of the demographic transition.

In contrast to the long-standing interest in the economic consequences of demographic change, there has been a more recent explosion of interest in demographic behavior. Few economists recognized the applicability of economic models to the kinds of social behavior that traditionally have been the bread and butter of sociologists and social demographers. Influenced most by the work of Gary Becker, economists are increasingly interested in marriage, divorce, childbearing, sexual behavior, and other social activities.

The broad reach of economic demography presents a considerable challenge for any effort to summarize the field. Since Spengler (1959) summarized economics and demography over 40 years ago, research has advanced on many fronts. This chapter will not attempt a comprehensive summary of this progress, however. The approach taken here is to identify some of the central ideas that are common to the field—in the section on conceptual frameworks—and then to focus in more detail on two important areas,

[1] University of Hawaii, Manoa and East-West Center. Contact for author: amason@hawaii.edu. Thanks to Ron Lee and Turro Wongkaren for their suggestions.

intergenerational transfers and population and development, in the section on theoretical models. This approach is employed, in part, because of the successful cross-fertilization of the approaches of economists, sociologists, and social demographers. Thus, it is safe to assume that the economic approach to many demographic issues is represented throughout this volume, in chapters devoted to fertility, mortality, and migration, for example. Those who are interested in a more detailed treatment of economic approaches to these subjects would also find the *Handbook of Population and Family Economics* (Rosenzweig and Stark 1997) to be useful.

CONCEPTUAL FRAMEWORKS

Economics can be divided into microeconomics and macroeconomics. Microeconomics is concerned primarily with the behavior of economic actors—firms, households, and individuals. Traditionally the aspects of individual behavior attracting the attention of economists were consumer behavior, investment behavior, and labor force behavior. Now childbearing, marriage, divorce, health-seeking behavior, sexual behavior, criminal behavior, and many other aspects of human behavior are routinely addressed by economists.

The microeconomics framework focuses on exchange. Each individual has resources at her disposal that come primarily in two forms—financial or material wealth and time. The individual exchanges her economic resources for goods and services to achieve the highest possible level of utility. The exchange can take many forms: time can be traded for money through work; financial resources can be traded for consumer goods and services; current resources can be traded for future resources, and so on. The terms under which exchange takes place is governed by prices (or wages) that are set in the marketplace in some circumstances but may be implicit in other circumstances.

The same principles that govern traditionally modeled forms of exchange apply to demographic behavior. Marriage can be modeled as an agreement between two individuals to exchange time, material resources, and love. Childbearing requires the exchange of time and goods for children. Migration involves exchange of the lost wages in the place of origin and the direct costs of moving for the new (and hopefully higher) wages in the place of destination. Age at death turns, in part, on decisions regarding the allocation of scarce resources among competing ends.

Although many economists have contributed to the economics of demographic behavior, Gary Becker has played a pivotal role. His book, *A Treatise on the Family* (1991), and his Nobel lecture (Becker 1993) provide a valuable exposition of the application of economics to demographic behavior.

Macroeconomics is concerned with longer-term aggregate growth and with shorter-term fluctuations in the economy, e.g., the rates of inflation and unemployment. Macroeconomic demography has focused primarily on the longer-term issues, although the effects of economic fluctuations on vital events—fertility, mortality, migration, divorce, and marriage—have received some attention by economists. By and large demographic variables are not thought to influence short-run fluctuations in the economy, in part because demographic variables, e.g., age-structure and population size, change much more gradually than the economic variables, e.g., the rate of inflation or the unemployment rate.

The distinction between macroeconomics and microeconomics has blurred over time. Increasingly, macroeconomic models are based implicitly or explicitly on the aggregation of individual responses. Some macroeconomic theories are based on the behavior of a representative agent, but many models acknowledge heterogeneity within the population. In particular, macroeconomic models recognize the dependence of behavior on age. An early example is the life-cycle saving model, which assumes that saving rates vary by age and thus aggregate saving is influenced by population age structure.

Samuelson (1958) developed a particularly influential macroeconomic model that addressed important issues that arise with intergenerational transfers. His model incorporates age structure and a population consisting of overlapping generations. Since this early effort, overlapping generation models have become part of the standard toolbox of macroeconomics and, as a result, demography and economics have become more closely linked.

Some of these models, including Samuelson's, are highly stylized in their treatment of demographic conditions and processes. It is not uncommon, for example, for populations in their models to consist of only three age groups. Often models assume that the death rate is the same at all ages—an interesting assumption as it implies that life expectancy does not decline as a cohort ages! These models typically sacrifice realism in order to achieve analytic tractability. Other macroeconomic models incorporate more realistic demography. Examples include Auerbach and Kotlikoff's (1987) study of U.S. fiscal policy, Lee's (1994b) model of intergenerational transfers, the Cutler et al. (1990) study of aging and U.S. economic growth, and the Boucekkine, de la Croix, and Licandro (2002) study of human capital, demographic change, and endogenous growth to name a few.

THEORETICAL MODELS

Two areas of research are emphasized in this section: intergenerational transfers and population and development. These areas are important and illustrate the application of economic theory to demographic issues.

Intergenerational Transfers

During the last two decades there have been enormous strides in measuring, modeling, and assessing the implications of intergenerational transfers at both the micro and macro levels. This research is important, in part, because all human populations have extended periods of dependency at the beginning of their lives. Human survival requires large transfers from adults to children. Increased transfers to children in the form of spending for health and education have played an essential role in modern economic development. As life expectancy has increased, an extended period of dependency has also emerged at older ages, and intergenerational transfers from working-age adults to the elderly have become increasingly important.

Economic research has laid a strong foundation for studying intergenerational transfers at the macro level. Following on the pioneering work of Samuelson (1958) and Willis (1988), a theoretical transfer framework has been developed by Lee and his collaborators (Bommier and Lee 2003; Lee 1994a, 1994b), which is discussed in detail in the "Research Exemplar" section below. "Generational accounting" is being used to evaluate the effects of public policy on future generations in many countries around the world (Auerbach, Gokhale, and Kotlikoff 1991; Auerbach, Kotlikoff, and Leibfritz 1999).

Significant advances at the microlevel have also been achieved. The increased availability of surveys and microlevel studies has greatly improved our ability to measure familial transfers and to discover why they occur (Altonji, Hayashi, and Kotlikoff 2000; Frankenberg, Lillard, and Willis 2002; Lillard and Willis 1997; McGarry and Schoeni 1997). Progress has been made in estimating and modeling bequests, a difficult issue (Attanasio and Hoynes 2000; Brown and Weisbenner 2002; Poterba 2000; Poterba and Weisbenner 2001). There have been important advances in modeling the allocation of resources within households, a step critical to estimating intrahousehold, intergenerational transfers (Deaton 1997; Lazear and Michael 1988). New innovative surveys are beginning to shed additional light on this issue (Chu 2000; Hermalin 2002).

The importance and form of transfers varies considerably from country to country and over time in individual countries. Almost universally, transfers from working-age adults to dependent children occur within households, although the extent to which education and health expenditures on children are privately or publicly funded varies considerably.

The situation is quite varied with respect to transfers to the elderly. Outside the industrialized countries of the West, most elderly coreside with their adult children. In Japan and South Korea, the extent of coresidence has declined very rapidly in the last few decades, but roughly half of the elderly live with children. In other Asian countries the great majority of elderly live with their children, and there is a surprising degree of stability in the aggregate. Taiwan is experiencing a gradual shift away from such arrangements, but in many other Asian countries this is not the case (East-West Center 2002). In Singapore, for example, 85% of those 60 and older lived with children in 1995 as compared with 88% in 1988, despite extraordinary economic and social change in virtually every other dimension of life (Kinsella and Velkoff 2001). The situation in Latin America is less thoroughly documented, but data for six Latin American countries show that living in multigeneration households has been the norm there as well (Kinsella 1990).

Extended living arrangements are less important in the West, but in some European countries the elderly are not living exclusively by themselves or with their spouses. In Greece and Spain, roughly 40% of those 65 and older were living in households with three or more persons. At the other extreme, only about 5% of the elderly of Sweden and Denmark lived in households with two or more persons (Kinsella and Velkoff 2001). In the U.S., the great majority of elderly do not live with their children, but this has not always been the case. The percentage 65 and older living with children in the U.S. declined from 64% in 1880 to 49% in 1940, 30% in 1960, and 18% in 1980 (Ruggles 1994). Given the importance of familial transfers, the intense focus by economists is hardly surprising.

FAMILIAL MODELS OF IG TRANSFERS.   Economic models of familial intergenerational transfers emphasize two motives. First, transfers may occur to satisfy distributional objectives. Altruistic models are based on the assumption that individuals care about others within the family (Becker 1974; Becker and Tomes 1976). Intergenerational transfers arise because parents care about their children (downward altruism), because children care about their parents (upward altruism), or both (two-sided altruism).

Second, transfers may be a nonmarket transaction between family members or others in a society. In this instance transfers involve an implicit contract or a *quid pro quo*. The form of these transactions can be relatively straightforward or quite complex. For example, grandparents may provide child care for their grandchildren and receive room and board, or adult children may provide personal care to their elderly parents with the understanding that they will receive a bequest. Parents may send their children to an expensive university with the understanding that, in return, they will receive old-age support from those children. When families insure their members against a variety of risks, this is also a form of exchange. Children may insure their parents against longevity risk. If parents die at an unexpectedly young age, children receive a bequest. If parents live longer than expected, outliving their resources, children provide support.

These alternative perspectives have led to a variety of hypotheses about why intergenerational transfers vary within and across societies and over time. If distributional objectives are important, changes in the distribution of earnings or implementation of public transfer programs will elicit changes in familial transfers. If nonmarket transactions are important, the development of market-based or public sector alternatives may lead to a diminished role for family-based transfers.

Barro (1974), Becker (1974, 1991), and Becker and Tomes (1976) develop altruistic models of intergenerational transfers that have been especially influential. In Barro's model, the behavior of individuals is guided by a utility function that is increasing in one's own consumption and the utility achieved by one's offspring. The utility of the offspring depends, in turn, on their own consumption and the utility of their offspring. Through this interlinking chain the current generation consumes and transfers resources to its children and is influenced by its concern, not only for its own children, but for all future generations.

An important implication of Barro's model is that familial transfers will neutralize fiscal policy. When a government exercises expansionary fiscal policy it stimulates the economy by increasing current spending financed by issuing debt. From the perspective of intergenerational transfers, the policy is an effort to stimulate spending by transferring resources to current generations from future generations. In Barro's model, however, the public policy is undone by altruistic households. They compensate future generations by increasing their saving and accumulating wealth, exactly offsetting the increase in public debt. Barro's model implies that public intergenerational transfers and private intergenerational transfers are perfect substitutes. A change in public transfers is matched dollar for dollar by a compensating change in private transfers.

In the Becker and Tomes framework the utility of parents depends on their own consumption, the number of children, and the quality per child. Quality is determined by spending per child (i.e., downward intergenerational transfers) and by an endowment, determined in turn by public sector policies, by luck, and by genetics. In the Becker and Tomes model an increase in household income leads to an increase in spending per child, but at a decreasing rate, because parents value higher-quality children. Becker and Tomes also show that "parents tend to invest more human capital in better-endowed children" and compensate more poorly endowed children with other kinds of transfers.

The decision by parents to invest in the human capital of their children is developed further in Becker (1991). Parents have two objectives in their transfer decisions. One is to maximize the family's total wealth by investing in the human capital of its members, especially its children. The second objective is distributional—allocating resources among family members, and across generations, in accordance with the preferences governing the parents' decision-making process. Some parents may feel very altruistic toward their children and allocate a large share of family resources to them; others may be more selfish.

It would be a matter of pure coincidence if the human capital investments that maximized family wealth produced an allocation of resources that satisfied the distributional preferences of the parents. If parents were especially altruistic, they would make additional transfers to their children, perhaps through a bequest. If parents were less altruistic (or had made especially large human capital investments in their children), they would expect their children to pay them back in some form of reverse intergenerational transfer—perhaps through old age support.

Transfers to children are the centerpiece of the Becker and Tomes model, but others have emphasized other features of intergenerational transfers. The old-age security hypothesis posits that children are the old-age security plan for parents. In countries with underdeveloped capital markets, accumulating financial wealth is not a viable option. As capital markets improve, parents can rely more on saving and less on children (Willis 1980). Protection against longevity risk will lead to bequests by elderly persons who die at a young age and support by children for elderly parents who live longer than expected (Kotlikoff and Spivak 1981). Monetary transfers from elderly parents to adult children may represent repayment for services provided to parents by children (Cox 1987).

Results from recent studies show that it is empirically difficult to distinguish alternative models of transfers, that there is every reason to believe that the motivation underlying transfers will vary from one setting to the next, and that transfers will often fill a multiplicity of purposes. In studies of interhousehold transfers in Malaysia and Indonesia, no single model explains transfers. The evidence there points to exchange, insurance, and repayments for educational "loans" as important motives for transfers (Frankenberg, Lillard, and Willis 2002; Lillard and Willis 1997). Intergenerational transfer arrangements in Taiwan are consistent with a variety of interpretations—but not the use of bequests to enforce old-age support (Lee, Parish, and Willis 1994). Altonji, Hayashi, and Kotlikoff (2000) conclude that in the U.S., money transfers respond to income difference and appear to be motivated by altruism rather than by implicit exchange. Time flows from children to parents are not accompanied by money flows from parents to children. However, the very low responsiveness of transfers to intergenerational income differences is at odds with the standard altruism model (Altonji, Hayashi and Kotlikoff 1992; Altonji, Hayashi, and Kotlikoff 2000).

RESPECTIVE ROLES OF THE FAMILY AND THE PUBLIC SECTOR.   Why do families get involved in some kinds of transactions and governments in others? And why does the balance between families and governments in low-income countries differ so much from that in the industrialized countries of the West? The family offers advantages for conducting transactions in realms where *identity* is important, in transactions, for example, that "involve consequences or obligations that extend over time" (Ben-Porath 1980). Families also suffer from disadvantages. Their small size limits the extent to which they can realize economies of scale in production. As insurers, families offer protection against moral hazard and adverse selection, but family members may face highly correlated risks reducing the extent to which pooling risks offers protection to family members. The role of the family may evolve as the effectiveness of enforcement of both private and social contracts changes, as markets develop that facilitate exchange between strangers, as individual and family characteristics such as income influence the potential gains and costs of the family, and as risks such as those associated with death, disability, and unemployment change.

Human capital investment is one area where identity is important, both because the returns to investment in human capital depend on characteristics of individuals that are difficult to observe and because human capital investments cannot be legally secured in the same way that a lender can protect himself from default on a loan to purchase a house, for example. Thus, education loans are unavailable in many countries or available only through publicly sponsored or subsidized programs.[2] Thus, the family continues to play a prominent, though not exclusive, role in human capital investment.

One of the difficulties the family faces is enforcement. If parents make large human capital investments in their children, what assurance do they have that the children will ever pay them back? Becker and Murphy (1988) address this issue and the circumstances under which it can lead to underinvestment in children and public intervention. One possibility is that social norms may operate with sufficient force to ensure that children will repay their parents. Another possibility is that parents are sufficiently altruistic that no payback is necessary. Through bequests parents can maintain control over the intergenerational distribution of family resources throughout their lives. But if social norms are insufficient and parents are not sufficiently altruistic, parents may choose to underinvest in the human resources of their children and/or parents may receive insufficient old-age support from their children.

There are a variety of ways under these circumstances that governments may intervene to ensure a more efficient and equitable distribution of resources. Governments may impose mandatory minimal levels of education or subsidize the costs of education by providing free public schooling or by subsidizing student loans. Thus the government can either mandate the intergenerational transfer or provide the transfer itself financed through its power of taxation. Similarly, some governments are mandating that children provide old-age support to their parents. Singapore is an example. Much more frequently governments provide direct support to seniors from taxes imposed on workers. Again, familial transfers are being mandated or public transfers are being made as a substitute for familial transfers.

An alternative perspective on government activity emphasizes political power. Preston's (1984) influential work first raised the possibility that generational shifts in political power were influencing the generational distribution of public resources. Razin, Sadka, and Swagel (2002) take a more formal approach, using a voting model to address the effects of aging on the size of transfers, and concluding, based on data for the U.S. and western European countries, that a rise in the dependency ratio leads to an increase in welfare spending.

In Preston's (1984) view, "we have made a set of private and public choices that have dramatically altered the age profile of well being." Measured along a variety of

---

[2] A dot-com company, "My Rich Uncle," has recently established a human capital market which allows students to sell a share of their future earnings to investors. It is too early to tell whether this effort will prove to be legal and financially successful. Thanks to Ron Lee for pointing this out to me.

dimensions, U.S. elderly made substantial gains relative to children as shifts in public policy during the 1970s substantially increased the resources of the elderly at the expense of workers and their children. In the view of Becker and Murphy (1988), increased spending on the elderly during the 1970s was essentially compensation for increased public spending on education beginning in the 1920s. Becker and Murphy's "back of the envelope" calculations indicate that the rate of return received by children, who were the beneficiaries of increased public spending, substantially exceeded the rate of return, realized through old-age support, of those who financed the increase in public spending on education. From Preston's cross-sectional perspective generational inequities appear to have increased, whereas from Becker and Murphy's longitudinal perspective public spending appears to have favored younger generations.

INTERGENERATIONAL TRANSFERS AND PUBLIC POLICY.   As population aging has accelerated, public policy with respect to intergenerational transfers has been the subject of an increased amount of attention by economists. One influential initiative has been the development of an accounting system—generational accounts—that provides an overall assessment of the generational effects of public policy. A second group of studies has focused more explicitly on Social Security reform.

Generational accounts were first introduced in 1991 by Auerbach, Gokhale, and Kotlikoff (1991). Generational accounts are used to evaluate current public policy from a generational perspective by comparing the net lifetime tax rate paid by different living cohorts, including the newborn generation, and the average rate paid by all future generations. For each cohort the taxes paid in each year are deducted from the public transfers received to determine *net* taxes at each age. Lifetime net taxes paid by a cohort are calculated as the present value of the net taxes paid at each age. The lifetime net tax rate is the ratio of the net taxes paid to the present value of labor income at each age during the cohort's lifetime.

For any living cohort, generational accounts are constructed—directly based on historical and projected taxes, transfers, and earnings assuming that current policy will continue unchanged. The generational account for all future generations combined is estimated indirectly, based on the debt that current generations leave for future generations to pay. The debt includes the standard national debt but also unfunded obligations that will require payments by future generations to generations that are currently alive. In 1995, for example, the estimated present value of the debt being shifted to future generations was $9.4 trillion versus a conventionally defined national debt of $2.1 trillion (Gokhale, Page, and Sturrock 1999).

Many industrialized countries face serious generational imbalances, with future generations expected to pay a substantially higher portion of their lifetime income in taxes than do current generations (Auerbach, Kotlikoff, and Leibfritz 1999). In the U.S., future generations will, on average, be required to pay 49% of their lifetime income as compared with 29% for the newborn generation (Gokhale, Page, and Sturrock 1999). Other countries face much greater generational imbalances. In the absence of reform, future generations in Japan will face a net tax rate of 386% of lifetime income as compared with 143% for the new-born generation (Takayama, Kitamura, and Yoshida 1999).

Why do countries face such large imbalances? In part, because they have accumulated large national debts. A more important source of generational imbalance is the impact of rapid population aging combined with public programs, primarily pension and health care programs, which provide substantial transfers to the elderly. These programs impose a net lifetime tax on each generation because the rate of return available from pay-as-you-go schemes is substantially less than the rate of return otherwise available—from the stock market, for example. Thus, each dollar "invested" in these transfer schemes effectively imposes a lifetime tax on all participants. The larger the size of the elderly population, the larger the size of such programs and their accompanying tax burden. The emergence of these huge implicit debts provides the impetus for Social Security reform.

The debate on Social Security reform deals with wide-ranging issues, only some of which are directly related to intergenerational transfers. Two important issues are considered here. The first is the effect of Social Security on saving. The second is the distribution of the benefits and costs from Social Security reform.

The effect of transfer system reform on saving is important for two reasons. First, if increases in transfer programs crowd out saving, capital accumulation and economic growth are undermined. Second, if transfer programs crowd out saving, they will have less effect on the economic status of the elderly.

The evidence about the effect of public pensions on saving is drawn mainly from the experience of western industrialized countries. Gale (1998) provides a recent review of theoretical and empirical issues. Whether Social Security transfer programs will depress saving rates was first explored by Feldstein (1974) and Munnell (1974), but the empirical evidence is quite mixed. Large effects have been estimated by Feldstein (1996), Gale (1998), Leimer and Richardson (1992), and Munnell (1974). Smaller offsets or mixed results are found by Bernheim and Levin (1989), Hubbard (1986), Hubbard and Judd (1987), King and Dicks-Mireaux (1982), and Dicks-Mireaux and King (1984). Some studies have concluded that Social Security does not depress saving at all or that the relationship is weak (Blinder, Gordon, and Wise 1980; Gullason, Kolluri, and Panik 1993; Leimer and Lesnoy 1982). Recent studies have considered the effect on saving of major reform, i.e., substantial privatization, of Chile's public pension system and concluded that the result was a substantial increase in saving rates (Coronado 2002; Holzmann 1997).

The Social Security–saving literature often neglects the possibility that changes in Social Security or other public transfer programs will induce a response in familial transfers rather than in private saving. As was first pointed out by Barro, this would neutralize the effect of public transfers on saving and capital (Barro 1974). To the extent that elderly do not make transfers to their children or, if they do, make them for exchange purposes (that is, in exchange for attention and assistance from their children), then the Barro argument would not apply. There is an extensive but inconclusive literature on these issues (see, for example, McGarry and Schoeni 1997).

Many of the current reform schemes propose phase-out of pay-as-you-go (PAYGO) Social Security and replacement with funded, privatized schemes. A contentious issue has been the extent to which establishing PAYGO systems or phasing them out benefits some generations at the expense of others. Some researchers have a quite optimistic take on this issue (Feldstein and Samwick 2001; Krueger and Kubler 2002), while others believe that any reform will require substantial redistributions. Transfer systems for old-age support generate large transfer wealth and corresponding implicit debts. The wealth is held by those now alive and is compensation for support provided to previous generations of retirees. The debt is owed by future generations.

The size of the implicit debt is very substantial. For the U.S. in the year 2000, the implicit debt (discounting at 3%) generated by Social Security (OASI) amounts to 1.7 times GDP, or 17 trillion, which is 46% of the total demand for wealth (Lee, Mason, and Miller 2003). Feldstein (1997: 9) estimates an implicit debt that is slightly lower. Many Latin American public pension programs also have large implicit debts. Bravo (2001) estimates implicit debt to GDP ratios arising from public pension program *circa* 1990 of 1 for Costa Rica, about 1.5 for Chile, Panama, and Cuba, about 2 for Brazil, and about 3 for Uruguay and Argentina. Familial transfer programs may also have large implicit debts. For Taiwan in 1960, the implicit debt generated by the family transfer system, as modeled by Lee, Mason, and Miller (2003), was about 0.9 times GDP.

If the obligations implicit in transfer systems are not honored, the costs of transition are borne entirely by those who are currently alive and fall most heavily on those who have already retired. If obligations are honored, the implicit debts must be repaid during a transition toward individual responsibility, prolonging the effects of the transfer system past the system's dissolution. Generations responsible for repaying the implicit debt face a double task: to make payments out of current income to honor past obligations by repaying the implicit debt and to save out of their current income to prefund their own retirements.

The size of the implicit debt varies considerably over the demographic transition and is strongly affected by the final stage of population aging. If the U.S. maintains its current Social Security system, the implicit debt relative to GDP will double between 2000 and 2100 due to population aging. The cost of delaying reform is substantial (Lee, Mason, and Miller 2003).

Population and Development

Economic research addresses many dimensions of development, e.g., economic structure, urbanization, social and institutional development. Recent research on population and development has emphasized a narrower concern—growth in income per capita (or per worker). A simple identity offers a device for organizing discussion of this literature. Income per capita can be expressed as the product of two terms, income per worker and the number of workers per capita: $Y/N \equiv Y/L \times L/N$. Expressed as growth rates, we have:[3]

$$\dot{y} \equiv \dot{y}^l + l - n \tag{1}$$

where $\dot{y}$ is the rate of growth of per capita income, $\dot{y}^l$ is the rate of growth of income per worker, l is the rate of growth of the labor force, and n is the rate of population growth. Growth in income or output per *worker*, the first term on the right-hand side of equation (1), has been the focus of most research on economic growth. Several recent studies extend analysis to growth in per capita income and the gap between labor force growth and population growth, $l-n$.

These studies explore what is known as the *demographic dividend*. We will discuss this recent literature first and then consider the effect of demographic factors on income or output per worker.

---

[3] This expression is obtained by taking the natural log of both sides and then the derivative with respect to time.

THE DEMOGRAPHIC DIVIDEND. The demographic transition is accompanied by an extended period during which the labor force grows more rapidly than the population. This generalization does not hold for all countries, but it does for many. The pattern can be seen in Figure 18.1, which plots the annual rate of growth of the labor force and the rate of growth of the population for countries of the world from 1960 to 1990 (Mason 2001a). The differences between the two growth rates are marked by diagonals in the figure.

In the countries early in their demographic transitions, the population growth rate and the labor force growth rate are both high and $l-n$ is close to zero. But as the demographic transition proceeds, the population growth rate declines more rapidly than the labor force growth rate and a gap emerges between the two—$l-n$ turns positive. Toward the end of the demographic transition, the gap becomes smaller and may turn strongly negative as population growth becomes increasingly concentrated among older age groups. The demographic dividend could then become a demographic burden.

If growth in output per worker is unaffected by the demographic transition, changes in $l-n$ yield equal changes in the rate of growth of per capita income—a demographic dividend. The effect is small in any one year but it persists for several decades. The global pattern shown in Figure 18.1 is for 30-year periods. A value of 0.5% per year for 30 years yields an increase in per capita income of 16%; a value of 1.0% per year for 30 years yields an increase in per capita income of 35%. Given that real per capita income growth for the world averaged 1.9% between 1960 and 1990, the demographic dividend potentially could explain a substantial portion of world economic growth.

Two sets of issues about the demographic dividend are immediately apparent. First, what accounts for the dividend and why is it higher in some countries than in others? Second, does the demographic dividend necessarily lead to higher growth in per capita income?

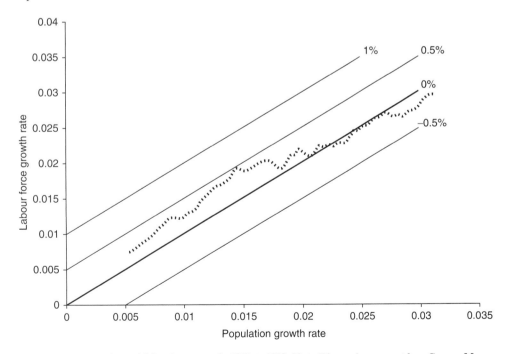

FIGURE 18.1. Population and labor force growth, 1960 to 1990. Note: Diagonals represent l–n. Source: Mason 2001a.

The labor force grows more rapidly than the population during the demographic transition for two reasons—favorable changes in age structure and, in some countries, increased female labor force participation.[4] The age structure effects can be substantial. An increase of 10 points in the percentage of the population in the working ages is not uncommon. The largest swings in the population age structure are found in countries that experience rapid fertility decline, such as those in East Asia. Slow demographic transitions, e.g., those that characterized many European countries and the U.S., produced modest swings. Latin American demographic change produced intermediate swings (Lee, Mason, and Miller 2001a).

Measured patterns of female labor force participation vary widely from region to region, reflecting differences in social, economic, and demographic conditions, differences in culture, but also differences in definition and data collection methods, especially in countries with large agricultural and informal sectors. In the 1960s and 1970s female labor force participation increased very substantially in the industrial market economies. Bloom and Freeman (1987) show, however, that for other major national groupings (low-income and, middle-income developing countries and major regional groupings) female labor force participation grew slowly or declined. In several highly successful East Asian economies rising female labor force participation rates had an important effect on labor force growth (Okunishi 2001).

The second question raised above is whether the demographic dividend automatically leads to more rapid growth in per capita income? Equation (1) is an identity, and there is no doubt that it holds. However, changes in population growth and labor force growth (and related demographic changes) may lead to changes in the growth of output per worker that either offset or reinforce the effects of the demographic dividend.

Analysis of output per worker has been greatly influenced by Solow's article on economic growth (Solow 1956). His neoclassical growth model describes a simple economy in which production is determined by the size of the labor force, the amount of physical capital, e.g., machinery, structure, and roads, and the level of technology. Output per worker can increase for two reasons: because of improvements in technology or because of *capital deepening*—an increase in capital per worker.

Capital deepening occurs because of an increase in the saving rate or a decline in the rate of growth of the labor force.[5] A higher saving rate leads to more investment and an increase in the capital stock relative to the labor force. A decline in labor force growth means that fewer entering workers must be "equipped" each year so that additional capital can be diverted to capital deepening. Solow shows that an increase in the saving rate or a decline in the labor force growth rate leads only to a transitory increase in the rate of capital deepening and the rate of growth of output per worker. Eventually, the economy will stabilize with output per worker growing at the rate of technological change. Output per worker will be on a higher path because of the higher saving rate or slower labor force growth rate, but growing at a rate determined entirely by technological change.

In the neoclassical growth model, long-run growth in output per worker is independent of l or n. In the long run, however, l and n must be equal. Thus, output per worker and output per capita grow at the same rate and neither is influenced by the rate

---

[4] These changes are offset to some extent by reduced labor force participation by school-age children and by older workers.

[5] Solow does not distinguish between the labor force growth rate and the population growth rate in his model.

of population growth or the rate of labor force growth. The short-run is quite a different matter. Throughout the demographic transition changes in l will affect the rate of growth of output per worker. To the extent that the demographic dividend arises because of an increase in l rather than a decline in n, the positive effects of the demographic dividend will be partially offset by negative effects on growth in output per worker. The size of the offset will vary depending on economic structure, the flexibility of labor markets, the extent to which the economy is integrated into the world economy, and a host of other factors.

In the simple neoclassical growth model demographic change also influences growth in output per worker indirectly through two channels—saving and technological change. A potentially important third channel, incorporated into extensions of the neoclassical growth model, is investment in human capital.[6] There are other potentially important demographic effects but most research has focused on innovation, saving, and human capital effects.[7]

INNOVATION.   In the standard neoclassical growth model, innovation is exogenous and typically assumed to raise output per worker by a constant amount each year (in the absence of capital deepening). Endogenous growth models explicitly model the development of new technology (Grossman and Helpman 1991; Lucas 1988; Romer 1990). In these models, the returns to innovation typically increase with the size of the economy. If population, labor force, the capital stock, and other production factors increase by an equal amount, the result is greater innovation and faster economic growth. Endogenous growth models have been the object of considerable attention in recent years, but some central features of these models are inconsistent with important empirical features of economic growth (Jones 1995). Consequently, it remains unclear how new efforts to model technological innovation are likely to influence understanding of the link between population growth and economic growth.

In contrast, the effect of population growth on technological innovation in the agricultural sector is well established. Given fixed technology and a fixed supply of agricultural land, the *law of diminishing returns* implies that an increase in the size of the agricultural labor force will lead to a decline in agricultural output per worker and lower agricultural wages, much in the manner originally hypothesized by Malthus.[8] The theory of induced innovation describes how agricultural practice evolves as population pressure leads to increased scarcity of agricultural land (Boserup 1965, 1981; Hayami 2001; Hayami and Ruttan 1987). In extensive studies of Asian agriculture, Hayami and Ruttan have shown that land scarcity led to the development of new high-yielding seed varieties and more intensive use of fertilizer. Output per hectare increased substantially, even though Asia is densely populated and its land heavily cultivated. Through induced innovation the law of diminishing returns is overturned—or at least weakened.

The success has been more pronounced in Asia than elsewhere. Food output per hectare increased by 2.9% per annum between 1963 and 1993 as compared with increases of 1.9% and 1.7% in Africa and Latin America, respectively, during the

---

[6] Mankiw, Romer, and Weil (1992) extend the model to include education or human capital. In this elaboration an increase in human capital per worker also leads to greater output per worker.

[7] See Kelley and Schmidt (2001) for a discussion of other channels through which population growth may influence economic growth.

[8] See Lee (1973) for a modern presentation of the Malthusian model and an analysis of its applicability to preindustrial England.

same period. Food output per capita achieved annual growth of 1.1% in Asia and 0.4% in Latin America, but declined by 0.2% annually in Africa (Hayami 2001: Table 4.2). Why Asia's agricultural sector adjusted so much more successfully to population growth than Africa's is an interesting issue, which we discuss in broad terms in the section on methodological challenges.

SAVING.   The idea that demographic factors influence saving and investment rates figured prominently in Coale and Hoover's study of Indian economic growth (Coale and Hoover 1958). Tobin (1967) provided an important elaboration on the neoclassical growth model that incorporated the effects of demographic variables on capital and income. Leff (1969) contributed several early, but much criticized, empirical studies. Recent studies are based on one of two models—the variable rate-of-growth model (Mason 1987; 1988) and the Fair and Dominguez (1991) specification.

Stripped to their essential elements, early models hypothesized that population age structure will affect aggregate saving rates because saving varies by age. In the life-cycle model, for example, working-age adults save in anticipation of retirement while the elderly dis-save in order to finance their retirement (Modigliani and Brumberg 1954). The Fair-Dominguez specification is based on the assumption that important variables, including the saving rate, can be described by a fixed age-saving profile. If saving varies by age for any reason, changes in age structure will influence the aggregate saving rate.

The variable rate-of-growth model (Mason 1987, 1988) is a more general formulation in that it considers both changes in the age composition of the population and changes in the age profile of saving that are induced by demographic change or other factors. This leads to a more complex saving model in which demographic factors interact with the rate of economic growth in determining the aggregate saving rate.

Several recent empirical studies have examined the population-saving link. Based on analysis of aggregate saving data, Kelley and Schmidt (1996), Williamson and Higgins (2001), and Toh (2001) conclude that changes in age-structure have had a very large effect on saving rates. Kelley and Schmidt find that the effects are greater in countries with rapidly growing economies as hypothesized by the variable rate-of-growth model, whereas Williamson and Higgins do not find a significant interaction. Deaton and Paxson (2000) employ a different empirical strategy, using household survey data to estimate age profiles of saving and simulating the effect of changing age structure using a variable rate-of-growth specification. They conclude that changes in age structure had an effect on saving rates but one that was more modest than found in studies of aggregate saving. Lee, Mason, and Miller (2000, 2001a, 2001b) simulate both changes in age structure and changes in age-profiles and reach an intermediate conclusion about the possible effects of changes in age structure.

In summary, the most recent evidence supports a link between demography and saving. According to these estimates the demographic dividend has led to higher saving rates. This would have boosted growth in output per worker and reinforced the effect on per capita income of the increase in $l-n$ in equation (1). The magnitude of the effect, however, remains a subject of controversy.

HUMAN CAPITAL.   There is extensive research on the contribution of human capital, education, and health to economic growth and the links to demographic variables. The literature is more diverse than the literature on saving and investment, but the neoclassical growth model can provide a useful conceptual framework. Mankiw, Romer, and Weil (MRW) (1992) take such an approach using secondary school enrollment as a proxy for investment in human capital. They conclude, as have many others, that increased investment in human capital yields high returns. The importance of health to economic development has also been firmly established, most recently by the WHO Commission on Macroeconomics and Health (World Health Organization 2001).

Most economic research on the links between demography and human capital investment are carried out in the fertility decision-making framework discussed in some detail above. In this framework, the number of children and investment in their human capital are jointly determined by changes in income and prices. A decline in the number of children does not *cause* an increase in human capital investment.

Of course, not all changes in childbearing reflect parental choice and, to the extent that unwanted births occur, they will, in the Becker framework, lead to a decline in expenditures per child. In a recent innovative approach Jensen and Ahlburg (2001) analyze the effects of unwanted births on health outcomes. They find that in two relatively low-income countries, the Philippines and Indonesia, where the trade-offs are harsher, unwantedness led to substantial increases in morbidity. In South Korea, where incomes are much higher, no measurable effects were found.

An alternative approach focuses on human capital investment in women of child-bearing age rather than on children. Declining child mortality has reduced the reproductive burden on women, and contraceptive innovations have increased their ability to regulate fertility. As a result of these and other changes, women have increased their participation in the formal labor force, where rewards are more closely linked to education. This has increased the incentives for women to invest more in education. The U.S. experience in this regard is described by Goldin and Katz (2002) in a study highlighted in the "Research Exemplars" section.

There are a number of comprehensive reviews of the literature on the connection between demography and human capital (Ahlburg and Jensen 2001; Kelley 1996; Montgomery and Lloyd 1996).

THE BOTTOM LINE.   Several recent studies have attempted estimates of the demographic dividend—the total contribution to growth in per capita income of changes in demographic factors. Although studies differ in their methodological approaches and in their details, the conclusions reached are broadly consistent. Bloom and Williamson (1998) conclude that demographic change between 1965 and 1990 accounted for about one-third of the growth in per capita income in developing countries. Mason (2001a) concludes that demographic factors accounted for 28% of Taiwan's growth in per capita output between 1965 and 1990. Kelley and Schmidt (2001) conclude that "fertility and mortality changes have each contributed around 22% to changes in output growth between 1965 and 1990. The evidence supports the view that the demographic transition has played an important, positive role in economic development.

METHODOLOGICAL CHALLENGES

An important methodological challenge for research on intergenerational transfers is to develop data and theoretical models that will support a broader and more comprehensive policy debate. Current policy research focuses almost exclusively on public transfers and primarily on public pension reform. The limited scope of the current policy debate is regrettable for two reasons. First, in some countries family support systems are eroding, and other countries may soon face similar trends. Second, familial transfers and public transfers are related—in some respects they are substitutes for each other. Thus, the effect of changes in public transfer policy depends in part on the response of familial transfers. The possibility that public support for the elderly might merely supplant family support has long been appreciated. However, current research efforts are focused almost entirely on family transfers or public policy and not the interaction between the two.

While it may seem unusual to think of family transfer programs as a policy variable, many governments are interested in maintaining and strengthening the family support system. Some countries have pursued explicit policies. Singapore passed the Maintenance of Parents Act in 1996, which established legal responsibilities of adult children for their parents (Singapore 2003). Under these circumstances it is as important to consider the implications of reform to familial support systems as to public support systems.

One of the recurring themes in research on population and development is that the economic, physical, and policy environments condition the effects of population change on economic growth. This was one of the important conclusions reached in the U.S. National Research Council's study of population and development undertaken in the mid-1980s (Johnson and Lee 1987). More recent studies have reinforced this conclusion (Ahlburg, Kelley, and Mason 1996; Bloom, Canning, and Sevilla 2002; Mason 2001b).

These studies show that a broad range of policy variables may *in principle* influence the development effects of population change, but the challenge remains to provide convincing empirical evidence on which set of policies will allow countries to exploit the demographic dividend.

RESEARCH EXEMPLARS

In this section, the major themes and methodological approaches of economic demography are illustrated through a more extensive discussion of two recent studies. The first, by Goldin and Katz (2002), considers how the development of oral contraceptives and the evolution of the U.S. legal system influenced education and marriage decisions by women. The second, by Lee (2000), develops a new method for analyzing intergenerational transfers and employs it to contrast traditional and modern industrial societies.

Claudia Goldin and Laurence F. Katz, "The Power of the Pill: Oral Contraceptives and Women's Career and Marriage Decisions"

Many observers have argued that the development of modern contraceptives, particularly the pill, has had an enormous influence on the lives of women in the U.S. The general point has been made, but there is surprisingly little solid empirical evidence about the effects of the pill—at least in research by economists. The reason in part is the difficulty in analyzing the effects of singular events. There is a before and an after, but the influence of any innovation is not felt immediately. Rather, they diffuse through a society at a pace that may be hindered or abetted by social norms, the legal system, and other institutions. Some groups may respond rapidly to new possibilities, while others may be very resistant to change. The Goldin and Katz (2002) paper is interesting both for its conclusions but also for its approach to such a difficult issue.

Goldin and Katz hypothesize that the development of the contraceptive pill reduced the costs of delaying marriage and pursuing long-duration professional education. This led to a rise in the age at marriage, an increase in premarital sexual activity, and an increase in the proportion of women pursuing advanced degrees and, subsequently, practicing in law, business, medicine, dentistry, and other professions.

The U.S. Food and Drug Administration approved the use of norethynodrel (Enovid) as an oral contraceptive for women in 1960, and its use quickly spread among married women. The use of the pill by single women spread much more slowly, however, because of legal and social impediments regarding the use of contraception by single women, particularly those who were minors. In 1969, the age of majority was 20 or older in 43 of the 50 U.S. states, and in all but a few states contraceptive services could not be provided to minors without parental consent. These laws were not strictly enforced and were sometimes circumvented, but contraceptive services were not readily available to single women. University health services, for example, did not offer contraceptives to all of their students until 1969 and later.

In 1971 the 26th Amendment to the Constitution was ratified, lowering the voting age from 21 to 18. The number of states with an age of majority of 20 or older declined to 32 in 1971 and to only 7 in 1974. In 1974, 27 states allowed women 16 or younger to obtain contraceptive services without parental consent as compared with only three states in 1969. In the view of Goldin and Katz, it was the new technology working in concert with the changing legal and social environment that affected the behavior of young single women.

Goldin and Katz propose a simple marriage model. Suppose the population consists of equal numbers of men and women who are unmarried but can marry either in period 1 or period 2. If woman i marries man j in period 1 the women gets Y_i (from her husband) and the man gets N_j (from his wife). If marriage is delayed until period 2, the gains from marriage for both the husband and wife are augmented by $\alpha_j - \lambda_0$, where α_j is the additional amount obtained if woman j delays marriage and invests in a career. And λ_0 is the cost of the delay. Through the marriage market, men and women choose their partners, the period of marriage, and whether a woman will pursue a career. Any women for whom $\alpha_j - \lambda_0 > 0$ will marry in period 2 and pursue a career. The introduction of the pill reduces the cost of delay from λ_0 to λ_p. This will induce an additional group of women to delay marriage and pursue a career. Given the lower cost of delay, these women will be more attractive marital partners and marry men with higher Y_i. Women for whom $\alpha_j - \lambda_p < 0$ will still choose to marry in the first period and forego a career. However, they will be worse off because their value in the marriage market will be diminished relative to women who choose careers, and hence they will form marital unions with men who have lower Y_i. Thus, the decline in the price of delay will lead to a higher mean age at marriage and an increase in the percentage of women pursuing careers.

Goldin and Katz call this the *direct* effect of the pill but also point to an *indirect* effect. The increase in the number of men and women postponing marriage will thicken the marriage market for those who delay marriage. The amount of information available to potential marital partners will increase, leading to a reduction of marital mismatch.

Goldin and Katz rely on a two-fold empirical strategy. First, they examine the timing of the increases in the age at marriage, premarital sex, and female enrollment in professional programs, showing that rapid increases closely followed changes in the legal environment for the nation as a whole. Second, they use a regression model to estimate the effect of restrictive laws on contraception for minors and abortion in the state of birth at the time that the individual was 18 years of age. They use a differences-in-differences specification by including dummy variables for both state of birth and year of birth. They analyze a 1% sample from the 1980 U.S. Census of women. The analysis is limited to college graduates or in some instances to women who had at least some college.

The results are quite interesting. Depending on the specification used they conclude that "improved access for minors generated a change of 24–37 percent of the 8.7-percentage-point decline" in the percentage married by age 23 that occurred between the 1940s birth cohort and the early 1950s birth cohort (Goldin and Katz 2002: 758). Improved access to the pill also has an important and statistically significant effect on the proportion of women in professional careers. "Improved pill access ... can explain an increase in the share of college women as lawyers and doctors of 1.2 to 1.6 percentage points as compared with an overall increase of 1.7 percentage points from 1970 to 1990" (Goldin and Katz 2002: 762). The development of the contraceptive pill and its increased availability to single women had a large, though not exclusive, effect on age at marriage and career choice of American women.

Ronald D. Lee, "Intergenerational Transfers and the Economic Life Cycle: A Cross-cultural Perspective"

In a series of studies, Lee and several colleagues have developed a conceptual framework for tracking intergenerational transfers at the aggregate level (Lee 1994a, 1994b; Lee and Lapkoff 1988). Lee (2000) uses that framework to analyze how transfers evolve as societies develop. He brings his analysis directly to bear on Caldwell's hypothesis that fertility declines as a consequence of the reversal in the direction of "wealth flows"—from children to parents in high-fertility societies; from parents to children in low-fertility societies.

Lee approaches the analysis and measurement of transfers indirectly. We know that transfers must occur because at some ages people consume much more than they produce. Lee considers an example of a group of Amazon Basin hunter-gather horticulturists who have been extensively studied by Kaplan (1994). Figure 18.2 charts the amount produced and the amount consumed per day, measured in calories, by the average person.

Young children are consuming much more than they are producing. Indeed, they do not begin to produce as much as they consume until they reach 20 years of age. Adults, on the other hand, are producing considerably more than they are consuming. Even those at the oldest ages are in a net surplus position. The differences between consumption and production are made up by transfers from those who are in a surplus position (adults in this case) to those who are in a deficit position (children). Among the Amazon Basin group, transfers are unambiguously in a downward direction, from adults to children.

A cursory examination of Figure 18.2 reveals that the surplus among adults appears to be substantially greater than the deficit among children. Does this mean that the total production is substantially greater than the total consumption? The

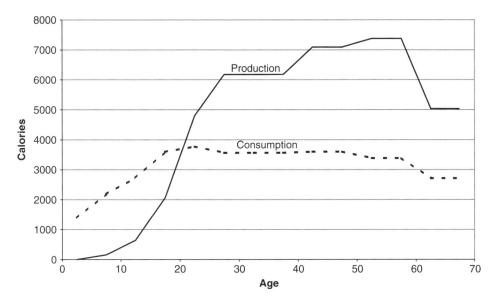

FIGURE 18.2. Interage resource reallocations for Kaplan's horticulturists (pooled). Source: Lee 2000.

answer is no. The values in Figure 18.2 are amounts per person and the age-distribution of the population is heavily weighted toward children. The weighted total consumption was equal to the weighted total of production. In hunter-gather societies there was no saving—people consumed what they produced.

The timing of production and consumption for the society can be summarized by their average ages, the population-weighted averages. For Kaplan's group the average age of consumption was 23.3 years and the average age of production was 34.3. If the average age of consumption is less than the average age of production, then transfers must be in a downward direction (Lee 1994b; Willis 1988).

Is the downward direction of transfers found for Kaplan's horticulturists typical of other traditional groups? What is the pattern for industrialized countries? Lee summarizes the results of other studies as shown in Figure 18.3. In this figure, the tail of the arrow is placed at the mean age of production and the point of the arrow at the mean age of consumption. For every preindustrial society the direction of transfers is strongly downward. For industrial societies the direction of the transfers are upward—from children to parents. The direction of transfers is upward in industrial societies because a large percentage of their populations consist of elderly who, unlike the Amazon horticulturists, are consuming substantially more than they are producing.

Lee finds that transfers reverse direction over the development process, but opposite to the direction hypothesized by Caldwell. In the high-fertility settings net transfers are from parents to children; in the low-fertility settings, from children to parents. As Lee points out, however, it is familial transfers, e.g., direct transfers between children and their parents, that matter in Caldwell's fertility theory. Total transfers include familial transfers and transfers that are effected by the state, e.g., public pensions, public education, and publicly financed health care programs. The decision by a couple to have another child might be influenced by the prospect that the child will provide old-age support to the couple, but it could hardly be influenced by the prospect that the child will pay taxes that fund programs for the elderly.

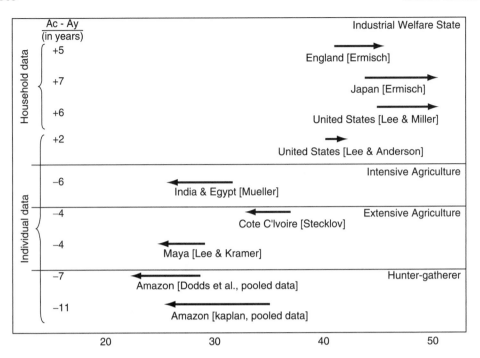

FIGURE 18.3. Summary of interage reallocations in various contexts. Source: Lee 2004.

Lee addresses this issue by separately considering public and familial transfers. In the most traditional settings, of course, all transfers are familial—or perhaps tribal or community-based. In modern Third World countries, public sectors are more developed, but in most countries they are small relative to the size of their economies. In many Latin America countries, the public sectors are larger because of the importance of public pension programs. In any event, however, most transfers are familial transfers and the direction of those transfers is downward, from parent to child.

In industrialized countries, however, public transfers are very large and upward in direction. In the U.S., public transfers for Social Security, Medicare, and Medicaid dominate familial transfers and account for the upward flow of total transfers. Figure 18.4 provides Lee's estimates of familial transfers in the U.S. Interhousehold transfers include bequests and *inter vivos* gifts and transfers. Intrahousehold transfers distinguish spending on higher education from other child costs. For each category Figure 18.4 shows the annual net transfer per household in the case of interhousehold transfers and per child in the case of intrahousehold transfers. The arrows point in the direction of the transfers and extend from the average age of the provider of the transfer to the average age of the recipient of the transfer, where the average ages are dollar weighted. Although total transfers in the U.S. are in the upward direction, familial transfers are in the downward direction. Based on the evidence available to this point, there is no reversal in familial transfers.

FUTURE PROSPECTS

The future of research on population economics will depend, first, on the environment in which research is conducted and, second, on the substantive issues of the day.

A. Interhousehold transfers

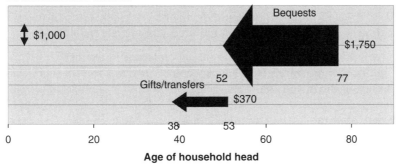

Age of household head

B. Within household transfers (per child)

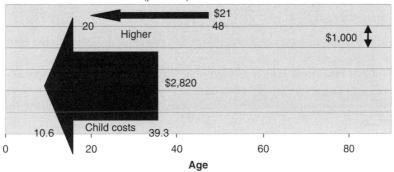

Age

FIGURE 18.4. Familial transfers in the U.S.

Turning first to the research environment, our ability to store, process, and share information is improving with remarkable speed. Many aspects of research are influenced by these developments. The complexity of models used by researchers has increased enormously. Economists are making greater use of microsimulation models and complex macrosimulation models. These approaches are providing a better understanding about heterogeneity and stochastic processes, for example.

Comparative research is facilitated by our ability to process large amounts of data at a low cost and also by the ease with which researchers around the globe can communicate and thus collaborate. The future holds rich possibilities for large, multi-country, collaborative efforts that should increase our understanding of how culture, history, and social and economic institutions condition the connections between economy and demography.

Perhaps the ease with which information is shared has encouraged more multidisciplinary research. If so, the future may hold more fruitful collaboration between economists and sociologists, historians, anthropologists, geographers, and physical scientists.

An important negative development has to do with the acquisition of information. Conducting surveys has become increasingly expensive and difficult in the West. Moreover, the environment for carrying out survey research is becoming increasingly restrictive. At some point in the future, impediments to collecting data may have a great influence on the kinds of research that we conduct.

No doubt the chapters in this volume identify many of the same issues that will be addressed in population research during the coming decades. Each of these issues has economic dimensions. Any short list would no doubt include the following:

1. Low fertility and possibly persistent subreplacement fertility
2. Continued improvements in life expectancy, perhaps to very high levels
3. Decline in the institution of marriage
4. Population aging
5. Population stabilization and decline
6. Recurring health crises
7. Changing reproductive technology
8. Shifting regional patterns

Three questions that are likely to attract more attention in future research on population and economics are:

1. How will developing countries adapt to the rapid and early aging that they are likely to experience?
2. Will the economic effects of aging be different when aging becomes a global rather than a regional phenomenon?
3. Will regional population shifts influence globalization forces over the coming decades?

Compared with western industrialized countries of the world, population aging in Latin America and Asia will be very rapid and occur at relatively low levels of development. How will this influence the ability of these countries to achieve generational equity and some modicum of economic security for the elderly? Perhaps the most important and complex task for these countries is to develop adequate political and economic institutions. Public pension programs are subject to political risk, for example, which in some settings undermines the effectiveness with which they can provide economic security to a growing elderly population. In a similar vein, the development of well-functioning, reliable financial markets is essential if the private sector is to provide a viable alternative to public pension programs. The financial crises in Latin America during the 1980s and in Asia in the 1990s provides ample testament to the fragility of personal wealth. The extended family continues to play a very important role in many countries, but is this a viable and sustainable approach to old-age security?

To this point population aging has been more of a national or regional phenomenon than a global one. The percentage of the world's population 65 and older increased only modestly during the last five decades, from 5.2% in 1950 to 6.9% in 2000. The U.N.'s low variant projection anticipates a much more substantial increase to 18.5% by 2050 (United Nations 2000). To an important extent the effects of aging in the industrialized West have been moderated by the emergence of a well-integrated global economy. The effects of worker shortages in the West, for example, are moderated by shifting production to China, India, and other countries with large working-age populations. But when China and India no longer have large growing workforces, how will their economies and the economies of the West be influenced by global population aging and population decline?

This brings us to the third issue: the relationship between regional population difference and globalization. The second half of the 20th century and the first half of the 21st century have been periods during which regional demographic shifts have been especially large. The More Developed Region's (MDR)[9] share of the world's population will decline from 32.3% in 1950 to 13.7% in 2050 under the U.N.'s low scenario. Equally dramatic are the shifts in age structure. The share of the working-aged population (15 to 64) is projected to rise from 55.0% in 1975 to 66.2% in 2050 in the Less Developed Region (LDR) while declining from 65.1% to 58.3% in the MDRs. How will these regional demographic shifts—and especially shifts in global distribution of the working age population—influence the flow of goods, money, and people across international boundaries? One can easily envision greater globalization and greater interest in the processes of globalization. But as history has shown, the push toward globalization will encounter strong isolationist forces with an outcome that remains uncertain.

[9] The More Developed Region (MDR) is comprised of Europe, North America, Australia/New Zealand, and Japan.

REFERENCES

Ahlburg, D. A., and E. R. Jensen. 2001. Education and the East Asian miracle. In *Population change and economic development in East Asia: Challenges met, opportunities seized*. Edited by A. Mason, 231–255. Palo Alto, Calif.: Stanford University Press.

Ahlburg, D. A., A. C. Kelley, and K. O. Mason. 1996. The impact of population growth on well-being in developing countries. Heidelberg: Springer-Verlag.

Altonji, J. G., F. Hayashi, and L. Kotlikoff. 1992. Is the extended family altruistically linked? Direct evidence using micro data. *American Economic Review* 82(5): 1177–1198.

Altonji, J. G., F. Hayashi, and L. Kotlikoff. 2000. The effects of income and wealth on time and money transfers between parents and children. In *Sharing the wealth: Demographic change and economic transfers between generations*. Edited by A. Mason and G. Tapinos, 306–357. Oxford: Oxford University Press.

Attanasio, O. P., and H. W. Hoynes. 2000. Differential mortality and wealth accumulation. *Journal of Human Resources* 35: 1–29.

Auerbach, A. J., J. Gokhale, and L. J. Kotlikoff. 1991. Generational accounts: A meaningful alternative to deficit accounting. In *Tax policy and the economy*. Edited by D. Bradford. Cambridge, Mass.: MIT Press for the National Bureau of Economic Research.

Auerbach, A. J., and L. J. Kotlikoff. 1987. *Dynamic fiscal policy*. Cambridge, Mass.: Cambridge University Press.

Auerbach, A. J., L. J. Kotlikoff, and W. Leibfritz. 1999. Generational accounting around the world. Chicago: University of Chicago Press.

Barro, R. J. 1974. Are government bonds net worth? *Journal of Political Economy* 82(6): 1095–1117.

Becker, G. S. 1974. A theory of social interactions. *Journal of Political Economy* 82: 1063–1093.

Becker, G. S. 1991. *A treatise on the family, enlarged ed.* Cambridge, Mass.: Harvard University Press.

Becker, G. S. 1993. Nobel lecture: The economic way of looking at behavior. *Journal of Political Economy* 101(3): 385–403.

Becker, G. S., and K. M. Murphy. 1988. The family and the state. *Journal of Law & Economics* XXXI (April):1–18.

Becker, G. S., and N. Tomes. 1976. Child endowments and the quantity and quality of children. *Journal of Political Economy* 84(4 pt. 2): S143–162.

Ben-Porath, Y. 1980. The F-connection: Families, friends, and firms and the organization of exchange. *Population and Development Review* 6(1): 1–30.

Bernheim, B. D., and L. Levin. 1989. Social Security and personal saving: An analysis of expectations. *American Economic Review* 79(2): 97–102.

Blinder, A. S., R. H. Gordon, and D. E. Wise. 1980. Reconsidering the work disincentive effects of social security. *National Tax Journal* 33(December): 431–442.

Bloom, D. E., D. Canning, and J. Sevilla. 2002. *The demographic dividend: A new perspective on the economic consequences of population change*. Santa Monica, Calif.: RAND.

Bloom, D. E., and R. B. Freeman. 1987. Population growth, labor supply, and employment in developing countries. In *Population growth and economic development: Issues and evidence*. Edited by D. G. Johnson and R. D. Lee, 105–147. Madison: The University of Wisconsin Press.

Bloom, D. E., and J. G. Williamson. 1998. Demographic transitions and economic miracles in emerging Asia. *World Bank Economic Review* 12(3): 419–456.

Bommier, A., and R. D. Lee. 2003. Overlapping generations models with realistic demography. *Journal of Population Economics* 16: 135–160.

Boserup, E. 1965. *The conditions of agricultural growth*. Chicago: Aldine.

Boserup, E. 1981. *Population and technological change: A study of long-term trends*. Chicago: University of Chicago Press.

Boucekkine, R., D. de la Croix, and O. Licandro. 2002. Vintage human capital, demographic trends, and endogenous growth. *Journal of Economic Theory* 104: 340–375.

Bravo, Jorge. 2001. Vieillessement de la Population et Systemes de Retraite: L'Amerique Latin dans une Perspective Internationale. *Les Dossier du CEPED* No. 62 (Paris, France, Mai)

Brown, J. R., and S. J. Weisbenner. 2002. Is a bird in hand worth more than a bird in the bush? Intergenerational transfers and savings behavior. *National Bureau of Economic Research (NBER) Working Paper No. w8753*.

Chu, C. Y. C. 2000. Panel study of family dynamics. Taipei, Taiwan: Academia Sinica.

Coale, A., and E. M. Hoover. 1958. *Population growth and economic development in low-income countries: A case study of India*. Princeton, N.J.: Princeton University Press.

Coronado, J. L. 2002. The effects of Social Security privatization on household saving: Evidence from Chile. *Contributions to Economic Analysis & Policy* 1(1): Article 7.

Cox, D. 1987. Motives for private income transfers. *Journal of Political Economy* 95: 508–546.

Cutler, D. M., J. M. Poterba, L. M. Sheiner, and L. H. Summers. 1990. An aging society: Opportunity or challenge? *Brookings Papers on Economic Activity* (1): 1–56.

Deaton, A. S. 1997. *The analysis of household surveys: A microeconometirc approach to development policy*. Baltimore and London: World Bank.

Deaton, A. S., and C. H. Paxson. 2000. Growth, demographic structure, and national saving in Taiwan. *Population and Development Review*. Vol. 26 (Supplement): 141–173.

Dicks-Mireaux, L., and M. A. King. 1984. Pension wealth and household savings: Tests of robustness. *Journal of Public Economics* 23(February/March): 115–139.

East-West Center. 2002. *The future of Asia's population*. Honolulu: East-West Center.

Fair, R. C., and K. M. Dominguez. 1991. Effects of the changing U.S. age distribution on macroeconomic equations. *American Economic Review* 81: 1276–1294.

Feldstein, M. 1974. Social Security, induced retirement, and aggregate capital accumulation. *Journal of Political Economy* 82(5): 905–926.

Feldstein, M. 1996. The missing piece in policy analysis: Social Security reform. *American Economic Review* 86(2): 1–14.

Feldstein, Martin. 1997. Transition to fully Funded Pension System: Five Economic Issues. *National Bureau of Economic Research (NBER) Working Paper No. w6149*.

Feldstein, M., and A. Samwick. 2001. Potential paths of Social Security reform. *NBER Working Paper No. w8592*.

Frankenberg, E., L. A. Lillard, and R. J. Willis. 2002. Patterns of intergenerational transfers in Southeast Asia. *Journal of Marriage and the Family* 64 (August): 627–641.

Gale, W. G. 1998. The effects of pensions on household wealth: A reevaluation of theory and evidence. *Journal of Political Economy* 106(4): 706–723.

Gokhale, J., B. R. Page, and J. R. Sturrock. 1999. Generational accounts for the United States: An update. In *Generational accounting around the world*. Edited by A. J. Auerbach, L. J. Kotlikoff, and W. Leibfritz. Chicago: University of Chicago Press.

Goldin, C., and L. F. Katz. 2002. The power of the pill: Oral contraceptives and women's career and marriage decisions. *Journal of Political Economy* 110: 730–770.

Grossman, G., and E. Helpman. 1991. *Innovation and growth in the global economy*. Cambridge, Mass.: MIT Press.

Gullason, E. T., B. R. Kolluri, and M. J. Panik. 1993. Social Security and household wealth accumulation: Refined microeconometric evidence. *Review of Economics and Statistics* 75(3): 548–551.

Hayami, Y. 2001. Induced innovation and agricultural development in East Asia. In *Population change and economic development in East Asia: Challenges met, opportunities seized*. Edited by A. Mason, 96–120. Palo Alto, Calif.: Stanford University Press.

Hayami, Y., and V. W. Ruttan. 1987. Population growth and agricultural productivity. In *Population growth and economic development: Issues and evidence*. Edited by D. G. Johnson and R. D. Lee. Madison: University of Wisconsin Press.

Hermalin, A. I. 2002. The well-being of the elderly in Asia: A four-country comparative study. Ann Arbor: University of Michigan Press.

Holzmann, R. 1997. Pension reform, financial market development, and economic growth: Preliminary evidence from Chile. *International Monetary Fund Staff Papers* 44(2): 149–178.

Hubbard, R. G. 1986. Pension wealth and individual saving: Some new evidence. *Journal of Money, Credit and Banking* 18(May): 167–178.

Hubbard, R. G., and K. L. Judd. 1987. Social Security and individual welfare: Precautionary saving, borrowing constraints, and the payroll tax. *American Economic Review* 77(4): 630–646.

Jensen, E. R., and D. A. Ahlburg. 2001. Child health and health care in Indonesia and the Philippines. In *Population change and economic development in East Asia: Challenges met, opportunities seized*, Edited by A. Mason, 255–279. Palo Alto, Calif.: Stanford University Press.

Johnson, D. G., and R. D. Lee. 1987. Population growth and economic development: Issues and evidence. In *Social Demography Series*. Madison: University of Wisconsin Press.

Jones, C. I. 1995. Time series tests of endogenous growth models. *The Quarterly Journal of Economics* 110(2): 495–525.

Kaplan, H. 1994. Evolutionary and wealth flows theories of fertility: Empirical tests and new models. *Population and Development Review* 20(4): 753–791.

Kelley, A. C. 1996. The consequences of rapid population growth on human resource development: The case of education. In *The impact of population growth on well-being in developing countries*. Edited by D. A. Ahlburg, A. C. Kelley, and K. O. Mason, 67–138. Heidelberg: Springer-Verlag.

Kelley, A. C., and R. M. Schmidt. 1996. Saving, dependency and development. *Journal of Population Economics* 9(4): 365–386.

Kelley, A. C., and R. M. Schmidt. 2001. Economic and demographic change: A synthesis of models, findings, and perspectives. In *Population matters: Demographic change, economic growth, and poverty in the developing world*. Edited by N. Birdsall, A. C. Kelley, and S. W. Sinding, 67–105. Oxford: Oxford University Press.

King, M. A., and L. Dicks-Mireaux. 1982. Asset holdings and the life cycle. *Economic Journal* 92: 247–267.

Kinsella, K. 1990. Living arrangements of the elderly and social policy: A cross-national perspective. In *US Census Bureau/CIR Staff Paper No. 52*. Washington, D. C.

Kinsella, K., and V. A. Velkoff. 2001. An aging world: 2001, international population reports. Washington, D. C.: U.S. Census Bureau.

Kotlikoff, L. J., and A. Spivak. 1981. The family as an incomplete annuities market. *Journal of Political Economy* 89(2): 372–391.

Krueger, D., and F. Kubler. 2002. Pareto improving Social Security reform when financial markets are incomplete? *National Bureau of Economic Research* (*NBER*) *Working Paper No.* w9410.

Lazear, E. P., and R. T. Michael. 1988. *Allocation of income within the household*. Chicago and London: University of Chicago Press.

Lee, R. D. 1973. Population in preindustrial England: An econometric analysis. *Quarterly Journal of Economics* 87(4): 581–607.

Lee, R. D. 1994a. The formal demography of population aging, transfers, and the economic life cycle. In *Demography of aging*. Edited by L. G. Martin and S. H. Preston, 8–49. Washington, D. C.: National Academy Press.

Lee, R. D. 1994b. Population age structure, intergenerational transfer, and wealth: A new approach, with applications to the United States. *Journal of Human Resources* 29(4): 1027–1063.

Lee, R. D. 2000. Intergenerational transfers and the economic life cycle: A cross-cultural perspective. In *Sharing the wealth: Demographic change and economic transfers between generations*, Edited by A. Mason and G. Tapinos, 17–56. Oxford: Oxford University Press.

Lee, R. D., and S. Lapkoff. 1988. Intergenerational flows of time and goods; Consequences of slowing population growth. *Journal of Political Economy* 96(3): 618–651.

Lee, R., A. Mason, and T. Miller. 2000. Life cycle saving and the demographic transition in East Asia. *Population and Development Review* 26: 194–219.

Lee, R. D., A. Mason, and T. Miller. 2001a. Saving, wealth, and population. In *Population does matter: Demography, poverty, and economic growth*. Edited by N. Birdsall, A. C. Kelley, and S. W. Sinding, 137–164. Oxford: Oxford University Press.

Lee, R. D., A. Mason, and T. Miller. 2001b. Saving, wealth, and the demographic transition in East Asia. In *Population change and economic development in East Asia: Challenges met, opportunities seized*. Edited by A. Mason, 155–184. Palo Alto, Calif.: Stanford University Press.

Lee, R., A. Mason, and T. Miller. 2003. From transfers to individual responsibility: Implications for savings and capital accumulation in Taiwan and the United States. *Scandinavian Journal of Economics* 105(3):339–357.

Lee, Y.-J., W. L. Parish, and R. J. Willis. 1994. Sons, daughters, and intergenerational support in Taiwan. *American Journal of Sociology* 99(4): 1010–1041.

Leff, N. H. 1969. Dependency rates and savings rates. *American Economic Review* 59(December): 886–895.

Leimer, D. R., and S. Lesnoy. 1982. Social Security and private saving: New time series evidence. *Journal of Political Economy* 90(3): 606–629.

Leimer, D. R., and D. H. Richardson. 1992. Social Security, uncertainty adjustments and the consumption decision. *Economica* 59(235): 311–335.

Lillard, L. A., and R. J. Willis. 1997. Motives for intergenerational transfers: Evidence from Malaysia. *Demography* 34(1): 115–134.

Lucas, R. E. 1988. On the mechanics of economic development. *Journal of Monetary Economics* 22: 3–42.

Mankiw, G., D. Romer, and D. Weil. 1992. A contribution to the empirics of economic growth. *Quarterly Journal of Economics* 107(2): 407–437.

Mason, A. 1987. National saving rates and population growth: A new model and new evidence. In *Population growth and economic development: Issues and evidence*. Edited by D. G. Johnson and R. D. Lee, 523–560. Social Demography Series, Madison: University of Wisconsin Press.

Mason, A. 1988. Saving, economic growth, and demographic change. *Population and Development Review* 14(1): 113–144.

Mason, A. 2001a. Population, capital, and labor. In *Population change and economic development in East Asia: Challenges met, opportunities seized*. Edited by A. Mason, 207–228. Palo Alto, Calif.: Stanford University Press.

Mason, A. 2001b. *Population change and economic development in East Asia: Challenges met, opportunities seized*. Palo Alto, Calif.: Stanford University Press.

McGarry, K., and R. Schoeni. 1997. Transfer behavior within the family: Results from the asset and health dynamics (AHEAD) study. *Journals of Gerontology Series B: Psychological and Social Sciences* 52B (special issue): 82–92.

Modigliani, F., and R. Brumberg. 1954. Utility analysis and the consumption function: An interpretation of cross-section data. In *Post-Keynesian economics*. Edited by K. K. Kurihara. New Brunswick, N. J.: Rutgers University Press.

Montgomery, M. R., and C. B. Lloyd. 1996. Fertility and maternal and child health. In *The impact of population growth on well-being in developing countries*. Edited by D. A. Ahlburg, A. C. Kelley, and K. O. Mason, 37–66. Heidelberg: Springer-Verlag.

Munnell, A. H. 1974. *The effect of Social Security on personal savings*. Cambridge, Mass.: Ballinger.

Okunishi, Y. 2001. Change labor forces and labor markets in Asia's miracle economies. In *Population change and economic development in East Asia: Challenges met, opportunities seized*. Edited by A. Mason, 300–331. Palo Alto, Calif.: Stanford University Press.

Poterba, J. 2000. The estate tax and after-tax investment returns. In *Does Atlas shrug? The economic consequences of taxing the rich*. Edited by J. Slemrod, 333–353. Cambridge, Mass.: Harvard University Press.

Poterba, J., and S. J. Weisbenner. 2001. The distributional burden of taxing estates and unrealized capital gains at the time of death. In *Rethinking estate and gift taxation*. Edited by W. G. Gale and J. Slemrod. Washington, D.C.: Brookings Institution.

Preston, S. H. 1984. Children and the elderly: Divergent paths for America's dependents. *Demography* 21(4): 435–457.

Razin, A., E. Sadka, and P. Swagel. 2002. The aging population and the size of the welfare state. *Journal of Political Economy* 110(4): 900–918.

Romer, D. 1990. Endogenous technological change. *Journal of Political Economy* 98: S71–S103.

Rosenzweig, M. R., and O. Stark. 1997. Handbook of population and family economics. In *Handbooks in economics*. Edited by K. J. Arrow and M. D. Intriligator Amsterdam: Elsevier.

Ruggles, S. 1994. The transformation of American family structure. *American Historical Review* 99(1): 103–128.

Samuelson, P. 1958. An exact consumption loan model of interest with or without the social contrivance of money. *Journal of Political Economy* 66: 467–482.

Singapore, A.-G.s.C. 2003. Singapore statutes online.

Solow, R. M. 1956. A contribution to the theory of economic growth. *Quarterly Journal of Economics* 70(1): 65–94.

Spengler, J. J. 1959. Economics and demography. In *The study of population: An inventory and appraisal*. Edited by P. M. Hauser and O. D. Duncan, 791–831. Chicago: The University of Chicago Press.

Takayama, N., Y. Kitamura, and H. Yoshida. 1999. Generational accounting in Japan. In *Generational accounting around the world*. Edited by A. J. Auerbach, L. J. Kotlikoff, and W. Leibfritz. Chicago: University of Chicago Press.

Tobin, J. 1967. Life cycle saving and balanced economic growth. In *Ten economic studies in the tradition of Irving Fisher*. Edited by W. Fellner, 231–256. New York: Wiley.

Toh, M. H. 2001. Savings, capital formation, and economic growth in Singapore. In *Population change and economic development in East Asia: Challenges met, opportunities seized*. Edited by A. Mason, 185–208. Palo Alto, Calif.: Stanford University Press.

United Nations. 2000. *World population prospects: The 2000 revision*. New York: United Nations.

Williamson, J. G., and M. Higgins. 2001. The accumulation and demography connection in East Asia. In *Population change and economic development in East Asia: Challenges met, opportunitites seized*. Edited by A. Mason, 123–154. Palo Alto, Calif.: Stanford University Press.

Willis, R. J. 1980. The old age security hypothesis and population growth. In *Demographic behavior: Interdisciplinary perspectives on decision-making*. Edited by T. Burch, 43–69. Boulder, Colo.: Westview Press.

Willis, R. J. 1988. Life cycles, institutions and population growth: A theory of the equilibrium interest rate in an overlapping-generations model. In *Economics of changing age distributions in developed countries*. Edited by R. D. Lee, W. B. Arthur, and G. Rodgers. Oxford: Oxford University Press.

World Health Organization, C.o.M.a.H. 2001. *Macroeconomics and health: Investing in health for economic development*. Geneva: World Health Organization.

CHAPTER 19

Historical Demography

ETIENNE VAN DE WALLE

The Study of Population: An Inventory and Appraisal (Hauser and Duncan 1959) included no chapter on "History and Demography," mostly, the editors claimed, because of "limitations of space." Their description of the discipline, however, pointed to its grave weaknesses at the time:

> To the demographer it may often seem that the historian's use of censuses and like sources is somewhat casual, which is perhaps because the historian's problems so often pertain to periods for which data coming up to standards of modern demography are wholly or partly lacking. There is a specialized sub-discipline of "historical demography" or "demographic history" whose practitioners work in periods antedating modern censuses and registration systems. Here they attempt to derive population estimates from whatever symptomatic data may be available. This is an exacting field of historiography which requires the combined skills of the expert in documentary criticism and the statistician. Significantly, it has been cultivated to a much greater extent by Europeans than by Americans. No doubt a good many American demographers share the following opinion of studies in historical demography: 'the possibilities of determining the size and characteristics of past populations with a sufficient degree of accuracy so as to make the data demographically very useful are small. ... The exact relationship of such summaries to population problems in the modern world would not appear very close' (50–51).

Hauser and Duncan were writing in 1959, at a watershed in the development of the discipline. In the chapter of the volume devoted to "Demography in France," Alfred Sauvy mentioned the name of Louis Henry several times, but never in the context of historical research, although Henry's path-breaking study of Genevan genealogies had been published in 1956. In 1956 Henry had produced, together with archivist Michel Fleury, a manual on the analysis of parish registers, and in 1958, with Etienne Gautier, a study of the parish of Crulai that would constitute the archetype of all subsequent parish monographs. Also in 1958, he laid down a plan to study a representative sample of rural parishes of France using nonnominal data. Thus, at the very time when *The Study of Population* was published, the field was being radically transformed, and two powerful new techniques of analysis had been presented: family reconstitution and the seeds of what would later be called population reconstruction, the aggregate analysis of parish records over time to reconstitute the age and sex distribution of the population.

CONCEPTUAL FRAMEWORKS

It is clear that whatever the worth of Hauser and Duncan's indictment of historical demography as they knew it, it did not characterize Henry's work. His main source of data consisted of parish records, not censuses, and he was acutely aware of the problems of data quality and bias. Moreover, he was a demographer using historical materials for whatever "useful" demographic information they could give; one example was the investigation of biological fertility, in the absence of the disturbing influence of contraceptive intervention that characterized contemporary high-quality sources of information on reproductive behavior. He was probably less interested in history than in the measurements of demographic variables that could be studied neither in the low-fertility and low-mortality populations of the western world, nor with the unreliable statistics of the less developed countries. As Henry put it, he wanted to "mine the past" for data that could not be obtained elsewhere. Ascertaining population size was not the primary objective of his investigations, nor were his goals the conventional measurements of mainstream demography: birth and death rates, life tables, distributions of the population by age and sex. His approach was based on individual observations treated in a cohort perspective, at a time when demography was dominated by the use of aggregate data at a period level. He proposed a method to use data on vital events to compute rates in the absence of an enumeration of the underlying population, in contrast with standard demographic techniques that combine lists of events and lists of people. The specific nature of his sources allowed him to study topics that had been barely broached before him, such as the proximate determinants of fertility and the components of the birth interval (Henry 1970).

Thus, historical demography was initially a technical discipline aiming at extracting measurements from archival sources consisting mostly of parish records of marriages and vital events in the past with the help of a toolbox of rigorous methods. The field has expanded vastly since then, both in the sources and in its focus on substantive topics. T. H. Hollingsworth (1969) has suggested that the use of the adjective in "historical demography" implies that it is an auxiliary science of history, a methodology to gather historical facts; whereas the history of population is not dependent on sophisticated techniques but can use a variety of approaches, such as induction from general principles, archeological evidence, or the consultation of contemporary authors. This distinction between historical demography and the history of population corresponds to the old distinction made by Hauser and Duncan between demography and population studies, and it is increasingly abandoned as artificial. Deaths, marriages, and births are social events of profound importance, and it is only artificially that they can be separated from their historical context. The same authors write on the two aspects of population in the same journals, and a combination of techniques and substance makes for the best research. The distinction will not be used in this chapter, where we will review some of the substantive focuses of studies on the determinants and consequences of population trends in the past. Perhaps more than in any other part of demography, however, the nature and the content of the available historical sources determine the type of studies that can be conducted. It is a data-based discipline, not one concerned primarily about issues. Hauser and Duncan's remark that the specialty remained a specialty of European researchers (that is, students of European history) remains true because of the depth of the European sources, although Japanese and Chinese sources are now making inroads into this monopoly.

The *Multilingual Demographic Dictionary* (IUSSP 1981) defines historical demography simply by its focus on populations of the past for which there are written sources. It excludes paleodemography, the study of nonwritten sources (e.g., skeletal remains) to investigate the preliterate past. It does not define "the past"; the time when it ends and the present commences is left to the decision of the researcher. A historical perspective is by definition comparative, and a comparison with the present facilitates the understanding of the past. To an extent that was greatly underestimated by Hauser and Duncan, the historical record is serving as a vast library of the human experience over time, a data bank to which new techniques are applied as they are developed, and a growing store of comparative material in which hypotheses on human behavior can be tested. Historical demography has ceased to be a toolbox of arcane techniques.

And yet its relation to history has remained a marginal one. Its focus is not on great men and important events, but on the obscure men and women of rural parishes whose "events" of record were baptisms, marriages, and burials, or on the mass of people enumerated in censuses with a few characteristics fitting predetermined broad categories. Because of its concentration on individual biographies and legal documents, traditional historiography had only skimmed the surface of a larger sociological reality. Even reputable historians shared some myths about the family characteristics of the past that historical demography helped to debunk. For example, it was commonly believed that the peasant populations of Europe lived in large extended family households, that women of the people had very large families, and that marriage occurred at a very young age. The study of documents from the past exposed these notions as stereotypes. The types of problems the new demographic historians have considered are illustrated by the titles of some of these articles or book chapters: "Did the Peasants Really Starve?" (Laslett 1965); "Did the Mothers Really Die?" (Schofield 1986). These are important questions, but hardly ones that traditional historians could have answered.

Historical demography has hugely contributed to a better understanding of underlying structures and tendencies over the long run. Because of that focus, it fit well in what became an important school of historians in the post–World War II period—the French *Annales* school and its followers all over the world. The new history of population was "serial" history, as opposed to "evential" history. To the extent that population structure and change influence economy and society, they have provided an indispensable backcloth for the description of the human past. The lasting impact of demography on history, after the initial excitement with technical innovations such as family reconstitution, has been in providing a window on the social structure of the past and on the dynamics of economic growth, urbanization, and consumption patterns. In turn, specialized areas of history, such as the history of technology, of disease, and of contraception, have proven indispensable for an understanding of the proximate determinants of population change.

METHODOLOGICAL CHALLENGES: THE
SOURCES AND THE TECHNIQUES

Family Reconstitution on the Basis of Nominal Records of Vital Events

Parish records had been used by historians and by demographers before Louis Henry. His essential contribution consisted in setting rules for determining, in the absence of direct information, the size and structure of the population "under observation"—e.g., a population exposed to particular risks such as marital fertility or infant and child mortality. The method consisted of reconstituting families (in the narrow sense of couples and their offspring) by linking nominal records over time. The Henry model was very widely accepted by others, both in France and abroad, and family reconstitution became the main technique used for investigating populations of the past. By 1980, there had been more than 500 parish monographs in France, most of them by students in university departments of history. Henry himself and his team reconstituted a large number of families in some 40 parishes as a nominal complement to his sample of nonnominal data; unfortunately, the results for the four "quadrants" of France were published separately in different journals (Henry 1972, 1978; Henry and Houdaille 1973; Houdaille 1976; for a recent description of the study and its methodology, see Séguy 2001). The earliest registers used in the reconstitutions go back to 1670. The availability and quality of the data decrease before the former date, but there have been attempts to extend family reconstitution in some parishes to earlier in the 17th or even the 16th century (Séguy 1999). Jean-Pierre Bardet (1983) attempted the study of a medium-sized city, Rouen, during the 17th and 18th centuries.

Family reconstitution was diffused outside of France. Jacques Charbonneau, a historian who had reconstituted families in a large parish of Normandy, Tourouvre-au-Perche, that was the place of origin of a large contingent of settlers in Canada, joined forces with demographer Jacques Légaré to attempt the complete reconstruction of the French population of Canada from its 17th-century beginnings (Charbonneau et al. 1993). In view of the large number of records to be linked, this project made use of automated computer methods, using a phonetic code of names. In England, E. A. Wrigley applied the Henry method of family reconstitution wholesale on a village of Devon, Colyton (Wrigley 1966). Wrigley and his colleagues (1997) would eventually publish the results of family reconstitution on a sample of 26 Anglican parishes. There are examples of the use of family reconstitution in parishes of other countries, such as Italy, Spain, Switzerland, and the lower countries; a few attempts have been made in the United States (Temkin-Greener and Swedlund 1978; Byers 1982; Logue 1985).

The family reconstitution method is labor-intensive and time-consuming. Before the era of computers, it relied on hand tabulation of individual records painstakingly copied on cards of different colors. Significant time could be gained by making use of already reconstituted families in the form of genealogies or population registers. Jacques Henripin (1954) had pioneered the use of genealogies in a study of Canada at the beginning of the 18th century, and Henry used them for his Genevan study. With Claude Lévy, he also analyzed the Dukes and Peers of France, showing that they had started to practice family limitation, like the Geneva bourgeoisie, in the 17th century (Lévy and Henry 1960). Jacques Houdaille (1988, 1989) used genealogies of the French lower nobility and bourgeoisie to document the progression of family limitation from higher to lower social classes. Similar studies were conducted among the ruling classes in Italian cities (see Livi-Bacci 1986), where the decline of fertility was also comparatively early. On the other hand, T. H. Hollingsworth's (1964) study of the English peerage showed little or no decline of fertility before the 19th century. John Knodel (1988) studied a large sample of village genealogies (*Ortsippenbücher*) in Germany.

There have been some attempts at family reconstitution in the U.S. using genealogies (Kantrow 1980). By far the largest American study (Bean, Mineau, and Anderton 1990) makes use of the nominative records collected and maintained by the Genealogical Society of Utah and supported by the Mormon Church. It uses family group sheets that list at least one member who was born or died in Utah or on the pioneer trail to that state. Genealogies, because of their roots in the study of cross-generational relationships, lend themselves to other uses, such as genetic investigations or the study of extended kinship networks. The historical genealogies of the Utah project are extended into the present through links with contemporary sources and used for epidemiological studies (Skolnick 1980). Post and associates (1997) have studied changes in the numbers of living parents and grandparents, siblings, aunts and uncles, and nephews and nieces in the Netherlands between 1830 and 1990.

Outside of Europe, Ts'ui-jung Liu initiated the study of Chinese genealogies. Seventeenth- and 18th-century Chinese data of good quality have been studied for the Qing imperial lineage from 1644 to 1911 (Liu, Lee, Reher, and Wang 2001). These sources focus on atypical, elite populations, and most often they provide no information on females or on deaths at the early ages. On the other hand, they have the potential to go back in time well beyond the periods covered in Europe. The published genealogy of the Wang clan has been used to investigate male mortality above age 20 over more than 1,500 years, suggesting that throughout the period mortality was very stable at levels close to those of the British peerage born in the second quarter of the 18th century (Zhao 1997).

The population register provides another source of data that uses already reconstituted families. Population registers consist of continuous sets of records that regularly update an initial census through the registration of additions and attritions (births, deaths, moves) to the population as they occur. They have the advantage of providing information on the structure of the population, while family reconstitution infers the denominator of rates by assuming the presence of certain persons in the parish studied. The Swedish population Registers started in 1749 and have been intensively analyzed by Swedish scholars (see, for example, Akerman 1973; Bengtsson, Fridlizius, and Ohlsson. 1981). They contain information on causes of death, including smallpox, since 1749 and, after vaccination became compulsory in 1816, "on whether an individual had been inoculated, vaccinated, previously been infected by smallpox, or had been neither infected nor treated by any preventive method" (Sköld 1996: 248). The Belgian population registers have existed since 1846; those of Verviers, a medium-sized industrial city, have been analyzed by George Alter (1988). Akira Hayami (1979) launched the study of the *shūmon aratame-chō* (religious faith investigation registers), the Japanese population registers. There are also household registration records in China that lend themselves to the study of peasant populations in the 18th and 19th centuries (Lee and Campbell 1997). The Japanese established population registers in Taiwan in 1905 (Wolf and Huang 1980).

Parish Records Used Aggregatively

Church records have been a perennial source of information for historians well before their statistical analysis was perfected, and there are many monographs that rely partly on them (for example, Demos 1971). Other historians have long used parish registers to compile the number of marriages, baptisms, and burials over time and to draw conclusions, based on their frequencies, on such subjects as the seasonality of events or the ratio of births to marriages as a rough indicator of fertility. The approach has been especially important in the study of mortality. The requirement of completeness and accuracy of the data are much less stringent than for family reconstitutions, since they do not have to be linked over time. Even incomplete records of deaths over time provide a reliable indication of the existence of food crises and the visit of epidemics.

Defective and incomplete parish registers can provide usable information for parts of the world where statistical data are scarce, for example, in Russia (Hoch 1998), Latin America (McCaa 2000), and even Africa (Notkola, Timaeus, and Siiskonen 2000). Studies at the local level have yielded long series of yearly or even monthly numbers of deaths with a sawtooth pattern of peaks well above the background level of mortality, corresponding to the existence of mortality crises of various kinds (for a European example, see Wrightson and Levin 1989). Such series have been compared over time for national and international aggregates (Appleby 1979; Livi-Bacci 1991; Post 1985). The seasonal pattern of death can throw light on the nature of epidemics. For example, the bubonic plague is a disease of the warmer parts of the year, as its vectors, the black rat and its flea, have originated in a subtropical region of Asia. Similarly, the age and sex of the deceased can provide interesting information on the patterns of mortality. Potential studies are not limited to Christian registers: Ann Bowman Jannetta (1987) has used Buddhist temple death registers in Japan to study epidemics and mortality between 1771 and 1852. These documents include information on the epidemic causes of death, particularly on smallpox and measles.

Parish records typically contain some information on the characteristics of the persons involved. Many parish monographs make use of this information as a complement to the results obtained from family reconstitution or from other sources on the structural characteristics of the population. Mention of the marital status of the mother of newborn children in a sample of ecclesiastical records provided the raw materials for the study of bastardy and illegitimacy in England (Laslett, Oosterveen, and Smith 1980). Marriage acts are especially informative, because they yield information of the survival of the parents of the bride and groom, the ability of the new couple and the witnesses to sign their name, and their occupations. Henry designed a representative sample of rural French parishes and proceeded to extract systematically all the available information on the parish records in an aggregative, nonnominal fashion. What is often called "the Louis Henry survey" covered France during the period between 1670 and 1829. One objective was the analysis of aggregate information on the population. This resulted in articles on such subjects as religious practice, the seasonality of conceptions, literacy, and illegitimacy. (See Séguy 2001: 77 for bibliographic references.) The main objective of the compilation, however, was the reconstruction of the 18th century by age and sex and the production of life tables on this basis (Blayo 1975). Jean-Noel Biraben has launched a similar study for an earlier period extending back to 1500 (Séguy 1999).

Henry's reconstruction of the population of France before the era of censuses was an early example of the method of back projection. Wrigley and Schofield (1981) adopted the method in order to reconstruct the population of England from 1541 to 1871 and to compute standard measures (for example, on the mortality of adults). Noël Bonneuil (1997) reconstructed the population of France by departments by combining backward projection from 1906 to 1856 with forward projection from 1806 to 1856. A project to reconstruct the population of Italy is in progress at the University of Bologna. Back projection is one example of a series of approaches that use the balance equation to estimate the values of lines and surfaces in the Lexis diagram. By relying on known values (for example, the age distribution at a certain date and the deaths by age in each year before the censuses) and making certain assumptions (for example, on the size of migration), it is possible to estimate other population values, such as the age distribution at earlier dates and the initial size of each birth cohort. A series of variants on this idea are described in Reher and Schofield (1993); the volume also includes a review by Ronald Lee expressing skepticism about the results of these efforts. Coale and Zelnick (1963) had used the same general principle to estimate the fertility of the white population of the United States, while also correcting successive censuses for underenumeration.

In a special chapter of Wrigley and Schofield's book, Lee (1981) used serial analysis to examine the relation between the long-term series of marriages, births, and deaths in the sample of parishes and wheat prices and meteorological data for England. Patrick Galloway (1988) applied the method to various preindustrial populations of Europe, and David Reher and Alberto Sanz-Gimeno (2000) to a combination of parish register and vital registration data in the 19th century. In a recent extension of this technique, Scott and Duncan (1998) have attempted to use time-series analysis of yearly data to explore the relation between local series of baptisms and burials on the one hand and national wheat prices and records of weather conditions for Britain on the other.

Microdata from Censuses

It was inevitable that the other principal source of demographic data, the census, be also analyzed anew on the basis of the nominal census lists remaining from the past. The individual data from some enumerations of past times have been made available for the first time. In other instances, the nominal lists on which the census had been taken have been processed again with electronic equipment and new analyses have been made with modern methods. Censuses provide information on the population structure, and when one exists for a hitherto unstudied locale, it may shed a great deal of light on the social conditions that prevailed. Censuses have been taken for taxation purposes since the highest antiquity—for example, under the Roman and Chinese empires—but in most instances only population totals have been reported, and most census listings have been lost. There is at least one remarkable exception: the dry sands of the Egyptian desert have preserved census returns on papyrus for some 300 households comprising close to 1,100 individuals, listed by name with mention of their age, relationship, and marital status. This provides one of the only pieces of detailed written quantitative evidence in the distant past (Bagnall and Frier 1994).

The *catasto* (land survey) of the city of Florence and the Tuscan countryside in 1427 provides the most remarkable example of a large enumeration of the past being opened up for research by the computer (Herlihy and Klapisch-Zuber 1985). It was taken for taxation purposes and constitutes the oldest surviving enumeration involving a full age and sex distribution of a large population. It contains a great deal of information about the wealth and occupations of household members during the Quattrocento, an important period of Italian history, and as such is of primary value to the social historian as well as the demographer. Of particular interest to the latter is the marital status distribution of the population, characterized by large age differences between the spouses. Florentine men married much younger women at a late age, and the remarriage of widows was uncommon: a pattern of nuptiality distinctly different from the western European one, but probably not unlike the pattern characteristic of Roman antiquity.

A great many nominal lists of inhabitants have been used, either in combination with parish records in family reconstitution studies, or for what they have to tell by themselves on the structure of the population (see, for example, Peter Laslett's [1977] seminal essay on Clayworth and Cogenhoe). A series of local enumerations in villages and cities has been analyzed for a particular purpose—the investigation of household structure in the past. Laslett has proposed a methodology to analyze census data and a typology of household forms that has been used in a wide variety of European and non-European contexts to explore patterns of residence (Laslett and Wall 1972; Wall, Robin, and Laslett 1983).

In the United States, the study of historical censuses has been facilitated by the systematic conservation of census lists; this is an area where American historical demography is in the forefront of data collection and analysis. In addition to the decennial censuses taken since 1790, a sizable number of colonial censuses have been preserved in manuscript form (Wells 1975), as well as state censuses of the 19th century. There has been a systematic effort to produce public use samples of all the federal censuses from 1880 to the present (Ruggles 1993). The interest in microdata from censuses stems in part from the development of methods that did not exist at the time the information was collected and processed. Equally important, perhaps, in the eyes of social historians is the creation of historical series of comparable data where the evolution of social phenomena and trends can be followed through time. This requires a return to primary records whose importance had not been appreciated at the time of data collection, and that had never been fully tabulated. Thus, the public use samples extracted from the censuses of 1900 and 1910 have been the object of sophisticated analyses of the occupational and ethnic composition of the population (Watkins 1994). The questions on children ever born and surviving have been used to probe the infant and child mortality at a particularly important moment in the mortality transition by using methods developed by William Brass to investigate the mortality of African countries with incomplete statistics at the aggregate level and by combining them with multivariate analysis at the individual level (Preston and Haines 1991). The development of multivariate techniques designed to analyze large amounts of complex information at the individual level has created a demand for this kind of source material.

Aggregate Analysis of Censuses

Published historical census data at the aggregate level have been used extensively either alone, or in combination with vital registration, to trace the evolution of vital trends or the changes in some structural characteristics of the population. Many 19th-century western censuses have standards of quality and completeness that have not yet been reached today in some countries of the developing world. The British Fertility Census of 1911 has provided the raw material for too large a number of studies to be listed here (a partial listing is given in Anderson 1998). The 1911 census included a series of questions that allowed the publication of a large number of tables showing the number of children born to women by age at the time of the census, by date of marriage, and by duration of marriage. This information has allowed the analysis of fertility trends during a particularly important phase of the fertility transition—by class, occupation, and rural/urban residence—for England, Wales, Scotland, and Ireland. Other national censuses of the 20th century contain less complete information on fertility, typically only the number of children ever born per woman. Several historical studies of fertility in the United States in the 19th century, when vital registration was not yet developed for the whole country, have used child/women ratios (for a review of this work, see Haines and Steckel 2000).

Most studies using aggregate census data for the 19th century, however, combine them with vital registration data that become standard parts of the statistical output of European nations. Most published censuses provide tabulations of the population by sex and marital status at least since midcentury, but vital registration rarely provides a detailed tabulation of birth by age and marital status of their mother. A large study designed by Ansley J. Coale to investigate the fertility transition in Europe at the subnational level (widely known as the Princeton European project) used indirect standardization to compute indices of overall, marital, and illegitimate fertility and of the proportion married to disentangle the effect of marital status from that of fertility control by other means. The index of marital fertility I_g, for example, relates the number of legitimate births registered in the years surrounding a census to the computed number that the married women enumerated in the census would have had if they had experienced the marital fertility of a high fertility standard population, the Hutterites of the early 20th century. The index of the proportion married I_m is weighted by the same fertility pattern, and total fertility I_f would be equal to the product of I_m and I_g but for the usually small effect of illegitimate fertility, I_h. These properties have led to the use of the Princeton indices well beyond the specific national studies executed under the project for Belgium (Lesthaeghe 1977), France (van de Walle 1974), Germany (Knodel 1974), Great Britain (Teitelbaum 1984), Italy (Livi-Bacci 1977), Portugal (Livi-Bacci 1971), Spain (Livi-Bacci 1968), and Russia (Coale, Anderson, and Härm (1974). Coale and Watkins (1986) summarized the results of the project. Other studies of the fertility decline in countries not covered by the Princeton project, but using the same methodology, have been published. There are also projects that use other fertility indices computed from vital registration, as for example studies by Patrice Galloway, Eugene Hammel, and Ronald Lee (1994) on Prussia and by J. Brown and T. Guinnane (2002) on Bavaria.

The combined use of previous national censuses and vital registration is limited mostly to the 19th and 20th centuries. They are particularly useful when there are more or less continuous series taken within unchanging national boundaries. A number of national monographs have assembled all the published information over time, thus providing series of demographic indices comparable to those of a more recent past (for example, Woods 2000).

Other Quantitative Sources: Tax Rolls, Court Records, Membership Lists, Tombstones, and Others

A great many sources that provide lists of people or lists of events or biographical materials lend themselves to quantitative analyses of various kinds. They are particularly useful for the investigation of periods where more conventional sources do not exist or of phenomena that have left few traces in these sources. Although inscriptions on Roman tombstones have been used to compute life tables, the materials suffer from unconquerable selection biases. Remarkably, an attempt to estimate age at marriage from such inscriptions has been more successful, showing very early ages for females and large differentials by sex, a pattern not unlike that found for Renaissance Florence (Hopkins 1965). Estimates of the mortality impact from 14th-century epidemics of the bubonic plague have been derived in England from land transfers recorded in manorial courts and in Italy from the annuity system used to accumulate funds for dowry payments. From institutional records, David Kertzer (1993) studied foundlings in 19th-century Italy, representing perhaps as much as 4 % of Italian births in the 1860s and suffering from extraordinarily high mortality. John Knodel (1988) used vaccination reports to estimate the proportion of south-German women nursing their children, an important determinant of fertility and mortality in the region. The list of such sources could be extended to many nominal or aggregate records that contain numerical information on people or events.

Whenever available, good biographical materials can be used to estimate mortality. It is possible, for example, to compute life tables for members of religious orders, starting from their age at a date of entry into the order, or for members of Congress starting at their election, provided records mention their date of death. Court records on rare events, such as attempted abortion or infanticide, are the only sources that enable the researcher to assess the frequency of these events, and the circumstances (e.g., the sex and marital status of the accused) under which they are attempted. In contrast to more sensationalist accounts based on the impressions of contemporary witnesses, in these sources they are rare events, committed typically by desperate unmarried mothers.

Medical, Religious, Legal, or Literary Evidence

The proximate determinants of fertility (e.g., the duration of breast-feeding or the use of contraception) must often be studied through unreliable literary evidence. Similarly, the study of medical sources provides evidence on diseases and their treatment. Although these sources are intrinsically biased, they provide a context in which the statistical evidence must be interpreted. For classic examples of the study of this type of evidence, see Nardi (1971) on abortion in the writings of antiquity, Noonan (1986) on contraception in the writings of the Christian tradition, or McNeil (1976) on the role on disease in human history.

THEORETICAL MODELS

There is a polarity in the organization of knowledge, between analysis and synthesis, between the sifting and organization of the hard data that were collected long ago for different purposes, and the models that are often based on intuition but serve to organize the facts as they are gathered. These models interpret historical events into intellectually satisfying constructs that are not necessarily grounded in sound evidence when they are proposed but that provide hypotheses to be tested in subsequent research. The progress of science is then determined by the success of efforts to either confirm the model or to bring the orthodoxy down and replace it with another one, more consistent with the facts. Whereas historical demography in its early years was dominated by the exploration of sources and the development of measurements, the emphasis has now shifted toward the investigation of whole social structures or demographic systems. The previous section of this chapter organized the discussion "horizontally" as it were, by looking at sources that may provide information on a variety of topics. This section and the next proceed "vertically," by considering large topics that have retained the attention of historical demographers and historians of population. This section considers the more properly demographic topics: fertility, mortality, and marriage. The next section describes some exemplars of more interdisciplinary research in the demographic structure of societies of the past, where historians of population have played a primary role.

Natural Fertility and the Fertility Transition

Louis Henry was led to the study of historical populations by his interest in the proximate determinants of natural fertility, i.e., the fertility of married couples that did not attempt to limit the number of their children by resorting to contraception or abortion. He did not invent the term *natural fertility*, which was commonly used before him to refer to the reproductive regime of high-fertility populations of the past. In early writings, Henry had called them "non-Malthusian populations" and qualified their fertility as biological; the terms were clearly inappropriate. He took an important step by providing a way of identifying natural fertility in statistical series, i.e., when the fertility of married couples was not a function of the number of children they already had. By comparing successive marriage cohorts of individuals in family reconstitutions, it was possible to distinguish clearly between the behavior of early cohorts where fertility was natural and that of later cohorts who practiced family limitation. The publication of Henry's (1961) result on natural fertility exerted an influence well beyond historical studies and laid the foundation for biometric models of the reproductive process and for the proximate determinant framework of fertility.

The dominant model in demography until then had been the theory of the demographic transition, a broad pattern of connected demographic changes in the course of modernization resulting from socioeconomic influences. One of the findings of the Princeton European project was that the decline of fertility took place under a wide variety of circumstances, at different levels of mortality, and in countries that had reached very different levels of socioeconomic development (Knodel and van de Walle 1979). This cast doubt on the theory of the demographic transition. The focus shifted to the timing of the fertility transition, the change from a regime of natural fertility to one of family limitation. A series of methodologies to measure the time of transition were proposed, based on the shape of the pattern of marital fertility (Coale and Trussell 1974) or on the average age of mothers at the time of their last birth (Knodel 1988; Wilson 1984). The Princeton European project proposed a dating of the fertility transition by computing the time when the index of marital fertility had declined by 10% from a predecline plateau (Coale and Watkins 1986). Such a predecline plateau of high fertility has been identified in most countries. For rural France, where the decline started before the existence of vital registration and censuses, David Weir (1994) connected the results of the family reconstitutions made by Louis Henry and his team with the 19th-century statistics and identified the end of the natural fertility regime at a time close to the

French Revolution. If France is excluded, close to 60% of the province-sized administrative areas of Europe experienced their marital fertility decline starting in the 30-year period from 1890 to 1920 (Coale and Treadway 1986:37). The concentration in time, in countries with vastly different economic and social conditions, suggested a common mechanism of ideational transmission rather than an adjustment to socioeconomic pressure.

A number of recent studies have attempted to rehabilitate the notion that marital fertility declined because of an adjustment to economic change, by using more sophisticated econometric models and a lower level of aggregation than the province (Galloway, Hammel, and Lee 1994; Brown and Guinnane 2002). The concept of natural fertility and the methods used for its measurement have been criticized for various reasons, for example, their lack of sensitivity that makes it very difficult to date the transition point with any precision. Low values of m, Coale and Trussell's indicator of the prevalence of parity-dependent family limitation, could be compatible with a significant proportion of the population practicing it (Okun 1994). Others have objected to the inability of the model to factor in the spacing of births (rather than the limitation of their number) that appears to characterize many reproductive regimes (Bean, Mineau, and Anderton 1990).

More importantly, controversy continues over the reality of the fertility transition. It has been asserted that there was not one fertility transition, i.e., a single historical movement, but many different transitions, each with its own motivations and characteristics, or even simply a continuous adaptation of fertility levels to local economic opportunities and the level of mortality. Simon Szreter (1996) hypothesized that the decline of fertility in England was the result of abstinence and spacing. There have been efforts to revive the theory of the demographic transition, by linking the secular decline of fertility to a decline of mortality whose effect was only appreciated with a very long lag by married couples (Chesnais 1992).

The concept of natural fertility started as a purely demographic concept, but it has become linked to the history of birth control. Two recent histories of contraception have deemphasized the innovation aspects of the fertility transition by claiming that women at all times had access to methods adequate for their needs (McLaren 1990; Riddle 1992). Janet Farell Brodie (1994), in an exemplary study of contraception and abortion in 19th-century America, has emphasized the extent to which the ideas and the paraphernalia of birth control were diffused in the public by pamphlets, commercial catalogs, advertising in newspapers, conferences, and word of mouth and were eventually stymied at the end of the century by legal interventions and a reversal of public opinion.

Crises of Mortality and the Epidemiologic Transition

Historical demography helped push back the date of reliable mortality data, particularly for infant and child mortality (Schofield, Reher, and Bideau 1991). Population reconstruction provided reliable life tables for the rural French and English population in the 18th century; official statistics for Sweden go back to 1750. These series show a steady decline of mortality from the high and fluctuating levels that prevailed at the earliest dates. In contrast, the decline of infant mortality is less obvious and does not start in earnest before the last decade of the 19th century (Vallin 1991). The prevailing general descriptive model of secular changes in mortality is that of the epidemiological transition from a stage of dominance by infectious and parasitic diseases to a situation where people die mostly in old age from chronic and degenerative diseases.

The statistical record before 1800 is dominated by peaks of exceptional mortality from crises caused by a mix of food shortages and epidemics (Livi-Bacci 1991). The history of such diseases as the bubonic plague (Biraben 1975), smallpox (Hopkins 1983), syphilis (Arrizabalaga, Henderson, and French 1997; Quetel 1990), or tuberculosis— even in the absence of precise quantitative information on causes of deaths—sheds light on the mechanisms of infection and on attempts at treatment in the past. In the 19th century, the frequency and intensity of crises diminish (Perrenoud 1991), although there are still occasional peaks of mortality in various countries from identifiable causes, such as the cholera epidemics of 1832 and 1856, the potato famine of 1846, and the 1870 smallpox epidemic. The Swedish data show a sharp decline in the frequency and mortality of smallpox epidemics in the 19th century as a result of the adoption of vaccination, the first successful use of preventive health measures against an infectious disease (Sköld 1996).

Two explanations have been given for the importance of infectious diseases in the past and for their decline. In a first explanation, the periodic visitation of diseases, and their establishment in an endemic form, was essentially an exogenous influence, an accident of epidemiology under favorable environmental circumstances. William McNeil (1976) illustrates this position. Disease pools developed in isolated parts of the world and were diffused with a devastating impact when interregional contacts increased, eventually to form a "common market of diseases." Infections such as smallpox and measles decimated the population at the time of first contact, but conferred immunity to their surviving victims and became childhood diseases. The epidemiological transition was the result of an increasing ability of preventive measures (e.g., smallpox vaccination) and the development of hygiene and public health (e.g., sewerage and clean water supply) to combat the infections.

The opposite position has represented the high levels of historical mortality as endogenous, the result of low standards of living and population pressure. The idea of a Malthusian equilibrium where population growth is kept within the bounds of subsistence by the positive check of mortality finds some support in the analysis of the record for Elizabethan England. By the 17th century, however, adjustments seem to occur through the preventive check on marriages (Wrigley and Schofield 1981: chapter 11). Thomas McKeown (1976) has argued that the decline of mortality in England during the 19th century, and hence the modern rise of population, was caused neither by medical innovations nor by an attenuation of the virulence of disease, and therefore must have been the result of better nutrition and an improvement in the standard of living. McKeown downplayed, and probably underestimated, the impact of smallpox inoculation and vaccination and of public health measures in the area of sanitation and water supply.

Whatever the reasons for the increase in expectation of life at birth during the 19th century in Europe and the United States, they do not seem to have operated on infant mortality, which remained practically unchanged before the last decade of the 19th century and then underwent a rapid decline. Although there is no consensus on the reason for this late decline of infant mortality, the most convincing analyses for England (Woods 2000), the United States (Preston and Haines 1991), and France (Rollet-Echalier 1990) suggest that the crucial element was a revolution in public and private attitudes toward the child, combined with new principles of hygiene in the home, including boiling milk and sterilizing bottles, which represented a breakthrough in the practice of artificial feeding.

The Western European Marriage Pattern and the Structure of Households

In 1965, John Hajnal published a pathbreaking study of European marriage patterns, in which he pointed out the existence of two distinct types of marriage separated roughly by an imaginary line going from Leningrad (as it was then called) to Trieste. The western European countries were characterized, around 1900, by late female marriage (typically above 25 years of age) and extensive celibacy. Eastern Europe, in contrast, had early marriages and high proportions marrying, resulting in higher levels of overall fertility. Hajnal attempted to trace back the temporal origins of the pattern and concluded that it had existed in many countries of western Europe at least since the 17th century. He associated it with an original pattern of household formation: "In Europe it has been necessary for a man to defer marriage until he could establish an independent livelihood adequate to support a family; in other societies the young couple could be incorporated in a larger economic unit, such as a joint family" (Hajnal 1965: 133). Alan Mcfarlane (1986) linked the European pattern of marriage with early capitalism, the dominance of market forces (particularly for the sale of land in private ownership), and the prevalence of wage labor. He believed that these conditions were attained in England by the 13th century and later in other European countries. Research has confirmed that the western European marriage pattern is distinctive, although there are other systems throughout the world where marriage is relatively late and the young couple sets up an independent home. Tokugawa Japan, offered such an example, although permanent celibacy was rare.

In theory, a marriage could only take place when a new couple had the economic resources to allow its independent establishment. The reconstruction of the English population by Wrigley and Schofield (1981) clearly demonstrated the role of nuptiality as the feedback mechanism regulating the growth of population in the 18th century so that it would not exceed the resources available for its support. Favorable real prices and agricultural wages would lead to earlier and more frequent marriages; times of scarcity would lead to the opposite result(for a recent review of the English nuptiality story in a long-term perspective, see Smith 1999). It has been argued that the development of cottage industry, and later the industrial revolution, by providing new opportunities for both male and female wage labor, must have led to younger and more universal marriage (Levine 1977). The evidence from the study of microdata from the 19th century is mixed on this, and the most recent research suggests that many factors regulated the contracting of unions during the 18th and 19th centuries in somewhat conflicting directions, depending on country, region, and the local economic organization (Devos and Kennedy 1999). These factors included the dominant forms of wage labor (e.g., day labor versus living-in servants), employer's control over housing, the intensity of human labor in the prevailing technology, the substitution of cheaper female workers for male workers in some types of production, and the elasticity of the marriage market with respect to increases in the standard of living. In the aggregate, and with some exceptions, the vast expansion of the industrial labor force and the steady increase in wages during the industrial revolution did not produce a commensurate increase in the proportions married before the 20th century in western countries (Coale and Treadway 1986).

The study of household structure from population listings, although at face value outside of the scope of demographic studies, provided one of the missing links in the reconstruction of past societies. It was initiated by Peter Laslett and his colleagues at the Cambridge Group for the History of Population and Social Structure. Household structure is a topic that had received little attention in traditional demography; the household was usually treated simply as a unit of enumeration in the census, without theoretical interest. The common misperception was that families of the past were very large and extended.

A large number of manuscript census listings from the past have been examined, and they show conclusively that with rare exceptions, the conjugal family unit (a man, his wife, and their children) constitutes the basic residential pattern of western populations and that this has been the dominant household structure among the common people of western Europe as far back as the evidence from enumerations will carry (Wall, Robin, and Laslett 1983). Households, as today, were typically limited to the conjugal pair and their children and were therefore small, and the marriage of the children entailed the founding of new households.

RESEARCH EXEMPLARS

From its beginnings in the study of the fertility and mortality of individuals, historical demography has evolved steadily toward the consideration of entire social structures and their dynamics in time and space. In this section, we consider two exemplars of research on opposite sides of this continuum between the micro- and macrodemographic focuses. The first example indicates how the study of individual records from village populations of the past can be made to yield surprisingly revealing evidence of individual behavior. The second illustrates the study of large populations as demographic systems where the impact of social and economic forces plays out in combination with marriage customs, rules of inheritance, and patterns of employment on a climatic and epidemiological backcloth.

Microdemography: Knodel and the German Family Genealogies

John Knodel, one of the members of the European fertility project who had analyzed the aggregate statistics for Germany during the 19th century (Knodel 1974), set out to explore the local features of fertility and mortality changes at the microlevel with the help of a remarkable source: village genealogies compiled by local German historians and genealogists on the basis of official statistics and church records and encompassing the vital events of all families that resided in a particular village. The data analyzed by Knodel comprise 14 villages and cover over 11,000 couples married between 1700 and 1899, and their 55,000 children (Knodel 1988: 20). They appear to be of high quality and completeness and allow remarkably detailed and sophisticated analysis on the basis of a large number of cases.

Knodel devotes a considerable part of his attention to issues of measurement and definition, looking for the best way of teasing out relevant sociological or biological indices to explain the findings. In addition to the measurement of fertility and child mortality that we shall discuss further below, his analyses pertain to such topics, among others, as the seasonality of vital events, maternal mortality, marriage, widowhood and remarriage, bridal pregnancies, prenuptial births and illegitimacy, along with their relevant differentials by region, social class, and religion. The approach focuses on individuals and families, and the social and economic structure of Germany is only treated in passing.

Infant and child mortality levels showed little evidence of a trend before 1900, but there were important differentials between the villages that are part of the sample. Infant mortality was highest in Bavarian villages and lowest in East Frisian villages, with Baden and Waldeck villages occupying an intermediary position. There was direct survey evidence, collected in the late 19th century to investigate mortality differentials, that women avoided breast-feeding their children in Bavaria and in other parts of southern Germany. This suggested that child feeding patterns provided an explanation of mortality differentials. Two analytical techniques confirmed such an explanation. First, the interval between confinements was considerably reduced in Waldeck and the East Frisian Villages when the first child had died during the first month of life, a circumstance that would interrupt suckling in populations that would commonly practice breastfeeding. In Bavaria, however, the reduction corresponded only to the expected duration of the nonsusceptible period after a birth (Knodel 1988: 547). A second confirmation of the role of infant feeding came with the use of a biometric technique devised by the French demographer Jean Bourgeois-Pichat in 1952 to isolate the effect of endogenous mortality (i.e., deaths linked to the lack of viability of the child and to the risks of delivery) from later mortality during the first year of life. The technique uses a mathematical scale to linearize the cumulated number of deaths by month; the intersect of the line with the vertical axis for age zero provides an estimate of endogenous mortality, while the slope measures exogenous mortality. For the German villages, endogenous mortality is rather uniform, but the points line up in the expected manner only for the East Frisian villages. For Waldeck, they deviate upward in a way that suggests excess mortality at the end of the first year, often associated with weaning after six to nine months. For Bavaria, on the contrary, the slope of the line is very steep and deviates downward; this would be a pattern in which mortality rises steeply during the early months of infancy but becomes more normal in later months (Knodel 1988: 52).

Knodel was initially drawn to the topic of breast-feeding by his concern for explaining differentials in natural fertility before the onset of the secular fertility transition. Bavaria, with its customary avoidance of nursing, had one of the highest fertility rates in Europe as well as very high mortality. Other factors affecting fecundity prior to the advent of birth control are less easy to identify, although there was a clear, and in some villages considerable, rise in fecundability between the mid-18th and the mid-19th century, perhaps as a result of changes in nutrition during that period (Knodel 1988: 285–286). This rise makes it more difficult to identify the time of the beginning of the fertility transition because it operates in the opposite direction of the effect of family limitation to maintain relatively stable levels of aggregate marital fertility (as measured for instance by the index I_g). Knodel uses other indexes to date the beginnings of family limitation: the Coale-Trussel m index of family limitation based on the age pattern of marital fertility; the age of mother at last birth; and parity progression probabilities. The analysis leads to the conclusion that the villages differed greatly in the date when family limitation appeared and that it became noticeable in some regions at the beginning of the 19th century (Knodel 1988: 317). There was little evidence of effective spacing of births (Knodel 1988: 348).

A recurrent theme in demography has been the relation between child mortality and reproductive behavior. The decline of fertility occurs generally earlier than that of child mortality, which remains high until the end of the century and is therefore unlikely to have been a factor in the fertility transition. As expected within a natural fertility framework, Knodel finds little evidence of replacement of a dead child before the decline of fertility. Toward the end of the period, he finds that the behavior of couples conforms to a parity-specific adaptation of reproductive behavior: those experiencing high mortality are less likely to use family limitation (Knodel 1988: 440–442).

Macrodemography: The Cambridge Group and the Social History of England

The descriptive work of Louis Henry and his colleagues and European epigones had shown that fertility in the past was high, that mortality was dominated by crises, that marriage was late and permanent celibacy frequent. Michael Flinn (1981) attempted a description of these elements as a "demographic system." The great merit of the Cambridge Group was to place that system in the historical context of an economy and a society, *The World We Have Lost* to use the title of Peter Laslett's influential work of 1965. "The fascination of work on population history stems from its central position in the fabric of social and economic life in the past" (Wrigley and Schofield 1981: 483). The true monument in this enterprise was the reconstruction of the English population between 1541 and 1871, which has served as the sturdy trunk on which various other studies of the socioeconomic structure of England could be grafted. It is significant that the work of the Cambridge Group that involved family reconstitution (Wrigley et al. 1997) was published much later and has received less attention. The project was an example of team work, not only by the close association of Wrigley and Schofield with other historians and demographers at the Cambridge Group, but also by their reliance on local historians for the collection and analysis of parish data and the use that independent researchers have made of their data.

Wrigley wrote about Malthus, and edited his complete works. In his work with Roger Schofield (1981), he followed in the footsteps of Malthus in exploring the interaction of the demographic and the socioeconomic systems and in demonstrating the relevance of behavior at the individual and family levels to explain the great secular waves of aggregate population growth in England. In the concluding chapter of *The Population History of England* (fittingly subtitled "a dynamic model of population and environment"), the authors present a schematic view of a homeostatic population equilibrium in the Malthusian tradition, first through the operation of the positive check of mortality, and second through that of the preventive check of marital restraint (Wrigley and Schofield 1981: 457–480). The central element in the model consists of a feedback loop where favorable food prices and the resulting real wages make it easier to contract marriages and hence increase fertility and population size. This in turn causes scarcity of food, increasing food prices and reducing real wages, thus reestablishing the equilibrium. Because the impact of nuptiality on fertility and population size takes a long time to work itself out, sizable lags are expected in the interaction of the variables. Moreover, there are secondary feedback loops that complicate the picture: through mortality in the early stage of the model corresponding to the Elizabethan period, and through the demand for labor outside of agriculture that becomes important during the stage corresponding to the industrial revolution. The examination of series of a real-wage index and crude marriage rates suggest indeed that the two series are correlated, with a lag.

The work raises the question of the uniqueness of the English situation. In an article published two years after the monumental *Population History of England,* Wrigley (1983) resolved the following "conundrums": Why was the growth of the English population during the 18th century faster than that of other countries of western Europe, and accelerating? Was it due to a decline of mortality or to a rise in fertility? The reconstruction of the population suggested that the expectation of life at birth had increased from 32.4 years in the 1670s and 1680s to 38.7 in the 1810s and 1820s, while the gross reproduction rate increased from 1.98 to 2.94. The fertility increase contributes two and a half times as much as the decline of mortality to the increase in the growth rate. To account for the fertility rise, the main proximate determinant was nuptiality.

The fundamental role played by nuptiality (both the age at marriage and the proportion never marrying) is indeed the most important finding, and it served as a unifying principle for many streams of research on the population of England and, consequently, of Europe, from Hajnal's European marriage pattern to Laslett's household constancy over time. It lies smack in the Malthusian tradition, and its focus is on secular changes.

FUTURE PROSPECTS

Historical demography has joined the mainstream of population studies. Techniques and explanatory frameworks have been exchanged liberally between historical demography and the rest of the field. The exchanges have been most active with the demography of developing countries, a topic that was also underrepresented in *The Study of Population* (Hauser and Duncan 1959). It is not uncommon to see scholars specializing alternatively in the study of a developing country and of a historical period of a western nation.

The field has clear limitations. It relies on unreliable data rife with bias. This means that an unusually large portion of the writing is devoted to methodological discussions and the description of esoteric techniques designed to circumvent bias. It also means that large segments of the population are unobservable and that some parts of the lives of individuals are better covered than others: the mortality of children and the fertile life of women. The classic family reconstitution techniques that use parish records typically only cover less than a third of the population consisting of stable families that spent all their life in the village. More than most other fields, historical demography is data-bound and must be content with the accidental inclusion of a variable in a data set collected for entirely different purposes. Although there have been occasional attempts to interview old people on a significant event of their youth (such as the use of contraception in past cohorts; see, for example, Fisher 2000) there is usually no way to design a questionnaire or assemble a panel the way it is increasingly done in the other social sciences with which demography is associated.

The reliance on data sets of the past means also that geographical coverage will be spotty. Some countries and some periods of history are inaccessible to the researcher and likely will remain so. This means, among other things, that no entirely satisfactory history of the world population can be written. The most satisfying attempt to do so was written by Massimo Livi-Bacci (1992), and it limits itself to general mechanisms and examples. Even the attempt to write a population history of Europe (Bardet and Dupâquier 1997), the continent where the sources are most abundant, is only partly successful because of the difficulty of integrating the points of views and the methodologies over the long term. Because of the particular nature of the North American sources, the field of historical demography remains small in the U.S. The journal *Demography* does not have a steady flow of articles on historical subjects, as do its European competitors, *Population Studies* and *Population*.

Perhaps the age of the pioneers is over and the most significant achievements of historical demography are behind us, as the most important sources have been analyzed and the general characteristics of past populations have been described. Of course, the field will continue to integrate the most advanced statistical methodologies, as witnessed by many of the chapters in a recent book on *Old and Recent Methods in Historical Demography* (Reher and Schofield 1993; see also Willigan and Lynch 1982). The history of population is going to evolve in the same way as the rest of demography. There is likely to be increasing cross-fertilization, with methods from historical demography carried over into mainstream demography of the present, and the new developments of demography adapted to the study of the limited records from the past.

It would be bold to try to predict exactly what approaches are likely to be used in the future and what discoveries will be made. In this section, we consider some possible directions of future research. First, explorations of new countries will take place and extensions back in time. The study of Chinese genealogies suggests that the past is not uniform, characterized by an undifferentiated regime dominated by the biological constraints of natural fertility and mortality from infectious diseases. The Chinese demographic regime, so it is argued, was grounded in collective social relations that are distinctly different from the individualistic behavior of Europe (Lee and Feng 1999). Infanticide was a significant check on population growth, and marital fertility appears to have been low, perhaps because of a higher degree of voluntary control. Other studies have suggested that mortality in China and Japan was less subject to the crises that buffeted the European regime (Zhao 1997; Jannetta 1987). A great attraction of historical demography is the opportunity it provides to investigate other data sets, other cultures, other epidemiological contexts. Each different data set may include its own fascinating set of questions, encountered nowhere else, that allow novel analyses. For example, the Taiwanese population registers recorded data on foot binding, which makes it possible to ascertain the ethnic group and the extent of female labor, as women with deformed feet cannot work in the fields (Wolf and Chuang 1994).

A second and related trend is the attention to a more comparative approach that would bring out the differences as well as the commonalities in widely separate countries. The Eurasian Project on the History of Population and Family, initiated by Akira Hayami in 1994, has been engaged in the comparative study of social organization and demographic processes at the family level in five research cites: southern Sweden, eastern Belgium, northern Italy, northeastern Japan and northeastern China (Bengtsson et al. 2004). Remarkably, the project has adopted a Malthusian paradigm, like that of the Cambridge group.

A third tendency is the design of studies that are less monographic than in the past but aim at examining particular substantive issues. A good example is a recent study of the relative impact of Protestantism and Catholicism on the demography of Alsace during the 19th century (McQuillan 1999). The study presents hypotheses based on the doctrinal differences between the traditional position of the Catholic Church toward the married state as an inferior status and Luther's recognition of sexuality as a fundamental human value. It attempts to test these hypotheses by using a combination of nominative and aggregate techniques in a carefully selected sample of villages. It investigates the history of pastoral practices and of the relations between church and state in the educational systems of the two communities. It concludes that doctrinal differences (particularly with respect to marriage) were less important in shaping the behavior of the Lutheran and Catholic communities than the openness of the hierarchies to modernity in the former and the conservatism of the latter. This accounts for a later decline of fertility in Catholic villages, a development that may have its parallels in other countries of mixed confessions like Ireland and Canada.

These are the new challenges. In the several decades that have elapsed since Duncan and Hauser made their pessimistic assessment in 1959, historical demography has gained an honorable status among the specialties that constitute the discipline of demography. The future of the discipline lies in its integration into a broader synthesis of the history of society and the family.

REFERENCES

Akerman, S., ed. 1973. *Aristocrats, farmers, proletarians. Essays in Swedish demographic history*. Upsala: Esselte Studium.

Alter, G. 1988. *Family and the female life course. The women of Verviers, Belgium, 1849–1880*. Madison: University of Wisconsin Press.

Anderson, M. 1998. Highly restricted fertility: Very small families in the British fertility decline. *Population Studies* 52: 177–199.

Appleby, A. B. 1979. Grain prices and subsistence crises in England and France, 1590–1740. *Journal of Economic History* 39: 865–887.

Arrizabalaga, J., J. Henderson, and R. French. 1997. *The great pox. The French disease in Renaissance Europe*. New Haven, Conn.: Yale University Press.

Bagnall, R. S., and B. W. Frier. 1994. *The demography of Roman Egypt*. Cambridge: Cambridge University Press.

Bardet, J. P. 1983. *Rouen et les Rouennais au XVIIe et XVIIIe siècles. Les mutations d'un espace social*. Paris: Société d'édition d'enseignement supérieur.

Bardet, J. P., and J. Dupâquier, eds. 1997, 1998. *Histoire des populations de l'Europe*. 2 vols. Paris: Fayard.

Bean, L. L., G. P. Mineau, and D. L. Anderton. 1990. *Fertility change on the American frontier. Adaptation and innovation*. Berkeley: University of California Press.

Bengtsson, T., C. Campbell, J. Z. Lee, et al. 2004. Life under pressure: *Mortality and living standards in Europe and Asia, 1700–1900*. Cambridge, MA: The MIT Press.

Bengtsson, T., G. G. Fridlizius, and R. Ohlsson. 1981. *Pre-industrial population change*. Stockholm: Almquist and Wiksell.

Biraben, J. N. 1975. *Les hommes et la peste en France et dans les pays européens et méditerranéens*. 2 vols. Paris: Mouton.

Blayo, Y. 1975. Le mouvement naturel de la population française de 1740 à 1860. *Population*, special issue:15–64.

Bonneuil, N. 1997. *Transformation of the French demographic landscape, 1806–1906*. Oxford: Clarendon Press.

Boserup. E. 1981. *Population and technological change. A study of long-term trends*. Chicago: The University of Chicago Press.

Bourgeois-Pichat, J. 1952. Essai sur la mortalite biologique de l'homme. *Population* 7:381–394.

Brodie, J. F. 1994. *Contraception and abortion in nineteenth-century America*. Ithaca: Cornell University Press.

Brown, J. C., and T. W. Guinnane. 2002. Fertility transition in a rural, Catholic population: Bavaria, 1880–1910. *Population Studies* 56:35–50.

Byers, E. 1982. Fertility transition in a New England commercial center: Nantucket, Massachusetts, 1680–1840. *Journal of Interdisciplinary History* 13:17–40.

Charbonneau, H., et al. 1993. *The first French Canadians: Pioneers in the St. Lawrence Valley.* Newark: University of Delaware Press.

Chesnais, J. C. 1992. *The demographic transition: Stages, patterns, and economic implications.* Oxford: Oxford University Press.

Coale, A., B. Anderson, and E. Härm. 1974. *Human fertility in Russia since the nineteenth century.* Princeton, N. J.: Princeton University Press.

Coale, A. J., and R. Treadway. 1986. A summary of the changing distribution of overall fertility, marital fertility, and the proportion married in the provinces of Europe. In *The decline of fertility in Europe.* Edited by A. J. Coale and S. C. Watkins, 31–181. Princeton, N. J.: Princeton University Press.

Coale, A. J., and T. J. Trussell. 1974. Model fertility schedules: Variations in the age structure of childbearing in human populations. *Population Index* 40: 185–258.

Coale, A. J., and S. C. Watkins, eds. 1986. *The decline of fertility in Europe.* Princeton, N. J.: Princeton University Press.

Coale, A. J., and M. Zelnick. 1963. *New estimates of fertility and population in the United States.* Princeton, N. J.: Princeton University Press.

Demos, J. 1971. *A little commonwealth: Family life in Plymouth Colony.* New York: Oxford University Press.

Devos, I., and L. Kennedy, eds. 1999. *Marriage and rural economy. Western Europe since 1400.* Turnhout, Belgium: Brepols.

Fisher, K. 2000. Uncertain aims and tacit negotiation: Birth control practices in Britain, 1925–50. *Population and Development Review* 26: 295–317.

Fleury, M., and L. Henry. 1956. *Nouveau manuel de dépouillement et d'exploitation de l'état civil ancien.* Paris: INED.

Flinn, M. 1981. *The European demographic system, 1500–1820.* Baltimore: Johns Hopkins University Press.

Galloway, P. R. 1988. Basic patterns of annual variations in fertility, nuptiality, mortality, and prices in pre-industrial Europe. *Population Studies* 42: 275–303.

Galloway, P. R., E. A. Hammel, and R. D. Lee. 1994. Fertility decline in Prussia, 1875–1910: A pooled cross-section time series analysis. *Population Studies* 48: 135–158.

Gautier, E., and L. Henry. 1958. *La population de Crulai, paroisse normande. Étude historique.* Paris: PUF.

Haines, M. R., and R. H. Steckel, eds. 2000. *A population history of North America.* Cambridge: Cambridge University Press.

Hajnal, J. 1965. European marriage patterns in perspective. In *Population in history.* Edited by D. V. Glass and D. E. C. Eversley, 101–143. London: Edward Arnold.

Hauser, P. M., and O. D. Duncan. 1959. *The study of population: An inventory and appraisal.* Chicago: The University of Chicago Press.

Hayami, A. 1979. Thank you Francisco Xavier: An essay in the use of micro-data for historical demography of Tokugawa, Japan. *Keio Economic Studies* 6.1.2: 65–81.

Henripin, J. 1954. *La population canadienne au début du XVIIIe siècle.* Paris: PUF.

Henry, L. 1956. *Anciennes familles genevoises. Étude démographique: XVIe-XXe siècle.* Paris: PUF.

Henry, L. 1958. Pour connaître la population de la France depuis Louis XIV. *Population* 13: 663–686.

Henry, L. 1961. Some data on natural fertility. *Eugenics Quarterly* 8:81–91.

Henry, L. 1970. *Manuel de démographie historique,* 2d ed. Geneva-Paris: Droz.

Henry, L. 1972. Fécondité des mariages dans le quart sud-ouest de la France de 1720 à 1829. *Annales ESC* 27: 612–640, 977–1023.

Henry, L. 1978. Fécondité des mariages dans le quart sud-est de la France de 1670 à 1829. *Population* 33: 855–883.

Henry, L., and J. Houdaille. 1973. Fécondité des mariages dans le quart nord-ouest de la France de 1720 à 1829. *Population* 28: 873–924.

Herlihy, D., and C. Klapisch-Zuber. 1985. *Tuscans and their families: A study of the Florentine Catasto of 1427.* New Haven, Conn.: Yale University Press.

Hoch, S. L. 1998. Famine, disease, and mortality patterns in the parish of Borshevka, Russia, 1830–1912. *Population Studies* 52: 357–368.

Hollingsworth, T. H. 1964. *The demography of the British peerage.* Supplement to *Population Studies* XVIII: 2.

Hollingsworth, T. H. 1969. *Historical demography.* Ithaca, N.Y.: Cornell University Press.

Hopkins, D. R. 1983. *Princes and peasants: Smallpox in history.* Chicago: The University of Chicago Press.

Hopkins, K. 1965. The age of Roman girls at marriage. *Population Studies* 18: 309–327.

Houdaille, J. 1976. La fécondité des mariages de 1670 à 1829 dans le quart nord-est de la France. *Annales de démographie historique 1976*: 341–391.

Houdaille, J. 1988. La bourgeoisie ancienne selon le dictionnaire généalogique d'André Delavenne. *Population* 43: 311–329.

Houdaille, J. 1989. La noblesse française 1600–1900. *Population* 44: 501–513.

International Union for the Study of Population (IUSSP). 1981. *Multilingual demographic dictionary*. Liège: Ordina Editions.

Jannetta, A. B. 1987. *Epidemics and mortality in early modern Japan*. Princeton, N. J.: Princeton University Press.

Kantrow, L. 1980. Philadelphia gentry: Fertility and family limitation among an American aristocracy. *Population Studies* 34:21–30.

Kertzer, D. I. 1993. *Sacrificed for honor. Italian infant abandonment and the politics of reproductive control*. Boston: Beacon Press.

Knodel, J. E. 1974. *The decline of fertility in Germany, 1871–1939*. Princeton, N. J.: Princeton University Press.

Knodel, J. E. 1988. *Demographic behavior in the past. A study of fourteen German village populations in the eighteenth and nineteenth centuries*. Cambridge: Cambridge University Press.

Knodel, J. E., and E. van de Walle. 1979. Lessons from the past: Policy implications of historical fertility studies. *Population and Development Review* 5: 217–245.

Laslett, P. 1965. *The world we have lost*. New York: Charles Scribner's Sons.

Laslett, P. 1977. Clayworth and Cogenhoe. In *Family life and illicit love in earlier generations*, 50–101. Cambridge: Cambridge University Press.

Laslett, P., and R. Wall. 1972. *Household and family in past time*. Cambridge: Cambridge University Press.

Laslett, P., K. Osterveen, and R. Smith, eds. 1980. *Bastardy and its comparative history*. London: Edward Arnold.

Lee, J., and C. Campbell, eds. 1997. *Fate and fortune in rural China: Social organization and population behaviour in Liaoning, 1774–1873*. Cambridge: Cambridge University Press.

Lee, J. Z., and Wang Feng. 1999. *One quarter of humanity. Malthusian mythology and Chinese realities*. Cambridge, Mass.: Harvard University Press.

Lee, R. 1981. Short-term variation: Vital rates, prices, and weather. In *The population history of England 1541–1871*. Edited by E. A. Wrigley and R. S. Schofield, 356–401. Cambridge: Cambridge University Press.

Lesthaeghe, R. J. 1977. *The decline of Belgian fertility*, 1800–1970. Princeton, N. J.: Princeton University Press.

Levine, D. 1977. *Family formation in an age of nascent capitalism*. New York:

Lévy, C., and L. Henry. 1960. Ducs et pairs sous l'ancien régime: Caractéristiques démographiques d'une caste. *Population* 15: 807–830.

Liu, T., J. Lee, D. V. Reher, and F. Wang. 2001. *Asian Population History*. Oxford: Oxford University Press.

Livi-Bacci, M. 1968. Fertility and nuptiality changes in Spain from the late 18th to the early 20th century. *Population Studies* 22: 83–102, 211–234.

Livi-Bacci, M. 1971. *A century of Portuguese fertility*. Princeton, N.J.: Princeton University Press.

Livi-Bacci, M. 1977. *A history of Italian fertility during the last two centuries*. Princeton, N.J.: Princeton University Press.

Livi-Bacci, M. 1986. Social-group forerunners of fertility control in Europe. In *The decline of fertility in Europe*. Edited by A. J. Coale and S. C. Watkins, 182–200. Princeton, N.J.: Princeton University Press.

Livi-Bacci, M. 1991. *Population and nutrition. Essay on the demographic history of Europe*. Cambridge: Cambridge University Press.

Livi-Bacci, M. 1992. *A concise history of world population*. Cambridge, Mass.: Blackwell.

Logue, B. J. 1985. The case for birth control before 1852: Nantucket reexamined. *Journal of Interdisciplinary History* 15:371–391.

McCaa, R. 2000. The peopling of Mexico from origins to revolution. In *A population history of North America*. Edited by M. R. Haines and R. H. Steckel, 241–304. Cambridge: Cambridge University Press.

Mcfarlane, A. 1986. *Marriage and love in England: Modes of reproduction 1300–1840*. Oxford: Basil Blackwell.

McKeown, T. 1976. *The modern rise of population*. London: Edward Arnold.

McLaren, A. 1990. *A history of contraception. From antiquity to the present day*. Oxford: Basil Blackwell.

McNeil, W. 1976. *Plagues and peoples*. New York: Doubleday.

McQuillan, K. 1999. *Culture, religion and demographic behaviour. Catholics and Lutherans in Alsace, 1750–1870*. Montreal: McGill-Queens University Press.

Nardi, E. 1971. *Procurato aborto nel mondo Greco Romano*. Milan: Giuffré.

Noonan, J. 1986. *Contraception: A history of its treatment by the Catholic theologians and canonists*, 2d ed. Cambridge, Mass.: Harvard University Press.

Notkola, V., I. M. Timaeus, and H. Siiskonen. 2000. Mortality transition in the Ovamboland region of Namibia, 1930–1990. *Population Studies* 54: 153–167.

Okun, B. S. 1994. Evaluating methods for detecting fertility control: Coale and Trussell's model and cohort parity analysis. *Population Studies* 48: 193–222.

Perrenoud, A. 1991. The attenuation of mortality crises in Europe and the decline of mortality. In *The decline of mortality in Europe*. Edited by R. Schofield, D. Reher, and A. Bideau, 18–37. Oxford: Clarendon Press.

Post, J. D. 1985. *Food shortage, climatic variability, and epidemic disease in preindustrial Europe. The mortality peak in the early 1740s*. Ithaca, N.Y.: Cornell University Press.

Post, W., F. van Poppel, E. van Imhoff, and E. Kruse. 1997. Reconstructing the extended kin-network in the Netherlands with genealogical data: Methods, problems, and results. *Population Studies* 51: 263–278.

Preston S. H., and M. R. Haines. 1991. *Fatal years. Child mortality in late nineteenth-century America*. Princeton, N.J.: Princeton University Press.

Quétel, C. 1990. *History of syphilis*. Baltimore: Johns Hopkins University Press.

Reher, D. S., and R. Schofield, eds. 1993. *Old and new methods in historical demography*. Oxford: Clarendon Press.

Reher, D. S., and A. Sanz-Gimeno. 2000. Mortality and economic development over the course of modernization: An analysis of short-run fluctuations in Spain, 1850–1990. *Population Studies* 54: 135–152.

Riddle, J. M. 1992. *Contraception and abortion from the ancient world to the Renaissance*. Cambridge, Mass.: Harvard University Press.

Rollet-Echalier, C. 1990. *La politique à l'égard de la petite enfance sous la IIIe république*. Paris: INED, PUF.

Ruggles, S. 1993. Historical demography from the census. Applications of the American census microdata files. In *Old and new methods in historical demography*. Edited by D. S. Reher and R. Schofield, 383–393. Oxford: Clarendon Press.

Schofield, R. 1986. Did the mothers really die? Three centuries of maternal mortality in "The world we have lost.". In *The world we have gained. Histories of population and social structure*. Edited by L. Bonfield, R. Smith, and K. Wrightson, 231–260. Oxford: Basil Blackwell.

Schofield, R., D. Reher, and A. Bideau, eds. 1991. *The decline of mortality in Europe*. Oxford: Clarendon Press.

Scott, S., and C. J. Duncan. 1998. *Human demography and disease*. New York: Cambridge University Press.

Séguy, I. 1999. J.-N. Biraben's survey of the population of France from 1500 to 1700. Presentation, sources, bibliography. *Population. An English Selection* 11: 133–154.

Séguy, I., ed. 2001. *La population de la France de 1670 à 1829. L'enquête Louis Henry et ses données*. Paris: INED.

Sköld, P. 1996. From inoculation to vaccination: Smallpox in Sweden in the eighteenth and nineteenth centuries. *Population Studies* 50: 247–262.

Skolnick, M. 1980. The Utah genealogical data base: A resource for genetic epidemiology. In *Cancer incidence in defined populations*. Edited by J. Cairns, et al., 285–297. New York: Cold Spring Harbor Laboratory.

Smith, R. M. 1999. Relative prices, forms of agrarian labour and female marriage patterns in England, 1350–1800. In *Marriage and rural economy. Western Europe since 1400*. Edited by I. Devos and L. Kennedy, 19–48. Turnhout, Belgium: Brepols.

Szreter, S. 1996. *Fertility, class and gender in Britain, 1860–1940*. Cambridge: Cambridge University Press.

Teitelbaum, M. S. 1984. *The British fertility decline: demographic transition in the crucible of the industrial revolution*. Princeton, N.J.: Princeton University Press.

Temkin-Greener, H., and A. C. Swedlund. 1978. Fertility transition in the Connecticut Valley: 1740–1850. *Population Studies* 32: 27–41.

Vallin, J. 1991. Mortality in Europe from 1720 to 1914. Long-term trends and patterns by age and sex. In *The decline of mortality in Europe*. Edited by R. Schofield, D. Reher, and A. Bideau, 38–67. Oxford: Clarendon Press.

van de Walle, E. 1974. *The female population of France in the nineteenth century*. Princeton, N.J.: Princeton University Press.

Wall, R., J. Robin, and P. Laslett, eds. 1983. *Family forms in historic Europe*. Cambridge: Cambridge University Press.

Watkins, S. C., ed. 1994. *After Ellis Island. Newcomers and natives in the 1910 census*. New York: Russell Sage Foundation.

Weir, D. 1994. New estimates of nuptiality and marital fertility in France, 1740–1911. *Population Studies* 48: 307–331.

Wells, R. V. 1975. *The population of the British colonies in America before 1776: A survey of census data*. Princeton, N.J.: Princeton University Press.

Willigan, J. D., and K. A. Lynch. 1982. *Sources and methods of historical demography*. New York: Academic Press.

Wilson, C. 1984. Natural fertility in pre-industrial England, 1600–1799. *Population Studies* 38: 225–240.

Wolf, A., and Chien-shan Huang. 1980. *Marriage and adoption in China, 1845–1945*. Palo Alto, Calif.: Stanford University Press.

Wolf. A., and Ying-chang Chuang. 1994. Fertility and women's labour: Two negative (but instructive) findings. *Population Studies* 48: 427–433.

Woods, R. 2000. *The demography of Victorian England and Wales*. Cambridge: Cambridge University Press.

Wrightson, K., and D. Levin. 1989. Death in Whickham. In *Famine, disease and the social order in early modern society*. Edited by J. Walter and R. Schofield, 129–165. Cambridge: Cambridge University Press.

Wrigley, E. A. 1966. Family limitation in pre-industrial England. *Economic History Review* 19: 82–109.

Wrigley, E. A. 1983. The growth of population in eighteenth-century England: A conundrum resolved. *Past and Present* 98: 121–150.

Wrigley, E. A., R. S. Davies, J. E. Oeppen, and R. S. Schofield. 1997. *English population history from family reconstitution 1580–1837*. Cambridge: Cambridge University Press.

Wrigley, E. A., and R. S. Schofield. 1981. *The population history of England 1541–1871*. Cambridge: Cambridge University Press.

Zhao, Z. 1997. Long-term mortality patterns in Chinese history: Evidence from a recorded clan population. *Population Studies* 51: 117–127.

CHAPTER 20

Ecological Demography

DUDLEY L. POSTON, JR.
and
W. PARKER FRISBIE

Hauser and Duncan's *The Study of Population* (1959) contains two chapters dealing with the interplay of ecology and demography. One is written by the biologist Peter W. Frank and the other by the demographer Otis Dudley Duncan. Frank's chapter draws on the principles of general ecology (referred to in his chapter as *population ecology*[1]) and shows their application to natality, mortality, age distribution, density, and several other demographic topics. Frank's examples are applied to *Homo sapiens* and to a variety of other species, such as Norway rats, fruit flies, butterflies, locusts, cockroaches, water fleas, and Pacific mackerels. Duncan's chapter argues that human ecology, in contrast to general ecology, provides a general "perspective, heuristic principles and concepts, and specific hypotheses of first-rate significance to the demographer" (1959: 678).

Duncan (1959) also provides one of the first theoretical expositions of the *ecological complex*, that is, the "collection of analytically distinguishable elements [of population, organization, environment, and technology], whose identification is part of the task of ecological theory" (1959: 684). In the literature of human ecology, Duncan's chapter is central and is one of the most cited theoretical treatments of the subject matter (for a recent review, discussion, and elaboration of the ecological complex, see Micklin and Sly [1998]).

This chapter is more consistent with Duncan's perspective than with Frank's, although it is narrower in orientation. It draws on human ecological theory as developed

---

[1] Frank's use of the term population ecology is different from that of Carroll and Khessina in this *Handbook*.

by Hawley (1950, 1968, 1986, 1998), Duncan (1959, 1961, 1964), Gibbs and Martin (1959), Schnore (1958, 1961), Namboodiri (1988, 1994), and several others (Micklin [1973], Poston et al. [1984], Micklin and Poston [1998], Micklin and Sly [1998], and Poston and Frisbie [1998]) and shows its relevance and application in analyses of the demographic processes of fertility, mortality, and migration.

Duncan notes that a difficulty in discussing the perspective of human ecology is that "even a provisional statement of [its] concerns will doubtless encounter strong objections from one or another group of scientists and thinkers who regard their studies of man as exemplifying the ecological viewpoint" (1959: 679). The next section of this chapter thus presents definitions of human ecology and ecological demography as the terms will be used in this chapter. A later section draws on current and past literature and illustrates the application of human ecology in the study of the demographic processes.

WHAT IS HUMAN ECOLOGY? WHAT IS ECOLOGICAL DEMOGRAPHY?

Human Ecology

Ecology may be defined as the "study of the interrelationships of organisms with their environment and each other" (*Encyclopedia Britannica* 1988: 959). One of the first statements was that of the Greek philosopher Theophrastus, who studied the "interrelationships between organisms and between organisms and their nonliving environment" (*Encyclopedia Britannica* 1988: 959). Ernest Haeckel used the term ecology in his study of plants, which was published in 1868. The term made its way into the English language with the translation of Haeckel's book in 1876. The term *human ecology* was first used by Robert Park and Ernest Burgess in their *Introduction to the Science of Sociology* (1924). For the first several decades after the term was introduced to sociologists, there was little agreement about its meaning and focus (Alihan 1938; Gettys 1940; Firey 1945). Amos Hawley's book, *Human Ecology: A Theory of Community Structure* (1950), which to this day is the definitive exposition of the field, sets out the subject matter of human ecology and its approach. According to Hawley, human ecology deals with "how growing, multiplying beings maintain themselves in a constantly changing but ever restricted environment" (1950: 66). For human populations, this requires examining the ways in which individuals act collectively to achieve more effective use of their habitat.

Despite this clear and unambiguous statement, some scholars ascribe to human ecology perspectives that are inconsistent with Hawley's thinking and that of McKenzie (1924, 1934, 1968), his predecessor and teacher. Three examples will suffice.

First, the sociobiologist Pierre van den Berghe notes that "sociologists who claim to be ecologists ... have reduced this specialty to a pedestrian kind of social geography (where) they largely plot social characteristics of people on maps" (1990: 174). Second, sociologists John Logan and Harvey Molotch write that "in human ecology, spatial relations are the analytical basis for understanding urban systems" (1987: 4). And, third, the social theorist Manuel Castells discusses the parallels between Marxian and ecological thinking and observes that the results obtained by ecology have no more value for establishing a theory of space than a mass of sociocultural correlations (1979: 122–123). Not only is Castells' comment incorrect, it also fails to capture the important materialistic and organizational similarities and differences between Marxist and ecological theory (for a statement, see Hawley [1984]).

These characterizations of human ecology as merely the study of spatial relations are due in part to the unfortunate statement of McKenzie (1924) in which he defined human ecology as the "study of the spatial and temporal relations of human beings as effected by the selective, distributive and accommodative forces of the environment." Hawley notes that although this simple, lucid statement inspired a great amount of empirical investigation, it caused human ecology to be regarded as little more than a descriptive study of spatial distributions, an outcome that McKenzie later noted was a misplacement of emphasis. Attention to spatial patterns, McKenzie recorded in his notes, should be subordinate and incidental to the analysis of sustenance relations (see Hawley's remarks in McKenzie [1968: xiii–xiv]).

There are other examples of the misuse or misunderstanding by social scientists of human ecology. Some refer to human ecology as studies using spatial rather than individual units of analysis (Robinson 1950), or as analyses of the physical features of geographical and built-up areas (Zorbaugh 1929; Suttles 1972), or as the factor analyses of the characteristics of aggregate units, i.e., factorial ecology (Berry and Rees 1969).

These illustrations exemplify Duncan's observation that "the term ecology is sometimes applied rather casually – even irresponsibly. [Frequently] studies adopting the label bear only a tenuous relationship to any systematic, scientific conception of the field" (1959: 680).

Human ecology is a field of study grounded in the four referential constructs of population, technology, organization, and environment. The unit of analysis is the human population, circumscribed more or less in a territorial fashion. Its major assumptions are that populations have unit character and integrity and that properties and attributes of these populations are more than the summation of their component parts.

Human ecology is concerned with the organizational aspects of human populations that arise from their sustenance-producing activities. These activities are necessary for the collective existence of the populations and must be adapted to the changing conditions confronting them. Included are an ever changing and mediating environment, their technological repertoires, and the size, composition, and distribution of the populations themselves (Duncan 1959; Frisbie and Poston 1975, 1978a, 1978b; Poston 1980, 1981).

Human ecologists address questions such as: What are the structural arrangements that characterize a population's sustenance-related endeavors? Under what conditions does one form of sustenance structure appear rather than another? What are the consequences for populations of varying configurations of sustenance-producing activities?

The answers lie in the fact that populations survive by virtue of collective organization. Human ecology is concerned with the determinants and consequences of sustenance organization, a consideration that addresses the interplay between human ecology and demography.

Much of the empirical literature of human ecology in recent decades focuses on demographic applications. The next section outlines the focus of ecological demography.

Ecological Demography

Human ecology offers demography an aggregate perspective for the analysis of the demographic processes. A fundamental tenet of human ecology is that a population redistributes itself through the vital processes and migration to achieve a balance or equilibrium between its size and life chances (Hawley 1968: 331; also see Davis [1963]). Duncan (1959: 708) also emphasizes the important ecological connections between organization and population size. Hawley (1950) notes that human populations will adjust their size through any of the demographic processes to maintain an equilibrium with their sustenance organization. Stated in another way, "demographic structure contains the possibilities and sets the limits of organized group life" (Hawley 1950: 78; see also Poston [1983]). Ecological demography is the application of human ecological theory to the analysis of the demographic processes.[2]

Although ecological theory provides an approach for the investigation of any of the three demographic processes, it is shown below that most empirical research has focused on population change due to net migration. The next section reviews major research in ecological demography.

ECOLOGICAL DEMOGRAPHY AND THE DEMOGRAPHIC PROCESSES

A principal theme in the human ecological literature since the publication of Hawley's *Human Ecology* (1950) is the relationship between changes in ecological and sustenance organization and the demographic processes. This owes to the already mentioned tenet of human ecology that populations redistribute themselves through fertility, mortality, and migration to maintain an equilibrium between size and opportunities for living. A basic premise is that a moving equilibrium is maintained between a population's size and the resource base from which its sustenance is drawn. The level at which a population survives is a function of this balance. According to Hawley, it is "the ratio of numbers to the opportunities for living" (1950: 149).

One thus arrives at the proposition that there is a reciprocal relationship between population size and organization for sustenance that operates through the influence of each on a population's level of living. Treating population size as dependent and sustenance organization as independent leads to the hypothesis that change in sustenance organization, to the extent that it produces change in the opportunities for living, will necessitate a change in population size. Analyses that have focused on this relationship are reviewed in this section, according to each of the three processes.

Ecological Analysis of Migration

As noted, of the three demographic processes, migration is the most efficient agent for effecting change in population size. The hypothesis often investigated in ecological studies of this genre is that variation among populations in levels of net migration is a function of differentials in sustenance organization. As particular sustenance functions in a population expand, new positions or niches are created; these niches are typically job opportunities, although other features of sustenance organization may be

---

[2] Namboodiri (1988) defines ecological demography somewhat more broadly. There is another subarea referred to as ecological demography that follows evolutionary and anthropological perspectives. For a discussion of this subject matter see Clark and Low (1991) and Low et al. (1992).

considered. Conversely, the diminution of certain sustenance functions results in a contraction of the number of niches and, hence, a reduction in the opportunities for employment. The net result of these developments, unless the effects of one cancel out those of the other, is a disturbance in the established equilibrium between population size and opportunities for living. Net migration is thus viewed as a population response, or as an effective method of returning to a condition of balance. Hawley writes that "readjustments to disequilibrium are effected primarily...through mobility. Population tends to distribute itself in relation to job opportunities, evacuating areas of diminishing opportunities and gravitating to areas of increasing opportunities" (1950: 167–168).

The ecological model is explicitly macrolevel. Ecological models of migration endeavor to recognize the characteristics of aggregates, such as countries or states/provinces, that lead to the net gain or loss of population through migration. Whereas microlevel analyses ask "Who moves and why?" ecological analyses ask "Where do migrants go and why?" Microlevel variables such as attitudes and motives do not play a role in ecological models. Psychological factors may have some effect on decisions to move, but a neglect of structural variables in order to concentrate on psychological variables overlooks the fact that attitudes and values are themselves components of behavior "and as such, should be explained rather than be used as the explanation" (Sly 1972: 616; see also Frisbie and Poston 1978b: 9). In this regard Hawley (1950: 320) writes:

> No doubt migration involves psychological elements, but it is also a manifestation of external changes. For an understanding of the general phenomenon, it is important to know not why the migrant thinks he has moved, but the conditions or characteristics common to all instances of migration and lacking in situations from which there is no migration.

An early test of this relationship is Sly's (1972) study of southern black migration from the "old cotton belt," a group of some 253 counties (with at least 25,000 acres in cotton as reported in the 1890 census) stretching in a belt from South Carolina to Texas. Migration patterns were hypothesized as responses to changes in organization, as well as in technology and the environment. Sly's ecological hypothesis was tested with data on southern black migration for the decades 1940 to 1950 and 1950 to 1960, and support was adduced for the ecological model.

Frisbie and Poston (1975) expanded on these results by noting that while there may be an overall relationship between sustenance organization and demographic behavior, the relationships will differ, depending on the particular kind of substance activity examined. They specified eight different components of sustenance organization for the nonmetropolitan counties of the U.S. in the circa-1960 time period. They hypothesized that "areas heavily dependent upon primary industry such as mining or agriculture (with the possible exception of large-scale agriculture) are likely to be population-decline areas; areas where services constitute the most significant form of sustenance activity are likely to be characterized by growing populations; areas dependent on transformation industry are expected to be intermediate in terms of growth potential" (1975: 776). Their hypotheses were upheld.

In a follow-up analysis, Frisbie and Poston (1976) hypothesized that the sustenance organizations of areas experiencing population growth in the 1960s should be more complex (that is, be characterized by more sustenance functions) than those experiencing population loss. As predicted, sustenance configurations for the growing counties were found to be more complex that those for the losing counties.

In two additional investigations that supported the ecological model, Frisbie and Poston (1978a, 1978b) investigated the relationships among sustenance organization components, sustenance differentiation, and the net migration behavior of the nonmetropolitan counties of the U.S. in the 1960 to 1970 period (see also Hirschl, Poston, and Frisbie [1998]).

Poston and White (1978) extended the above analyses by introducing a variable that mediates the association between sustenance organization and population/migration change, namely, the potential supply of labor in the population, that is, the indigenous labor force supply (see also, Pursell 1972; Bradshaw 1976; Bowles 1976). It turns out that the effect of indigenous labor force supply on migration is independent of the effects of other aspects of sustenance organization (see also Ervin [1987]).

The studies cited are but a selection of numerous investigations that have examined the extent to which migration appears to be a demographic response to changes in ecological and economic organization (cf., Gibbs 1964; Stinner and DeJong 1969; Tarver 1972; Brown 1975; 1998; 2002; Beale 1975; Fuguitt and Beale 1976; Sly and Tayman 1977; Wardwell 1977; Shin 1979; Krout 1982; London 1986, 1987; Ervin 1987; Saenz and Colberg 1988; Poston, Hirschl, and Frisbie 1991).

Ecological Analyses of Fertility and Mortality

Less prominent among human ecological studies of demographic behavior are investigations that focus on fertility and mortality. This section examines this limited literature.

An ecological explanation of fertility behavior focuses on the sustenance organization of human populations and ascertains the extent to which differences in their organizational forms and structures are related to differences in their fertility behavior.

One way of viewing this relationship involves thinking of fertility behavior as a means of increasing or decreasing the size of the population in much the same way as migration. To illustrate, the population's sustenance organization could become more complex and new positions would be created. The population would need to respond demographically and provide members to fill these niches, so that the initial equilibrium between population size and organization could be maintained.

Fertility behavior is not the most efficient demographic response because of the time lag between the creation of the new members and their eventual employment in sustenance activities. Sly writes that in the "short run, migration appears to be the most efficient response. It can increase (or decrease) population more rapidly than can changing fertility and is more efficient in that it can be more selective" (1972: 618).

It is likely that sustenance organization complexity influences fertility behavior in a different way than that just discussed. Rather than the two being related positively, they are related negatively. In the first place a high fertility pattern is dysfunctional for an increasingly complex sustenance organization because so much of the sustenance produced must be consumed directly by the population. High fertility should reduce the absolute amount of uncommitted sustenance resources, thereby limiting the population's flexibility for adapting to environmental, technological, and other kinds of changes and fluctuations. Low fertility is more consonant with the needs and requirements of an expansive sustenance organization. More sustenance would be available for investment back into the system in a low-fertility population than in a population with high fertility. Large quantities of sustenance normally consumed by the familial and educational institutions in a high-fertility population would hence be available as mobile or fluid resources in a low-fertility population. Sustenance organization in this latter instance would thus have the investment resources available for increasing complexity, given requisite changes in the environment and technology. One would thus hypothesize a negative relation between organizational complexity and fertility.

An early ecological study of fertility is Kasarda's (1971) comparative analysis of nations between 1930 and 1969. Reasoning that the level of fertility in a society should be associated with its type of sustenance organization, he investigated the degree to which female labor force participation in nonagricultural occupations, the number of unpaid family workers, and the degree of youth labor force participation served as intervening variables between the less proximate effects of industrialization, urbanization, and education. His findings suggest that most of the intervening variables are associated with fertility. Moreover, with regard to the ecological theory of fertility, he shows that the less proximate factors affect fertility through the intermediate variables (1971: 314).

In a later ecological study of fertility, London (1987) focuses on the explicitly human ecological aspects of economic development and their influences on fertility. He examines the relationship between measures of the division of labor (Gibbs and Poston 1975) and the crude birth rate among the provinces of Thailand for the 1960 to 1970 period. He hypothesizes that the greater the complexity of the division of labor, the lower the fertility. At the bivariate level he finds support for his hypothesis.

In an extension of the above analysis, London and Hadden (1989) examine the utility of three different fertility theories, namely, human ecological theory, "wealth flows" theory, and political economic theory, as explanations of fertility differentials among the provinces of Thailand. They find that "hypotheses derived from [these] three different theoretical perspectives received support ... [suggesting] that no existing 'theory' by itself can fully explain a phenomenon as complex as fertility decline" (1989: 34).

Poston and Chang (2005) use an ecological model and other theoretical perspectives in their study of female and male fertility rates among the counties of Taiwan in 1995. Their ecological model focuses on ecological organization; they reason that the more complex the organization, the lower the fertility. The ecological model works as expected in explaining variation in female fertility rates but does not do as well in accounting for male fertility differences among the counties.

A review of the literature of ecological demography finds several analyses of mortality (for example, Gibbs 1959; Davis 1963; Friedlander 1969). The study by Gibbs (1959) of the relationship between changes in mortality and fertility and changes in sustenance organization is representative of this genre. He is interested in ascertaining whether human populations avoid an increase in mortality by reducing their fertility when confronted with organizational changes leading to decreases in sustenance. He examines changes in the crude death and birth rates for 45 countries circa 1921 to 1937 (the years of worldwide economic depression). His expectations are generally supported by the data.

Having reviewed relevant literature in ecological demography, the next section focuses explicitly on migration and endeavors to illustrate how demographic studies of internal migration can be theoretically informed by the rubrics of the ecological complex: organization, population, technology, and environment. Each of the rubrics is discussed separately.

FOUR HUMAN ECOLOGICAL CONCEPTS
AND THE ANALYSIS OF MIGRATION

This section[3] discusses the conceptual and theoretical development of the four rubrics of the ecological system and proposes the kinds of relationships anticipated between each and population change due to internal migration.

Organization

It is not an overstatement to say that organization is the fundamental element of the subject matter of human ecology. This is so because it is social organization that mediates the balance between population size, growth, and distribution and the natural environment upon which it depends (Micklin 1973). Human ecology is concerned with the organizational aspects of human populations arising from their sustenance-producing activities (Frisbie and Poston 1978b: 14). In fact, the two broad goals of human ecology are to establish (1) the causes and (2) the consequences of particular characteristics of sustenance organization in human populations (Gibbs and Martin 1959: 33). The latter goal is of particular importance in ecological analyses of migration.

There is major agreement regarding the centrality of organization within human ecology (Duncan 1959; Hawley 1950; Gibbs and Martin 1959; Micklin 1973; Poston, Frisbie and Micklin 1984; Namboodiri 1994; Poston and Frisbie 1998). However, despite its central position in human ecology and in the ecological theory of migration, the idea of sustenance organization was for decades in a primitive state of development both conceptually and empirically. Indeed, most of the research on sustenance organization that ecologists conducted in the 1950s and 1960s treats the concept as if it referred solely to the division of labor. This occurs even though there is little in the extant theoretical treatments of the concept to warrant such a limitation.

The notion of organization in human ecology is multifaceted. Attention here will thus be directed to some of the characteristics of sustenance organization and will suggest their relationships with migration. A major dimension of sustenance organization involves what Hawley refers to as the "arrangement of differentiated parts suited to the performance of a given function or set of functions" (1950: 178). This is sustenance differentiation, i.e., the extent to which the population is differentiated in its sustenance activity.

Sustenance differentiation consists of two elements: (1) the number of activities and (2) the degree of uniformity in the distribution of the population across the activities. A high degree of sustenance differentiation obtains when there is a relatively large number of activities characterizing the population and when the population members are evenly distributed across these activities (Gibbs and Poston 1975). Scholars since Durkheim (1893 [1960]) have included this dimension as a major component of the division of labor. There are many measures of sustenance differentiation, six of which have been elaborated by Gibbs and Poston (1975).

A positive relationship is expected to obtain between sustenance differentiation and migration. Increases in sustenance differentiation should result in an expansion in the

---

[3] This section draws in part on materials in Poston and Frisbie (1998).

number of ecological niches, so that the original balance between population size and life chances must be reestablished, with net in-migration serving as the most efficient mechanism. One would hypothesize that the greater the degree of sustenance differentiation, the greater the population growth attributable to migration.

Another dimension of sustenance organization is functional interdependence; it can be combined with sustenance differentiation to form the other side of the division of labor (Gibbs and Poston 1975). The degree of functional interdependence in a population depends on (1) the number of exchange linkages, (2) the variety of products involved, and (3) the volume of exchange flows (Eberstein and Frisbie 1982). Empirical indicators of functional interdependence are often based on commodity-flow data. It is reasonable to assume that the greater the degree of involvement of an area in the society-wide web of interdependence, the more that area will be a major point of confluence for goods, services, and financial resources, all of which should lead to an expansion of the population via migration.

A third dimension of sustenance organization is the volume of sustenance produced by the population, i.e., the degree of productivity of the particular configuration of sustenance activities. Research on U.S. migration patterns (Poston and Frisbie 1984) uses data from the censuses of business and agriculture to tap five aspects of sustenance productivity: retail services productivity, wholesale services productivity, personal services productivity, agricultural productivity, and mining productivity. How should each component be related to net migration? Although these are only five examples of a larger number of components of sustenance organization, discussion of them and their linkages with migration illustrates the applicability of sustenance components in ecological analyses of migration.

It may be hypothesized that productivity in retail services is positively related to migration, because growth in retail services is often linked closely to employment growth and associated economic opportunities. Consequently, areas that are highly productive of retail sustenance should be characterized by in-migration. In contrast, areas with significant amounts of wholesale sustenance productivity are expected to have more out-migration than in-migration, because increases in wholesale volume need not necessarily be associated with increases in employment in wholesaling. Frisbie and Poston (1978b: 50) write that "wholesalers may be able to absorb expanding business by the addition of a comparatively few employees, accompanied by a much greater degree of mechanization."

Similarly, areas high in personal services productivity should be characterized more by net losses due to migration. Included among personal services are amusement and recreation services and hotel and motel employment. Services that support recreation and leisure time activities may be linked to economic opportunities, especially in areas that offer amenities such as a mild climate (Kasarda 1980). However, personal services occupations are often low-paying, so there is no necessary reason to expect a positive effect on migration (Poston 1981: 146).

A positive relationship should exist, however, between agricultural productivity and migration. Agricultural productivity is usually measured as the dollar amount of agricultural products marketed per farm with sales above a particular amount, say, $10,000 or $25,000. Accordingly, areas "in which commercial agriculture is pursued successfully [can be expected to] enjoy an expansion of job opportunities [and positive net migration] as a complex of ancillary agribusiness establishments develops" (Frisbie and Poston 1978b: 48–49). Therefore, unlike the frequently demonstrated negative relationship between small-scale agricultural activity and net migration, in this case one would expect a positive association.

The last sustenance productivity variable is mining. A negative association is expected with net migration because of the reduced demand for labor in an extractive industry such as mining (which typically comprises metal, bituminous coal, and lignite mining, as well as oil and gas extraction), once such areas are past the initial exploration and "boom" stage (Frisbie and Poston 1978b: 46).

A fourth dimension of sustenance organization is the degree of efficiency of the sustenance organization. Given the level of sustenance produced, how efficiently does this occur? How much effort is required to produce the sustenance, whatever its volume? Ideally, such a variable would be operationalized by developing a ratio of the amount of sustenance produced to the amount of energy consumed in the production process. Unfortunately, data of this type are not available below the national level. In earlier research Poston and Frisbie (1984) examined the efficiency of the manufacturing component, operationalized as the value added by manufacturing per manufacturing establishment. The numerator reflects the dollar value of the shipments after accounting for the manufacturing inputs. As conceptualized and operationalized, manufacturing efficiency is more capital intensive than labor intensive. Almost by definition, the greater the efficiency, the less the requirement for personnel inputs. Accordingly, one would hypothesize that the relationship between manufacturing efficiency and net migration is inverse.

A final structural characteristic or dimension of sustenance organization is the degree to which population members are engaged in sustenance-related pursuits (Poston and Johnson 1971; Martin and Poston 1972, 1976). What patterns of utilization of population members characterize the organization of one ecological unit versus another, especially with regard to ascribed statuses? How fully realized are the potential contributions of population members? To what extent do inequalities exist in the population by ascribed statuses? The degree to which populations differentiate by ascribed statuses in allocating sustenance roles to their members is an important dimension of sustenance organization, especially if the analyst is interested in sustenance productivity and other input-related functions.

To some extent, differentiation by ascribed, rather than achieved, status may have a direct effect on the likelihood of an area's gain or loss due to net migration. This is most likely when the focus is on race- or sex-specific migration, because if issues of ascribed status significantly affect the distribution of workers across employment categories, they may act as a deterrent to the in-movement of minorities and females. On a more general level, if an unreasonable reliance on ascribed status as an allocative mechanism undermines the most productive use of labor, sustenance productivity will be negatively affected, which, in turn, will inhibit movement into the area. Conversely, in Saudi Arabia and other Middle Eastern countries, female labor is very limited and results in very heavy immigration of expatriate labor.

Population

It goes without saying that of the four ecological concepts, population is the most advanced in terms of conceptual and operational detail. This is easily understood since an entire specialization, demography, is devoted to the study of population characteristics and dynamics (see many of the chapters in this *Handbook*). However, with few exceptions (Poston and White 1978; Frisbie and Poston 1978b; Namboodiri 1994), ecologists seldom examine dimensions of the population as influences on population redistribution. Yet it is well known from demographic research that such population variables as age, race, and sex composition have predictable effects on net migration (see chapter 1, "Age and Sex," in this *Handbook*).

In an earlier section of this chapter, attention was directed to the research of Poston and White (1978) introducing the need to consider the size of the potential labor force already in the population as a mediating influence of the relationship between other ecological variables and migration.

In other research on nonmetropolitan migration, Frisbie and Poston (1978b) examine the extent to which demographic variables such as racial composition and age structure influence migration, despite the already demonstrated relationships between various components of sustenance organization and nonmetropolitan net migration. They suggest that if, "as seems to be the case from available evidence, blacks continue to leave nonmetropolitan areas where historically the minority was heavily concentrated, and if whites are not apt to move to these areas in numbers great enough to offset the loss of blacks, it would appear plausible to hypothesize an inverse relationship between percent nonwhite and net migration change" (Frisbie and Poston 1978b: 67). Regarding age structure, they note that numerous nonmetropolitan counties with many elderly residents grow through net migration. However, despite the prevalence of these "retirement" counties, they hypothesize that "one would expect a negative relationship between median age and net migration for no other reason than the fact that migration is selective of young adults" (Frisbie and Poston 1978b: 68). Their analyses supported both hypotheses.

Technology

Of the four basic ecological categories, technology is the most critical for the adaptation of human populations. Lenski (1970: 102–103) writes that technology is the "prime mover" in the process of social change and adaptation for at least three reasons: (1) it sets the boundaries for feasible social and economic options; (2) technological change appears to be more easily accepted by the population than change in organization or ideology; (3) it is "easier to compare the effects of alternative tools or techniques than it is to compare the effects of alternative systems of social organization or alternative ideologies" (Lenski 1970: 102).

The concept is prominent in ecological and other macrolevel sociological theories. And there is a consensus in definitions of technology. Frisbie and Clarke (1979:593) note the following:

> A fair degree of convergence is evident in efforts to theoretically circumscribe the concept. Lenski (1970: 37) defines technology as 'the information, techniques, and tools by means of which men utilize the material resources of their environment.' Similarly, Sjoberg (1965: 214) describes technology as 'the tools, the sources of energy and the knowledge connected with the use of both tools and energy that a social system employs.' On a slightly less abstract level and using somewhat different terminology, Ogburn (1955: 383) conceives of technology as the 'kinds of capital equipment, quantity of capital goods, manner and use of non-human resources, scientific discovery, invention (and) machines.' Finally, Duncan notes that the 'concept of

"technology" in human ecology refers not merely to a complex of art and artifact ... but to a set of techniques employed by a population to gain sustenance from its environment and to facilitate the organization of sustenance-producing activity' (1959: 682).

Three dimensions figure prominently in the above definitions: material features (tools, capital equipment, machines); information (knowledge, techniques, scientific discovery); and energy. These are the same three ecosystem "commodity" flows that Duncan (1964) identifies as basic to the survival of populations. However, the problem with trying to apply these three dimensions to national subareas, such as counties, states, or provinces, is that, like the larger concept of technology of which these are a part, the dimensions have been conceived at the societal level of analysis. It is difficult to contend that the level of technology, as just defined, varies in any significant way at the subsocietal level. For example, not all county populations make use of the same tools, techniques, and information, but the technology available, while its actual application may be concentrated in a few areas, tends to have a society-wide impact in urban industrial nations. In a sense, then, the level of technology is a constant for population groups such as the counties, states, or provinces of countries. The fact that one county might differ from another in its energy consumption per capita, or in regard to some other measure of technology, is due not so much to differentials in levels of, or access to, technology, as from variations in climate, natural resources, and social organization that require or make feasible the application of given technologies. Thus, at the subsocietal level it is necessary to focus primarily on particular applications of technology that bear directly on the substantive question of interest, rather than on the level or availability of technology.

Scholars have given only minimal attention to the issue of empirically applying the technology component of the ecological complex to the study of populations below the societal level. As a consequence, there are few guidelines to suggest even a point of departure in specifying particular technological applications with significant consequences for migration patterns. An exception is the strategy followed by Sly (1972) in his study of black male migration from southern cotton-belt counties. In that research, Sly brings the technological dimension to bear in highly specific terms by incorporating into his analysis particular technological variables (viz., farm gasoline consumption and the use of tractors) that could be expected to have an impact on the particular population of interest. The implication is that in attempting to explain variations in migration among counties, it is necessary to narrow the focus to those specific technological factors that bear directly or indirectly on the ability of counties to attract population.

A first approximation toward conceptualization may be made by noting that one of the long-recognized technological keys to the establishment and growth of population aggregates is the presence and development of adequate transportation facilities. More than 100 years ago, Cooley (1894 [1930: 75–83]) observed that population and wealth will tend to come together wherever there is a break or an interruption in routes of transportation. The development of transportation facilities partially determines industrial concentration and influences the expansion of local populations (Hawley 1981). Since the availability of transportation is a major determinant of the ease of access of a population to its environment, a population's ability to compete with other populations, and the efficiency of sustenance extraction, the first dimension of technology to be considered should involve mobility facilitating technology.

Two empirical indicators of this dimension of technology are the presence of an interstate highway crossing a county (or state or province) and the intersection in the area of two or more interstate highways. While these measures may be "obvious," the obviousness of their influence does not imply either triviality or simplicity of effect. In fact, there is a large literature that testifies both to the importance and complexity of the impact of interstate arteries on subarea population change in general and change due to migration in particular (Dickinson 1964; Wheat 1969; Gauthier 1970; Fuguitt and Beale 1976; Briggs 1980; Lichter and Fuguitt 1980).

Although there is some disagreement regarding the actual magnitude of the effects of interstate highways on population redistribution and net migration, most theoretical discussions point to a positive relationship that may be indirect as well as direct. Briggs (1980) presents a rationale underlying the expectation of a relationship between the presence of interstate highway crossings and intersections and net migration. He finds that the interstate highway system facilitates the total amount of movement by lowering the time-cost of travel and "channels this movement along fewer paths" (1980: 22), thereby favoring those areas which lie at the intersection of these paths. One would also expect that major highways will have an indirect effect, because they "give impetus to fundamental changes in the sustenance organization or economic activity [especially] in non-metropolitan areas, resulting in a demographic response, namely, in-migration" (Lichter and Fuguitt 1980: 494). One reason for anticipating a positive effect on net migration is that interstate highway links stimulate local economies as services develop to serve travelers (Briggs 1980), as industry finds it possible to locate or expand in these more easily accessible places, and as local market expansion is facilitated (Lichter and Fuguitt 1980).

Research based on the theories of McKenzie, Hawley, and other ecologists shows that centrality in the airline network of the United States has effects that parallel those found with respect to interstate highways. Although not focusing specifically on net migration, the work of Irwin and Kasarda demonstrates that being a hub in the airline network is significantly related to employment growth in metropolitan areas, and "that changes in network position are a cause rather than a consequence of this employment growth" (Irwin and Kasarda 1991: 524).

A second kind of technological application deals with the acquisition of sustenance. At a minimum, ecologists need to develop indicators of this dimension that reflect technological inputs affecting both primary and transformative sustenance activities. One such set of indicators indexes those features of agricultural technology that previous research shows to affect county net-migration patterns.

It is commonplace to assume that areas for which agricultural enterprise constitutes a major economic base are apt to experience migration losses as agricultural production becomes increasingly mechanized and productive and capital intensive. However, previous research demonstrates that (1) where production is highly land intensive or (2) where large volume and capital-intensive production of food and fiber predominate, positive net migration is a likely outcome (Frisbie and Poston 1978b). The explanation of these findings is, in the first instance, that highly land-intensive agriculture has also tended to be labor intensive, and the greater the number of persons who can be productively engaged per land unit, the greater the likelihood of population growth due to migration. In the second case, capital-intensive, commercial agriculture, which corresponds neither to the land-intensive nor land-extensive type of utilization but which involves large volume and heavily mechanized production, creates an expansion of job opportunities and, thus, positive net migration as a complex of ancillary agribusiness establishments develop. It is also reasonable to assume that large-volume producers will be more likely to require full-time labor, which with respect to both the number of workers and their skill level, is beyond the resources of small-scale "family" agricultural enterprise.

A useful measure of technological inputs into the first type, i.e., land-intensive production, is tons of fertilizer applied per acre farmed. In the case of large-scale, commercial agriculture, an important indicator of applied technology is expenditures on machinery per acre. In regard to both of these "application-specific" technology measures, the argument suggests a positive relationship with migration.

Perhaps the most obvious operationalization of agricultural technology is expenditures on gasoline and petroleum products per farm. At first glance, one might expect that this variable also would be related positively to population growth due to migration. However, areas with high expenditures on gasoline and petroleum consumed in farm production are likely areas specializing in land-extensive agriculture. Frisbie and Poston (1978b) observe that this type of activity has to do mainly with the production of livestock on rangeland often incapable of generating a crop directly available for human consumption. Such land is productive principally "because ruminants are able to convert forage to meat or milk and the land area required per animal unit is likely to be quite large ... in areas devoted to ranching ... [And in this type of environmental setting] less labor is needed to make optimum use of rangeland than is involved in growing crops" (Frisbie and Poston 1978b: 48). Consequently, counties in which land-extensive, agricultural technology contributes significantly to sustenance extraction are unlikely to provide substantial employment opportunities. Such areas are thus expected to experience population decline via net out-migration. Accordingly, one would hypothesize that a negative association should exist between expenditures on gas and petroleum per farm and migration.

Regarding the transformative component of sustenance acquisition, a useful indicator of the employment of available technology is new capital expenditures. These include expenditures "for permanent additions and major alterations to manufacturers' operating plants, as well as for new machinery and equipment purchases that were chargeable to fixed-asset accounts, ... Expenditures include the cost of plant equipment for replacement purposes, as well as for additions to productive capacity" (U.S. Bureau of Census 1978: xliii). Not included are costs of land, mineral rights, maintenance, or repairs.

Thus, new capital expenditures will index at least the hardware and capital-equipment dimension of technology in the manufacturing sector, i.e., the capital goods, equipment, and machines that figure prominently in the definitions of technology cited above. Of course, it is possible that capital may be substituted for labor, so that high levels of new capital expended might well mean a leveling off, if not an outright reduction in, local employment opportunities. If so, the absolute magnitude of capital expenditures is expected to be inversely related to migration. Indeed, precisely such a zero-order negative association with net migration is observed in counties of the South in research by Poston and Frisbie (1984).

Finally, it is noted that the causal direction of the relationship between new capital investments and migration may be a matter for debate. For example, if firms in the manufacturing sector correctly anticipate that future labor costs will be insupportably high, new capital expenditures aimed at substituting for labor might result. One reason for expecting higher labor costs is out-migration. However, it is not clear that such a sequence of events is at all probable. In fact, Hawley argues that "migration flows from

areas of low rates of capital investment to areas of high rates of capital investment"
(Hawley 1950: 330). Hence, one should anticipate a positive relationship between net
migration and the rate of new capital expenditures with the predominant causal path
being from the latter variable to the former.

Environment

In human ecological terms, the environment is defined as "whatever is external to and
potentially or actually influential on a phenomenon under investigation" (Hawley 1968:
330). The concept of environment occupies a central position in the general theoretical
framework of human ecology mainly because the environment is the ultimate source of
sustenance for a population (Hawley 1968: 330). However, little empirical research in
sociological human ecology takes the environment directly into account, perhaps
because of its breadth. That is, by definition, the environment "has no fixed content
and must be defined anew for each different object of investigation" (Hawley 1968:
330). In fact, some hold that the environment is the "least well conceptualized of the
variables constituting the ecological complex" (Berry and Kasarda 1977: 14).

However, close scrutiny of the ecological treatment of the environment reveals an
implicit specificity not apparent in the above general definition. The environment
comprises not everything external to the phenomenon of interest, but only those
externalities that, by virtue of the limits they set on the acquisition of sustenance, affect
the life chances of an organized population with a given technological repertoire. In
other words, "the environment is viewed as a set of limiting conditions, which may be
narrow or broad, depending upon the technological devices and modes of organization
that prevail in a given population" (Schnore 1958: 628; see also Michelson [1970: 24–
25]). Therefore, the human ecologist must logically narrow the arena of inquiry to those
factors that, in light of existing technology, serve as limiting (or enabling) resources for
the adaptation and growth of populations. The following paragraphs are intended to
further sharpen this focus. It will be useful first to describe the sort of factors that are
not included under the environmental rubric.

It is apparent that the outcomes of a population's organizational and technological
operations on the environment and the adaptations or maladaptations thereby achieved
often have been mistaken for the environment itself. Consequently, indicators of the
state of a population's life chances, or quality of life, sometimes have been loosely
categorized as "environmental." With such a definition of the environment, one might
include such things as the prevalence of crime and other deviant activities, mortality and
morbidity rates, unemployment rates, industrial structures, levels of education and
income, and so forth. For example, one often hears that some environments are more
violent or criminal than others. In the same way, one might speak of a political or
economic or cultural environment or "climate." Regardless of the stylistic elegance of
such phrases, this indulgence in metaphor quickly and easily destroys the precision
required in empirical analysis. Put differently, the issue is much more than merely
semantic, since the logical result leads to the conclusion that everything is the
environment, except the population under study.

Therefore, it is not useful to consider social and economic activities (or aberrations)
of local populations to be part of their environment. Certain of these activities, for
example, employment in given industries, are best viewed as aspects of ecological

organization. Others, such as crime and deviance, rates of mortality and morbidity, unemployment, education, and income levels, are best conceived as indicators of different aspects of life chances that emerge from a population's organized efforts to adapt to the environment. In a very real sense, the latter variables tend to indicate the degree of success or failure of the adaptive process. In short, they may reveal a disequilibrium between population and life chances. As such, they should be useful in helping to account for variation in migration and thus should be included in models designed to explain migration. But they should not be conceptualized as aspects of the environment.

Inevitably, efforts to circumscribe a concept involve decisions of both exclusion and inclusion. To this point, discussion has concentrated on the types of factors that should be excluded from the environmental rubric. Attention is now directed to those factors that may reasonably be included within the bounds of the concept of the environment. Although a certain degree of arbitrariness is unavoidable in setting conceptual boundaries, such circumscription is necessary for orderly analysis.

Despite the difficulties that arise in attempts to give conceptual and operational substance to the concept, it is clear that the ecological environment has two broad and distinct dimensions: the physical and the social. Hawley writes:

> Environment ... includes not only the physical and biotic elements of an occupied area but also the influences that emanate from other organized populations in the same and in other areas. In certain circumstances the latter acquire a more critical importance than the former (1981: 9).

Specifically, Hawley has distinguished two dimensions, the biophysical and the ecumenic. The "former includes physiographic features, climate, soil characteristics, plant and animal life, mineral and other materials," and so forth. In contrast, the ecumenic refers to the "ecosystems or cultures possessed by peoples in adjacent areas and beyond" (Hawley 1986: 14).

Attention is first directed to these broad typological considerations and then toward finer-grained distinctions. The physical environment, of course, refers to such things as climate, natural resources, and topography. In addition, one may distinguish aspects of the man-made physical environment (Michelson 1970: 1976), such as types of buildings and other physical structures. The social, or in Hawley's words, the ecumenic, environment refers to other populations and organizations that influence the populations being investigated.

Cross-sectional analyses have found certain climatological aspects of the physical environment to be associated with population redistribution (Poston and Mao 1996, 1998; Poston and Musgrave 1999; Walther and Poston 2004). Measures pertaining to temperature have been key in these and related considerations of climate; sometimes temperature serves as the only consideration (Karp and Kelly 1971; Graves 1980; Poston and Mao 1996; 1998). A temperature index typically involves the measurement of average daily temperature during a cold month such as January, or a warm month such as July; the two measurements are highly related (Poston and Musgrave 1999).

In recent research, Poston, Gotcher, and Gu (2004) analyze the states of the United States regarding the effects of physical climate on three migration rates for the 1995 to 2000 period, namely, in-migration, out-migration, and net migration. They gather data on 11 climate variables and use factor analysis to reduce them to the three dimensions of temperature, humidity, and wind. They show that the temperature and humidity dimensions are significantly associated with one or more of the three migration rates.

They also show that the effects on migration of the climate variables are sustained even after controlling for the effects on migration of factors dealing with ecological organization, the social environment, and population.

The above analyses are cross-sectional. When undertaking longitudinal investigations of changes in migration, a logical difficulty emerges. The climate of any area changes very slowly and over extremely long periods of time. Thus, while there may be some year-to-year fluctuations in temperature or rainfall in analytical units such as counties, states, or provinces of a country, climate is, for all practical purposes, invariant. To employ change in climate as a substantive explanation of population change due to migration in, for example, a one- or two-decade interval amounts to attempting to explain variation with a constant.

Although measures of the physical climate have been shown to have some utility in cross-sectional studies of migration, it is also useful to draw on natural environmental factors that show more temporal variation when affected by technology and organization. Thus, playing an important role in the measurement of the physical environment should be variables such as air quality (e.g., mean levels of suspended particulates of sulphur dioxide), mean annual inversion frequency, and a water quality index (Liu 1976).

There are also aspects of the man-made physical environment that may affect both net and gross migration patterns. Foremost is the availability and nature of housing stock, although one may debate the direction of the causal influence. That is, one might argue that population growth is a cause rather than a consequence of the construction of housing. However, evidence from the sociological literature suggests the primary causal flow to be from new housing to population change and not vice versa. To illustrate, regarding suburban growth, Guest (1978: 254) concludes that "population growth is primarily determined by the creation of new additional housing units." And Marshall (1979: 991) suggests "that population redistribution is largely a function of the redistribution of dwelling units," a conclusion congruent with research by Schnore (1965), Duncan, Sabagh, and Van Arsdol (1962), Guest (1973), and Krivo and Frisbie (1982).

Regarding the social, or ecumenic, environment, two entities have substantial influence. First, the ecological linkages of sustenance exchange are mediated and controlled through large, dominant metropolitan centers, a finding that has been shown to obtain in the United States and in China (Vance and Sutker 1954; Duncan et al. 1960; Poston, Tian, and Jia 1990; Poston and Gu 1993). Although usually applied mainly to urban areas, one can argue that no section of large industrialized countries is isolated from metropolitan influence (Hawley 1971). Indeed, the factor "most frequently demonstrated to be related to changes in the number of inhabitants of counties, as well as cities, is that of propinquity to large urban centers" (Frisbie and Poston 1975: 780; see also Fuguitt and Thomas 1966, Fuguitt 1971, DeAre and Poston 1973, Frisbie and Martin 1973). Virtually all prior research leads to the conclusion of a positive effect on migration of an area's proximity to a metropolitan area. Several measures of the latter variable are available. Size and proximity to the nearest metropolitan area, as measured by an index of proximity developed by Hathaway and his colleagues (1968), are used as one indicator. An alternative operationalization, construction of a dummy variable scored 1 if the area is adjacent to a metropolitan area and 0 if not, is also relevant.

McCarthy and Morrison (1979) find convincing evidence of the significance of urban influence on population change in general and migration in particular. They note

618

Dudley L. Poston, Jr. and W. Parker Frisbie

that a nonmetropolitan county might be affected by the commuting of local population to metropolitan centers as well as by "urban influence" per se. Urban influence may be interpreted in two different, but interrelated, senses: (1) the economic and organizational dominance of metropolitan areas adjacent to the county and (2) the influence of urban populations within the county. After careful examination and comparison of the relationship between commuting and information on counties' adjacency to metropolitan areas, McCarthy and Morrison conclude that "knowing a county is not adjacent to a metropolitan area is tantamount to knowing that very few of its residents commute to metropolitan labor markets" (1979: 23).

Of course, population aggregates and organizations other than those immediately adjacent to the geographical unit of analysis may also exercise a social environmental, or ecumenic, influence, as understood by human ecologists. Hence, a second social environmental influence on geographical units is that emanating from extra-local, especially federal, governments. For instance, a generally positive relationship is expected between the proportion of the area's population employed by the government and population change due to migration, if for no other reason than the job opportunities associated with this extra-local source of employment. With regard to another measure of government influence, the proportion of local revenue attributable to governmental sources, it is also reasonable to expect a positive relationship with migration, because increased extramural revenues should lead to a general improvement of quality of life. Conversely, there is growing evidence that significant numbers of persons have begun to migrate from places where extensive governmental services are provided at least partly because of the heavy influence of government in their daily lives and the higher taxes associated with provision of those services (Kasarda 1980). Areas in which federal monies constitute a disproportionately large share of local revenues are apt to be depressed areas incapable of generating sufficient funds for their own maintenance. Under either interpretation, areas with high levels of federal governmental revenue inputs would not appear to be attractive destinations for migrants. Thus, it is plausible to expect that high levels of federal employment should be associated with positive migration change, while federal revenue proportions have an opposite effect.

CONCLUSION

This chapter has several objectives: (1) to provide a general outline of the ecological orientation; (2) to distinguish human ecology from ecological demography; (3) to discuss and review the explicit focus of ecological demography, namely, the application of human ecological theory to empirical investigations of the demographic processes; and (4) to show the importance and relevance of human ecology specifically for the study of the demographic process of migration.

It was necessary to first set out the general orientation of sociological human ecology, mainly because of the fact that even today, despite the immense number of publications providing evidence to the contrary, the field is still misunderstood by many sociologists and social scientists to be either a descriptive exercise or any kind of aggregate analysis. It was shown in the first and second sections of this chapter that some still believe that human ecology represents spatial or aggregate investigations of human phenomena. This representation minimizes considerably the rich sociological context of human ecology and indicates misunderstanding, perhaps even ignorance, of its orientation and subject matter.

The broad theoretical purview of human ecology has been distinguished from the narrower focus of ecological demography. Human ecology is concerned with the organizational aspects of human populations that arise from their sustenance producing activities. For the purposes of this chapter, it was noted that human ecology offers demography a specific aggregate perspective for the analysis of the demographic processes. The third section reviewed in detail the relevant literature of ecological demography.

The final section of the chapter outlined and articulated the theoretical and empirical ties between one demographic process, net migration, and the four basic referential constructs of population, organization, environment, and technology. In a review of the empirical and theoretical literature spanning more than five decades, it was shown that demographic models of migration benefit from use of the ecological per-spective. Accentuated were the explicitly sociological features of the ecological perspec-tive in a demonstration of its fruitful employment in demographic investigations. The strictly spatial studies that so many have thought to be ecological not only are not ecological, they are usually not sociological. Moreover, they are theoretically lacking and are of little utility for demographic investigations.

It is the contention of this chapter that human ecology holds great potential for informing demographic study, particularly if it maintains its sociological emphasis on sustenance organization. We believe that the materials presented and developed here support such a conclusion.

REFERENCES

Alihan, M. A. *Social ecology: A critical analysis.* 1938. New York: Columbia University Press.

Beale, C. L. 1975. The revival of population growth in nonmetropolitan America. USDA Economic Research Service, ERS-605.

Berry, B. J. L., and J. D. Kasarda. 1977. *Contemporary urban ecology.* New York: Macmillan.

Berry, B. J. L., and P. H. Rees. 1969. The factorial ecology of Calcutta. *American Journal of Sociology* 74: 445–491.

Bowles, G. K. 1976. Potential change in the labor force in the 1970–1980 decade for metropolitan and nonmetropolitan counties in the United States. *Phylon* 37: 263–269.

Bradshaw, B. S. 1976. Potential labor force supply, replacement, and migration of Mexican American and other males in the Texas-Mexico border region. *International Migration Review* 10: 29–45.

Briggs, R. 1980. *The impact of interstate highway system on nonmetropolitan growth,* Final Report. Washing-ton, D.C.: U.S. Department of Transportation.

Brown, D. L. 1975. Socioeconomic characteristics of growing and declining metropolitan counties, 1970. USDA Economic Research Service, ERS-306.

Brown, D. L. 1998. Enhancing the spatial policy framework with ecological analysis. In *Continuities in sociological human ecology.* Edited by M. Micklin and D. L. Poston, Jr., 195–213. New York: Plenum Press.

Brown, D. L. 2002. Migration and community: Social networks in a multilevel world. *Rural Sociology* 67: 1–23.

Castells, M. 1979. *The urban question: A Marxist approach.* Cambridge, Mass.: MIT Press.

Clark, A. L., and B. S. Low. 1991. Testing evolutionary hypotheses with demographic data. *Population and Development Review* 27: 633–660.

Cooley, C. H. 1894 [1930]. The theory of transportation. In *Sociological theory and social research.* Edited by R. C. Angell, 75–83. New York: Holt, Rinehart, and Winston.

Davis, K. 1963. The theory of change and response in modern demographic history. *Population Index* 29: 345–366.

DeAre, D., and D. L. Poston, Jr. 1973. Texas population in 1970: Trends and variations in the populations of nonmetropolitan towns. *Texas Business Review* 47: 1–6.

Dickinson, R. E. 1964. *City and region.* London: Routledge & Kegan Paul.

Duncan, B., G. Sabagh, and M. Van Arsdol. 1962. Patterns of city growth. *American Journal of Sociology* 67: 418–429.

Duncan, O. D. 1959. Human ecology and population studies. In *The study of population.* Edited by P. M. Hauser and O. D. Duncan, 678–716. Chicago: University of Chicago Press.

Duncan, O. D. 1961. From social system to ecosystem. *Sociological Inquiry* 31: 140–149.

Duncan, O. D. 1964. Social organization and the ecosystem. In *Handbook of modern sociology.* Edited by R. E. L. Faris, 37–82. Chicago: Rand-McNally.

Duncan, O. D., R. W. Scott, S. Lieberson, B. Duncan, and H. H. Winsborough. 1960. *Metropolis and region.* Baltimore: Johns Hopkins Press.

Durkheim, E. 1893 [1960]. *The division of labor in society.* New York: The Free Press.

Eberstein, I. W., and W. P. Frisbie. 1982. Metropolitan function and interdependence in the U.S. urban system. *Social Forces* 60: 676–700.

Encyclopedia Britannica, 15th ed., Vol. 14. 1988. Chicago: Encyclopedia Britannica.

Ervin, D. J. 1987. The ecological theory of migration: Reconceptualizing indigenous labor force. *Social Science Quarterly* 68: 866–875.

Firey, W. 1945. Sentiment and symbolism as ecological variables. *American Sociological Review* 10: 140–148.

Frank, P. W. 1959. Ecology and Demography. In *The Study of Population.* Edited by P. M. Hanser and O. D. Duncan, 652–677. Chicago: University of Chicago Press.

Friedlander, D. 1969. Demographic responses and population change. *Demography* 6: 359–381.

Frisbie, W. P., and C. J. Clarke. Technology in evolutionary and ecological perspective: Theory and measurement of the societal level. *Social Forces* 58: 591–613.

Frisbie, W. P., and W. A. Martin. 1973. Texas population in 1970: Trends in county population gain and loss. *Texas Business Review* 47: 188–196.

Frisbie, W. P., and D. L. Poston, Jr. 1975. Components of sustenance organization and nonmetropolitan population change: A human ecological investigation. *American Sociological Review* 40: 773–784.

Frisbie, W. P., and D. L. Poston, Jr. 1976. The structure of sustenance organization and population change in nonmetropolitan America. *Rural Sociology* 41: 354–370.

Frisbie, W. P., and D. L. Poston, Jr. 1978a. Sustenance differentiation and population redistribution. *Social Forces* 57: 42–56.

Frisbie, W. P., and D. L. Poston, Jr. 1978b. *Sustenance organization and migration in nonmetropolitan America.* Iowa City: Iowa Urban Community Research Center, University of Iowa.

Fuguitt, G. V. 1971. The places left behind: Population trends and policy for rural America. *Rural Sociology* 36: 449–470.

Fuguitt, G. V., and C. L. Beale. 1976. Population change in nonmetropolitan cities and towns. USDA Economic Research Service, AER-323.

Fuguitt, G. V., and D. W. Thomas. 1966. Small town growth in the United States: An analysis by size, class and by place. *Demography* 3: 513–527.

Gauthier, H. L. 1970. Geography, transportation, and regional development. *Economic Geography* 46: 612–619.

Gettys, W. E. 1940. Human ecology and social theory. *Social Forces* 18: 469–476.

Gibbs, J. P. 1959. Demographic adjustment to a decrease in sustenance. *Pacific Sociological Review* 2: 61–66.

Gibbs, J. P. 1964. A note on industry changes and migration. *American Sociological Review* 29: 266–270.

Gibbs, J. P., and W. T. Martin. 1959. Toward a theoretical system of human ecology. *Pacific Sociological Review* 2: 29–36.

Gibbs, J. P., and D. L. Poston, Jr. 1975. The division of labor: Conceptualization and related measures. *Social Forces* 53: 468–476.

Graves, P. E. 1980. Migration and climate. *Journal of Regional Science* 20: 227–237.

Guest, A. M. 1973. Urban growth and population densities. *Demography* 10: 53–70.

Guest, A. M. 1978. Suburban social status: Persistence or evolution? *American Sociological Review* 43: 251–264.

Haeckel, E. 1876. *The history of creation, or, the development of the earth and its inhabitants by the action of natural causes: A popular exposition of the doctrine of evolution in general, and of that of Darwin, Goethe and Lamarck in particular.* Translated from the German by E. R. Lankester. London: Henry S. King & Co.

Hathaway, D. E., J. A. Beegle, and W. K. Bryant. 1968. *People of rural America*. Washington, D.C.: U.S. Government Printing Office.

Hawley, A. H. 1950. *Human ecology: A theory of community structure*. New York: Ronald Press.

Hawley, A. H. 1968. Human ecology. In *International encyclopedia of the social sciences*. Edited by D. L. Sills, 328–337. New York: Crowell, Collier and Macmillan.

Hawley, A. H. 1971. *Urban society*. New York: Ronald Press.

Hawley, A. H. 1981. Human ecology: Persistence and change. In *The state of sociology: Problems and prospects*. Edited by J. F. Short, 119–140. Beverly Hills, Calif.: Sage.

Hawley, A. H. 1984. Human ecological and Marxian theories. *American Journal of Sociology* 89: 904–917.

Hawley, A. H. 1986. *Human ecology: A theoretical essay*. Chicago: University of Chicago Press.

Hawley, A. H. 1998. Human ecology, population, and development. In *Continuities in sociological human ecology*. Edited by M. Micklin and D. L. Poston, Jr., 11–25. New York: Plenum Press.

Hirschl, T. A., D. L. Poston, Jr., and W. P. Frisbie. 1998. The effects of public and private sustenance organization on population redistribution in New York state. In *Continuities in sociological human ecology*. Edited by M. Micklin and D. L. Poston, Jr., 251–267. New York: Plenum Press.

Irwin, M., and J. D. Kasarda. 1991. Air passenger linkages and employment growth in U.S. metropolitan areas. *American Sociological Review* 56: 524–537.

Karp, H. H., and K. D. Kelly. 1971. *Toward an ecological analysis of intermetropolitan migration*. Chicago: Markham.

Kasarda, J. D. 1971. Economic structure and fertility: A comparative analysis. *Demography* 8: 307–317.

Kasarda, J. D. 1980. The implications of contemporary distribution trends for national urban policy. *Social Science Quarterly* 61:373–400.

Krivo, L., and W. P. Frisbie. 1982. Measuring change: The case of suburban status. *Urban Affairs Quarterly* 17: 419–445.

Krout, J. A. 1982. The changing impact of sustenance organization activities on nonmetropolitan net migration. *Sociological Focus* 15: 1–13.

Lenski, G. E. 1970. *Human societies*. New York: McGraw-Hill.

Lichter, D. T., and G. V. Fuguitt. 1980. Demographic response to transportation innovation: The case of the interstate highway. *Social Forces* 59: 492–512.

Liu, B. C. 1976. *Quality of life indicators in U.S. metropolitan areas: A statistical analysis*. New York: Praeger.

Logan, J. R., and H. L. Molotch. 1987. *Urban fortunes: The political economy of place*. Berkeley: University of California Press.

London, B. 1986. Ecological and political-economic analyses of migration to a primate city: Bangkok, Thailand, ca. 1970. *Urban Affairs Quarterly* 21: 501–526.

London, B. 1987. Ending ecology's ethnocentrism: Thai replications and extensions of ecological research. *Rural Sociology* 52: 483–500.

London, B., and K. Hadden. 1989. The spread of education and fertility decline: A Thai province level test of Caldwell's 'Wealth Flows' Theory. *Rural Sociology* 54: 17–36.

Low, B. S., A. L. Clark, and K. A. Lockridge. 1992. Toward an ecological demography. *Population and Development Review* 18: 1–31.

Marshall, H. 1979. White movement to the suburbs: A comparison of explanations. *American Sociological Review* 44: 975–994.

Martin W. T., and D. L. Poston, Jr. 1972. The occupational composition of white females: Sexism, racism and occupational differentiation. *Social Forces* 50: 349–355.

Martin, W. T., and D. L. Poston, Jr. 1976. Industrialization and occupational differentiation: An ecological analysis. *Pacific Sociological Review* 19: 82–97.

McCarthy, K. F., and P. A. Morrison. 1979. *The changing demographic and economic structure of nonmetropolitan areas in the United States*, Report No. R-2399-EDA. Santa Monica, Calif.: RAND Corporation.

McKenzie, R. D. 1924. The ecological approach to the study of the human community. *American Journal of Sociology* 30: 287–301.

McKenzie, R. D. 1934. The field and problems of demography, human geography and human ecology. In *The fields and methods of sociology*. Edited by L. L. Bernard. New York: R. Long & R. R. Smith.

McKenzie, R. D. 1968. *Roderick D. McKenzie on human ecology: Selected writings*. Edited by A. H. Hawley. Chicago: University of Chicago Press.

Michelson, W. 1970. *Man and his environment*. Reading, Mass.: Addison-Wesley.

Micklin, M. 1973. Introduction: A framework for the study of human ecology. In *Population, environment and social organization: Current issues in human ecology*. Edited by M. Micklin. Hinsdale, Ill.: Dryden Press.

Micklin, M., and D. L. Poston, Jr., (eds.:). 1998. *Continuities in sociological human ecology*. New York: Plenum Press.

Micklin, M., and D. F. Sly. 1998. The ecological complex: A conceptual elaboration. In *Continuities in sociological human ecology*. Edited by M. Micklin and D. L. Poston, Jr., 51–66. New York: Plenum Press.

Namboodiri, K. 1988. Ecological demography: Its place in sociology. *American Sociological Review* 53: 619–633.

Namboodiri, K. 1994. The human ecological approach to the study of population dynamics. *Population Index* 60: 517–539.

Ogburn, W. F. 1955. Technology and the standard of living in the United States. *American Journal of Sociology* 60: 380–386.

Park, R. E., and E. W. Burgess. 1924. *Introduction to the science of sociology*. Chicago: University of Chicago Press.

Poston, D. L., Jr. 1980. An ecological analysis of migration in metropolitan America, 1970–75. *Social Science Quarterly* 61: 418–433.

Poston, D. L., Jr. 1981. An ecological examination of southern population redistribution, 1970–75. In *The population of the South: Structure and change in social demographic context*. Edited by D. L. Poston, Jr., and R. H. Weller, 137–154. Austin: The University of Texas Press.

Poston, D. L., Jr. 1983. Demographic change in nonmetropolitan America in the 1960s and 1970s: Population change versus net migration change. *The Rural Sociologist* 3: 28–33.

Poston, D. L., Jr., and C. F. Chang. 2005. Bringing males in: A critical demographic plea for incorporating males in methodological and theoretical analyses of human fertility. *Critical Demography*, forthcoming.

Poston, D. L., Jr., and W. P. Frisbie. 1984. *Ecological models of migration: A final report of Research Grant RO1 HD 15337*. Submitted to the National Institute of Child Health and Human Development, National Institutes of Health. Austin, Texas: The University of Texas at Austin, Population Research Center.

Poston, D. L., Jr., and W. P. Frisbie. 1998. Human ecology, sociology and demography. In *Continuities in sociological human ecology*. Edited by M. Micklin and D. L. Poston, Jr., 27–50. New York: Plenum Press.

Poston, D. L., Jr., W. P. Frisbie, and M. Micklin. 1984. Sociological human ecology: Theoretical and conceptual perspectives. In *Sociological human ecology: Contemporary issues and applications*. Edited by M. Micklin and H. M. Choldin. Boulder, Colo.: Westview.

Poston, D. L., Jr., D. J. Gotcher, and Y. Gu. 2004. The effect of climate on migration: United States, 1995–2000. Presented at the Annual Meeting of the Population Association of America, Boston, March 31–April 3.

Poston, D. L., Jr., and B. C. Gu. 1993. The giant cities of China: Patterns of dominance and integration. In *Progress in human ecology*. Edited by B. Hamm, Chapter 7. New Delhi: Vedams Books International.

Poston, D. L., Jr., T. A. Hirschl, and W. P. Frisbie. 1991. Sustenance organization and population redistribution in New York State: A human ecological analysis. In *Community, society and migration: Noneconomic migration in America*. Edited by P. C. Jobes, W. F. Stinner, and J. M. Wardwell, 193–220. Lanham, Md.: University Press of America.

Poston, D. L., and G. C. Johnson. 1971. Industrialization and professional differentiation by sex in the metropolitan Southwest. *Social Science Quarterly* 52: 331–348.

Poston, D. L., Jr., and M. X. Mao. 1996. An ecological investigation of interstate migration in the United States, 1985–1990. *Advances in Human Ecology* 5: 303–342.

Poston, D. L. Jr., and M. X. Mao. 1998. Interprovincial migration in China, 1985–1990. *Research in Rural Sociology and Development* 7: 227–250.

Poston, D. L. Jr., and M. Musgrave. 1999. The effect of climate on internal migration in the United States and China. Presented at the Open Meeting of the Human Dimensions of Global Environmental Change Research Community, Shonan Village Center, Kanagawa Prefecture, Japan, June 25.

Poston, D. L., Jr., Y. Tian, and Z. Jia. 1990. The urban hierarchy of China. In *Urbanization and geographical distribution of population*. Edited by B. D. H. Doan, 100–130. Pusan, Korea: Social Survey Research Center, Pusan National University.

Poston, D. L., Jr., and R. White. 1978. Indigenous labor supply, sustenance organization and population redistribution in nonmetropolitan America: An extension of the ecological theory of migration. *Demography* 15: 637–641.

Pursell, D. E. 1972. Determinants of male labor mobility. *Demography* 9: 257–281.

Robinson, W. S. 1950. Ecological correlations and the behavior of individuals. *American Sociological Review* 15: 351–357.

Saenz, R., and E. Colberg. 1988. Sustenance organization and net migration in small Texas nonmetropolitan communities, 1960–1980. *Rural Sociology 53*: 334–345.

Schnore, L. F. 1958. Social morphology and human ecology. *American Journal of Sociology* 63: 620–634.

Schnore, L. F. 1961. The myth of human ecology. *Sociological Inquiry* 31: 128–139.

Schnore, L. F. 1965. *The urban scene*. New York: The Free Press.

Shin, E. H. 1979. Correlates of intercounty variation in net migration rates of blacks in the Deep South, 1960–1970. *Rural Sociology* 44: 39–55.

Sjoberg, G. 1965. Cities in developing and in industrial societies: A cross–cultural analysis. In *The study of urbanization*. Edited by P. M. Hauser and L. F. Schnore, 213–263. New York: Wiley.

Sly, D. F. 1972. Migration and the ecological complex. *American Sociological Review* 37: 615–628.

Sly, D. F., and J. Tayman. 1977. Ecological approach to migration R-examined. *American Sociological Review* 42: 783–795.

Stinner, W. R., and G. F. DeJong. 1969. Southern Negro migration: Social and economic components of an ecological model. *Demography* 5: 455–473.

Suttles, G. 1972. *The social construction of communities*. Chicago: University of Chicago Press.

Tarver, J. 1972. Patterns of population change among southern nonmetropolitan towns: 1950–1970. *Rural Sociology* 37: 53–72.

U.S. Bureau of the Census. 1978. *County and city databook, 1977*. Washington, D.C.: U.S. Government Printing Office.

van den Berghe, P. L. 1990. Why most sociologists don't (and won't) think evolutionarily. *Sociological Forum* 5: 173–185.

Vance, R. B., and S. S. Sutker. 1954. Metropolitan dominance and integration. In *The urban South*. Edited by R. B. Vance and N. J. Demerath, 114–134. Chapel Hill: University of North Carolina Press.

Walther, C. S., and D. L. Poston, Jr. 2004. Patterns of gay and lesbian partnering in the larger metropolitan areas of the United States. *Journal of Sex Research*: 41: 201–214.

Wardwell, J. M. 1977. Equilibrium and change in nonmetropolitan growth. *Rural Sociology* 42: 156–179.

Wheat, L. F. 1969. The effects of modern highways on urban manufacturing growth. *Highway Research Record* 277: 9–24.

Zorbaugh, H. 1929. *The Gold Coast and the slum*. Chicago: University of Chicago Press.

CHAPTER 21

Biodemography

James R. Carey and James W. Vaupel

Biodemography may be compared to a tree with two main branches, each with many smaller branches, and with deep historical roots. This is a tree that currently is relatively small but burgeoning rapidly. Although still a modest subfield within demography, biodemography may be one of the fastest growing areas of demography and one of the most innovative and stimulating. There are two main branches today:

1. Biological-demographic research directly related to human health, with an emphasis on health surveys—a field of research that might be called biomedical demography (or "epidemography," because it is a cross between demography and epidemiology).
2. Research at the intersection of demography and biology (as opposed to bio-medicine), a field referred to as biological demography.

The first branch involves demographers engaging in collaborative research with epidemiologists. This collaboration is very important, for both fields and for deeper understanding of human health. Researchers in the second branch face an even bigger challenge. Demographic and epidemiological concepts and methods are fairly similar, but the underlying paradigms of demography and biology are less related.

Both of the two main branches of biodemography have many smaller branches. As in any innovative, rapidly growing interdisciplinary field, these smaller branches form tangles and thickets. Consequently, it is difficult to present a coherent structure for evolving research in biodemography. One way to proceed is to make use of the hierarchical ordering of knowledge within biology. This hierarchical ordering provides a basis for ordering the research subdivisions that range from the molecular and cellular to the ecological and evolutionary. This ordering of biodemography by levels is useful because, as the eminent physiologist George Bartholemew (1964:8) noted over four decades ago: "each level [of biological integration] offers unique problems and insights, and... each level finds its explanations of mechanism in the levels below, and its significance in the levels above." For example, the results of studies on different apolipoprotein E (APOE) gene alleles shed important light on molecular mechanisms for different risks of ischemic heart disease, Alzheimer's disease, and other chronic conditions, thus providing information on a person's individual risk of these chronic diseases and, in turn, informing the design of population surveys and model construction for epidemiological forecasting (Ewbank 2004).

This organizational concept is used in Table 21.1 to summarize what are believed to be the main disciplinary subareas of biodemographic research within each of three broad levels of biological organization: Level I (molecular to physiological), Level II (individual to kin), and Level III (population to evolution). Although several of the research categories in Table 21.1 are arbitrary and the range of research examples cited in each is incomplete, the information contained in this table likely captures the emerging scope and complexity of the field and highlights the considerable potential for scientific synergy through interdisciplinary research.

The subdisciplines listed within each of the three levels have the potential to be

TABLE 21.1. **Emerging Research Agenda for Biodemography with Crosscutting Themes from Both Biological Demography and Biomedical Demography**

Level/sublevels	Concept/example(s)
Level I: Molecular to physiological biodemography	
	Level I is concerned with processes at the lower levels of biological organization, from the molecular to the physiological (Finch et al. 2000); includes basic research on aging and longevity with model organisms as well as the results of studies such as clinical assays involving determination of hand-grip and lung capacity and body fluids such as urine and blood; demographic approach to health analysis includes some indicators of "biology" which are biological risk factors (Crimmins and Seeman 2000).
Molecular	Advances in technology will likely make it possible to carry out molecular screening of a large number of molecules in body fluids or tissue samples that may identify genetic variation or be markers of disease processes (Burns et al. 1998; Halter and Reuben 2000); molecular techniques provide tools for investigating questions about the evolution of humans, including phylogenetic relationships among subpopulations; demographic implications of medically assisted reproduction and preimplantation diagnostics (McClure 1996); medical implications of human genome project (Collins 1999), and demographic outcome.
Genetic	Use of twins or other related individuals to control for unobserved heterogeneity associated with genetics; analyses of data on the genetics of individuals or gene frequencies for populations including exploration of genes that may explain geographical differences in individual response to medications (Wallace 1997); demographic implications of preimplantation and fetal diagnosis (Holzgreve and Hahn 2003); determination of the risk of specific diseases in individuals; research on the genetic basis for common diseases and mortality will benefit from application of multistate modeling. Also research on the determinants of health and behaviors could expand to include controls for genetic differences (Ewbank 2000); genetic determinants of longevity in model organisms including nematodes (Johnson 1990; Kenyon 1997) and *Drosophila* (Curtsinger et al. 1992; Harshman 2003; Helfand and Inouye 2002).

Genomic	Includes research on origins of human populations and ancient migration streams, the role of evolution in human history, differences in migration patterns of males and females, historical demography of cultures with ancient roots (Cavalli-Sforza et al. 1994; Owens and King 1999). Genome-level basis for disease patterns in human populations; study of population-level genomics—the interface between population genetics, molecular biology, and demography (Black et al. 2001; Harpending 2003; Harpending and Rogers 2000).
Cellular	Assays can be used on cells to indicate their health and level of functioning (Halter and Reuben 2000). For example, specific cells can be isolated from blood or tissue samples for testing functional capability such as white blood cells responsible for initiating inflammation, red blood cells for their ability to produce clotting proteins and skin, muscle and fat cells to shed light on their functional characteristics.
Organ	Clinical measurements of body fluids provide important information on the functioning of many organs. For example, blood levels of thyroid hormones provide measures of over- or underfunction of the thyroid gland (Halter and Reuben 2000); noninvasive technology documents cardiac arrhythmias and fluctuations in blood pressure; sleep monitoring equipment can be used to document nocturnal activity and sleep patterns; simple mechanical devices are available to estimate pulmonary (lung) function.
Physiological	Longevity response of animals to caloric restriction requires an understanding of how animals modulate their metabolic rates when subjected to food shortages (Feder et al. 2000); physiology-to-gene approaches where goal is to find the genetic basis for physiological response underlying longevity; gene-to-physiology approach where goal is to examine the performance and fitness implication of discrete genes or products they encode (e.g., alcohol dehydrogenase on ethanol tolerance); understanding of allostatic load, which is the cost of chronic exposure to fluctuating or heightened neural or neuroendocrine response resulting from repeated or chronic environmental challenge that an individual reacts to as being particularly stressful (McEwen and Stellar 1993); late-life influence of prenatal environment (Barker 1994).

Level II: Individual-, cohort- and kinship-level biodemography

	Level II is concerned with processes involving biological organization of whole organism and three levels or types of groupings—the cohort, which is a group experiencing the same event (e.g., birth, marriage); the family, which consists of nuclear, stem, and extended family and thus grades into more extensive kinship relations, including ablineal and colineal kin.
Individual	Integration of different kinds of ages, including biological (e.g., functional capabilities), social (i.e., roles and habits relative to others), and psychological (e.g., adaptive capacities such as memory, learning, and emotions) age in life course analysis (Settersten and Mayer 1997); whereas life course currently refers to the "social processes extending over the individual life span" (Settersten and Mayer 1997), a biodemographic agenda will incorporate an understanding of biological processes as well since the biological (reproduction) and social (marriage, family creation) are inextricably intertwined; rescaling the life cycle as life expectancy increases (Lee and Goldstein 2003).
Birth & reproduction	Encompasses interconnections of the biology of reproduction and the demography of individuals and family formation (Bulatao and Casterine 2001; Wachter and Bulatao 2003). Includes genetic influences on fertility (Kohler and Rodgers 2003; Rutter 2003), basic questions regarding pair-bonding in monogamous species (Young 2003), mediation of physiological and behavioral processes (Cameron 2003), fertility patterns and behavioral controls in nonhuman primates (Altmann and Alberts 2003), evolution of primate reproductive rates (Ross and Jones 1999); evolutionary perspectives on human fertility and mating patterns (Campbell 2003; Gangestad 2003; Kaplan et al. 2003; Lam 2003; Worthman 2003), and general syntheses of human fertility and reproduction (Bachrach 2001; Hobcraft 2003; Wachter 2003); biological basis for regional and global fertility declines (Bongaarts 2001; Caldwell 2001).

Continued

TABLE 21.1. Emerging Research Agenda for Biodemography with Crosscutting Themes from Both Biological Demography and Biomedical Demography—*Cont'd*

Level/sublevels	Concept/example(s)
Mortality & longevity	Trajectories of mortality at postreproductive and advanced ages (Vaupel 1997; Vaupel 2003; Vaupel et al. 1998); models examining relationship between mortality cause-elimination and human life expectancy (Olshansky et al. 1990); reliability theories of aging and longevity (Gavrilov and Gavrilova 2001); the elderly in nature (Austad 1997; Carey and Gruenfelder 1997; Kaplan 1997; Lee 1997), evolutionary theory and senescence (Johnson and Shook 1997; Partridge 1997; Rose 1997; Tuljapurkar 1997); interspecies differences in life span distribution (Horiuchi 2003); comparative life table analysis (Deevey 1947), primate life tables (Gage 1998), and comparative demography of life spans (Carey and Judge 2000).
Birth-Death Interactions	Revisitation of cost of reproduction concepts (Bell and Koufopanou 1986; Carey 2003b; Reznick 1985); fundamental relationship between early reproduction and late-life mortality (Müller et al. 2001; Müller et al. 2002); effect of child's death on birth spacing, fertility, and fertility transition (Montgomery and Cohen 1998).
Morbidity/frailty	Medical demography—the study of chronic disease, disability, and mortality in mature and aging populations, including interaction of disability dynamics and mortality (Manton and Stallard 1994); evolutionary (Darwinian) medicine—approaches to human health based on knowledge of human evolutionary history (Trevathan et al. 1999; Williams and Nesse 1991); natural history of disease stages and the life cycle; comorbidity; cause-elimination models (Palloni 2001); general need to develop sets of proximate biological factors related to health outcomes based on knowledge of biology and the relationship between bioindicators, demographic variables and health outcomes (Crimmins et al. 1996; Lollar and Crews 2003); use of studies on both captive and free-ranging animal populations for investigating the maintenance of allostasis, the cascade of events leading to allostatic load (McEwen and Stellar 1993), and biopsychosocial, predisease pathways to diverse health outcomes (Singer and Ryff 2001); morbidity and aging in nonhuman species, including primate gerontology (DeRousseau 1994) and insect frailty studies (Papadopoulos et al. 2002).
Migration/movement	Integration of conceptual and empirical framework developed in ecology for dispersal (movement affecting spatial pattern) and migration (mass directional movement) to demography including biological and behavioral basis for age-specific patterns of migration and dispersal (Rogers 1984, 1985; Begon et al. 1996).
Family and kin	Desired family size and the course of fertility (Bacci 2001; Vogler 2000); patterns of availability and access of elderly to kin (Wolf 1994); two-sex demography (Pollak 1986); biodemography of parental care (Clutton-Brock 1991) and parental behavior (Numan 1998); family and population implications of reprogenetics—modification of germline DNA (Kollek 2003); comparative socioecology of kinship bonding and mating systems (Foley 1999).

Level III: Population, ecological, and evolutionary biodemography

	Level III is concerned with levels of organization and processes above the individual, including populations (groups of individuals coexisting at a given moment), ecological (interrelationship of organisms and their surroundings), and evolutionary (the descent, with modifications, of different lineages from common ancestors). biodemography is inextricably linked to all of these organizational groupings since vital rates and population processes underlie the dynamics of change at all levels.
Population principles	Theory of population dynamics (Preston et al. 2001) and applications to humans (Keyfitz 1977; Shryock and Siegel 1976) and nonhuman species (Caswell 1989); theoretical basis for evolution of life span and aging (Orzack 2003); demography of growth rate (Mangel 2003).

Human populations	Sociobiological and anthropological perspectives on health (Nguyen and Peschard 2003); evolution of human life span (Kaplan et al. 2003; Kaplan and Lancaster 2003); anthropological demography (Hill and Kaplan 1999), including questions regarding birth and death rates of indigenous peoples, population sex ratios in indigenous societies, ages at onset, termination of reproduction and cultural comparisons between foragers versus pastorals (Ellison 2001; Hill and Hurtado 1996); extraordinary longevity in human populations (Robine 2003; Robine and Saito 2003; Wilmoth and Robine 2003); limits to world population (Cohen 1995).
Nonhuman populations	Life history theory in biodemographic contexts (Caswell 1989; Cole, 1954; Tuljapurkar 1990); studies of geographical structure involving both demography and genetics to examine the distribution of genotypes within and between populations (Roderick 1996; Slatkin 1987); use of social insects as models and concepts of sociobiology (Wilson 1971; Wilson 1975) to gain fundamental insights into social aspects of aging, longevity, fertility, and intra- and intergenerational transfer (Lee 2003; Rueppell et al. 2004); ecological correlates of life span and hazard rates (Gaillard et al. 2003; Ricklefs and Scheuerlein 2003; Wachter 2003); senescence and mortality in field and laboratory populations of plants (Roach 2001; Roach 2003)
Ecological biodemography	Conservation biodemography (Young and Clarke 2000b) and biodemography of invasive species (Sakai et al. 2001), including minimum viable populations (Soule 1987), demography of harvesting (Carey 1993; Getz and Haight 1989); metapopulation analysis (Hastings and Harrison 1994; Thrall et al. 2000), demographic toxicology (Stark and Banks 2003), demographic effects of habitat fragmentation (Young and Clarke 2000a).
Evolutionary biodemography	Understanding the processes of evolution informs every area of biology, including biodemography; concerned with the interface of demography, genetics, and evolution in age-structured populations (Charlesworth 1994); evolution of life history traits and trade-offs between birth and death (Stearns 1992); accounting for the evolution of short or long life span (Carey 2003a); post-Darwinian longevity (Vaupel 2003); understanding the underlying demography related to the unbroken chains of descent of all organisms from viruses to redwoods to humans (Meagher and Futuyma 2001).

mutually informing both within and between categories and levels. There are also a number of instances where closely related concepts have been independently derived in population biology and demography. For example, the early work by Andrei Rogers (1984, 1985) on multiregional demography is conceptually identical with recent work on metapopulation analysis in conservation biology (Hastings and Harrison 1994). The studies involving "geographical structure" in wild populations of animals (Roderick 1996) are similar to studies concerned with many of the same questions and use many of the same genetic tools as those in epidemiological demography (Ewbank 2000; Finch and Tanzi 1997; Finch, Vaupel, and Kinsella 2000; Wallace 1997, 2000). Although applied in different contexts, in a basic way the use of the concept of natural selection (Meagher and Futuyma 2001) has parallels with the concept of demographic selection (Vaupel, Manton, and Stallard 1979), since both involve a winnowing process.

The remainder of this chapter is structured as follows. The first section is an extended discussion of the branch of biodemography referred to here as biological demography. Next is a shorter description of the other main branch, referred to here as biomedical demography. The bulk of this chapter thus focuses on biological demography. Currently the biomedical branch is at least as prominent as the biological branch, with at least as many demographers actively involved. And the biomedical branch is certainly path-breaking, with substantial results to date and much promise. In the section dealing with this branch, some of the key researchers and main publications are presented. This chapter, however, emphasizes biological demography because the concepts and methods of biomedical demography are quite accessible elsewhere to demographers, whereas the concepts and methods of biological demography are much more foreign and difficult to understand. Moreover, it is felt that understanding biological thinking in demography requires an appreciation of a set of biological-demographic principles. A major portion of the chapter thus is devoted to an exposition of these principles as well as a justification and rationale for why it is useful and important to think in terms of such principles.

BIOLOGICAL DEMOGRAPHY

Conceptual Framework

Biological demography is an emerging interdisciplinary science concerned with identifying a universal set of population principles, integrating biological concepts into demographic approaches, and bringing demographic methods to bear on population problems in different biological disciplines. Whereas biomedical demography brings survey techniques, biomedical information, modeling strategies, and statistical methods to bear on questions about the health of different *human populations*, biological demography brings experimental paradigms, model systems, evolutionary perspectives, and comparative techniques to bear on questions about the demographic characteristics of different *species*. Biomedical demographers ask questions about the shape of the trajectory of human mortality at advanced ages. In contrast, biological demographers ask the more general question of whether the slowing of mortality at advanced ages is a universal life table characteristic of species as diverse as nematodes, fruit flies, mice, and humans. Biological demography not only situates the population traits of humans within the broader demographic context of all living organisms, it also provides a scientific framework for asking basic questions that differ from, but are complementary to, those asked in conventional demography.

Because of the range of the subdisciplines in biology and of the subspecialties in demography, the term *biological demography* does not fully reflect the diversity of its main intellectual lineages, including gerontology, population biology, and demography (Hauser and Duncan 1959a); the complexity of its deep historical roots (Malthus 1798; Pearl 1922); or the scope of the questions commonly addressed by biological demographers (Carey and Tuljapurkar 2003; Vaupel et al. 1998; Wachter and Finch 1997). Although biological-demographic researchers use mathematical and statistical modeling techniques similar to those used in classic demography, they also use experimental methods to address questions about the nature of mortality, fertility, development, and aging in such model organisms as fruit flies and rodents. Thus, unlike most research in classic demography, biological-demographic research exploits the hierarchical ordering of knowledge that unites and drives the biological sciences.

Biological demography embraces all the research at the intersection of demography and biology. It hence includes studies of fertility, migration, and mortality. To date, however, the main emphasis has been on studies of survival and longevity, with some emerging research on fertility and on the links between fertility and mortality. Whereas the traditional paradigm that frames biological gerontology is concerned with questions at the molecular, cellular, and/or physiological levels, the biological-demographic paradigm of aging integrates research at the organismal level—the quintessence of biological relevance because all discoveries at lower levels of biological organization concerning aging must ultimately be tested at the level of the whole organism. And unlike traditional research in both classic demography and the biology of aging, biological demography draws from population biology and thus emphasizes evolutionary and ecological concepts, life history theory, and comparative methods. This multidisciplinary synthesis represents a unique research paradigm concerned with both proximate questions (e.g., those concerned with the *mechanisms* of aging) as well as with ultimate ones (e.g., those concerned with the evolutionary and ecological *function* of a particular life span). Thus biological-demographic research embraces many questions about both aging and life span that do not fall within the bounds of either traditional demography or gerontology.

Contribution to Mainstream Demography

Biological demography can strengthen traditional demography in at least three ways. *First*, the concepts, principles, and theories developed in biological demography can enhance the coherence and the development of a higher unity of order and process. This higher unity cannot occur without viewing the human life course in the context of other components or processes. Biological demography has the potential for integrating biology into the pedagogical framework of classic demography in much the same way as basic biology is integrated into biomedicine. The focus on humans is retained, but the epistemological foundations are strengthened, the biological scope is expanded, and the demographic perspectives are broadened.

Second, results from experimental biological demography should provide better explanations of the life table patterns observed in human populations that are not evident in the absence of broader biological concepts. For example, biological-demographic principles link senescence and sexual reproduction. The principles suggest explanations of sex differentials in life expectancies, why older individuals may grow older more slowly, whether limits to the life span are related, whether post-reproductive life is common or rare, how sociality affects life span, and if and how post-reproductive life spans in other species increase fitness.

Third, the biological-demographic principles should provide a more secure foundation for making predictions about the trajectory of mortality at older ages, the nature of life span limits (or the lack thereof), and the magnitude and sign of the gender gap. In general, every discipline including demography is faced with the perennial struggle to define and renew itself and to ensure its relevance in an ever changing world. Like other social sciences, demography is slowly coming to terms with important truths that the biological sciences have proved beyond any doubt: that all aspects of humans—mind, behavior, body—are products of biological evolution (Foster 2000). It follows that this program in particular, and biological demography in general, should help demography maintain a robust, energetic, and creative presence in modern science.

As Preston (1990) points out, instead of demographers asking why life expectancy at birth for the world as a whole has doubled in this century, demographers might ask the more biological question: why has no one ever been recorded as living past age 122. Instead of asking why childbearing is increasingly delayed in the United States, demographers might ask why the reproductive life span for women is essentially confined to ages 15 to 50. Or instead of asking why the gender gap favors females by 4 to 10 years in developed countries, demographers might ask whether a female longevity advantage is present in the majority of nonhuman species.

HISTORICAL OVERVIEW

Early History

Demography has multiple points of contact with biology, as well as mathematics, statistics, the social sciences, and policy analysis. Many of the chapters in this *Handbook* make manifest these contacts. Although population biology and demography share common ancestors in both Malthus (1798) (i.e., populations grow exponentially but resources do not) and Darwin (1859) (i.e., selection on birth and death rates result from the struggle for existence), the more contemporary biology-demography interface appeared in the research of two distinguished demographers in the early decades of the 20th century— Alfred J. Lotka (1880–1949) and Raymond Pearl (1879–1940). Lotka developed concepts and methods that are still of fundamental importance in biological demography; his two most significant books are *Elements of Physical Biology* (Lotka 1924) and *Theorie Analytique des Associations Biologiques* (1934). Pearl pioneered biological-demographic research on several species, including flatworms, the aquatic plant *Ceratophyllum demersum*, the fruit fly *Drosophila melanogaster*, and humans (1924; 1925). He founded two major journals, the *Quarterly Journal of Biology* and *Human Biology*, and helped found both the Population Association of America (PAA) and the International Union for the Scientific Investigation of Population Problems (which later became IUSSP—the International Union for the Scientific Study of Population).

Following the pioneering work of Lotka and Pearl in the 1920s and 1930s there was, until the 1970s, little interest among demographers in integrating biology into any part of the discipline. There were a few chapter entries on population studies in such crosscutting disciplines such as demography and ecology (Frank 1959), demography and anthropology (Spuhler 1959), and genetics and demography (Kallmann and Rainer 1959) in Hauser and Duncan's (1959b) *The Study of Population*. These and other similar chapters served more as illustrations of how demographic methods were used by different disciplines than as sources of knowledge for demography.

Convergence of Ideas

In the early 1970s a group of population biologists and demographers, including Nathan Keyfitz, launched the journal *Theoretical Population Biology* (*TPB*). The journal was intended to be a forum for the interdisciplinary discussion of "the theoretical aspects of the biology of populations, particularly in the areas of ecology, genetics, demography, and epidemiology" (*TPB* 2004: General Information). This description is still used by the publisher to describe the journal, although the audience is described as "population biologists, ecologists, and evolutionary ecologists," with no mention of demographers (or epidemiologists) (*TPB* 2004: General Information). Some demographers over the years have published articles in *TPB*, but the journal, which has thrived and is now published eight times per year, has become dominated by population biologists and evolutionary ecologists. As the more mathematical aspects of biological demography develop, *TPB* may finally be able to attain its original goal.

In the late 1970s IUSSP members expressed concern that demography was at risk of isolating itself and becoming more a technique than a science. Nathan Keyfitz lamented that "demography has withdrawn from its borders and left a no man's land which other disciplines have infiltrated" (Keyfitz 1984a: Foreword). Hence in 1981 a workshop titled *Population and Biology* was organized at the Harvard University Center for Population Studies (Keyfitz 1984b) to explore the possible impact of biological "laws" on social science (Jacquard 1984; Lewontin 1984; Wilson 1984), the selective effects of marriage and fertility (Leridon 1984), the autoregulating mechanisms in human populations (Livi-Bacci 1984), and the concepts of morbidity and mortality (Cohen 1984). That no notable papers or concepts emerged from this meeting between biologists and demographers, many of whom were among the most prominent scientists in their respective fields, was itself significant. The good intentions of top scientists are not enough to integrate two fields with fundamentally different disciplinary histories, professional cultures, and epistemological frameworks. To make progress it is imperative to layout a clear set of important (and ultimately fundable) questions that lie at the disciplinary interface. This is particularly important for integrating disciplines with disparate historical roots, such as demography with its roots in the social and analytical sciences and biology with its roots in the natural and experimental sciences.

In the mid-1980s two separate meetings were organized that brought scientists together to address the more circumscribed and focused questions that lie at the interface between biology and demography. The first workshop was organized by Sheila Ryan Johannson and Kenneth Wachter at the University of California, Berkeley, in 1987, supported by the National Institute on Aging (NIA), and titled *"Upper Limits to Human Life Span."* Although there were no publications or proceedings from this workshop, it was important historically because it was the first meeting to bring biologists and demographers together to focus expressly on a circumscribed topic of great importance to demographers, biologists, and policy makers—aging and longevity. This workshop set the stage for virtually all of the subsequent developments in the biological demography of longevity and aging.

The second workshop during the late 1980s that helped frame biological demography was organized in 1988 at the University of Michigan by Julian Adams, Albert Hermalin, David Lam, and Peter Smouse and titled *Convergent Issues in Genetics and Demography*. An edited volume emerging from this workshop (Adams 1990) included sections on the use of historical information, including pedigree and genealogical data in genetics and demography, on the treatment and analysis of variation in the fields of genetics and demography, on epidemiology as a common ground for the convergence of demography and genetics, and on issues in genetics and demography that have attracted the attention of scientists in both fields such as two-sex models, minimum viable population size, and sources of variation in vital rates. This workshop was significant because it revealed the importance of organizing research at the interface of biology and demography around a circumscribed topic, in this case genetics.

Recent Coalescence

The Berkeley and Ann Arbor workshops set the stage for the organization of a cluster of three highly successful workshops held between 1996 and 2001. The first was a workshop on the *Biodemography of Longevity* that was organized and chaired by Ronald Lee of the Committee on Population of the U.S. National Research Council and held in Washington, D.C., in April 1996. This meeting was one of the seminal developments in biological demography because of the new insights and perspectives that emerged on the nature of aging and the life span from the interchange of demographic and biological ideas. The workshop led to the book *Between Zeus and the Salmon: The Biodemography of Longevity*, edited by Kenneth Wachter and Caleb Finch (1997). This volume includes papers on the empirical demography of survival, evolutionary theory and senescence, the elderly in nature, postreproduction, the human life course and intergenerational relations, the potential of population surveys in genetic studies, and synthetic views on the plasticity of human aging and life span.

The second workshop, organized and chaired by Kenneth Wachter and Rodolfo Bulatao, focused on fertility and was designed to complement the workshop on the biological demography of longevity. Like the others preceding it, this workshop brought together demographers, evolutionary biologists, geneticists, and biologists to consider questions at the interface of the social sciences and the life sciences. Topics included in the resulting volume (Wachter and Bulato 2003) were the biological demography of fertility and family formation; genetic and ecological influences on fertility; education, fertility and heritability; mating patterns, energetics and sociality of human reproduction.

A recent workshop concerned with biological demography was organized by James Carey and Shripad Tuljapurkar and titled *Life Span: Evolutionary, Ecological, and Demographic Perspectives*. It was held in 2001 on the Greek Island of Santorini. This workshop was a follow-up to the earlier one on biological demography but with a greater emphasis on life span rather than aging. The edited volume from this workshop (Carey and Tuljapurkar 2003) included papers on conceptual and theoretical perspectives on life span and its evolution, ecological and life history correlates, and genetic and population studies of life span in nonhuman species and in humans.

At the beginning of the 21st century biological demography is reemerging as a locus of cutting-edge demographic research. It is clearly accepted that fertility, mortality, and morbidity have a basic biological component. Moreover, biology is fundamentally a population science, and there is growing recognition that biological studies can benefit greatly from demographic concepts and methods. From a biologist's perspective, biological demography envelops demography because it embraces research pertaining to any nonhuman species, the populations of genotypes and biological measurements related to age, health, physical functioning, and fertility. Within this vast territory, several research foci are noteworthy and are briefly described in the next section.

GENERAL BIOLOGICAL DEMOGRAPHIC PRINCIPLES

Inasmuch as scientific principles and hard data are bound together in close etiological and epistemological relationships, the usefulness of the store of data from biological demography is enhanced through the synthesis of these data using a dialectic that combines demographic and biological concepts. The objective in this section is to summarize a number of general principles that have been identified in recent research in biological and comparative demography (Carey 2003b; Carey and Judge 2001).

Conventional demography, defined by Pressat (Pressat 1985: 54) as "the study of populations and the processes that shape them," is a science that depends for its data on observation and the recording of events occurring in the external world, rather than on experiments under controlled conditions. One of the overriding constraints of any of the observational social sciences such as demography and sociology was referred to by

Hauser and Duncan (1959a) as "the problem of historicism"—the question of the extent to which generalizations drawn from human data localized in time and space can lead to general principles rather than simply to descriptions of situations unique to a particular time and location. This constraint preempts the use of human data alone as a source for the derivation of the most basic principles.

Principles of Senescence

Timiras (1994) notes that despite some minor interpretative differences, the terms aging and senescence are often used interchangeably, even though *aging* refers to the process of growing old regardless of chronological age, whereas *senescence* is a process restricted to the state of old age characteristic of the late years of an organism's life span. Senescence in this context is defined as "the deteriorative process characterized by increased vulnerability, functional impairment, and probability of death with advancing age" (Timiras 1994: 3). In this section we describe two principles of senescence that are fundamental to biological demography because they provide the biological, evolutionary, and conceptual foundation for its constituent disciplines—whereas demography is concerned with the determinants of probabilities of death, biology is concerned with the determinants of vulnerability.

NATURAL SELECTION SHAPES SENESCENCE RATE.   All systems, from the simplest kind of equipment to the most complicated species of life, experience senescence, at least in their component parts. Whether or not the entity as a whole suffers senescence, however, depends on the balance between the forces of wear and tear, on the one hand, and the counterbalancing forces of repair and rejuvenation, on the other. For living organisms, this balance is determined by natural selection, by Darwinian evolution.

   Evolutionary models of life history characteristics in general and of senescence in particular fall into two types (Partridge and Barton 1993): optimization models and nonadaptive age-specific mutation models. In optimization models the forces of evolution are assumed to yield the best-possible design of a species' life history, the design that maximizes Darwinian fitness. Williams (1957) proposed an optimization model of senescence, the so-called antagonistic-pleiotropy model. The basic idea is that some genes have a favorable or unfavorable effect on fertility or survival at younger ages, with an opposite effect on mortality at older ages. A small positive (or negative) effect at younger ages may be more important than a large opposite effect at older ages if few individuals survive to these ages and if their reproduction is low. Williams' model is often formulated in terms of mutations that have a positive effect at some particular age and a negative effect at some other age (Charlesworth 1994). Williams' idea, however, is more general. It is simply an example of the kind of thinking about trade-offs that underlies all optimization modeling. Williams thought that his model implied senescence; he did not consider the logical possibility that such an optimization model might lead to negative senescence, i.e., to the decline in mortality with age (Vaupel et al. 2004). The "disposable soma" model (Kirkwood 1992; Kirkwood and Rose 1991) is a related example of this kind of thinking applied to senescence.

   In the second class of models, evolutionary forces act in a nonadaptive way, as follows. Evolution acts on randomly occurring mutations. Some of these mutations may have age-specific effects. In particular, some mutations may only be harmful at older ages. There is little selective pressure to remove such mutations from the population because the individuals who have them have produced most of their offspring before they have reached old age. Hence, such mutations tend to accumulate, resulting in senescence. Charlesworth (1994) provides a general discussion of mutation-selection balance, i.e., of models of the opposing forces of deleterious mutation and subsequent Darwinian selection. Hamilton (1966) developed an influential mutation-accumulation model of senescence.

ALL SEXUAL ORGANISMS SENESCE.   Hamilton's (1966) mutation accumulation model led him to conclude that senescence cannot be avoided by any organism and that senescence is an inevitable outcome of evolution. This view, combined with arguments made by Weissman in the 1880s and 1890s about the senescence of somatic cells and the immortality of germ cells, was developed by Bell (1988), who postulated a deep connection between the two invariants of life—birth and death—by demonstrating that protozoan lineages senesce as the result of an accumulated load of mutations. This senescence can be arrested by the recombination of micronuclear DNA with that of another protozoa through conjugation. Conjugation (sex) results in new DNA and in the apoptotic-like destruction of old operational DNA in the macronucleus. Thus, rejuvenation in the replicative DNA and senescence of operational DNA is promoted by sexual reproduction. When this line of thinking is extended to multicellular organisms, sex and somatic senescence can be inextricably linked (Clark 1996). In multicellular, sexually reproducing organisms, the function of somatic cells (i.e., all cells constituting the individual besides the germ cells) is to promote the survival and function of the replicative DNA—the germ cells (Clark 1996). Prior to bacteria, the somatic DNA was the germ line DNA; prior to multicellular animals, the somatic cell was the germ cell. Like the macronuclei in the paramecia, the somatic cells senesce and die as a function of their mitotic task of ensuring the survival and development of the germ cells. The advent of sex in reproduction allowed exogenous repair of replicative DNA (Bell 1988), while in multicellular organisms the replication errors of somatic growth and maintenance are segregated from that DNA passed on to daughter cells and are discarded at the end of each generation. Senescence, according to Bell and Clark, is built into the life history of all sexually reproducing organisms. The death rate can be altered by modifying senescence, but death itself can never be eliminated. This evolutionary argument concerning senescence is one of the fundamental canons in the emergence of all sexually reproducing organisms.

Recently, however, the canon has been questioned. There is a deep inconsistency between Hamilton's view that senescence is inevitable even "in the farthest reaches of almost any bizarre universe" (Hamilton 1966: 12) and the Weissman-Bell-Clark emphasis on senescence in sexually reproducing species. In plants there is no distinction between the soma and the germ line, but at least for some plants mortality rises with age. Single-celled organisms that do not sexually reproduce certainly tend to have short lives: they can hardly be termed immortal except in the sense that the species survives. Furthermore, fundamental objections have been raised regarding Hamilton's model and its resulting conclusions (Lee 2003; Vaupel et al. 2004). It seems clear that the component parts of any individual suffer wear and tear, but, as discussed above, under some circumstances the organism as a whole can experience constant or even declining mortality if the damaged parts can be repaired or discarded and replaced. Hence the assertion that all (sexual) organisms suffer senescence is no longer the truism it was once deemed to be. Research on this issue is one of the most exciting current topics in biological demography.

Principles of Mortality

The single most important function of the life table is age-specific mortality—the fraction of individuals alive at age x that die prior to age $x + 1$. There are at least three reasons that this function is more important than, for example, cohort survival or life expectancy (Carey 2003b):

1. Death is an event constituting a change of stage from living to dead, whereas survival is a continuation of the current state. Life table parameters are based on probabilities of measurable events rather than "nonevents" like survival. This is important because death can be disaggregated by cause whereas survival cannot.
2. Age-specific mortality is algebraically independent of events at all other ages; thus changes in age patterns can often be traced to underlying physiological and/ or behavioral changes at the level of the individual. With the exception of period survival, this is not true for the other life table parameters.
3. Several different mathematical models of mortality (e.g., Gompertz 1825) have been developed that provide simple and concise means for expressing the life table properties of cohorts with a few parameters. In the following section we describe some mortality concepts that we believe are both general and relevant to understanding mortality in humans.

MORTALITY DECELERATES AT ADVANCED AGES.   Slowing or deceleration of mortality at older ages has been observed in every large-scale life table study of insects (e.g., *Drosophila*, houseflies, Medflies, and bruchid beetles), and similar patterns have been observed in human populations (Carey 2003b). There are three reasons why this general principle is important (Carey et al. 1992): (1) it provides a conceptual and empirical point of departure from the Gompertz model of ever increasing, age-specific mortality; (2) it forces demographers and gerontologists to rethink the idea that senescence can be operationally defined and measured by the increase in mortality rates with age; and (3) it suggests that there is no definite limit to the life span.

MORTALITY IS SEX-SPECIFIC.   The prevailing wisdom in gerontology is that the female advantage in life expectancy is a universal law of nature. Carey and associates (1995) examined whether a female longevity advantage exists for the Medfly and discovered that the answer was not clear. They showed that males exhibit a higher life expectancy at eclosion, but females are four times more likely than males to be the last to die. They concluded that there were at least three reasons why it is impossible to state unequivocally that either males or females are "longer-lived" (Carey et al. 1995). First, longevity can be characterized in different ways (e.g., life expectancy at eclosion [day 0], life expectancy at day 30, age when 90% of the original cohort is dead [life endurancy], maximal life span, and so forth); one measure of longevity often favors one sex, whereas another measure favors the other sex. Second, there is considerable variation among cohorts for a given longevity measure. For example, neither male nor female longevity is greater in all groups regardless of the measure used. And finally, relative longevity for the two sexes depends on the environment in which they are maintained or the treatment to which they were subjected. Expectation of life for males and females is similar if flies were maintained in solitary confinement but favored males if the flies were maintained in grouped cages. The overall conclusion was that sex-specific mortality responses and, in turn, male–female life expectancy differences cannot be predicted a priori. Moreover, a female longevity advantage is not universal across species.

MORTALITY TRAJECTORIES ARE FACULTATIVE.   The term *facultative* is used in biology to describe life history traits that have alternative conditions that often vary with environmental conditions. For example, clutch size in some birds, diapause in insects, and diet selection in many animals are all considered facultative. We suggest that the term also applies to the mortality patterns in the Medfly and most other species because there exists no unique pattern; the specific trajectories frequently depend on environmental conditions. One of the most compelling findings emerging from the collection of life table studies on the Medfly, and one that was not evident even after the first large-scale study was completed, is that female mortality patterns are extraordinarily plastic. The reason this elasticity was not evident in the first series of studies is because none involved manipulations that altered the physiology and behavior of the flies. It is now apparent that manipulations that affect the components of a fly's life history, such as irradiation, diet, or mating, have a profound effect on the trajectory of mortality in females and less of an effect on male trajectories.

SELECTION SHAPES MORTALITY TRAJECTORIES.   The concept of subgroups endowed with different levels of frailty is known as demographic heterogeneity, and the winnowing process as the cohort ages is referred to as demographic selection (Vaupel, Manton, and Stallard 1979). As populations age, they become more selected because groups with higher death rates die out in greater numbers than those with lower death rates, thereby transforming the population into one consisting mostly of individuals with low death rates (Vaupel, Manton, and Stallard 1979). The actuarial consequence of cohorts consisting of subsets, each possessing a different level of frailty, is that the mortality trajectory of the whole may depart substantially from Gompertz rates even though each of the subgroups displays Gompertz mortality rates. Vaupel and Carey (1993) fitted observed *C. capitata* mortality patterns with mixtures of increasing Gompertz curves and demonstrated that 12 subgroups were sufficient to capture the observed pattern of Medfly mortality using a range of frailty values and initial proportions of subgroups. As cohorts age, demographic selection appears to winnow the frail, leave the robust, and thus shape the mortality trajectory.

Principles of Longevity

Longevity refers to the period between birth and death of an individual. It is operationalized in several different ways, including *expectation of life at birth*—the average number of years (days, weeks, etc.) that a newborn will live; *median life span*—the age at which half of an initial cohort is dead (or alive); *life endurancy*—the age at which 90% of the original cohort is dead, and *record life span*—the age at which the longest-lived, observed individual died. As a life history trait, longevity covaries with other traits, including body size, brain size, ability to fly, armored animals, subterranean habits, and sociality (Sacher 1978).

LONGEVITY IS ADAPTIVE.   In evolutionary biology an "adaptation" is a characteristic of organisms whose properties are the result of selection in a particular functional context. Just as different bird beaks are adaptations for exploiting different niches that must be balanced with other traits such as body size and flight propensity, the longevity of an animal is also an adaptation that must be balanced with other traits, particularly with reproduction. Variations in the relationship between reproduction and longevity can only make sense when placed within the context of demographic factors, duration of the infantile period, number of young, and the species' ecological niche, that is, the organism's overall life history strategy. Indeed, the longevity potential of a species is not an arbitrary or random outcome of evolutionary forces but rather an adaptive one that must fit into the broader life history of the species.

Longevity is positively correlated with body size between orders (e.g., the smaller rodents are shorter lived than the larger primates) though not necessarily within orders (e.g., longevity is not correlated with body size in seals and walruses [pinnipeds] or in small bats) (Carey and Judge 2000). Longevity is also positively correlated with certain unique traits, including flight ability (birds and bats), possession of armor (turtles and armadillos), and subterranean lifestyle (moles and mole rats). Analysis reveals that life spans differ by a factor of over 50 in mammals, reptiles, amphibians, and fish and by over 15-fold in birds. It also provides an important biological and evolutionary context for human longevity. To illustrate, primates are long-lived mammals, great apes (gorillas and chimpanzees) are long-lived primates, and humans are long-lived great apes. Indeed, analysis reveals that human longevity exceeds nearly all other species both relatively and absolutely. This finding is important because it suggests that extended longevity should be considered along with features such as large brain, bipedalism, and language as a key trait of our species.

LIFE SPAN IS INDETERMINATE.   Maximal length of life remains as one of the most compelling concepts in demography and gerontology. The validity of this concept is viewed by many as self-evident because different species exhibit different life expectancies; all individuals eventually die before the age of infinity, and, therefore, each species must possess unique and finite maximal ages. Kannisto (1991; 1996) notes that the problem with this idea is that our knowledge of the nature of mortality makes it difficult to accept the notion that there is a single age that some individuals may reach but that none has any chance of surviving. He views the only valid alternative as the existence of an asymptote to which the probability of dying tends and that may or may not be near 100%. Manton and Stallard (1984) note that declines in the age-specific rates of increase of mortality for male and female cohorts in the United States are inconsistent with a fixed life span limit. Wilmoth and Lundström (1996: 89) state "we have established the important empirical fact that the upper limits of the human age distribution have been rising steadily during the past century or more and show no sign thus far of possessing a fixed upper bound." In general, it may be concluded from recent research that it is possible to estimate Medfly life expectancy, but these flies, and most likely other species as well, do not appear to have a characteristic life span. The concept of an *indeterminate* life span implied by Medfly data is fundamentally different from the concept of a *limitless* life span.

REPRODUCTION IS A FUNDAMENTAL LONGEVITY DETERMINANT. Most organisms, from yeast and plants to invertebrates, birds, and mammals, suspend reproduction during periods unfavorable for reproduction by entering a different physiological mode. Such waiting strategies for prolonging survival while maintaining reproductive potential have been extensively documented in the physiological, ecological, and natural history literature. For example, when food is scarce, yeast enter a stationary phase, tardigrades form tuns, nematodes go into a dauer stage, mollusks and earthworms undergo a quiescence, fruit flies experience a reproductive diapause, long-lived queens among ants and wasps hibernate, some fish reabsorb their ovaries, amphibians and reptiles aestivate, mice retard their ovariole depletion, some birds (hummingbirds and swifts) become torpid, and plants suspend their physiological and reproductive activities. Recent research on Medfly aging (Carey 2003b) reveals that female Medflies may experience two physiological modes of aging with different demographic schedules of fertility and survival. These include a waiting mode, in which both mortality and reproduction are low, and a reproductive mode, in which mortality is low at the onset of egg laying but accelerates as eggs are laid. Medflies that switch from a waiting to a reproductive mode due to a change in diet (from sugar to full protein diet) survive longer than those kept in either mode exclusively. The switch from waiting mode to reproductive mode initiates egg laying and reduces the level of mortality below current rates but increases the rate of aging. Understanding this relationship between longevity and reproduction in Medflies is important because it links the reproductive fate of individuals with environmental conditions and points toward important causal mechanisms that may be related to, and mediated by, the rate of ovarian depletion and/or gonadal activity(Carey 2003b).

THE HERITABILITY OF INDIVIDUAL LIFE SPAN IS MODEST. Life span heritability is defined as the proportion of the variance among individual ages of death that is attributable to differences in genotype. Contrary to popular myth, parental age of death appears to have minimal prognostic significance for offspring longevity (McGue et al. 1993). Finch and Tanzi (1997) note that the heritability of life span accounts for less than 35% of its variance in short-lived invertebrates (nematode and fruit flies), mice, and humans. Although McGue and associates (1993) find evidence for genetic influences, environmental factors are clearly shown to account for a majority of the variance in age at death. For example, these researchers report that the average age difference at death for twins is 14.1 and 18.5 years for identical (monozygotic) and fraternal (dizygotic) twins, respectively, and 19.2 years for two randomly chosen individuals. The study by Herskind and co-workers (1996) followed more than 2,800 twin-pairs with known zygosity from birth to death. It showed that about 25% of the variation in life span in this population could be attributed to genetic factors. Generally, traits that are most essential to the survival of an organism, including survival itself, show little heritability due to strength of selection and fixation.

Biological-Demographic Principles and the Human Primate

Most of the biological-demographic principles concerning senescence, mortality, and longevity presented in the previous section are general and thus apply to a large number of species. There are also actuarial characteristics in all species, including humans, that are specific to that species, or to a narrow group to which the species belongs. Such species-level characteristics are superimposed on the more general patterns. For example, general mortality patterns in humans include a decline after infancy, increases through the reproductive life span (the overall U-shaped trajectory known among demographers as the age curve of mortality), and a sex differential. However, the specific level pertains to details of the mortality experience unique to humans, including the actual probabilities of death by age, inflection points of age-specific mortality, the cause-specific probabilities of death, and the age-specific pattern of the sex differential. The observed actuarial patterns are a combination of the evolutionary components of the trajectory (which will be common to a large number of species with overlapping life history characteristics) and the proximate age and sex-specific factors contributing to mortality and survival under certain conditions.

Many life history traits largely unique to humans are widely documented in anthropology and human biology. These include bipedalism, large brains, complex language, tool use, and a prolonged juvenile period. However, the extraordinary absolute longevity of humans, as well as longevity relative to body size, is a life history trait that is not fully recognized and appreciated. The purpose of this section is to identify and describe three biological-demographic principles that link the primate evolutionary past with modern human longevity. A substantial part of this section is based on recent research by Judge and Carey (2000).

BODY AND BRAIN SIZE PREDICT EXTENDED HUMAN LONGEVITY.   As discussed above, most species, including humans, do not have a definite maximum life span. The oldest age reached in a population depends on the size of the population and on environmental conditions. If, however, mortality rises steeply with age, as is the case for humans, primates more generally, and most mammals, and if population sizes are roughly comparable, on the order, say, of thousands or millions, then as a crude but useful approximation, it is possible to characterize the maximum likely life span of individuals in such a population as, say, "50 to 55 years" or "about 30 years" (Vaupel 2003). The following discussion uses this notion of approximate (maximum) life span.

Brain size is correlated with both body size and life span in mammals as a whole and within the Primate order. Relative brain size and relative life span (residual brain and life span after controlling for body mass) are highly correlated. Judge and Carey (2000) examined longevity records for 133 species of primates with respect to adult female body size and adult brain size and placed human life span in context relative to extant primates and estimates for early (extinct) hominids. The great apes have long lives that slightly exceed the life span predicted by body and brain size. However, the closest relatives of humans, namely, gorillas and chimpanzees, are exceeded in their positive deviation from the expected by five other Old World primate genera. No Old World nonhuman genus approaches the positive deviation from expected life span demonstrated by New World monkeys of the genus *Cebus* (i.e., capuchin monkeys). *Cebus* exhibit life spans that rival those of chimpanzees, even though chimps are roughly 15 times larger. The 25-year life span predicted by *Cebus* body and brain size is much exceeded by the 45 to 50-year life spans actually observed.

LONG-LIVED MONKEYS HAVE LIFE SPANS PROPORTIONAL TO HUMAN CENTENARIANS.
Centenarian humans are not out of the scope of primate longevity, especially given the

large numbers of human observations; that is, high numbers increase the probability of sampling the extreme right tail of the distribution. *Cebus* monkeys exhibit relative life span potentials similar to humans and converge in traits such as a relatively large brain, generalized ability to exploit a wide range of ecological niches over a broad geographical distribution, fruit-based omnivorous diet, and polygynous mating systems (Judge and Carey 2000). Although *Cebus* are female philopatric (females remain in their natal groups while males disperse), it is not known whether human ancestors were male or female philopatric. If human ancestors had the potential for 72 to 90-year life spans for one to two million years, one might wonder why prolonging the life span to 100 years under modern conditions of ecological release has not been easier?

POST-REPRODUCTION EXPECTED FROM PRIMATE PATTERNS.   Hammer and Foley (1996) use body and raw brain volume estimates from fossil crania to predict early hominid longevity using a multivariate regression of log body weight and brain volume. Estimates based on regressions of anthropoid primate subfamilies, or limited to extant apes, indicate a major increase in longevity between *Homo habilis* (52 to 56 years) and *H. erectus* (60 to 63 years), occurring roughly 1.7 to 2 million years ago. Their predicted life span for small-bodied *H. sapiens* is 66 to 72 years. From a catarrhine (Old World monkeys and apes) comparison group, Judge and Carey (2000) predict 91 years when contemporary human data are excluded from the equation. For early hominids to live as long or longer than predicted was probably extremely rare; the important point is that the basic Old World primate design resulted in an organism with the potential to survive longer than a contemporary mother's ability to give birth. Notably, Hammer and Foley's predicted life span of *H. habilis* exceeds the age of menopause in extant women by 7 to 11 years, and that of *H. erectus* exceeds menopause by 15 to 18 years. This suggests that postmenopausal survival is not an artifact of modern lifestyle but may have originated between one and two million years ago coincident with the radiation of hominids out of Africa.

Williams (1957) first suggested that menopause may be the evolutionary result of a human life history that requires extended maternal care of offspring. Diamond (1992) notes that menopause probably resulted from two distinctly human characteristics: (1) the exceptional danger that childbirth poses to mothers and (2) the danger that a mother's death poses to her offspring. Perinatal mortality tends to increase with maternal age, and the death of an older mother endangers not only her current infant but earlier-born infants still dependent on her for food, protection, and other forms of care. However, more recently, Hawkes and co-workers (1998) argue that it is postreproductive longevity that has evolved rather than an early cessation of female reproduction; the reproductive spans of human and other ape females are not appreciably different. Rather, kin selection for older relatives subsidizing the reproduction of younger female kin may have been a primary mechanism extending human life span (the "grandmother hypothesis"). This subsidization also allowed humans a later age at maturity and, as a result, a longer period of time for growth and learning.

AN EMERGING BIOLOGICAL-DEMOGRAPHIC PARADIGM

The view many demographers have of biology is similar to the view of many sociologists who believe that "biology" and the "social" are locked in an explanatory zero-sum game in which any ground ceded to the former diminishes the value of the later (Freese et al. 2003). But even if sociologists (and by extension demographers) banish "biological" explanations of social behavior from their forums, swelling interest in the topic would still exist elsewhere in the academy, as would a curiosity among the general public (Freese et al. 2003). What separates biological perspectives in sociology (sociobiology) and demography (biodemography) from their more conventional alternatives is not whether biological perspectives on sociological or demographic questions are correct but how useful specifically biologically minded thinking and experimental methods are for understanding human demography.

In the perennial struggle of all disciplines, including demography, to define and renew themselves and to ensure their relevance in an ever changing world, each discipline is always faced with decisions about whether to move in new directions. As Foster (2000) notes, demography, like other social sciences, is slowly coming to terms with important truths that the biological sciences have proved beyond any doubt, namely, that both the human mind and human behaviors are as much products of biological evolution as is the human body. Wilson (1998) notes that human beings may be unique in their degree of behavioral plasticity and in their possession of language and self-awareness, but all of the known human systems, biological and social, taken together form only a small subset of those displayed by the thousands of living species. We believe that the integration of biology into demography through the emerging field of biological demography will provide a deeper understanding of demographic processes and will thus offer insights about which patterns are common to a broad range of organisms and which demographic patterns are uniquely human.

Model System

Inasmuch as demography is concerned with whole-animal phenomena such as births and death, model systems (e.g., nematode worms fruit flies, laboratory rodents) can be brought to bear on fundamental questions about the nature of fertility and mortality. However, in mainstream demography a stumbling block to the serious use of model systems in studying aging has been the mistaken belief that, because causes of death in humans are unrelated to causes of death in nonhuman species (particularly in invertebrates such as nematodes and fruit flies), little can be learned from the detailed knowledge of age-specific mortality in these model species. This perspective is based on a theory familiar to most demographers, namely, the "theory of the underlying cause" in public health and medicine, which states that if the starting point of a train of events leading to death is known (e.g., cancer), death can be averted by preventing the initiating cause from operating (Moriyama 1956). For aging research the problem with this perspective is that death is seen as a single force, that is, the skeleton with the scythe. A more apt characterization that applies to deaths in all species is given by Kannisto, who notes that deaths are better viewed as the outcome of a crowd of "little devils"—individual potential or probabilistic causes of death that sometimes hunt in packs and reinforce each other's efforts, and at other times are independent (Kannisto 1991). Inasmuch as underlying causes of death are frequently context-specific, they are difficult to distinguish from immediate causes; their postmortem identification in humans is often arbitrary and, in invertebrates, virtually impossible. Thus, studying the causes of death often provides little insight into the nature of aging. If aging is a varying pattern of vulnerability to genetic and environmental insults, then the most important use of model species in both teaching and research on the demography of aging is to interpret their age patterns of mortality as proxy indicators of frailty. That is, different model systems can be used to address questions at different levels of demographic generality.

Levels of Specificity

The demographic profiles of humans have characteristics typical of a wide variety of organisms due to a similarity in evolutionary selection pressures. For example, the characteristic of higher male than female mortality during the prime reproductive ages is typical among sexually reproducing animals of a large number of vertebrate and invertebrate species. The pattern is an evolutionary result of sexual selection on males and, as such, is a *general characteristic* of a large number of species. Other observed general characteristics include the variable rate of change in mortality with age (rates that decline after the earliest stage and then increase with age) and a slowing of mortality at the most advanced ages (Vaupel et al. 1998). Given such generalities, there are also characteristics of mortality profiles that pertain more specifically to a particular species (or other taxonomic group). Such species-level characteristics are imposed on some general pattern.

The mortality experience for humans can thus be considered at two levels. The *general level* exhibits a decline after infancy, increases through the reproductive life span (the overall U-shaped trajectory), and a sex differential. The *specific level* pertains to details of the mortality experience unique to humans, including the actual probabilities of death by age, inflection points of age-specific mortality, the cause-specific probabilities of death, and the age-specific pattern of the sex differential. The observed mortality pattern is a combination of the evolutionary components of the trajectory (which will be common to a large number of species with overlapping life history characteristics) and the proximate age- and sex-specific factors contributing to mortality under certain conditions. For example, under contemporary conditions male reproductive competition selects for riskier behavior and results in deaths due to accidents and homicides during early adulthood. The general and specific components of any population's mortality schedule can only be determined through studies using model systems. This requires use of experimental demography and comparative biology.

Emerging Areas of Biological-Demographic Research: Selected Examples

EVOLUTIONARY DEMOGRAPHY.   How long do individuals in different species live? How fecund are they? How big do they become? Such questions about the age-trajectories of mortality, fertility, and growth are of fundamental interest to biological demographers, as well as to life-history biologists and evolutionary theorists. Although there is a vast empirical literature about these age-trajectories, there are remarkably few species for which reliable life tables are available. Furthermore, considerable work needs to be done to develop theory. Demographers can contribute to this work, as evidenced by contributions by Tuljapurkar (1990; 1997), Wachter (1999), Lee (2003), and James Vaupel and co-workers (2004). Lotka, as discussed earlier, pioneered research in evolutionary demography, but following his seminal contributions in the 1920s and 1930s, most demographers turned to other topics. The recent resurgence of interest in evolutionary demography (now nicknamed evo-demo) suggests that this area may become one of the most interesting and important branches of all demography. Its potential is enhanced by the fundamental importance of demography in evolution, as briefly explained in the following paragraph.

Nothing in biology, Dobzhansky has asserted, makes sense except in the light of evolution (Dobzhansky 1973). An equally valid overstatement is that nothing in evolution can be understood except in the light of demography. Evolution is driven by population dynamics governed by age-schedules of fertility and survival. Lotka emphasized this in his pathbreaking research. Since the work of Lotka, models of the evolution of fertility, mortality, and other life-history patterns have been based on stable population theory. Lotka's (1928) equation:

$$\int_0^\omega e^{-ra} l(a) m(a) da = 1 \tag{1}$$

specifies the intrinsic growth rate, r, of a closed population, typically of females, as a function of the proportion, $l(a)$, of newborns surviving to age a and age-specific maternity (or fertility), $m(a)$. If a new subspecies emerges as a result of mutation, then the subspecies is assumed to have an evolutionary advantage if its intrinsic growth rate is greater than that of other subspecies.

Closely related to evolutionary demography is the field of research at the intersection of demography and life-history theory. Life-history theory in biology is concerned with explaining evolutionary fitness in relationship to species-specific characteristics such as age at maturity, age at fecundity, clutch or litter size, size at birth, and age-specific survival rates across species. Biological demography is thus inextricably linked to life history theory because the analysis of a species' life history traits must ultimately be considered relative to their effects on birth and/or death rates. Whereas demographers concerned with human populations usually consider birth and death separately (for an exception, see Montgomery and Cohen 1998), life history theorists consider the fitness implications of particular sets of age-specific birth and death rates as defined by the intrinsic rate of population increase (as discussed above; also see Fisher 1958). The seminal papers on life history theory in the population biology, ecology, and evolution literature include papers on the population consequences of life history traits (Cole 1954), the use of the Lotka equation to evaluate insect populations (Birch 1948), and the sensitivity of changes in different life history traits such as age of first reproduction and total fecundity on the intrinsic rate of increase (Lewontin 1965). Recent papers by Ricklefs and Scheuerlein (2003), Gaillard and co-workers (2003), and Harshman (2003) consider life history traits in the context of life span and aging. Recent papers by Kaplan and his anthropology colleagues (1997; Kaplan, Lancaster, and Robson 2003; Kaplan and Lancaster 2003) exemplify how life history theory can be brought to bear on important questions concerned with human demography, embodied capital, and the evolution of extraordinary life span.

GENETIC AND GENOMIC DEMOGRAPHY.   Biological-demographic concepts may also be brought to bear on questions in genetics and genomics in at least two broad contexts. The first is concerned with human demographic history. The genome of the human species preserves a record of population dynamics, that is, changes in size and of subdivisions into partially isolated demes (Harpending 2003). Genetic studies suggest that the human species is derived from a small population of perhaps several thousand individuals who underwent a dramatic demographic expansion during the last interglacial period approximately 100,000 years ago (Harpending 2003; Stringer and Andrews 1988). There are several issues in human demography and genetics for which the genetic evidence of a small founding population and subsequent rapid growth are important, including:

1. Genetic evidence provides clear support for the "Garden of Eden" model of modern human origins in which humans are the outcome of a speciation event in a small population.
2. Human demographic history is the underlying determinant of the distribution of genetic diversity in human species. Thus diversity should be recent rather than ancient and localized rather than dispersed throughout human species.
3. A history of rapid expansion and colonization of most of the earth suggests that our species has from the beginning been ecologically disruptive (Reich and Goldstein 1998).

The second context in which biological-demographic concepts can be brought to bear on genetics and genomics is in biomedical and health aspects of contemporary populations (Ewbank 2000). This research is discussed in the section on biomedical demography.

PALEODEMOGRAPHY. Anthropology and demography have natural affinities, since both fields are concerned primarily with humans and with vital events including birth and death (Spuhler 1959; Weiss 1973). Skeletal remains are the source of information about prehistoric populations regarding sex, age at death, lifetime morbidity, and nutrition. Hence, a main focus on paleodemography is determining how to extract more information from bones. This requires a sophisticated understanding of biology as well as a facility with methods of using physical indicators to determine sex and estimate age at death and other variables. A promising recent advance is the development, by Ursula Wittwer-Backofen and Jutta Gampe, of methods to count annual rings deposited in teeth as a way of determining age at death (personal communication). Roughly similar methods can be used to estimate the age of animals in the wild, with teeth used for mammals and otoliths (ear bones) for fish. Lesions in bones and minerals in teeth and bones can shed light on health and nutritional histories. Information about human population development for the long period during which written records were scarce or nonexistent thus hinges on biological information.

ECOLOGICAL BIODEMOGRAPHY. Four studies concerned with the biodemography of wild populations of organisms underscore the importance of ecological studies. The first is one on field aging rates of the Virginia opossum, *Didelphis virginiana* (Austad 1993). The study was designed to test the hypothesis "that populations historically subjected to low rates of environmentally imposed mortality will ultimately evolve senescence that is retarded in relation to that of populations historically subjected to higher mortality rates" (Austad 1993: 696). Because islands have reduced predation relative to the mainland, theory predicts that rates of aging will be lower in the insular population. Consistent with this prediction, Austad (1993) reports reduced senescence for island populations based on physiological measures of aging.

A second series of studies was conducted by Reznick and associates, who developed a model system for studying the ecology and evolution of longevity in guppies, a small freshwater fish from the northeastern coast of South America and some neighboring Caribbean islands (Reznick et al. 1997). Reznick manipulated field predation rates of adults and, over evolutionary time, observed accelerated maturation rates, increased allocation to reproduction, and changes in the size and interval of litters. Reznick's most generalized finding is that environment shapes life span in guppies. The life span of guppies recovered from streams that supported predator populations, whether naturally or through deliberate introductions, was shorter than those in streams in which predators were not present.

The third biodemographic study is by Tatar, Grey, and Carey (1997). This work characterized differences in senescence among populations of grasshoppers that occur along an altitudinal gradient in the Sierra Nevada, California. Experimental males from five populations of the grasshopper *Melanoplus sanguinipes/devastator* sibling species complex were collected along the altitudinal gradient. The researchers found that differences in the physiological capacity to survive in a sheltered, common environment revealed genetic differences in underlying rates of senescence, providing maternal effects do not affect the rate of aging in offspring.

A fourth study of aging in the wild was by Roach on the perennial plant, *Plantago lanceolata*, using an initial cohort of 10,000 individuals in a natural field environment (Roach 2003). In order to separate the effects of the environment- and age-dependent factors on mortality, additional cohorts were planted in the field over the next three years for a total of 27,000 plants. The results demonstrate that demographic patterns in natural populations are strongly influenced by seasonal and yearly environmental variation, particularly temperature and rainfall. Her study also demonstrates that there is an interdependence of demographic patterns across life stages. Cohorts established in different years showed different patterns of mortality, and the history of mortality within a cohort was critical to late-age demographic patterns. This study also showed that age-dependent patterns of mortality may be masked by age-independent environmental factors and that to study aging in a natural population requires one to account for these other influences on mortality. A covariate regression analysis was used to determine the age-dependent risk of mortality for this field population (Roach and Gampe, unpublished). Several factors, including microsite spatial location, temperature, rainfall, reproduction, size, and genetics, were all found to significantly influence mortality. When all of these factors were accounted for in the regression model, there was no evidence of an increased risk of dying with age. These results suggest that increasing size after reproductive maturity may allow species to escape from demographic senescence. An additional greenhouse study contrasting field-grown plants with 1,000 plants grown in the greenhouse demonstrates the remarkable plasticity of mortality patterns (Roach 2001). Over a period of four years, mortality was 6% in the greenhouse and 91% for similarly aged plants in the field. Given these contrasting patterns of mortality, individuals in natural populations will thus clearly never experience the extreme old ages of individuals studied under controlled environmental conditions.

BIOMEDICAL DEMOGRAPHY

As noted at the outset of this chapter, biodemography pertains to two different fields, namely biological demography and biomedical demography. These two fields are as distinct as biology is from biomedicine. This chapter has emphasized the concepts and findings of biological demography, in part because the concepts and findings are less familiar to most demographers. The last few pages of this chapter will now turn to the other branch of biodemography.

The number of demographers working in the area of biomedical demography is at least as large as the number working in biological demography. Grant funding is substantially greater and publications are at least as numerous. The field of biomedical demography is innovative and important, with the potential for making contributions that help improve public health. The field can essentially be characterized as the interface between demography and epidemiology. Demography and epidemiology intersect and overlap. Demographers more frequently focus on how diseases and disabilities influence the structure and dynamics of a population, whereas epidemiologists are typically concerned with how population patterns of a specific disease of interest shed light on the etiology, prevention, and cure of the disease. Many demographers have acquired a substantial knowledge of the biology of various diseases and disabilities and have developed models of morbidity and mortality. Some relate disease and disability patterns and trends in a population to consequences for health care systems. Demographers and epidemiologists often collaborate on designing better surveys, questionnaires, and health measurements.

The field of biomedical demography emerged over the past two decades and is now flourishing. This development was fostered by funding from the Behavioral and Social Science branch of the U.S. National Institute on Aging. The head of this branch, Richard Suzman, deserves credit for recognizing and supporting the role of demographers in biomedical research. Other sources of inspiration and funding have been the Italian National Institute on Aging, headed by Claudio Franceschi, and the epidemiology and demography program at the University of Southern Denmark, currently under the leadership of Kaare Christensen and Bernard Jeune.

A key event in the history of biomedical demography was a National Research Council workshop in 2000 called *Cells and Surveys: Should Biological Measures be Included in Social Science Research?* The workshop was organized and chaired by Caleb Finch, James Vaupel, and Kevin Kinsella (Finch et al. 2000). The workshop sought to address questions such as the following: What can social science in general and demography in particular reasonably expect to learn from biomedical information? Which genetic, pedigree, historical, and environmental data ought to be collected in order to be most useful to a wide range of scientists? The volume published from this workshop (Finch et al. 2000) includes chapters on the use of bioindicators in demographic and social research, the potential of using genetic information in demography, research on aging human subjects, the relevance of animal models for human populations, value-added survey research, and consent and privacy issues.

Currently, several major research projects are underway that are headed or co-headed by biomedical demographers. In the United States the three most notable are the Health and Retirement Survey (HRS), the National Long Term Care Survey (NLTCS), and the MacArthur Study of Successful Aging. Soldo played a major role in designing the HRS, Manton has long directed the NLTCS, and Crimmins, Haywood, and Singer have worked with the MacArthur data. The very large Chinese Longitudinal Survey of Healthy Longevity was devised by Zeng and Vaupel. Vaupel (and colleagues) participated in the design, funding, and analysis of large longitudinal studies of aging among older Danish twins, very old Sardinians, and elderly Russians living in Moscow and St. Petersburg. Weinstein and Goldman are the leaders of the Taiwan Study of the Elderly (Weinstein and Willis 2000).

A main contribution of biomedical demographers has been the development of models. Manton has played a leadership role in the elaboration of dynamic models for analyzing complicated longitudinal data. The numerous publications of Manton and colleagues are summarized (Manton and Yashin 2000). Also notable are the modeling contributions of Ewbank (2000) and the work of biological demographers (Carey et al. 1998; Müller et al. 1997).

Demographers over the past half century have increasingly become involved with the design of surveys and the analysis of survey data, especially pertaining to fertility or morbidity and mortality. Recently, various kinds of physical measurements (height and weight), physiological measurements (of blood pressure and cholesterol levels), nutritional status (assessed by the analysis of blood or urine and other methods), physical performance (hand-grip strength or ability to pick a coin up from the floor), and genetic makeup (as determined by analysis of DNA) have been added to surveys, including those conducted by Christensen, Goldman, Weinstein, Zeng, and others. Such biological measurements can be used as covariates in demographic analyses in much the same way that social and economic information is used. These kinds of analyses are an important activity of biomedical demographers (Finch et al. 2000).

In particular, there has been a rapid growth of interest in using genetic information in medical-demographic research (Ewbank 2000). Of particular interest is the information from DNA about specific genes, as in research by Ewbank (2001), and Yashin (Yashin et al. 2000). Information from DNA about genetic polymorphisms (i.e., mutations) can be used to determine the genetic structure of a population and to make inferences about the influence of migration and inbreeding on the population. A central goal of such "molecular demography" is to identify genetic polymorphisms that affect mortality, morbidity, functioning, fecundity, and other sources of demographic change. Much of this research to date, as illustrated by analyses conducted by Ewbank, Vaupel, and Yashin (cited above), has focused on finding genetic variants that influence longevity. This relationship can be studied by analyzing changes with age in the proportion of survivors who have some specific allele (i.e., version of a gene). If in a given cohort the allele becomes more frequent with age, that allele may be associated with lower mortality.

It should not be forgotten, however, that much can be learned about genetics even if DNA is unavailable. The genetic and common environment components of these variations in life spans, fertility, and other demographic characteristics can be analyzed in humans using demographic data on twins, siblings, cousins, and other relatives of various degree. These data are available in genealogies and in twin, household, parish, and other population registries. Required is information about the proportion of genes shared by two individuals and about shared nongenetic influences. Analysis of variance methods, correlated frailty approaches, and nested event-history models have been applied by demographers. Kohler and Rodgers (2003) have studied how much of the variation in number of children can be attributed to genetic variation in family size preferences among potential parents, and Anatoli Yashin has analyzed genetic variation as it is related to susceptibility to various diseases and to mortality in general (Yashin and Iachine 1997; Yashin et al. 2001).

In sum, both the biomedical-demography branch of biodemography and the biological-demography branch are vibrant areas of demographic research that are rapidly growing and that have great potential to enrich and enlarge the domain of demography. Not only can demographers learn much from biologists and epidemiologists, they are also capable of contributing much to research on life in general, as opposed to humans in particular, and to research on population health.

REFERENCES

Adams, J. 1990. Introduction: Genetics and demography and historical information. In *Convergent issues in genetics and demography*. Edited by J. Adams, D. A. Lam, A. I. Hermalin, and P. E. Smouse, 3–13. New York: Oxford University Press.

Altmann, J., and S. C. Alberts. 2003. Intraspecific variability in fertility and offspring survival in a nonhuman primate: Behavioral control of ecological and social sources. In *Offspring: Human fertility behavior in biodemographic perspective*. Edited by K. W. Wachter and R. A. Bulato, 140–169. Washington D.C.: National Academies Press.

Austad, S. N. 1993. Retarded senescence in an insular population of Virginia opossums (*Didelphis Virginiana*). *Journal of Zoology* 229: 695–708.

Austad, S. N. 1997. Postreproductive survival. In *Between Zeus and the salmon: The biodemography of longevity*. Edited by K. W. Wachter and C. E. Finch, 161–174. Washington, D.C.: National Academies Press.

Bacci, A. L. 2001. Comment: Desired family size and the future course of fertility. In *Global fertility transition*. Edited by R. A. Bulatao and J. B. Casterline, 282–289. New York: Population Council: Supplement to Population and Development Review 27.

Bachrach, C. 2001. Comment: The puzzling persistence of postmodern fertility preferences. In *Global fertility transition*. Edited by R. A. Bulatao and J. B. Casterline, 332–338. New York: Population Council: Supplement to Population and Development Review 27.

Barker, D. P. J. 1994. *Mothers, babies and diseases in after life*, 1st ed. London: BMJ Publishing Group.

Bartholomew, G. A. 1964. The roles of physiology and behaviour in the maintenance of homeostasis in the desert environment. In *Homeostasis and feedback mechanisms*. Edited by G. M. Huges, 7–29. Cambridge: Cambridge University Press.

Begon M., J. L. Harper, C. R. Townsend. 1996. Ecology: Individuals, Populations and Communities, 3rd ed., Blackwell Science Ltd, Oxford.

Bell, G. 1988. *Sex and death in Protozoa*. Cambridge: Cambridge University Press.

Bell, G., and V. Koufopanou. 1986. The cost of reproduction. In *Oxford surveys in evolutionary biology*. Edited by R. Dawkins and M. Ridley, 83–131. Oxford: Oxford University Press.

Birch, L. C. 1948. The intrinsic rate of natural increase of an insect population. *Journal of Animal Ecology* 17: 15–26.

Black, W. C., C. F. Baer, M. F. Antolin, and N. M. DuTeau. 2001. Population genomics: Genome-wide sampling of insect populations. *Annual Review of Entomology* 44: 441–469.

Bongaarts, J. 2001. Fertility and reproductive preferences in post-transitional societies. In *Global fertility transition*. Edited by R. A. Bulatao and J. B. Casterline, 260–281. New York: Population Council: Supplement to Population and Development Review 27.

Bulatao, R. A., and J. B. Casterine. 2001. *Global fertility transition*. New York: Population and Development Review.

Burns, M. A., B. N. Johnson, S. N. Brahmasandra, et al. 1998. An integrated nanoliter DNA analysis device. *Science* 282: 484–487.

Caldwell, J. C. 2001. The globalization of fertility behavior. In *Global fertility transition*. Edited by R. A. Bulatao and J. B. Casterline, 116–128. New York: Population Council: Supplement to Population and Development Review 27.

Cameron, J. L. 2003. Hormonal mediation of physiological and behavioral processes that influence fertility. In *Offspring: Human fertility behavior in biodemographic perspective.* Edited by K. W. Wachter and R. A. Bulato, 104–139. Washington, D.C.: National Academies Press.

Campbell, B. 2003. Pubertal maturation, andrenarche, and the onset of reproduction in human males. In *Offspring: Human fertility behavior in biodemographic perspective.* Edited by K. W. Wachter and R. A. Bulato, 260–288. Washington D.C.: National Academies Press.

Carey, J. R. 1993. *Applied demography for biologists.* New York: Oxford University Press.

Carey, J. R. 2003a. Life span: A conceptual overview. In *Life span: Evolutionary, ecological, and demographic perspectives.* Edited by J. R. Carey and S. Tuljapurkar, 1–18. New York: Population Council: Supplement to Population and Development Review 29.

Carey, J. R. 2003b. *Longevity. The biology and demography of life span.* Princeton, N.J.: Princeton University Press.

Carey, J. R., and C. Gruenfelder. 1997. Population biology of the elderly. In *Between Zeus and the salmon: The biodemography of longevity.* Edited by K. W. Wachter and C. E. Finch, 127–160. Washington, D.C.: National Academies Press.

Carey, J. R., and D. S. Judge. 2000. *Longevity records: Life spans of mammals, birds, reptiles, amphibians and fish.* Odense, Denmark: Odense University Press.

Carey, J. R., and D. S. Judge. 2001. Principles of biodemography with special reference to human longevity. *Population: An English Selection* 13: 9–40.

Carey, J. R., P. Liedo, H.-G. Müller, J.-L. Wang, and J. W. Vaupel. 1998. A simple graphical technique for displaying individual fertility data and cohort survival: Case study of 1000 Mediterranean fruit fly females. *Functional Ecology* 12: 359–363.

Carey, J. R., P. Liedo, D. Orozco, M. Tatar, and J. W. Vaupel. 1995. A male-female longevity paradox in Medfly cohorts. *Journal of Animal Ecology* 64: 107–116.

Carey, J. R., P. Liedo, D. Orozco, and J. W. Vaupel. 1992. Slowing of mortality rates at older ages in large Medfly cohorts. *Science* 258: 457–461.

Carey, J. R., and S. Tuljapurkar. 2003. *Life span: Evolutionary, ecological and demographic perspectives.* New York: Population and Development Review.

Caswell, H. 1989. *Matrix population models.* Sunderland, Mass.: Sinauer.

Cavalli-Sforza, L. L., P. Menozi, and A. Piazza. 1994. *The history and geography of human genes.* Princeton, N.J.: Princeton University Press.

Charlesworth, R. 1994. *Evolution in age-structured populations,* 2nd ed. Cambridge: Cambridge University Press.

Clark, W. 1996. *Sex and the origins of death.* Oxford: Oxford University Press.

Clutton-Brock, T. H. 1991. *The evolution of parental care.* Princeton, N.J.: Princeton University Press.

Cohen, J. E. 1984. Demography and morbidity: A survey of some interactions. In *Population and biology.* Edited by N. Keyfitz, 199–222. Liege, Belgium: Ordina Editions.

Cohen, J. E. 1995. *How many people can the earth support?* New York: W. W. Norton & Company.

Cole, L. C. 1954. The population consequences of life history phenomena. *Quarterly Review of Biology* 29: 103–137.

Collins, F. S. 1999. Shattuck lecture–medical and societal consequences of the Human Genome Project. *New England Journal of Medicine* 341: 29–37.

Crimmins, E. M., M. D. Hayward, and Y. Saito. 1996. Differentials in active life expectancy in the older population of the United States. *Journal of Gerontology: Social Sciences* 51B: S111–S120.

Crimmins, E. M., and T. Seeman. 2000. Integrating biology into demographic research on health and aging (with a focus on the Macarthur Study of Successful Aging). In *Cells and surveys: Should biological measures be included in social science research?* Edited by C. E. Finch, J. W. Vaupel, and K. Kinsella, 9–41. Washington, D. C.: National Academies Press.

Curtsinger, J. W., H. H. Fukui, D. R. Townsend, and J. W. Vaupel. 1992. Demography of genotypes: Failure of the limited life-span paradigm in *Drosophila Melanogaster.* *Science* 258: 461–463.

Darwin, C. 1859. *On the origin of species.* Cambridge, Mass.: Harvard University Press (reprinted 1964).

Deevey, E. S. J. 1947. Life tables for natural populations of animals. *Quarterly Review of Biology* 22: 283–314.

DeRousseau, J. C. 1994. Primate gerontology: An emerging discipline. In *Biological anthropology and aging.* Edited by D. E. Crews and R. M. Garruto, 127–153. New York: Oxford University Press.

Diamond, J. 1992. *The third chimpanzee.* New York: Harper Perennial.

Dobzhansky, T. 1973. Nothing in biology makes sense except in the light of evolution. *The American Biology Teacher* 35: 125–129.

Ellison, P. T. 2001. *On fertile ground: A natural history of human reproduction.* Cambridge, Mass.: Harvard University Press.

Ewbank, D. 2000. Demography in the age of genomics: A first look at the prospects. In *Cells and surveys: Should biological measures be included in social science research?* Edited by C. E. Finch, J. W. Vaupel, and K. Kinsella, 64–109. Washington, D. C.: National Academies Press.

Ewbank, D. C. 2004. The Apoe gene and differences in life expectancy in Europe. *Journal of Gerontology: Biological Sciences* 59A: 16–20.

Feder, M. E., A. F. Bennett, and R. B. Huey. 2000. Evolutionary physiology. *Annual Review of Ecology and Systematics* 31: 315–341.

Finch, C. E., and R. E. Tanzi. 1997. Genetics of aging. *Science* 278: 407–411.

Finch, C. E., J. W. Vaupel, and K. Kinsella. 2000. *Cells and surveys: Should biological measures be included in social science research?* Washington, D. C.: National Academies Press.

Fisher, R. A. 1958. *The genetical theory of natural selection,* 2nd ed. New York: Dover Publications.

Foley, R. A. 1999. Hominid behavioural evolution: Missing links in comparative primate socioecology. In *Comparative primate socioecology.* Edited by P. C. Lee, 363–386. Cambridge: Cambridge University Press.

Foster, C. 2000. The limits to low fertility: A biosocial approach. *Population and Development Review* 26: 209–234.

Frank, P. W. 1959. Ecology and demography. In *The study of population.* Edited by P. M. Hauser and O. D. Duncan, 652–677. Chicago: University of Chicago Press.

Freese, J., J. C. A. Li, and L. D. Wade. 2003. The potential relevances of biology to social inquiry. *Annual Review of Sociology* 29: 233–256.

Gage, T. B. 1998. The comparative demography of primates: With some comments on the evolution of life histories. *Annual Review of Anthropology* 27: 197–221.

Gaillard, J.-M., A. Loison, M. Festa-Bianchet, N. G. Yoccoz, and E. Solberg. 2003. Ecological correlates of life span in populations of large herbivorous mammals. In *Life span: Evolutionary, ecological, and demographic perspectives.* Edited by J. R. Carey and S. Tuljapurkar, 39–56. New York: Population Council: Supplement to Population and Development Review 29.

Gangestad, S. W. 2003. Sexually antagonistic coevolution: Theory, evidence and implication for patterns of human mating and fertility. In *Offspring: Human fertility behavior in biodemographic perspective.* Edited by K. W. Wachter and R. A. Bulato. Washington, D.C.: National Academies Press.

Gavrilov, L. A., and N. S. Gavrilova. 2001. The reliability theory of aging and longevity. *Journal of Theoretical Biology* 213: 527–545.

Gerdes, L. U., B. Jeune, K. Andersen-Ranberg, H. Nybo, and J. W. Vaupel. 2000. Estimation of apolipoprotein E genotype-specific relative mortality risks from the distribution of genotypes in centenarians and middle-aged men: Apolipoprotein E gene is a 'frailty gene' not a 'longevity gene'. *Genetic Epidemiology* 19: 202–210.

Getz, W. M., and R. G. Haight. 1989. *Population harvesting.* Princeton, N.J.: Princeton University Press.

Gompertz, B. 1825. On the nature of the function expressive of the law of mortality. *Philosophical Transactions* 27: 513–585.

Halter, J. B., and D. B. Reuben. 2000. Indicators of function in the geriatric population. In *Cells and surveys: Should biological measures be included in social science research?* Edited by C. E. Finch, J. W. Vaupel, and K. Kinsella, 159–179. Washington, D. C.: National Academies Press.

Hamilton, W. D. 1966. The moulding of senescence by natural selection. *Journal of Theoretical Biology* 12: 12–45.

Hammer, M., and R. Foley. 1996. Longevity, life history and allometry: How long did hominids live? *Human Evolution* 11: 61–66.

Harpending, H. 2003. Humans: Demographic history. In *Nature: Encyclopedia of the human genome.* Edited by D. N. Cooper, 383–387. London: Nature Publishing Group.

Harpending, H. C., and A. R. Rogers. 2000. Genetic perspectives on human origins and differentiation. *Annual Review of Genomics and Human Genetics* 1: 361–385.

Harshman, L. E. 2003. Life span extension of *Drosophila melanogaster:* Genetic and population studies. In *Life span: Evolutionary, ecological, and demographic perspectives.* Edited by J. R. Carey and S. Tuljapurkar, 99–126. New York: Population Council: Supplement to Population and Development Review 29.

Hastings, A., and S. Harrison. 1994. Metapopulation dynamics and genetics. *Annual Review of Ecology and Systematics* 25: 167–188.

Hauser, P. M., and O. D. Duncan. 1959a. The nature of demography. In *The study of population.* Edited by P. M. Hauser and O. D. Duncan, 29–44. Chicago: University of Chicago Press.

Hauser, P. M., and O. D. Duncan. 1959b. *The study of population*. Chicago: University of Chicago Press.

Hawkes, K., J. F. O'Connell, N. G. B. Jones, H. Alvarez, and E. L. Charnov. 1998. Grandmothering, menopause, and the evolution of life history traits. *Proceedings of the National Academy of Sciences USA* 953: 1336–1339.

Helfand, S. L., and S. K. Inouye. 2002. Rejuvenating views of the ageing process. *Nature Genetics* 3: 149–150.

Herskind, A. M., M. McGue, N. V. Holm, T. I. A. Sorensen, B. Harvald, and J. W. Vaupel. 1996. The heritability of human longevity: A population-based study of 2872 Danish twins Paris Born 1870–1900. *Human Genetics* 97: 319–323.

Hill, K., and A. M. Hurtado. 1996. *Ache life history: The ecology and demography of a foraging people*. New York: Aldine De Gruyter.

Hill, K., and H. Kaplan. 1999. Life history traits in humans: Theory and empirical studies. *Annual Review of Anthropology* 28: 397–430.

Hobcraft, J. N. 2003. Reflections on demographic, evolutionary, and genetic approaches to the study of human reproductive behavior. In *Offspring: Human fertility behavior in biodemographic perspective*. Edited by K. W. Wachter and R. A. Bulato, 339–357. Washington D.C.: National Academies Press.

Holzgreve, W., and S. Hahn. 2003. Fetal diagnosis. In *Nature: Encyclopedia of the human genome*. Edited by D. N. Cooper, 177–480. London: Nature Publishing Group.

Horiuchi, S. 2003. Interspecies differences in the life span distribution: Humans versus invertebrates. In *Life span: Evolutionary, ecological, and demographic perspectives*. Edited by J. R. Carey and S. Tuljapurkar, 127–151. New York: Population Council: Supplement to Population and Development Review 29.

Jacquard, A. 1984. Concepts of genetics and concepts of demography: Specificities and analogies. In *Population and biology*. Edited by N. Keyfitz, 29–40. Liege, Belgium: Ordina Editions.

Johnson, T. E. 1990. Increased life-span of age-1 mutants in *Caenorhabditis elegans* and lower Gompertz rate of aging. *Science* 249: 908–912.

Johnson, T. E., and D. R. Shook. 1997. Identification and mapping of genes determining longevity. In *Between Zeus and the salmon: The biodemography of longevity*. Edited by K. W. Wachter and C. E. Finch, 108–126. Washington, D.C.: National Academies Press.

Judge, D. S., and J. R. Carey. 2000. Post-reproductive life predicted by primate patterns. *Journal of Gerontology: Biological Sciences* 55A: B201–B209.

Kallmann, F. J., and J. D. Rainer. 1959. Physical anthropology and demography. In *The study of population*. Edited by P. M. Hauser and O. D. Duncan, 759–790. Chicago: University of Chicago Press.

Kannisto, V. 1991. Frailty and survival. *Genus* 47: 101–118.

Kannisto, V. 1996. *The advancing frontier of survival. Life tables for old age*. Odense, Denmark: Odense University Press.

Kaplan, H. 1997. The evolution of the human life course. In *Between Zeus and the salmon: The biodemography of longevity*. Edited by K. W. Wachter and C. E. Finch, 175–211. Washington, D.C.: National Academies Press.

Kaplan, H., J. Lancaster, and A. Robson. 2003. Embodied capital and the evolutionary economics of the human life span. In *Life span: Evolutionary, ecological, and demographic perspectives*. Edited by J. R. Carey and S. Tuljapurkar, 152–182. New York: Population Council: Supplement to Population and Development Review 29.

Kaplan, H. S., and J. B. Lancaster. 2003. An evolutionary and ecological analysis of human fertility, mating patterns, and parental investment. In *Offspring: Human fertility behavior in biodemographic perspective*. Edited by K. W. Wachter and R. A. Bulato, 170–223. Washington D.C.: National Academies Press.

Kenyon, C. 1997. Environmental factors and gene activities that influence life span. In *C. Elegans Ii*. Edited by D. L. Riddle, T. Blumenthal, B. J. Meyer, and J. R. Priess, 791–813. Cold Spring Harbor, N.Y.: Cold Spring Harbor Press.

Keyfitz, N. 1977. *Applied mathematical demography*. New York: Springer-Verlag.

Keyfitz, N. 1984a. Introduction: Biology and demography. In *Population and biology*. Edited by N. Keyfitz, 1–7. Liege, Belgium: Ordina Editions.

Keyfitz, N. 1984b. *Population and biology*. Liege, Belgium: Ordina Editions.

Kirkwood, T. B. L. 1992. Comparative life spans of species: Why do species have the life spans they do? *American Journal of Clinical Nutrition* 55: 1191S–1195S.

Kirkwood, T. B. L., and M. R. Rose. 1991. Evolution of senescence: Late survival sacrificed for reproduction. *Phil. Trans. Royal Society of London* 332: 15–24.

Kohler, H., and J. L. Rodgers. 2003. Education, fertility and heritability: Explaining a paradox. In *Offspring: Human fertility behavior in biodemographic perspective*. Edited by K. W. Wachter and R. A. Bulato, 46–90. Washington D.C.: National Academies Press.

Kollek, R. 2003. Reprogenetics: Visions of the future. In *Nature: Encyclopedia of the human genome*. Edited by D. N. Cooper, 27–35. London: Nature Publishing Group.

Lam, D. 2003. Evolutionary biology and rational choice in models of fertility. In *Offspring: Human fertility behavior in biodemographic perspective*. Edited by K. W. Wachter and R. A. Bulato, 322–338. Washington, D.C.: National Academies Press.

Lee, R. D. 1997. Intergenerational relations and the elderly. In *Between Zeus and the salmon: The biodemography of longevity*. Edited by K. W. Wachter and C. E. Finch, 212–233. Washington, D.C.: National Academies Press.

Lee, R. D. 2003. Rethinking the evolutionary theory of aging: Transfers, not births, shape senescence in social species. *Proceedings of the National Academy of Sciences* 100: 9637–9642.

Lee, R. D., and J. R. Goldstein. 2003. Rescaling the life cycle: Longevity and proportionality. In *Life span: Evolutionary, ecological, and demographic perspectives*. Edited by J. R. Carey and S. Tuljapurkar. New York: Population Council: Supplement to Population and Development Review 29.

Leridon, H. 1984. Selective effects of sterility and fertility. In *Population and biology*. Edited by N. Keyfitz, 83–98. Liege, Belgium: Ordina Editions.

Lewontin, R. C. 1965. Selection for colonizing ability. In *The genetics of colonizing species*. Edited by H. G. Baker and G. L. Stebbins, 77–94. New York: Academic Press.

Lewontin, R. C. 1984. Laws of biology and laws in social science. In *Population and biology*. Edited by N. Keyfitz, 19–28. Liege, Belgium: Ordina Editions.

Livi-Bacci, M. 1984. Introduction: Autoregulating mechanisms in human populations. In *Population and biology*. Edited by N. Keyfitz, 109–116. Liege, Belgium: Ordina Editions.

Lollar, D. J., and J. E. Crews. 2003. Redefining the role of public health in disability. *Annual Review of Public Health* 24: 195–208.

Lotka, A. J. 1924. *Elements of physical biology*. Baltimore: Williams & Wilkins.

Lotka, A. J. 1928. The progeny of a population element. *American Journal of Hygiene* 8:875–901.

Lotka, A. J. 1934. *Theorie analytique des associations biologiques. Part I. Principes*. Paris: Hermann et Cie.

Malthus, T. R. 1798. The first essay.

Mangel, M. 2003. Environment and longevity: The demography of the growth rate. In *Life span: Evolutionary, ecological, and demographic perspectives*. Edited by J. R. Carey and S. Tuljapurkar, 57–70. New York: Population Council: Supplement to Population and Development Review 29.

Manton, K. G., and E. Stallard. 1984. *Recent trends in mortality analysis*. Orlando, Fla.: Academic Press.

Manton, K. G., and E. Stallard. 1994. Medical demography: Interaction of disability dynamics and mortality. In *Demography of aging*. Edited by L. G. Martin and S. H. Preston, 217–278. Washington, D.C.: Naitonal Academies Press.

Manton, K. G., and A. I. Yashin. 2000. *Mechanisms of aging and mortality: The search for new paradigms*. Odense, Denmark: Odense University Press.

McClure, M. E. 1996. The "art" of medically assisted reproduction: An embryo is an embryo is an embro. In *Birth to death: Science and bioethics*. Edited by D. C. Thomasma and T. Kushner, 35–49. Cambridge: Cambridge University Press.

McEwen, B., and E. Stellar. 1993. Stress and the individuals: Mechanisms leading to disease. *Archives of Internal Medicine* 153: 2093–2101.

McGue, M., J. W. Vaupel, N. Holm, and B. Harvald. 1993. Longevity is moderately heritable in a sample of Danish twins born 1870–1880. *Journal of Gerontology* 48: B237–B244.

Meagher, T. R., and D. J. Futuyma. 2001. Executive document: Evolution, science, and society. *The American Naturalist* 158: 1–45.

Montgomery, M. R., and B. Cohen. 1998. *From birth to death: Mortality decline and reproductive change*. Washington, D.C.: National Academies Press.

Moriyama, I. M. 1956. Development of the present concept of cause of death. *American Journal of Public Health* 46: 436–441.

Müller, H. G., J. R. Carey, D. Wu, and J. W. Vaupel. 2001. Reproductive potential determines longevity of female Mediterranean fruitflies. *Proceedings of the Royal Society, London B* 268: 445–450.

Müller, H.-G., J.-M. Chiou, J. R. Carey, and J.-L. Wang. 2002. Fertility and lifespan: Late children enhance female longevity. *Journal of Gerontology: Biological Sciences* 57A: B202–B206.

Müller, H.-G., J.-L. Wang, W. B. Capra, P. Liedo, and J. R. Carey. 1997. Early mortality surge in protein-deprived females causes reversal of sex differential of life expectancy in Mediterranean fruit flies. *Proceedings of the National Academy of Sciences* 94: 2762–2765.

Nguyen, V.-K., and K. Peschard. 2003. Anthropology, inequality, and disease: A review. *Annual Review of Anthropology* 32: 447–474.

Numan, M. 1998. Parental behavior, mammals. In *Encyclopedia of Reproduction.* Edited by E. A. J. D. N. Knobil, 684–694. San Diego: Academic Press.

Olshansky, S. J., B. A. Carnes, and C. Cassel. 1990. In search of Methuselah: Estimating the upper limits to human longevity. *Science* 250: 634–639.

Orzack, S. H. 2003. How and why do aging and life span evolve? In *Life span: Evolutionary, ecological, and demographic perspectives.* Edited by J. R. Carey, and S. Tuljapurkar. New York: Population Council: Supplement to Population and Development Review 29.

Owens, K., and M.-C. King. 1999. Genomic views of human history. *Science* 286: 451–453.

Palloni, A. 2001. Increment-decrement life tables. In *Demography: Measuring and modeling population processes.* Edited by S. H. Preston, P. Heuveline, and M. Guillot, 256–272. Malden, Mass.: Blackwell Publishers.

Papadopoulos, N. T., J. R. Carey, B. I. Katsoyannos, N. A. Kouloussis, H.-G. Müller, and X. Liu. 2002. Supine behaviour predicts time-to-death in male Mediterranean fruit flies. *Proceedings of the Royal Society of London: Biological Sciences* 269: 1633–1637.

Partridge, L. 1997. Evolutionary biology and age-related mortality. In *Between Zeus and the salmon: The biodemography of longevity.* Edited by K. W. Wachter and C. E. Finch, 78–95. Washington, D.C.: National Academies Press.

Partridge, L., and N. H. Barton. 1993. Optimality, mutation and the evolution of ageing. *Nature* 362: 305–311.

Pearl, R. 1922. *The biology of death.* Philadelphia: J. B. Lippincott.

Pearl, R. 1924. *Studies in human biology.* Baltimore: Williams & Wilkins.

Pearl, R. 1925. *The biology of population growth.* New York: Alfred A. Knopf.

Pollak, R. A. 1986. A reformulation of the two-sex problem. *Demography* 23: 247–259.

Pressat, R. 1985. *The dictionary of demography.* Oxford: Blackwell.

Preston, S. 1990. Sources of variation in vital rates: An overview. In *Convergent issues in genetics and demography.* Edited by J. Adams, D. A. Lam, A. I. Hermalin, and P. E. Smouse, 335–352. New York: Oxford University Press.

Preston, S. H., P. Heuveline, and M. Guillot. 2001. *Demography: Measuring and modeling population processes.* Malden, Mass.: Blackwell.

Reich, D., and D. Goldstein. 1998. Microsatellite data support an early population expansion in Africa. *Proceedings of the National Academy of Sciences* 95: 8119–8123.

Reznick, D. 1985. Costs of Reproduction: An evaluation of the empirical evidence. *Oikos* 44: 257–267.

Reznick, D. N., F. H. Shaw, F. H. Rodd, and R. G. Shaw. 1997. Evaluation of the rate of evolution in natural populations of guppies (Poecilia reticulata). *Science* 275: 1934–1937.

Ricklefs, R. E., and A. Scheuerlein. 2003. Life span in the light of avian life histories. In *Life span: Evolutionary, ecological, and demographic perspectives.* Edited by J. R. Carey and S. Tuljapurkar, 71–98. New York: Population Council: Supplement to Population and Development Review 29.

Roach, D. A. 2001. Environmental effects on age-dependent mortality: A test with a perennial plant species under natural and protected conditions. *Experimental Gerontology* 36: 687–694.

Roach, D. A. 2003. Age specific demography in *Plantago*: Variation among cohorts in a natural population. *Ecology* 84: 749–756.

Robine, J.-M. 2003. Life course, environmental change, and life span. In *Life span: Evolutionary, ecological, and demographic perspectives.* Edited by J. R. Carey and S. Tuljapurkar, 229–238. New York: Population Council: Supplement to Population and Development Review 29.

Robine, J.-M., and Y. Saito. 2003. Survival beyond age 100: The case of Japan. In *Life span: Evolutionary, ecological, and demographic perspectives.* Edited by J. R. Carey and S. Tuljapurkar, 208–228. New York: Population Council: Supplement to Population and Development Review 29.

Roderick, G. K. 1996. Geographic structure of insect populations: Gene flow, phylogeography, and their uses. *Annual Review of Entomology* 41: 325–352.

Rogers, A. 1984. *Introduction to multiregional mathematical demography.* New York: John Wiley & Sons.

Rogers, A. 1985. *Regional population projection models.* Beverly Hills, Calif.: Sage Publications.

Rose, M. R. 1997. Toward an evolutionary demography. In *Between Zeus and the salmon: The biodemography of longevity.* Edited by K. W. Wachter and C. E. Finch, 96–107. Washington, D.C.: National Academies Press.

Ross, C., and K. E. Jones. 1999. Socioecology and the evolution of primate reproductive rates. In *Comparative primate socioecology*. Edited by P. C. Lee, 73–110. Cambridge: Cambridge University Press.

Rueppell, O., G. V. Amdam, R. E. Page, Jr., and J. R. Carey. 2004. From genes to societies. Science Aging Knowledge Environment 5, pp. pe5.

Rutter, M. L. 2003. Genetic influences on fertility: Strengths and limitations of quantitative inferences. In *Offspring: Human fertility behavior in biodemographic perspective*. Edited by K. W. Wachter and R. A. Bulato, 18–45. Washington, D.C.: National Academies Press.

Sacher, G. A. 1978. Longevity and aging in vertebrate evolution. *Bioscience* 28: 497–501.

Sakai, A. K., F. W. Allendorf, J. S. Holt, et al. 2001. The population biology of invasive species. *Annual Review of Ecology and Systematics* 32: 305–332.

Settersten, R. A. J., and K. U. Mayer. 1997. The measurement of age, age structuring, and the life course. *Annual Review of Sociology* 23: 233–261.

Shryock, H. S., and J. S. Siegel. 1976. *The methods and materials of demography*. New York: Academic Press.

Singer, B. H., and C. D. Ryff. 2001. *New horizons in health: An integrative approach*. Washington D.C.: National Academy Press.

Slatkin, M. 1987. Gene flow and the geographic structure of natural populations. *Science* 236: 787–792.

Soule, M. E. 1987. *Viable populations for conservation*. Cambridge: Cambridge University Press.

Spuhler, J. N. 1959. Physical anthropology and demography. In *The study of population*. Edited by P. M. Hauser and O. D. Duncan, 728–758. Chicago: University of Chicago Press.

Stark, J. D., and J. E. Banks. 2003. Population-level effects of pesticides and other toxicants on arthropods. *Annual Review of Entomolgy* 48: 505–519.

Stearns, S. C. 1992. *The evolution of life histories*. Oxford: Oxford University Press.

Stringer, C. B., and P. Andrews. 1988. Genetic and fossil evidence for the origin of modern humans. *Science* 239: 1263–1268.

Tatar, M., D. W. Grey, and J. R. Carey. 1997. Altitudinal variation for senescence in *Melanoplus* grasshoppers. *Oecologia* 111: 357–364.

Thrall, P. H., J. J. Burdon, and B. R. Murray. 2000. The metapopulation paradigm: A fragmented view of conservation biology. In *Genetics, demography and viability of fragmented populations*. Edited by A. G. Young and G. M. Clarke, 75–96. Cambridge: Cambridge University Press.

Timiras, P. 1994. Introduction: Aging as a stage in the life cycle. In *Physiological basis of aging and geriatrics*. Edited by P. Timiras, 1–5. Boca Raton, Fla.: CRC Press.

Trevathan, W. R., E. O. Smith, and J. J. McKenna. 1999. *Evolutionary medicine*. New York: Oxford University Press.

Tuljapurkar, S. 1990. *Lecture notes in biomathematics: Population dynamics in variable environments*. New York: Speinger-Verlag.

Tuljapurkar, S. 1997. The evolution of senescence. In *Between Zeus and the salmon: The biodemography of longevity*. Edited by K. W. Wachter and C. E. Finch, 39–77. Washington, D.C.: National Academies Press.

Vaupel, J. W. 1997. Trajectories of mortality at advanced ages. In *Between Zeus and the salmon: The biodemography of longevity*. Edited by K. W. Wachter and C. E. Finch, 17–37. Washington, D.C.: National Academies Press.

Vaupel, J. W. 2003. Post-Darwinian longevity. In *Life span: Evolutionary, ecological, and demographic perspectives*. Edited by J. R. Carey and S. Tuljapurkar, 258–269. New York: Population Council: Supplement to Population and Development Review 29.

Vaupel, J. W., A. Baudisch, M. Dolling, D. A. Roach, and J. Gampe. 2004. The case for negative senescence. *Theoretical Population Biology*, 65: 339–351.

Vaupel, J. W., and J. R. Carey. 1993. Compositional interpretations of Medfly mortality. *Science* 260: 1666–1667.

Vaupel, J. W., J. R. Carey, K. Christensen, T. E. Johnson, A. I. Yashin, N. V. Holm, I. A. Iachine, V. Kannisto, A. A. Khazaeli, P. Liedo, V. D. Longo, Y. Zeng, K. G. Manton, and J. W. Curtsinger. 1998. Biodemographic trajectories of longevity. *Science* 280: 855–860.

Vaupel, J. W., K. G. Manton, and E. Stallard. 1979. The impact of heterogeneity in individual frailty on the dynamics of mortality. *Demography* 16: 439–454.

Vogler, G. P. 2000. The value of sibling and other "relational" data for biodemography and genetic epidemiology. In *Cells and surveys: Should biological measures be included in social science research?* Edited by C. E. Finch, J. W. Vaupel, and K. Kinsella, 110–132. Washington, D. C.: National Academies Press.

Wachter, K. 1999. Evolutionary demographic models for mortality plateaus. *Proceedings of the National Academy of Sciences* 96: 10544–10547.

Wachter, K. W. 2003. Hazard curves and life span prospects. In *Life span: Evolutionary, ecological, and demographic perspectives.* Edited by J. R. Carey and S. Tuljapurkar, 270–291. New York: Population Council: Supplement to Population and Development Review 29.

Wachter, K. W., and R. A. Bulato. 2003. *Offspring: Human fertility behavior in biodemographic perspective.* Washington, D.C.: National Academies Press.

Wachter, K. W., and C. E. Finch. 1997. *Between Zeus and the salmon: The biodemography of longevity.* Washington, D.C: National Academies Press.

Wallace, R. B. 1997. The potential of population surveys for genetic studies. In *Between Zeus and the salmon: The biodemography of longevity.* Edited by K. W. Wachter and C. E. Finch, 234–244. Washington, D.C.: National Academies Press.

Wallace, R. B. 2000. Applying genetic study designs to social and behavioral population surveys. In *Cells and surveys: Should biological measures be included in social science research?* Edited by C. E. Finch, J. W. Vaupel, and K. Kinsella, 229–249. Washington, D. C.: National Academies Press.

Watcher, K. W. 2003. Biodemography of fertility and family formation. In *Offspring: Human fertility behavior in biodemographic perspective.* Edited by K. W. Wachter and R. A. Bulato, 1–17. Washington, D.C.: National Academies Press.

Weinstein, R. B. W., and R. J. Willis. 2000. Stretching social surveys to include bioindicators: Possibilities for the health and retirement study, experience from the Taiwan Study of the Elderly. In *Cells and surveys: Should biological measures be included in social science research?* Edited by C. E. Finch, J. W. Vaupel, and K. Kinsella, 250–275. Washington, D. C.: National Academies Press.

Weiss, K. M. 1973. *Demographic models for anthropology.* Washington, D.C.: Society for American Archaeology.

Williams, G. C. 1957. Pleiotropy, natural selection, and the evolution of senescence. *Evolution* 11: 398–411.

Williams, G. C., and R. M. Nesse. 1991. The dawn of Darwinian medicine. *The Quarterly Review of Biology* 66: 1–22.

Wilmoth, J. R., and H. Lundstrom. 1996. Extreme longevity in five countries. *European Journal of Population* 12: 63–93.

Wilmoth, J. R., and J.-M. Robine. 2003. The world trend in maximum life span. In *Life span: Evolutionary, ecological, and demographic perspectives.* Edited by J. R. Carey and S. Tuljapurkar, 239–257. New York: Population Council: Supplement to Population and Development Review 29.

Wilson, E. O. 1971. *The insect societies.* Cambridge, Mass.: The Belknap Press of Harvard University Press.

Wilson, E. O. 1975. *Sociobiology: The new synthesis.* Cambridge, Mass.: The Belknap Press of Harvard University Press.

Wilson, E. O. 1984. New approaches to the analysis of social systems. In *Population and biology.* Edited by N. Keyfitz, 41–52. Liege, Belgium: Ordina Editions.

Wilson, E. O. 1998. *Consilience.* New York: Alfred A. Knopf.

Wolf, D. A. 1994. The elderly and their kin: Patterns of availability and access. In *Demography of aging.* Edited by L. G. Martin and S. H. Preston, 146–194. Washington D.C.: Naitonal Academies Press.

Worthman, C. M. 2003. Energetics, sociality, and human reproduction: Life history theory in real life. In *Offspring: Human fertility behavior in biodemographic perspective.* Edited by K. W. Wachter and R. A. Bulato, 289–321. Washington, D.C.: National Academies Press.

Yashin, A. I., G. DeBenedictis, J. W. Vaupel, Q. Tan, K. F. Andreev, I. A. Iachine, M. Bonafe, S. Valensin, M. DeLuca, L. Carotenuto, and C. Frenceschi. 2000. Genes and longevity: Lessons from studies of centenarians. *Journal of Gerontology: Biological Sciences* 55A: B319–B328.

Yashin, A. I., and I. A. Iachine. 1997. How frailty models can be used for evaluating longevity limits: Taking advantage of an interdisciplinary approach. *Demography* 34: 31–48.

Yashin, A. I., S. V. Ukraintseva, et al. 2001. Have the oldest old adults ever been frail in the past? A hypothesis that explains modern trends in survival. *Journal of Gerontology: Biological Sciences* 56A: B432–B442.

Young, A. G., and G. M. Clarke. 2000a. Conclusions and future directions: What do we know about the genetic and demographic effects of habitat fragmentation and where do we go from here? In *Genetics, demography and viability of fragmented populations.* Edited by A. G. Young and G. M. Clarke, 361–366. Cambridge: Cambridge University Press.

Young, A. G., and G. M. Clarke. 2000b. *Genetics, demography and viability of fragmented populations.* Cambridge: Cambridge University Press.

Young, L. J. 2003. The neural basis of pair bonding in a monogamous species: A model for understanding the biological basis of human behavior. In *Offspring: Human fertility behavior in biodemographic perspective*. Edited by K. W. Wachter and R. A. Bulato, 91–103. Washington, D.C.: National Academies Press.

CHAPTER 22

Mathematical Demography

Kenneth C. Land,
Yang Yang, and Zeng Yi

INTRODUCTION

Mathematical demography is a specialization in demography concerned with the articulation, analysis, and empirical application of theoretical models or representations of populations and demographic processes via the use of mathematics, including mathematical statistics. It has its roots in actuarial science, biology, mathematics, and statistics, fields with which it retains strong ties today (see, e.g., Jordan 1975; Keyfitz 1977a, 1977b; Lotka 1924[1956]; Smith and Keyfitz 1977).

The topics that can be covered in a survey of mathematical demography are numerous and diverse. Therefore, any survey of the field in the confines of a chapter in this *Handbook* must be selective. After some introductory materials on the theory of models and the nature of demographic phenomena and data, this chapter reviews the essential concepts and mathematics of the two basic classic population models that constitute the core of mathematical demography, namely, the life table/stationary population model and the stable population model. Recent contributions that extend these models are also reviewed in various ways. The third major topic reviewed is model schedules or age-specific rates of demographic events such as births and deaths, summary demographic indices, such as the total fertility rate and life expectancy, and recent developments in tempo adjustment formulas based thereon. Space limitations do not permit a detailed exposition of recent contributions to mathematical demography that generalize and extend the classic life table/stationary and stable population theories. After laying out the basics of these models, however, many recent contributions are cited, and the ways in which they build upon the classic models are described.

Models in Science and in Demography

This chapter first reviews some elements of the modern theory of models (Casti 1992a, 1992b; Land 1971, 2001). This theory defines formal models in generic terms and shows the universality of the uses of formal modeling systems across the sciences. The objective is to position the models studied in mathematical demography within this general framework.

Following Casti (1992b), a general definition of *models* is that they are tools by which individuals order and organize experiences and observations.

An implication of this definition is that many of the verbal characterizations of population phenomena that are used in demography are indeed models. They have stimulated research over the years and will continue to do so. As an example, Notestein's (1945) verbally stated *demographic transition model* stimulated demographers to focus attention on trends in birth and death rates and their relationship to economic development and improvements in health and longevity.

If models are tools for ordering experiences, what are "formal models"? *Formal models* encapsulate some slice of experiences and observations within the relationships constituting a formal system such as formal logic, mathematics, or statistics (cf., Casti 1992a). A *formal demographic model* thus is a way of representing aspects of demographic phenomena using a formal apparatus that provides a means for exploring the properties of the demographic phenomena mirrored in the model. Demographers construct formal models to assist in bringing a more clearly articulated order to their experiences and observations, as well as to make more precise predictions about certain aspects of the populations. Since most of the remaining discussion pertains to formal demographic models, the adjective "formal" will no longer be used with "models."

Some notation is useful. Consider a particular subset D of demographic phenomena and suppose that D can exist in a set of distinct *abstract states* $\Omega = \{\omega_1, \omega_2, \ldots\}$. The set Ω defines the *state space* of D. Whether or not a demographer can determine the state of D in a particular moment of study depends on the experiences, observations, or measurements (*observables*) at the demographer's disposal. As a simple example, suppose D is a human population in which two sexes are distinguished. Then a reasonable set of abstract states that distinguishes a two-sex population might be

$$\Omega = \{\omega_1 = \text{male}, \omega_2 = \text{female}\}.$$

Next, consider the concept of an observable. An *observable* of D is a rule f associating a real number to each ω in the state space Ω, i.e., an observable is a measuring instrument. More formally, an observable is a map $f: \Omega \to R$, where R denotes the set of real numbers. Using the example of a two-sex population and the usual "dummy variable" coding rule, one could define

$$f(\omega_1) = 0 \text{ and } f(\omega_2) = 1$$

as observables.

Generally, a full accounting of the complexities of population phenomena would require an infinite number of observables $f_\alpha: \Omega \to R$, where the subscript α ranges over a possibly uncountable index set. Thus, a complete accounting of demographic and related population phenomena D would be described by a large set Ω and the possibly *infinite set of observables* $F = \{f_\alpha\}$. But it is usually not necessary in demography to deal with such a large set of observables in order to build useful demographic models.

In brief, in building demographic models, demographers throw away most of the possible observables that could affect demographic phenomena and focus attention on *a proper subset A of F*, which may or may not capture the full complexity and nuances of demographic phenomena.

A *demographic model D^** may now be characterized as an abstract state–space Ω together with a finite set of observables $f_i: \Omega \to R$, $i = 1, 2, \ldots, n$. Symbolically,

$$D^* = \{\Omega, f_1, f_2, \ldots, f_n\}.$$

But there is more to the notion of a demographic model than just the list of observables by which it is characterized. The essential "systemness" of D^* is contained in relationships that link the observables. These relationships are termed the *equations of state* for D^*. Formally, the equations of state can be written as

$$\Phi_i(f_1, f_2, \ldots, f_n) = 0, \quad i = 1, 2, \ldots, m,$$

where the Φ_i (.) are mathematical relationships expressing the dependency relations among the observables. This can be more compactly written as

$$\Phi(f) = 0. \tag{1}$$

There are two forms in which the equations of state that define demographic models are used. The first is to state relationships among observables that produce a *descriptive model* or *definition* of a demographic index or rate. Many demographic models, from population life tables used to estimate the years of life expected to be lived in a population to a formula for calculating the total fertility rate, are used in this descriptive or definitional sense. A second way in which the equations of state are used in demography is to state causal relationships among observables that produce an *explanatory model* in which variations across time or demographic space in certain observables are explained by variations in other observables.

To represent explanatory demographic models, Eq. (1) must be further developed. Suppose that the last m observables $f_{n-m+1}, \ldots, f_m$, called *endogenous* (i.e., determined within the system under consideration), are functions of the remaining observables $f_1, f_2, \ldots, f_{n-m}$, which are *exogenous* (i.e., determined outside the system under consideration). In other words, suppose that m functional relations are defined, with some finite number r of numerical parameters, $\beta_1, \beta_2, \ldots, \beta_r$, for determining values of the endogenous observables as a function of the exogenous observables. Here the notation

$$\beta \equiv (\beta_1, \beta_2, \ldots, \beta_r)$$

will denote the vector of parameters and the notation

$$x \equiv (f_1, f_2, \ldots, f_{n-m})$$

and

$$y \equiv (f_{n-m+1}, f_{n-m+2}, \ldots, f_n)$$

will denote vectors of the exogenous and endogenous observables, henceforth *variables*, respectively. The equations of state become

$$y = \Phi_\beta\,(x). \tag{2}$$

This last expression, perhaps formulated with stochastic/random components, is in a form that encompasses many explanatory demographic models.

As an example of the application of these formal notations to the definition of a common demographic index, consider the mathematical model that underlies the definition of a common measure of fertility used in demography, the total fertility rate (TFR), a period fertility rate used more often than any other. The TFR is defined as the average number of births a woman would have if she were to live through her reproductive years (usually ages 15 to 49) and bear children at each age at the rates observed in a particular year or period. The actual childbearing of cohorts of women is given by the completed or cohort fertility rate (CFR), which measures the average number of births 50-year-old women had during their reproductive years.

Formally, let $f_p(t, a)$ denote the age-specific fertility rates for women aged a at time t, and let $f_c(t, a)$ represent the age-specific fertility rates at age a for cohorts of women born at time t. Then the equation of state (1) for the *period total fertility rate* for time t is

$$\text{TFR}(t) = \int f_p(t, a)da \tag{3}$$

and the equation for the *cohort fertility rate* for the cohort born at time T is

$$\text{CFR}(t) = \int f_c(t, a)da. \tag{4}$$

In applications, the integrals are replaced by finite summations and the sums are taken over the reproductive ages.

One question has been avoided to this point: What differentiates models from theories? These terms sometimes are distinguished and sometimes are used interchangeably. Usually, scientific theories are regarded as more general than scientific models. A *theory* is a *family of related models*, and a *model* is a formal manifestation of a particular theory (cf., Casti 1992b). In the presentation later of the life table/stationary population model, this distinction will be illustrated.

What Good are Models?

Consider next some uses of models in demography. What good are they? One list of the benefits of models was presented by the mathematical demographer Nathan Keyfitz over three decades ago (Keyfitz 1971a). Keyfitz noted that the development of demography had been greatly influenced by the demand for the prediction of future population; this stimulated the development of demographic models such as the life table and stable population models. He then identified the following benefits of models: Models focus research by identifying theoretical and practical issues. Models help in assembling and explaining data. Models permit the design of experiments, simulations, and other research studies out of which causal knowledge can be obtained. Models systematize comparative study across space and time. Models reveal formal analogies between problems that on their surface are quite different. And models help in the making of predictions. To the list provided by Keyfitz, the following benefits of models can be added: Models provide a "lens" through which patterns can be detected in demographic data that otherwise cannot be perceived. Models help to improve demographic measurement. And, in particular, models provide a locus for defining, developing, and interpreting summary measures of demographic events and phenomena.

The Nature of Demographic Phenomena and Data

In their discussion of the evolution of demography into a cumulative and integrated science, Morgan and Lynch (2001) identified four factors intrinsic or internal to the discipline that have facilitated this evolution. They are summarized here because they may be viewed as the basis on which the extraordinary development and application of mathematical models in demography has proceeded.

The first is the fact that *demographic phenomena are relatively easily measured*. Births and deaths, the core events studied by demography, are biologically based and thus are anchored in an unmistakable and universal reality. While the meaning of these events is socially constructed by the individuals involved and the cultures in which they participate, their actual occurrence is universally recognized. The same may be said for sex and age (or other dimensions of time), which are key variables in the study of human populations. That is, their social significance may vary, but the fact that there are objective sexes in a population or age (or duration since some event) is unchallenged. (See chapter 1, "Age and Sex," in this *Handbook* for more discussion.) Morgan and Lynch (2001) note that another topic studied by demographers, migration, may be less well developed due to the greater difficulty in defining migration. (See chapter 11, "Internal Migration," in this *Handbook*.)

A second key feature is that *demographic phenomena are inherently quantifiable*. This is due to the fact that births and deaths are categorical (in fact, they are dichotomous) and thus easily counted. Intermediate instances of birth and death are few and rare. The consequence is that repeated measurement and intersubjective agreement among observers would likely be high. This is not to say that demographic measurement is easy for a large population—only that it is relatively straightforward.

Third, the *presence of accounting identities* has facilitated the successful development of demography as a science. Traditional demography focuses on the description of the composition of human populations by age, sex, and other characteristics and the study of change therein (dynamics). The basic methods of demography are centered on the well-known *population accounting or balancing equation*:

$$P_t \equiv P_{t-1} + B_{t-1,t} - D_{t-1,t} + NM_{t-1,t}. \tag{5}$$

where P_t denotes the size of a population at accounting time (e.g., year) t, and $B_{t-1,t}$, $D_{t-1,t}$, and $NM_{t-1,t}$ denote, respectively, the flows into or out of the population from time $t-1$ to t by births, deaths, and net migration. Land and Schneider (1987) note that this identity is an instance of the general law of conservation of mass in physics. It also is an example of the equations of state (1), a functional relationship linking the observables of a demographic model of a population. Using identity (5), demographers can perform quality checks on their data and engage in indirect estimation when only fragments of data are available.

The fourth factor is the presence of *structural features or relationships among key concepts*. Not only can births and deaths be unambiguously identified and counted in human populations, and not only can the counts be related to each other via the basic demographic accounting equation (5), they also can be used to define populations at risk of one event or another and the corresponding dynamics or rates of occurrence of the events. These, in turn, can be used to build life table/stationary population models, stable population models, and related models to describe and/or explain the corresponding population processes. This chapter now turns to an exposition of some of the basics of these models.

LIFE TABLE/STATIONARY POPULATION THEORY AND EXTENDED MODELS

Classic Single-Decrement Population Life Table Theory/Models

Classic single-decrement population life table theory is a simple descriptive mathematical theory that demographers use to represent the age-specific mortality patterns to which a population is subject and to summarize those patterns in the form of estimates of years of life expected to be lived on average in a population. It also is the simplest mathematical theory of the age structure of a population, called a stationary population, subjected to certain patterns of fertility and mortality. The following detailed statement of the basic concepts and mathematics of this theory builds on expositions by Jordan (1975), Keyfitz (1977b), Preston, Heuveline, and Guillot (2001), and Schoen (1988). The theory consists of an interrelated set of mathematical functions that apply to entire families of functions. Thus, in keeping with the distinction between mathematical theories and mathematical models made earlier, the life table/stationary population theory is first presented. For purposes of empirical estimation of a life table for a particular population, the mathematical functions of the theory must be given specific algebraic expressions, as will be described later. These specific algebraic expressions transform life table theory into specific life table models that then can be estimated by corresponding methods. In the exposition that follows, however, the terms *theory* and *models* will not always be distinguished. Instead, conventional terminology will be adopted and the term model will be used in most places.

THE SURVIVAL FUNCTION. The normal mortality pattern observed among human lives, illustrated graphically in Figure 22.1, is familiar to demographers. The elimination

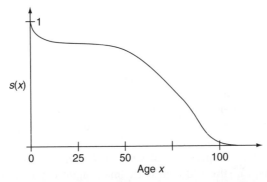

FIGURE 22.1. Graphic representation of the human survival function.

of lives by death is rapid in infancy, slows down during childhood, then increases throughout adolescence and middle life, accelerating as the end of the life span is approached. The life table is a mathematical model for expressing these facts. One approach to developing the life table model is via the survival function.

Definition: The probability that a new life, aged 0, will survive to attain age x will be regarded as a function of x and referred to as the *survival function, s(x)*.

Properties of s(x): On the basis of general knowledge of the normal mortality pattern described above, the following three properties may be postulated for $s(x)$:

1. $s(x)$ is *a decreasing function* as x increases, since the probability of surviving to age x is greater than the probability of surviving to age $x + t$, $t > 0$;
2. Since the focus here is on normal patterns of human mortality, it is convenient and reasonable to assume that $s(x)$ is *a continuous function of* x.
3. At $x = 0$, $s(x) = 1$ and at the upper end of the life span, denoted ω (omega), $s(x) = 0$.[1]

THE LIFE TABLE.   The main device for exhibiting mortality data in demography is the *life table* or the *mortality table*. The l_x and d_x functions of the life table have the following definitions:

$$l_x = l(0) \cdot s(x) \qquad (6)$$

$$= l_0 \cdot s(x), \text{ where } l(0) = l_0 \text{ is a positive constant,}$$

$$d_x = l_x - l_{x+1}. \qquad (7)$$

The value of l_0 is called the *radix* of the table, usually taken to be some large round number like $10^5 = 100,000$; d_x is the *annual decrement* of the table.

The interpretation of l_x as a "number living" or "number surviving" and of d_x as a "number dying" is a convenient aid in visualizing many of the relations that follow. But it should be remembered that neither l_x nor d_x has any absolute meaning; the sizes of both depend on the value of the radix chosen to construct the table. Note also that l_x, from property (2), is a continuous function of x, although tabulated values appear in life tables only for integral values of x.

The approach taken here to the definition of the life table is *classic* in the sense that it does not derive the survival function from the definition of a stochastic process governing the sample paths (life histories) of the individual members of a birth cohort. Rather, it begins by postulating properties of the survival function and supposes that the probabilities applying to the birth cohort group-as-a-whole will be exactly applicable to each individual in the cohort, so that one only needs to compute the expected values of the various life table functions. In this sense, it often is called a *deterministic model*. Generally, this deterministic approach to the concepts and functional relationships that define life table theory applies when the population base on which mortality events are defined and recorded is sufficiently large so that there are few irregularities in

---

[1] The designation of a terminal age ω is merely a convenient simplifying device. No empirical fact supports the assumption that a life can survive for n years but not for n years and one second. Thus, it would be more realistic to say that the values of $s(x)$ are negligible for $x \geq \omega$. However, the more precise condition $s(\omega) = 0$ is retained because of its convenience in the subsequent mathematical analysis.

the data due to random or stochastic fluctuations. How large is "sufficiently large?" Opinions on this topic vary, but most demographers are comfortable with application of the deterministic model of the life table to the full human age range from birth to the end of life to a population base of at least 10,000 person-years of exposure per year, or an average of about 10,000 persons observed per year. For populations or longitudinal panels of individuals followed over time that are smaller, most demographers would recommend the use of a statistically based survival model approach to the definition and estimation of a life table model, as described later.

It is evident that the intensity of mortality varies at each *moment* of age, and it is important to have some way of measuring this *instantaneous* variation. The *slope* of the empirical $s(x)$ described above is related to the number of deaths at that point [since $l_x = l_0 \cdot s(x)$, the $s(x)$ graph may be thought of as an l_x curve with a change in the vertical scale], for the steeper the curve the greater the number of deaths. Since the slope is measured by the derivative, it is natural to turn next to the derivative of l_x.

THE FORCE OF MORTALITY. The mortality index just described is known as the *force of mortality/hazard function* and is denoted by the symbol μ_x. Its definition is

$$\mu_x = -\frac{Dl_x}{l_x} = -\frac{1}{l_x}\frac{d}{dx}l_x = -\frac{d}{dx}\ln l_x. \tag{8}$$

Properties of μ_x:

1. μ_x is a measure of mortality at the precise moment of attaining age x.
2. μ_x expresses this mortality in the form of an annual rate; this is because the derivative of l_x is

$$Dl_x = \lim_{h \to 0}\frac{l_{x+h} - l_x}{h},$$

so μ_x from (8), may be written

$$\mu_x = \lim_{h \to 0}\frac{l_x - l_{x+h}}{h \cdot l_x} = \lim_{h \to 0}\frac{{}_h q_x}{h}, \tag{9}$$

where q_x denotes the (conditional) probability that (x) will die within 1 year. The expression ${}_h q_x / h$ may be regarded as an annual rate of mortality based on the mortality during the age interval x to $x + h$.

3. The value of μ_x normally exceeds 1 at both ends of the life-span[2].

Empirical Force Function: Corresponding to the typical empirical bathtub-shaped survival curve, the empirical force of mortality typically looks like that shown in Figure 22.2.

Derivation of Life Table Functions from μ_x: From a mathematical point of view, μ_x is the most basic life table function in the sense that once given its values (functional

---

[2] Consider the first 24 hours of life, for example, the value of ${}_{1/365} q_0$ may exceed $1/365$ so that the ratio ${}_h q_0 / h$ exceeds 1. Since there are no survivors at age ω, we may write ${}_{\omega - x} q_x = 1$, which is true for all x. But if x is an age such that $\omega - x$ is less than 1, it follows that $\frac{{}_{\omega - x} q_x}{\omega - x} > 1$, and hence values of μ_x exceeding 1 will occur in the year of age $\omega - 1$ to ω.

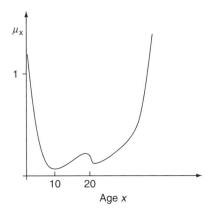

FIGURE 22.2. Graphic representation of the human force of mortality function.

form), all other life table values may be derived. The values of the force of mortality itself are independent of the life table radix, which implies that there is only one instantaneous rate of mortality. To demonstrate these derivations, recall that

$$\mu_x = -D \ln l_x.$$

Replace x by y and integrate both sides between the limits 0 and x:

$$\int_0^x \mu_y dy = -\int_0^x D \ln l_y dy$$

$$= -\ln l_y |_0^x = -\ln \frac{l_x}{l_0},$$

so that the survival function can be written:

$$l_x = l_0 e^{-\int_0^x \mu_y dy}. \tag{10}$$

There is a similar expression for the (conditional) probability that (x) will survive to age $x + n$

$$_n p_x = \frac{l_{x+n}}{l_x} = \frac{l_0 e^{-\int_0^{x+n} \mu_y dy}}{l_0 e^{-\int_0^x \mu_y dy}} = e^{-\int_x^{x+n} \mu_y dy}. \tag{11}$$

The probability $_n q_x$ may then be expressed as

$$_n q_x = 1 - e^{-\int_0^n \mu_{x+1} dt}. \tag{12}$$

Alternatively, noting that

$$l_y \mu_y = -D l_y,$$

integrating between the limits of x and $x + n$ yields

$$\int_x^{x+n} l_y \mu_y dy = -\int_x^{x+n} D l_y dy$$

$$= -l_y |_x^{x+n} = l_x - l_{x+n} = _n d_x \tag{13}$$

which defines the *annual decrement* when $n = 1$. Letting $y = x + t$, $0 \leq t \leq n$, and integrating from 0 to n, this last expression becomes

$$_n d_x = l_x - l_{x+n} = \int_0^n l_{x+t} \mu_{x+t} dt. \tag{14}$$

Dividing by l_x gives the following expression for $_n q_x$:

$$_n q_x = \frac{_n d_x}{l_x} = \frac{l_x - l_{x+n}}{l_x}$$

$$= \frac{1}{l_x} \int_0^n l_{x+t} \mu_{x+t} dt = \int_0^n {}_t p_x \mu_{x+t} dt. \tag{15}$$

The relationship between the central death rate and the force of mortality can be seen by writing out the integral expressions for the numerator and denominator

$$m_x = \frac{\int_0^1 l_{x+t} \cdot \mu_{x+t} dt}{\int_0^1 l_{x+t} dt} \tag{16}$$

From this, it is apparent that m_x is the weighted mean value of the force of mortality over the year of age x to $x + 1$ where the weights are the number of lives attaining each age $x + t$ in the interval. Depending on the specific functional form of the force function, $\mu_{x+1/2}$ is a more or less appropriate estimate for this average value.

The Person-Years Function: Two life table functions then can be defined:

$$_n L_x = \int_x^{x+n} l_y dy = \int_0^n l_{x+t} dt \tag{17}$$

and

$$T_x = \int_x^\infty l_y dy = \int_0^\alpha l_{x+t} dt$$
$$= \sum_{y=x}^\alpha L_y = \sum_{t=0}^\alpha L_{x+t} \tag{18}$$

where if $n = 1$

$$_1 L_x = L_x.$$

As a consequence of the definitions, note that

$$\frac{dL_x}{dx} = l_{x+1} - l_x = -d_x$$

and

$$\frac{dT_x}{dx} = -l_x.$$

Considering that l_x represents the mortality experience of a birth cohort as it ages, the integral $_n L_x$ is the *person-years* lived by that cohort between ages x and $x + n$. Similarly, T_x represents the *total person-years* in prospect for the group numbering l_x who have attained age x on the radix l_0. Note that the upper bounds in the two integrals defining T_x could be replaced by ω and $\omega - x$, respectively, if an upper bound on the life table has been set beyond which no one survives.

The Life Expectation Function: The *complete expectation of life at age x* is defined as:

$$e_x = \frac{T_x}{l_x} = \frac{1}{l_x} \int_0^\infty l_{x+t} dt = \int_0^\infty {}_t p_x dt \tag{19}$$

The life expectation function may be interpreted as representing the *expected average future lifetime* remaining at age x.

THE STATIONARY POPULATION.   There are two ways of viewing the functions of the life table. The first, as just reviewed, is to view the table as tracking the survival of a birth cohort. This is the *cohort life table* view. An alternative perspective leads to a view of the life table as *a model of the age structure of a population* subject to certain conditions. In particular, following Jordan (1975), suppose that a population produces l_0 annual births, l_0 being the radix of a given life table, and suppose that these births are uniformly distributed over each calendar year. Let the deaths among the population occur in accordance with the given life table, and let there be no migration into or out of the population. Then, after the birth and death process has continued for a period of years at least equal to the terminal age of the life table, the total population and its age distribution remain constant (stationary).

To see the validity of this proposition, consider first the consequences of the assumption that the l_0 annual births are uniformly distributed over each calendar year. Clearly, this means that there will be l_0 births uniformly distributed over any year of time, and that in any fraction of a year h, however small, there will be $h\,l_0$ births. It follows that there will be l_x lives attaining age x in any year and $h\,l_0$ lives attaining age x in any time interval h, as survivors of the births which occurred in the corresponding periods of time x years ago.

Consider next the incidence of deaths. Each of the $h\,l_y$ lives attaining age x in any interval h is subject to the force of mortality μ_y, and hence the differential expression $h\,l_y\,\mu_y dy$ represents the number of lives dying at exact age y in that interval. Then the number dying between ages x and $x + 1$ in any interval h will be given by $\int_x^{x+1} h l_y \mu_y dy = h d_x$. Two consequences are: (1) letting h equal 1, the number dying between ages x and $x + 1$ in any year of time will be d_x; (2) since the number dying between ages x and $x + 1$ in any fraction of a year h is proportional to h, it is clear that the deaths between ages x and $x + 1$, and hence all deaths, occurring in any period of time are uniformly distributed over that period.

It may now be seen that such a population is indeed stationary. For the total of the deaths at all ages in any interval h is $\int_0^\omega h l_y \mu_y dy = h l_0$, which is the same as the number of births occurring in the interval. Since the interval h is an arbitrarily small period of time, it may be concluded that each life which leaves the population by death is simultaneously replaced by a new birth.

Furthermore, the distribution of the total population by ages is stationary. Consider the lives which are aged x last birthday at any time. These are the lives which have attained integral age x but not age $x + 1$. In any interval h, the number of lives which leave this group by attaining age $x + 1$ is $h l_{x+1}$, and the number which leave the group by death is hd_x, making a total decrement of $hl_{x+1} + hd_x = hl_{x+1} + h(l_x - l_{x+1}) = hl_x$. Thus, the total decrement is exactly equal to the number entering the group during the interval by attaining age x. In other words, when a life leaves this age group, either by death or by attaining age $x + 1$, its place is simultaneously taken by a life entering from the next lower age group. Under these circumstances, the number living at a given age last birthday is always constant.

Now $\frac{1}{r} l_{x+m/r}$ represents the number of lives attaining exact age $x + m/r$ in any interval of time $1/r$ and therefore approximates the number of lives between exact ages $x + m/r$ and $x + (m + 1)/r$ at any moment of time. Hence the number of lives between exact ages x and $x + 1$ at any moment of time is

$$\lim_{r \to \infty} \sum_{m=0}^{r-1} \frac{1}{r} l_{x+\frac{m}{r}} = \int_0^1 l_{x+t} dt = L_x.$$

Thus, L_x is the constant number of lives between exact ages x and $x + 1$ at any moment of time. Similarly, T_x is the number of lives aged x and over at any moment of time.

SUMMARY OF PROPERTIES OF THE STATIONARY POPULATION.   This conception of the life table may be compared with the cohort-survivorship group interpretation. In particular, the following interpretations and relationships characterize the stationary population:

1. l_x represents the number of lives attaining age x in any year of time;
2. d_x represents the number of deaths between ages x and $x + 1$ in any year of time;
3. l_0 = number of births per year = $\sum_{x5} d_x$ = total deaths per year;
4. $_nL_x$ = number of persons living in the population between ages x and $x + n$ at any moment in time;
5. T_x = number of lives aged x and over at any moment in time;
6. T_0 = total size of the population;
7. $_nL_x/T_0$ = proportion of the population ages x to $x + n$ at any moment in time;
8. T_x/T_0 = proportion of the population aged x or older at any moment in time;
9. $L_0/T_0 = 1/e_0$ = birth rate = death rate
10. $_nm_x$ = ratio of the number of deaths between ages x and $x + n$ in any year of time to the number living between those ages at any moment in time.

Although the stationary population model is admittedly artificial, the theory is applicable when the stationary conditions are approximately realized. In addition, more realistic mathematical models of human populations, such as the stable and piecewise-stable population models described below, are generalizations of the stationary population model.

Estimation of Complete and Abridged Population Life Tables

It is difficult to find a mathematical expression, involving a small number of parameters, which will fit the force of mortality function for human populations closely over its entire range (see, however, the section below on model schedules). For this reason, traditional methods of estimation of population life tables have been dominated by three considerations.

First, the data available to demographers to use in the estimation of population life tables are limited and aggregated. Demographers typically do not have access to complete life history information giving details on birth dates, death dates, and populations exposed to risk at every point in some historical period. Rather, the usually available data consist of age-specific estimates of populations exposed to risk from censuses and age-specific enumerations of deaths from a vital statistics register. As explained in the next section, these are used to construct occurrence/exposure death rates from which demographers estimate life tables. Indeed, as noted by Preston and colleagues (2001), all of the various model specifications and estimation methods for constructing population life tables that have been developed can be viewed as devices for transforming occurrence/exposure data on death rates into age-specific probabilities of dying (i.e., the q_x's), from which the other life table functions can be calculated.

Second, there is no simple, universally accepted family of parametric mortality force functions (or survival functions) that can be used to estimate the life table over the entire age range of human life. Thus, one cannot simply conjoin the death rates with a parametric force function in say, a least squares curve-fitting procedure and obtain an accurate fit to the death rates throughout the age range.

Third, the preeminent interest of demographers in population life table estimation is the accurate estimation of the expectation of life function. For this, demographers place a high premium on the preservation of local irregularities in the death rates, provided they are based on population-level data and considered to be accurate.

DATA AVAILABLE FOR THE ESTIMATION OF POPULATION LIFE TABLES. Given complete, continuous-time observations on all births and deaths for all persons in a population exposed to the risk of mortality, it is possible to produce direct estimates of the life table survival function, l_x, and/or the central mortality rates, m_x (see Elandt-Johnson and Johonson 1980). However, the aggregate, population-level data available to demographers usually fall far short of this ideal situation. The more typical circumstance is that vital statistics and census agencies provide data for the computation of occurrence/exposure rates for a sequence of age intervals $[x_0, x_0 + n), \ldots, [x_i, x_i + n), \ldots, [x_i, x_\omega)$. By *occurrence/exposure rates* is meant rates of the form

$$_nM_x = \frac{_nD_x}{_nK_x} \tag{20}$$

where $_nD_x$ denotes the number of deaths occurring (enumerated) to members of the population who are aged x to $x + n$ at last birthday during the period of observation, and $_nK_x$ denotes the average number of persons living in the population during the observation period and thus exposed to the risk of mortality. In this definition, n typically is 1 or 5 years, except for the first and last age intervals, where it may be shorter or longer respectively. In *period data*, rates of the form of Eq. (20) are computed for each age interval from, say, calendar-year deaths in the numerator and an estimate of the midyear population size (the average population exposed to the risk of mortality during the year) in the denominator. In *cohort data*, rates of the form of Eq. (20) are computed each year or each five years from estimates of the numerator and denominator as an initial one-year or five-year birth cohort ages through time.

ESTIMATION OF COMPLETE (UNABRIDGED) LIFE TABLES. A *complete* or *unabridged life table* is a table in which single-years-of-age define the estimation-age-intervals, i.e., the age intervals over which the table is estimated, except for an open-ended interval at the upper end of the table that may begin at age 85 or 95 or 100, depending on the availability of accurate data at the oldest ages.

Complete life tables usually are estimated for national populations, for example the United States population, by using census counts of the population in decennial census years and averages of death enumerations for three years surrounding the census year, e.g., 1979 to 1981, 1989 to 1991, 1999 to 2001. In the calculation of such tables, major empirical questions usually pertain to the accuracy of the age information in the census enumeration. Such information is subject to problems of age heaping, digit preference, and other inconsistencies. (See chapter 1 in this *Handbook* for more discussion.) Consequently, much of the methodology involved in the construction of these life tables involves methods of data adjustment to remove obvious inconsistencies. After adjustment, the death and population enumerations are usually combined into the conventional five-year age groups (5 to 9, 10 to 14, 15 to 19, ..., 80 to 84) for the nonextreme ages. After grouping, the death and census enumerations typically are interpolated back to single years of age by one of a variety of osculatory interpolation methods (see Keyfitz 1977b; Keyfitz and Flieger 1971).

The product of this sequence of (1) data adjustment, (2) grouping into five-year age groups, and (3) interpolation is a series of single-year-of-age death counts and a corresponding series of single-year-of-age population estimates that are "smoother" than the observed series. These, in turn, will produce mortality rates that are smoother than those calculated from observed deaths and population counts. The ultimate justification is the assumption in the life table model that the survival curve is continuous.

Based on these considerations, assume in this section that the available data constitute a smooth series of deaths by single years of age at last birthday:

$$D_0, D_1, D_2, \ldots, D_x, \ldots, D_{84}$$

and a smoothed series of single age population estimates:

$$K_0, K_1, K_2, \ldots, K_x, \ldots, K_{84}$$

from which we obtain a corresponding smoothed series of occurrence/exposure death rates:

$$M_0, M_1, M_2, \ldots, M_x, \ldots, M_{84}.$$

With these data, there are two well-known life table models/methods for converting the occurrence/exposure rates to life table mortality probabilities. Each could be described as a "local" method of life table estimation, since each approximates the mortality force function (equivalently, the survival function) by functions that are continuous within age intervals but piecewise discontinuous between age intervals. This produces a life table that is faithful to the "local behavior" of the death rates and that yields an accurate estimate of the expectation of life function.

Method 1: Piecewise-Constant Force of Mortality (Equivalently, Piecewise-Exponential Survival Function) Model. At the level of the force of mortality function, this model begins by assuming that μ_{x+t} is constant within single ages:

$$\mu_{x+t} = \mu_x \quad (0 \le t < 1) \tag{21}$$

This amounts to approximating the force function by a function that is constant within single ages but that differs between ages—called a *piecewise-constant force function*—as shown in Figure 22.3.

An immediate consequence of this assumption is that the definition of the life-table central mortality rate (16) simplifies to

$$m_x = \frac{\int_0^1 l_{x+t} \cdot \mu_x dt}{\int_0^1 l_{x+t} dt} = \frac{\mu_x \int_0^1 l_{x+t} dt}{\int_0^1 l_{x+t} dt} = \mu_x \tag{22}$$

Following the *general estimation algorithm format* of Schoen (1975), Schoen and Land (1979), and Land and Schoen (1982), the results may be summarized as the following estimation algorithm:
Data-Model Orientation Equation:

$$M_x = m_x = \mu_x \tag{23}$$

Flow Equation:

$$l_{x+1} = l_x e^{-M_x}. \tag{24}$$

Person-Years Equation:

$$L_x = [l_x - l_{x+1}]/M_x = [l_x - l_{x+1}]M_x^{-1} \tag{25}$$

Note that all of the columns of a complete life table can be calculated from these three equations.

Method 2: Piecewise-Hyperbolic Force Function (Equivalently, Piecewise-Linear Survival Function) Model. In one of the first attempts to describe algebraically the mortality experience of human lives, the 18th-century mathematician Abraham de Moivre (1725) proposed that the survivorship curve (l_x) of a life table could be represented by a single straight line. His hypothesis, that from an arbitrary number of births equal numbers would die each year until the entire cohort had expired, is of course unrealistic for any extended segment of the human age range. Nonetheless, a spin-off is in wide use today, that is, the assumption that between any two ages which are one unit apart, deaths tend to occur uniformly.

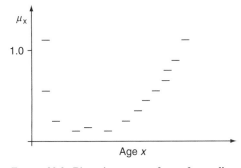

FIGURE 22.3. Piecewise-constant force of mortality.

A mathematical statement of the "uniform distribution of deaths" hypothesis is that the survival function decreases linearly with time (t) into an interval:

$$l_{x+t} = l_x + bt, \quad (0 \le t < 1) \tag{26}$$

with $b < 0$ (since l_{x+t} is a decreasing function). Because Eq. (26) is equivalent (after rearranging) to

$$l_{x+t} - l_x = bt, \tag{27}$$

it can in fact be seen that $b = -d_x = -(l_x - l_{x+1})$ by setting $t = 1$. Thus, Eq. (27) can be rewritten as

$$l_{x+t} = l_x - t \cdot d_x, \quad (0 \le t < 1) \tag{28}$$

and, since it is not required that the annual decrement be equal across single ages x, it follows that this is a *piecewise-linear survival function* specification. To derive the underlying mortality force function to which this survival curve applies, the definitional equation (8) given earlier may be applied:

$$
\begin{aligned}
\mu_{x+t} &= \frac{-1}{l_{x+t}} \frac{d}{dt} l_{x+t} = \frac{-1}{l_x - t \cdot d_x} \frac{d}{dt} [l_x - t \cdot d_x] \\
&= \frac{-1}{l_x - t \cdot d_x} [0 - 1 \cdot d_x] = \frac{d_x}{l_x - t \cdot d_x}, \quad (0 \le t < 1)
\end{aligned}
\tag{29}
$$

Algebraically, this function is of the form $a/(b + ct)$, for a, b, and c constants, i.e., this life table model specifies a *piecewise-hyperbolic force of mortality function*.

Again, this model leads to the following estimation algorithm:
Data-Model Orientation Equation:

$$M_x = m_x \tag{30}$$

Flow Equation:

$$l_{x+1} = p_x l_x = \left[\frac{1 - \frac{1}{2} M_x}{1 + \frac{1}{2} M_x} \right] l_x \tag{31}$$

Person-Years Equation:

$$L_x = \frac{1}{2}(l_x + l_{x+1}). \tag{32}$$

INITIATING AND TERMINATING THE COMPLETE LIFE TABLE. A final topic is how to initiate the life table at the early ages and terminate it at the last ages. When occurrence/exposure rates are available and accurate for ages 0 to 5 (i.e., M_0, M_1, M_2, M_3, M_4), one converts these to life-table survival and/or death probabilities via Eqs. (23), (24) or (30), (31). However, the force of mortality usually is considered to be changing so rapidly in these early years of life as to require more elaborate procedures, especially for q_0 (equivalently p_0).

For this reason, and because standard occurrence/exposure mortality rates for age 0 mix deaths and/or population estimates for two calendar years of births, a variety of *separation factors* have been developed to produce accurate estimates of q_0 from which to initiate the life table; see Keyfitz (1977b), Shryock and Siegel (1975), and Preston et al. (2001) for details.

For the oldest ages in the open-ended interval, the usual orientation equation is applied:

$$_\infty M_x =_\infty m_x. \tag{33}$$

This avoids the necessity of defining the oldest age to which a person can live. Inaccuracies in age reports for older people discourage further refinement. Furthermore, death registrations contain different error structures (in the numerator of $_\infty M_x$) from those in census counts (in the denominator of $_\infty M_x$).

Combining Eq. (33) with the definition $m_x = (l_x - l_\infty)/_\infty L_x$ and the fact that $l_\infty = 0$, it follows that $_\infty M_x = l_x/_\infty L_x$, and thus

$$_\infty L_x = \frac{l_x}{_\infty M_x}, \tag{34}$$

where x is the start of the terminal age. With $l_\infty = 0$, we obtain $_\infty q_x = 1$. Also, the expectation of life at age x becomes

$$e_x = \frac{_\infty L_x}{l_x} = \frac{1}{_\infty M_x}, \tag{35}$$

so that the expectation of life is the reciprocal of the terminal death rate.

THE ESTIMATION OF ABRIDGED POPULATION LIFE TABLES.   For most demographic research purposes, it is not necessary to calculate a complete life table. Rather, an *abridged life table*, that is, a life table defined on estimation age intervals larger than 1 year, say 5 or 10 years, provides sufficient accuracy for most purposes and is less cumbersome. Assume that the available data are in the form of a sequence of occurrence/exposure rates

$$_1 M_0,\ _4 M_1,\ _n M_5, \cdots,_n M_x, \cdots,\ _\infty M_{85}$$

where n is 5 or 10 years. Note that the only single age treated separately is age 0; then ages 1 to 4 are grouped; then the 5 or 10 age groupings; and finally the open-ended last age interval.

To estimate an abridged population life table, one could apply either of the piecewise exponential or linear survival function models/methods described above for complete tables. However, whereas both of these piecewise methods are accurate for the estimation of complete tables, they lose accuracy when applied to the estimation of abridged tables. Therefore, demographers have developed several additional methods for the estimation of abridged tables. These methods may be viewed as "adjustments" or "corrections" to the basic piecewise-exponential and piecewise-linear survival function models for the construction of complete life tables.[3] Several of these adjusted methods are now described.

---

[3] The assumption of the data-model orientation equation in the estimation algorithms for complete life tables (e.g., Eq. [30]) is referred to as a *sectional stationarity assumption*. For abridged life table estimation, this assumption may be relaxed to a *sectional stability assumption*. For more details, see Keyfitz (1968, 1970).

Three adjustment methods may be viewed as modifications of the piecewise-exponential life table model. This is due to the fact that the empirical tenability of the basic assumption of the exponential model (that the force of mortality is constant within age intervals) is less adequate as the estimation age intervals of the life table increase beyond single ages. Thus, each of these three methods modifies this assumption. The modification then produces correction factors for the flow and person-years equations of the piecewise-exponential algorithm stated earlier (Keyfitz and Frauenthal 1975; Greville 1943; and Reed and Merrell 1939). In fact, the Keyfitz-Frauenthal method can be viewed as a generalization of the Greville method, which in turn is a generalization of the Reed-Merrell method. Since the correction factor introduced by the Keyfitz-Frauenthal method allows for the most variability from age interval to age interval, it also is the most computationally intensive and, of the three methods, generally provides the most accurate abridged table estimates.

Two additional abridged life table estimation methods can be viewed as modifications of the piecewise-linear survival function model. The description of these methods requires one to define the concept of the *average number of years lived in the interval x to x + n by those dying in the interval, denoted* $_na_x$. This concept was introduced by Chiang (1960, 1968, 1972) in a reformulation of the classic linear survival function model. It is an application of the expectation of life function to the age interval x to $x + n$ and thus has the definition

$$_na_x = \frac{\int_0^n t l_{x+t} \mu_{x+t} dt}{\int_0^n l_{x+t} \mu_{x+t} dt}. \tag{36}$$

Note that the piecewise-linear l_x (uniform distribution of deaths) specification leads to

$$_na_x = \frac{_nL_x - n \cdot l_{x+n}}{_nd_x} = \frac{\frac{n}{2}(l_x + l_{x+n}) - n \cdot l_{x+n}}{l_x - l_{x+n}} = \frac{n}{2}, \tag{37a}$$

i.e., under the linear survival function specification the average number of years lived in the x to $x + n$ interval by those who die in the interval is $n/2$. But, in general, Eq. (37a) does not hold. Indeed, there is a general formula for transforming the central mortality rates, $_nm_x$, of the life table to the age-specific probabilities of dying, $_nq_x$ that uses Chiang's $_na_x$ (see Preston et al. 2001):

$$_nq_x = \frac{n \cdot_n m_x}{1 + (n -_n a_x)_n m_x} \tag{37b}$$

For the piecewise-linear l_x model, with $_na_x = n/2$, Eq. (37b) implies:

$$_nq_x = \frac{n \cdot_n m_x}{1 + \frac{n}{2}_n m_x} = \frac{2n \cdot_n m_x}{2 + n \cdot_n m_x}, \tag{37c}$$

which is equivalent to:

$$_np_x = \frac{1 - \frac{n}{2}_n m_x}{1 + \frac{n}{2}_n m_x}. \tag{37d}$$

Using the data-model orientation equations of the piecewise-linear l_x model (Eq. (30), one then can use either Eq. (37b) or Eq. (37c) to transform the observed $_nM_x$ into estimates of the survival function.

Again, however, these equations hold only for the piecewise-linear l_x model, and, in general, if one wants to use Eq. (36) in the construction of an abridged life table, one must either (1) borrow estimates of $_na_x$ from another population that one assumes is applicable (see, e.g., Elandt-Johnson and Johnson 1980; Preston et al. 2001) or (2) estimate the $_na_x$ empirically. Each of these methods has limitations. For instance, when estimates of $_na_x$ are borrowed from another population, e.g., by using $_na_x$'s from an unabridged life table that is calculated for data surrounding decennial census years (when age-specific population estimates are most accurate) together with data on observed $_nM_x$'s and Eq. (37b) to calculate an abridged life table for an intercensal year, the implicit assumption is that there has been no change in the survival curve in the intervening years. This may be more accurate than the direct application of the piecewise-linear l_x model via Eqs. (37c) or (37d). But it nonetheless is an approximation. As noted, an alternative approach is to estimate the $_na_x$ empirically. Two methods that have been proposed for this purpose are the piecewise-quadratic survival function method of Schoen (1978) and Land and Schoen (1982) and the iterative method of Keyfitz (1968, 1970) that is based on the model specification that l_{x+t} is a cubic function over the interval x to $x + n$.

INITIATING THE ABRIDGED TABLE.   An innovation in abridged life table estimation introduced by Keyfitz (1970) is a short-cut method for treating the youngest ages in the life table. This consists of assuming, for each of the three age intervals 0, 1 to 4, 5 to 9, a value for $_na_x$. For age 0, Keyfitz estimated the empirical regression

$$a_0 = 0.07 + 1.7M_0 \tag{38}$$

from data on a number of countries in which day, month, and year of birth were available. For ages 1 to 4, he found that $_4a_1$ may be set equal to 1.5 years without much loss in accuracy; for ages 5 to 9, $_5a_5$ can be set to 2.5 years. Under the (sectional stationarity) data-model orientation equations specified earlier, this yields two equations in each of the first three age intervals

$$l_{x+n} = l_x -_n M_x \cdot_n L_x \tag{39}$$

$$_nL_x = (l_x - l_{x+n})_na_x + nl_{x+n} \tag{40}$$

which can be solved simultaneously for the unknown $_nL_x$ and l_{x+n}. Coale and Demeny (1983) have conducted similar empirical studies across many populations; an adaptation of their findings is given by Preston and associates (2001).

Example: Abridged Life Tables for U.S. Males, 1994.   Table 22.1 displays abridged period life tables for U.S. males in 1994 based on the *Vital Statistics of the United States 1994* released by the National Center for Health Statistics (NCHS). Panel A is constructed under the piecewise-linear survival function model using the methods for the 0 to 1 and 85+ age intervals described above. Panel B is constructed under the Schoen-Land Piecewise-Quadratic Survival Function Model using the same procedures for the first and last age intervals.

For Panel A, the columns are the following:

$_nm_x$: $_n M_x = \frac{_nD_x}{_nK_x}$, where $_nD_x$ and $_nK_x$ were obtained from the life table of the *Vital Statistics of the United States*, and $_nM_x =_n m_x$ (Orientation Equation);

TABLE **22.1. Abridged Life Tables for United States Males, 1994**

Panel A Piecewise-Linear Survival Function Model: U.S. Males, 1994

Age x	$_nm_x$	$_na_x$	$_nq_x$	$_np_x$	l_x	$_nd_x$	$_nL_x$	T_x	e_x
0	0.008857	0.085057	0.008786	0.991214	100,000	879	99,196	7,232,035	72.320347
1	0.000467	1.500000	0.001867	0.998133	99,121	185	396,023	7,132,839	71.960615
5	0.000229	2.500000	0.001142	0.998858	98,936	113	494,400	6,736,815	68.092357
10	0.000308	2.500000	0.001538	0.998462	98,823	152	493,737	6,242,416	63.167363
15	0.001262	2.500000	0.006292	0.993708	98,671	621	491,805	5,748,678	58.260800
20	0.001645	2.500000	0.008189	0.991811	98,051	803	488,246	5,256,873	53.613845
25	0.001781	2.500000	0.008864	0.991136	97,248	862	484,084	4,768,627	49.035870
30	0.002361	2.500000	0.011733	0.988267	96,386	1,131	479,101	4,284,544	44.452075
35	0.002956	2.500000	0.014671	0.985329	95,255	1,397	472,780	3,805,442	39.950159
40	0.003790	2.500000	0.018772	0.981228	93,857	1,762	464,882	3,332,662	35.507775
45	0.004911	2.500000	0.024258	0.975742	92,095	2,234	454,892	2,867,781	31.139248
50	0.007354	2.500000	0.036105	0.963895	89,861	3,244	441,196	2,412,889	26.851247
55	0.011202	2.500000	0.054483	0.945517	86,617	4,719	421,287	1,971,693	22.763376
60	0.018080	2.500000	0.086491	0.913509	81,898	7,083	391,780	1,550,407	18.931010
65	0.027170	2.500000	0.127208	0.872792	74,814	9,517	350,279	1,158,627	15.486701
70	0.040832	2.500000	0.185250	0.814750	65,297	12,096	296,246	808,348	12.379492
75	0.061032	2.500000	0.264762	0.735238	53,201	14,086	230,791	512,102	9.625796
80	0.098104	2.500000	0.393908	0.606092	39,115	15,408	157,057	281,311	7.191826
85+	0.190799	5.241114	1.000000	0.000000	23,708	23,708	124,254	124,254	5.241114

Panel B Piecewise-Quadratic Survival Function Model: U.S. Males, 1994

Age x	$_nm_x$	$_na_x$	$_nq_x$	$_np_x$	l_x	$_nd_x$	$_nL_x$	T_x	e_x
0	0.008857	0.085057	0.008786	0.991214	100,000	879	99,196	7,224,020	72.240196
1	0.000467	1.500000	0.001866	0.998134	99,121	185	396,023	7,124,823	71.879753
5	0.000229	2.500000	0.001142	0.998858	98,936	113	494,400	6,728,800	68.011345
10	0.000308	3.493513	0.001538	0.998462	98,823	152	493,888	6,234,401	63.086259
15	0.001262	2.669589	0.006293	0.993707	98,671	621	491,910	5,740,513	58.178069
20	0.001645	2.546252	0.008190	0.991810	98,050	803	488,282	5,248,602	53.529591
25	0.001781	2.605065	0.008866	0.991134	97,247	862	484,173	4,760,320	48.950572
30	0.002361	2.598266	0.011736	0.988264	96,385	1,131	479,210	4,276,148	44.365152
35	0.002956	2.601436	0.014675	0.985325	95,254	1,398	472,918	3,796,938	39.861153
40	0.003790	2.605368	0.018779	0.981221	93,856	1,763	465,060	3,324,021	35.416101
45	0.004911	2.664741	0.024277	0.975723	92,094	2,236	455,247	2,858,960	31.044057
50	0.007354	2.675823	0.036151	0.963849	89,858	3,248	441,739	2,403,713	26.750173
55	0.011202	2.692393	0.054598	0.945402	86,609	4,729	422,135	1,961,974	22.653119
60	0.018080	2.643413	0.086706	0.913294	81,881	7,100	392,673	1,539,839	18.805870
65	0.027170	2.614451	0.127580	0.872420	74,781	9,541	351,146	1,147,166	15.340300
70	0.040832	2.577242	0.185782	0.814218	65,241	12,121	296,838	796,019	12.201282
75	0.061032	2.555457	0.265542	0.734458	53,120	14,106	231,119	499,181	9.397217
80	0.098104	3.249195	0.329092	0.670908	39,014	12,839	130,876	268,062	6.870844
85+	0.190799	5.241114	1.000000	0.000000	26,175	26,175	137,187	137,187	5.241114

U =	0.002112
V =	0.161284
W =	0.003270
X =	0.029572
Y =	0.341311
Z =	0.037550

Data source: U.S. Vital Statistics, 1994.

Note: See Chart 1 of Schoen (1978) for details of the calculation of survival function, lx, using the weights U to Z.

$_na_x$: for age 0, $a_0 = 0.07 + 1.7M_0$, (Eq. (38));

for ages 1–4, $_4a_1 = 1.5$;
for ages 5–9, $_5a_5 = 2.5$;

for ages 10–84, $_5a_x = \dfrac{n}{2} = \dfrac{5}{2} = 2.5$, (Eq.(37));

for ages 85 and above, $_\infty a_{85} = e_{85}$;

l_x: for ages 0, 1 to 4, and 5 to 9, the simultaneous equations (39) and (40) are solved, i.e., $l_{x+n} = l_x - _nM_x \cdot _nL_x$, where

$$_nL_x = \frac{n \cdot l_x}{1 + (n - _na_x)_nM_x};$$

for instance, if age $= 0$,

$$_1L_0 = \frac{1 \cdot l_0}{1 + (1 - a_0)_1M_0} = \frac{100000}{1 + (1 - .085).009} = 99,196;$$

$$l_1 = l_0 - _1M_0 \cdot _1L_0 = 100000 - .009*99196 = 99,121;$$

similar procedures apply for l_5, $_4L_1$, and $_5L_5$, with q_0 computed by application of Eq. (37b) and $p_0 = 1 - q_0$;

for other age categories, the Piecewise-Linear Flow Equation gives:

$l_{x+n} = _np_x \cdot l_x = [\frac{1 - \frac{n}{2} _nM_x}{1 + \frac{n}{2} _nM_x}]l_x;$

$_nL_x$: for the first three age categories, see calculations shown above;
for ages 10 to 84, use the Piecewise-Linear Person-Year Equation:

$_nL_x = \frac{n}{2}(l_x + l_{x+n});$
for ages 85+, use Eq. (34): $_\infty L_x = \frac{l_x}{_\infty M_x};$

$_nd_x$: $_n d_x = l_x - l_{x+n};$

$_np_x$: for ages under 85, $_np_x = \frac{1 - \frac{n}{2} _nM_x}{1 + \frac{n}{2} _nM_x}$, (Flow Equation);
for ages 85 +, $_\infty p_{85} = 0$;
$_nq_x$: for ages under 85, $_nq_x = 1 - _np_x$;
for ages 85+, $_\infty q_{85} = 1$;

$_nT_x$: $T_x = \sum_{t=0}^{\infty} L_{x+1};$

e_x^0: for ages under 85, $e_x = \frac{T_x}{l_x}$;
for ages 85 +, $e_x = \frac{_\infty L_x}{l_x} = \frac{1}{_\infty M_x}.$

In Panel B the assumption of the piecewise-linear survival function model is modified by the piecewise-quadratic survival function: $l_{x+t} = l_x + bt + ct^2$ (Land and Schoen 1982: 301–309). Several columns are calculated differently as follows:
$_na_x$: the same with Panel A for the first three and the last age categories;
for ages 10 to 84,

$$_na_x = \frac{n^2}{240}\left[\frac{l_x(_nM_{x+n} + 38_nM_x +_n M_{x-n}) + l_{x+n}(14_nM_{x+n} + 72_nM_x - 6_nM_{x-n})}{l_x - l_{x+n}}\right]$$

l_x and $_nL_x$: the above expression for $_na_x$ yields corresponding expressions for flow and person-years equations that are given in Chart 1 of Schoen (1978)[4].

$_nq_x$: for age under 85, $_nq_x = \frac{_nd_x}{l_x}$;

    for age 85 +, $_\infty q_{85} = 1$;

$_np_x$: for age under 85, $_np_x = 1 -_n q_x$;

    for age 85 +, $_{85} = 0$.

Substantively, it can be seen that the assumption of the piecewise-linear l_x model that deaths within an age interval occur, on average, halfway through the interval results in an underestimation of the a_x for many age intervals. This, in turn, translates into slightly underestimated q_x's throughout much of the age range from childhood to the end of life (see Eqs. (37a–d))—which leads to a slightly larger e_0 estimated from the piecewise-linear survival function model in Panel A than from the piecewise-quadratic survival function model in Panel B. For these data, however, both models yield quite accurate estimates of e_0.

Multiple-Decrement Life Tables

The life table models just described may be extended and generalized in various ways. This section describes three extensions and generalizations to processes by which an individual can exit the life table in two or more ways, to processes that allow for entrances or increments into living states as well as exits or decrements from those states, and to situations in which only sample-level data are available with which to estimate the life table, rather than population-level data, and for which we therefore need to make a more careful use of statistical methods of estimation and inference. The exposition here is limited to a general sketch of the basic ideas of these additional life table models.

A first extension is to *multiple-decrement life* tables, which incorporate the simultaneous operation of several causes of decrement or exit to a particular body of lives. For example, one may be concerned with an insurance coverage in which disability and mortality are distinct causes of claim and the interacting effects of exposure to both causes of decrement must be analyzed. Or one may wish to study a mortality experience in terms of its component causes of death, such as cancer, heart disease, or accidents, treating each cause of death as a separate decrement.

To model such multiple-decrement processes, the state-space of the single-decrement life table model must be elaborated to incorporate the multiple modes of exit from the key defined state of the life table, being alive at age x. This is shown in Figure 22.4. Panel (a) of Figure 22.4 illustrates the state-space of the single-decrement life table, which consists of two states, namely, being alive at age x and being dead. To connect these two states, Panel (a) has a single arrow directed from the alive state to the dead state, which represents the operation of the age-specific force of mortality or decrement

---

[4] Schoen (1978) has demonstrated empirically that an abridged life table estimated according to the quadratic survival function is more accurate than those estimated by several other abridged table methods, including the Keyfitz-Frauenthal method.

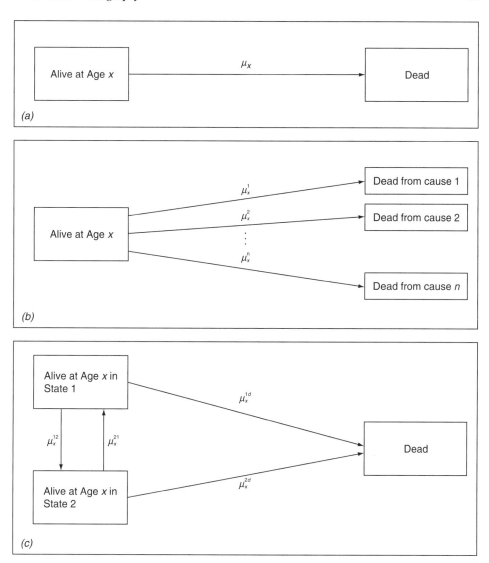

FIGURE 22.4. State space of the multiple decrement life table models.

of the life table at each age x. Because the force of mortality varies with age, the underlying mathematical model of this single-decrement process is that of a *time (age)-inhomogeneous stochastic process* (Land and Schoen 1982:278). This model specifies a simple, single-element state-space, consisting simply of being alive at age x, for those individuals in the life table model who have not yet exited or died. The only other state of this model is what is termed an absorbing state (because no returns to the living state are possible), which consists of having exited the table to the dead state.

By comparison, Panel (b) of Figure 22.4 shows a graphic representation of the state-space and forces of mortality for a multiple-decrement life table that has n possible forms of exit from the table. It can be seen that the major changes in the graphic representation of the life table model from Panel (a) to Panel (b) are that the absorbing or dead state now has been refined or disaggregated into n subcategories, and the single force of decrement of Panel (a) now is correspondingly disaggregated to allow for an instantaneous risk of decrement from the alive state to each of the absorbing or cause-specific death states. Detailed expositions of the mathematics of population multiple-decrement life tables and corresponding methods of estimation from occurrence/exposure rates can be found in Preston, Keyfitz, and Schoen (1972); Jordan (1975); Elandt-Johnson and Johnson (1980); Schoen (1988); and Preston et al. (2001).

Multistate Life Table and Projection Models

Panel (c) of Figure 22.4 is a graphic representation of a second generalization of the single-decrement life table, namely, to a *multistate* or *increment-decrement life table*. Rather than decomposing the dead or exit state of the life table into multiple causes or types of exit, the multistate life table disaggregates the single alive-at-age-x of the life table into multiple possible states that may be occupied by individuals alive. The multistate life table represented in Panel (c) of Figure 22.4 is for a simple two-living-state table. The two living states could take the form, for example, of two regions between which migration is possible in a biregional migration table, or the states of currently married or currently divorced in a nuptiality table, or the states of being in or out of the labor force in a labor force participation table, or the states of active or disabled in an active/disabled table. And, of course, the state-space could be refined to incorporate more than two living states at each age x. It can be seen that the major changes in the graphic representation of the life table model from Panel (a) to Panel (c) are the following: The alive at age x state now has been refined or disaggregated into two subcategories, and the single force of decrement from the alive state of Panel (a) now is correspondingly disaggregated to allow for an instantaneous risk of decrement from each alive state to the other alive state at each age x, with decrements to the receiving state referred to as increments to that state. At the same time, individuals alive in either state of the table are subjected at each age x to the risk of exit from the table to the dead state. A key property of multistate life tables is that, within the time period of the age intervals that define the table, they permit individuals alive in the table to exit or decrement from the state they occupied at the beginning of the age interval to another state and then to increment or return back to the original state. For life table models of demographic processes in which individuals may make multiple transitions within age intervals such as from nonmarried to married and back to nonmarried again, this is an indispensable property.

The multistate life table model has roots in mathematics, biostatistics, and actuarial science that date back to Du Pasquier (1912), Fix and Neyman (1951), and Sverdrup (1965). But its development and extensive empirical application by demographers mainly began in the 1970s. The generalization of the single-decrement population life table was initiated in the 1970s for applications to population-level (i.e., census and vital statistics) data on multiregional migration (Rogers 1975) and nuptiality on marriage and divorce (Schoen 1975; Schoen and Land 1979).

Hoem and Fong (1976) introduced an application to working life tables that used large-sample survey data rather than population-level data. Even for large-sample surveys, however, sample sizes for the estimation of age-specific transition probabilities may become small. The result is more age-to-age variability in the estimated transition probabilities. Accordingly, Hoem and Fong introduced a method of smoothing the age-specific estimates of transition probabilities by moving averages across the age intervals. Moving average and related methods of graduation or smoothing estimates of transition probabilities across age intervals subsequently has been used extensively for the estimation of labor force participation life tables by Schoen and Woodrow (1980), voting in U.S. presidential elections by Land, Hough, and McMillen (1986), and tables of school life by Land and Hough (1989).

A particularly active area of methodological development and empirical application of multistate life tables has been the estimation of years of active/disability-free/health life as contrasted to inactivity/disability/unhealthy years among the elderly population. The initial definition of active life expectancy in terms of a lack of limitations in activities of daily living was given by Katz and colleagues (1983). The standard life table method for estimating active life expectancy used by these authors is a *prevalence-rate-based life table* method of decomposing the $_nL_x$ column of a population life table into years lived in an active state and years lived in an inactive or disabled state, a method presented by Sullivan (1971; for a recent exposition, see Molla, Wagener, and Madans 2001). Due to its minimal data requirements (the existence of a population life table appropriate for the particular population for which estimates are desired and a set of age-specific prevalence rates or proportions of persons identified as either in the active or inactive states), the Sullivan method has been widely applied and remains useful today (see Crimmins, Saito, and Ingegneri 1997; Cambois, Robine, and Hayward 2001).

However, Rogers, Rogers, and Branch (1989) noted that one critical assumption of prevalence-rate-based life table methods is that transitions can only occur in one direction among the living statuses, specifically, from the active to the inactive state in active life expectancy tables. Using data on age-specific transition rates among the active and inactive statuses from longitudinal panel surveys of the elderly, they applied multistate life table methods to the estimation of active life expectancy. Subsequent research (Crimmins, Saito, and Hayward 1993) indicates that the Sullivan method for estimating active life expectancy generally yields estimates that do not differ greatly from those obtained by multistate models. Nonetheless, when data on transitions among living states are available, the methodological and empirical research accumulated over the past two decades suggests that multistate life table models should be applied.

Research by Zeng, Gu, and Land (2004) demonstrates that the disabled life expectancies based on conventional multistate life table methods are significantly underestimated due to an assumption of no functional status changes between the ages of individuals in a longitudinal panel at the date of the last wave in which they were interviewed and their subsequent death. Zeng and colleagues (2004) present a new method to correct the bias and apply it to 1998 and 2000 longitudinal survey data of about 9,000 oldest old Chinese aged 80 to 105. The results show that estimates of active life expectancy can be improved if data on the disability status of the elderly in the month or so prior to death are available. These data permit a more accurate estimation of individuals' functional status in the time period between a last wave of panel interviews and death. Zeng and associates (2004) also applied and extended methods developed by Molla and associates (2001) (based on Chiang 1960 and Keyfitz 1977b) to estimate standard errors of status-based active life expectancy (i.e., active life expectancy for persons with different functional status at initial age).

Benefiting from methodological advances in multidimensional demography (Rogers 1975; Willekens et al. 1982; Land and Rogers 1982; Schoen 1988), Bongaarts (1987) developed a multistate nuclear-family-status life table model. Zeng extended Bongaarts's nuclear-family-status life table model into a general multistate family household simulation macro model that includes both nuclear and three-generation family households (Zeng 1986, 1988, 1991). The multistate life table macro models developed by Bongaarts and Zeng are female-dominant one-sex models and assume that input rates are constant.

Based on Bongaarts' and Zeng's one-sex life table models, Zeng, Vaupel, and Wang (1997, 1998) developed a two-sex multistate dynamic macro projection model known as "ProFamy" that permits demographic schedules to change over time and uses as inputs only conventional data that are available from ordinary surveys, vital statistics, and censuses. Zeng, Land, Wang, and Gu (2005) extended the ProFamy model by adding cohabitation and race dimensions to all computation and estimation procedures. In addition to statuses defined by the number of coresiding children and parents and parity, the extended ProFamy family household projection model includes seven marital/union statuses: (1) never-married and not cohabiting, (2) married, (3) widowed and not cohabiting, (4) divorced and not cohabiting, (5) never married and cohabiting, (6) widowed and cohabiting, and (7) divorced and cohabiting. The ProFamy model has been used to generate U.S. household projections by race (Zeng et al. 2005), household automobile consumption forecasts in Austria (Prskawetz, Jiang, and O'Neill 2002); German households and living arrangement projections (Hullen 2000, 2003), and family household projections in smaller areas (e.g., Hullen 2001; Heigl 2001; Jiang and Kuijsten 1999a, 1999b; Yang and Zeng 2000).

The classic headship-rate method for projections of households is not linked to demographic rates, projects a few household types without size, and does not deal with household members other than heads. By comparison, the multistate ProFamy new method uses demographic rates as input and projects more detailed household types, sizes, and living arrangements for all members of the population. Projections using ProFamy and observed U.S. demographic rates in the 1990s show that the discrepancies between the projections and 2000 census observations are reasonably small, thus validating the new method.

Hazard Regression Models and Survival Curves from Longitudinal Studies

This section extends and generalizes the classic single-decrement population life table model by taking its basic survival process ideas and applying statistical methods of parameter estimation and hypothesis testing to them. While there are prior roots in the use of life table models for the estimation of survival curves following medical treatment in biostatistics (Berkson and Gage 1952) and in the application of panel regression models in sociology (Coleman 1964), the major paper that initiated this extension of life table/ survival model ideas is the classic article on the intersection of regression models with life table concepts by Cox (1972). This article presented the use of regression models to control for multiple covariates simultaneously in the estimation of life tables and introduced the *proportional hazards regression model* and the partial likelihood method for its estimation from sample data. These developments are so associated with Cox's article that proportional hazards regression models are now known as *Cox regression models*.

Cox's paper has generated a voluminous literature on survival models and methods in biostatistics and related disciplines over the past three decades, as shown in the works of Allison (1995), Hosmer and Lemeshow (1999), Ibrahim, Chen, and Sinha (2001), Kalbfleisch and Prentice (2002), Klein and Moeschberger (1997), Lawless (2003), Therneau and Grambsch (2000), and Yamaguchi (1991). In addition to providing a procedure for bringing statistical methods of inference to bear on the use of sample data to estimate the life table model, a key feature of these models is that they provide a means to transform the life table as a primarily descriptive model, as in equation (1) above, and into an explanatory model, as in equation (2), in which heterogeneity in variations among individuals in survival times are explained, at least in part, in terms of certain exogenous variables or regression covariates. Regarding terminology, when a regression model for survival data is applied to a nonrepeatable process, such as time of survival to death, it is termed a *hazard regression model*; when the regression model is applied to a process that allows for multiple occurrences like entries into, and exits from, the labor force over the adult life course, it is termed an *event history model*. The event history terminology was introduced by Tuma, Hannan, and Groeneveld (1979). A recent account of event history models and statistical methods of estimation and inference is given in Singer and Willet (2003).

The proportional hazard regression model approach, and, more generally, the statistical approach to the estimation of single-decrement life tables from sample data, was introduced to demographers by Menken et al. (1981) and Trussell and Hammerslough (1983). Extensions to multistate hazard regression models and multistate life tables and associated empirical applications by demographers followed. Hoem and Funck-Jensen (1982) laid out the probability theoretical foundations of multistate life tables and indicated how regression models could be used to account for population heterogeneity in this context. Hayward and Grady (1990) applied regression models to longitudinal sample data on processes of work and retirement among a cohort of older men to estimate a multistate hazard/life table model. Land, Guralnik, and Blazer (1994) combined panel regression models to estimate hazards and expected transition probabilities to use in a multistate estimation of disability processes and active life expectancy among the elderly.

A related approach using longitudinal panel data and hazard regression models for the estimation of multistate life tables builds on the random walk model of human mortality and aging of Woodbury and Manton (1983) and the generalized latent-class model known as the grades-of-membership (GoM) model (Woodbury and Clive 1974; Manton, Stallard, and Singer 1994; Manton, Woodbury, and Tolley 1994). Applications of this combined random walk/GoM model to longitudinal panel data for the estimation of the interaction of mortality and disability dynamics and of active life expectancy have been made by Manton, Stallard, and Corder (1997) and Manton and Land (2000).

STABLE POPULATION THEORY
AND ITS EXTENSIONS

Classic Stable Population Theory

Deterministic models of population growth exist in two forms: (1) those that use a continuous time variable and a continuous age scale (Lotka 1907; Sharpe and Lotka 1911) and (2) those using a discrete time variable and a discrete age scale (Bernadelli 1941; Lewis 1941; and Leslie 1945; Sykes 1969). Both have advantages. The discrete formulation is closer to demographic practice in population projections. But the continuous formulation is closer to continuous life table/stationary population theory. Thus, the classic single-sex stable continuous-time population theory is now presented.

Recall that the continuous-time formulation of the stationary population model requires that the number of births equal the number of deaths over any finite time interval. When it is not required that births equal deaths, but instead that each is assumed to occur according to rates that are forever fixed, the more interesting continuous-time model of a stable population is obtained, due to the work of Lotka (1907) and Sharpe and Lotka (1911). In this model, the births of a current generation are associated with those of the preceding generation to define several important constants that describe the ultimate growth and composition of such a population.

THE RENEWAL EQUATION AND STABLE GROWTH.   The continuous single-sex model of population dynamics is expressed as an integral equation. To obtain $B(t)$, the number of female births at time t, women aged x to $x + dx$ at time t "at risk" of childbirth are the survivors of those born x years ago. Denote the number of females born x years ago by $B(t - x)$ and the life table survival probability (for surviving from birth to age x) by $p(x)$. Then this quantity is $B(t - x)p(x)dx$, where $x \leq t$. At time t, these women give birth to

$$B(t - x)p(x)m(x)dx \qquad (41)$$

female children per year, where $m(x)\ dx$ is the annual rate of female childbearing among women aged x to $x + dx$.

Integrating Eq. (41) over all ages x and adding $G(t)$ to include births to women already alive at an initial time point (time zero) yields the *Lotka integral equation*:

$$B(t) = G(t) + \int_0^t B(t - x)p(x)m(x)dx, \qquad (42)$$

where (Keyfitz 1977b):

$$G(t) = \int_{\alpha-t}^{\beta-t} K(x + t)m(x + t)dx$$

$$= \int_{\alpha-t}^{\beta-t} k(x)\frac{p(x + t)}{p(x)}m(x + t)dx, \qquad (43)$$

α and β being, respectively, the lower and upper bounds of the childbearing ages, and $k(x)dx$ denoting the number of women aged x to $x + dx$ at time zero. For $t \geq \beta$, $G(t)$ is zero; hence Eq. (42) reduces to

$$B(t) = \int_0^t B(t - x)p(x)m(x)dx, \text{ for } t \geq \beta. \qquad (44)$$

Because Eqs. (42) and (43) show how a population of individuals born $t - x$ years ago gives rise to a new cohort of individuals at time t, this often is called *Lotka's renewal equation*.

On replacing $B(t)$ and $B(t - x)$ by Qe^{rt} and $Qe^{r(t-x)}$, respectively, and noting that $m(x)$ is nonzero only in the childbearing ages $\alpha \leq x \leq \beta$, the *characteristic equation* is obtained:

$$\Psi(r) = \int_\alpha^\beta e^{-rx} p(x) m(x) dx = \int_\alpha^\beta e^{-rx} \Phi(x) dx = 1, \tag{45}$$

where the product $p(x) \, m(x)$, denoted by $\Phi(x)$, is called the *net maternity function*. To solve the integral equation in (45), the value of r for which $\Psi(r)$ is unity needs to be determined.

The terms inside the integral in Eq. (43) are always nonnegative, and e^{-rx} is a decreasing function of r, which guarantees the existence of a real root, i.e., a quantity that is a real number and for which $\Psi(r) = 1$. Differentiating $\Psi(r)$ with respect to r, the first derivative is always negative for all real values of r. Hence $\Psi(r)$ is a monotonically decreasing function. Thus, the curve of $\Psi(r)$ can cross the horizontal line of unity height only once, i.e., these can be only on real root of Eq. (45), as illustrated in Figure 22.5.

In addition to the real root, the characteristic equation (45) can be satisfied by complex values of r. These complex roots occur in complex conjugate pairs. To see this, suppose the complex number $u + iv$ is a root, where $i = \sqrt{-1}$. Euler's theorem indicates that the exponential of a complex number can be written

$$e^{rx} = e^{ux+ivx} = e^{ux}[\cos(vx) + isun(vx)],$$

and hence (45) is

$$\Psi(r) = \int_\alpha^\beta e^{-ux}[\cos(vx) - i\sin(vx)]\Phi(x)dx = 1. \tag{46}$$

Since there is no imaginary portion of the right-hand side, that on the left must vanish, i.e.

$$\int_\alpha^\beta e^{-ux}\sin(vx)dx = 0. \tag{47}$$

Thus, since the sin function is a symmetric function for which $\sin(vx) = \sin(-vx)$, it follows that $u - iv$ must also be a root of (45). It can be demonstrated that the real root r must be larger than the value of u in any complex root $u \pm iv$, that is, $r_1 > u$ (Lotka 1998).

For any r_k that is a root of (45),

$$B(t) = Q_k e^{r_k t}, \tag{48}$$

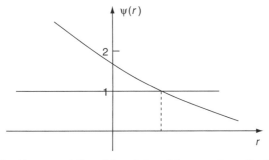

FIGURE 22.5. Graphic representation of the solution of the renewal equation for its real root.

is a solution, and, assuming the roots are distinct, they may be summed to give the general solution

$$B(t) = \sum_{k=1}^{\infty} Q_k e^{r_k t}$$

$$= Q_1 e^{r_1 t} + \sum_{k=2}^{\infty} Q_k e^{u_k t}[\cos{(v_k t)} + i\sin{(v_k t)}]. \tag{49}$$

Since each complex root is accompanied by its complex conjugate, which is multiplied by the conjugate coefficient, the imaginary terms in the series on the right of Eq. (49) will cancel out, and a real trigonometric series remains. This is necessary for the solution to make sense, because the representation of counts of a real population of births could hardly include imaginary terms.

Consider next the problem of evaluating the Q_k to fit a given initial condition defined by $G(t)$. One begins by taking Laplace transforms of both sides of Eq. (46), often denoting $p(x)m(x)$ by $\Phi(x)$ the net maternity function:

$$B^*(r) = G^*(r) + B^*(r)\Phi^*(r), \tag{50}$$

where

$$B^*(r) = \int_0^{\infty} e^{-rt} B(t) dt,$$

$$G^*(r) = \int_0^{\infty} e^{-rt} G(t) dt,$$

and

$$\Phi^*(r) = \int_0^{\infty} e^{-rt} \Phi(t) dt.$$

It follows that (50) may be reexpressed as

$$B^*(r) = \frac{G^*(r)}{1 - \Phi^*(r)}. \tag{51}$$

When the integrals defining the Laplace transforms on the right-hand side of Eq. (51) exist (i.e., equal some definite finite real number), then their inverse transforms also exist, and $B(t)$, the inverse of $B^*(r)$ on the left-hand side of Eq. (51), is the solution to the integral equation Eq. (42). Feller (1941) showed that this solution is unique on the condition that $B^*(r)$ can be expressed in partial fractions

$$B^*(r) = \frac{G^*(r)}{1 - \Phi^*(r)} = \frac{Q_1}{r - r_1} + \frac{Q_2}{r - r_2} + \ldots + \frac{Q_k}{r - r_k} + \ldots \tag{52}$$

and that $\sum Q_k$ converges absolutely, the r_k being the roots (finite or infinite in number) of $\Phi^*(r) = 1$, which is identical with the characteristic equation $\Psi(r) = 1$ of Eq. (45). Inverting the terms of the expansion of Eq. (52) results in Eq. (49) once again. To determine the coefficients of the partial fractions in Eq. (52), one takes the derivatives:

$$Q_k = \lim_{r \to r_k} \frac{(r - r_k)G^*(r)}{1 - \Phi^*(r)} = \frac{G^*(r)}{-d\Phi^*(r)/dr}\Big|_{r=r_k},$$

which yields the following solution for the constants

$$Q_k = \frac{\int_0^\beta e^{-r_k t} G(t)dt}{\int_0^\beta x e^{-r_k x} p(x)m(x)dx}. \tag{53}$$

For the maximal root, this relationship may be expressed more meaningfully as

$$Q = \frac{V}{A}, \tag{54}$$

where

$$V = \int_0^\beta e^{-rt} G(t)dt \tag{55}$$

is called the called the *total reproductive value* of a (single-sex) population and

$$A = \frac{\int_\alpha^\beta x e^{-rx} p(x)m(x)dx}{\int_\alpha^\beta e^{-rx} p(x)m(x)dx} = \int_\alpha^\beta x e^{-rx} p(x)m(x)dx \tag{56}$$

is the *mean age of childbearing in the stable population.*

This completes the specification of the components of solution (57) for $B(t)$. For sufficiently large values of t, all terms beyond the first become negligibly small relative to the first, because $r_1 > u_k$ for all $k > 1$. Hence, ultimately

$$B(t) \cong Qe^{r_1 t}. \tag{57}$$

Thus, after a sufficiently long period of time the "waves" corresponding to the complex terms of Eq. (49)—if any—will "wear off," and the birth trajectory will be purely exponential, as in Figure 22.6.

In brief, the birth trajectory in the continuous-time stable population model is an exponentially damped sinusoidal curve in which the sinusoidal waves, caused by "echoes" of past fluctuations in births that have left their imprint on the age structure of the initial ($t = 0$) population, gradually decline to insignificance and the exponential

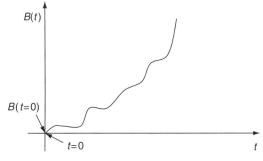

FIGURE 22.6. Illustration of the wearing off of population waves.

growth (at rate r) becomes dominant. This is the ultimate *stable growth* birth trajectory implied by the stable population model. Its defining parameter, r, is called the *intrinsic rate of growth* of the stable population, i.e., it is the rate at which the population ultimately will grow after the sinusoidal waves of its initial age structure wear off. This tendency for the effect of the initial age structure of a population to wear off after a sufficiently long period of time is the basis for the well-known *ergodic theorems* of stable population theory (Arthur 1982; Cohen 1979; Keyfitz 1977b; Lopez 1961; McFarland 1969; Sykes 1969; Parlett 1970).

NUMERICAL SOLUTION OF THE CHARACTERISTIC EQUATION.   The solution of the characteristic equation developed in the preceding section is theoretical. To apply it in practice, the integral

$$\int_0^5 e^{-r(x+t)} p(x+t) m(x+t) dt, \ x = \alpha, \ldots, \beta - 5$$

usually is evaluated as the product of $e^{-r(x+2.5)}$, $L(x)/l(0)$, and $F(x)$, where $F(x)$ is the observed birthrate among women aged x to $x+4$ at last birthday. Thus, $\Psi(r)$ is approximated by

$$\sum_{x=\alpha}^{\beta-5} e^{-r(x+2.5)} \frac{L(x)}{l(0)} F(x), \tag{58}$$

with the summation taken over childbearing ages x, which are multiples of 5. Consequently, assuming that the childbearing ages lie between $\alpha = 10$ and $\beta = 50$, Eq. (45) may be solved numerically by determining that value of r for which

$$e^{-12.5r} \frac{L(10)}{l(0)} F(10) + e^{-17.5r} \frac{L(15)}{l(0)} F(15) + \ldots + e^{-47.5r} \frac{L(45)}{l(0)} F(45) = 1. \tag{59}$$

Several iterative methods have been proposed to find the r that satisfies (59). Of these, the method of *functional iteration* described by Keyfitz (1977b) is one of the most efficient. To apply that method, one begins by multiplying both sides of Eq. (59) by $e^{-27.5r}$ and chooses an arbitrary initial value for r, with which the resulting expression on the left-hand side of the equation is evaluated. Taking 1/27.5 of the natural logarithm of this quantity, an improved approximation of r may be obtained with which the same expression is evaluated; this continues until two consecutive approximations differ by less than a small prescribed amount.

To illustrate, applying the method of functional iteration to the 1995 life table for U.S. females and the fertility data in Table 22.2, results in $r = -0.00846$. The same computations carried out with comparable 1968 data by Keyfitz (1977b) yield an r of 0.005715, indicating a considerable decline in fertility, since mortality experienced a decline during the two decades [$e_0^0 = 74.0$ in 1968; $e_0^0 = 78.9$ in 1995]. Given a numerical approximation of r, one may apply the following expression to evaluate the *mean age of childbearing* in the stable population model:

$$A = \sum (x + 2.5) e^{-r(x+2.5)} \frac{L(x)}{l(0)} F(x) \tag{60}$$

TABLE 22.2. Stable Population Parameters and Indices for United States Females, 1995

Age	Stationary population L(x)	Birth rate F(x)	Net maternity function Φ (x)	Moments of net maternity function	
				First	Second
10	495,268	0.00059	0.00291	0.03634	0.45425
15	494,466	0.02163	0.10697	1.87205	32.76090
20	493,251	0.04394	0.21674	4.87673	109.72646
25	491,839	0.04515	0.22208	6.10709	167.94502
30	489,978	0.03350	0.16414	5.33461	173.37496
35	487,380	0.01410	0.06873	2.57736	96.65110
40	483,739	0.00273	0.01320	0.56114	23.84831
45	478,577	0.00013	0.00062	0.02950	1.40143
Total		0.16178	0.79540	21.39483	606.16245

Reproduction rates		
Net reproduction rate	NRR/R (0)	= 0.79540
Gross reproduction rate	GRR	= 0.80888
Stationary population		
Mean age of childbearing	μ	= 26.90
Variance of age of childbearing	σ^2	= 38.48
Stable population		
Intrinsic rate of growth	r	= −0.00846
Intrinsic birth rate	b	= 0.00870
Intrinsic death rate	d	= 0.01715
Mean age of childbearing	A	= 27.32
Mean age	a	= 46.50
Mean length of generation	T	= 27.06

Comparison of age composition

	1995	stable
0–14	0.2076	0.1380
15–64	0.6447	0.5890
65+	0.1476	0.2729
	1.0000	1.0000

Data source: U.S. Census Bureau and Vital Statistics.

Table 22.2 reports numerical values of r and A for 1995 together with several other quantities defined in the next two subsections.[5]

THE NET MATERNITY FUNCTION.   Net maternity functions of various countries at different points in time show a regularity that demographers have tried to capture by means of curve fitting. Lotka proposed a normal probability function, and Keyfitz (1977b) compared the fits of the normal curve with those provided by alternative probability functions (see also Hoem et al. 1981). Such a view of the net maternity function leads naturally to an examination of its moments:

[5] For exemplary applications of life tables/stationary population and stable population models to the comparative study of the population dynamics of many national populations with a focus on population growth and aging, see Keyfitz and Flieger (1990).

$$R(n) = \int_{\alpha}^{\beta} x^{n}\Phi(x)dx, \, n = 0, 1, 2, \ldots.$$

The first three moments are of principal interest because they define the following demographic parameters:

Net Reproduction Rate:

$$NRR = R(0) = \int_{\alpha}^{\beta} x^{0}p(x)m(x) = \int_{\alpha}^{\beta} x^{0}\Phi(x)dx$$

$$= \int_{\alpha}^{\beta} e^{-0 \cdot x}\Phi(x)dx = \Psi(0); \tag{61}$$

Mean Age of Childbearing in the Stationary Population:

$$\mu = \frac{\int_{\alpha}^{\beta} xp(x)m(x)dx}{\int_{\alpha}^{\beta} p(x)m(x)dx}$$

$$= \frac{\int_{\alpha}^{\beta} x\Phi(x)dx}{\int_{\alpha}^{\beta} \Phi(x)dx} = \frac{R(1)}{R(0)}; \tag{62}$$

Variance of Age at Childbearing in the Stationary Population:

$$\sigma^{2} = \frac{\int_{\alpha}^{\beta} (x - \mu)^{2}p(x)m(x)dx}{\int_{\alpha}^{\beta} p(x)m(x)dx}$$

$$= \frac{\int_{\alpha}^{\beta} (x - \mu)^{2}\Phi(x)dx}{\int_{\alpha}^{\beta} \Phi(x)dx} \tag{63}$$

$$= \frac{R(2)}{R(0)} - \mu^{2}$$

The net reproduction rate gives the number of (female) children expected to be born to a (female) baby now born if the current schedule of fertility and mortality is maintained. A related measure, which does not consider the effects of mortality, is the *gross reproduction rate*:

$$GRR = \int_{\alpha}^{\beta} m(x)dx. \tag{64}$$

Example: As another example, Table 22.2 presents the net maternity function for United States females in 1996. Observe that the related parameters may be computed as follows:

$$NRR = R(0) = \sum_{x=10}^{45} \frac{L(x)}{l(0)} F(x) = 0.7954;$$

$$GRR = 5 \sum_{x=10}^{45} F(x) = 0.8089$$

$$\mu = \frac{\sum_{x=10}^{45}(x+2.5)L(x)F(x)}{\sum_{x=10}^{45}L(x)F(x)} = \frac{21.3948}{0.7954} = 26.90;$$

$$\sigma^2 = \frac{606.1625}{0.7954} - (26.90)^2 = 38.48$$

Lotka showed how these three parameters may be used to obtain a numerical approximation of r, the intrinsic rate of growth using an iterative solution. This is referred to as the *method of normal fit* by Keyfitz and Flieger (1971). Its application to the data in Table 22.2 yields the same r of -0.00846.

RELATIONS UNDER STABILITY.   The age composition of a population that is undisturbed by migration is determined by the regime of fertility and mortality to which it has been subjected (Keyfitz 1969). If this regime has remained unchanged for a sufficiently long time period, the initial age composition of the population is "forgotten" in that its influence on the current age composition disappears entirely. Such a *stable population* is characterized by (1) a proportionally fixed age composition and (2) increases at a constant intrinsic rate of growth r.

Let $c(x, t)$ denote the proportional age composition of a female population at time r. The number at age x at time t, denoted $k(x, t)$, are survivors of $B(t - x)$ births x years ago, i.e.,

$$k(x,t) = B(t - x)p(x).$$

Integrating this quantity over all ages of life, the total female population is obtained. Thus, the proportion of this population which is at age x at time t is of density

$$c(x,t) = \frac{k(x,t)}{\int_0^\omega k(x,t)dx} = \frac{B(t - x)p(x)}{\int_0^\omega B(t - x)p(x)dx}. \qquad (65)$$

If $c(x, t)dx$ is the proportion of females aged x to $x + dx$ at time t, the *crude death rate* at time t of this population is

$$d(t) = \int_0^\omega c(x,t)\mu(x)dx; \qquad (66)$$

and the *crude birth rate* at time t is

$$b(t) = \int_\alpha^\beta c(x,t)m(x)dx; \qquad (67)$$

which also may be found by setting $x = 0$ in the numerator of Eq. (64):

$$b(t) = c(0,t) = \frac{B(t)}{\int_0^\omega B(t - x)p(x)dx}. \qquad (68)$$

Definitions (65) through (68) apply to any population, stable or not. However, in a stable population, they yield simplified analytic expressions. To see this, recall that at stability $B(t) = Qe^{rt}$. Substituting this into Eqs. (65) and (68) results in a stable population with the proportional age composition

$$c(x,t) = \frac{Qe^{r(t-x)}p(x)}{\int_0^\omega Qe^{r(t-x)}p(x)dx} = \frac{e^{-rx}p(x)}{\int_0^\omega e^{-rx}p(x)dx} = c(x), \tag{69}$$

and birthrate

$$b(t) = \frac{Qe^{rt}}{\int_0^\omega Qe^{r(t-x)}p(x)dx} = \frac{1}{\int_0^\omega e^{-rx}p(x)dx} = b, \tag{70}$$

from which is obtained

$$c(x) = be^{-rx}p(x). \tag{71}$$

Since under stability t has disappeared from the expressions for $c(x, t)$ and $b(t)$, these quantities are independent of time and may be denoted simply as $c(x)$ and b, respectively. Usually, $c(x)$ is called the *stable age composition* and b the *intrinsic birth rate*. The *intrinsic death rate*, d, may be found by subtracting the intrinsic rate of growth from the intrinsic birth rate:

$$d = b - r. \tag{72}$$

Since the net reproduction rate $R(0)$ is a measure of the level of intergenerational increase, it is concluded that

$$e^{rT} = R(0), \tag{73}$$

where T is the *mean length of a generation*. Taking natural logarithms of both sides and simplifying results in

$$T = \frac{1}{r} \ln R(0). \tag{74}$$

The *mean age of the stable population* is

$$a = \frac{\int_0^n xe^{-rx}p(x)dx}{\int_0^\omega xe^{-rx}p(x)dx} = \int_0^\omega xc(x)dx. \tag{75}$$

To illustrate, consider the numerical application of these concepts to the data of Table 22.2. When $r = -0.00846$

$$b = \frac{1}{\sum_{x=0}^{85} e^{-r(x+2.5)}L(x)/l(0)} = 0.0087,$$

$$d = b - r = 0.0172,$$

$$T = \frac{1}{r} \ln (0.7954) = 27.06,$$

$$a = \frac{\sum_{x=0}^{85} (x + 2.5)e^{-r(x+2.5)}L(x)}{\sum_{x=0}^{85} e^{-r(x+2.5)}L(x)} = 46.50,$$

To obtain the proportions of the stable population that are in various age groups, one defines

$$C(x) = \int_x^{x+5} c(a)da = b \int_x^{x+5} e^{-ra}p(a)da, \tag{76}$$

and evaluates it numerically for each 5-year age group as

$$C(x) = be^{-r(x+2.5)}\frac{L(x)}{l(0)}$$

$$= \frac{e^{-r(x+2.5)}L(x)}{\sum_{x=0}^{85} e^{-r(x+2.5)}L(x)}.$$

After grouping into three age intervals, these proportions are given at the bottom of Table 22.2 in comparison with the age structure of the 1995 population. The stable-equivalent population exhibits an older and smoother[6] age distribution than that of the stationary population.

Nonstable Population and Variable-r Extensions of Stable Population Theory

The classic stable population model described above is a generalization of the stationary population model, which permits age-specific growth rates to be nonzero. The assumption of constancy of age-specific growth rates under stable population theory can be further relaxed to accommodate growth rates that vary with age. This generalizes to the nonstable population model, which is applicable to any population. Since the demographic relations in this general model are associated with varying growth rates by age, they are termed as variable-r relations (Preston et al. 2001). The most important development of the nonstable population model and variable-r method for demographic estimation dates back to the 1980s. Preston and Coale (1982) derived various extensions of the relations connecting major demographic parameters in stationary and stable populations to more general conditions. Much of their work is based on the following relation first shown by Bennett and Horiuchi (1981):

$$k(x,t) = B(t)e^{-\int_0^x r(a,t)da}p(x,t) \tag{77}$$

where $k(x, t)$ is the number of persons age x at time t; $B(t)$ is the number of births at time t; $p(x, t)$ is the life table survival probability from age 0 to age x at time t and $p(x,t) = e^{-\int_0^x \mu(a,t)da}$ with $\mu(x,t)$ being the force of mortality function at time t. Preston and Coale expanded this equation to include migration by adding the term, $e(x, t)$, or the net out-migration function, to $r(x, t)$. Thus, the formulation has been generalized from a closed population to an open population. For the convenience of exposition, t is dropped for the following equations, and all functions pertain to the time t.

The establishment of Equation (77) immediately leads to the following relations, which bear a remarkable resemblance to three fundamental formulas that characterize a stable population. Substituting Eq. (77) in Eq. (68), the *crude birth rate* of the population becomes

---

[6] The smoothness is observed for five-year age grouping from 0 to 85+.

$$b = \frac{B}{\int_0^\omega k(x)dx} = \frac{B}{\int_0^\infty Be^{-\int_0^x r(a)da}p(x)dx} = \frac{1}{\int_0^\infty e^{-\int_0^x r(a)da}p(x)dx}. \tag{78}$$

In a similar fashion, Eq. (77) and (78) may be substituted in Eq. (69) to obtain the *age composition* of the population:

$$c(x) = \frac{k(x)}{\int_0^\infty k(x)dx} = \frac{Be^{-\int_0^x r(a)da}}{\int_0^\infty Be^{-\int_0^x r(a)da}p(x)dx} = be^{-\int_0^x r(a)da}p(x) \tag{79}$$

Substituting Eq. (79) into Eq. (67) yields the *characteristic equation* for any population:

$$1 = \int_\alpha^\beta e^{-\int_0^x r(a)da}p(x)m(x)dx \tag{80}$$

It is easy to demonstrate the connection of this formulation with that in the stable population model. If all age-specific growth rates are constant, that is, $r(a) = r$ at all a, then $e^{-\int_0^x r(a)da} = e^{-rx}$. Eqs. (78) and (79) then become precisely the corresponding functions in the stable population expressed in Eqs. (70) and (71), and Eq. (80) becomes the characteristic equation expressed in Eq. (45) for the stable population model. Table 22.3 shows a brief comparison of these major demographic relations for the stationary population, the stable population, and any nonstable population. As noted before, the variable r or $r(x)$ function is the age-specific growth rate plus the age-specific rate of out-migration, wherever applicable.

The basic relations shown above give rise to other variable-r relations that go beyond the analogs of the classic stable population relations (Preston and Coale 1982; Preston et al. 2001). They connect all major demographic functions to one another through the set of age-specific growth rates that are readily observable and can be utilized as a growth correction which allows all of the relationships of a stationary population to be reestablished. Therefore, variable-r extensions of the basic classic stable population relations find many useful applications in demographic estimation. Space limitations allow only a brief discussion of several such applications in studies of birth rates and fertility, mortality, multiple decrements, and estimation using discrete demographic data. More detailed expositions are available in Preston and Coale (1982) and Preston et al. (2001).

First, the birth rate can be estimated straightforwardly using Eq. (78) and given intercensal growth rates and a life table prevailing for the corresponding time period.

TABLE 22.3. **Demographic Relations in Stationary, Stable, and Any Population**

	Stationary population	Stable population	Any population
Crude birth rate	$b = \dfrac{1}{\int_0^\infty p(x)dx}$	$b = \dfrac{1}{\int_0^\infty p(x)e^{-rx}dx}$	$b = \dfrac{1}{\int_0^\infty p(x)e^{-\int_0^x r(a)da}dx}$
Proportionate age distribution	$c(x) = bp(x)$	$c(x) = be^{-rx}p(x)$	$c(x) = be^{-\int_0^x r(a)da}p(x)$
Characteristic equation	$1 = \int_\alpha^\beta p(x)m(x)dx$	$1 = \int_\alpha^\beta e^{-rx}p(x)m(x)dx$	$1 = \int_\alpha^\beta e^{-\int_0^x r(a)da}p(x)m(x)dx$

This offers an advantage of estimating the birth rate based on imperfect demographic data because it does not require a reported age distribution and therefore minimizes the bias introduced by a highly distorted age distribution at young ages in some populations (Preston and Coale 1982). Preston and Coale (1982) also observed that the period net reproduction rate can be estimated directly from the set of $r(x)$'s and the proportionate distribution of mothers' age at childbirth, $v(x) = B(x)/B$:

$$NRR = \int_{\alpha}^{\beta} p(x)m(x)dx = \int_{\alpha}^{\beta} v(x)e^{\int_0^x r(a)da} dx \qquad (81)$$

Illustrative applications of this method to 1976 Swedish data (Preston and Coale 1982) and 1995 to 2000 Japanese data (Preston et al. 2001) show results that are nearly identical with those produced by the traditional method when single-age intervals are used or the person-years function used in the traditional method is the same as that computed by the intercensal survivorship ratios. Note that it is assumed that the population is closed to migration and the age-specific rates of net emigration have been added to growth rates before Eq. (81) is applied.

Intercensal mortality conditions for a closed population also can be inferred using Eq. (77) from two census age distributions. Preston and Bennett (1983) show that such estimates produce good results for high-quality census data. By multiplying both sides of Eq. (77) by the death rate at age x, $\mu(x)$ and integrating over the entire age range, Preston et al. (2001) connect the number of deaths with the number of births in any population:

$$B = \int_0^{\infty} D(x)e^{\int_0^x r(a)da} dx, \qquad (82)$$

where the number of deaths, $D(x)$, is growth-corrected by the variable r function. This expands to yet another expression where the population at any age y is written as a function of the number of decrements above age y:

$$N(y) = \int_y^{\infty} D(x)e^{\int_x^y r(a)da} dx \qquad (83)$$

Bennett and Horiuchi (1981) show the utility of this system of equations in checking the completeness of death registration in some populations. If the census count at age y implied by the number of deaths above age y and age-specific growth rates is too low, this suggests either that deaths above age y are underregistered or that the population count is inflated, the latter of which is less likely. Preston and associates (1996) further demonstrate, in their estimation of African-American mortality rates at older ages, that the incompleteness of death records does not disturb the reconstruction of life table functions using variable-r relations. The key insight here is that the observed number of deaths by age can be applied with a growth correction using the variable-r method and then used to infer the age distribution of deaths in the life table. And the remaining columns of the life table follow. This approach, which uses only the set of age-specific growth rates, is also useful if deaths are based on a sample of the population or if population data are subject to large distortions due to persistent age misreporting. An example is Merli's (1998) estimation of intersensal mortality in Vietnam from 1979 to 1989.

Another application of variable-r relations arises from the generalization of Eq. (77) to multiple-decrement situations by introducing the rate of decrement from cause i, $\mu^i(x)$, to adjust the growth rate $r(x)$ (Preston and Coale 1982). After some simple transformations using $\mu^i(x)$, two basic elements of a multiple-decrement life table are obtained: the observed number of decrements from cause i, $D^i(x)$ and the probability of a newborn succumbing to cause i, l_0^i/l_0, which are linked through the following equation:

$$\frac{l_0^i}{l_0} = \frac{\int_0^\infty D^i(x)e^{\int_0^x r(a)da}dx}{B},$$ (84)

where the probability of succumbing to cause i can be calculated from $D^i(x)$ with variable-r correction, which is divided by the number of births. The advantage of this correction is displayed in an application to the estimation of the "case-fatality ratio" in epidemiology (Preston 1987a). If the actual population is stationary (that is, $r(x) = 0$), the case-fatality ratio is simply estimated as the ratio of annual deaths from the cause of interest to annual diagnoses. In a growing population (that is, when $r(x) > 0$ at all x); however, this ratio will underestimate the true case-fatality ratio, which is directly inferred from Eq. (84). Therefore, the estimation procedure using the growth correction displaces the one without (see Preston et al. 2001: 180). Other applications have been made to make estimates of marital survival (Preston and Coale 1982; Preston et al. 2001).

The above demographic relations have been presented mainly in continuous form and must be adapted to discrete time intervals for empirical applications because demographic data normally come in age intervals with lengths of multiples of 5 or 10. Preston and associates (2001) show that the geometric mean of population counts at both ends of the interval and the mean growth rate over the interval provide good approximations when the growth rate function is relatively regular during the period. A second approximation using five-year age intervals, introduced by Preston (1987a), equals the midpoint of an interval with the sum of counts in the five-year interval divided by five. Applications of this method have mainly occurred in single decrement survival processes and include the estimation of intercensal survival of a population (Preston and Bennett 1983; United Nations 1983), survival (Preston 1987a), and marital survival from multiple decrements (Preston 1987b). Using an intercensal approach, Preston and Strong (1986) also investigate survival from a single decrement in a multiple-decrement process.

Applications of variable-r methods also extend to the use of modeling age patterns of mortality and the iterative intracohort interpolation procedure for estimating intercensal age distributions as a refinement of the basic variable-r procedure (Coale 1984); see Preston et al. (2001) for details on these developments.

Population Momentum and Family Household Momentum

Extensions and applications of the stable population model/theory not only pertain to age composition and age-specific growth rates but also involve the effect of changes in these on changes in population size. Characterizing and modeling the momentum of population growth is another valuable application of the stable population model. *Population momentum* generally refers to the phenomenon by which an existing population age structure that is a legacy of past fertility and mortality conditions future population growth. Keyfitz (1971b) first articulated this notion by applying stable population theory to study relations between population size and age composition. He showed that even if the fertility rates of a growing stable population were immediately reduced to replacement level (i.e., $NRR = 1.0$) and maintained thereafter until the new equilibrium of a stationary population of fixed size and age composition is attained, the population would continue to grow, often by sizable amounts if it was a population with a young age structure. And any such population has a built-in growth potential in its age structure.

Note that Preston and Coale's (1982) derivation of the variable-r method shows how age-specific growth rates are linked to population momentum through the net reproduction rate. Eq. (81) indicates that if the $NRR = 1.0$, it is necessary that the mean of $e^{\int_0^x r(a)da}$ weighted by $v(x)$ (mothers' ages at childbirths) be 1.0 for $a \in [\alpha,\beta]$, which is achieved when the sum of $r(x)$ over the childbearing interval is 0.0. That is, the imposition of the replacement-level fertility results in the sum of age-specific growth rates approximating zero on average throughout the childbearing years.

Since its introduction by Keyfitz (1971b), population momentum has evolved into an influential demographic concept that bears critical policy implications for controlling population growth in many parts of the world that are undergoing the demographic transition from high to low rates of birth and death. Several structural efforts have been made to refine his original formulation. Keyfitz (1985) himself developed a basis for a more general expression by finding the exact form of the annual number of births in the eventual stationary population. Following this path, Preston and Guillot (1997) gave the formula for the momentum factor by relating the age structure of the eventual population with that of the initial population. Links between population momentum and aging have also been specified. Kim and Schoen (1997) articulate how population momentum coincides with population aging. Meanwhile, the age above which all of the population growth occurs has been identified to be near the middle of the reproductive life span (Kim, Schoem, and Sarma 1991; Kim and Schoen 1993; Preston 1986). Empirically, analyses show the value of the population momentum factor for the major regions of the world (Preston and Guillot 1997), and that momentum may account for most of the future growth in the world's population (Bongaarts and Bulatao 1999; National Research Council 2000).

The assumptions on which Keyfitz's (1971b) formulation of the momentum factor is based are hypothetical and therefore have limited usage in actual population projections. Some of the assumptions are modified by recent improvements (a complete exposition is given by Schoen and Jonsson 2003). In Keyfitz's framework, replacement-level fertility is achieved by a sudden decrease in fertility of the initial population to the replacement level. As he acknowledges, few populations experience instantaneous declines in fertility. Instead, the achievement of replacement-level reproduction takes place gradually and often over a number of years or decades. Keyfitz also requires that the fall in fertility be proportional at all ages by the factor $1/NRR$ with the scalar multiple (NRR) pertaining to the before-decline value. This ignores changes in the age pattern of fertility associated with changes in fertility levels. In addition, he does not raise the possibility that fertility transition can also be nonlinear. Historical time patterns of fertility changes show examples of both linear and exponential declines for a number of countries (United Nations 2000).

Attempts to generalize Keyfitz's initial contribution have proven fruitful in accommodating a gradual transition to replacement-level fertility. Schoen and Kim (1998) model momentum by imposing a gradual instead of a sudden decline in growth rates of births. There are also techniques to approximate long-term birth trajectories under declining fertility. A general way for determining the birth trajectory produced by a flexible pattern of decline in vital rates is provided by Li and Tuljapurkar (1999, 2000). Goldstein (2002) generalizes the expressions given by Keyfitz (1971b) and Frauenthal (1975) to a simpler result that focuses on the initial level of fertility and the speed of the decline. Goldstein and Stecklov (2002) used the Li-Tuljapurkar relationship to replace traditional population projections and got high correspondence between the two. These analytical extensions produce approximations that perform well under relatively short durations of population momentum (for up to 40 to 50 years), but tend to increasingly deviate from "true" (projected) trends in both hypothetical and actual populations as the duration of fertility decline lengthens (Schoen and Jonsson 2003). Furthermore, they cannot be applied to more general transition regimes that result in constant (stable) but nonzero growth.

In an effort to directly model changing vital rates and the gradual decline in fertility, Schoen and Kim (1994) and Kim and Schoen (1996) developed an analytical framework of a "quadratic hyperstable" (QH) model, wherein a population is generated by monotonic transitions (either increasing or decreasing) of the set of age-specific birth rates and grows by a quadratic exponential function. An age composition that changes over time is also specified. This dynamic model generalizes the stable population model by allowing fertility rates to change over time, accommodates stable-to-stable fertility transitions, and provides significantly more precise estimates of momentum of any length.

Schoen and Jonsson (2003) further extend the quadratic hyperstable population model to a new form which associates exponentially changing fertility to the resultant exponential quadratic birth sequence. Since the new QH model can be used to analyze long-term effects of monotonic transitions between any two sets of constant vital rates, it is a significant generalization of the stable population model. The Schoen-Jonsson QH model is a special case of the QH model, with new procedures to capture monotonic transitions between any levels of fertility. Schoen and Jonsson begin by specifying the QH model in a discrete form using a sequence of Leslie projection matrices that are generated by monotonically increasing/decreasing net maternity functions. This gives the birth trajectory whose structure resembles that of the Coale-Trussell Model Fertility Schedules (Coale and Trussell 1974). The advantage of this approach is that it offers a flexible pattern of change that not only applies to the proportional distribution of births by age of the mother required by early models, but also allows fertility to change monotonically in a specified fashion. They derive an exponentiated quadratic birth trajectory of the QH population in closed form.

Schoen and Jonsson apply the QH model to solve for the momentum associated with gradual transitions in fertility to replacement level. They consider both the transition to stationarity and any stable-stable transition. They first use the equation of an exponentiated quadratic birth trajectory to determine the cumulative change in the size and structure of the QH population over the period of fertility decline. Then they hold fertility constant at replacement level to find the ultimate stationary population. By doing so, they find two factors that determine the relative size of the eventual birth cohort. The first factor is essentially the same factor presented in different ways in previous works by Li and Tuljapurhar (1999), Goldstein (2002), and Schoen and Kim (1998), that is, a continuation of the initial stable growth for half the period of decline. The second is an offsetting factor previously overlooked. It takes into account the changing age composition of the population experiencing the declining fertility rate that is no longer stable. Therefore, it is a factor that reflects the interaction between the changing age composition, age pattern of fertility, and the level of fertility. Considering this factor reduces the growth in the number of births. Using the same approach, they model the transition from an initial stable population to another stable population and provide explicit expressions to bridge between any two stable rates.

Schoen and Jonsson apply the theoretical model to populations with high fertility (Singapore 1957) and moderate fertility (Mexico 1983). They compare the effects of both linear declines and exponential declines in NRR on population momentum using the Li-Tuljapurhar (1999) method, the Goldstein (2002) models, and the new QH model. The results indicate that both the Li-Tuljapurhar and Goldstein approximations lose accuracy for declines longer than 50 or so years, and they tend to overestimate the growth because they do not reflect the offsetting growth factor mentioned above. The QH model, on the other hand, proves successful for estimating momentum values over any length of the transition regardless of the beginning fertility level because it reinforces the role of the interaction between the two factors in moderating the growth.

Keyfitz's original concept of population momentum has also led to the discovery of a new type of momentum—the momentum of family/household types. Using data from national surveys and vital statistics, census micro files, and the "ProFamy" multistate household family projection method (discussed above), Zeng and associates (2005) prepared projections of U.S. elderly (ages 65 and over) households from 2000 to 2050. Medium projections, smaller and larger family scenarios with corresponding combinations of assumptions of marriage/union formation and dissolution, fertility, mortality, and international migration were performed to analyze future trends of U.S. households and their possible higher and lower bounds, as well as the enormous racial differentials.

Under a constant scenario with everything (marriage union formation and dissolution, fertility, mortality, migration, and so forth) after 2000 assumed to remain the same as in 2000, they found that the proportional distributions of household types/size and living arrangements of the elderly change considerably until 2020 or so and remain more or less stable afterward (except the percent of the oldest-old (ages 85 and over) living alone continues to increase substantially after 2020). Why would distributions of households and elderly living arrangements change considerably from 2000 to 2020 while the demographic parameters remain constant in the same period? The answer of Zeng and associates (2004) is that *family/household momentum* plays an important role.

The cohorts who were younger in 2000 experienced and will experience stabilized (or constant) higher rates of marriage/union disruption and lower marriage/union formation than the cohorts who were older in 2000 and had already completed most of their family life course. The profiles of households and elderly living arrangements in 2000 represent the mixed cumulative life course experiences of younger and older cohorts in the past few decades. Although the marriage/union formation and dissolution rates are assumed to remain constant during the period of 2000 to 2050, the distributions of households and elderly living arrangements would change considerably because the older cohorts, who had more traditional family patterns, will be replaced by the younger cohorts with modern family patterns. Family household momentum is similar to the population momentum concept of Keyfitz (1971b), in which population size could continue to increase after the fertility is equal to or even below the replacement level. The ProFamy method/program and the family household projections provide empirical evidence for the first time to numerically illustrate the concept of family household momentum.

MODEL SCHEDULES, SUMMARY INDICES, AND QUANTUM/TEMPO ADJUSTMENTS

Modeling Demographic Schedules

In almost all models of mathematical demography such as the single-decrement, multiple-decrement, multiple increment-decrement life tables, multistate population and family household simulation and projection models, and the stable population model and its extensions, age-sex-specific demographic rates are needed. The age-sex-specific demographic rates, ordered across the full age range from birth to death, are termed *demographic schedules*. The classic examples of demographic schedules are age-sex-specific mortality rates, age-specific fertility rates, age-sex-specific marriage and divorce rates, and age-sex-specific migration rates.

The most commonly used demographic schedules of age-specific rates of fertility and marriage are defined as the number of events occurring in an age interval divided by the total number of persons of the same age. Without transformation, however, these age-specific rates often cannot be used for computing status transitions for constructing life tables and family household simulations and projections, because their denominators do not distinguish the at-risk and not-at-risk populations for experiencing the events; they may be biased in measuring the period quantum and changes in period tempo (to be discussed below). Thus, more sophisticated age-specific occurrence/exposure rates, which are defined as the number of events occurred in the age interval divided by the person-years lived at risk of experiencing the event within the age interval, are required (see Eq. (22) for the case of mortality).

For many years, statisticians and demographers tried to establish analytical formulas for describing the patterns of human mortality, fertility, marriage, divorce, and migration. Examples of such efforts in modeling mortality schedules are the Gompertz, Logistic, Weibull, Heligman & Pollard, Quadratic, and Kannisto models (Thatcher, Kannisto, Vaupel 1998; Zeng and Vaupel 2003). Rogers (1986) proposes parametric models to describe the demographic schedules of migration, mortality, and nuptiality. Coale and McNeil (1972) develop a double-exponential first-marriage model, including age-specific model standard schedules of frequency distribution of first marriage and three parameters: the proportion eventually ever married, the lowest age at first marriage, and the average age at first marriage. Coale and Trussell (1974) propose a fertility double-exponential model, including model standard schedules of age-specific natural fertility and age-specific deviation from natural fertility due to birth control and parameters of total natural fertility level and level of birth control; a statistical version of the Coale-Trussell model was developed by Brostrom (1985), Trussell (1985), and Xie and Pimentel (1992).

As an illustrative example in modeling demographic schedules, this section summarizes the relational Gompertz fertility model originally proposed by Brass (1968, 1974, 1975, 1978; see also Booth 1984; Paget and Timaeus 1994) and its extension by Zeng et al.

(2000). Define H(x) as the cumulated fertility rate up to exact age x. Define the total fertility rate (TFR) as in Eq. (3), that is, as the sum of age-specific fertility rates over all ages. The model then assumes that H(x)/TFR follows the Gompertz distribution:

$$H(x)/TFR = \exp(A \exp(Bx))$$ (85)

where A and B are constants. Using the complementary log-log transformation

$$-\ln(-\ln(H(x)/TFR)) = -\ln(-A) - B\,x$$
$$Y(H(x)/TFR) = -\ln(-A) - B\,x$$ (86)

where Y stands for the complementary log-log transformation of H(x)/TFR.

Observed data from various populations show that the linear relationship expressed in equation (86) yields a reasonably good fit, except at extreme ages (Pollard and Volkovics 1992). To improve the fit, Brass introduces the standard fertility schedule and derives the following Relational Gompertz Fertility Model, which substantially improves the empirical fittings, including those at extreme ages, as compared to the original Gompertz fertility model expressed in Eq. (86):

$$Y(H(x)/TFR) = \alpha + \beta\, Y_s(H_s(x)/TFR_s)$$ (87)

where $H_s(x)$ is the cumulated fertility rate up to exact age x in the standard fertility schedule and TFR_s is the total fertility rate of the standard schedule. A_s and B_s are constants.

Equation (87) establishes that the Y transformation of an observed schedule is a linear function of the Y transformation of the Standard Schedule, and the two parameters α and β can be estimated using Ordinary Least Squares (OLS) regression or other estimation procedures. The TFR summary index can be estimated directly or indirectly from the empirical fertility data. Its standard schedule can be easily established by using the observed rates in the population under study or, if the data are poor in the population under study, by using rates from another demographically similar population.

Studies by Brass and others produce clear statistical meanings for the parameters α and β. The α parameter determines the age location (i.e., early or late) of the fertility distribution, and the β parameter determines the spread or degree of concentration of the distribution. More specifically, the smaller the α, the later the process, and when α is equal to 0, the age location of the schedule is identical to the standard. The smaller the β, the more dispersed the curve of the schedule, and when β is equal to one, the spread or the degree of the concentration of the schedule is identical to the standard (United Nations 1983). Despite their clear statistical meanings, however, it is remarkably difficult to estimate or project α and β directly for purposes of projecting or simulating demographic rates for the future years for four main reasons. First, there are no observed values of α and β from demographic data resources (such as vital statistics, surveys, or censuses) for past years that can be used as a basis for future trend extrapolation. Second, estimates of α and β are not compatible across time and regions (Zeng et al. 2000). Third, it is difficult to connect changes in the values of α and β with the quantity of changes in timing and concentration of the demographic process. For example, if one tells policy makers or the public that α will decrease by 0.2 and β will decrease by 0.1 in the fertility schedule in 10 years, few understand the demographic meaning of the terms. Fourth, linking α and β with socioeconomic and human behavior variables, such as changes in women's education and labor force participation, for future trends extrapolation is even more implausible. In sum, α and β are demographically unmeasurable, uninterpretable, incompatible across time and regions, and unpredictable. It is, therefore, important to find a way to link α and β with variables that are demographically measurable, interpretable, and predictable. The simple method proposed and tested by Zeng and associates (2000) is intended to solve this problem. This research is what Rogers (1986: 60) anticipated in his statement "[a]lthough the model schedule parameters are not always demographically interpretable, future research is likely to link them to variables that are."

Define M as the median age, i.e., the exact age at which 50% of the events have occurred, and N and O as first and third quartiles, i.e., the exact age at which 25% and 75% of the events have occurred, respectively. Define M_S, N_S, and O_S as the median age, the first, and the third quartiles of the standard schedule. Zeng and associates (2000) then propose the following estimator to link the parameter β with the interquartile range:

$$\beta = (O_S - N_S)/(O - N), \tag{88}$$

where $(O_S - N_S)$ is the interquartile range of the standard schedule that is known and may be denoted as I_S. Let $(O - N)$, the interquartile range of the schedule to be estimated or projected, be denoted by I. Now only the value of I needs to be estimated, rather than both the O and N values. Then an analytical formula for estimating β can be expressed as follows:

$$\beta = I_S/I \tag{89}$$

After β is estimated, the estimation of α is straightforward. Following equation (87), and setting x equal to the median age (M) of the schedule to be estimated or projected: $Y(H(M)/TFR) = \alpha + \beta Y_S(H_S(M)/TFR_S)$. $Y(H(M)/TFR)$ is equal to $\ln(-\ln(0.5))$. $Y_S(H_S(M)/TFR_S)$ can be obtained from the standard schedule by linear interpolation if M is not an integer. Thus, α can be quickly estimated. Once α and β are estimated, H(x) and f(x) can be computed based on equation (87) for H(x) and using $f(x) = H(x + 1) - H(x)$. The single-year age-specific rates f(x) can thus be derived using the above proposed method based on the three parameters of total rate, median age, interquartile range, and a standard schedule. The three parameters are all demographically interpretable, measurable, and predictable, and the standard schedule can be easily established based on the proper data. The method has been successfully tested on 180 reliable observed demographic schedules in various countries and periods and to nearly 10,000 simulated schedules with various combinations of possible values (including the extremes) of α and β (Zeng et al. 2000).

The method that uses median age and interquartile range instead of α and β as input proposed by Zeng and associates (2000) relaxes the traditional unrealistic assumption in population projections that the curve of the fertility schedule moves to the right or left in a parallel way. Instead, using this method, one assumes that the demographic events would be delayed or advanced, while the curve becomes more spread or more concentrated or, more specifically, that young people delay the events more than older persons, or vice versa. It is also useful for formulating assumptions about future demographic trends for purposes of policy analysis and planning. It can be used to indirectly estimate demographic schedules when the detailed age-specific data are not currently available, which is useful for developing countries and subregion studies in developed countries.

Model Standard Schedules and Summary Demographic Indices

Despite their remarkable success, model demographic schedules as discussed above have not been fully satisfactory, especially for applications in many developing countries where the empirical data needed to estimate the model parameters are not readily available. Since the 1950s, population studies for developing countries have progressed rapidly, and demographers have realized that it is extremely important to establish reasonable models of mortality for such efforts because many developing countries do not have reliable life tables. Given the fact that analytical formulas cannot describe well the different age patterns of human mortality, demographers have tried to find a set of model standard schedules of life tables to represent various mortality patterns and levels. The result is model life tables. Empirically based model life tables are identical to ordinary real life tables in every way, except that they relate to no particular single place or time. Since the 1950s, at least nine different sets of empirical model life tables have been published. The two most widely used families of model life tables are discussed here.

The initial version of the Coale and Demeny (1966) regional model life tables was derived from a set of 192 life tables by sex recorded for human populations that were chosen from an original set of 326 life tables from Europe (206), Latin America (33), Asia (32), Oceania (22), North America (18), and Africa (15). Coale-Demeny regional model life tables are of four "families of regions" called "North," "South," "East," and "West." The North model table is based on nine life tables from Norway, Sweden, and Iceland. It is characterized by relatively low infant and old age mortality but high adult mortality caused by an unusually high incidence of tuberculosis. The South model table is derived from 23 Mediterranean life tables from Portugal, Spain, Sicily, and southern Italy. It has high mortality under age 5, particularly among infants, low adult mortality, and high mortality over age 65. The East model table was generated from 31 primarily Central European life tables from Austria, Germany, Bavaria, Prussia, north Italy, Poland, and Czechoslovakia. It has high infant and high old-age mortality, relative to childhood and adult rates. The West model table is regarded as describing an "average" mortality pattern and is by far the most frequently used. Coale and Demeny (1966; 1983) recommend its use when no reliable information on the age pattern of mortality is available. The West models are based on a diverse array of about 130 life tables which were considered to be accurate but which did not fit into any of the other three groups. They include life tables from the Netherlands, Finland, France, England and Wales, Japan, Ireland, Israel, Australia, Canada, and South Africa. In 1985, a second version of the model life tables was published by Coale and Demeny (1985). The upper boundary of the life tables in the second version was raised to age 100 instead of age 80 in the 1966 version.

In 1982, the United Nations published a set of model life tables based entirely on empirical life tables from developing countries. As many accurate life tables were collected from developing countries as possible. After careful data quality evaluation, 36 male and 36 female life tables from 10 Latin American countries, 11 Asian countries and 1 African country were selected. These life tables were then divided into five groups: "Latin American," "Chilean," "South Asian," "Far Eastern," and "General." The "General" pattern was produced as an average of all the original empirical model life tables. The different patterns have roughly the following characteristics:

1. Latin American: relatively high infant, child, and adult mortality and relatively low old-age mortality

2. Chilean: extremely high infant mortality
3. South Asian: high mortality under 15 and over 55, but relatively low mortality at adult ages
4. Far Eastern: very high mortality at old ages
5. General: average mortality pattern

As discussed above, almost all of the internationally published fertility and nuptiality models (e.g., Coale and McNeil 1972; Coale and Trussell 1974; Brass 1968; Zeng et al. 2000) aim to model age-specific rates of fertility and marriage, which are defined as the number of events occurring in an age interval divided by the total number of persons of the same age. These age-specific rates, however, cannot be used for computing status transitions for constructing multistate life tables and family household projections or simulation because their denominators do not distinguish between the at-risk and not-at-risk populations experiencing the events. Furthermore, similar to the situation in many developing countries a couple of decades ago, when reliable life tables were not available, the age-sex-specific occurrence/exposures rates of marriage/union formation and dissolution and age-parity-marital/union-status-s occurrence/exposures rates of fertility, which are needed for family household projections or simulations, are not readily available for many developing countries and some developed countries. These occurrence/exposure rates at the national level can be estimated from national surveys which collected fertility and marriage histories data but are usually not available for local or small areas. Therefore, there is an imperative need to establish model standard schedules of the age-sex-specific occurrence/exposure rates of marriage/union formation and dissolution and age-parity-specific occurrence/exposure rates of marital and non-marital fertility. The basic ideas and approach for establishing such model standard schedules of marriage/union formation and dissolution and fertility may be similar to those used for creating the model life tables, but intensive innovative investigations are called for in future studies.

Model standard schedules of marriage/union formation and dissolution, fertility, and mortality model life tables have three practically useful properties. First, they can serve as a standard for smoothing the observed age-specific demographic rates with poor quality. Second, they can be used to perform indirect estimation in case the directly observed rates are not complete. Third, they can be used to project future age-sex-specific demographic rates for population and family household projections or simulations.

Age-sex-specific demographic schedules are useful in analysis and modeling, but they should be accompanied by summary indices, because the numerous age-sex-specific numbers cannot concisely represent the *quantum* or *level* and *tempo* or *timing* (of the rates by age) of demographic processes. Thus, *summary demographic indices* are necessary in demographic studies. Furthermore, as Keyfitz (1972) points out, demographic projections based on trend extrapolation of each age-sex-specific rate can result in an excessive concession to flexibility and readily produce erratic results. Accordingly, demographers focus on forecasts of the summary indices in population and family household projections or simulations. Demographers define and estimate various summary indices depending on the purpose of their studies and data availability. Two of the most commonly used summary indices are the period life expectancy and the period Total Fertility Rate.

It has been noted earlier that the period life expectancy (mathematically defined in Eq. [20]) is the average life span of a hypothetical cohort subjected to the observed period age-specific death rates. Similarly, demographers interpret the conventional period TFR(t) (i.e., the observed period total fertility rate in year t, mathematically defined in Eq. [3]) as the total number of births an average member of a hypothetical female cohort would have during her reproductive life if the hypothetical cohort *exactly* (with no changes in quantum, tempo, and shape of the schedule) experienced the observed period age-specific fertility rates. This interpretation is equivalent to imagining that the observed period age-specific fertility rates are *constantly* extended a sufficient number of years into the future (e.g., 35 years), so that a hypothetical cohort would have gone through the whole reproductive life span (e.g., ages 15 to 50). The observed period TFR(t) is the total number of births an average member of the hypothetical cohort would have during her whole reproductive life. A topic of recent interest among mathematical demographers has been the development of formulas for adjustment of standard period life expectancy and period TFR(t) for changes in quantum and tempo.

Quantum/Tempo Adjustment Formulas

THE BONGAARTS-FEENEY QUANTUM ADJUSTMENT FORMULA. It is well known in demography that the observed period TFR(t) is biased if cohort tempo is changing (Ryder 1956, 1959, 1964, 1980, 1983; Keilman 1994; Keilman and Van Imhoff 1995). The demographic literature on fertility measures includes many criticisms of and alternatives to the period TFR(t), but there has been no agreement on its replacement. An important recent development was initiated by Bongaarts and Feeney (1998), who derive a simple and effective *quantum adjustment formula*[7]:

$$\text{TFR}^*(t) = \text{TFR}(t)/(1 - r(t)) \qquad (90)$$

where $\text{TFR}^*(t)$ is the adjusted period order-specific total fertility rate that reduces bias caused by changes in the timing of fertility, $\text{TFR}(t)$ is the observed period order-specific total fertility rate in year t, and $r(t)$ denotes the observed annual changes in order-specific period mean age at childbearing in year t.[8] To simplify the notation, subscripts for the order of births are suppressed, but it should be kept in mind that all of the derivations and discussion refer to order-specific fertility.[9] Similar to the conventional interpretation of the classic period TFR(t), as stated above, Bongaarts and Feeney (1998: 287–289) assume, in deriving their quantum adjustment formula, that the observed period age-parity-specific fertility rates are extended a sufficient number of years into the future (e.g., 35 years), with changing period tempo, but assuming a constant quantum and an invariant shape of the schedule.

One important question, however, needs to be addressed: Does the Bongaarts-Feeney (abbreviated as B-F hereafter) formula work when its underlying assumption of

[7] Bongaarts and Feeney (1998: 287) refer to their formula as a "tempo adjustment formula." A more complete description is that it is a formula for adjusting the quantum for tempo effects. While this phrasing may seem trivial, it is an important distinction in view of the tempo adjustment formula presented later in this Section.
[8] The annual change $r(t)$ is defined as the difference of the mean age at experiencing the event between two successive years. The unit of $r(t)$ is "years old/per year."
[9] If one does not distinguish the orders of births, errors in the estimates may likely occur. For example, when people reduce their fertility they do so primarily by reducing childbearing at higher birth orders. As a result, the mean age at childbearing for all births without order specification declines even when the timing of individual births does not change (Bongaarts and Feeney 1998; Bongaarts 1999).

an invariant shape of the fertility schedule and its implied equal changes in timing of births across reproductive ages do not hold, as is likely the case in the real world? Bongaarts and Feeney (1998) present a successful test of their adjustment method by comparing the completed fertility of true cohorts born from 1904 to 1941 in the United States with the weighted averages of the adjusted period $TFR^*(t)$ over the years during which the true cohorts were in the childbearing ages. But they do not perform a sensitivity analysis directly targeting the underlying assumption about the invariant shape of the schedule and its implied assumption about equal changes in timing of births at all reproductive ages. Consequently, there are questions raised about the sensitivity of the B-F formula to the likely violation of its assumption (Kim and Schoen 2000; Van Imhoff and Keilman 2000; Kohler and Philipov 2001). If the B-F method is very sensitive to the likely violation of its underlying assumption, it should not be used unless an appropriate correction is made.

Zeng and Land (2001) present a sensitivity analysis of the B-F method, based on fertility data in the U.S. from 1918 to 1990 and in Taiwan from 1978 to 1993, and the Brass Relational Gompertz fertility model and its extension (as discussed earlier). Zeng and Land (2002) conclude that the adjusted $TFR^*(t)$ using the B-F formula, which assumes an invariant shape of the fertility schedule, usually does not differ significantly from an adjusted $TFR^*(t)$ that allows systematic changes (with constant rate) in the shape of the fertility schedule. This finding is consistent with an analysis by Kohler and Philipov (2001) in which they show that the biases in the B-F formula are quite small if a constant rate of increase in the variance of the fertility schedule prevails over time. This finding implies that the B-F method is usually not sensitive to its underlying assumption on invariant shape of the fertility schedules and equal changes in timing across ages. That is, it is generally robust for producing reasonable estimates of the adjusted period $TFR^*(t)$ that reduce distortion caused by tempo changes, except in abnormal conditions. The B-F method may be sensitive to substantial nonsystematic changes (i.e., large and time-varying changes in the tempo and shape of the schedule). Another important point is that the adjusted $TFR^*(t)$ using the B-F method neither represents actual cohort experiences in the past nor forecasts any future trend. Rather, as compared to the conventional $TFR(t)$, it merely provides an improved reading of the period fertility measure that reduces the tempo distortion, and it is a hypothetical cohort measure, similar to the period life table measures in a general sense.

The word "improved" is used above to indicate that the adjusted $TFR^*(t)$ using the B-F method is relatively more reasonable than the conventional $TFR(t)$ in measuring the period fertility level because it reduces the tempo distortion. But the observed period $TFR(t)$, whose denominator is the age-specific total number of women in the population, also does not distinguish those who are at risk and those who are not at risk of giving birth of the particular order (van Imhoff and Keilman 2000). This is one of the reasons why the observed period TFR is distorted by changes in the timing of fertility and needs to be adjusted. However, the adjusted $TFR^*(t)$ using the B-F method still is not entirely free of distortion; it is not only based on certain simplifying assumptions, but also on the restricted data of period fertility rates whose denominator does not distinguish the at-risk and not-at-risk populations. For example, if a substantial number of women postponed their first (or second) births a few years ago and now give birth in the current year, the observed total fertility rate of first (or second) births would not be low (say, 0.8). However, if other women delay births substantially and this resulted in a large annual increase in mean age at childbearing of first (or second) birth (say, 0.3

year), the adjusted TFR of first (or second) births using the B-F method in this case could be unreasonably high (say, 1.14). The fact that the adjusted U.S. TFR of second births by the B-F method in the year 1944 exceeded one (Zeng and Land 2001) might be a concrete example of such cases.

Zeng and Land (2001) recommend the application of the B-F method to adjust the observed parity-specific period TFR when the timing of fertility is changing under normal conditions. However, the application of the B-F method under abnormal conditions is problematic. In particular, when observed annual changes in the timing of fertility exceed 0.25, and the annual changes in the interquartile range exceed 0.1 and have large fluctuations, one must be cautious in applying the B-F method, since the adjustments may be incorrect. Zeng and Land (2001) also recommend presentation of both observed period TFR and the adjusted TFR using the B-F method. The observed TFR reveals the implications of fertility for population growth (or decline), and the adjusted TFR reflects a better reading of the period fertility level, reducing the distortion caused by changes in tempo.

THE ZENG-LAND TEMPO ADJUSTMENT FORMULA.   Zeng and Land (2002) show that, under conditions of changing tempo, not only are observed period total fertility rates biased, but also observed changes in the period tempo of fertility are biased. Zeng and Land (2002) derive a *tempo adjustment formula* as follows for adjusting the bias in observed changes in the period tempo of fertility, based on the same assumptions as those imposed in the B-F method:

$$r^*(t) = r(t)/(1 - r(t)). \tag{91}$$

where $r(t)$ are *observed changes* in the period tempo, and the $r^*(t)$ are *adjusted changes* in the tempo in year t, reducing the bias caused by changes in the timing of childbearing.

Eq. (91) implies that, similar to the fact that the observed period quantum is distorted by changing tempo, observed changes in period tempo are distorted also.[10] The relative error rate of the observed annual changes in period tempo can be computed as:

$$\text{Relative bias} = [r(t) - r^*(t)]/r^*(t) = -r(t). \tag{92}$$

The relative bias of the observed annual change in period tempo as an estimate of the actual change in tempo is of the same magnitude as the annual change itself with an opposite sign. For example, if the observed annual change in the period tempo of fertility is 0.1 years, it underestimates the actual value of the annual increase by 10% (the actual value is 0.111). If the observed annual change in period tempo of fertility is −0.09 years, it overestimates the actual value of the annual decrease by 9% (the actual value is −0.0826). As compared to the conventionally observed TFR(t) and r(t), both the B-F adjusted quantum (TFR*(t)) and Zeng-Land adjusted changes in tempo (r*(t)) do better; they adjust the bias in the observed quantum and changes in tempo due to changes in fertility timing.

---

[10] Even under conditions similar to scenario 4 of Bongaarts and Feeney (1998), which assumes that TFR(t) changes over time, Eqs. (91) and (92) still are valid.

AN EXTENSION OF RYDER'S TRANSLATIONAL EQUATION.   In the process of deriving the tempo adjustment formula, Zeng and Land (2002) also derive an alternative quantum adjustment formula using r*(t) as input:

$$TFR^*(t) = TFR(t)(1 + r^*(t)) \qquad (93)$$

Zeng and Land (2002) show analytically that the relationship between the adjusted $TFR^*(t)$ and the observed period $TFR(t)$, using $r^*(t)$ and $r(t)$ as the input respectively and the B-F formula, can be easily generalized to real cohorts (instead of only hypothetical cohorts), provided the assumptions of constant quantum, constant changes in tempo and invariant shape of the schedule hold for all real cohorts concerned. In this generalized case, the mathematical proof of Eqs. (90), (91), (92), and (93), as well as the general relationship expressed in these four equations, still hold, but the symbolic terms need to be changed as:

$$CFR = TFR(1 + r_c) \qquad (94)$$

where CFR is the constant cohort complete fertility rate, TFR is the constant period total fertility rate, and r_c is the constant changes in cohort tempo, which are defined as the difference of the mean age at childbearing between two successive cohorts. Eq. (94) may be referred to as a *period-cohort quantum equation*.

$$CFR = TFR/(1 - r_p) \qquad (95)$$

where r_p denotes the constant annual changes in period tempo, defined as the difference of the mean age at childbearing between two successive years.

Based on Eqs. (94) and (95), a relationship between r_c and r_p can be derived:

$$r_c = r_p/(1 - r_p) \qquad (96)$$

Eq. (96) may be referred to as a *period-cohort tempo equation*.

The period-cohort quantum Eq. (94) and Eq. (95) can be regarded as alternatives to Ryder's *basic translation equation*. Using the notation defined in this chapter, Ryder's basic translation equation (Ryder 1956, 1964) can be expressed as: $CFR = TFR/(1 - r_c)$, which differs from the period-cohort quantum equations expressed in Eqs. (94) and (95). The discrepancy between Ryder's basic translation equation and the period-cohort quantum Eqs. (94) and (95) is due to different assumptions. Ryder assumes that fertility rates at each age change according to its own polynomial, ignored all moments of order higher than 1, and then approximated the age-specific polynomial as a straight line (Ryder 1964). Zeng and Land assume that all cohorts postpone or advance the births by an equal amount as compared with the immediate preceding cohort and that the shape of the cohort age-specific schedules is assumed to be invariant, but the curve shifts to the right or left when the timing changes. As tested by Zeng and Land (2001), the assumptions of the invariant shape of the fertility schedule and equal changes in cohort tempo usually are not sensitive to the estimates except in abnormal conditions.

The numerical difference between using Ryder's basic translation equation and the period-cohort quantum Eqs. (94) and (95) is rather small if r_c is small. However, the period-cohort quantum equations, as expressed in Eqs. (94) and (95), have led to a derivation of the period-cohort tempo Eq. (96). This is an extension of the Ryder's basic translation equation and expands demographic knowledge to an analytical expression of the relationship between period and cohort changes in tempo. Furthermore, the period-cohort quantum and period-cohort tempo equations are based on simpler and more reasonable assumptions and are derived in a much easier way, as compared to Ryder's basic translation equation.

The Zeng-Land extension not only expands knowledge of relationships among formulas in mathematical demography but is also useful in modeling the quantum-tempo of periods and cohorts for population and family household projection or simulation. For example, the period-cohort and quantum-tempo relationships expressed in Eqs. (94), (95), and (96) may be used in component population projections, which begin with estimates of an initial age distribution and projections of age-specific fertility, mortality and migration rates. Following trend extrapolation or expert opinion approaches, one may first project (or assume) the future cohort TFR and changes in mean age at childbearing. Using Eqs. (94), (95), and (96), one can then estimate the future period TFR and changes in the period mean age at childbearing to formulate the needed period projection matrices. Such estimates or projections of period TFR and period age at childbearing based on understandings of the cohort trends and taking into account the important effects of changes in cohort tempo on the period quantum and period tempo certainly make more sense than just solely extrapolating the distorted period rates.

Finally, the analytical formulas concerning the quantum/tempo adjustments and relationships discussed in this chapter may be extended to other nonrepeatable demographic events, such as first marriage, order-specific divorce, and leaving the parental home. The relationships of period, cohort (or hypothetical cohort) quantum, and tempo changes analyzed here and other related studies may also turn out to be useful in examining quite different topics, such as the effect of delayed retirement in a public pension system on the system's finance.

CONCLUSION

This chapter illustrates how mathematics is used by demographers to develop theories and models of populations and has surveyed much of the literature of this specialty. Specifically, this chapter reviews some of the essential concepts and mathematics of the two basic classic population models that constitute the core of mathematical demography—the life table/stationary population model and the stable population model. Despite the fact that these core models have been quite thoroughly studied for decades, both continue to be subjects of active research in mathematical demography. Extensions of the classic single-decrement life table model to multistate and stochastic representations continue to be areas of methodological research and empirical application. In the case of stable population theory, the topics of population momentum and related generalizations of the classic model are foci of continued research interest. The third major topic reviewed is model schedules or age-specific rates of demographic events such as births and deaths, summary demographic indices, such as the total fertility rate and life expectancy, and recent developments in tempo adjustment formulas based thereon. The implications of quantum/tempo adjustment formulas for population models and summary demographic indices also are subjects of current debate and research interest.

Even in a long chapter, however, there are many topics of importance in mathematical demography that cannot be included. A few of these are the following. First, two-sex models: all of the models reviewed here are one-sex models. Especially for the study of marriage and divorce (or more generally, union formation and dissolution) processes, fertility, and long-range population projections, it is important to take into account the interaction of the sexes; Schoen (1988) includes a review of the essential concepts and models for interacting populations. Another topic not reviewed that is receiving increasing attention is the cross-disciplinary integration of biological and demographic models (Yashin and Iachine 1997). The incorporation of genetic data into demographic surveys (Finch, Vaupel, and Kinsella 2001) and its use in the study of the biodemography of aging and longevity (Wachter and Finch 1997) will stimulate this cross-disciplinary fertilization and evolution of the models of demography.

In brief, mathematical demography is indispensable to the development of formal representations of the structure of populations and population processes. It will continue to evolve and generate new contributions, generalizations, and extensions.

REFERENCES

Allison, P. D. 1995. *Survival analysis using the SAS system: A practical guide*. Cary, N.C.: SAS Institute.

Arthur, W. B. 1982. The ergodic theorems of demography: A simple proof. *Demography* 19:439–445.

Bennett, N. G., and S. Horiuchi. 1981. Estimating the completeness of death registration in a closed population. *Population Index* 42: 207–221.

Berkson, J., and R. P. Gage. 1952. Survival curve for cancer patients following treatment. *Journal of the American Statistical Association* 47: 501–515.

Bernadelli, H. 1941. Population waves. *Journal of the Burma Research Society* 31: 1–18.

Bongaarts, J. 1987. The projection of family composition over the life course with family status life tables. In *Family demography: Methods and applications*. Edited by J. Bongaarts, T. Burch, and K. W. Wachter. Oxford: Clarendon Press.

Bongaarts, J. 1999. Completing the demographic transition. *Population and Development Review* 25: 515–529.

Bongaarts, J., and G. Feeney. 1998. On the quantum and tempo of fertility. *Population and Development Review* 24: 271–291.

Booth, H. 1984. Transforming Gompertz's function for fertility analysis: The development of a standard for the relational Gompertz function. *Population Studies*, 38: 495–506.

Brass, W. 1968. Note on Brass method of fertility estimation. In *The demography of tropical Africa*. Edited by W. Brass et al., Chapter 3, Appendix A. Princeton, N.J.: Princeton University Press.

Brass, W. 1974. Perspectives in population prediction: Illustrated by the statistics of England and Wales. *Journal of the Royal Statistical Society*, 137, Series A: 532–583.

Brass, W. 1975. Methods of estimating fertility and mortality from limited and defective data. Chapel Hill, N.C.: International Program for Population Statistics.

Brass, W. 1978. The relational Gompertz model of fertility by age of women (mimeographed). London: London School of Hygiene and Tropical Medicine.

Brostrom, G. 1985. Practical aspects on the estimation of the parameters in Coale's M Model for Marital Fertility. *Demography* 22: 625–631.

Cambois, E., J.-M. Robine, and M. D. Hayward. 2001. Social inequalities in disability-free life expectancy in the French male population. *Demography* 38: 513–524.

Casti, J. L. 1992a. *Reality rules. I. Picturing the world in mathematics—the fundamentals*. New York: Wiley-Interscience.

Casti, J. L. 1992b. Reality *rules. II. Picturing the world in mathematics—the frontier*. New York: Wiley-Interscience.

Chiang, C.-L. 1960. A stochastic study of the life table and its applications. II. Sample variance of the observed expectations of life and other biometric functions. *Human Biology* 32: 221–238.

Chiang, C.-L. 1968. *Introduction to stochastic processes in biostatistics.* New York: Wiley.

Chiang, C.-L. 1972. On constructing current life tables. *Journal of the American Statistical Association* 67: 538–541.

Coale, A. J. 1984. Life table construction on the basis of two enumerations of a closed population. *Population Index* 50: 193–213.

Coale, A. J., and P. Demeny. 1966. *Regional model life tables and stable populations.* Princeton, N.J.: Princeton University Press.

Coale, A. J., and P. Demeny. 1983. *Regional model life tables and stable populations,* 2d ed. New York: Academic Press.

Coale, A. J., and D. R. McNeil. 1972. The distribution by age of the frequency of first marriage in a female cohort. *Journal of American Statistical Association,* 67: 743–749.

Coale, A. J., and T. J. Trussell 1974. Model fertility schedules: Variations in the age structure of childbearing in human populations. *Population Index* 40: 185–258.

Cohen, J. E. 1979. Ergodic theorems in demography. *Bulletin (New Series) of the American Mathematical Society* 1: 275–295.

Coleman, J. S. 1964. *Introduction to mathematical sociology.* New York: Free Press.

Cox, D. R. 1972. Regression models and life-tables (with discussion). *Journal of the Royal Statistical Society B* 34: 187–220.

Crimmins, E. M., Y. Saito, and M. D. Hayward. 1993. Sullivan and multistate methods of estimating active life expectancy: Two methods, two answers. In *Calculation of health expectancies: Harmonization, consensus achieved and future perspectives.* Edited by J. M. Robine, C. D. Mathers, M. R. Bone, and I. Romieu, 155–160. Montrouge, France: John Libbey Eurotext.

Crimmins, E. M., Y. Saito, and D. Ingegneri. 1997. Trends in disability-free life expectancy in the United States. *Population and Development Review* 23: 555–572.

de Moivre, A. 1725. *Annuities on lives: Or, the valuation of annuities upon any number of lives; as also, of reversions.* London: Millar.

Du Pasquier, L. G. 1912. Mathematische Theorie der Invaliditats-Versicherung. *Mitt. Ver. Schweitzer. Versicherungsmath.* 7:1–7.

Elandt-Johnson, R. C., and N. L. Johnson. 1980. *Survival models and data analysis.* New York: Wiley.

Feller, W. 1941. On the integral equation of renewal theory. *Annals of Mathematical Statistics* 12: 243–267.

Finch, C. E., J. W. Vaupel, and K. Kinsella, Eds. 2001. *Cells and surveys.* Washington, D.C.: National Academies Press.

Fix, E., and J. Neymann. 1951. A simple stochastic model of recovery, relapse, death and loss of patients. *Human Biology* 23: 205–241.

Frauenthal, J. C. 1975. Birth trajectory under changing fertility conditions. *Demography* 12: 447–454.

Goldstein, J. R. 2002. Population momentum for gradual demographic transitions: An alternative approach. *Demography* 39:6 5–73.

Goldstein, J. R., and G. Stecklov. 2002. Long-range population projections made simple. *Population and Development Review* 28: 121–141.

Greville, T. N. E. 1943. Short methods of constructing abridged life tables. *Record of the American Institute of Actuaries 32* (Part I): 29–42.

Hayward, M. D., and W. R. Grady. 1990. Work and retirement among a cohort of older men in the United States. *Demography* 27: 337–356.

Heigl, A. 2001. Demographic fact book. *http://www.hypovereinsbank.de/media/pdf/rese_chan_defabo_Welt.pdf.*

Hoem, J. M., and M. S. Fong. 1976. *A Markov chain model of working life tables.* Working Paper No. 2. Copenhagew: Laboratory of Actuarial Mathematics, University of Copenhagen, Denmark.

Hoem, J. M., and U. Funck-Jensen. 1982. Multistate life table methodology: A probabilist critique. In *Multidimensional mathematical demography.* Edited by K. C. Land and A. Rogers. New York: Academic Press.

Hoem, J. M., D. Madsen, J. L. Nielsen, E.-M. Ohlsen, H. O. Hansen, and B. Rennermalm. 1981. Experiments in modelling recent Danish fertility curves. *Demography* 18: 231–244.

Hosmer, D. W., and S. Lemeshow. 1999. *Applied survival analysis: Regression modeling of time to event data.* New York: Wiley.

Hullen, G. 2000. Projections of living arrangement, household and family structures using ProFamy. Warschau, Deutsch-polnisch-ungarisches Demographentreffen, October 2000.

Hullen, G. 2001. New macrosimulations of living arrangements and households in Germany. Paper presented at Population Association of America, 2001 Annual Meeting, March 2001, pp. 7–31.

Hullen, G. 2003. Living arrangements and households: Methods and results of demographic projection. A book (reader) published by the German Federal Institute for Population Research (BIB), with Foreword by Charlotte Hohn, Director of BIB. http://www.gert-hullen.privat.t-online.de/manuskripte/materialien_hu_29072003.pdf.

Ibrahim, J. G., M.-H. Chen, and D. Sinha. 2001. *Bayesian survival analysis*. New York: Springer-Verlag.

Jiang, L., and A. Kuijsten. 1999a. Effects of changing households on environment—Case studies in two regions of China. Paper presented at workshop Population and environment: Modeling and simulating this complex interaction. Organized by Max Planck Institute for Demographic Research at Rostock, Germany, August 12–13, 1999.

Jiang, L., and A. Kuijsten. 1999b. Household projections for two regions of China. Paper presented at the European Population Conference, The Hague, The Netherlands, August 30–September 3, 1999.

Jordan, C. W., Jr. 1975. *Life contingencies*, 2d ed. Chicago: The Society of Actuaries.

Kalbfleisch, J. D., and R. L. Prentice. 2002. *The statistical analysis of failure time data*, 2d ed. New York: Wiley.

Katz, S., L. G. Branch, M. H. Branson, J. A. Papsidero, J. C. Beck, and D. S. Greer. 1983. Active life expectancy. *New England Journal of Medicine* 309: 1218–1224.

Keilman, N. 1994. Translation formulae for non-repeatable events. *Population Studies* 48: 341–357.

Keilman, N., and E. V. Imhoff. 1995. Cohort quantum as a function of time-dependent period quantum for non-repeatable events. *Population Studies* 49: 347–352.

Keyfitz, N. 1968. A life table that agrees with the data. II. *Journal of the American Statistical Association* 63: 1253–1268.

Keyfitz, N. 1969. Age distribution and the stable equivalent. *Demography* 6: 261–269.

Keyfitz, N. 1970. Finding probabilities from observed rates, or how to make a life table. *The American Statistician* 24: 28–33.

Keyfitz, N. 1971a. Models. *Demography* 8: 571–580.

Keyfitz, N. 1971b. On the momentum of population growth. *Demography* 8: 71–80.

Keyfitz, N. 1972. On future population. *Journal of American Statistical Association*, 67: 347–363.

Keyfitz, N. 1977a. *Applied mathematical demography*. New York: Wiley.

Keyfitz, N. 1977b. *Introduction to the mathematics of population with revisions*. Reading, Mass: Addsion-Wesley.

Keyfitz, N. 1985. *Applied mathematical demography*, 2d ed. New York: Wiley.

Keyfitz, N., and W. Flieger. 1971. *Population: Facts and methods of demography*. San Francisco: Freeman.

Keyfitz, N., and W. Flieger. 1990. *World population growth and aging*. Chicago: The University of Chicago Press.

Keyfitz, N., and J. Frauenthal. 1975. An improved life table method. *Biometrics* 21: 889–899.

Kim, Y. J., and R. Schoen. 1993. Crossovers that link populations with the same vital rates. *Mathematical Population Studies* 4: 1–19.

Kim, Y. J., and R. Schoen. 1996. Populations with quadratic exponential growth. Mathematical Population Studies 6: 19–33.

Kim, Y. J., and R. Schoen. 1997. Population momentum expresses population aging. *Demography* 34: 421–428.

Kim, Y. J., and R. Schoen. 2000. Changes in timing and the measurement of fertility. *Population and Development Review* 26: 554–559.

Kim, Y. J., R. Schoen, and P. S. Sarma. 1991. Momentum and the growth-free segment of a population. *Demography* 28: 159–176.

Kohler, H. P., and M. Philipov. 1999. Variance effects in the Bongaarts-Feeney formula. *Demography* 38 (1): 1–16.

Klein, J. P., and M. L. Moeschberger. 1997. *Survival analysis: Techniques for censored and truncated data*. New York: Springer-Verlag.

Land, K. C. 1971. Formal theory. *Sociological Methodology* 1971: 175–220.

Land, K. C. 2001. Models and indicators. *Social Forces* 80: 381–410.

Land, K. C., J. M. Guralnik, and D. G. Blazer. 1994. Estimating increment-decrement life tables with multiple covariates from panel data: The case of active life expectancy. *Demography* 31: 297–319.

Land, K. C., G. C. Hough, Jr., 1989. New methods for tables of school life, with applications to U.S. data from recent school years. *Journal of the American Statistical Association* 84: 63–75.

Land, K. C., G. C. Hough, Jr., and M. M. McMillen. 1986. Voting status life tables for the United States, 1968–1980. *Demography* 23: 381–402.

Land, K. C., and A. Rogers, eds. 1982. *Multidimensional mathematical demography*. New York: Academic Press.

Land, K. C., and S. H. Schneider. 1987. Forecasting in the social and natural sciences: Some isomorphisms. In *Forecasting in the social and natural sciences*. Edited by K. C. Land and S. H. Schneider, 7–31. Boston: D. Reidel.

Land, K. C., and R. Schoen. 1982. Statistical methods for Markov-generated increment-decrement life tables with polynomial gross flow functions. In *Multidimensional mathematical demography*. Edited by K. C. Land and A. Rogers, 265–346. New York: Academic Press.

Lawless, J. F. 2003. *Statistical models and methods for lifetime data*, 2d ed. Hoboken, N.J.: Wiley.

Lewis, E. L. 1941. On the generation and growth of a population. *Sankhya* 6: 93–96.

Leslie, P. H. 1945. On the use of matrices in certain population mathematics. *Biometrika* 33: 183–212.

Li, N., and S. Tuljapurkar. 1999. Population momentum for gradual demographic transitions. *Population Studies* 53: 255–262.

Li, N., and S. Tuljapurkar. 2000. The solution of time-dependent population models. *Mathematical Population Studies* 7: 311–329.

Lopez, A. 1961. *Problems in stable population theory*. Princeton, N.J.: Office of Population Research.

Lotka, A. J. 1907. Relation between birth rates and death rates. *Science* 26: 21–22.

Lotka, A. J. 1924 [1956]. *Elements of mathematical biology*. New York: Dover. [Originally published as *Elements of physical biology* by Williams and Wilkins, New York.]

Lotka, A. J. 1998. *Analytical theory of biological populations*. Translated and with an Introduction by D. P. Smith and H. Rossert. New York: Plenum Press.

Manton, K. G., and K. C. Land. 2000. Active life expectancy estimates for the U. S. elderly population: A multidimensional continuous-mixture model of functional change applied to completed cohorts, 1982–1996. *Demography* 37: 253–265.

Manton, K. G., E. Stallard, and L. S. Corder. 1997. Changes in the age dependence of mortality and disability: Cohort and other determinants. *Demography* 34: 135–157.

Manton, K. G., E. Stallard, and B. H. Singer. 1994. Methods for projecting the future size and health status of the U.S. elderly population. In *Studies of the economics of aging*. Edited by D. Wise, 41–77. Chicago: National Bureau of Economic Research and University of Chicago Press.

Manton, K. G., M. A. Woodbury, and H. D. Tolley. 1994. *Statistical applications using fuzzy sets*. New York: Wiley.

McFarland, D. D. 1969. On the theory of stable population: A new and elementary proof of the theorems under weaker assumptions. *Demography* 6: 301–322.

Menken, J., J. Trussell, D. Stempel, and O. Babakol. 1981. Proportional hazards life table models: An illustrative analysis of socio-demographic influences on marriage dissolution in the United States. *Demography* 18:181–200.

Merli, G. 1998. Mortality in Vietnam, 1979–1989. *Demography* 35: 345–360.

Molla, M. T., D. K. Wagener, and J. H. Madans. 2001. *Summary measures of population health: Methods for calculating healthy life expectancy*. Atlanta: Centers for Disease Control and Prevention.

Morgan, S. P., and S. M. Lynch. 2001. Success and future of demography: The role of data and methods. *Special issue on population health and aging: Strengthening the dialogue between epidemiology and demography*. *Annals of the New York Academy of Sciences* 954: 35–51.

National Research Council. 2000. *Beyond six billion: Forecasting the world's population*. Edited by J. a. R. A. B. Bongaarts. Washington, D.C.: National Academies Press.

Notestein, F. 1945. Population—The long view. In *Food for the world*. Edited by Theodore W. Schultz, 36–57. Chicago: The University of Chicago Press.

Paget, W. J., and I. M. Timaeus, 1994. A relational Gompertz model of male fertility: Development and assessment. *Population Studies* 48: 333–340.

Parlett, B. 1970. Ergodic properties of population. I. The one-sex model. *Theoretical Population Biology* 1: 191–207.

Pollard J. H., and E. J. Volkovics. 1992. The Gompertz distribution and its applications. *Genus* 48 (3–4): 15–28.

Preston, S. H. 1986. The relation between actual and intrinsic growth rates. *Population Studies* 40: 343–351.

Preston, S. H. 1987a. Relations among standard epidemiologic measures in a population. *American Journal of Epidemiology* 126: 336–345.

Preston, S. H. 1987b. Estimation of certain measures in family demography based upon generalized stable population relations. In *Family demography: Methods and their application*. Edited by J. Bongaarts, 40–62. Cambridge: Cambridge University Press.

Preston, S. H., and N. Bennett. 1983. A census-based method for estimating adult mortality. *Population Studies* 37: 91–104.

Preston, S. H., and A. J. Coale. 1982. Age structure, growth, attrition and accession: A new synthesis. *Population Index* 48: 217–259.

Preston, S. H., I. T. Elo, I. Rosenwaike, and M. Hill. 1996. African-American mortality at older ages: Results of a matching study. *Demography* 35: 1–21.

Preston, S. H., and M. Guillot. 1997. Population dynamics in an age of declining fertility. *Genus* 53: 15–31.

Preston, S. H., P. Heuveline, and M. Guillot. 2001. *Demography: Measuring and modeling population processes.* Malden, Mass.: Blackwell.

Preston, S. H., N. Keyfitz, and R. Schoen. 1972. *Causes of death: Life tables for national populations.* New York: Seminar Press.

Preston, S. H., and M. Strong. 1986. Effects of mortality declines on marriage patterns in developing countries. In *Consequences of Mortality Trends and Differentials.* United Nations Population Study, No. 95, 88–100. New York: United Nations.

Prskawetz, A., L. Jiang, and B. C. O'Neill. 2002. Demographic composition and projections of car use in Austria. Working Paper of Max Planck Institute for Demographic Research, Germany. http//www.demogr.mpg.de/; click "Staff Publications" to search for author's name.

Reed, L. G., and M. Merrell. 1939. A short method for constructing an abridged life table. *American Journal of Hygiene* 30: 33–62.

Rogers, A. 1975. *Introduction to multiregional mathematical demography.* New York: Wiley.

Rogers, A. 1986. Parameterized multistate population dynamics and projections. *Journal of American Statistical Association*, 81: 48–61.

Rogers, A., R. G. Rogers, and L. G. Branch. 1989. A multistate analysis of active life expectancy. *Public Health Reports* 104: 222–225.

Ryder, N. B. 1956. Problems of trend determination during a translation in fertility. *Milbank Memorial Fund Quarterly* 34(1): 5–21.

Ryder, N. B. 1959. An appraisal of fertility trends in the United States. In *Thirty years of research in human fertility: Retrospect and prospect*, 1959, 38–49. New York: Milbank Memorial Fund.

Ryder, N. B. 1964. The process of demographic translation. *Demography* 1: 74–82.

Ryder, N. B. 1980. Components of temporal variations in American fertility. In *Demographic patterns in developed societies.* Edited by R. W. Hiorns, 15–54. London: Taylor Francis.

Ryder, N. B. 1983. Cohort and period measures of changing fertility. In *Determinants of fertility in developing countries.* Edited by R. A. Bulatao and R. D. Lee, with P. E. Hollerbach and J. Bongaarts, 737–756. New York: Academic Press.

Schoen, R. 1975. Constructing increment-decrement life tables. *Demography* 13: 313–324.

Schoen, R. 1978. Calculating life tables by estimating Chiang's a. *Demography* 15: 625–635.

Schoen, R. 1988. *Modeling multigroup populations.* New York: Plenum.

Schoen, R., and S. H. Jonsson. 2003. Modeling momentum in gradual demographic transitions. *Demography* 40: 621–635.

Schoen, R., and Y. J. Kim. 1994. Hyperstability. Paper presented at the annual meeting of the Population Association of America, Miami, May 5–7.

Schoen, R., and Y. J. Kim. 1996. Stabilization, birth waves, and the surge in the elderly. *Mathematical Population Studies* 6: 35–53.

Schoen, R., and Y. J. Kim. 1998. Momentum under a gradual approach to zero growth. *Population Studies* 52: 295–299.

Schoen, R., and K. C. Land. 1979. A general algorithm for estimating a Markov-generated increment-decrement life table with applications to marital status patterns. *Journal of the American Statistical Association* 74: 761–776.

Schoen, R., and K. Woodrow. 1980. Labor force status life tables for the United States, 1972. *Demography* 17: 297–322.

Sharpe, F. R., and A. J. Lotka. 1911. A problem in age-distribution. *Philosophical Magazine*, Ser. 6, 21: 435–438.

Shryock, H. S., and J. S. Siegel. 1975. *The methods and materials of demography.* 2 vols. Washington, D.C.: U.S. Government Printing Office.

Singer, J. D., and J. B. Willet. 2003. *Applied longitudinal data analysis: Modeling change and event occurrence.* New York: Oxford University Press.

Smith, D., and N. Keyfitz, eds. 1977. *Mathematical demography: Selected papers.* New York: Springer-Verlag.

Sullivan, D. F. 1971. A single index of mortality and morbidity. *HSMHA Health Report* 86: 347–354.

Sverdrup, E. 1965. Estimates and test procedures in connection with stochastic models for death, recoveries, and transfers between different states of health. *Skandinavisk Aktuarietidskrift* 40: 184–211.

Sykes, Z. M. 1969. On discrete stable population theory. *Biometrics* 25: 285–293.

Thatcher, A. R., V. Kannisto, and J. W. Vaupel. 1998. *The force of mortality at ages 80 to 120*. Odense, Denmark; Odense University Press. Online at *http://www.demogr.mpg.de/Papers/Books/Monograph5/ForMort.htm*.

Therneau, T. M., and P. M. Grambsch. 2000. *Modeling survival data*. New York: Springer.

Trussell, J. 1985. *Mm* (computer program). Princeton, N.J.: Office of Population Research.

Trussell, J., and C. Hammerslough. 1983. A hazards-model analysis of the covariates of infant and child mortality in Sri Lanka. *Demography* 20: 1–26.

Tuma, N. B., M. T. Hannan, and L. P. Groeneveld. 1979. Analysis of event histories. *American Journal of Sociology* 84: 820–854.

United Nations. 1983. *Manual X: Indirect techniques for demographic estimation*. New York: United Nations.

United Nations, Statistical Division. 2000. *Demographic yearbook, historical supplement*, March 17. New York: United Nations.

Van Imhoff, E., and N. Keilman. 2000. On the quantum and tempo of fertility: Comment. *Population and Development Review* 26: 549–553.

Wachter, K. W, and C. E. Finch, eds. 1997. *Between Zeus and the salmon: The biodemography of longevity*. Washington, D.C.: National Academies Press.

Willekens, F. J., I. Shah, J. M. Shah, and P. Ramachandran. 1982. Multistate analysis of marital status life tables: Theory and application. *Population Studies* 36: 129–144.

Woodbury, M. A., and J. Clive. 1974. Clinical pure types as a fuzzy partition. *Journal of Cybernetics* 73: 1073–1080.

Woodbury, M. A., and K. G. Manton. 1983. A theoretical model of the physiological dynamics of circulatory disease in human populations. *Human Biology* 55: 417–441.

Xie, Y., and E. E. Pimental. 1992. Age patterns of marital fertility: Revising the Coale-Trussell method. *Journal of the American Statistical Association* 87: 977–994.

Yamaguchi, K. 1991. *Event history analysis*. London: Sage.

Yang, C., and Y. Zeng. 2000. Household projections for Taiwan. *Taiwanese Journal of Sociology* 24: 239–279.

Yashin, A. I., and I. I. Iachine. 1997. How frailty models can be used for evaluating longevity limits: Taking advantage of an interdisciplinary approach. *Demography* 34: 31–48.

Zeng, Y. 1986. Changes in family structure in China: A simulation study. *Population and Development Review* 12: 675–703.

Zeng, Y. 1988. Changing demographic characteristics and the family status of Chinese women. *Population Studies* 42: 183–203.

Zeng, Y. 1991. *Family dynamics in China: A life table analysis*. Madison: The University of Wisconsin Press.

Zeng, Y., D. Gu, and K. C. Land. 2004. A new method for correcting underestimation of disabled life expectancy and application to Chinese oldest-old. *Demography* 41: 335–361.

Zeng, Y., and K. C. Land. 2001. A sensitivity analysis of the Bongaarts-Feeney new method for adjusting bias in observed period total fertility rates. *Demography* 38: 17–28.

Zeng, Y., and K. C. Land. 2002. Adjusting period tempo changes—with an extension of Ryder's basic translation equation. *Demography* 39: 269–285.

Zeng, Y., K. C. Land, Z. Wang, and D. Gu. 2005. U. S. Family Household Dynamics and Momentum—Extension of ProFamy Method and Application. Forthcoming in *Population Research and Policy Review*, 24(4).

Zeng, Y., and J. W. Vaupel. 2003. Oldest old mortality in China. *Demographic Research* 8: 215–244.

Zeng, Y., J. W. Vaupel, and Z. Wang. 1997. A multidimensional model for projecting family households—with an illustrative numerical application. *Mathematical Population Studies* 6: 187–216.

Zeng, Y., J. W. Vaupel, and Z. Wang. 1998. Household projection using conventional demographic data. *Population and Development Review*, Supplementary Issue: *Frontiers of Population Forecasting* 24: 59–87.

Zeng, Y., Z. Wang, Z. Ma, and C. Chen. 2000. A simple method for estimating α and β: An extension of Brass relational Gompertz fertility model. *Population Research and Policy Review* 19: 525–549.

CHAPTER 23

Political Demography

Michael S. Teitelbaum

This chapter addresses the complex relationships between demographic and political forces. The scope is both international and internal to states, and includes both directions of putative causation: how demographic change affects politics, and how political forces affect demographic patterns.

CONCEPTUAL FRAMEWORKS

Political demography addresses both the political determinants and the political consequences of demographic change. It is a subject of rapidly increasing importance in both academic and policy arenas, but one that lies somewhat uncomfortably at the boundaries of demography and political science. As such it has been underattended by both demographers and political scientists. The best definition of political demography is Weiner's (1971):

> Political demography is the study of the size, composition, and distribution of population in relation to both government and politics. It is concerned with the political consequences of population change, especially the effects of population change on the demands made upon governments, on the performance of governments, on the distribution of political power within states, and on the distribution of national power among states. It also considers the political determinants of population change, especially the political causes of the movement of people, the relationship of various population configurations to the structure and functions of government, and public policies directed at affecting the size, composition, and distribution of populations. Finally, in the study of political demography it is not enough to know the facts and figures of population—that is fertility, mortality, and migration rates; it is also necessary to consider the knowledge and attitudes that people and their governments have toward population issues (597).

Notwithstanding a convincing case made by Weiner that political demography deserves serious attention, most political scientists have expressed rather little interest in, and made few contributions to, studies of two of the three major demographic forces, namely fertility and mortality. However, some have made quite significant contributions to the study of the third, migration, both within and across international boundaries, but particularly with regard to international migration. In part this is because of the important security dimensions that can arise when large-scale international population movements affect the cohesion of societies and generate social and political conflict both within and between countries. Moreover, international migration is by definition a function of the world system of sovereign states, is addressed by a variety of international treaties and organizations, and is heavily affected by policies adopted by national governments.

The important topics in political demography include, but are not limited to, the following:

- The impacts of differing rates of national population growth on military manpower
- The political and policy consequences of changes in population size, age structure, and density, including differentials among ethnic and religious communities and their impacts on domestic social and political relations, central-local relations, regional income disparities, and political representation
- The political consequences of migration both within and across national borders
- Government policies designed to affect the size, composition, distribution, and growth rate of a population

THEORETICAL MODELS

Theoretical writings in political demography have a remarkably long history and impressive pedigree. Those who have addressed political demography (though not necessarily calling it such) include many of the leading theorists of politics and society, including those of ancient China, as well as Plato, Aristotle, and Ibn Khaldun (Teitelbaum 1988). More recently, political theorists/practitioners such as Thomas Jefferson drew close connections between population density and the nature of civic life and politics.

In the domain of economics, economic theorists from the 16th century onward have described demographic patterns as critical elements of economic prosperity and political stability. Mercantilist theorists of 16th- and 17th-century Europe advised the monarchs of the day that they could increase the power and wealth of their realms by increasing the fertility and constraining the emigration of their subjects.

Their intellectual opponents, the free-market physiocrats, argued instead that land, not population, was the principal source of wealth. Utopian thinkers of the 18th century rejected both mercantilist and physiocratic views, arguing that what really mattered was not population size or land area, but equitable distribution of resources.

The classic economists who dominated late 18th- and early 19th-century economic theory, including Adam Smith, David Ricardo, and Thomas Malthus, theorized that agricultural returns to increasing labor and capital inputs would diminish and that free markets would regulate population increase in an automatic manner. Malthus in particular focused on the negative impact he perceived of unrestrained population growth on the increasing poverty of the lower classes. He argued for delayed marriage and celibacy outside of marriage rather than interventions such as contraception and abortion, which he considered to be "unnatural" and "vice" (Teitelbaum 1988).

By the late 19th century, Marxist-Leninist theorists were proclaiming that any level of population could be sustained so long as a socialist system led to the equitable distribution of wealth and income.

During the 1930s, many students of politics and economics developed causal theories that attributed the Great Depression in part to the generally low fertility rates then being experienced, and worried too about the impending generational conflict they foresaw if younger cohorts continued to be smaller than older ones. Meanwhile, politicians on both the left and right saw strategic and military dangers resulting from the same low fertility. The U.S.S.R. under Stalin, Germany under Hitler, and Italy under Mussolini all adopted a variety of policies and programs designed to encourage their populaces to increase their fertility rates.

Following the end of World War II, American scholars (economists, demographers, biologists) began to write both theoretical and empirical analyses describing the *potential* negative impacts of rapid population growth in developing countries on economic development, political stability, and human welfare.

Longstanding Marxist-Leninist views on population, described above, were sustained until the 1980s and 1990s but were then rejected by Chinese Communist leaders, who concluded that unrestrained population growth threatened the very future of socialism. It is bemusing to note that at almost the same time, political theorists of the American "New Right" came to embrace (perhaps unknowingly) many of the earlier Marxist-Leninist (and mercantilist and utopian) arguments that population issues per se mattered rather little; for these New Right intellectuals, poverty was a result of political intervention in the economy ("economic statism") and could be alleviated only by the establishment of a correct "free market" economic system. In such a system, population size would be self-regulating.

METHODOLOGICAL CHALLENGES

Despite the importance, both theoretical and practical, of the issues addressed under the rubric of political demography, it has been underattended by both demographers and political scientists. Most demographers might perhaps be forgiven for their inattention, since the focus of their work is appropriately upon matters internal to the demographic system of fertility, mortality, migration, and age composition. Moreover, numerous demographers of considerable prominence have addressed matters under the rubric of "population policy" that involve substantial components of political decision making. For instance, see chapter 28, "Population Policy," in this *Handbook*.

The similar inattention of political scientists is somewhat more puzzling, if it is true that demographic forces have important political dimensions. Yet to many political scientists, the causal relationships between demography and politics have seemed elusive, with numerous other variables always intervening. While it might be the case that a high proportion of young people tended toward political turbulence, such turbulence could be more directly explained by reference to the disruptions of industrialization or to the high rates of unemployment rather than to age composition itself. In addition, during the postwar period, western political scientists focused their attention appropriately on the security implications of the Cold War, a subject in which demographic variables seemed trivial (but see discussion below).

Moreover, to many political scientists and others interested in social and political theories, the field of demography is sometimes seen as largely atheoretical and excessively empirical, attending primarily to improved measurement via censuses and vital statistics. Indeed, it is fair to say that many social scientists are largely ignorant of demographic theory and methods and see demographers as technical and dull number crunchers.

This is far from the truth, of course. To the contrary, demography (along with related fields such as epidemiology and actuarial science) has developed some of the most sophisticated and highly mathematical models of any discipline that seeks to address the complexities of human behavior. The subfield known as "formal demography" deploys the calculus and complex equations to model the ways in which changes in fertility and mortality affect the size, age structure, and "intrinsic" rates of change in a highly abstracted human population. Almost all demographers routinely employ age-standardized or synthetic rates of fertility, such as the period total fertility rate, and also address the combined effects of fertility and mortality via measures such as the net reproduction rate. The "life table" developed by actuaries and demographers offers a formal summary of hypothetical probabilities of dying at each age, drawn from empirical data or sophisticated techniques of estimation.

At the same time, it is fair to say that no demographic models to date have succeeded in correctly forecasting long-term changes in fertility, at least in human populations in which voluntary control of childbearing is widely used. The theories and forecasts put forward by Malthus in the early 19th century, while influential during that period, have long been repudiated as empirically incorrect by all but a handful of demographers. From the 1930s to the 1970s, most demographers embraced a formulation known as "demographic transition theory," which purported to show that social and economic trends provide a sufficient explanation of the fundamental shift in Western Europe from high fertility/high mortality to low fertility/low mortality over the preceding two centuries. However, during the 1970s, when the Princeton Fertility Study first sought to rigorously test demographic transition theory empirically using laboriously-assembled sets of comparable historical data, the theoretical superstructure proved to be inadequate to explain the timing and pace of fertility declines across Europe. Given this, political scientists might be forgiven for concluding that demography "lacks theory," at least in terms of theory that could explain and predict human fertility trends.

There is a further methodological challenge facing those who wish to analyze the political effects of demographic changes. Phrased simply, the political consequences of demography depend as much on *perceptions* of demographic change as on demographic reality. Perceptions may vary dramatically over time and may differ substantially between elites and publics. Hence efforts to relate quantitative data on demographic change to political behavior must themselves contend with the intervening variables of how change is reflected in public and elite opinion. The realities matter to be sure, but so too do the perceptions.

Finally, there are inevitable methodological problems associated with efforts to understand the political determinants of population change. For example, since the 1950s many governments of developing countries have adopted policies to slow rapid population growth. Most of these have focused on the subsidized provision of safe and effective methods of voluntary fertility control (though in a few cases, e.g., in India under the Emergency, and allegedly in some regions of China, verging into coercion). While analysts of voluntary family planning programs conclude that many, though not all, such programs have been effective in accelerating and amplifying fertility declines, some critics assert that in methodological terms the fertility declines recorded may have taken place without such programs and hence cannot be demonstrated to have been caused by them.

Similarly, few would dispute that some large migratory movements across international borders have resulted from political decisions of governments (e.g., the departure of hundreds of thousands of Kosovars to Albania and Macedonia in 1999). Yet there are other cases of mass movements (e.g., Cubans and Haitians to the U.S.) which some ascribe to political factors, while others argue that the causes are purely economic or environmental.

RESEARCH EXEMPLARS

As noted earlier, until recently only a few researchers have focused their attention upon the intersections between demographic and political change, although a number of notable pioneers such as Weiner and Zolberg have long offered valuable analyses and insights. Happily, over the past 15 years or so there has been a vigorous surge of attention to such matters. An incomplete list of publications that illustrates the value of such efforts would include the following: Anderson and Fienberg's (2001) analysis of the politics of census taking; Brubaker's (1996) study of nationalism in Europe; Huntington's (1996) book on the "clash of civilizations"; Kaufmann's (1998) discussion of 20th-century partitions and population transfers; Kennedy's (1994) forward look at the challenges in the 21st century; Nichiporuk's (2000) assessment of the links between security and demographic trends; Petersen's (1987) analysis of the politics of collecting ethnic data; Russell's (1988) study of migration policy and politics in Kuwait; Teitelbaum and Winter's (1985, 1998) analyses of the political effects of low fertility and of fertility when accompanied by high migration; Weil's (1998) assessment of the role of the state in immigration; Weiner's (1971) pioneering analysis of political demography; the various analyses in the volume on demography and national security edited by Weiner and Russell (2001); Weiner and Teitelbaum's (2001) study of political demography and demographic engineering; and Zolberg, Suhrke and Aguayo's (1989) study of refugee patterns and conflict.

FUTURE PROSPECTS

There are several questions of import in political demography that could constructively be addressed in greater detail in future research in this area. The key analytical questions are the following: Does population size matter? Does age structure matter? Does population composition matter? and Do demographic interactions between immigration and fertility matter? In the last section of this chapter, each of these analytical questions will be examined.

Does Size Matter?

As noted earlier, one time-honored perception is that a state's international power (military, economic, political) is directly related to the size of its population. Such views go back to antiquity but in modern times have found their most pervasive acceptance among intellectuals and political leaders of all political persuasions in France. In the aftermath of the crushing defeat of the Franco-Prussian War of the 1870s, French elites began to attribute their nation's military and economic failures to what they described as the disastrous imbalance of low French fertility vis-à-vis the rapid demographic growth of Germany (an ironic twist when compared to more recent French-German demographic trends). As early as the 1890s, French intellectuals, including Emile Zola, founded the National Alliance for the Growth of the French Population (Teitelbaum and Winter 1985: 27–38).

These concerns took on added momentum as the clouds of war gathered in the first decade of the 20th century. Following World War I, Premier Georges Clemenceau spoke as follows during the 1919 parliamentary debate on ratification of the Treaty of Versailles:

> The treaty does not say that France must undertake to have children, but it is the first thing which ought to have been put in it. For if France turns her back on large families, one can put all the clauses one wants in a treaty, one can take all the guns of Germany, one can do whatever one likes, France will be lost because there will be no more Frenchmen (Teitelbaum and Winter 1985: 27).

By the 1930s the French government decided that demographic stagnation required France to emphasize mechanized rearmament and to retreat behind its Maginot Line. Paul Reynaud, a prominent minister in the government of the day, argued for mechanized rearmament by noting that "there is only one factor that dominates all: the demographic factor" (Teitelbaum and Winter 1985: 37).

Such concerns have persisted among current French leaders, now expressed in both French and European terms. President Jacques Chirac, then Mayor of Paris, was quoted as follows in 1984 interview in the left-wing newspaper *Liberation*:

> Two dangers stalk French society: social democratization and a demographic slump.... If you look at Europe and then at other continents, the comparison is terrifying. In demographic terms, Europe is vanishing. Twenty years or so from now, our countries will be empty, and no matter what our technological strength, we shall be incapable of putting it to use" (*Liberation* 1984: 1).

Such concerns were by no means limited to France. During the 1930s, Germany under the Nazis and the Soviet Union under Stalin adopted strong policies to raise fertility rates for explicitly military and strategic reasons.

In other industrialized countries, such as Australia and Canada, strategic concerns about low fertility led to policies favoring population expansion but with characteristics different from those in Europe. During World War I, Australian Prime Minister William ("Billy") Hughes admonished Australians to "populate or perish." During World War II, Prime Minister Curtin warned that, given its location near densely populated Asian nations, Australian security required a population of 30 million. The basis for Curtin's target of 30 million is lost in the mists of history. But given that its population at the time was 7 million, it was evident that increasing fertility could not suffice. Hence most Australian political elites embraced policies that actively promoted and financed large-scale immigration, initially from the U.K. and later from other European countries, in concert with the "White Australia" policies that originated in the early 1900s (Lines 1992: 199).

In Canada, Prime Minister Wilfrid Laurier was enthusiastically predicting as early as 1904 that there would be 60 million Canadians—a ten-fold increase—within the lifetimes of those in his audience (Gooderham 1995: A1). Since then, numerous Canadian politicians have long proclaimed that the population of Canada should grow to at least 30 million. Like the identical target number in Australia, the origins of this Canadian target are uncertain, but it is rarely challenged (Trempe 1998). Like Australia, Canada has focused its efforts in this direction on an active immigration recruitment policy. However, in the 1980s an expert group convened by the government called for costly financial incentives to raise fertility, justified in strategic terms. The expert group asked rhetorically "whether the goal of maintaining the population was not as important as that of national defence. Perhaps as much could be spent for the first as for the second; in the long term, there is no point in 'defending' a population that is disappearing" (Government of Canada 1984: 5–8).

In the United States such concerns have tended to be more muted. A few advocates, mainly from the New Right (Simon 1981), argue that the West "is committing slow-motion demographic suicide" in both military and economic terms. The most persistent proponent of this view is Ben Wattenberg, a political journalist at the conservative American Enterprise Institute. In a book evocatively titled *The Birth Dearth*, and described by its author as "this alarmist tract" (Wattenberg 1989: 10), as well as in many of his nationally syndicated columns, Wattenberg argues that higher fertility in countries of the "industrial Communist world" would lead to their ascendancy over the West by 2085. In a book review published in the *Congressional Record* in 1987, I wrote as follows about the utility of such very long-term projections:

> One wonders . . . what political scientists would make of forecasts that hold national characters and military alliances constant for a full century; put another way, if Wattenberg had been writing 100 years ago, when the Czar ruled Russia and Britain ruled the waves, what would he have predicted about the relative strength of NATO and the Warsaw Pact in 1987? (Teitelbaum 1987).

Few books with long time horizons have been proven so wrong so quickly. The Warsaw Pact (and eventually the Soviet Union itself) dissolved into political and economic chaos within only a few years of its 1987 publication. Yet however dubious, Wattenberg's claims were embraced by American political leaders of considerable stature, with enthusiastic endorsements from the then-Senator Daniel P. Moynihan, former U.N. Representative Jeanne J. Kirkpatrick, and former Presidential candidate Malcolm S. Forbes, Jr. (Wattenberg 1989: 177).

To the extent that empirical evidence is available on this subject, the findings are decidedly mixed. In terms of raw military power, it is evident that within given levels of economic development, governments of more populous states would on average be able to tap more of the resources needed for such power than would those of small states. However, only two prosperous and developed countries (United States and Japan) rank among the most populous 10 countries. The other populous countries are all relatively low-income countries, i.e., China, India, Indonesia, Brazil, Pakistan, the Russian Federation, Bangladesh, and Nigeria.

Certainly the governments of all of these countries can command larger national budgets than would be available if they had the same per capita income but smaller populations. In addition, many (China, India, Brazil, Pakistan, and the Russian Federation) have trained substantial cadres of skilled scientists and engineers needed for the development of sophisticated weaponry. All of them therefore have the capability of developing nuclear, biological, and chemical weaponry, as well as medium- and long-range missiles to deliver them, if they are prepared to devote significant fractions of their national budgets to such purposes. Smaller countries with lower per capita incomes are less able to move in such directions, although North Korea offers a sobering counterpoint.

Yet, as demonstrated by cases such as Iraq and Israel, even some quite small countries with access to economic and human resources can succeed in such technologies, either on their own or via alliances with other countries. Indeed, the case of Israel demonstrates that an advanced state with a very small population base is capable of creating its own homegrown high-tech defense capabilities that can make it at least the equal of far more populous neighboring states.

Some have argued that countries with larger populations are not only stronger, but also tend to be more aggressive toward their neighbors, in the spirit of the 1930s *lebensraum* claims of German and Japanese expansionists that large-population countries have a need and a right to control additional territory (Rager 1941). However, in empirical terms there is no consistent pattern of this type, even though most large countries do indeed command substantial military forces. The same agnosticism seems in order about claims that countries with higher demographic growth rates or population densities tend to be more aggressive toward their neighbors.

Does Age Structure Matter?

The age structure of a population, of critical interest to demographers (see chapter 1 in this *Handbook*), has been less than well understood by political scientists. While age structure can in principle be affected by fertility, mortality, and migration, fertility is quantitatively the most important by far. Other things equal, a high fertility rate will produce a youthful age composition, while low fertility yields an older age structure. Any population in transition from high to low fertility rates will experience a shift in its age structure from more to less youthful—known as population or demographic "aging." Increases in fertility will shift the age structure in the opposite direction.

Mortality reduction also affects age structures but with less force. Declines in infant and child mortality lead to increased proportions of children and youth, while mortality reduction among the elderly does the opposite. High mortality rates tend to decline more rapidly among the young. Once low mortality levels are achieved, further declines tend to be concentrated among older age groups. Hence there is not a uniform age structure impact of mortality declines, and such effects tend to be modest relative to the effects of fertility changes.

Finally, migration can affect age structures, given that migrants tend usually to be concentrated among young adults. Yet such migrants are also typically accompanied by their young children and sometimes by their elderly parents. Hence the effects of migration on age structure are, like those of mortality change, less concentrated than are fertility changes in their impacts on age structure.

The fact that over the past half century most of the world's countries have experienced fertility declines means that the age structures of most countries have been shifting toward declining proportions of children and increasing proportions of older residents. When such trends last occurred, during the 1930s and 1940s, some commentators developed what might be termed the hypothesis of demographic senescence (Teitelbaum and Winter 1985: 108–110). It was argued that populations with "older" age compositions are afflicted by a lack of political vigor, creativity and ambition, economic vitality, social dynamism, military prowess. In the aftermath of the disasters of World War II, two prominent French political intellectuals, Robert Debré (whose son Michel Debré was to be the first Premier of the Fifth Republic) and the eminent demographer Alfred Sauvy opined as follows:

> The terrible failure of 1940, more moral than material, must be linked in part to this dangerous sclerosis. We saw all too often, during the occupation, old men leaning wearily towards the servile solution, at the time that the young were taking part in the national impulse towards independence and liberty. This crucial effect of our senility, is it not a grave warning? (Debré and Sauvy 1946: 58).

In another setting, Sauvy vividly characterized an aging society in memorable terms, as one comprised of "old people, living in old houses, ruminating about old ideas" (Teitelbaum 1978: xx–xxi).

In the depths of the Great Depression, in 1938, Myrdal expressed concern that an older age structure would make it harder for younger people to advance in their careers and would thereby reduce society's impetus toward progress:

> When on account of the changed age structure individual opportunities to rise socially are blocked, people will get discouraged. They will lose their dynamic interest in working life. Society will lose the mental attitude that goes with progress. Interest in security will be substituted for an earlier interest in social advancement (Myrdal 1940: 165).

A related possibility is that shifts toward older age structures produced by fertility declines in developing countries will tend toward reductions in pressures that have been stimulating political instability domestically and emigration internationally. On this argument, the "youth bulge" that has characterized high-fertility developing countries explains in some measure the political turmoil many of them have experienced, given the fact that young adults (and especially males) are more prone to radical or revolutionary political movements. Certainly mass protests by young people have contributed to bringing down governments in Jakarta, Manila, and Tehran and were decisive in separating Bangladesh from Pakistan. Similarly, international migrants have long been concentrated heavily among young adults, and hence on this argument the past decades' surge in such migrations should be expected to wane as the age structures of origin countries shift away from their recent youth bulge compositions.

Does Population Composition Matter?

In addition to age, other aspects of population composition are deemed important in cultural or political terms. The relative size of a social group is surely a factor in its political power, particularly in democratic systems. Moreover, even if such power is not actually redistributed, ethnic, socioeconomic, and geographical groups often *perceive* differences in their relative size and growth rates as factors affecting the distribution of power.

Typically, certain groups increase their numbers more rapidly than others. Such differentials may be attributed to differences in fertility, mortality, or migration rates. In some cases, leaders of such groups affirmatively encourage their followers toward high fertility or immigration rates for the very purpose of accruing greater political power. Though demographic changes are usually gradual, sustained over extended time periods they can produce substantial shifts in relative numbers.

Such changes do not automatically result in comparable shifts in the distribution of political power. As in most such subjects, there are many other variables that are influential, including the cohesiveness of a social group, the skills of its leadership, its financial resources, or its ability to deny needed goods and services to others. Moreover, the "mix" of such variables depends heavily upon the kind of political system in which the group operates—whether it is democratic or not, the kind of system of political representation it has, or how important elections are in the political system.

Because compositional changes tend to be gradual, they are often accommodated by gradual political adjustments. However, such shifts have become problematic in political or security terms when political adjustments to them have been blocked (e.g., in Lebanon in the 1940s, 1950s, and 1960s), when they are seen to be unusually rapid and hence threatening, or when they result from unlawful or illegitimate processes, such as illegal immigration. In such cases, bloody ethnic strife can result, as in the civil wars in Lebanon and the former Yugoslavia, ethnic strife in the northeastern states of India, and the violence and mass genocides in Rwanda, Burundi, and Zaire. Centrifugal political forces have also occurred, as in the case of the former Soviet Union, which for several decades before it dissolved in 1991 had experienced some of the largest fertility differentials among regional and ethnic groups in the country.

Do Demographic Interactions between Immigration and Fertility Matter?

When there are large inflows of immigrants into an area where indigenous fertility is low, rapid transformations usually occur in the composition of the population. The political implications of such changes are in the direction of turbulence, but the outcomes are indeterminate, depending on such factors as the history of relations among the relevant social groups; the degree to which the immigrants identify themselves with the majority or a minority group; and the extent to which the laws and practices of the destination country favor or disfavor the immigrant groups.

Consider the historical case of the European settlement of North America. In less than one century, mass immigration from Europe and increased mortality among the indigenous population shifted the territory's demographic composition from predominantly Native American to European. While the native population opposed this rapid demographic transformation, they lacked the capacity to restrain the continuing influxes.

In the 21st century, rapid internal demographic transformations are possible in many settings in industrialized countries, in part because indigenous fertility rates have declined to very low levels while substantial inflows of immigrants are occurring. Efforts to increase fertility rates are often urged, but the historical record suggests that these are likely to be rather unsuccessful. Yet modern industrialized societies, unlike Native American tribes, do have the organizational and technical capacity to restrain migratory movements. Whether they seek to do so is essentially a question to be determined by the relative political influences of those who benefit from immigration and those who lose.

SUMMARY AND CONCLUSIONS

Political demography addresses some of the most fundamental questions related to the scientific study of both population and political behavior. What are the political consequences of population change, including the distribution of political power among and within states? To what extent do political factors determine population change, including the effects of widespread public policies to affect the size, composition, and distribution of populations and political forces that affect the mass movements of people both internal to states and across international borders.

These subjects have attracted the attention of many of the leading theorists of politics and society since antiquity. Moreover, the issues are of sometimes passionate concern to political leaders and journalists of the present day.

As such, political demography warrants more concerted and thoughtful attention by both demographers and political scientists. In view of the excesses that characterize much of the public debate, it is critical that academic writings on the subject be both well informed about the political and demographic substance and objective and nuanced in interpreting the often partial and conflicting evidence available.

REFERENCES

Anderson, M. J., and S. E. Fienberg. 2001. *Who counts?: The politics of census-taking in contemporary America*. New York: Russell Sage.

Brubaker, R. 1996. *Nationalism reframed: Nationhood and the national question in the new Europe*. Cambridge: Cambridge University Press

Debré, R., and A. Sauvy. 1946. *Des Francais pour la France: La probleme de la population*. Paris: Gallinard.

Gooderham, M. 1995. Canada pulling in the welcome mat. *San Francisco Chronicle* 22 (March): A1.

Government of Canada. 1984. *Demographic aspects of immigration. Report of a Meeting in Montreal 14 December 1984*. Montreal: Government of Canada.

Huntington, S. 1996. *The clash of civilizations and the remaking of world order*. New York: Simon and Schuster.

Kaufmann, C. 1998. When all else fails: Ethnic population transfers and partitions in the twentieth century. *International Security* 23(2): 120–156.

Kennedy, P. 1994. *Preparing for the twenty-first century*. New York: Vintage Books.

Liberation. 1984. Interview with Jacques Chirac. 30 October.

Lines, W. J. 1992. *Taming the great south land: A history of the conquest of nature in Australia*. Sydney: Allen & Unwin.

Myrdal, G. 1990 [reprinted 1962]. *Population: A problem for democracy*. Gloucester, Mass: Peter Smith.

Nichiporuk, B. 2000. The security dynamics of demographic factors. Document MR-1088-WFHF/RF/ DLPF/A. Santa Monica: RAND Corporation.

Petersen, W. 1987. Politics and the measurement of ethnicity. In *The politics of numbers*. Edited by W. Alonso and P. Starr. New York: Russell Sage.

Rager, F. A. 1941. Japanese emigration and Japan's population pressure. *Pacific Affairs*, Sept.: 300–321.

Russell, S. S. 1988. Politics and ideology in migration policy formulation: The case of Kuwait. *International Migration Review* 23: 24–47.

Simon, J. 1981. *The ultimate resource*. Princeton, N.J.: Princeton University Press, 1981.

Teitelbaum, M. S. 1978. Aging populations. *Encyclopaedia Britannica Yearbook 1978*. New York, Encyclopaedia Britannica.

Teitelbaum, M. S. 1987. Review of the birth dearth. *Congressional Record* 133 (125), July 28.

Teitelbaum, M. S. 1988. Demographic change through the lenses of science and politics. *Proceedings of the American Philosophical Society* 132 (2): 173–184.

Teitelbaum, M. S., and J. M. Winter. 1985. *The fear of population decline*. Orlando and London: Academic Press.

Teitelbaum, M. S., and J. M. Winter. 1998. *A question of numbers: High migration, low fertility, and the politics of national identity*. New York: Hill and Wang.

Trempe, R. 1998. Personal communication to the author. June 16.

Wattenberg, B. J. 1989. *The birth dearth: What happens when people in free countries don't have enough babies?*, 2 ed. New York: Pharos Books.

Weil, P. 1998. *The state matters: Immigration control in developed countries*. New York: United Nations.

Weiner, M. 1971. Political demography: An inquiry into the political consequences of population change. In *Rapid population growth: Consequences and policy implications*, chapter XV. Baltimore: Johns Hopkins University Press.

Weiner, M., and S. S. Russell, eds. 2001. *Demography and national security*. New York: Berghahn Books.

Weiner, M., and M. S. Teitelbaum. 2001. *Political demography, demographic engineering*. New York: Berghahn Books.

Zolberg, A. R., A. Suhrke, and S. Aguayo. 1989. *Escape from violence: Conflict and the refugee crisis in the developing world*. New York: Oxford University Press.

PART IV

APPLIED DEMOGRAPHY

The term *applied demography* covers the myriad ways in which demographic data and research findings may be used to address problematic issues faced by human groups. The extent of use is reflected in Kreager's (1993: 522) contention, "Today we are accustomed to population data entering into almost every aspect of social analysis and policy, from the minimal facts of our citizenship and legal status to the implications of childrearing, income, and voting patterns for issues like social security, education, and health care." The subfield of applied demography is a programmatic response to the longstanding recognition of "population problems" (Davis 1967; Desai 2004; Hauser 1942; Micklin 1992; Notestein 1945, 1953; Thompson and Lewis 1965).

Hauser and Duncan's *The Study of Population* did not feature issues of applied demography. No section or chapter title in their book reflects such an orientation. Rather, the focus of their volume is an evaluation of demography as a science. There is an occasional reference to problematic aspects of demographic conditions and trends, e.g., uneven population distribution (Bogue 1959: 398), but generally little concern that the discipline of demography ought to give greater attention to identification or resolution of population problems.

The editors of the present *Handbook* recognize that any current assessment of the discipline would be incomplete without significant attention to its applied components. While this *Handbook* does not cover the entire field of applied demography (see Siegel 2002), the chapters of Part IV provide a representative sample of the ways in which demographic knowledge may be used to inform and guide efforts to resolve societal problems.

Chapter 24 by Potter and Mundigo reviews the history and organization of fertility planning programs that typically operate in developing nations where there is a desire to reduce high rates of population growth. In Chapter 25 Smith and Morrison outline the relatively new subfields of small area and business demography, showing how demographic information and methods are used to guide business decisions and commercial development. The next two chapters cover different facets of demographic approaches to health issues. In chapter 26 Kawachi and Subramanian elaborate the intersection of demography and epidemiology, here labeled health demography, while in chapter 27 Hayward and Warner take an alternative approach to population health, focusing on quality of life issues. The final chapter of Part IV, chapter 28 by May addresses the formulation and implementation of population policies aimed at guiding and regulating demographic conditions and events.

The chapters in Part IV not only demonstrate that demographic information and techniques have important practical uses, but also show that the once assumed chasm between demographic theory and practice is, and probably always has been, a myth. As Stycos (1977: 107) notes, "if theory without policy is for academics, policy without theory is only for gamblers." Stated otherwise, theoretical and applied demography are best viewed as interdependent dimensions of demographic science.

REFERENCES

Bogue, D. J. 1959. "Population Distribution." pp. 383–399 in *The Study of Population: An Inventory and Appraisal*, edited by P. M. Hauser and O. D. Duncan. Chicago: University of Chicago Press.

Davis, K. 1967. "Population Policy: Will Current Programs Succeed?" *Science* 158:730–739.

Desai, S. 2004. "Population Change." pp. 69–86 in *Handbook of Social Problems: A Comparative International Perspective*, edited by G. Ritzer. Thousand Oaks, CA: Sage Publications.

Hauser, P. M. 1942. "Population and Vital Phenomena." *American Journal of Sociology* 48(3):309–322.

Kreager, P. 1993. "Histories of Demography: A Review Article." *Population Studies* 47(3):519–539.

Micklin, M. 1992. "LDC Population Policies: A Challenge for Applied Demography." *Journal of Applied Sociology* 9(1):45–63.

Notestein, F. W. 1945. "Population: The Long View." pp. 36–57 in *Food for the World*, edited by T. W. Schultz. Chicago: University of Chicago Press.

Notestein, F. W. 1953. "Economic Problems of Population Change." Presented at Eighth International Conference of Agricultural Economics.

Siegel, J. S. 2002. *Applied Demography: Applications to Business, Government, Law, and Public Policy*. San Diego: Academic Press.

Stycos, J. M. 1977. "Population Policy and Development." *Population and Development Review* 3(1/2):103–112.

Thompson, W. S. and D. T. Lewis. 1965. *Population Problems*. New York: McGraw-Hill.

CHAPTER 24

Fertility Planning

JOSEPH E. POTTER AND AXEL I. MUNDIGO

SUBSTANTIVE ISSUES

The 20th century was witness to major demographic changes, both in the industrial North and the less developed South. Population growth rates in the North oscillated as fertility declined to below replacement levels in many countries during the Great Depression and then rose during the course of the postwar "baby boom." In the South, as death rates declined faster than birth rates in the 1950s and 1960s, population growth rates exploded. Yet, as the century came to an end, there were signs that fertility was declining almost everywhere, and the specter of runaway population growth was no longer a major concern. Many countries in the North as well as a few from the South moved into a new and worrisome demographic pattern, characterized by below-replacement fertility. In some European countries, this pattern has given rise to fears of eventual depopulation and uncertainty as to how to deal with a rapidly aging population.

How did all these changes in human fertility come about? Certainly, much of the change was due to new behavior patterns that came into being along with aspirations for social mobility, health, education, and consumption. The introduction of effective methods of contraception and improved service delivery systems also helped to cement a major ideational change, one whereby couples, regardless of education or income, saw the advantages of reducing their family size. Fertility planning became a universally accepted part of a couple's reproductive behavior and lifelong decisions. Following an initial period of polemical debates, often driven by ideological and religious arguments, in most societies family planning came to be accepted as a human right and frequently formed an integral part of government health services and/or population policies. What brought about this change? What difference has it made? What are the present and future challenges with regard to fertility planning? These are the questions to be explored in this chapter.

Evolution of an Idea

The perception that individual couples could modify their fertility behavior to suit their own personal goals, especially to maximize economic resources and ensure household prosperity, gained force during the 19th century. Northern European populations were the first to effectively control their family size. France seemed to have initiated the trend toward lower fertility even earlier, a trend that continued throughout the 19th century. Spengler (1938: 110) remarked that moderate fertility was considered as a welcome trend in France, the result of "intellectual progress, order and foresight." Similarly, in the western and northwestern countries of Europe "the [fertility] decline initiated in the 1870's and 1880's proceeded without interruption, except for the years immediately after World War I, and gathered momentum in the 1920's" (Glass 1969: 25). Eventually, the low levels of fertility began to worry many countries and the 1930s saw the first pronatalist policies adopted by France, Belgium, and Italy and later by the Nazi regime in Germany. How did these changes in the control of human fertility begin? What social mechanisms were set into motion that so effectively spread the notion of fertility planning? Who were the main actors involved? Answers to these and other questions are important to understanding the global convergence in the 21st century of the idea that fertility planning is a right and that reproductive goals are a personal choice.

The impetus toward achieving a smaller family size and adopting a behavior consonant with this goal can, in broad terms, be explained by the combined forces of industrialization and modernization that pummeled the social fabric of Europe and North America during the 19th century. What actually happened within families was many times a combination of later age at marriage and a cessation of childbearing at progressively earlier marital durations (Ryder 1959: 411). While delayed marriage played an important role in some contexts, it was clear that families were also resorting to contraception in order to achieve their family size goals. As Coale (1969: 8) has noted, "the initial method of birth control was withdrawal or coitus interruptus." The use of this method requires awareness of its effectiveness and mechanism combined with a flexible attitude toward sexual intercourse that permits the interruption of the act. A strong commitment by the couple, especially by the male, to avoid another pregnancy is also essential (Santow 1993; Schneider and Schneider 1992). This points to an important element in these early efforts to control fertility: the active role of the male in reproductive decisions and behavior. Furthermore, besides withdrawal the other commonly used method was the condom, also a male method. Both methods require self-discipline and concentration: withdrawal at a critical preorgasmic moment and the condom either interrupting the sexual act or in preparation for it by placing the condom on the penis before insertion. Women had only very rudimentary alternatives, such as the insertion of sponges or douching after intercourse. In most settings, male dominance of fertility planning would see an abrupt end in the latter half of the 20th century with the appearance of new and more technologically sophisticated methods of contraception.

While the development of a secular, cogent attitude toward fertility planning was born in the industrializing North during the 19th century it later spread rapidly to the low-income areas of the South as modernization and mass media communications spread new ideas. The initial expansion of the notion that fertility planning was a feasible, positive measure was helped by early pamphleteers and controversies about them that gave birth control a great deal of publicity. These initial efforts planted the seed from which emerged today's large-scale family planning organizations that promote and assist countries in setting up effective networks of clinics and services.

Pioneers

England was the birthplace of the first locally organized movement to make public the advantages of fertility planning. Contraceptive availability at the time was scarce or nonexistent, the available methods were rudimentary, and the information poor or inaccurate. In effect there were few effective means by which couples could achieve their family size desires. In 1823, a series of publications known as "handbills" appeared with the intent of informing working people of the advantages of using coitus interruptus and sponges. Their authorship has been attributed to Francis Place, founder of the birth control movement in England. Conservative groups who labeled them as "diabolical handbills" immediately denounced them (Bogue 1969: 18). Half a century later, in 1876, also in England, a Mr. Bradlaugh and his friend, Mrs. Besant, published a pamphlet innocuously titled "The Fruits of Philosophy." This pamphlet openly advocated birth control and provided explicit details on the use of methods then available. A trial ensued as the Victorian morality was offended by the pamphleteers' open and explicit approach to the subject. Amid great publicity both authors were sentenced to six months' imprisonment. Although the sentence was not carried out, the "cause célèbre" nature of this trial contributed to the dissemination of birth control information and to the launching of national movements in Belgium, Australia, India, and the United States (Hodgson and Watkins 1997). In some ways, the commotion resulting from the opposition to "The Fruits of Philosophy" served to successfully expand the information and public debate on birth control in Europe and the United States, a situation akin to the controversies that Vatican opposition to the pill would cause 100 years later.

As in Europe, the discussion of fertility planning in the United States was the effort of visionary individuals who advocated the advantages of smaller families. Among the first to achieve wide notoriety in the promotion of contraception was Margaret Sanger, the founder of the American birth control movement and a leader in the intellectual battles about the meaning of population growth in the modern world. She organized the first World Population Conference, held in Geneva in 1927. The following year, with Raymond Pearl as President, she launched the International Union for the Scientific Study of Population—IUSSP—with headquarters in Paris (Bogue 1969: 28). She initiated what may be called a social movement for birth control, but she was also responsible for focusing the attention of academics and medical practitioners on the implications of runaway population growth. The IUSSP became instrumental in the promotion of academic research and also in the organization of world population conferences that attracted the attention of governments and international bodies. Surprising as it may seem, the resulting development of private voluntary family planning programs and international organizations to support them, such as the International Planned Parenthood Federation, were the outcome of individual initiatives, initially supported by liberal and forward looking philanthropies. It was not until the last half of the 20th century that governments became aware of the effects of rapid population growth and became the major proponents of fertility planning.

Technological Change

The contraceptive revolution that began in the 1960s greatly changed sexual behavior patterns and reproductive decision making within couples, giving women for the first time a fully reliable means to plan and control their fertility. However, discussion of contraception from a medical standpoint was not new. The first reference to methods to prevent births appeared in ancient Chinese medical texts, dating to around 2700 B.C. It is known that during the period of classical Greece and the Roman Empire, philosophers debated the issue of birth control. Soranus (98–138 A.D.), the greatest gynecologist of antiquity, wrote about contraceptives and their difference from abortifacients, describing a number of occlusive pessaries, vaginal plugs, and the use of astringent solutions (Taylor 1976: 324–325). Soranus's writings influenced western medical gynecological practice until well into the Middle Ages. But an important barrier emerged that impeded the spread of contraceptive knowledge and practice—the Catholic Church. St. Thomas Aquinas (1225–1274) declared contraception to be a vice against nature, an opinion which became the basis for the Church's prohibition of the use of contraception by its members. This prohibition became doctrine and was reaffirmed several times, most recently by Pope Paul VI, in his now famous encyclical *Humane Vitae*, issued in July 1968. *Humanae Vitae* was a product of the times, a response to the debate that emerged in the 1960s as a result of the scientific breakthrough that dramatically challenged the Church's position on birth control—the pill—coincidentally developed by a devout Catholic, John Rock.

When John Rock's first publications (with Pincus and Garcia) about the effectiveness of a contraceptive pill were issued in 1956 and 1958, a new era in reproductive behavior was set off. The pill revolutionized fertility planning: it greatly contributed to the separation of sexual behavior from reproductive outcomes, and women had available to them reliable means with which to effectively plan their childbearing. The pill was a female-controlled method that differed from previous options in that it was a pharmacological method. The pill contains steroid hormones that check the stimulation of the ovaries by setting in motion a feedback mechanism, which temporarily inhibits the secretion of hypothalamic releasing factors and gonadotropins to allow for cyclical activity. With combined and sequential contraceptives, the pills are omitted to allow for the monthly menstrual bleeding to take place. (For more details about the chemical action of the contraceptive pill see Taylor 1976: 381–399.)

The review of this new medical development by the U.S. Food and Drug Administration (FDA) generated great publicity. Rock was interviewed on every major television network, and stories of his scientific breakthrough appeared in *Time* and *Newsweek*. During the FDA review, one of the panel members suggested that the Vatican would never approve the contraceptive pill. John Rock quickly responded: "Young man, don't you sell my Church short" (Gladwell 2000: 52).

At the Vatican, Paul VI was engrossed in an internal controversy as his Pontifical Commission on Birth Control, which had been expected to complete its deliberations and to have made a recommendation by the time of the 1964 Belgrade Conference, and was not able to issue a definitive pronouncement. The Pontifical Commission was split in its views, but a majority of its members advocated a liberal position on birth control. At this juncture, the Pope had a unique opportunity to resolve the issue of contraception by accepting the Commission's majority opinion that supported a more tolerant Church position. Instead, he decided to side with the more conservative Vatican elements that opposed artificial contraception. The conservative forces won the battle, and contraception was condemned as sinful, except when practiced by abstention during the fertile period of the menstrual cycle, i.e., the rhythm method. Paul VI made public his encyclical *Humanae Vitae* in 1968, a document that caused great consternation among Catholics the world over. In the years preceding its publication, speculation among Catholics was that the Vatican would take a more laissez-faire attitude on this issue. As Gary Wills (2000: 87) has noted: "Paul VI's actions in the years leading to Humanae Vitae looked so contradictory as to seem perverse." Paul VI's decision was influenced by his own view of the papacy and how history would see him:

> The Pope was a man obviously torn by doubts, tormented by scruples, haunted by thoughts of perfection, and above all dominated by an exaggerated concern—some called it an obsession—about the prestige of his office as Pope. (Wills 2000: 94)

The Catholic Church, having reaffirmed its traditional opposition to birth control, became in some regions an important influence on the government attitudes and policies on family planning. At the very least, the Church's position led to heated debates on fertility planning in countries with a significant Catholic population. It also greatly undermined John Rock's hope that the pill would come to be seen as a natural way to regulate human fertility by acting on the body's hormonal makeup.

The invention of the pill was soon followed by the development of other highly effective methods of contraception. These included injectables, the IUD, and eventually progestin-only pills, subdermal implants, and the levonorgestrel IUD. Perhaps equally important was the development of simplified and effective methods for performing female and male sterilization. The development, testing, and regulatory approval of these and other methods of contraception have involved an enormous amount of effort and funding from both the public and private sectors in countries around the world. We will examine what is known about the use of both modern and more traditional methods of contraception in the following section.

RESEARCH FINDINGS

The combination of increased concern for population growth, the growing availability of effective contraception, and the rapid implementation of service programs around the world gave rise to a massive and unusually well-coordinated international effort to collect survey data on fertility and contraceptive use. The first fertility surveys were conducted in the United States and Europe, but they were soon followed in the 1960s by surveys in developing countries to assess both the use of and the demand for contraception. The early rounds of these surveys, often referred to as KAP (for knowledge, attitude, and practice) surveys, were carried out by or on behalf of private family planning organizations but often with support from international organizations, including the Population Council and United Nations agencies such as the Latin American Demographic Center (CELADE).

In the mid-1970s, an ambitious effort to collect and analyze data on reproductive practices, the World Fertility Survey (WFS), was launched under the auspices of the International Statistics Institute. Headquartered in London, the WFS was responsible for carrying out surveys in 61 countries between 1975 and 1986 (Gille 1987). These surveys all used a common core questionnaire that permitted comparative analysis. The project was funded by USAID and the UNFPA, had a staff of 50 to 60 professionals led by Sir Maurice Kendall, and involved the participation of leading demographers from around the world. The WFS was followed by further international survey projects, most notably the Contraceptive Prevalence Surveys (CPS) and the Demographic and Health Surveys (DHS) that were funded by USAID and headquartered in the United States (Anderson and Cleland 1984; Fisher and Way 1988; Zlidar et al. 2003). As of this writing, DHS has provided technical assistance for more than 170 surveys in 69 countries throughout Africa, Asia, the Near East, Latin America, and the Caribbean. Another important series of surveys was carried out at the U.S. Centers for Disease Control and Prevention (CDC). The CDC Division of Reproductive Health conducted 35 surveys in 25 countries between 1985 and 2000 (Morris 2000). In addition to these internationally sponsored surveys, some countries carried out their own surveys, sometimes on an even larger scale, as was the case in China and Mexico.

While there has been some argument as to how much all the data collected by these surveys has contributed to knowledge concerning the social and economic determinants of fertility (Caldwell 1985; Davis 1987), there is no doubt they have provided an accurate and detailed accounting of three of the four main "proximate determinants" of fertility, including contraceptive practice, breast-feeding, and marriage during the course of the fertility transitions that have taken place during the last three or four decades (Bongaarts 1982). They have also yielded comparable estimates of the shifts in ideal family size and the prevalence of unwanted fertility (Westoff 1988a, 1988b). The one area where survey research has often failed to produce reliable estimates is with respect to abortion, both spontaneous and induced, especially in those countries where abortion is sanctioned on either moral or legal grounds.

Due to the vast amount of survey data collected since the 1960s, it is possible to obtain a fairly accurate assessment of the changes in the patterns of contraceptive use, as well as in the changes in fertility over nearly a half century. Figure 24.1 presents an

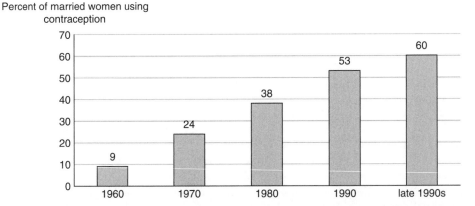

FIGURE 24.1. Contraceptive use in less developed countries 1960 to late 1990s. Source: Population References Bureau and the United Nations Population Division.

overview of the dramatic growth in contraceptive prevalence in less developed countries (LDCs), based on United Nations estimates. Estimates of the Total Fertility Rate (TFR), as well as of the percentage of married women currently using any contraceptive method as well as the percentage using a modern contraceptive method, are shown for the major regions and subregions of the world in Table 24.1. At the turn of the century the prevalence of contraceptive use in LDCs was 60% as compared to 68% in more developed countries (MDCs). The corresponding levels of the TFR in 2002 were estimated to be 1.6 in MDCs and 3.1 in LDCs.

While Table 24.1 shows a reasonably small difference in contraceptive prevalence between MDCs and LDCs, there are striking differences among LDC regions in both the TFR and contraceptive prevalence. For example, the TFR for sub-Saharan Africa remains high at 5.6, and the contraceptive prevalence rate is low at 19%. The corresponding figures for Asia are 2.6% and 64%, and for Latin America and the Caribbean, 2.7% and 70%. And, of course, within these major regions there are further differences among subregions and even greater differences across countries. Nevertheless, these TFRs and contraceptive prevalence rates show that, with the exception of sub-Saharan

TABLE 24.1. Fertility and contraceptive use: 2002, main world regions

Region	Total Fertility Rate	Percent Married Women Using Contraception: All Methods	Modern Methods
World	2.8	61	55
More Developed	1.6	68	58
Less Developed	3.1	60	54
Less Developed excl.China	3.5	48	41
Africa	5.2	26	20
Sub-Saharan Africa	5.6	19	13
Northern Africa	3.5	49	43
Western Africa	5.8	14	8
Eastern Africa	5.7	21	16
Middle Africa	6.4	11	4
Southern Africa	3.1	53	52
North America	2.1	76	71
Latin America & Caribbean	2.7	70	62
Central America incl.Mexico	3.1	65	57
Caribbean	2.6	61	57
South America	2.5	74	65
Asia	2.6	64	59
Asia excl. China	3.1	52	44
Western Asia	3.9	51	30
South Central Asia	3.3	49	42
Southeast Asia	2.7	57	50
East Asia	1.7	82	81
Europe	1.4	67	52
Northern Europe	1.6	70	67
Western Europe	1.5	77	73
Eastern Europe	1.2	64	42
Southern Europe	1.3	64	47
Oceania	2.5	59	56

Source: Population Reference Bureau. 2002 Population Data Sheet.

Africa, fertility is now well below and in many cases less than half what it was 30 years ago, and the use of contraception, particularly modern contraception, is now widespread.

While the trend toward the adoption of contraception and reduced fertility has been almost universal, the actual methods of contraception practiced in different countries vary widely. The magnitude of this variation can be seen in Table 24.2, which shows contraceptive use by method for 31 countries selected from among those for which the United Nations and the Population Reference Bureau have compiled this information (United Nations 2002; Population Reference Bureau 2002). The percentages refer to use of contraception by married women of childbearing age and are from the most recent available survey. The percentages highlighted in bold print are for the most prevalent method, methods for which the prevalence is 60% of that of the most prevalent method, or simply a method with a prevalence greater than 10%. While the countries have been selected to show the diversity in world experience, the picture of substantial differences in method mix is nonetheless representative of the larger universe of data. So too is the tendency in many of the countries for the bulk of contraceptive use to be concentrated on one or two methods rather than being spread over a larger number.

It is clear that the most prevalent methods are not the same across these countries. For example, while female sterilization is an important (highlighted) method in 19 of the countries shown in Table 24.1, its prevalence is below 5% in eight of the countries, all of which have a relatively large percentage (over 50%) of married women practicing contraception. Male sterilization is less frequently practiced than female sterilization in all of these 31 countries but is an important method in South Korea and the United States. Other methods also show a wide range in prevalence: the pill from less than 2% in four countries to more than 20% in seven countries, reaching a maximum of 47% in Belgium. Use of injectables varies from 23% in South Africa to very low figures in 18 countries, the condom from 43% in Japan to less than 3% in 11 countries, vaginal barrier methods are used by more than 5% of married women only in Japan and Indonesia, rhythm is practiced by over 10% of married women in Sri Lanka, Vietnam, and Peru. And, finally, withdrawal is the most widely practiced method in Turkey and Romania.

While there are certain patterns in the data on use of particular methods, they do not yield easy generalizations. There is often a substantial variation in the method mix within a particular region. For example, the pill is the most widely used method in Thailand but is little used in South Korea. The method mix for the latter is dominated by female sterilization and condom, whereas in North Korea, the IUD is by far the most widely used method. Likewise, there is no consistent variation in the types of methods used in a country according to either the level of fertility or development. Finally, though not shown in the table, a prospective view of the evolution of contraceptive use through time based on earlier surveys shows little consistent variation. If anything, a country's method mix tends to become narrower rather than wider as the use of contraception increases through time.

Of course, each of these societies has a particular history, culture, medical system, and set of relations with other societies, and explanations for the individual patterns can be sought in those particularities. For example, Bulut et al. (1997) look, albeit unsuccessfully, for an explanation of the high use of withdrawal in Turkey in terms of the reproductive morbidity experienced in the population. Goldberg and Serbanescu (1995) have considered how the economic and political history of Romania and the Czech Republic account for the low use of modern methods in those countries. But perhaps the most intriguing is Coleman's (1981) study of the factors underlying the high use of condoms in Japan. He ends up suggesting that "a large proportion of Japanese married couples who are using condoms are not particularly pleased with the method" (1981: 36) and that "Japanese couples' extensive reliance on condoms results largely from the unavailability of other methods, in a cultural context of embarrassment and passivity toward contraception" (1981: 29). In an era of globalization in which goods and ideas are thought to travel more freely than ever before, however, the variation found in Table 24.2 seems anomalous. How could assessments of the convenience or effectiveness of the different methods vary so widely? Programs promoting the use of certain methods could, of course, have an influence, and we will come back to the topic of how this surely occurred in both China and Mexico. But, neither program influence nor laws restricting access to particular methods, such as the restrictions the medical profession placed on hormonal contraception in Japan, could account for a large portion of the variation shown in Table 24.2.

TABLE 24.2. **Percent of Married Women of Reproductive Age using Contraception, by Method, Latest Survey, Selected Countries**

Country and year	Female steriliza-tion	Male steriliza-tion	Pill	Injectable	IUD	Condom	Vaginal barrier	Rhythm	With-drawal	Any method
Africa										
Egypt 2000	1.4	–	9.5	6.1	**35.5**	1.0	0.4	0.6	0.2	56.1
Cabo Verde 1998	**12.8**	0.0	**18.2**	7.7	4.3	3.0	0.1	4.9	2.0	52.9
Kenya 1998	6.2	–	**8.5**	**11.8**	2.7	1.3	0.8	6.1	0.6	39.0
South Africa 1998	**15.8**	2.1	**10.6**	**23.2**	1.8	1.7	0.0	0.3	0.6	56.1
Asia										
Jordan 1997	4.2	–	6.5	0.7	**23.1**	2.4	0.6	4.9	7.6	52.6
Turkey 1998	4.2	0.0	4.4	0.5	**19.8**	8.2	0.6	1.1	**24.4**	63.9
Bangladesh 1999–00	6.7	0.5	**23.0**	7.2	1.2	4.3	0.5	5.4	4.0	53.8
India 1998–99	**34.2**	1.9	2.1	–	1.6	3.1	–	3.0	2.0	48.2
Kazakhstan 1999	2.8	0.0	2.4	0.6	**42.0**	4.5	0.4	4.6	2.9	66.1
Nepal 2001	**15.0**	6.3	1.6	8.4	0.4	2.9	0.6	1.1	2.6	39.0
Sri Lanka 1993	**23.5**	3.7	5.5	4.5	3.0	3.3	0.0	**15.2**	5.0	66.1
Indonesia 1997	3.0	0.4	**15.4**	**21.1**	8.1	0.7	6.0	1.1	0.8	57.4
Philippines 2000	**10.6**	0.2	**13.7**	2.5	3.3	1.3	0.5	9.5	4.8	47.0
Thailand 1996–97	**22.0**	2.0	**23.1**	**16.4**	3.2	1.8	1.3	–	–	72.2
Vietnam 2001	5.7	0.4	7.4	0.5	**41.2**	5.8	0.1	**12.4**	–	73.9
Hong Kong 1992	**18.9**	0.9	**17.1**	1.7	5.1	**34.5**	1.5	5.1	1.5	86.2
China 1997	**33.5**	7.7	1.7	0.4	**36.4**	3.4	0.2	–	–	83.8
Japan 2000	3.0	0.6	0.8	–	1.5	**43.1**	6.1	3.7	**15.3**	55.9
Korea, North 1990-92	4.1	0.3	0.1	0.0	**48.5**	0.0	0.0	8.9	0.0	61.8
Korea, South 1997	**24.1**	**12.7**	1.8	–	**13.2**	**15.1**	–	–	–	80.5
Latin America & Caribbean										
Brazil 1996	**40.1**	2.6	**20.7**	1.2	1.1	4.4	0.1	3.0	3.1	76.4
Colombia 2000	**27.1**	1.0	**11.8**	4.0	**12.4**	6.1	1.7	6.0	6.3	76.2
Dominican Rep. 1996	**40.9**	0.1	**12.9**	1.1	2.5	1.4	0.3	1.8	1.9	63.7
El Salvador 1998	**32.4**	–	8.1	8.9	1.5	2.5	0.7	3.1	2.6	59.7

(Continued)

TABLE 24.2. (*Continued*)

Country and year	Female steriliza- tion	Male steriliza- tion	Pill	Injectable	IUD	Condom	Vaginal barrier	Rhythm	With- drawal	Any method
Mexico 1997	**30.6**	1.2	6.9	3.2	**14.2**	3.8	–	–	–	68.5
Peru 2000	**12.3**	0.5	6.7	**14.8**	9.1	5.6	1.5	**14.4**	3.2	68.0
Oceania										
Australia 1995	**12.8**	9.7	**26.7**	–	2.0	**11.7**	1.7	2.0	–	66.7
North America										
United States 1995	**23.8**	**13.2**	**15.6**	1.4	0.7	**13.3**	3.6	2.3	2.3	76.4
Europe										
Belgium 1991–92	**10.9**	7.0	**46.7**	–	5.0	4.7	0.1	2.1	2.0	78.4
France 1998		8.5	**38.0**	–	**21.2**	5.3	0.9	–	–	79.5
Czech Republic 1997	7.2	–	**23.2**	–	**13.9**	12.7	0.7	1.7	7.3	67.0
Romania 1999	2.5	–	7.9	–	7.3	8.5	3.3	5.6	**28.7**	63.8

Source: United Nations Population Division, World Contraceptive Use 2001 (ST/ESA/SER. A/210); Population Reference Bureau, Family Planning WorldWide 2002 Data Sheet.

The social process through which individuals and couples in a society come to rely on certain contraceptive methods and reject the use of others is not well understood. However, it is clear that this is a domain in which the past matters and in which uncertainty and misinformation can play important roles. Throughout, but especially in the early stages of the adoption process, it is common for potential users of a method to be concerned about the health consequences of the methods available to them. Fear that a method will be damaging to one's health can range from "scientifically founded" concerns, such as those of contracting pelvic inflammatory disease from using the IUD, to worries that a method will prove to be life threatening based on lay conceptions of how the body works and/or rumors circulating in the community. Because of these concerns, medical advice and counseling play a key role in the adoption process (Potter 1999). Moreover, it is highly likely that because of the difficulty of knowing a great deal about a large number of methods, potential users tend to pay attention to, and be influenced by, what other people they know are doing to prevent pregnancy and how that practice or method has worked out for them. This tendency to follow rather than lead is also common among the doctors, nurses, and others who may prescribe or counsel regarding contraception.

Because both users and providers are influenced by what their peers are doing, the choices that a society makes early on in the transition tend to be self-reinforcing. Users not only find it easier to learn about the methods that are most widely practiced, but they probably find these same methods the easiest to obtain. Providers also have more information available about, and readier access to, frequently used methods. Moreover, they also have more experience with the requisite procedures and with monitoring the possible side effects. Last but not least, doing what others are doing in a given situation is the best defense against any possible claim of malpractice (Phelps 1992). In such a path-dependent system, it is not clear that the best technologies will always win out or that a potential user will really have much choice regarding which method to use in a given situation. Rather, the same learning through social networks that tends to speed the adoption of contraception in a community will also lead to a socially prescribed or influenced set of choices regarding method (Bongaarts and Watkins 1996; Potter 1999). In many countries, programs to promote the use of contraception were part and parcel of the process leading to increased use of modern contraception and a particular method mix.

IMPLEMENTATION STRATEGIES

The Logics for Intervention

After World War II, the world's population increased substantially, mostly as a result of the decline in death rates in poor countries. As awareness of this change grew in the 1950s and 1960s, population was often portrayed as a serious crisis threatening economic growth in the less developed regions of the world. However, then as now, the arguments in favor of governments adopting specific policies to reduce fertility and promote contraceptive practice have proven controversial. The remarkable aspect of this enduring discussion is that the challenges to neo-Malthusian logics have emerged from quite different quarters over the last four decades.

The link between academic arguments and government actions to reduce population growth has never been particularly tight, and it is likely that many population policies were adopted out of sheer astonishment at the fact or prospect of increasing numbers. Nevertheless, as developing countries began to adopt fertility planning policies, they felt the need to explain them internally to their political constituencies and to the public at large. One of the earliest and most influential arguments for reducing fertility was published in *Population Growth and Economic Development in Low-Income Countries* by Ansley J. Coale and Edgar M. Hoover (1958). Coale (1969: 22) had concluded that "rapid growth does tend to diminish the amount of capital available for increasing the average productivity of the work force and increasing the average per capita income [of the citizenry]." He went to assert that: "Any low-income country that succeeds in initiating an immediate reduction in fertility would in the short run enjoy a reduction in the burden of child dependency that would permit a higher level of investment and more immediately productive uses of investment" (Coale 1969: 84). In short, rapid population growth hindered the economic prospects in low-income, largely agrarian societies. It also condemned families to an endless cycle of poverty. Coale (1969: 333) concluded that: "Without regard to the question of how many people can be fed with given agricultural resources, it is clear that a reduction of fertility from high levels has immediate economic advantages.... The economic advantages of reduced fertility thus begin immediately and cumulate for an indefinite period into the future." In a couple of generations, countries that adhered to this advice and reduced fertility could double the income per capita of the population through personal and public savings that could be applied to economic investments and to health and educational improvements. Coale and Hoover's book ended with a careful analysis of India's situation at mid-20th century and a somewhat less detailed examination of Mexico, both reaching the same conclusion: fertility decline would lead to improved economic prospects.

Coale and Hoover's measured message was accompanied by a number of more strident arguments that urged countries to act quickly to reduce population growth. Zero Population Growth advocates blamed the United States for the size and growth rate of its population and the attendant impact on global pollution and environmental decay. Paul Ehrlich published his popular book, *The Population Bomb,* in 1968, which contributed to making "the population problem" a topic of general public debate. Furthermore, other important analyses were coming out from major scientific and policy groups: the American Assembly had issued *The Population Dilemma* (1963) and the Club of Rome was preparing its ambitious report, *The Limits to Growth* (1974). The International Conference on Family Planning Programs, sponsored by the Population Council and the Ford Foundation in 1965, led to *Family Planning and Population Programs,* an edited volume (Berelson et al. 1966) reviewing the population situation in many countries around the world. Some intellectuals and advocates of a New International Economic Order (NIEO) were reluctant to accept the notion that population was, by itself, an impending crisis and rejected neo-Malthusian claims that portrayed family planning and the reduction of demographic growth as a panacea for intractable social ills. These critics argued for the need for structural change as a solution to population issues in the developing world, and denounced international efforts supported by the United States to implement family planning programs in third world countries. The largest and most important forum where the conflicting points of view met head on was the World Population Conference (WPC) held in Bucharest, Romania, in 1974.

The WPC was the first major intergovernmental meeting on this topic organized by the United Nations. Three different views of the impact of population on development were presented: "Asian and European countries, along with the US, took the position that rapid population growth intensified problems of economic and social development and therefore merited urgent attention...[M]any Latin American and African countries...expressed the view that population was not an important variable in development [while] another group of countries argued that population growth was desirable" (Singh 1998: 8). Remarkably, amidst these differing positions coupled with concerns regarding the injustices in the world economic system, it proved possible to forge a consensus document, the World Population Plan of Action (WPPA), which recognized that connections between population and development might vary across settings, but established the right of couples to decide freely and responsibly on the number of their offspring and advocated the integration of population into social and economic planning (Finkle and Crane 1975).

The WPPA served as a legitimate basis for generating international support for family planning programs among rich countries and for adopting population policies to address high fertility in a considerable number of poor countries. The United States had hoped for an even stronger statement that would have recognized the need to establish "national goals together with a world goal of replacement level fertility by the year 2000," a phrase that had been used by Caspar Weinberger, the head of the U.S. delegation (Singh 1998: 11). This was also a time when support for international family planning enjoyed bipartisan support in the Congress. Lyndon Johnson was the first U.S. president to endorse the logic for efforts to reduce population growth in poor countries, but support for these efforts was also strong in the succeeding Nixon and Ford administrations.

By the time of the next United Nations–sponsored conference on population, held in Mexico City in 1984, there had been a radical change in the U.S. position on population growth and support for family planning programs. The Reagan administration had moved away from the view that world population growth was an urgent issue and toward the position that population was a neutral phenomenon. This shift was consonant with the "revisionist" findings of a number of academic studies that would be incorporated in a study by the U.S. National Academy of Sciences, *Population Growth and Economic Development: Policy Questions* (Committee on Population 1986). It also fit well with the administration's increasing involvement in domestic politics regarding abortion. James Buckley, a conservative senator, was appointed head of the U.S. delegation to the Mexico City conference, where he downplayed the importance of population growth, emphasized the importance of free markets for economic prosperity, and signaled that the U.S. would not allow any support that it provided for fertility planning to finance or support abortion.

While the Mexico City conference covered some new ground and demonstrated the increasing commitment of developing countries to national policies related to population and family planning, it basically served to reaffirm the WPPA adopted in Bucharest (Finkle and Crane 1985). By the time of the next United Nations–sponsored conference, enough changes had taken place regarding the way that policies related to fertility planning were viewed that it was decided that an entirely new program of action should be considered for adoption at the International Conference on Population and Development (ICPD), which was to be held in Cairo in 1994 (Finkle and McIntosh 1995). Not the least of these changes was the rise of feminism anticipated by Stycos (1971).

Feminism brought a rationale to the population debate that was entirely different from the earlier logic: the impact that reducing fertility would have on economic development. Rather, it called for attention to women's health and for the integration of maternal and child health services. It also began to look into the legal aspects of reproductive matters (Dixon-Mueller 1993; Cook 1989) and to argue for the rights of women to health, choice, and self-determination. From the start, feminist groups had questioned the focus on women as instruments of demographic policy. Feminists also claimed that most family planning programs only paid attention to women's contraceptive needs without considering their related health needs, and that contraceptives given without medical supervision exposed women to unnecessary health risks (Seltzer 2002). Consequently a new justification for family planning based on health took hold that would eventually evolve into an entirely new way of conceptualizing fertility planning. The name adopted for this approach was reproductive health, a term that had been used by WHO for some years but which had never been formally approved by any U.N. body (Singh 1998). There was an extensive set of prior discussions that preceded the ICPD concerning the new logic for fertility planning, and the discussion continued through the conference itself. In these discussions, the United States had again radically shifted its position and was at the forefront of the initiative to revamp and reinvigorate international attention to population issues. The principal opponents of the changes being proposed were the Holy See, nations strongly allied with the Vatican, and some Islamic countries that maintained conservative positions regarding women's rights.

The reproductive health concept that was finally embodied in the ICPD programme of action linked human rights, women's health, and fertility planning into one overarching paradigm. There were four elements that distinguished this statement from earlier ones:

1. Fertility planning should be integrated within a wider set of services related to sexual and reproductive health, including the treatment of sexually transmitted

diseases (STDs), the reduction of maternal mortality, and the promotion of maternal health; these services should address the needs of both men and adolescents as well as women.

2. Demographic targets and quotas for the recruitment of new contraceptive acceptors were no longer acceptable components of population policy.

3. The empowerment of women and gender equality were paramount.

4. NGOs should play an important role in providing reproductive health services since they often have a comparative advantage in comparison with governments based on their more direct involvement in grassroots movements, informal organizations, and networks (Singh 1998).

Much has been made of the 1994 Cairo Conference. It has been said to have "codified views long advocated by women's health activists the world over. Their humanistic and feminist goals became cornerstones of Cairo's landmark accord, which recognized the rights of all people to reproductive health, called for special attention to women's empowerment and to clients' needs, and repudiated reliance on contraceptive services as the tool for achieving demographic targets" (Haberland and Measham 2002: 1; United Nations 1994). As we enter the 21st century, the concept of reproductive health has become widely accepted as a guiding tool to design service programs, to fine tune population policies, and to expand demographic research to areas formerly the exclusive domain of epidemiologists. For the research community, it has brought new and tough challenges, particularly to generate appropriate information on a variety of women's illnesses, including reproductive tract infections, which is needed to assist government planners in the design and implementation of effective services to deal with these issues. For program administrators, it has meant reformulating goals and developing new ways to assess progress.

Paradoxically, during the years following the Cairo ICPD, new evidence has been assembled showing that fertility decline can, and often does, have an important impact on economic development. Indeed, a considerable fraction of the salutary economic performance of the countries of Southeast Asia and East Asia since the 1960s has recently been attributed to the "demographic dividend" that resulted from the shifts in the age distribution that resulted from the steep fertility declines in those regions (Bloom and Williamson 1998; Bloom, Canning, and Malaney 2000). The new analyses place less emphasis on population growth as a whole and much more on the dependency ratio, which is temporarily depressed by fertility decline before it ultimately results in a proportionate increase in the proportion of elderly. One of the main questions posed by this perspective is whether the fertility declines that began in the 1970s in Latin America will yield an equally positive contribution to economic performance, or whether the Asian success story was due to a series of policies and contextual factors that are not likely to exist in other regions.

Implemention Strategies: Case Studies

India pioneered fertility planning policies by establishing a national family planning program in 1952. Since then family planning programs and policies designed to improve and provide access to contraceptive methods have increased substantially. In 1976 there were 94 countries providing direct support to family planning services; 10 years later the number had increased to 116, with another 23 providing indirect support (through nongovernmental agencies), and by the end of the 20th century those numbers had increased to 145 and 34, respectively. Only 14 countries remained that provided no support for contraceptive services to their populations. African countries that were slower in adopting family planning policies had made, toward the end of the 1990s, an impressive gain: 50 of 53 countries were providing contraceptive services to their people (Seltzer 2002: 17).

CHINA.   China's birth planning program is one of the most successful and the most controversial effort to introduce modern contraception to a huge population. It was designated to reduce fertility to below replacement levels within the relatively short span of three decades. What led to the adoption of this fertility planning policy? How has it evolved through time? What will be its future in an international environment in which there is greater concern for human rights than for controlling population growth?

In 1970, the total fertility rate of China was 5.75 children per woman, a very high level for a country that at the time had 800 million people, relatively low levels of mortality, and very low per capita income (U.N. 1973: 112). The country was recovering from the devastation of years of misguided and erratic industrial and social policies, many of which had failed. The Great Leap Forward (1959 to 1961) was a disastrous industrialization drive that nearly destroyed the agricultural basis of the country and led to rapid deterioration of living standards, coupled with famines, high mortality, and a temporary reduction of fertility. The Cultural Revolution (1965 to 1975) led to an increase in fertility and social chaos, as many of the professional elites, including teachers, physicians, and other people with high technical capacity were sent to work in the countryside. As China emerged from these difficult times, its leadership began to consider the reality of its population size and the implications of continued rapid population growth for the future development of the nation.

China's effort to reduce its population growth by lowering its fertility was set in motion in 1971 when the State Council issued its first comprehensive population policy (State Directive No. 51), which soon became known by its slogan: *wan xi shao* (later [pregnancies]—longer [intervals]—fewer [children]). Although voluntary, the campaign included strong material incentives for limiting family size and was vigorously promoted throughout the politico-organizational structure of China, from central committees to grassroots levels (Mundigo 1992). By 1979, the goals of the policy were drastically refined when the government launched the "one-child family policy" to sharply limit fertility (Greenhalgh 1986, 1992). The policy evolved rapidly from a voluntary to a compulsory phase in which pregnancies that were not authorized had to be terminated, which rapidly increased abortion rates throughout the country (Mundigo 1992, 1999). This one-child policy became an integral component of China's development plans, deemed essential to the achievement of the "four modernizations" (industry, agriculture, science/technology, and defense).

Using societal goals as justification, China in 1982 and 1983 once again strengthened its birth planning policy requiring women with one child to have an IUD inserted; sterilization became mandatory for families with two or more children. In 1983, despite widespread resistance (Greenhalgh 1992), a massive nationwide sterilization campaign was undertaken during which an estimated 20 million women and men were sterilized. Fines and losses of privileges were imposed on couples who did not comply with the policy. The new penalties had a strong effect, which overshadowed long-held beliefs about the economic benefits of having a large family. Still exempted from the policy at this time were ethnic minorities with populations under 10 million living in their native regions (Rigdon 1996), some rural community groups, and people living in harsh environments, such as mountains. These groups were given flexibility with regard to family size but usually two children was the limit; only in very exceptional situations was a third birth allowed.

In 1984, the government issued Central Document No.7, which provided details on when and where flexibility was to be exercised, which couples could have a second birth, and which condemned abuses in the implementation of the policy by local cadres. Document No. 7 had opened "a small hole to close up a large one," allowing second births among rural families with "practical difficulties" as long as the second child did not compromise local plans and targets, nor the achievement of population stabilization at 1.2 billion people advocated by the central government (Greenhalgh 1986:492). As a greater a number of births than expected resulted, the government issued Central Document No. 13 in 1986, closing some of the loopholes that had been created by Document No. 7 and, once again, tightening the policy (Li et al. 1990). These various changes included strengthening the organizational structure of the cadres responsible for the effective implementation of the birth planning program and issuing detailed regulations to set up administrative units in every commune, neighborhood, factory, or production brigade. In production brigades, a leader was designated as the person responsible for monitoring birth planning activities within the unit.

In the early 1990s, the policy was once again modified and strengthened: exemptions allowed to the minorities no longer applied and conditions allowing people to have a second child were clarified. In May 1991, the Central Committee of the Communist Party and the State Council issued a new document called "Decision on Strengthening Birth Planning Work and Strictly Controlling Population Growth" that reflected the continuing efforts of Chinese policy makers to fine-tune the policy. It called for greater attention to implementing the policy in rural areas, where it had faltered because of flexible regulations and the reluctance of local cadres to monitor the program by pressuring their fellow villagers (Greenhalgh, Chuzhu, and Nan 1994: 366). The importance of population policy remained undiminished in the 1990s, as is reflected in a 1993 speech by Mme. Peng Peiyun, Minister-in-Charge of the State Birth Planning Commission, in which she announced the decline in China's birth rate (Peiyun 1993: 402):

1. While focusing our main efforts on accelerating the development of the national economy, we must continue to carry out the birth planning program more effectively to control population growth, improve the quality of human resources, and thus create a favorable population environment for the construction of socialist modernization.
2. We should abide by the principle of the 'three no-changes,' that is, the present family planning policy should not be changed, the target already set for controlling population growth should not be changed, and the practice for top leaders of the Communist Party organizations and governments at all levels to be personally in charge of the family planning program should not be changed.

Needless to say, China's authoritarian, forceful, and demographically oriented approach to fertility planning was, by the early 1990s, completely out of step with the developments taking place in the international community during the preparations for the Cairo ICPD. The program was drawing increasing amounts of criticism, not only from feminists but also from conservatives who used the Chinese case to discredit international family planning efforts and organizations. Within China, partly as a result of the substantial relaxation of government control of people's daily lives that came with the move toward a more open market-oriented society, there was increasing concern for the difficulties that arose in administering the program, for the abuses it generated, and for the consequences that continued below-replacement level fertility would have for the age distribution (Kaufman 2003). From the time of the ICPD until the present, considerable efforts to experiment with ways to reform the program have been undertaken, and there are indications, but no guarantee, that these reforms will be extended in the future.

One problem stemming from the strict limitations on the number of births incorporated in the Chinese policy was the heavy toll on the treatment and survival of baby girls in areas where son preference was still strong. Moreover, thanks to the widespread availability of ultrasound machines at county and township hospitals and family planning clinics, there was a burgeoning amount of sex-selective abortion in spite of regulations forbidding using the technology for this purpose. Another type of abuse had to do with the collection of fines for excess births, which became an important source of revenue for local governments, with local officials sometimes encouraging excess births so that they could proceed to collect the corresponding fines (Erli 2001).

Perhaps the main innovation that has been introduced in the Chinese program since 1990 is the concept of informed choice of contraceptives (*zhixing xuanzi*) (Kaufman, Erli, Kaining, and Zhenming 2003). This was first implemented in the course of a project to introduce several new long-term contraceptives, including Norplant and a late-model IUD (Ping 1995, cited in Kaufman et al. 2003). Following the Cairo ICPD, two major experimental projects were launched in China to test the viability of new models of service delivery that relied on meeting people's reproductive health needs rather than enforcing contraceptive practice. One of these was developed within China's State Family Planning Commission, while the other was funded by the UNFPA with the stipulation that birth planning targets had to be suspended in the 32 experimental counties in which the project was to be undertaken. The project developed by the State Family Planning Commission was initiated in 1995 in six carefully chosen counties and cities on the more highly developed east coast, and was later expanded to 11 counties by the end of 1997, to 200 by 1998, and over 800 in early 2000 (Kaufman et al. 2003). In this project the goals were to expand the range and quality of services provided by family planning clinics and to demonstrate that realigning the family planning program with people's needs and interests would not result in additional births.

While these projects have proven to be highly successful, they have also encountered resistance within the larger government bureaucracy charged with implementing China's birth planning policy. Recent legislative decisions in China underscore the continued importance of fertility planning in the context of internal and international changes. The March 2000 decision set out the rationale for the Chinese birth planning effort into the 21st century, asserting the need to continue efforts to limit population growth with specific goals for the decade 2000 to 2010. The 2001 Law "legalizes institutions for the state planning of population and births and at the same time places legal restraints on them" (Winckler 2002: 393). For the birth planning program, it specifies program incentives, expanded health services, and legal responsibilities, in each case balancing state power and citizen protection. Citizens are rewarded for keeping to the letter of the law and officials are punished if they fail to comply with its mandate. Article 19 of the law makes clear that another objective is to minimize the use of abortion. Sterilization, although not mentioned, is implicitly included as a voluntary option. Citizens who do not comply with the law are expected to pay a "social compensation fee," which is equivalent to the cost to society for bearing an additional child not authorized under current legislation. Generally speaking, the 2001 law has set a course for the Chinese birth planning program that pays increased attention to the Cairo recommendations and to the need for comprehensive reproductive health services. Program officials have received special training on the scope of reproductive health services, including sexual health. Men are increasingly objects of program attention (there was a Men's Health Day in 2000) and there is also greater concern with the spread of HIV/AIDS. These enormous changes show recognition by Chinese authorities that the future of the program, as it becomes increasingly market oriented and voluntaristic, depends on responding to the real needs of the Chinese citizenry.

MEXICO.   Mexico's population in the early 1970s was among the fastest growing in the world. The TFR was near seven, its crude birth rate exceeded 40 births per thousand population, and the population growth rate was about 3.5% per annum. Mexico's population in 1940 was 20 million, and by 1970 it had more than doubled to 50 million. During the intervening decades, optimism about the future, a growing industrial infrastructure, urbanization, and gains in the amount of land under cultivation had sustained a pro-growth ideology that included demographic expansionism. A General Law of Population, adopted in 1947, encapsulated the government's pronatalist attitude advocating universal marriage and promoting large families. Moreover, before 1970, contraception was not easily available (the sale of contraceptives was illegal until 1973), and government family planning services were nonexistent. Two private associations with limited outreach offered family planning services, the Association Pro-Maternal Health, founded in 1959, and the Foundation for Population Studies (FEPAC), an International Planned Parenthood Federation affiliate that started in 1965 (Aparicio 1988: 27).

But by the early 1970s, the economic model upon which Mexico had so successfully relied since the 1930s was showing clear signs of strain and no longer seemed able to accommodate the rapidly increasing population. Agricultural production had slowed, and the amount of land available for expanding cultivation was nearly exhausted. For the first time Mexico had to import basic staple foods and grains. Mexico's public sector expenditures rose rapidly, and the government began to use foreign loans to compensate for the loss in domestic revenue as production in most sectors lagged. Urban marginality and rural unemployment or underemployment threatened existing social stability, with the disadvantaged sectors growing rapidly in proportions, particularly in larger urban agglomerations (Alba and Potter 1986).

With the publication of the results of the 1970 census, demographic data became available in Mexico in the early 1970s that both facilitated and hardened population projections. These all indicated that even if fertility were to be reduced over the coming decades, the population would double within 20 years—this at a time when it was estimated that at least two million Mexicans were permanently unemployed (Cabrera 1972). In fact, the earlier projections prepared by Benitez-Zenteno and Cabrera (1966) had been instrumental in alerting government officials to the implications of the demographic situation and in setting in motion debate on this issue in Mexico.

The projections had convinced Victor Urquidi, the President of the Colegio de Mexico, that the problem needed to be understood at official levels, where there was little technical capacity to deal with this new and possibly controversial issue (Urquidi 1970, 1973). Urquidi, working in close association with Manuel Bartlett, then Under-Secretary of the Interior (Secretaria de Gobernación), assisted the government in putting together the official documentation that tied together the argument for a population policy. In 1973, President Luis Echeverría Alvarez decided to take action after becoming convinced that controlling population growth was important and that he could obtain the necessary political support from his cabinet, which in turn had been stimulated by Urquidi's lectures and discussions in government circles. The president invited a group of his top advisers (Mario Moya Palencia, then Secretary of the Interior, Bartlett, and Urquidi) to work on the final draft of the document that eventually became the 1974 General Law on Population which would set the country on a path toward fertility planning. The Law was clearly important for Mexico but also had international ramifications. Antonio Carrllo Flores, a former Minister of Foreign relations in Mexico, had been named Chair of the planning committee for the 1974 WPC in Bucharest, where Mexico's new policy would be showcased, providing a policy precedent that other Latin American countries watched carefully.

Indeed, the 1974 Law was a quintessential example of the Bucharest-era logic for integrating population in development planning and establishing a National Population Council (CONAPO) that was to coordinate the efforts of a large number of ministries. If CONAPO's secretariat, located in the Ministry of the Interior, was not always as influential as one might have expected in terms of influencing the decisions of other ministries, it certainly served to educate cabinet ministers regarding the country's demographic dynamics. And it was from this same group of ministers that the next president was usually chosen. Also important was the role that CONAPO played in disseminating an enormous barrage of public service announcements that heralded the advantages of small families.

The 1974 Law established the government's responsibility for providing Mexicans with the contraceptive services with which they could freely decide on the number and spacing of their children, again very much in line with the 1974 WPPA. Government family planning services were first provided through the existing clinic and hospital infrastructure of the main public health institutions, especially the Ministry of Health (SSA) and the Mexican Social Security Institute (IMSS), which were for the most part located in urban areas. These services were provided free of charge and seemed to meet a well-established if somewhat latent demand for fertility limitation.

The approach to service provision in the next administration that began in 1976 with the inauguration of José López Portillo as president was more ambitious. It involved the development of targets for the number of contraceptive acceptors to be recruited by the various institutions and extended services to rural areas beyond the reach of the existing infrastructure. Here it was believed that there might be greater resistance to the idea and practice of fertility planning, both because of the role of children in subsistence agriculture and the much lower levels of education of the rural population (Alba and Potter 1986). All in all, the efforts to expand and direct the provision of services in line with the National Family Planning Plan adopted in October 1977 were remarkably successful given that they were implemented all over the country through extremely large government institutions. Surveys showed large increases in contraceptive use and substantial decline in fertility, especially in urban areas, along with continued unmet demand for contraception (Brambila 1998). On the other hand, concerns were also being raised regarding the extent to which the program was respecting its intended voluntary nature, which had been carefully laid out in the original law and the accompanying constitutional amendment. There was a clear emphasis in the program on promoting the use of the most effective methods requiring the least amount of compliance, the IUD and female sterilization, and on accepting these methods immediately postpartum (Potter, Mojarro, and Nuñez 1987).

Debates and developments like those we have mentioned as leading to the ICPD program of action also ran their course in Mexico in the late 1980s and early 1990s. There was criticism of the government population program from feminist NGOs on the left and conservative religious and pro-life groups on the right. In 1995 CONAPO took on a leading role in incorporating a feminist perspective into policy pronouncements and formulations with respect to population and, more broadly, also made a major effort to ensure that informed consent was respected with regard to the acceptance of sterilization, the IUD, and other contraceptive methods. But where CONAPO came to play an absolutely crucial role during the first years of the new century was in preserving the government's role in the provision of contraceptive services in the new administration of President Vicente Fox.

Fox was the first person from a party other than the PRI to be elected president in 60 years, His party was the most conservative of those vying for power and, from its inception, had been associated with the Catholic Church. A wide spectrum of individuals and organizations, including a number of feminist NGOs that had long been critical of the government's policies in previous PRI administrations, were concerned that the Fox administration would move to limit the government's role in providing family planning services and further restrict the already very limited legal access to abortion that existed in Mexico. As it turned out, despite a number of challenges, President Fox stood by the national population policy and indeed became a vociferous advocate of the need for Mexico to benefit from the demographic dividend generated by the fertility decline of the preceding quarter century. In 2003, the TFR was estimated to be not far above replacement level, and the population growth targets set nearly 30 years earlier had been realized (CONAPO 2003).

In summary, the cases of China and Mexico certainly represent major historical markers of changes that occurred in the world in the 1970s that promoted of the idea of fertility planning backed by effective national programs and anchored by policy rationales tied to long-term development plans. While both policies clearly have considerable momentum, they have also responded to the changes that have taken place in the international environment. Almost no one would question the effectiveness of either policy. However, the elusive question of what would have happened had they not been implemented is not easily answered. It is to research and argument on this elusive counterfactual that we turn in the next section.

IMPLEMENTATION RESULTS

The proliferation of family planning programs and their legitimization by governments during the past 50 years has played a key role in the fertility transitions in the developing world. However, the exact contribution of these programs in determining changes in demographic behavior has been the subject of considerable debate. The argument over the importance of family planning programs as a means of bringing about and sustaining fertility decline crystallized during the 1970s, perhaps nowhere more starkly than in an exchange between demographers Amy Tsui and Donald Bogue (1978) and Paul Demeny (1979). Tsui and Bogue pointed to the magnitude of the impending growth in world population, but then noted that family programs were proving to be effective instruments for inducing rapid fertility declines and that if they were implemented on a sufficient scale in the world, population growth rates could fall much more quickly than was then envisaged by United Nations population projections. Demeny questioned the strength of the evidence for program impact and argued forcefully that the real problem lay with the demand for children in most of the world's poor countries. He concluded that the most effective policies would be those that brought about changes in the incentives for childbearing.

With the accumulation of both data and experience over the next two decades, empirical analysis of the magnitude of the effects of family planning programs on fertility progressed considerably but still yielded conflicting results, or at least results on the basis of which analysts reached differing conclusions. One main approach was to examine the variation in fertility across countries and assess the degree to which it was associated with the level of social and economic development, on the one hand, and with the amount of "family planning program effort," on the other. A number of such studies carried out over the years by Ross and colleagues showed that program effort was a significant predictor of lower fertility (e.g., Mauldin and Ross 1991). However, these results were challenged by Pritchett (1994), who argued that they were flawed both by the limited indices of development included in the models and by the potentially circular influence that the demand for small families might have in eliciting program effort. Pritchett showed that once actual measures of the demand for children were included in such cross-national regression models, the size of the effect of program effort fell considerably. Bongaarts (1994: 619) replied that, among other limitations, Pritchett's critique suffered from having ignored the "much broader and powerful influence that programs can have by reducing non-economic costs of contraceptive use, such as lack of knowledge, fear of side effects, and social and familial disapproval."

Another and much less easily assailable type of evidence regarding the demographic influence of family planning programs comes from the two large-scale experiments that have been undertaken to assess their impact. The first and most well known of these was carried out in in the Matlab region of Bangladesh by the International Centre of Diarrhoeal Disease Research (ICDDRB). In this study, half of the villages in a very large area were provided with intensive family planning services that included household visits to every married, fecund woman in the community by a full-time project employee who provided information and services. In the comparison area, services were restricted to those usually provided by the government. The project began in October 1977 and quickly resulted in a noticeable differential in both contraceptive use and the TFR. By 1980, the difference in the TFR between the treatment and the comparison areas had reached 1.6 births, a differential that was maintained over the next decade (Koenig et al. 1992). In addition to the effect on fertility and contraceptive use, the intervention was also shown to have a negative impact on abortion rates due to the lower incidence of unintended pregnancies (Rahman, DaVanzo, and Razzaque 2001).

The second large-scale experiment to assess the impact on fertility of providing family planning and reproductive health services was the Navrongo Community Health and Family Planning Project conducted in rural area of Northern Ghana beginning in 1994. The project, implemented in three phases, sought to develop and test culturally appropriate systems of family planning service delivery and to generate demand for and improve the provision of health services in the target communities. Five distinct geographical areas were provided with different combinations of family planning and health services (community-based primary care and family planning services, regular clinical services with upgraded facilities and staff training, as well as no intervention). Sizable program impacts were observed for the community-based components on both contraceptive use and immunization (Debpuûr et al. 2002). Moreover, the experiments showed success in introducing and stimulating critical ideational change in rural communities of northern Ghana known for their high fertility and low acceptance of family planning. The project has been able to mobilize village chiefs, elders, and women's organizations and has also reassured men that family planning is acceptable to their respected leaders, thus breaking down some of the traditional barriers that in many pretransitional contexts are responsible for maintaining high fertility levels (Debpuûr et al. 2002: 154–155).

Implementation of the project also seems to have made contraception and family planning services more accessible and more visible than in other communities in the region. The project has fostered more receptive attitudes to the concept of reproductive behavior and choice in a traditional setting. In areas where a nurse-outreach approach was used, the impact in enhancing women's preferences to limit childbearing was clear, although the impact on reported contraceptive use, while statistically significant, was too small to induce appreciable fertility differentials. Overall, the experimental approaches used in the Navrongo Project have lowered fertility among all age groups, but this change appears to have taken place in the absence of a major increase in contraceptive use.

If the large amount of data and analysis of family planning programs that have been conducted during the last four decades has yielded differing conclusions with regard to program impact, the question itself now seems to be receding in importance. This shift is in part due to the expanded range of concerns that result from a focus on reproductive health rather than contraceptive prevalence. However, it is also due to the amount of fertility decline that has taken place throughout the world as an increasing number of developing or formerly developing countries have reached levels of fertility that are either close to, or actually below, replacement. In the concluding section we will turn to two of the most important questions regarding fertility planning that will demand attention in the first three decades of the new millennium.

NEXT STEPS

At the dawn of the 21st century, there is still much progress to be made with respect to fertility planning. While use of contraceptives has increased enormously in many parts of the world, the quality of the services provided to the many individuals and couples who use them, particularly those in the most disadvantaged groups, is far from ideal. In addition to direct evidence regarding the limitations of current service programs, the wide variation across countries in the mix of contraceptives used and the fact that in most countries couples make use of just one or two methods are indicative of both real and subjective constraints on access to a wide variety of contraceptive technologies.

Second, even within countries with a high prevalence of use (including some developed countries such as the United States), unwanted pregnancy is a common phenomenon among sexually active adolescents who often lack access to the information and services for the prevention of pregnancy and sexually transmitted diseases. As was highlighted in the program of action adopted at the ICPD, these are important issues that deserve attention and resources.

We would like to end this chapter by focusing on two very large reproductive issues on which there is much less agreement about what needs to be done. The first of these is below-replacement-level fertility. In many industrialized countries, current fertility has fallen to levels that in the long run and in the absence of immigration would lead to population decline. In Europe as a whole, the TFR is now 1.4, which implies a population loss of about one third from one generation to the next and an age distribution with an unprecedented percentage of the population past the now custom-ary age of retirement. In some countries, the TFR is well below 1.4, implying even faster rates of decline and an even more elderly age distribution. At this juncture, while the affected countries have certainly taken note of the phenomenon, there is no consensus that below-replacement-level fertility represents an important threat to social welfare, nor any well-developed understanding of the factors that have led individuals and couples to postpone and limit fertility to such a degree. This phenomenon is not restricted to European countries and has emerged in a number of East and Southeast Asian countries such as Thailand and South Korea, where fertility declined from high levels in the 1960s. Whether or not it will constitute the end-point for the fertility transitions taking place in the rest of Asia and Latin America is a question now clearly coming in to view (Bongaarts 2003).

Demeny (2003a, 2003b) has pointed to a number of factors that may have led to the current indifference regarding below-replacement fertility. First is the apparent disson-ance with concern for rapid population growth in developing countries and domestic actions that would serve the opposite aim: it is hard to view diminished population growth rates as helpful in one context but harmful in another. Second, due the current age distribution, population decline has yet to become manifest in many countries with low fertility. Third is the assumption that there are effective ways to deal with or forestall the problems that might result from an aging population and decreasing numbers, either by way of institutional adjustments or by way of increased immigration. Finally, there seems to be an expectation that, sooner or later, fertility will spontan-eously rebound in a self-correcting response to the current imbalance. In the view of some (e.g., Morgan 2003), below-replacement fertility is the kind of social problem that a society would like to have: something brought on by the enhancement of the status of women and ever higher living standards and levels of education. On the other hand, others have noted that such behavioral patterns often become self-reinforcing and gain a momentum of their own with each passing year (Kohler, Billari, and Ortega 2002).

If below-replacement fertility were to persist at levels that eventually came to be seen as a major threat to social welfare, what corrective steps might be taken? Unfor-tunately, there are few if any examples of successful pronatalist policies that might serve as a guide. Any option that involved restricting access to the means of fertility control would be unacceptable, and so too might be redistributive policies that favored large families with "non-means tested or even regressive allocation of family and child benefits" (Demeny 2003b). Considering the key role of neo-Malthusianism in the debate over population policy (Hodgson and Watkins 1997), it is paradoxical that, in the future, the stimulus for a radical rethinking of population policy on demographic grounds may arise in the most democratic of societies and where fertility is deemed to be too low rather than too high.

The second major challenge for fertility planning in the coming decades comes at the opposite end of the development spectrum. The region of the world where access and choice of contraception is still problematic and will remain so for a long time is sub-Saharan Africa. African societies are confronting the dilemma of rapid population growth generated by high fertility, along with the reality or the prospect of huge increases in mortality, especially of those in the reproductive years, resulting from the epidemic of HIV/AIDS that has hit Africa far harder than any other region of the world. Of the roughly 40 million people living with HIV/AIDS in 2001, more than 70% were in sub-Saharan Africa, a region that accounts for less than 11% of the world's population. The number of new infections is still rising in most but not all African countries, even those with the highest prevalence rates.

Most countries in that region are afflicted with low and often declining living standards that are mutually related both with the epidemic and with patterns of reproduction that involve early and sustained exposure to the risk of sexually transmitted disease. One of the many questions that arises in the attempt to come to terms with this desperate situation concerns the role of family planning programs in bringing about change in reproductive patterns and treating and preventing HIV/AIDS. Some have voiced concern that the epidemic has the potential to disrupt the substantial progress that family planning programs and national population policies have made in the region (Caldwell and Caldwell 2002). However, others have argued that "more integrated programmes of sexual and reproductive health care and STD/HIV/AIDS control should be developed which jointly offer certain services, expand outreach to new population groups, and create well-functioning referral links to optimize the outreach and impact of what are to date essentially vertical programmes" (Askew and Berer 2003).

What seems to be clear, though, is that the challenges related to fertility planning in sub-Saharan Africa differ substantially from those encountered, for the most part successfully, in Asia and Latin America in earlier decades. First, the nature of the demand for fertility planning seems to be substantially different. In Asia and Latin America, the first goal of most of the early adopters of contraception was fertility limitation within marriage, whereas in Africa the bulk of the early demand is for either the prevention of pregnancy prior to marriage or for birth spacing within marriage (Caldwell and Caldwell 2002). Second, the HIV/AIDS epidemic obviously requires an even greater emphasis on education regarding reproductive risks and the mechanisms of the sexual transmission of disease, with serious consideration given to the options of dual protection or abstinence. A third difference, related to both the epidemic and to the importance of sex outside of marriage, is the need for privacy and confidentiality, since stigma is paramount concern for women on both fronts. Last but not least, services will have to be developed and sustained by health systems that are as yet among the most sparse and precarious in the world.

What lies ahead for the world in fertility planning is a peculiar dichotomy. In the developed industrial world—the so-called North—couples have become, despite religious opposition from fundamentalist groups or the Vatican—extremely efficient contraceptors and have adopted very low family size ideals, in some cases reproducing below their own aspirations. In the South, generally speaking, and especially in countries in the middle range of economic development, most individuals and couples have adopted lower family size ideals and are well on their way to achieving them. The great exception is sub-Saharan Africa, where the situation remains uncertain as high fertility and low survival trends threaten the very subsistence of those societies. How some African countries will recoup from the loss of people at the peak of their productive lives, and what reproductive and fertility patterns will emerge as the orphans of today grow to adulthood, is surely the most frightening issue in the contemporary fertility panorama.

REFERENCES

Alba, F., and J. E. Potter. 1986. Population and development in Mexico since 1940: An interpretation. *Population and Development Review* 12(1):47–75.

American Assembly. 1963. The population dilemma. *Englewood Cliffs, N. J.: Prentice-Hall.*

Anderson, J. E., and J. G. Cleland. 1984. The world fertility survey and contraceptive prevalence surveys: A comparison of substantive results. *Studies in Family Planning* 15(1):1–13.

Aparicio, R. 1988. Niveles, tendencias e impacto demográfico de la anticoncepción. In *Memorias de la reunión sobre avances y perspectivas de la investigación social en planificación familiar en México.* México, D.F.: Secretaría de Salud.

Askew, I., and M. Berer. 2003 The contribution of sexual and reproductive health services to the fight against HIV/AIDS: A review. *Reproductive Health Matters* 11(22):51–73.

Benitez-Zenteno, R., and G. Cabrera. 1966. *Proyecciones de la población de México: 1960–80.* México, D.F.: Banco de México SA.

Berelson, B., R. K. Anderson, O. Harkavy, J. Maier, W. P. Mauldin, and S. J. Segal, eds. 1966. *Family planning and population programs.* Chicago: University of Chicago Press.

Bloom, D., D. Canning, and P. Malaney. 2000. Demographic change and economic growth in Asia. *Population and Development Review* 26:257–290.

Bloom, D., and J. Williamson. 1998. Demographic transitions and economic miracles in emerging Asia. *World Bank Economics Review* 12:419–456.

Bogue, D. 1969. *Principles of demography.* New York: Wiley.

Bongaarts, J. 1982. The fertility-inhibiting effects of the intermediate fertility variables. *Studies in Family Planning* 13:179–189.

Bongaarts, J. 1994. The impact of population policies: comment. *Population and Development Review* 20:616–620.

Bongaarts, J. 2003. Completing the fertility transition in the developing world: The role of educational differences and fertility preferences. *Population Studies* 57(3):321–336.

Bongaarts, J., and S. C. Watkins. 1996. Social interactions and contemporary fertility transitions. *Population and Development Review* 22(4):639–682.

Brambila, C. 1998. Mexico's population policy and demographic dynamics: The record of three decades. In *Do population policies matter?: Fertility and politics in Egypt, India, Kenya, and Mexico 1998.* Edited by A. Jain, 157–191. New York: The Population Council.

Bulut, A., V. Filipi, T. Marshall, H. Nalbant, N. Yolsal, and W. Graham. 1997. Contraceptive choice and reproductive morbidity in Istanbul. *Studies in Family Planning* 28(1):35–43.

Cabrera, G. 1972. Consideraciones sobre el crecimiento demográfico de México. *Planificación* 8.

Caldwell, J. C. 1985. Strengths and limitations of the survey approach for measuring and understanding fertility change. In *Reproductive change in developing countries 1985.* Edited by J. Cleland and J. Hobcraft, 45–63. Oxford: Oxford University Press.

Caldwell, J. C., and P. Caldwell. 2002. Africa: The new family planning frontier. *Studies in Family Planning* 33(1):76–84.

Coale, A. J. 1969. The decline of fertility in Europe from the French Revolution to World War II. In *Fertility and family planning 1969.* Edited by S. J. Behrman, L. Corsa, and R. Freedman. Ann Arbor: University of Michigan Press.

Coale, A. J., and E. M. Hoover. 1958. *Population growth and economic development in low-income countries.* Princeton, N.J.: Princeton University Press.

Coleman, S. 1981. The cultural context of condom use in Japan. *Studies in Family Planning* 12(1):28–39.

Committee on Population. 1986. *Population growth and economic development: Policy questions*. Commission on Behavioral and Social Sciences and Education, National Research Council. Washington, D.C.: National Academies Press.

CONAPO. 2003. *Prontuario demográfico de México 2000–2003*. México, D.F.: Consejo Nacional de Población.

Cook, R. 1989. Antiprogestin drugs: Medical and legal issues. *Family Planning Perspectives* 21(6):267–272.

Davis, K. 1987. The world's most expensive survey. *Sociological Forum* 2(4):829–834.

Demeny, P. 1979. On the end of the population explosion. *Population and Development Review* 5(1):141–162.

Demeny, P. 2003a. Population policy. In *Encyclopedia of population 2003*. Edited by P. Demeny and G. McNicoll, 752–763. New York: MacMillan Reference.

Demeny, P. 2003b. Population policy dilemmas in Europe at the dawn of the twenty-first century. *Population and Development Review* 29(1):1–28.

Debpuûr, C., J. F. Phillips, E. F. Jackson, A. Nazzar, P. Ngom, and F. N. Binka. 2002. The impact of the navrongo project on contraceptive knowledge and use, reproductive preferences, and fertility. *Studies in Family Planning* 33(2):141–164.

Dixon-Mueller, R. 1993. *Population policy and women's rights*. Westport, Conn.: Praeger.

Ehrlich, P. R. 1968. *The population bomb*. New York: Ballantine Books.

Erli, Z. 2001. From a number-centered officer to a quality of care advocator: A personal story. Paper presented at the Asia Pacific Conference on Reproductive Health, Manila, Philippines.

Finkle, J. L., and B. Crane. 1975. The politics of Bucharest: Population, development, and the new international economic order. *Population and Development Review* 1(1):87–114.

Finkle, J. L., and B. Crane. 1985. Ideology and politics at Mexico City: The United States at the 1984 International Conference on Population. *Population and Development Review* 11(1):1–28.

Finkle, J. L., and C. L. McIntosh. 1995. The Cairo Conference on Population and Development: A new paradigm? *Population and Development Review* 21(2):223–260.

Fisher, A., and A. A. Way. 1988. The demographic and health surveys program: An overview. *International Family Planning Perspectives* 14(2):15–19.

Gille, H. 1987. Origins and nature of the world fertility survey. In *The World Fertility Survey: An assessment 1987*. Edited by J. Cleland and C. Scott, 7–28. Oxford: Oxford University Press.

Gladwell, M. 2000. *John Rock's error: What the co-inventor of the pill didn't know: Menstruation can endanger women's health. The New Yorker*.

Glass, D. V. 1969. Fertility trends in Europe. In *Fertility and family planning*. Edited by S. J. Behrman, L. Corsa, and R. Freedman. Ann Arbor: University of Michigan Press.

Goldberg, H. I., and F. Serbanescu. 1995. Unintended pregnancy and unmet need for contraception in two countries of Eastern Europe. Paper presented at the Annual Meeting of the American Public Health Association, October 30–November 2, San Diego, Calif.

Greenhalgh, S. 1986. Shifts in China's population policy. *Population and Development Review* 12(3):491–516.

Greenhalgh, S. 1992. Negotiating birth control in village China. *Working Paper No. 38, Research Division*. New York: The Population Council.

Greenhalgh, S., Z. Chuzhu, and L. Nan. 1994. Restraining population growth in three Chinese villages. *Population and Development Review* 20(2):365–396.

Haberland, N., and D. Measham. 2002. *Responding to Cairo: Case studies of changing practice in reproductive health and family planning*. New York: Population Council.

Hodgson, D., and S. C. Watkins. 1997. Feminists and neo-Malthusians: Past and present alliances. *Population and Development Review* 23(3):469–523.

Kaufman, J. 2003. Myths and realities of China's population program. *Harvard Asia Quarterly* 7(1):21–25.

Kaufman, J., Z. Erli, Z. Kaining, and X. Zhenming. 2003. Quality of care in China: Scaling up a pilot project into a national reform program. Paper prepared for workshop *From Pilot Projects to Policies and Programs: Strategies for Scaling Up Innovations in Health Service Delivery*, Bellagio, Italy.

Koenig, M. A., U. Rob, M. A. Khan, J. Chakraborty, and V. Fauveau. 1992. Contraceptive use in Matlab, Bangladesh in 1990: Levels, trends, and explanations. *Studies in Family Planning* 23:352–364.

Kohler, H., F. C. Billari, and J. A. Ortega. 2002. The emergence of lowest-low fertility in Europe during the 1990s. *Population and Development Review* 28(4):641–680.

Li, V. C., G. C. Wong, Q. Shu-hua, C. Fu-Ming, L. Pu-Quan, and J. Sun. 1990. Characteristics of women having abortion in China. *Social Science and Medicine* 31(4):445–453.

Mauldin, W., and J. Ross. 1991. Family planning programs: Efforts and results, 1982–1989. *Studies in Family Planning* 22(6):350–367.

Meadows, D. H., et al. 1974. *The limits to growth*. New York: Universe Books.

Morris, L. 2000. History and current status of reproductive health surveys at CDC. *American Journal of Preventive Medicine* 19(1S): 31–34.

Morgan, S. P. 2003. Is low fertility a twenty-first-century demographic crisis? *Demography* 40:589–603.

Mundigo, A. 1992. The determinants of impact and utilization of fertility research on public policy: Mexico and China. In *The role of family planning programs as fertility determinant 1992*. Edited by J. Ross and J. Phillips. London: Oxford University Press.

Mundigo, A. 1999. Population and abortion policies in China: Their impact on minority nationalities. *Human Evolution* 14(3):207–230.

Peiyun, P. 1993. Accomplishments of China's family planning program: A statement by a Chinese official. *Population and Development Review* 19(2):399–403.

Phelps, C. E. 1992. Diffusion of information in medical care. *Journal of Economic Perspectives* 6(3):23–42.

Population Reference Bureau. 2002. *Family planning worldwide:* 2002 data sheet. Washington, D. C.: Population Reference Bureau.

Potter, J. E. 1999. The persistence of outmoded contraceptive regimes: The cases of Mexico and Brazil. *Population and Development Review* 25(4):703–739.

Potter, J. E., O. Mojarro, and L. Nuñez. 1987. The influence of health care on contraceptive acceptance in rural Mexico. *Studies in Family Planning* 18(3):144–156.

Pritchett, L. 1994. Desired fertility and impact of population policies. *Population and Development Review* 20(1):1–52.

Rahman, M., J. DaVanzo, and A. Razzaque. 2001. Do better family planning services reduce abortion in Bangladesh? *The Lancet* 358(9287):1051–1056.

Rigdon, S. M. 1996. Abortion law and practice in China: An overview with comparisons to the United States. *Social Science and Medicine* 42(4):543–560.

Ryder, N. B. 1959. Fertility. In *The study of population*. Edited by P. M. Hauser and O. D. Duncan. Chicago: University of Chicago Press.

Santow, G. 1993. Coitus interruptus in the twentieth century. *Population and Development Review* 19(4):767–792.

Schneider, J., and P. Schneider. 1992. Going forward in reverse gear: Culture, economy, and political economy in the demographic transitions of a rural Sicilian town. In *The European experience of declining fertility, 1850–1970: The quiet revolution 1992*. Edited by J. R. Gillis, L. A. Tilly, and D. Levine, 146–174. Cambridge and Oxford: Blackwell.

Seltzer, J. R. 2002. *The origins and evolution of family planning programs in developing countries*. Santa Monica, Calif.: Population Matters/Rand.

Singh, J. S. 1998. *Creating a new consensus on population: The International Conference on Population and Development*. London: Earthscan.

Spengler, J. 1938. *France faces depopulation*. Durham, N.C.: Duke University Press.

Stycos, J. M. 1971. *Ideology, faith and family planning in Latin America*. New York: McGraw-Hill.

Taylor, H. C. 1976. *Human reproduction: Physiology, population and family planning*. Cambridge, Mass: MIT Press.

Tsui, A. O., and D. J. Bogue. 1978. Declining world fertility: Trends, causes, implications. *Population Bulletin* 33(4). Washington, D.C.: Population Reference Bureau.

United Nations. 1973. Demographic yearbook, 1972. (ST/Stat/Ser.R/1). New York: United Nations.

United Nations. 1994. *Report of the international conference on population and development*. Doc. A/Conf.171/13, New York: United Nations.

United Nations. 2002. *World contraceptive use 2001 (chart)*. ST/ESA/SER. A/210. New York: United Nations.

Urquidi, V. 1970. *Pérfil general: Economía y población. El pérfil de Mexico en 1980*. Mexico, D.F.: Siglo XXI.

Urquidi, V. 1973. Población y desarrollo. *Gaceta Médica de Mexico* 105(5).

Westoff, C. F. 1988a. Is the KAP-gap real? *Population and Development Review* 14(2):225–232.

Westoff, C. F. 1988b. The potential demand for family planning: A new measure of unmet need and estimates for five Latin American countries. *International Family Planning Perspectives* 14(2):45–53.

Wills, G. 2000. *Papal sin: Structures of deceit*. New York: Doubleday.

Winckler, E. A. 2002. Chinese reproductive policy at the turn of the millennium. *Population and Development Review* 28(1):379–418.

Zlidar, V. M., R. Gardener, S. O. Rutstein, L. Morris, H. Goldberg, and K. Johnson. 2003. New survey findings: The reproductive revolution continues. *Population Reports,* Series M, No. 17.

CHAPTER 25

Small-Area and Business Demography

STANLEY K. SMITH AND PETER A. MORRISON

INTRODUCTION

A chain of supermarkets decides to launch a new line of ethnic foods. Where should it concentrate its marketing efforts? A school district is plagued by increasingly crowded elementary schools. Is this a temporary phenomenon or a continuing long-run trend? A hospital considers adding an obstetrics unit. Will anticipated service demand cover the additional costs? A metropolitan transportation agency plans to expand its rapid transit system. Where should new routes and transit stops be added? A manufacturer needs to build a new plant. Where can it find enough skilled workers to staff that plant? Answering questions like these lies at the heart of small-area and business demography.

Small-area and business demography are distinct but closely related fields of applied demography. Both focus mainly on practical applications of demographic methods and materials, designed to help managers, administrators, and government officials analyze and solve the problems faced by their organizations (Siegel 2002). Each draws on many of the same concepts, data sources, and techniques, but not all small-area analyses pertain to the world of business, and business demography is not confined just to small areas. This chapter reviews the objectives and distinctive features of small-area demography, the evolution and practice of business demography, and the primary tools used in both fields. It presents several illustrations from these two decision-oriented fields and offers observations about recent developments and future prospects. Although the primary focus is the United States, many of the issues discussed have their counterparts in other nations as well.

SMALL-AREA DEMOGRAPHY

Small-area demography refers to demographic applications and analyses at local or regional scales. The term *small area*, however, has no exact or universally recognized definition. It may refer to any subnational area for which area-specific samples from national surveys are too small to provide estimates with acceptable levels of precision (e.g., Rao 1999). More frequently, small areas refer to counties and subcounty areas such as cities, ZIP code areas, traffic analysis zones, census tracts, and individual blocks (e.g., Murdock and Ellis 1991). We use the latter definition here. Small areas vary in size from less than an acre to thousands of square miles, and from a mere handful of residents (or none at all) to many millions.

Objectives of Small-Area Analysis

Most small-area analyses have one of three basic objectives: to advance knowledge, to inform public policy, or to support business decision making. We consider all three but focus primarily on the latter two.

ADVANCE KNOWLEDGE.   Some small-area studies are undertaken to advance the understanding of social, economic, demographic, environmental, epidemiological, and other conditions and trends. States, provinces, cities, and other small areas are used as units of analysis to investigate the causes and consequences of these conditions and trends. Examples include investigations of whether differences in government tax and expenditure policies affected interprovincial migration in Canada (Day 1992); how poverty, urbanization, and geographic location affected the incidence of cholera among regions in Mexico (Borroto and Martinez-Piedra 2000); whether residents of zones surrounding the site of an industrial accident in Italy experienced higher-than-normal cancer rates (Bertazzi et al. 2001); and whether differences in geographic, industrial, educational, and demographic characteristics affected county population growth rates in the United States between 1840 and 1990 (Beeson, DeJong, and Troesken 2001). Although they may have policy or business implications, these and similar studies are undertaken primarily for the scientific purpose of advancing knowledge.

INFORM PUBLIC POLICY.   Small-area analyses are also undertaken to inform public policy. Small-area data can be used to allocate government funds, determine eligibility for entitlement programs, delineate political and electoral boundaries, monitor the effectiveness of public policies, select sites for public facilities, and develop program budgets. Examples include using population estimates by traffic analysis zone for political redistricting (Serow et al. 1997); using block-level population and household projections for choosing sites for fire stations (Tayman, Parrott, and Carnevale 1997); constructing school enrollment projections by grade for a public school district (McKibben 1996); and calculating teenage birth rates by ZIP code to identify areas in need of adolescent pregnancy prevention programs (Gould et al. 1998). These studies may advance scientific understanding, but their primary purpose is to improve governmental decision making.

SUPPORT BUSINESS DECISION MAKING. Small-area analyses also support business decision making, primarily in the areas of site selection, marketing, sales forecasting, strategic planning, litigation support, and human resources. Examples include evaluating an array of small-area demographic and socioeconomic data in order to select store locations for a large supermarket chain (Morrison and Abrahamse 1996); projecting the number of births in a hospital's service area to predict the future demand for obstetric services (Thomas 1997); constructing life tables for employees of a large corporation to determine potential health care costs (Kintner and Swanson 1997); and developing small-area estimates and projections as part of a company's bank loan application (Murdock and Hamm 1997). Many topics of business demography parallel those of public policy but focus on private rather than public sector decision making.

Distinctive Problems of Small-Area Analysis

Several problems distinguish small-area analyses from those with a larger geographic scale. First is shifting geographic boundaries. For nations, states, and most counties, boundaries remain constant over time. For subcounty areas, however, boundaries change frequently: Cities annex adjoining areas, census tracts are subdivided, ZIP code areas are reconfigured, service areas are redefined, and new statistical areas are formed. When small-area data are used for time series analyses, the consistency of historical data series must be evaluated and adjustments made as needed. Achieving consistency is often time consuming and sometimes impossible.

Second is data availability. Many types of data are not tabulated for areas below a certain level of geography. For example, vital statistics in the United States are generally tabulated for states and counties but not for subcounty areas. Consequently, analyses that are feasible at higher levels of geography often cannot be done at lower levels or must rely on proxy variables. Data availability is even more problematic in many less developed countries (Cleland 1996).

Third is data reliability. Even the best data sources are flawed. Errors affect data quality more severely for small areas than large areas, where they are often mutually offsetting. In addition, survey data are frequently less reliable for small areas than large areas because sample sizes are smaller and survey responses more variable.

Finally, location-specific events and characteristics are more likely to affect population growth in small areas than in large areas. Events such as the closing of a military base, the construction of a large housing development, the addition of a major employer, and changes in zoning requirements have more impact on population growth in small areas than in large areas because their effects are less likely to be offset by the effects of other events. Physical characteristics such as flood plains and the availability of vacant land are more likely to affect growth trends in small areas than in large areas because fewer alternative locations are available. Seasonal populations such as "snowbirds" and migrant farm workers potentially comprise a larger proportion of the total population in small areas than in large areas; these populations typically follow different growth trends and have different socioeconomic and demographic characteristics than the rest of the population. These and other location-specific factors can complicate analyses at any geographic scale, but small areas are by far the most vulnerable to their influence.

BUSINESS DEMOGRAPHY

Business demography involves the application of demographic concepts, data, and techniques to the practical concerns of business decision makers. It is an eclectic, loosely organized field, driven by tangible problems rather than by the quest to advance knowledge or to improve measurement. Specific applications have evolved in response to new data sources, computer technology, and analytical methods, as well as to changes in the business environment itself. Since many applications focus on small areas, a substantial overlap exists between business demography and small-area demography.

Evolution of the Field

Businesses have based decision making on demographic data and techniques for more than a century (Pol and Thomas 1997). The emergence of business demography as a distinct field, however, is quite recent. The release of 1970 census data in machine-readable form gave rise to an electronic data industry, which began with a mere handful of companies in the early 1970s and grew to more than 70 companies by the mid-1980s (Russell 1984). The number of data vendors subsequently declined as demographic data became more widely available, but these firms were replaced by other demographically oriented firms specializing in survey research, trend analysis, marketing, mapping, and software development, as well as the provision of census data and the production of population estimates and projections. Today, many businesses routinely base decisions on the advice of consultants and employees skilled in collecting, analyzing, and interpreting demographic data.

Responding to these developments, the Population Association of America formed a Committee on Business Demography in 1982. In 1985, this committee joined with the Committee on State and Local Demography to begin publishing the *Applied Demography* newsletter; by 2004, its subscriber base exceeded 400. During this period, two commercially oriented magazines (*American Demographics* and *Business Geographics*) were launched, reporting on developments in demographic trends and business applications. Business demography thus has coalesced into a visible and well-established field, although it remains somewhat loosely defined and organized.

The Practitioners

Professionally, business demographers fall into three distinct groups. First are analysts employed by private companies, whose work focuses primarily on the business activities of their employers (e.g., human resources, market analyses, customer profiles, site selection). Second are analysts with firms that contract out to clients needing demographic data and analysis (e.g., to develop estimates and projections of the population residing within five miles of a specific location). These firms serve a variety of government agencies and business enterprises. Third are individual consultants who work on specific projects for particular clients. Private consulting is a full-time activity for some, but a part-time pursuit for most.

Not all practitioners have formal training in demography. Many have backgrounds in economics, geography, marketing, statistics, survey research, real estate, or other disciplines. Even those with formal demographic training often acquire many of their job skills primarily through work experience rather than academic training. Few academic demography programs deal with business issues, and few business schools offer training in demographic applications.

The skills needed by business demographers extend beyond the scope of what academic training programs normally provide. In addition to applying general demographic knowledge and skills, business demographers must be able to:

- Explain and interpret demographic realities to audiences with little knowledge of demographic perspectives and techniques.
- Identify important effects and potential issues that demographic changes may pose for a specific firm or industry.
- Construct demographic assumptions about the future that serve the needs of business decision makers.
- Be conversant with a range of disciplinary frameworks and theories (e.g., economics, finance, marketing, psychology, sociology, and geography) that inform decision making within a specific business context.

In their day-to-day work, most business executives focus on concerns in areas such as marketing, product development, human resources, and strategic planning. Rarely do they have the time or expertise needed to analyze the underlying demographic forces that affect these concerns. Demographers can contribute to business decision making by offering new perspectives on business problems (for example, distinguishing among age, period, and cohort effects that shape and reshape a market). They can inform, advise, and even serve as catalysts for organizational change. By exposing executives to new concepts and perspectives, demographers can elevate management thinking from an operational to a strategic level (e.g., Kintner and Swanson 1997; Pol and Thomas 1997; Rives 1997; Siegel 2002).

TOOLS

The tools of small-area and business demography are the same as those demographers use generally: basic demographic concepts, measures, and techniques; computer hardware and software; and data from a variety of sources. What sets them apart is that—in small-area and business demography—they are used primarily for decision-making purposes. In many applications, the development and interpretation of population estimates and projections plays a particularly important role.

Demographic Concepts, Measures, and Techniques

The demographic concepts, measures, and techniques used most frequently in small-area and business demography focus on population characteristics (e.g., age, sex, race, education, income), consumer units (e.g., individuals, households, families), demographic events (e.g., births, deaths, marriages, divorces, migration), and the distribution of demographic events and characteristics across geographic areas (e.g., counties, census tracts, ZIP code areas). In addition, small-area and business demographers often extend common demographic concepts and measures to fit the needs of specific projects. For example, they may conduct cohort analyses of magazine subscribers, construct life tables for automobiles, or develop age-standardized rates of beer consumption (Siegel 2002). They also combine demographic and consumer data to yield new products such as *lifestyle clusters* based on the classification of neighborhoods by demographic characteristics and consumer preferences (e.g., Mitchell 1995; Weiss 1988).

Since most of these concepts, measures, and techniques are covered elsewhere in this volume, we do not review them here. However, given the importance of population estimates and projections for so many purposes, we briefly describe and evaluate several commonly used estimation and projection methods. Later in this chapter, we provide a number of illustrations showing how demographic concepts, measures, and techniques can be applied to specific topics in small-area and business demography.

Computer Hardware and Software

Exponential increases in computing power and data storage capacity in recent years have greatly expanded the possibilities for organizing, integrating, and analyzing data. Powerful software packages have largely automated statistical analysis and reporting. Computer networks enable analysts to share information and transfer data globally through the Internet. Advances in reporting and displaying spatial information through geographic information systems have been especially influential because many analyses call for data grouped into customer service areas, traffic analysis zones, school districts, and other uniquely defined regions. Discussions of the role of computer technology in small-area and business demography can be found in Bryan and George (2004), Gobalet and Thomas (1996), and Smith, Tayman, and Swanson (2001).

Data Sources

The data used in small-area and business demography come primarily from three sources: censuses, administrative records, and sample surveys.

CENSUSES.   Most industrialized countries enumerate their entire populations once every 5 or 10 years. Censuses are not as frequent or as reliable in most less developed countries, but they have become increasingly widespread and comprehensive over the last 50 years (Cleland 1996). Censuses provide the most reliable source of demographic data throughout the world.

The United States has conducted a census every 10 years since 1790. Under current practices, the starting point for each decennial census is a list of housing units from the preceding census, which has been updated using delivery data from the U.S. Postal Service, information from local government agencies, and a variety of administrative records. Most housing units are mailed census forms that the occupants are asked to fill out and return by mail; in some rural areas, the forms are delivered by census enumerators. Follow-up visits are made to housing units from which no form was returned, and a variety of procedures are used to develop complete and accurate information. About five of six households receive short-form questionnaires collecting a limited amount of population and housing data; about one of six receives a long-form questionnaire collecting information on a broader set of variables (see Table 25.1).

TABLE 25.1. Data Collected in 2000 Census, United States

All households (short-form questionnaire)
Population: Name, relationship to householder, sex, age, date of birth, race, and Hispanic origin.
Housing: Number of people in household, telephone number, and tenure (ownership status).
Sample of households (long-form questionnaire)
Population: Same as short form, plus marital status, school enrollment, educational attainment, ethnic origin (ancestry), language spoken at home, place of birth, citizenship, year of entry into the U.S., place of residence five years ago, disability status, living with grandchildren, military service, employment status, employment history, place of work, transportation to work, occupation, industry, and income.
Housing: Same as short form, plus type of housing unit, year built, length of residence in current unit, number of rooms, number of bedrooms, plumbing facilities, kitchen facilities, telephone in unit, type of heating fuel, number of motor vehicles, size of lot, presence of home business, annual cost of utilities, monthly rent or mortgage payment, second mortgage, real estate taxes, property insurance, and value of property.

Source: Smith, Tayman, and Swanson 2001: 37.

Each housing unit is assigned a specific geographic location based on its latitude and longitude. Natural and man-made features such as rivers, streets, and city boundaries are also assigned locations. Population and housing data are then grouped into specific geographic areas using the Topologically Integrated Geographic Encoding and Referencing (TIGER) system developed by the U.S. Census Bureau. Census results are tabulated for a variety of geographic areas, including states, counties, cities, ZIP code areas, census tracts, block groups, and blocks. Discussions of issues and procedures related to the decennial census can be found in Anderson (1988), Anderson and Fienberg (1999), Edmonston and Schultze (1995), and Skerry (2000).

ADMINISTRATIVE RECORDS. Censuses provide accurate and comprehensive data, but only infrequently. What data sources can be used for the years after or between censuses? One possibility is administrative records kept by federal, state, and local government agencies for purposes of registration, licensing, and program administration. Data on births, deaths, marriages, and divorces are called *vital statistics*. Most industrialized countries maintain accurate records of these events, but records are far from complete in many less developed countries (Cleland 1996). Other administrative records include school enrollments, building permits, drivers' licenses, Medicare enrollees, voter registration lists, and property tax records. These records provide information on a variety of demographic events and population characteristics. Since they are available on an annual or even a monthly basis in many countries, they can be used to construct population estimates and to conduct a variety of demographic analyses.

A population register is a system of data collection in which population characteristics are continuously recorded (Wilson 1985). A universal register attempts to include the entire population, whereas a partial register is limited to specific groups such as school children, registered voters, or Social Security recipients. Universal registers are maintained in only a few countries, but partial registers can be found in many countries throughout the world. Since migration plays a major role in small-area population growth, registers that capture moves from one place to another are particularly important. Although some European countries maintain migration registers (Rees and Kupiszewski 1999), most countries do not.

The full benefits of population registers (or administrative records in general) can be realized only if data are accurate and up-to-date; if individuals can be linked from one register to another through a personal identification number; and if the political climate permits such linkages to be made. These conditions are met in only a few countries. Denmark and Finland have produced census statistics based solely on administrative records, and Norway and Sweden are moving rapidly in this direction (Longva, Thomsen, and Severeide 1998). Problems with one or more conditions have prevented the use of administrative records to supplement or replace regular censuses in the United States, Great Britain, and many other countries (Redfern 1989; Scheuren 1999).

An additional drawback of administrative records is that they are not available for many small areas. Some are available only for states and counties. Others are available for some subcounty areas (e.g., cities) but not for others (e.g., census tracts, traffic analysis zones, school districts). If individual records are geocoded by latitude and longitude, of course, administrative records can be tabulated to fit any level of geography.

SAMPLE SURVEYS.   Administrative records cover only some of the variables that are of interest to demographers, economists, sociologists, geographers, epidemiologists, planners, and other analysts dealing with small-area data. Sample surveys are often employed to collect data on variables not covered by administrative records.

In the United States, the Current Population Survey (CPS) is a monthly survey of about 50,000 households conducted by the U.S. Census Bureau. It collects information on marital status, fertility, migration, income, education, employment, occupation, and other characteristics, in addition to basic demographic variables such as age, sex, and race. Data from the CPS are currently tabulated for regions, states, and large metropolitan areas, but not for smaller geographic areas. Even for these larger areas, small sample sizes sometimes result in unreliable data and misleading trends.

This is a common problem when survey data are used for small-area estimates and analyses. Although the problem can be alleviated to some extent by using techniques that "borrow strength" from other areas or data sources (e.g., Ghosh and Rao 1994; Rao 1999), small sample sizes often limit the reliability of survey estimates for small areas.

The American Community Survey (ACS) may overcome this problem (U.S. Census Bureau 2003). Begun on an exploratory basis in 1996, this survey collects the same types of data as the long-form questionnaire of the decennial census. If carried out as planned, the ACS will be fully implemented by 2004 with some three million households surveyed each year. Starting in 2005, the ACS is expected to provide annual estimates of demographic, social, economic, and housing characteristics for every state and for all cities and counties with 65,000 or more residents. For smaller places, it will take three to five years to accumulate a large enough sample to produce reliable estimates. Under current plans, estimates will be made down to the block-group level for the entire nation by the end of the decade and the ACS will replace the long-form questionnaire in the 2010 census. These plans, of course, are subject to change.

Estimates and Projections

Censuses, administrative records, and sample surveys provide the primary data used in demographic analyses. For many purposes, however, these data must be transformed into population estimates or projections. Population estimates refer to past time periods for which census data are not available (e.g., years after or between censuses); they are typically based on methods that combine data from censuses, administrative records, and/or sample surveys. Population projections refer to the future and are based on historical trends and assumptions regarding future trends.

ESTIMATES.   Estimates refer to the size and/or characteristics of the population of a specific geographic area at a specific point in time. Businesses use population estimates to develop consumer profiles, to choose sites for new stores or branch offices, and to identify underserved markets. Federal, state, and local governments use them to establish electoral boundaries, to plan service delivery, and to determine the need for various types of public facilities. Researchers use them to study social trends, environmental conditions, and geographic movements. They are used as population size controls for sample surveys, as denominators for many types of rates, and as a basis for distributing public funds. Clearly, the development of accurate, timely population estimates is critical for many purposes.

Intercensal estimates refer to estimates computed for dates between two previous censuses; *postcensal* estimates refer to those developed for dates after the most recent census. Intercensal estimates can be based on mathematical interpolations between the two end points or can be tied to data series that reflect intercensal population changes. Postcensal estimates can be based on the extrapolation of historical trends or can be tied to data that reflect postcensal population changes. Most applications call for postcensal estimates, which reflect the most recent information available to data users; accordingly, in this chapter we focus on this type of estimate. Detailed descriptions of population estimation methods can be found in Bryan (2004); Murdock and Ellis (1991); Rives et al. (1995); and Siegel (2002).

Postcensal estimates of total population are usually based on methods that incorporate symptomatic indicators of population change. (A symptomatic indicator is a variable that changes in conjunction with changes in population.) Population estimates are most frequently based on housing unit, component, and regression methods.

The *housing unit* method is the most commonly used method for making small-area population estimates in the United States (U.S. Bureau of the Census 1990) and has been widely used in other countries as well (e.g., Simpson et al. 1996). In this method, the population of an area is calculated as the number of occupied housing units (i.e., households) times the average number of persons per household, plus the number of persons living in group quarters facilities (e.g., college dormitories, prisons, nursing homes) or without traditional housing (e.g., the homeless), according to the following formula:

$$POP_t = (HH_t \times PPH_t) + GQ_t$$

where *POP* is the total population, *HH* is the number of households, *PPH* is the average number of persons per household, *GQ* is the population residing in group quarters facilities or nontraditional housing, and t is the estimation date (Smith 1986). The number of households can be estimated from data on building permits, electricity customers, property taxes, and other records that reflect changes in the housing stock. PPH can be estimated from previous values and variables associated with changing household size. The residual population can be estimated from public records or data provided by the administrators of group quarters facilities.

Component methods are based on the demographic balancing equation in which the population in year t is expressed as the population counted in the most recent census (POP_0), plus the number of births (B) and in-migrants (IM) and minus the number of deaths (D) and out-migrants (OM) since that census:

$$POP_t = POP_0 + B - D + IM - OM$$

Two of the best-known component methods are the *Component II* and *Tax Returns* methods developed by the U.S. Census Bureau (e.g., Murdock, Hwang, and Hamm 1995; Starsinic et al. 1995). These methods are similar in that both are used solely for estimating the population less than age 65 (estimates of the population aged 65 and older are based on changes in Medicare data); both use vital statistics data to measure the natural increase of the population ($B - D$); and both use foreign immigration data from the U.S. Immigration and Naturalization Service. Where they differ is in the data and techniques used to estimate the domestic portion of net migration ($IM - OM$).

The Component II method bases estimates of domestic net migration on changes in school enrollments for grades 1 to 8; these estimates are converted into migration rates for all persons less than age 65 using migration data from the most recent decennial census. The Tax Returns method (formerly called the *Administrative Records* method) bases estimates of domestic net migration on address changes listed on federal income tax returns. Addresses are matched for different years and the number of persons represented by each return is determined by the number of exemptions claimed (excluding exemptions for age 65+ and blindness). For both methods, estimates of the group quarters population are developed separately.

A number of methods use regression techniques in which population estimates are based on symptomatic indicators of population change (e.g., O'Hare 1976; Feeney, Hibbs, and Gillaspy 1995). Commonly used symptomatic indicators include school enrollments, electricity customers, building permits, registered voters, drivers' licenses, tax returns, births, and deaths. The most widely used regression method is *Ratio-Correlation*, in which all variables are expressed as changes in proportions over time. Using county estimates as an illustration, the dependent variable in the regression equation is the percentage change in the county's share of state population between the two most recent censuses (e.g., 1990 and 2000). The independent variables are the percentage changes between those two censuses in the county's share of state totals for the symptomatic indicators. The regression coefficients are applied to percentage changes in county shares for the symptomatic indicators between the most recent census and the estimation date (e.g., April 1, 2000, and July 1, 2005); this provides an estimate of the percentage change in the county's share of the state population. A county's population can then be estimated by applying its newly estimated population share to an independent estimate of the state's population.

These methods can be used alone or in combination with each other. For many years, the U.S. Census Bureau used the Tax Returns method for city estimates and the Component II, Ratio-Correlation, and Tax Returns methods for county estimates. Since 1996, it has used the Housing Unit method for city estimates and the Tax Returns method for county estimates. Currently, the U.S. Census Bureau controls county estimates to a national total, but calculates state estimates as the sum of each state's county estimates (U.S. Census Bureau 2004).

All these estimation methods have been widely used and extensively studied. Each has an established track record for producing reasonably accurate estimates (e.g., Bryan, 2004; Shahidullah and Flotow 2001; Smith 1986; Smith and Mandell 1984). In theory, all except the ratio methods can be used at any level of geography (since ratio methods express smaller areas as proportions of larger areas, they typically are used only for subnational estimates). In practice, however, the component and regression methods are used primarily for state and county estimates because the data needed to apply them for subcounty areas are seldom available. In contrast, the Housing Unit method can be used at virtually any level of geography, from states down to counties, cities, census tracts, and even individual blocks.

In general, population estimates tend to be more accurate for more populous places than less populous places, and for places registering moderate growth rates than for places that are either growing or declining rapidly. Evaluations of 1980 and 1990 estimates produced by the U.S. Census Bureau showed mean absolute percentage errors of about 2% for states and 4% for counties (Long 1993). Errors for 2000 county estimates were slightly smaller than those reported for 1980 and 1990 (Davis 2001). For subcounty estimates, mean absolute percentage errors were found to be 15.2% for 1980 and 12.4% for 2000 (the U.S. Census Bureau did not release an evaluation of 1990 subcounty estimates). Errors varied tremendously by size: In both years, places with fewer than 100 residents had mean absolute percentage errors of about 35%, whereas places with more than 100,000 residents had mean absolute percentage errors of about 4% (Galdi 1985; Harper, Devine, and Coleman 2001).

Estimates of demographic characteristics such as age, sex, and race are typically based on the cohort-component method, in which birth, death, and migration rates are applied separately to each age/sex/race group in the population (e.g., Siegel 2002). Estimates for particular population subgroups are sometimes based on data from administrative records, such as when Medicare data are used to estimate the population aged 65+ (e.g., Bryan 2004). Since estimates of demographic characteristics are more variable than estimates of total population, they are typically controlled to independent estimates of total population.

At the national and state levels, estimates of socioeconomic characteristics such as income, employment, and education can be based on sample surveys. For local areas, however, place-specific survey data are seldom available; when they are, they often provide unreliable estimates because sample sizes are too small or sample strata cross geographic boundaries (Siegel 2002). For these places, estimates can be based on synthetic techniques in which proportions derived from other data sources or larger areas are applied to population estimates for smaller areas. For example, a city's labor force could be estimated by applying labor force participation rates by age, sex, and race from a state or national survey to population estimates by age, sex, and race for that city. In contrast to estimates of total population, little research has considered the accuracy of estimates of demographic and socioeconomic characteristics for small areas.

PROJECTIONS.   Population projections also serve many purposes. They can measure the relative contributions of mortality, fertility, and migration to population growth. They can illustrate the likely range of future demographic scenarios and the sensitivity of population growth to changes in particular assumptions. Most important, they can provide an objective basis for anticipating and accommodating future population change. Population projections have been used to forecast Medicare costs (Miller

2001), welfare obligations (Opitz and Nelson 1996), health care expenditures (Kintner and Swanson 1997), water consumption (Texas Water Development Board 1997), housing demand (Mason 1996), and many other phenomena of interest to decision makers.

Many different approaches to projecting future populations have been devised, ranging from the conceptually simple and straightforward to the highly complex and data-intensive. Some are objective and replicable; others are subjective, intuitive, or vaguely defined. Some provide projections of demographic characteristics and components of growth; others provide projections only of total population. Discussions of national, regional, and global projections can be found in Bongaarts and Bulatao (2000) and O'Neill et al. (2001). Discussions of state and local projections can be found in Davis (1995), Pittenger (1976), and Smith, Tayman, and Swanson (2001).

Most objective methods can be grouped into three basic categories: trend extrapolation, structural, and cohort-component. *Trend extrapolation* methods express the future as a continuation of historical trends. Some methods are very simple, such as those in which past growth rates are projected to remain constant. Others are much more complex, such as those based on time series models. Trend extrapolation methods are often applied to the population as a whole, but can also be applied to particular population subgroups (e.g., a racial or ethnic group), individual components of growth (e.g., births or birth rates), or data expressed as ratios (e.g., county shares of state population). The defining characteristic of trend extrapolation methods is that a variable's projected values are based solely on its historical values.

Structural models provide population projections based on variables that are expected to have an impact on population change (e.g., wage rates, job opportunities, educational levels). Some structural models are relatively simple, involving only a single equation and a few explanatory variables; others are much more complex, containing many equations, variables, and parameters. Some focus on total population change; others differentiate among components of growth. The defining characteristic of structural models is that the projected values of a variable are based not only on its own historical values, but also on projected values of other variables. Whereas trend extrapolation models tell us virtually nothing about the causes of population change, structural models provide explanations as well as projections.

The *cohort-component* method accounts separately for births, deaths, and migration, the three components of population growth. Most applications subdivide the population into age/sex groups; some further subdivide by race, ethnicity, or other demographic characteristics. Projections of each component can be based on the extrapolation of past trends, projected trends in other areas, structural models, or some other technique. The cohort-component method is used more frequently than any other projection method because it can incorporate many different data sources, assumptions, and application techniques and because it provides projections of demographic characteristics as well as projections of the total population.

The choice of a projection method depends on the availability of resources and the purposes for which the projections will be used. Simple extrapolation methods require few resources and can be applied quickly at virtually any level of geography, but provide only limited demographic detail and have little usefulness as analytical tools. More complex extrapolation methods require more data and modeling expertise, but share most of the other attributes of simple extrapolation methods. Cohort-component models are more data-intensive, time-consuming, and costly than trend extrapolation methods, but provide a much higher level of demographic detail and are more useful as analytical tools. Structural models are often the most data-intensive, time-consuming, and costly, but provide a variety of interrelated projections and offer the greatest analytical usefulness. Choosing a projection method for any particular project requires balancing the need for geographic, demographic, and socioeconomic detail against time, money, and data constraints.

No single method or category of methods has been found to produce projections of total population that are consistently more accurate than those produced by any other method or category of methods (e.g., Long 1995; Smith and Sincich 1992; White 1954). In general, mean absolute percentage errors tend to increase as population size declines, as growth rates deviate in either direction from moderate but positive levels, and as the projection horizon extends further into the future. For economic variables, many studies have found that combining projections based on a variety of methods, data sets, or assumptions leads to greater forecast accuracy than can be achieved using a single projection by itself (Armstrong 2001). Although there have been few studies to date, we believe the same may be true for projections of demographic variables.

For 10-year horizons, typical mean absolute percentage errors for population projections have been found to be about 6% for states, 12% for counties, and 18% for census tracts; for 20-year horizons, errors are roughly twice as large (Smith, Tayman, and Swanson 2001). Clearly, there is much greater uncertainty in projecting future populations than in estimating current or past populations. Given this uncertainty, population projections prepared by the U.S. Census Bureau and many other demographic agencies generally contain several alternative series based on different methods, different combinations of assumptions, or the development of formal confidence limits. Delineating alternative future scenarios strengthens decision making by underscoring the uncertainties inherent in population projections.

ILLUSTRATIONS

Demographers address a varied and ever expanding range of practical concerns in the public policy and business arenas. Accurate forecasts of residential energy needs, school enrollments, medical expenditures, and home ownership trends depend partly on foreseeing changes in population size, distribution, and composition. Human resource planning requires data on the characteristics of the available labor force and the employer's specific personnel needs. Site analyses call for comparative information on the demographic composition of populations clustered in and around competing locations. Sound financial planning relies on information regarding the effects of demographic changes on wealth accumulation, consumption, and investment. Technical issues arising in adversarial contexts require the testimony of experts with an understanding of demographic data and methods and a familiarity with any legal requirements that may apply. The following examples illustrate the diverse nature of the topics addressed by small-area and business demographers.

Catering to Home Buyers

The home-building industry is highly decentralized. A typical builder constructs just a few dozen homes a year in one or two communities. Business volume depends on short-term factors such as interest rates, consumer confidence, and local housing market conditions. Accordingly, builders tend to be inattentive to longer-term demographic trends and are notoriously weak in their marketing strategies. When homes sell in a region, builders are likely to build more of the same type until like-minded builders collectively saturate the local market. Typically, a builder's major concern is simply to sell newly built homes quickly and profitably.

A demographic perspective can provide builders with valuable marketing insights, particularly in volatile times. For example, demographers can highlight the degree of diversity found within the baby boom generation. Prospective home buyers may include individuals, childless married couples, single adults paired up with coinvestors, and other domestic units that hardly resemble the traditional family of American nostalgia. Compared with families with children, such home buyers have distinctive needs and preferences (e.g., houses that are maintenance-free and contain such adult-oriented features as home offices, hobby rooms, and flexible internal space that can be adapted to fluid living arrangements). Demographic insights can help builders cater to the highly varied needs of prospective home buyers and target distinct segments within the overall market.

Newspaper Readership

Newspaper publishers and editors recognize that they must adapt to powerful societal and demographic changes that are transforming advertising markets, reading habits, and readers' interests. Increasingly, large cities tend to be populated by ethnic pluralities. To gain circulation (and advertising dollars), publishers need to focus more news stories on specific groups who collectively account for substantial proportions of the residents of a city (e.g., Latinos and particular Asian nationalities). Furthermore, many readers live alone, are divorced or remarried, or are cohabiting. Among married couples, fewer have children at home but more anticipate future eldercare obligations. Accompanying these diverse lifestyles are new interests and activities.

Demographers can identify the changing demographics of newspaper circulation and readership, helping publishers cater to the collections of small audiences with shared interests who comprise an increasingly segmented readership (e.g., Morrison 1995). They also can devise and calibrate specialized tools for segmenting a customer base. For example, the surnames of a newspaper's subscribers can be used to distinguish those who are likely to be Latino, Korean, or Chinese (e.g., Abrahamse, Morrison, and Bolton 1994; Lauderdale and Kestenbaum 2000).

Site Evaluation and Selection

For many businesses, geographic proximity to consumer markets is imperative because most retail transactions are made at specific locations. Geographic location can be equally critical to the provision of public services. In both the private and public sectors, then, small-area demography plays a central role in site evaluation and selection: Pediatricians seek office locations near families with young children; school boards try to predict where the next wave of families with young children will move; banks seek branch locations in high-income suburban areas; hotels search for areas with large numbers of tourists or business travelers; and supermarkets, hardware stores, and health clinics look for sites in the midst of densely populated areas. Demographic analysis can inform decision making by evaluating a proposed site or weighing the comparative merits of several competing sites (e.g., Johnson 1997; Murdock and Hamm 1997; Voss 1997).

Tayman, Parrott, and Carnevale (1997) illustrate an application of site evaluation and selection in the public sector. These analysts chose locations for new fire stations in a growing metropolitan area. They used a model combining methods from demography, geography, and urban planning and compared potential sites by evaluating small-area data on projected population and household growth, road networks, travel times, land use plans, and access to "critical sites" such as hospitals, schools, and nursing homes. This case study—involving a problem both broad in scope and requiring more than demographic expertise alone—typifies the kind of situations encountered by many public-sector demographers.

Morrison and Abrahamse (1996) illustrate a business application of site evaluation and selection. These analysts screened several thousand square miles within metropolitan southern California to identify the 10 best store locations for a large supermarket chain catering to one-stop shoppers. Using a variety of demographic factors that were expected to enhance sales, the analysts selected locations based on potential sales volume. To pinpoint the density of geographic concentrations of food expenditures, they devised a model positing that the fraction of customers drawn to any given store from an area x miles away is determined by the number of people living in the area, its distance from the store, and the personal characteristics of supermarket shoppers. To identify consumers likely to be attracted to the convenience of one-stop shopping, they used census tract data on the proportion of families with two employed adults (whose work schedules would necessitate convenience). Other factors judged to be important were the proportions of large households (conducive to family-centered meals at home) and long-time homeowners (who would have lower mortgage payments and hence higher disposable incomes). These factors were shown to enhance the conventional distance-decay models that are typically used for choosing optimal sites.

Forecasting School Enrollment: Myth versus Reality

Not all changes in school enrollment trends are demographically induced. Seemingly minor policy changes often have a major impact on the size and direction of enrollment changes, particularly where the effects of policy changes happen to coincide with spurious demographic events. McKibben (1996) chronicled an instance where an obscure change in state educational policy led to the mistaken public perception that a local school district was on the cusp of a long-term growth cycle. By lowering the minimum age for a child to enroll in kindergarten, the state board of education—through a simple change in policy—had introduced a one-time inflation of kindergarten cohort size. Community residents, reading media reports on a national "baby boomlet," discovered its apparent manifestations locally at the kindergarten level and strenuously opposed the local school board's plan to close several rural elementary schools.

In fact, there was no "baby boomlet" in their district. McKibben's team of analysts uncovered both the policy and its effect and produced an enrollment forecast that was not confounded by the artificial appearance of growth. Using local data and the cohort-component method, they developed population and school enrollment projections that better informed the public debate and strengthened the planning process, helping avert unwarranted and costly plans to keep unneeded schools open.

Spatial Analysis and Public Health

Small-area demographic analysis supported by geographic information systems (GIS) opens up a host of potential contributions to the field of public health. Gobalet and Thomas (1996) described several case studies in which demographic techniques and perspectives strengthened the planning of health education campaigns and services. In one, a county public health department sought to identify areas in which public health interventions might reduce unnecessary hospitalizations among elderly residents with an above-average risk of developing acute but preventable conditions. The point of departure was an index of indicators believed to describe factors placing a senior citizen at risk of—among other things—reduced independence, increased morbidity, and premature death. The indicators (based on decennial census data) included high rates of linguistic isolation, living alone, and poverty. Together, these indicators identified census tracts with high index values (designated *Senior Risk Zones*, or SRZs).

The question these analysts wished to answer was whether seniors residing in SRZs were in fact more prone to early disability, untreated health problems, and unnecessary hospitalization than other seniors, as hypothesized in the model. To answer this question, they obtained hospital discharge data on diagnoses and patient addresses. The data, however, were available only by ZIP code, not by census tract. Using GIS, the analysts converted ZIP code data into census tract estimates and compared diagnoses with risk-index values for areas both inside and outside the SRZs. The analysis demonstrated that SRZs were, indeed, areas where preventable hospitalizations among seniors were disproportionately concentrated, making them potentially useful tools for targeting public health intervention.

Political Redistricting

Officials in states, counties, cities, school districts, and other jurisdictions that elect representatives are required by law to redraw election district lines using new data from each successive decennial census. Redistricting is a politically sensitive process that is subject to exacting legal standards. Demographers can play a central role in this process by providing the data and analysis needed to ensure that political jurisdictions comply with legal mandates. Because redistricting typically bestows an advantage on one group at the expense of another, constructing new boundaries often foments controversy and sometimes leads to acrimonious legal proceedings (Morrison 1997).

Legal challenges brought under Section 2 of the Federal Voting Rights Act generally arise when minority groups claim that their voting strength is diluted by the way particular boundaries are drawn. The concept of *dilution* focuses attention on counting those members of the population who are entitled to vote and distributing this population geographically into voting districts. Typically, the resources that demographers use for such purposes are census data for small geographic units (e.g., census tracts and block groups), in which age and citizenship are shown separately for each minority group.

Since categories are not always neatly delineated, measurement can be difficult. For example, *Black* and *Hispanic* are not mutually exclusive categories, and the term *Asian* obscures separate nationalities that may exhibit genuine political differences (e.g., Chinese and Vietnamese). The opportunity to designate more than one racial category in the 2000 census further complicated the issue, making it more difficult to evaluate changes in racial composition over time. Since demographers have been trained to respect definitional subtleties and to recognize data limitations, they can deal successfully with many of the nuances that arise in redistricting.

Conforming to Legally Mandated Standards

Demographic data, concepts, and techniques can also be used to evaluate affirmative action goals for equalizing employment opportunities. Courts of law addressing employment discrimination disputes need an accurate picture of each minority group's proportion in a pool of prospective employees. The demographic and socioeconomic factors conditioning those proportions vary from place to place. Here, demographers may be called upon to delineate the racial and ethnic composition of a pool of workers eligible to be hired or promoted and to defend their measures and conclusions in adversarial settings.

Suppose that City X has a population that is 30% Hispanic, but only 15% of the city's employees are Hispanic. Does that disparity mean that employment opportunities have been less available to Hispanic than to non-Hispanic job seekers? Turning the question around, if employment opportunities were equally available to Hispanics, what would be their expected proportion among qualified job seekers in a city that is 30% Hispanic? It would be naive to imagine that a group's proportion of qualified job seekers would be precisely equal to its proportion of the overall population because age/sex structures, labor force participation rates, and other characteristics differ considerably from one racial/ethnic group to another.

Changes in any of these characteristics increase the complexity of the analysis. For example, suppose that Hispanics made up 15% of City X's population a decade ago and that the very same individuals who worked for the city then are still its employees. Under such conditions, today's 30% Hispanic share would be incorrect as a benchmark for analyzing people hired 10 or more years ago. However, would 15% be the correct benchmark?

As this hypothetical example suggests, a group's presence in the current population may not represent its actual availability in either the current or the previous pool of qualified job seekers. The legal, technical, and philosophical issues related to legally mandated standards are highly complex. Their resolution requires not only knowledge of the law and the ability to apply demographic data and techniques, but experience and wisdom as well. (For related literature on the interplay of demography and the law, see Morrison, 1993, 1998, 1999a; Smith 1993.)

Costs of Health Benefits

Applications of business demography to the structure and dynamics of large corporate workforces have strategic implications for managing the cost of health benefits. Most

Americans receive health benefits through employers, making groups of employees (and their families) the basis for health care financing. How do changes in workforce size affect the cost of health benefits? Does reducing the workforce by a certain percentage reduce health care costs by the same percentage? Do employers have complete control over the number of persons receiving company-sponsored health benefits?

To answer these questions, Kintner and Swanson (1996) analyzed three possible sources of change in the health benefits group associated with salaried employees at General Motors (GM): (1) flows into and out of GM related to employment processes; (2) flows into and out of the health benefits group related to demographic processes; and (3) transfers from active employment to retirement or layoff.

The GM health benefits group includes employees and their dependents. Employees become eligible for benefits through hiring; they lose benefits through quits, discharges, and deaths. Employees also leave this group through layoff or retirement (but may still be eligible for health benefits). Figure 25.1 summarizes the flows into and out of the health benefits group. Additions include new hires and their families, plus births and marriages to employees already belonging to the group. The group loses members through quits, deaths, divorces, and lost eligibility. Transfers occur through retirement and layoffs.

Kintner and Swanson estimated these flows using record-matching techniques and identified the relative contributions of employment and demographic processes to changing group size. Their analysis revealed the limits that GM faces in controlling the size of its health benefits group. GM's use of window retirement packages for downsizing gives it some control, as does its control over hiring and firing. Nevertheless, demographic processes unrelated to turnover or transfers tend to have a substantial impact on changes over time in the size and composition of GM's health benefits group.

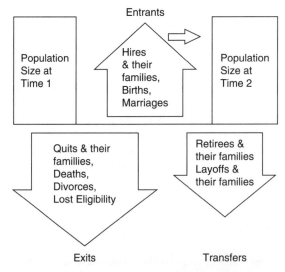

FIGURE 25.1. Flows into and out of health benefits group.

Labor Force Characteristics

A company may operate several production facilities which were started at different stages in its history. One byproduct of such sequential expansion may be a workforce whose age structure varies across facilities, with attendant human resource implications. As part of a consulting project, one of the authors of this chapter (Morrison) studied a company that operated several production facilities across the nation. Some opened as early as the 1940s; others, as late as the 1980s. Each plant depended heavily on a small cadre of experienced engineering and maintenance employees to repair mechanical breakdowns, which impose costly reductions in output.

This company had compiled age data for its overall workforce but had never examined them separately by facility. Doing so revealed that the workforce at some plants exhibited distinctive age structures. Figure 25.2 shows the age structures for two of the company's plants. Plant A has an age structure similar to that of the entire company. Plant B, by contrast, began operations 40 years ago and has a disproportionately older work force. The majority of Plant B's employees are nearing retirement age, foreshadowing the impending loss of many highly experienced employees—precisely those employees whose skills would be most difficult to replace.

These elementary demographic insights carry several important messages about how the company might prepare for the future. To cushion against the expected future losses of worker skills through retirement, a prudent manager might view existing skills as assets whose value will sharply appreciate in the years ahead. A forward-looking

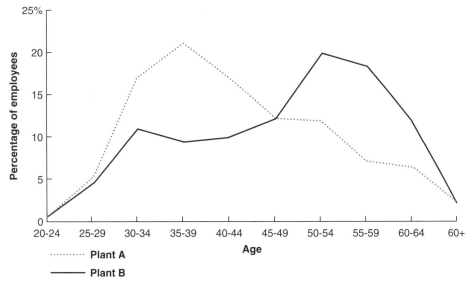

Work-Force Woes
Employee age structures at two of a company's production plants show distinctive age patterns–and impending loss of experienced workers at Plant B.

FIGURE 25.2. Workforce woes.

company might try to conserve those assets, perhaps by establishing an "unretirement bank" of retirees who would be willing to work part-time when the need arose. Plant B is an obvious pilot site in which to test such an innovation, perhaps as a first step toward instituting it across the company.

Spotting Hidden Market Opportunities

Demographers are sometimes called upon to highlight the long-term significance of impending population shifts for consumer markets. Characterizing market evolution with reference to changing age structure, household makeup, and spatial distribution introduces new perspectives on potential opportunities. The following example illustrates how a demographic perspective might inform business thinking on the potential market for a relatively new product, the low-speed electric neighborhood vehicle (Morrison 1999b).

Neighborhood vehicles (NVs) encompass a wide range of lightweight contraptions for transporting people within settings that are sheltered from conventional automobile traffic. Unlike golf carts (ubiquitous in retirement communities), NVs travel faster and afford passenger-cargo configurations that can be adapted to fit the varied needs of households at different stages in the life cycle. For example, the same NV platform might suit the needs of four passengers (e.g., grandparents with visiting children or grandchildren) or two passengers (e.g., a childless couple with six bags of groceries).

The most likely locations for NVs are master-planned residential communities, either gated or otherwise separated from regular automotive traffic. Such communities represent several distinct markets that might form distinctive niches for NVs—for example, retirement communities populated by older adults; golf and leisure communities populated by empty-nesters; and new towns (e.g., Columbia, Maryland, and Celebration, Florida) populated by a broad spectrum of locally oriented suburbanites. Other potential markets would include sprawling health or industrial parks, college campuses, and controlled-access national parks.

Although the market for NVs was not highly developed at the end of the 20th century, three ongoing developments are likely to spark consumer interest. First is the proliferation of compact communities, both residential and commercial, within which new types of personal transportation are required. The common denominator in such communities is the need to shuttle around conveniently in settings that are unsuitable for automobiles or public transportation. Second is the growing proportion of one- and two-person "empty-nest" households, which aligns well with the capacity limits of the NV. These households might desire NVs as an alternative to a second car or as a discretionary indulgence analogous to a snowmobile or powerboat. Third is the rapidly expanding elderly population, which will initially promote the spread of leisure communities for relatively young, active retirees, but will eventually lead to large numbers of people with health and mobility limitations.

Presently, the customer base for NVs is spatially and demographically concentrated, but it is likely to grow rapidly in future years. Distinct market niches will likely materialize that can be targeted with different variants of an NV built on a common platform. Demographic insights can spark new ideas and nurture a strategic business vision for this nascent industry.

CONCLUSIONS

Small-area and business demography are closely intertwined because they use many of the same demographic concepts, data sources, and statistical techniques, and they address many of the same practical questions faced by decision makers. Several recent developments have driven—and will continue to drive—the advancement of both fields.

First, small-area data have become increasingly prevalent in many countries. These data are generally based on administrative records, but sample surveys also have played a role (e.g., the American Community Survey). Often, they are spatially referenced, allowing for the aggregation of individual-level data into a variety of customized geographic areas (e.g., consumer market areas, school districts, traffic analysis zones). New or enhanced data sources permit analyses that were impossible only a few years ago.

Proprietary databases derived from customer records have also become more common. Many businesses have developed automated data registries for individual customers. Examples include airline frequent-flier programs that track individual travel behavior; supermarket bar code scanners that track each shopper's purchases; and purchase histories recorded by credit card companies. These data afford unprecedented opportunities for targeting consumers based on personal characteristics and purchase histories. "You are where you live"—the marketer's dictum from the 1980s—has been replaced by "You are what you just bought." Data from both public and private sources will become increasingly available in the coming years, at ever smaller geographic scales.

Second, computer power has increased exponentially. Applications that once required expensive mainframe computers and highly developed programming skills are now feasible using inexpensive personal computers and standard software. The technology for storing, retrieving, and matching data has advanced rapidly, permitting many new applications. The Internet has facilitated the collection of data from widely divergent sources, promoted the sharing of information across vast distances, and provided businesses and government agencies with a powerful marketing tool. The end of these advances is not in sight.

Third, the development of geographic information systems (GIS) has greatly facilitated the collection, organization, manipulation, and analysis of spatially referenced data. This may be the single most important recent development affecting small-area and business demography. GIS can be used to select sites, develop population or customer profiles, track changes in health status, target areas to participate in government programs, screen potential markets, launch new products, and improve the visual presentation of information (e.g., Borroto and Martinez-Piedra 2000; Gobalet and Thomas 1996; Gould et al. 1998). Advances in satellite imagery and global positioning systems have made it possible to use GIS to track population, housing, and other trends over time and space (e.g., Harvey 2000; Lo 1995; Webster 1996). These advances are particularly useful for places lacking reliable administrative records. The growth of GIS databases may also facilitate the development of new methods for projecting future growth, such as spatial diffusion models that base changes in one geographic area on what happened earlier in nearby areas (e.g., Morrill, Gaile, and Thrall 1988).

These three developments have greatly enhanced the value of small-area and business demography for decision making. Several potential barriers, however, could limit future advances. The most formidable arises from concerns about privacy and the confidentiality of data. The collection of personal information is widely viewed as an invasion of privacy. Other concerns include the loss of confidentiality that may occur when data are shared among government agencies and private businesses or used for purposes other than those for which they were collected. These concerns have tended to limit the collection and use of administrative records data in the United States, Germany, the United Kingdom, and several other countries (e.g., Doyle et al. 2001; Redfern 1989; Scheuren 1999). Since the linkage of personal records from several data sets is essential for many purposes, concerns about privacy and confidentiality could prevent the most effective use of data for both public and private sector decision making. As illustrated by recent discussions regarding the use of linked data for national security purposes, this promises to be a topic of vigorous debate during the coming years.

Not all applications of business demography pertain to small areas. As markets have globalized, business interests have focused increasingly on the emergence of massive groups of consumers in countries like India and China. Given their large populations and rapid economic growth, these countries provide huge but largely untapped consumer markets. Anticipating the future growth of these markets poses distinctive problems amenable to demographic analysis (e.g., Morrison, Levin, and Seever 1996). Although many applications of business demography have focused on ever smaller geographic areas and demographic subgroups, we believe future applications will address these broader horizons as well.

REFERENCES

Abrahamse, A. F., P. A. Morrison, and N. M. Bolton. 1994. Surname analysis for estimating local concentration of Hispanics and Asians. *Population Research and Policy Review* 13:383–398.

Anderson, M. J. 1988. *The American census: A social history*. New Haven, Conn.: Yale University Press.

Anderson, M. J. and S. E. Fienberg. 1999. *Who counts? The politics of census-taking in contemporary America*. New York: Russell Sage Foundation.

Armstrong, J. S. 2001. Combining forecasts. In *Principles of forecasting: A handbook for researchers and practitioners*. Edited by J. S. Armstrong, 417–439. Norwell, Mass.: Kluwer Academic Publishers.

Beeson, P. E., D. N. DeJong, and W. Troesken. 2001. Population growth in U.S. counties, 1840–1990. *Regional Science and Urban Economics* 31:669–699.

Bertazzi, P. A., D. Consonni, S. Bachetti, M. Rubagotti, A. Baccarelli, C. Zocchetti, and A. C. Pesatori. 2001. Health effects of dioxin exposure: A 20-year mortality study. *American Journal of Edipemiology* 153:1031–1044.

Bongaarts, J., and R. A. Bulatao. 2000. *Beyond six billion: Forecasting the world's population*. Washington, D.C.: National Academy Press.

Borroto, R. J., and R. Martinez-Piedra. 2000. Geographical patterns of cholera in Mexico, 1991–1996. *International Journal of Epidemiology* 29:764–772.

Bryan, K. N., and R. George. 2004. Geographic information systems. In *The methods and materials of demography*, 2d ed., Edited by J. S. Siegel and D. A. Swanson, Appendix D. San Diego: Elsevier Academic Press.

Bryan, T. 2004. Population estimates. In *The methods and materials of demography*, 2d ed., Edited by J. S. Siegel and D. A. Swanson, San Diego: Elsevier Academic Press.

Cleland, J. 1996. Demographic data collection in less developed countries 1946–1996. *Population Studies* 50:433–450.

Davis, H. C. 1995. *Demographic projection techniques for regions and smaller areas*. Vancouver, Canada: UBC Press.

Davis, S. T. 2001. Evaluating county population estimates: The big picture, hard to enumerate counties, and counties with special treatment. Paper presented at the annual meeting of the Southern Demographic Association, Miami Beach, Fla.

Day, K. M. 1992. Interprovincial migration and local public goods. *Canadian Journal of Economics* 25:123–144.

Doyle, P., J. I. Lane, J. J. M. Theeuwes, and L. V. Zayatz. 2001. *Confidentiality, disclosure, and data access: Theory and practical applications for statistical agencies.* Amsterdam: Elsevier Science.

Edmonston, B., and C. Schultze, eds. 1995. *Modernizing the U.S. census: Panel on census requirements in the year 2000 and beyond.* Washington, D.C.: National Academies Press.

Feeney, D., J. Hibbs, and R. T. Gillaspy. 1995. Ratio-correlation method. In *Basic methods for preparing small-area population estimates.* Edited by N. W. Rives, W. J. Serow, A. S. Lee, H. F. Goldsmith, and P. R. Voss, 118–136. Madison: Applied Population Laboratory, University of Wisconsin.

Galdi, D. 1985. Evaluation of 1980 subcounty population estimates. *Current Population Reports*, Series P-25, Number 963. Washington, D.C.: U.S. Bureau of the Census.

Ghosh, M., and J. N. K. Rao. 1994. Small area estimation: An appraisal. *Statistical Science* 9:55–76.

Gobalet, J. G., and R. K. Thomas. 1996. Demographic data and geographic information systems for decision making: The case of public health. *Population Research and Policy Review* 15:537–548.

Gould, J. B., B. Herrchen, T. Pham, S. Bera, and C. Brindis. 1998. Small-area analysis: Targeting high-risk areas for adolescent pregnancy prevention programs. *Family Planning Perspectives* 30:173–176.

Harper, G., J. Devine, and C. Coleman. 2001. Evaluation of 2000 subcounty population estimates. Paper presented at the annual meeting of the Southern Demographic Association, Miami Beach, Fla.

Harvey, J. 2000. Small area population estimation using satellite imagery. *Statistics in Transition* 4:611–633.

Johnson, K. M. 1997. Selecting markets for corporate expansion: A case study in applied demography. In *Demographics: A casebook for business and government.* Edited by H. J. Kintner, T. W. Merrick, P. A. Morrison, and P. R. Voss, 129–143. Santa Monica, Calif.: RAND.

Kintner, H. J., and D. A. Swanson. 1996. Ties that bind: A case study of the link between employers, families, and health benefits. *Population Research and Policy Review* 15:509–526.

Kintner, H. J., and D. A. Swanson. 1997. Estimating vital rates from corporate databases: How long will GM's salaried retirees live? In *Demographics: A casebook for business and government.* Edited by H. J. Kintner, T. W. Merrick, P. A. Morrison, and P. R. Voss, 265–297. Santa Monica, Calif.: RAND.

Lauderdale, D., and B. Kestenbaum. 2000. Asian American ethnic identification by surname. *Population Research and Policy Review* 19:283–300.

Lo, C. P. 1995. Automated population and dwelling unit estimation from high-resolution satellite images: A GIS approach. *International Journal of Remote Sensing* 16:17–34.

Long, J. F. 1993. Postcensal population estimates: States, counties, and places. Technical Working Paper No. 3, U.S. Census Bureau, Washington, D.C.

Long, J. F. 1995. Complexity, accuracy, and utility of official population projections. *Mathematical Population Studies* 5:203–216.

Longva, S., I. Thomsen, and P. I. Severeide. 1998. Reducing costs of censuses in Norway through use of administrative registers. *International Statistical Review* 66:223–234.

Mason, A. 1996. Population and housing. *Population Research and Policy Review* 15:419–435.

McKibben, J. N. 1996. The impact of policy changes on forecasting for school districts. *Population Research and Policy Review* 15:527–536.

Miller, T. 2001. Increasing longevity and Medicare expenditures. *Demography* 38:215–226.

Mitchell, S. 1995. Birds of a feather. *American Demographics* 17:40–48.

Morrill, R., G. L. Gaile, and G. I. Thrall. 1988. *Spatial diffusion.* Newbury Park, Calif.:Sage Publications.

Morrison, P. A. 1993. More than meets the eye. *Chance* 6:24–30.

Morrison, P. A. 1995. Broadening client perspectives on business concerns. *Applied Demography* 10:1–3.

Morrison, P. A. 1997. Empowered or disadvantaged? Applications of demographic analysis to political redistricting. In *Demographics: A casebook for business and government.* Edited by H. J. Kintner, T. W. Merrick, P. A. Morrison, and P. R. Voss, 17–32. Santa Monica, Calif.: RAND.

Morrison, P. A. 1998. Demographic influences on Latinos' political empowerment: Comparative local illustrations. *Population Research and Policy Review* 17:223–246.

Morrison, P. A. 1999a. Unveiling the demographic "action" in class-action lawsuits: Two instructional cases. *Population Research and Policy Review* 18:491–505.

Morrison, P. A. 1999b. Gauging future prospects for a neighborhood vehicle: Where demographic analysis fits in. Paper presented at the annual meeting of the Southern Demographic Association, San Antonio, Tex.

Morrison, P. A., and A. F. Abrahamse. 1996. Applying demographic analysis to store site selection. *Population Research and Policy Review* 15:479–489.

Morrison, P. A., M. H. Levin, and P. M. Seever. 1996. Tracking growth of emerging consumer markets worldwide: Where demographic analysis fits in. Paper presented at the Sixth International Conference on Applied and Business Demography, Bowling Green, Ohis.

Murdock, S. H., and D. R. Ellis. 1991. *Applied demography*. Boulder, Colo.: Westview Press.

Murdock, S. H., and R. R. Hamm. 1997. A demographic analysis of the market for a long-term care facility: A case study in applied demography. In *Demographics: A casebook for business and government*. Edited by H. J. Kintner, T. W. Merrick, P. A. Morrison, and P. R. Voss, 218–246. Santa Monica, Calif.: RAND.

Murdock, S. H., S. Hwang, and R. R. Hamm. 1995. Component methods. In *Basic methods for preparing small-area population estimates*. Edited by N. W. Rives, W. J. Serow, A. S. Lee, H. F. Goldsmith, and P. R. Voss, 10–53. Madison: Applied Population Laboratory, University of Wisconsin.

O'Hare, W. 1976. Report on a multiple regression method for making population estimates. *Demography* 13:369–379.

O'Neill, B. C., D. Balk, M. Brickman, and M. Ezra. 2001. A guide to global population projections. *Demographic Research* 4:203–288.

Opitz, W., and H. Nelson. 1996. Short-term population-based forecasting in the public sector: A dynamic caseload simulation model. *Population Research and Policy Review* 15:549–563.

Pittenger, D. B. 1976. *Projecting state and local populations*. Cambridge, Mass.: Ballinger.

Pol, L. G., and R. K. Thomas. 1997. *Demography for business decision making*. Westport, Counn.: Quoram Books.

Rao, J. N. K. 1999. Some recent advances in model-based small area estimation. *Survey Methodology* 25:175–186.

Redfern, P. 1989. Population registers: Some administrative and statistical pros and cons. *Journal of the Royal Statistical Society, Series A* 152:1–41.

Rees, P., and M. Kupiszewski. 1999. Internal migration: What data are available in Europe? *Journal of Official Statistics* 15:551–586.

Rives, N. W. 1997a. Strategic financial planning for hospitals: Demographic considerations. In *Demographics: A casebook for business and government*. Edited by H. J. Kintner, T. W. Merrick, P. A. Morrison, and P. R. Voss, 251–264. Santa Monica, Calif.: RAND.

Rives, N. W., W. J. Serow, A. S. Lee, H. F. Goldsmith, and P. R. Voss, eds. 1995. *Basic methods for preparing small-area population estimates*. Madison: Applied Population Laboratory, University of Wisconsin.

Russell, C. 1984. The business of demographics. *Population Bulletin* 39. Washington, D.C.: Population Reference Bureau.

Scheuren, F. 1999. Administrative records and census taking. *Survey Methodology* 25:151–160.

Serow, W. J., E. W. Terrie, B. Weller, and R. W. Wichmann. 1997. The use of intercensal population estimates in political redistricting. In *Demographics: A casebook for business and government*. Edited by H. J. Kintner, T. W. Merrick, P. A. Morrison, and P. R. Voss, 33–54. Santa Monica, Calif.: RAND.

Shahidullah, M., and M. Flotow. 2001. An evaluation of the accuracy of 2000 population estimates for counties in Illinois. Paper presented at the annual meeting of the Southern Demographic Association, Miami Beach, Fla.

Siegel, J. S. 2002. *Applied demography*. San Diego: Academic Press.

Simpson, S., I. Diamond, P. Tonkin, and R. Tye. 1996. Updating small area population estimates in England and Wales. *Journal of the Royal Statistical Society, Series A* 159:235–247.

Skerry, P. 2000. *Counting on the census?* Washington, D.C.: Brookings Institution Press.

Smith, S. K. 1986. A review and evaluation of the housing unit method of population estimation. *Journal of the American Statistical Association* 81:287–296.

Smith, S. K. 1993. Expert testimony in adversarial legal proceedings: Some tips for demographers. *Population Research and Policy Review* 12:43–52.

Smith, S. K., and M. Mandell. 1984. A comparison of population estimation methods: Housing unit versus component II, ratio correlation, and administrative records. *Journal of the American Statistical Association* 79:282–289.

Smith, S. K., and T. Sincich. 1992. Evaluating the forecast accuracy and bias of alternative population projections for states. *International Journal of Forecasting* 8:495–508.

Smith, S. K., J. Tayman, and D. A. Swanson. 2001. *State and local population projections: Methodology and analysis*. New York: Kluwer Academic/Plenum Publishers.

Starsinic, D. E., A. S. Lee, H. F. Goldsmith, and M. A. Sparr. 1995. The Census Bureau's administrative records method. In *Basic methods for preparing small-area population estimates*. Edited by N. W. Rives,

W. J. Serow, A. S. Lee, H. F. Goldsmith, and P. R. Voss, 54–69. Madison: Applied Population Laboratory, University of Wisconsin.

Tayman, J., B. Parrott, and S. Carnevale. 1997. Locating fire station sites: The response time component. In *Demographics: A casebook for business and government*. Edited by H. J. Kintner, T. W. Merrick, P. A. Morrison, and P. R. Voss, 203–217. Santa Monica, Calif.: RAND.

Texas Water Development Board. 1997. Water for Texas: A consensus-based update to the state water plan. Vol. II, Technical Planning Appendix. Document No. GF-6-2. Austin, Tex.

Thomas, R. K. 1997. Using demographic analysis in health services planning: A case study in obstetrical services. In *Demographics: A casebook for business and government*. Edited by H. J. Kintner, T. W. Merrick, P. A. Morrison, and P. R. Voss, 159–179. Santa Monica, Calif.: RAND.

U.S. Census Bureau. 1990. State and local agencies preparing population and housing estimates. *Current Population Reports*, Series P-25, Number 1063. Washington, D.C.

U.S. Census Bureau. 2003. American Community Survey Operations Plan. (www.census.gov/acs/www/downloads/opsplanfinal).

U.S. Census Bureau. 2004. State and Country Total Population Estimates. (www.census.gov/popest/topics/methodology).

Voss, P. R. 1997. Targeting wealthy ex-Wisconsinites in Florida: A case study in applied demography. In *Demographics: A casebook for business and government*. Edited by H. J. Kintner, T. W. Merrick, P. A. Morrison, and P. R. Voss, 109–128. Santa Monica, Calif.: RAND.

Webster, C. J. 1996. Population and dwelling unit estimates from space. *Third World Planning Review* 18:155–176.

Weiss, M. J. 1988. *The clustering of America*. New York: Harper & Row.

White, H. 1954. Empirical study of the accuracy of selected methods of projecting state populations. *Journal of the American Statistical Association* 49:480–498.

Wilson, C. 1985. *The dictionary of demography*. Oxford: Basil Blackwell.

CHAPTER 26

Health Demography

ICHIRO KAWACHI AND S.V. SUBRAMANIAN

WHAT IS HEALTH DEMOGRAPHY?

In their 1992 book *The Demography of Health and Health Care* (part of the Plenum Series on Demographic Methods and Population Analysis), Louis Pol and Richard Thomas declared there was neither a widely accepted definition of *health demography* nor a distinct group of professionals who called themselves health demographers (Pol and Thomas 1992). They went on to note that most of those involved with health demography were not professionally trained demographers, but epidemiologists, sociologists, and other social scientists who happened to apply demographic concepts in the health field. Pol and Thomas provided the following definition of health demography:

> Health demography is perhaps best defined as the application of the content and methods of demography to the study of health status and health behavior... Thus health demography concerns itself with the manner in which such factors as age, marital status, and income influence both the health status and health behaviors of populations and, in turn, how health-related phenomena affect demographic attributes (Pol and Thomas 1992: 1).

A decade later, there is still no organized body of professionals who call themselves health demographers. On the other hand, demographers and epidemiologists (along with sociologists, medical geographers, and even a few economists) have begun to converge on an emerging field that has been referred to as "the social determinants of population health" (Marmot and Wilkinson 1999; Berkman and Kawachi 2000; Eckersley, Dixon, and Douglas 2001). Frustrated with the progressively narrow concern for identifying "risk factors" for disease (including the search for genetic markers) as a way of understanding and addressing problems of public health, some epidemiologists have called for broadening the usual inventory of determinants of health to include variables such as socioeconomic status, race/ethnicity, and social support, all of which are intended to capture some aspect of social organization rather than simply characteristics of individuals (Berkman and Kawachi 2000). By advocating for the movement of these classic demographic variables to a central role in research on the health of populations, these *social* epidemiologists (as they call themselves) represent one end of the potential spectrum of health demographers.

At the same time, social demographers have rediscovered the role of social context in human behavior, and "with encouragement from their sociologic neighbors, have begun to recognize the severe shortcomings of a purely variable-based view of the world" (Palloni and Morenoff 2001: 140). The foundation for a viable discipline of health demography therefore rests in the convergence of two disciplines, demography and epidemiology, particularly those branches of each that emphasize the effects of social contexts and group membership.

As will be shown below, demography and epidemiology share a common historical origin dating back to the 17th century. However, during the course of their respective development and refinement, the two fields have diverged and become specialized to the extent that few professional epidemiologists today would claim to be a demographer, and vice versa. Practitioners in each field are trained in separate and distinct programs, learn from different textbooks, resort to different analytical methods, attend separate conferences and professional meetings, and publish their work in specialized journals (with notable exceptions such as the interdisciplinary journal, *Social Science & Medicine*).

Even when they are analyzing the same phenomena in the field of population health, for instance, the mortality crisis in Eastern Europe following economic transformation, or racial and ethnic disparities in birth outcomes, epidemiologists and demographers tend to adopt different study designs, different conceptual frameworks to select and define variables, different assumptions and tests of causality—indeed, different *languages* to define the problem and describe the data. Nonetheless, there are more apparent similarities than differences between the concerns of the two disciplines when it comes to tackling the fundamental questions of population health. In this chapter we will examine the differences and contrasts between epidemiology and demography in addressing the substantive concerns of health demography. We will also point to intersections and areas of convergence between the two that hold promise for delineating health demography as a viable interdisciplinary endeavor.

HISTORICAL LINKS BETWEEN DEMOGRAPHY AND EPIDEMIOLOGY

Epidemiology and demography share a common linguistic heritage (Rockett 1999). The term *epidemiology* derives from the Greek roots *epi* (upon) and *demos* (people) and *logos* (study). Meanwhile, *demos* and another Greek root, *graphein* (to write, draw) combine to form the term demography. Given these roots, it is not surprising that the two disciplines share a common agenda centered on the study of *populations* as opposed to individuals. Interestingly, the population focus of epidemiology became progressively obscured with the rise in popularity of so-called *risk factor* epidemiology (concerned with identifying individual causes of specific diseases) in the mid-20th century and, more recently, molecular epidemiology (concerned with identifying individual genetic susceptibility to disease).

In addition to their shared linguistic heritage, however, epidemiology and demography also share a historical past. John Graunt (1620–1674) is credited with laying the groundwork for both epidemiology and demography when, for the first time, he demonstrated systematic regularity in births and deaths across age, gender, and geographical areas (Graunt 1662 [1975]). William Farr is considered to be one of the intellectual founders of both epidemiology and demography. Indeed, prior to 1850, what we recognize today as distinct and separate concerns of epidemiology and demography were very much interwoven (Susser and Bresnahan 2001). For example, questions concerning the prevalence of diseases and rates of mortality were seldom divorced from considerations of the living conditions of the population as well as changing population composition. Similarly, beginning with Malthus, questions of population change were seldom considered in isolation from the effects of such change on population health.

Susser and Bresnahan (2001) trace the rift between modern epidemiology and demography back to the identification of the tubercle bacillus (1882) and the rise of germ theory. Parallel with the ascendancy of germ theory, the focus of epidemiologists moved away from the study of populations toward the identification of specific pathogens that caused specific diseases. The separation of epidemiology from demography was further heightened during the era of chronic disease epidemiology, which stretched from the identification of cigarettes as the cause of lung cancer (circa 1950) to the end of the 20th century. As methods for investigating risk factors for individual diseases became established in modern epidemiology, "demography gradually disappeared from epidemiology textbooks and training" (Susser and Bresnahan 2001: 13). As for demography, "the study of health has played a small role in demography," despite the shared history of the use of population-based mortality data by demographers and epidemiologists (Weinstein et. al. 2001: 312).

Despite more than a century of divergence between the disciplines, however, the concepts and methods of demography have never ceased to be relevant for those seeking to understand the determinants of population health. As Pol and Thomas (1992) argued, there is hardly an aspect of demography that does *not* have some relevance. Demographers and epidemiologists use the same tools to define and measure population health, for example, life tables, direct and indirect standardization of mortality rates, disability-adjusted life years, and so on. Other demographic variables, such as fertility, migration, and population characteristics (size, distribution), have numerous implications for population health. Finally, both epidemiologists and demographers concur that major compositional characteristics of the population, e.g., age, sex, race, socioeconomic status, religion, and family structure, are among the most fundamental determinants of population health.

Two trends in the late 20th century—the aging of the population and the widening disparities in health across socioeconomic groups—have encouraged the gradual reengagement of the two disciplines. As the population ages, demographers have turned to health itself as an outcome, including implications for health care need and utilization. This increased concern with health as an outcome of interest to demographers has been paralleled by a renewed interest from epidemiologists in the *population*-level and social determinants of health (Berkman and Kawachi 2000; Weinstein, Hermalin, and Stoto 2001). In particular, practitioners of the emerging (or perhaps more accurately, resurgent) subdiscipline of epidemiology, who call themselves *social* epidemiologists, now acknowledge the limitations of a narrowly biomedical perspective in understanding the determinants of population health (Berkman and Kawachi 2000). The movement of social epidemiology has brought about an expanded understanding of the determinants of population health, including variables such as socioeconomic status, family structure, and residential segregation. Health demography increasingly involves an integration of the substantive concerns, concepts, and tools developed in both social epidemiology and demography.

SUBSTANTIVE ISSUES

Social Epidemiology and Demography: A Common Agenda

A definitive program of research for health demography would be premature, given the lack of any training program, textbook, or professional association to represent such a field. Nevertheless, we have identified some basic principles that guide the practice of both demographers and social epidemiologists investigating the social determinants of health. We discuss each of these in turn:

1. Focus on population health, as opposed to individual health.
2. Recognizing the importance of contextual influences on health (including multi-level approaches to study design and analysis)
3. Adopting a life-course perspective on health.
4. Concern for integrating both biological markers and psychosocial pathways in studying the determinants of health.

The Population Health Perspective

Prior to defining what we mean by a "population perspective," a word or two is warranted on the differing approaches of demographers and epidemiologists toward studying "health." As Jack Caldwell (2001) noted:

> Demography has maintained its primary focus on population, births, and deaths. All are definable within a fairly high degree of precision, a criterion about which demographers feel strongly. . . . When demographers purport to write on health, most of their output is usually on mortality change. One reason is that these conditions cannot be defined exactly, a situation that has been worsened by WHO's all-inclusive definition of *good health*. Another reason is the source of data. If demographers work alone through censuses or surveys, they must depend upon self diagnosis or the reporting of symptoms by respondents, and such reporting is often inaccurate (22).

Caldwell's skepticism notwithstanding, a growing number of demographers have been turning their attention toward a broader definition of health beyond simply counting the dead (or living). Without going to the opposite extreme of admitting everything under the WHO definition, health demographers have increasingly turned to more complex outcomes such as cause-specific mortality, disability, self-rated health, health services use, and health behaviors. Problems remain with the accuracy of self-reported health outcomes, but in many large-scale population-based surveys, both demographers and epidemiologists have begun to complement self-reports with biological markers of physiological change (Goldman 2001). Some of these biomarkers (such as salivary cortisol measurements) have only recently become widely available.

With regard to the *focus* of analysis, Caldwell (2001) again drew a sharp distinction between demographers and epidemiologists:

> Demographic analysis tends to seek background or fundamental influences—using social and economic data—not on the individual but on entire societies.... Epidemiologic studies are the most population-based of all medical research, but nevertheless, they are not usually embedded in whole populations seen over long periods of time in their social and economic context (31).

Happily, social epidemiologists have heeded this critique. Indeed, one of the guiding principles of social epidemiology (articulated in the first textbook with that title (see Berkman and Kawachi 2000) is the recognition that individuals are embedded in societies and populations, as well as in history. Applying the population perspective to epidemiological research means asking "Why is this *population* healthy, while another is not?" As Geoffrey Rose (1994) pointed out, the answer to that question may be different from the question that is typically posed in risk factor epidemiology: "Why is this *individual* healthy (or sick), while someone else is not?" For example, the classic case-control study design in epidemiology in the 1950s and 1960s led to the demonstration that individual smokers were at 15 to 20 times the risk of developing lung cancer compared to nonsmokers. However, no case-control study could have succeeded in identifying the correct cause of lung cancer *if everyone in the population had smoked*.

The classic epidemiological approach of identifying individual risk factors falls short both conceptually and methodologically in the task of explaining population patterns and distributions of health. For example, over 300 individual risk factors have now been identified for coronary heart disease. With knowledge of these individual risk factors, epidemiologists can now predict who is at increased risk of developing a heart attack in the future. Such an approach is exemplified by the Framingham Risk Charts. However, this individually oriented approach cannot tell us why some *populations* have much lower rates of heart attack compared to others, for example, why Japanese men have much lower rates of heart attack than American males, even though they smoke twice as much. The answer to the population question requires a population perspective, including knowledge of the distribution of risk factors in the population, as well as the interactions between individual risk factors and with potential contextual influences. Lacking an explicit population perspective, risk factor epidemiology is ill equipped for investigating what Caldwell called the "background or fundamental influences" on health.

The Geographical and Contextual Perspective

Both demographers and social epidemiologists now recognize that the determinants of health operate at multiple levels or contexts. This multilevel approach to population health is crucial not only to health demography, but it is also reflected in conceptual and methodological developments in allied fields, including ecoepidemiology (Susser and Susser 1996a, 1996b; Schwartz, Susser, and Susser 1999), medical geography (Jones and Moon 1993), and medical sociology (Macintyre 2000; Macintyre and Ellaway 2000). Medical geography, in particular, has always been concerned with the role of places and localities (Jones and Moon 1993, 1987; Moon 1990; Kearns 1993). While geographical variations in population health status have been used in epidemiology for descriptive and planning purposes, geographical contexts have seldom been part of the explanation for health status and health disparities, at least until recently.

Indeed, contextual influences on population health may be place-based (e.g., the impact of residing in particular geographical localities), or they may be defined by some other extraindividual, *social organizational* characteristics (such as cultural norms, political systems, labor market structure, population dynamics) that could be spatially or nonspatially described.

Historically, interest in geographical variations in health, and in ecological variables in particular, waned in the social sciences following the powerful demonstration of the ecological fallacy by Robinson (1950) and others. Also, in the health sciences, analyses involving ecological variables became discredited along with the emerging dominance of risk factor epidemiology (Macintyre and Ellaway 2000). For example, ecological analyses were given scant attention (a mere two mentions in the index) in seminal textbooks such as the first edition of Rothman's *Modern Epidemiology* (1986). Unfortunately, in their distaste for committing the ecological fallacy, epidemiologists threw the proverbial baby out with the bath water. Indeed, the problem was not ecology. Rather, the real issue that Robinson (1950) brought to the table was the genuine risk of making individual inferences based on ecological associations. With such distinctions not being clearly articulated, a separate fallacy, termed the *atomistic or individualistic fallacy*, has been coined to refer to the epidemiologist's tendency to assume that health was solely determined by individual risk factors and behaviors (Schwartz 1994; Diez-Roux 1998). Within the social sciences, this trend has been reversed with the renewed interest in contextual influences on health, led by medical geographers, demographers, sociologists, and social epidemiologists (Kawachi and Berkman 2003).

Health demography, as an interdisciplinary subject, should be concerned with the constitutive role of places and contexts (whether defined as neighborhoods, workplaces, political systems, or regional economies). This would entail defining "area/place effects"; identifying a typology of contextual effects; and developing a research and training agenda that emphasizes the notion of contextual heterogeneity. Indeed, health scientists pursuing what may be called the "social determinants of health" research within public health have provided a basis to develop these ideas.

To begin with, area—or place—effects refer to the health effects of variables that tell us something about the places or contexts, and not simply about the individuals who inhabit them. Macintyre (1997) provides a useful distinction for considering place-effects, referred to as collective and contextual place-effects.

A collective effect refers to aggregated group properties that exert an influence on health over and above individual characteristics, for example, living in areas with a high proportion of people who have certain individual characteristics (e.g., based on age, social class, income, or race). A contextual effect, meanwhile, reflects the broader political or institutional context, for example, the presence or absence of opportunity structures that are intrinsic to places, such as the presence of infrastructure resources or the economic and legal policies of states. These variables have also been referred to as "integral" variables.

Meanwhile, by putting the notion of contextual heterogeneity at the center of the "social determinants to health," medical geographers have provided a useful framework, drawing on multilevel methodological perspectives (Subramanian, Jones, and Duncan 2003). At the most basic level, operationalizing the idea of contextual heterogeneity requires us to distinguish compositional (individual) explanations from contextual (including collective) explanations of geographical variations in health outcomes.

The compositional explanation for area differences would ascribe the variations in health outcomes to the characteristics of individuals who reside in them. If this is true, then similar types of people (based on their age, sex, race, socioeconomic status, and so on) will experience similar health outcomes no matter where they live. On the other hand, if place makes a difference, then similar types of people can be expected to achieve different levels of health depending on where they live.

We can, and should, however, go beyond the simplistic notions of "context and composition." If places make a difference for population health outcomes, then the degree to which they may matter can be anticipated to be quite different for different types of individuals. Such contextual heterogeneity could be manifested in at least two ways. First, place variations may be greater for one population group than another. Thus, if between-context differences are greater for low (compared to high) socioeconomic status (SES) groups, this would suggest that where low SES groups reside is crucial for their health, while for high SES groups it may not really matter where they live. The second dimension related to contextual differences is an intrinsic interest in monitoring places. Thus, for instance, places that are worse off for low SES may or may not be worse off for the high SES groups, suggesting that the contextual geography of health cannot be summarized in one map; rather the map may vary depending on one's SES.

If contextual differences exist, independent of individual, compositional factors, then explaining such differences using variables that relate to contexts (not individuals) is critical to the development of causal models of contextual effects. In summary, the interest in contextual analysis lies not simply in evaluating health achievements based on "who you are in relation to where you are." Rather, it is posing the question in terms of "who you are *depends* on where you are." The methodological implications for incorporating contextual perspectives to social inequalities in health are discussed in a later section.

The Life Course Perspective

Parallel with the growing interest in the dimension of place and contexts, researchers have increasingly sought to understand the patterns of population health and health disparities along the dimension of *time*. The life course approach relates to how health status at any given age, for a given birth cohort, reflects not only contemporary conditions but also embodiment of prior living circumstances, *in utero* onward (Krieger 2000). Detailed presentations of this perspective have been articulated elsewhere (Kuh and Ben Shlomo 1997; Hertzman 1999).

Three distinct pathways have been hypothesized to be relevant to the life course approach (Hertzman 1999). First, one path includes *latent effects* in which the early life environment affects adult health independent of intervening experience. A frequently cited example is the association between markers of intrauterine development (for example, birth weight) and adult diseases, such as hypertension, coronary heart disease, and cancers of the prostate and breast (Davey Smith, Gunnell, and Ben-Shlomo 2001). However, a growing body of research indicates that factors associated with a child's early life environment, such as maternal attachment, parent-child interactions, and child abuse, have wide-ranging and lasting effects on health behaviors and physical outcomes in adulthood (Taylor, Repetti, and Seeman 1997; Felitti et al. 1998). According to Hertzman (1999):

Specific biological factors (e.g., low birth weight) or developmental opportunities (e.g., adequate exposure to spoken language) at critical/sensitive periods in (early) life have a lifelong impact on health and well-being, regardless of subsequent life circumstances. The fact that crucial elements of emotional control, peer social skills, language development, and the understanding of relative quantity all have critical periods in the first five years of human life adds biological plausibility to the latency model (86).

A second type of life course effect, referred to as *pathway effects*, posits that the early life environment sets individuals onto life trajectories that in turn affect health status over time. An example is the tracking of socioeconomic disadvantage from childhood through to adult life. Finally, a third type of life course effect, referred to as the *cumulative model*, posits that the intensity and duration of exposure to unfavorable environments accumulate over time and produce adverse effects on health status, in a dose-response manner. For example, the effects of poverty on physical and psychological health are much more pronounced among individuals who suffer repeated spells of economic hardship, as opposed to single episodes (Lynch, Kaplan, and Shema 1997; McDonough et al. 1997). A cumulative life course approach, therefore, lends itself to the recommendation that investigators assess wealth, permanent income, and long-term economic deprivation, as opposed to single-time measures of income or poverty (Williams and Collins 1995).

Integrating Biological Markers and Psychosocial Pathways

The life course perspective discussed in the previous section has led naturally to the search for specific biological *mechanisms* that link early life environments to physical and psychological health outcomes. Demographers and social epidemiologists alike have begun to address the possibility of mapping the linkages between early life circumstances and subsequent health outcomes by incorporating biological markers into study designs. Early life circumstances "imprint" themselves on the central nervous system via brain development and alterations in neurochemistry. In turn, because the central nervous system "talks" to a variety of other physiological systems, including the immune, hormone, and clotting systems, biological measurements of these systems can help to establish the causal chains extending from early life circumstances to differential resilience and vulnerability to disease later in life (Kelly, Hertzman, and Daniels 1997).

Incorporating biological markers into social science surveys is likely to become an important part of the health demographer's research strategy for other compelling reasons. As Goldman (2001) argues, if exposures to different social environments are causally related to health, then scientists ought to be able to demonstrate how stressful working conditions, unsafe neighborhoods, poverty, and racial discrimination, as well as a host of other exposures throughout the life course, express themselves in terms of differences in biological and physiological parameters that matter to health.

Two broad classes of biological markers are of potential interest to health demographers: primary mediators of the stress process and markers of secondary outcomes. The former class of biomarkers is exemplified by the organizing concept of "allostatic load" introduced by McEwen and others (McEwen 1998; McEwen and Seeman 1999). *Allostatic load* is defined as the "wear and tear" exacted on the body's physiological systems as a result of chronic stressors (such as living in poverty or residing in unsafe neighborhoods). So far, four primary mediators of this process have been proposed, including cortisol, noradrenalin, epinephrine, and dihydroepiandrosterone (DHEA) (McEwen and Seeman 1999). These primary mediators have widespread influences throughout the body that potentially account for the differential resilience and vulnerability of individuals in response to adverse social circumstances. For example, cortisol is a quintessential "stress hormone" associated with activation of the hypothalamus-pituitary-adrenal (HPA) axis. The dysregulation of cortisol secretion is implicated in a wide range of disease processes, from elevated blood pressure and higher central adiposity to glucose intolerance, immune suppression, and cognitive decline (McEwen 1998). Cortisol measurement has been incorporated into surveys and study designs via 12-hour urine collections and, more recently, noninvasive and relatively inexpensive saliva specimens.

In empirical work, elevated markers of allostatic load have been linked "upstream" to adverse early life circumstances and lower socioeconomic position, as well as "downstream" to mortality risk, functional decline, and cognitive decline (Seeman et al. 1997).

In contrast to biological markers like cortisol (which represents one of the primary mediators of the allostatic process), biomarkers of *secondary outcomes* refer to those that tap into the cumulative responses to the primary mediators in various tissue/organ systems (McEwen and Seeman 1999). For example, waist-hip ratios and glycosylated hemoglobin levels both reflect the effects of sustained elevations in blood glucose and the insulin resistance that develops as a result of elevated cortisol and sympathetic nervous system activity over time. Elevated blood pressure is yet another secondary outcome resulting from the cumulative effects of allostasis. Other secondary biological markers have been proposed for the immune and clotting systems (McEwen 1998).

In sum, the substantive concerns of the emerging field of health demography have significant implications for the design of future studies conducted by both demographers and social epidemiologists. As suggested by Goldman (2001), future prospective studies should

> begin at birth, follow respondents at regular intervals throughout the life cycle, obtain detailed life histories concerning social, SES, psychological and health dimensions, consider not only the individual and family but the broader social environment, and include biological measurements along the way (134–135).

METHODOLOGICAL ISSUES

Addressing the substantive concerns of health demography requires not only novel study designs, but also departures from the traditional methods of analyzing data. In this section, we contrast the standard methodological concerns of demographers and epidemiologists, then go on to highlight multilevel statistical methodology as an emerging area of convergence between the two disciplines.

Social Epidemiology and Social Demography Contrasted

Palloni and Morenoff (2001) provide a useful summary of major methodological differences between demography and epidemiology. First, epidemiologists are taught during their training to view randomized clinical trials as the "gold standard" of evidence. No doubt this claim stems from famous instances in which observational data (such as the apparently protective effect of beta-carotene intake on lung cancer risk) were later overturned or contradicted by clinical trial evidence (beta-carotene supplementation seems to increase the risk of lung cancer). Clinical trials are feasible, indeed desirable, where the independent variable consists of a simple "exposure" that can be exogenously manipulated (such as swallowing a beta-carotene pill). However, relatively few questions of interest to the health demographer (for example, the relationship between minority ethnic status and low birth weight) have this characteristic.

When clinical trials are not feasible, epidemiologists would still prefer study designs with tight control over potential confounding factors. For example, in examining the relationship between smoking and lung cancer, a traditionally trained epidemiologist would prefer a study design that afforded the tightest possible control over social class. Thus, the classic British Doctors' Study, one of the first to demonstrate a link between cigarette smoking and lung cancer, consisted solely of male physicians (Doll and Hill 1956). As Palloni and Morenoff (2001) have noted, "in general, the study designs favored by epidemiologists are more conducive to the identification rather than the explanation of causal factors" (143). However, the price paid by epidemiologists is their propensity to overcontrol for social and behavioral factors. The interest of the health demographer clearly cannot be focused on isolating the causal effect of cigarette smoking on lung cancer, stripped of its social context.

In contrast, social demographers, being less concerned with identifying the causal role of single risk factors, tend to "lean heavily toward study designs requiring ... representative samples, a richer stock of characteristics of individuals or social contexts" (Palloni and Morenoff 2001: 143). *Social* epidemiologists would heartily concur with these sentiments (Berkman and Kawachi 2000).

A second area of contrast between demographers and epidemiologists is in their use of analytical methods. While both epidemiologists and demographers tend to draw on the same repertoire of regression models, the interpretation of regression coefficients in social demography draws on "complex models that, more often than not, consider simultaneous causality and incorporate networks of causal relations (simultaneous equation models), recognize latent constructs made up of multiple indicators (latent and structural equation models and models with multiple indicators), and involve nested processes (choice based models, selection models)" (Palloni and Morenoff 2001: 144). By contrast, it is still relatively rare to see such complexity acknowledged in epidemiological models:

> Odds ratios in epidemiology emerge from and are couched in the most simplistic of linear representations, with little concern for the existence of simultaneity, nested processes, sequence of causal stages, and potential differences between latent constructs and indicators (Palloni and Morenoff 2001: 144).

To be fair to epidemiologists, recent developments in causal thinking within epidemiology have begun to show serious attention to the problems of endogeneity, simultaneity, and selection, through implementation of graphic models (causal diagrams), potential-outcome (counterfactual) models, and structural-equations models (Greenland and Brumback 2002). These methods have yet to make inroads in *social* epidemiology, however. Meanwhile, a potential area of methodological convergence between social demographers and social epidemiologists is the emerging consensus that we need to move beyond single-level models if we are to address questions of social embeddedness and the role of social contexts in shaping health behaviors and health outcomes.

Multilevel Statistical Methods

Traditional epidemiological and demographic methods, while extremely useful, are not adequate for the task of implementing the population, contextual, and life course perspectives raised in the preceding section. In this section, we do not intend to repeat the well-established set of either the classic demographic methods (such as life table methodology, population projection methodology, etc.) or the classic epidemiological methods (such as case-control and cohort study designs, etc.).[1]

Analysis of data in traditional epidemiological and demographic studies tends to be carried out at a single level, be it individual or aggregate. Since they operate at a single scale, these analytical approaches are incapable of handling the substantive concerns raised in the previous sections, specifically those related to integrating geographical and temporal perspectives into understanding socioeconomic inequalities in population health (Subramanian, Jones, and Duncan 2003). While choosing to work at the aggregate level leaves the investigator prone to the charge of committing the ecological fallacy (Robinson 1950) or, more precisely, aggregation bias (Roberts and Burstein 1980), choosing to work exclusively at the individual level risks committing the individualistic fallacy (Alker 1969). Critical to overcoming these problems is the explicit recognition of multiple sources/levels of variation that contribute to population differences in health. One way to accommodate multiple sources/levels of variations is to exploit the idea of nesting, so that individuals (one source/level) are seen to be nested within contexts or places or ecologies (second source/level). Such a nested framework anticipates two related assumptions vital for the health demographic perspectives outlined earlier:

1. If we structure individuals to be nested within their contexts, we implicitly assume that individuals from one area are more alike than different.
2. If we explicitly recognize the different levels that structure the outcome, it also suggests that variances that can be attributed to different levels can be simple or complex.

While these concerns are both of substantive importance, as we argued above, there are also statistical implications. As is well recognized, single-level regression models make two assumptions that are incompatible and problematic with the contextual, life course, and multilevel perspectives that we outlined earlier. The first assumes that each individual observation is independent of the other or, in formal terms, there is no "clustering." The second relates to the "homoscedasticity" assumption, i.e., that variation around the average relationships is constant. The presence of clustered data can seriously undermine statistical significance testing. For example, the effect of cluster sampling on the actual α level of a t-test performed at a nominal α level of 0.05, with a small intraclass correlation (ρ) of 0.05 and cluster size of 10, the operating α level was found to be 0.11 (Barcikowski 1981). With large ρ and large cluster sizes, the operating α level increases rapidly. Clearly, in such situations, not taking into account the clustered nature of the data can produce spurious levels of statistical significance (Tate and Wongbundhit 1983).

---

[1] For an excellent discussion of the classic demographic methods, the reader is referred to the textbook by Preston and colleagues (Preston, Heuveline, and Guillot 2001); for epidemiological methods, see the textbook by Rothman and Greenland (1998), as well as Moon and colleagues (2000).

One way to deal with the clustering is to view data structures in a hierarchical manner. We refer to hierarchy as consisting of units grouped at different levels. To give an example, a health demographer may be interested in examining the effect of residential segregation (by class or race) on individual health outcomes (e.g., the risk of infant mortality or low birth weight) (Acevedo-Garcia and Lochner 2003). In this case, we can think of a two-level structure where individuals are level 1 (lower level) units that are clustered within metropolitan areas of varying degrees of residential segregation at level 2 (higher level). Although empirical studies of residential segregation and health outcomes have seldom adopted this design, data structures of this type are crucial in sorting out the compositional effects of areas from their contextual effects, as well as for determining the relative importance of the different levels for health status. In ecological studies, an observed association between racial segregation (e.g., as assessed by the index of dissimilarity for a metropolitan area) and infant mortality may be consistent with either a compositional effect (i.e., a high proportion of black residents within a metropolitan area giving rise to high infant mortality rates) or to a contextual effect (i.e., something about residential segregation *per se* resulting in high risk of infant mortality), or both.

Recent developments in multilevel statistical methods have provided a unified and realistic approach to address the issues of clustering and to model complex variance structures simultaneously at multiple levels (Bryk and Raudenbush 1992; Longford 1993; Goldstein 1995). Multilevel modeling procedures account for the clustering and dependency in the outcome by partitioning the total variance into different components. In the simplest case, the response variation can be partitioned into a lower-level component and a higher-level residual component, with the latter representing the "source" of the clustering in the response. Indeed, it is this partitioning of the variance that provides important clues regarding the levels "where the action lies."

Besides the technical advantages that this methodology offers, the multilevel analytical approach provides one very useful way of addressing the substantive issues outlined above (Leyland and Goldstein 2001; Subramanian, Jones, and Duncan 2003). As the name suggests, the approach anticipates that determinants of health status occur simultaneously on several levels, e.g., individuals, neighborhoods, regions, and states. Consequently, multilevel techniques are essentially about modeling heterogeneity at each of the desired levels of the conceptual model through a range of variables that tell us something about each of the levels. Importantly, these methodological and substantive perspectives are supported by a robust technical estimation process (Goldstein 1995). In the following discussion we briefly summarize the statistical nature of a basic multilevel model.[2]

Consider again our example of isolating the effect of residential segregation on low birth weight (a risk factor for infant mortality). A two-level simple multilevel model with a continuous response with a single level-1 continuous predictor treated as a fixed effect can be written as:

$$y_{ij} = \beta_0 + \beta_1 x_{ij} + (u_{0j} + e_{0ij}) \tag{1}$$

In Equation 1, y_{ij} is a continuous response (birth weight) for individual i in metropolitan area j. The fixed parameters β_0 is the population mean (intercept), and β_1 estimates the

---

[2] A more detailed statistical and methodological exposition of multilevel models can be found elsewhere (Subramanian, Jones, and Duncan 2003).

overall relationship between y_{ij} and x_{ij}. The random parameter u_{0j} is the specific effect of metropolitan area j, while e_{0ij} is the residual for individual i from the metropolitan area j. It is assumed that the random parameters are independent and are normally distributed at each level. Thus, $\boldsymbol{u}_{0j}$ is distributed with a population mean of zero and a population variance of $\boldsymbol{\sigma}_{u0}^2$ (the between metropolitan population variance) and the level-1 residuals e_{0ij} are also assumed to have a mean zero and variance $\boldsymbol{\sigma}_{e0}^2$ (the between individual within metropolitan area population variance). The total variance in y_{ij}, therefore, can be written as:

$$\text{Var}\,(\boldsymbol{y}_{ij}) = \boldsymbol{\sigma}_{u0}^2 + \boldsymbol{\sigma}_{e0}^2 \tag{2}$$

For the above, the ICC coefficient $(\boldsymbol{\rho}_u)$ can be defined as:

$$\boldsymbol{\rho}_{\mathrm{u}} = \boldsymbol{\sigma}_{u0}^2 / \boldsymbol{\sigma}_{u0}^2 + \boldsymbol{\sigma}_{e0}^2 \tag{3}$$

The ICC, therefore, is the proportion of variance accounted for by the metropolitan areas. Since variance components at level 2 and level 1 are unrelated to the population mean and have similar distributional assumptions, it is possible to add the different variance components and apportion the percentage variance to each level. While this basic multilevel model allows us to disentangle the composition and contextual sources of variation, it can be easily extended to explore the contextual heterogeneity and cross-level interactions between ecological and individual variables (Subramanian, Jones, and Duncan 2003).

Any research on population health that takes context and place seriously is intrinsically multilevel and cannot be otherwise. Multilevel methods consider most data structures within a nested framework, and such nesting could be hierarchical and/or nonhierarchical. Seen this way, repeated/longitudinal analysis (whether it is people or places that are repeatedly measured), multivariate analysis (when there is more than one interrelated outcome), and cross-classified analysis (when we do not have neat hierarchical nesting) are simply special cases of a multilevel framework (Subramanian, Jones, and Duncan 2003).[3]

TRENDS AND DIFFERENTIALS IN MORTALITY AND MORBIDITY

In the previous sections, we highlighted some key substantive and methodological issues relevant to health demography research conducted at the individual (micro) level, e.g., the salience of incorporating a life course perspective, the use of biological markers in longitudinal studies, and the relevance of contextual influences on individual health. In this section we summarize the trends and differentials in mortality and morbidity at the population (macro) level. We focus the discussion on three topics: (1) the concept of the epidemiological transition (and its critique); (2) the measurement of mortality and morbidity at the population level; and (3) trends and differentials in global health status.[4]

---

[3] For a detailed exposure to the methodological possibilities available through a multilevel framework for routinely collected health-related data see the compilation by Leyland and Goldstein (2001).
[4] Readers are referred to chapter 9, "Infant Mortality," and chapter 10, "Adult Mortality," for more specific and detailed accounts of ongoing research in health demography.

The Epidemiological Transition

One area of common interest to both demographers and epidemiologists is to describe and forecast global patterns of health. Originally, demographers found it useful to describe stages in the "demographic transition" to refer to the change from high fertility and high mortality rates in "traditional" societies to a pattern of low fertility and low mortality rates in "modern" societies (Thompson 1929; Notestein 1945). Subsequently, Omran (1971) extended this framework to describe three stages in the "mortality transition" consisting of: (1) the age of pestilence and famine, associated with the predominance of mortality from epidemic infectious diseases, malnutrition, and complications of pregnancy and childbirth; (2) the age of receding pandemics, during which mortality fell and life expectancy increased[5]; and (3) the age of noncommunicable diseases, during which mortality came to be dominated by chronic degenerative diseases such as heart disease, stroke, and cancer. A fourth stage in the mortality transition was later added by Olshansky and Ault (1986) and by Rogers and Hackenberg (1987), describing an era of delayed mortality from degenerative diseases, as well as the resurgence of "old" infectious diseases (e.g., tuberculosis) and the emergence of new infectious diseases (e.g., HIV/AIDS). Patterns of mortality and morbidity in this fourth stage have been explained largely on the basis of individual lifestyle (Rogers and Hackenberg 1987), although this interpretation has been questioned on the grounds that it overemphasizes individual determinants of health while underplaying the importance of broader social and economic factors (Beaglehole and Bonita 1997).

Demographic and epidemiological research continues to be informed by the concept of the epidemiological transition. However, both the epidemiological transition, and the related but broader concept of the "health transition" (Caldwell 1990), have been criticized on the grounds that they are descriptive frameworks rather than true theories that yield predictions about patterns of population health (Wallace 2001). Beaglehole and Bonita (1997) provide a cogent critique of the epidemiological transition model. For example, they point out that the model fails to explain differences in mortality rates between countries and has limited ability to predict changing patterns of disease with "modernization." Contemporary examples of mortality change, such as the mortality crisis in post-Soviet Russia (McKee 2001), do not fit well into the orderly progression of stage suggested by the model. In fact, it has become evident that the various stages in the health transition can overlap within any given country and that they do not necessarily progress in a linear fashion. Moreover, the categorization of diseases into infectious and noncommunicable diseases ignores major causes of mortality and morbidity, such as traffic accidents, unintentional injuries, and violence. Finally, Beaglehole and Bonita noted a tendency to analyze the transition in isolation from the background social and economic forces that propel population-level changes in health status.

In summary, according to Beaglehole and Bonita (1997), "although the health transition theory is a useful descriptive tool, it remains a blunt instrument with only limited predictive power" (10). Health demographers therefore face a challenge in further developing and refining the construct into a theory that is testable and

---

[5] In Western Europe and North America, the second stage of the mortality transition has been dated from the beginning of the 18th century until the early 20th century, with the 1918 to 1920 influenza pandemic being the last major pandemic (Mackenbach 1994).

applicable to both developing and industrialized countries, as well as historical and contemporary contexts.

Measurement of Mortality and Morbidity

Mortality and cause-of-death statistics based on death certificates continue to be the mainstay of health assessment in both demography and epidemiology. However, those outside the field often overlook the complexities of mortality data collection. As Sir Austin Bradford Hill (1984) remarked:

> In making comparisons between death rates from different causes of death at different times or between one country and another, it must be realized that one is dealing with material which the distinguished American statistician Raymond Pearl long ago described as, 'fundamentally of a dubious character,' though of vital importance in public health work (259).

It still remains the case that complete cause-specific death registration data are routinely available for only a minority of the world's countries. Less than one-third of the global population is covered by national vital registration systems, and there is wide regional variation in coverage, ranging from 80% population coverage in the European region to less than 5% coverage in the Eastern Mediterranean and African regions of the World Health Organization (Bonita and Mathers 2003). On the other hand, recent improvements in sample registration systems and surveys have improved coverage, especially for under-five child mortality and maternal mortality. For example, data collection on child mortality has improved with cross-country surveys such as the Demographic and Health Surveys (DHS) and the Multiple Indicator Cluster Survey (MICS) program of UNICEF. Bonita and Mathers (2003) estimate that national vital registration systems together with sample registration data currently cover about 74% of global mortality. Survey data and indirect demographic techniques provide information on child and adult mortality for the remaining 26% of estimated global mortality.

The assessment of morbidity is even more complex than the measurement of mortality, since it must frequently rely on the self-reports of symptoms and illnesses by survey respondents. For instance, it is widely recognized that even the self-report of the commonly used single item on general health perception ("How would you rate your overall health? Excellent, Very Good, Good, Fair, or Poor?") can be biased. The problem is related to unmeasured differences in expectations and norms for health, based on culture, educational attainment, age, gender, and other respondent characteristics. In developing countries in particular, the socioeconomic gradient in poor self-rated health often runs in the "wrong" direction, with more educated groups reporting higher levels of morbidity, even though their objective health status (e.g., as measured by mortality rates) is clearly superior to lower socioeconomic groups (Sen 2002).

The accuracy of self-reported morbidity in surveys can be improved by validating specific diagnoses against medical records and pathology reports. Obviously, these procedures are time-consuming and expensive and limit the size of the survey. An alternative is to use data from hospitals or clinics or even restrict survey respondents to health professionals (such as in the Harvard Nurses' Health Study). However, as pointed out by Caldwell (2001), such approaches go "far toward destroying the concept of a *population*, which is basic to the way demographers see the world" (22–23; emphasis in the original).

In recent years, the World Health Organization has pioneered cross-country survey-based approaches to measuring disability. Based on the International Classification of Functioning, Disability and Health (ICF), the WHO carried out a Multi-Country Survey Study in over 60 countries during 2000–2001. A health module was administered to assess six core domains of health status, including pain, affect, cognition, mobility, self-care, and usual activities (including household and work-related activities) (Üstün et al. 2001). The WHO survey included case vignettes and some used selected measures to calibrate respondents' self-assessments of their health. Statistical methods were developed to correct potential biases in self-reported data (Murray et al. 2002b). Over half were household interview surveys, two were telephone surveys, and the remainder postal surveys. The results of the WHO Multi-Country Survey for the first time provide measures of disability prevalence and health status that are comparable across a broad set of countries (Bonita and Mathers 2003). It represents an important step toward standardizing the measurement of morbidity and disability across populations.

Finally, the World Health Organization has taken the lead in refining summary measures of population health status that combine measures of survival and morbidity into a single metric (Murray et al. 2002a). Two classes of measures have received particular attention: the disability-adjusted life-year (DALY), which is a "health gap" measure that combines time lost due to premature mortality with time lived with disability and healthy life expectancies (HALE), which measures the equivalent number of years of life lived in full health extrapolated from comparable cross-national data (World Health Organization 2000). Both sets of measures have been widely debated. In particular, critics have pointed out the data demands and complexity of making the calculations that involve numerous assumptions (Almeida et al. 2001). The weighting of disability states as well as the social values implicit in the weighting of life years at different ages has been similarly contested. Such debates notwithstanding, health demographers (and policy planners) increasingly recognize the limitations of assessing population health status through measures of mortality or life expectancy *alone* (i.e., ignoring morbidity).

Global Trends and Differentials in Mortality and Morbidity

Improvements in global health status, as measured by gains in life expectancy, have been accompanied by widening differentials both between and within countries. Life expectancy at birth currently ranges from 81.4 years for women in the established market economies of Western Europe, North America, Japan, Australia, and New Zealand, down to 48.1 years for men in sub-Saharan Africa (Bonita and Mathers 2003). While mortality rates have declined markedly for specific causes of death (such as coronary heart disease) in wealthy countries, other regions of the world have witnessed equally spectacular reversals in life expectancy. For example, between 1991 and 1994, life expectancy at birth in the former Soviet republics fell by 4 years for males and by 2.3 years for females (McKee 2001). Between 1994 and 1998, life expectancy for Russian men improved, but declined significantly again over the next three years (Bonita and Mathers 2003). Worldwide, about 37 million people are currently living with HIV/AIDS, of whom 95% reside in developing countries. The impact of HIV/AIDS has been catastrophic in sub-Saharan Africa, where between 2000 and 2005, the United Nations Development Program has projected that the decline in life expectancy due to the disease will amount to 34 years in Botswana, 26 years in Zimbabwe, 19 years in South Africa, and 17 years in Kenya (United Nations Development Program 2002).

According to the World Health Organization, about 56 million deaths occurred worldwide in 2000, of which 10.9 million (20%) were deaths among children aged less than five years of age (WHO 2001). Of the under-five child deaths in the world, 99.3% occurred in developing countries. Developing countries also share a disproportionate burden of premature deaths at young adult ages (15 to 59 years). Just over 30% of all deaths in developing countries occur at these ages, compared with 15% in richer countries. By contrast, 70% of deaths in developed countries occur beyond age 70 (Bonita and Mathers 2003).

Contrary to the linear progression from infectious diseases to noncommunicable diseases implied by the epidemiological transition, many countries confront a so-called "double burden" of diseases, with high prevalence of both old and new infectious diseases in addition to emerging epidemics of chronic noncommunicable diseases such as heart disease, stroke, diabetes, and cancer. Of the 56 million deaths worldwide in 2000, 32.8 million (or 59%) were due to noncommunicable diseases, which killed twice as many people as infectious, maternal, perinatal, and nutritional causes combined (17.8 million, or 31% of all deaths). Injuries killed an additional 5.1 million people in 2000, or about one-tenth of the world's total deaths (Bonita and Mathers 2003).

There is enormous heterogeneity in health status even within developing countries. In China (which accounts for one-sixth of the world's population), fewer than 10% of all deaths occur before age five, compared with 40% in Africa (accounting for one-tenth of the global population). Conversely, 45% of deaths in China occur beyond age 70, compared with only 10% in Africa (Bonita and Mathers 2003).

Within individual countries also, differentials in mortality have been recorded since the very beginning of vital records registration. In several countries, such as the United Kingdom (Drever and Bunting 1997) and the United States (Pappas et al. 1993), these differentials have not only persisted in spite of technological advances in medicine and the rising standard of living, but they also seem to have widened in recent decades.

The magnitude of the health differentials is striking, even in wealthy countries. Within the United States, for example, a black male born in the District of Columbia can expect to live 57.9 years, lower than the life expectancy of the male citizens of Ghana (58.3 years), Bangladesh (58.1 years), or Bolivia (59.8 years). By contrast, an Asian American woman born in Westchester County, New York, can expect to live on average for 90.3 years (Murray et al. 1998).

The challenge for health demographers, then, is not only to refine methods for documenting and monitoring population health, but also to develop new theories and conceptual models to account for the causes of health variations both within and between countries.

NEXT STEPS

In this chapter, we have attempted to set forth what we view as the key conceptual, substantive, and methodological challenges to the advancement of health demography as an interdisciplinary science. We have argued, along with others (Susser and Bresnahan 2001), that despite nearly two centuries of divergence and specialization, demographers and epidemiologists are poised on the brink of a major bridging across disciplinary boundaries, concerns, and methods. Indeed, such convergence was the theme of a recently edited issue of the *Annals of the New York Academy of Sciences*

(Weinstein, Hermalin, and Stoto 2001). Demographers are already assimilating the techniques and measures that used to belong in the domain of medical epidemiologists, such as the assessment of specific disease diagnoses in population surveys or the collection of biological specimens in longitudinal studies (Goldman 2001). For their part, epidemiologists, especially *social* epidemiologists, have begun to move toward population-based, as opposed to clinical, samples, and to incorporate an expanded understanding of the determinants of health in their work, which includes not just the traditional "risk factors" (such as genetic susceptibility or lifestyle behaviors) but, in addition, *social* determinants such as socioeconomic status, social support, and neighborhood contexts (Berkman and Kawachi 2000; Kawachi and Berkman 2003).

The cross-fertilization of demography and epidemiology is happening at a crucial stage in the evolution of human health. New threats and challenges to global health, such as the AIDS pandemic, the worldwide aging of the population, and the widening economic gulf between rich and poor countries associated with globalization, demand analytical approaches and strategic responses that are simultaneously rooted in the historical concerns of demographers with whole *populations*, as well as the more individual and biological focus of epidemiologists.

At the population (macro) level, health demographers will continue to be engaged by improving systems of measuring, monitoring, and forecasting mortality and morbidity. Much work remains to be carried out in refining the theory of health transition, to turn it into a genuine theory capable of yielding testable predictions about patterns and trends in population health. The measurement of morbidity still lags behind the measurement of mortality for all but the most economically advanced societies. Quantitative techniques for summary indices of health status (combining morbidity measures with survival) are still in their relative infancy, in part because of lack of data as well as lack of agreement about how to weight different health states and life years at different stages of the life span.

At the individual (micro) level, health demographers will continue to be challenged by the task of developing better conceptual models of the determinants of health. This task involves not only expanding the repertoire of the individual determinants of health, e.g., contextual influences such as income inequality (Kawachi, Kennedy, and Wilkinson 1999) and neighborhood environments (Kawachi and Berkman 2003), but also incorporating the dimension of time (the life course) and elucidating the biological pathways and mechanisms that connect population-level forces to individual health.

The subject matter of health demography is not new. We concur with Pol and Thomas (1992), who observed that

> This emerging discipline actually represents a synthesis and reformulation of concepts and substantive data developed in a variety of other fields...(most obviously) the convergence of traditional demography with aspects of biostatistics and epidemiology (2).

After a long period of separation, the fields of demography and epidemiology are finally converging. The dynamic interplay between the changing size and composition of the population as well as its changing health patterns across different multilevel contexts lie at the core of the inquiry of health demography. The foundational basis for this new field not only draws on the natural and historical overlaps between epidemiology and demography (Weinstein, Hermalin, and Stoto 2001), but also on a renewed appreciation of the need to integrate research across multiple levels of analysis, from the societal and population level down to the individual, biological, and molecular levels (Shonkoff and Phillips 2000).

REFERENCES

Acevedo-Garcia, D., and Lochner, K. 2003. Residential segregation and health. In *Neighborhoods and health*. Edited by I. Kawachi and L. F. Berkman, 265–281. New York: Oxford University Press.

Alker, H. A., Jr. 1969. A typology of ecological fallacies. In *Quantitative ecological analysis*. Edited by M. Dogan and S. Rokkan, 69–86. Cambridge: Massachusetts Institute of Technology.

Almeida, C., Braveman, P., Gold, M. R., et al. 2001. Methodological concerns and recommendations on policy consequences of the World Health Report 2000. *Lancet* 357:1685–1691.

Barcikowski, R. S. 1981. Statistical power with group mean as the unit of analysis. *Journal of Educational Statistics* 6:267–285.

Beaglehole, R., and Bonita, R. 1997. *Public health at the crossroads. Achievements and prospects*. Cambridge: Cambridge University Press.

Berkman, L. F., and Kawachi, I. 2000. *Social epidemiology*. New York: Oxford University Press.

Bonita, R., and C. D. Mathers. 2003. Global health status at the beginning of the twenty-first century. In *Global public health: A new era*. Edited by R. Beaglehole, 24–53. Oxford: Oxford University Press.

Bryk, A. S., and S. W. Raudenbush. 1992. *Hierarchical linear models: Applications and data analysis methods*. Newbury Park, England: Sage Publications.

Caldwell, J. C. 1990. Introductory thoughts on health transition. In *What we know about health transition: The cultural, social and behavioural determinants of health*. Edited by J. Caldwell, S. Findley, P. Caldwell, G. Santow, W. Cosford, J. Braid, D. Boers-Freeman, xi–xiii. Canberra: Australian National University.

Caldwell, J. C. 2001. Demographers and the study of mortality. Scope, perspectives, and theory. In *Population health and aging: Strengthening the dialogue between epidemiology and demography*. Edited by M. Weinstein, A. I. Hermalin, and M. A. Stoto, 19–34. *Annals of the New York Academy of Sciences* Vol. 954:19–34.

Davey Smith, G., D. Gunnell, and Y. Ben-Shlomo. 2001. Life-course approaches to socio-economic differentials in cause-specific adult mortality. In *Poverty, inequality and health. An international perspective*. Edited by D. Leon and G. Walt, 88–124. Oxford: Oxford University Press.

Diez-Roux, A. V. 1998. Research forum: Bringing context back into epidemiology: Variables and fallacies in multilevel analysis. *American Journal of Public Health* 88(2):216–222.

Doll, R., and A. B. Hill. 1956. Lung cancer and other causes of death in relation to smoking: A second report on the mortality of British doctors. *British Medical Journal* 2:1071–1081.

Drever, F., and J. Bunting. 1997. Patterns and trends in male mortality. In *Health inequalities: Decennial supplement, DS Series No. 15*. Edited by F. Drever and M. Whitehead. London: The Stationery Office.

Eckersley, R., J. Dixon, and B. Douglas. 2001. *The social origins of health and well-being*. Cambridge: Cambridge University Press.

Felitti, V. J., et al. 1998. Relationship of childhood abuse and household dysfunction to many of the leading causes of death in adults. The Adverse Childhood Experiences (ACE) Study. *American Journal of Preventive Medicine* 14:245–258.

Goldman, N. 2001. Social inequalities in health. Disentangling the underlying mechanisms. In *Population health and aging: Strengthening the dialogue between epidemiology and demography*. Edited by M. Weinstein, A. I. Hermalin, and M. A. Stoto, 118–139. *Annals of the New York Academy of Sciences*, Vol. 954, 118–139.

Goldstein, H. 1995. *Multilevel statistical models*. London: Arnold.

Graunt, J. 1662 [1975]. *Natural and political observations mentioned in a following index, and made upon the bills of mortality*. New York: Arno Press.

Greenland, S., and B. Brumback. 2002. An overview of relations among causal modeling methods. *International Journal of Epidemiology* 31:1030–1037.

Hertzman, C. 1999. The biological embedding of early experience and its effects on health in adulthood. *Annals of the New York Academy of Sciences* 896:85–95.

Hill, A. B. 1984. *A short textbook of medical statistics*, 11th ed. London: Hodder & Stoughton.

Jones, K., and G. Moon. 1987. *Health, disease and society*. London: Routledge.

Jones, K., and G. Moon. 1993. Medical geography: Taking space seriously. *Progress in Human Geography* 17(4):515–524.

Kawachi, I., and L. F. Berkman. 2003. *Neighborhoods and health*. New York: Oxford University Press.

Kawachi, I., B. P. Kennedy, and R. G. Wilkinson. 1999. *Income inequality and health. The society and health population reader*. New York: The New Press.

Kearns, R. A. 1993. Place and health: Toward a reformed medical geography. *Professional Geographer* 45:139–147.

Kelly, S., C. Hertzman, and M. Daniels. 1997. Searching for the biological pathways between stress and health. *Annual Review of Public Health* 18:437–462.

Krieger, N. 2000. Discrimination and health. In *Social epidemiology*. Edited by L. F. Berkman and I. Kawachi, 36–75. New York: Oxford University Press.

Kuh, D. L., and Y. Ben Shlomo. 1997. *A life course approach to chronic disease epidemiology: Tracing the origins of ill health from early to adult life*. Oxford: Oxford University Press.

Leyland, A. H., and H. Goldstein. 2001. *Multilevel modelling of health statistics*. Chichester, England: John Wiley & Sons.

Longford, N. 1993. *Random coefficient models*. Oxford: Clarendon Press.

Lynch, J. W., G. A. Kaplan, and S. J. Shema. 1997. Cumulative impact of sustained economic hardship on physical, cognitive, psychological, and social functioning. *New England Journal of Medicine* 337:1889–1895.

Macintyre, S. 1997. What are spatial effects and how can we measure them? In *Exploiting National Surveys and Census Data: The Role of Locality and Spatial Effects*. Edited by A. Dale. Manchester: Centre for Census and Survey Research, University of Manchester, pp. 1–28.

Macintyre, S. 2000. The social patterning of health: Bringing the social context back in. *Medical Sociology Newsletter* 26:14–19.

Macintyre, S., and A. Ellaway. 2000. Ecological approaches: Rediscovering the role of physical and social environment. In *Social epidemiology*. Edited by L. F. Berkman and I. Kawachi, 332–348. New York: Oxford Press.

Mackenbach, J. P. 1994. The epidemiologic transition theory. *Journal of Epidemiology and Community Health* 48:329–332.

Marmot, M., and R. G. Wilkinson. 1999. *The social determinants of health*. Oxford: Oxford University Press.

McDonough, P., G. J. Duncan, D. Williams, and J. House. 1997. Income dynamics and adult mortality in the United States, 1972 through 1989. *American Journal of Public Health* 87(9):1476–1483.

McEwen, B. S. 1998. Protective and damaging effects of stress mediators. *New England Journal of Medicine* 338:171–179.

McEwen, B. S., and T. S. Seeman. 1999. Protective and damaging effects of mediators of stress: Elaborating and testing the concepts of allostasis and allostatic load. *Annals of the New York Academy of Sciences* 896:30–47.

McKee, M. 2001. The health consequences of the collapse of the Soviet Union. In *Poverty, inequality and health. An international perspective*. Edited by D. Leon and G. Walt, 17–36. Oxford: Oxford University Press.

Moon, G. 1990. Conceptions of space and community in British health policy. *Social Science and Medicine* 30:165–171.

Moon, G., et al. 2000. *Epidemiology: An introduction*. Buckingham, England: Open University Press.

Murray, C. J. L., C. M. Michaud, M. T. McKenna, and J. S. Marks. 1998. *U.S. patterns of mortality by county and race, 1965–1994*. Cambridge, Mass.: Harvard University Burden of Disease Unit, Harvard Center for Population and Development Studies, and the Centers for Disease Control and Prevention.

Murray, C. J. L., J. A. Salomon, C. D. Mathers, and A. D. Lopez. 2002a. *Summary measures of population health: Concepts, ethics, measurement and applications*. Geneva: World Health Organization.

Murray, C. J. L., A. Tandon, J. Salomon, and C. D. Mathers. 2002b. New approaches to enhance cross-population comparability of survey results. In *Summary measures of population health: Concepts, ethics, measurement and applications*. Edited by C. J. L. Murray, J. A. Salomon, C. D. Mathers, and A. D. Lopez. Geneva: World Health Organization.

Notestein, F. W. 1945. Population—the long view. In *Food for the world*. Edited by T. W. Schultz, 36–57. Chicago: University of Chicago Press.

Olshansky, S. J., and A. B. Ault. 1986. The fourth stage of the epidemiologic transition: The age of delayed degenerative diseases. *Milbank Memorial Fund Quarterly* 64(3):355–391.

Omran, A. R. 1971. The epidemiologic transition: A theory of the epidemiology of population change. *Milbank Memorial Fund Quarterly* 49(1):509–538.

Palloni, A., and J. D. Morenoff. 2001. Interpreting the paradoxical in the Hispanic paradox. In *Population health and aging: Strengthening the dialogue between epidemiology and demography.* Edited by M. Weinstein, A. I. Hermalin, and M. A. Stoto, 140–174. *Annals of the New York Academy of Sciences,* Vol. 954.

Pappas, G., S. Queen, W. Hadden, and G. Fisher. 1993. The increasing disparity in mortality between socio-economic groups in the United States, 1960 and 1986. *New England Journal of Medicine* 329:103–109.

Pol, L. G., and R. K. Thomas. 1992. *The demography of health and health care.* Netherlands: Kluwer Academic/Plenum Publishers.

Preston, S. H., P. Heuveline, and M. Guillot. 2001. *Demography: Measuring and modeling population processes.* Oxford: Blackwell.

Roberts, K. H., and L. Burstein. 1980. *Issues in aggregation.* San Francisco: Jossey-Bass.

Robinson, S. 1950. Ecological correlations and the behaviour of individuals. *American Sociological Review* 15: 351–357.

Rockett, I. R. H. 1999. Population and health: An introduction to epidemiology. *Population Bulletin* 54(4): 3–43.

Rogers, R. G., and R. Hackenberg. 1987. Extending epidemiologic transition theory: A new stage. *Social Biology* 34:234–243.

Rose, G. 1994. *The strategy of preventive medicine.* New York: Oxford University Press.

Rothman, K. J. 1986. *Modern Epidemiology.* Boston: Little, Brown and Company.

Rothman, K. J., and Greenland, S. 1998. *Modern Epidemiology, 2nd edition.* Philadelphia: Lippincott, Williams & Wilkins.

Schwartz, S. 1994. The fallacy of the ecological fallacy: The potential misuse of a concept and the consequences. *American Journal of Public Health* 84:819–824.

Schwartz, S., E. Susser, and M. Susser. 1999. A future for epidemiology? *Annual Review of Public Health* 20:15–33.

Seeman, T. E., B. H. Singer, J. W. Rowe, R. I. Horwitz, and B. S. McEwen. 1997. Price of adaptation—Allostatic load and its health consequences: MacArthur Studies of Successful Aging. *Archives of Internal Medicine* 157:2259–2268.

Sen, A. 2002. Health: Perception versus observation. *British Medical Journal* 324:860–861.

Shonkoff, J. P., and D. A. Phillips. 2000. *From neurons to neighborhoods: The science of early child development.* Washington, D.C.: National Academies Press.

Subramanian, S. V., K. Jones, and C. Duncan. 2003. Multilevel methods for public health research. In *Neighborhoods and health.* Edited by I. Kawachi and L. F. Berkman, 65–111. New York: Oxford University Press.

Susser, E., and M. Bresnahan. 2001. Origins of epidemiology. In *Population health and aging: Strengthening the dialogue between epidemiology and demography.* Edited by M. Weinstein, A. I. Hermalin, and M. A. Stoto, 6–18. *Annals of the New York Academy of Sciences,* Vol. 954.

Susser, M., and E. Susser. 1996a. Choosing a future of epidemiology. I. Eras and paradigms. *American Journal of Public Health* 86(5):668–673.

Susser, M., and E. Susser. 1996b. Choosing a future of epidemiology. II. From black box to Chinese boxes and eco-epidemiology. *American Journal of Public Health* 86(5):674–677.

Tate, R., and Y. Wongbundhit. 1983. Random versus nonrandom coefficient models for multilevel analysis. *Journal of Educational Statistics* 8:103–120.

Taylor, S. E., R. Repetti, and T. Seeman. 1997. What is an unhealthy environment and how does it get under the skin? *Annual Review of Psychology* 48:411–447.

Thompson, W. S. 1929. Population. *American Journal of Sociology* 34(6):959–975.

United Nations Development Program. 2002. *Human development report 2002.* New York: Oxford University Press.

Üstün, T. B., S. Chatterji, M. Villanueva, et al. 2001. Multi-country household survey study on health and responsiveness, 2000–2001. GPE discussion paper No. 37. Geneva: World Health Organization.

Wallace, R. B. 2001. Bridging epidemiology and demography. theories and themes. In *Population health and aging: Strengthening the dialogue between epidemiology and demography.* Edited by M. Weinstein, A. I. Hermalin, and M. A. Stoto, 63–75. *Annals of the New York Academy of Sciences,* Vol. 954.

Weinstein, M., A. I. Hermalin, and M. A. Stoto. 2001. *Population health and aging: Strengthening the dialogue between epidemiology and demography.* New York: Annals of the New York Academy of Sciences, Vol. 954.

Weinstein, M., A. I. Hermalin, M. A. Stoto, V. J. Evans, D. Ewbank, J. Haaga, M. Ibrahim, and J. Madans. 2001. Greater collaboration across the disciplines: Challenges and opportunities. In *Population health and aging: Strengthening the dialogue between epidemiology and demography.* Edited by M. Weinstein, A. I. Hermalin, and M. A. Stoto, 311–321. *Annals of the New York Academy of Sciences*, Vol. 954.

Williams, D. R., and C. Collins. 1995. U.S. socioeconomic and racial differences in health. *Annual Review of Sociology* 21:349–386.

World Health Organization. 2000. *World health report 2000. Health systems: improving health performance.* Geneva: World Health Organization.

World Health Organization. 2001. *World health report 2001.* Geneva: World Health Organization.

CHAPTER 27

The Demography of Population Health

MARK D. HAYWARD AND DAVID F. WARNER

Demographic regimes of low fertility and low mortality in developed nations have been in place for over half a century (Hayward and Zhang 2001). The result is populations with advanced age structures and slow or even negative growth rates. Italy, Greece, Sweden, and Japan, for example, are fast approaching a situation where approximately one in five persons will be 65 years of age or older, and these countries will continue to age (Kinsella and Velkoff 2001). Already, Greece, Italy, and Sweden have populations where there are more elderly than youth aged 0 to 14.

Below-replacement levels of fertility and declining mortality over an extended period of time have led some European and American demographers to warn of impending population declines (Davis, Bernstam, and Ricardo-Campbell 1987), and this prediction has come to fruition. Population declines have occurred recently in Italy and Greece as well as Eastern European nations such as Estonia, Latvia, Hungary, Romania, Russia, and Belarus. Projections by the United Nations predict that the populations of most of Europe and Japan will decline in size over the next five decades (United Nations 1996a, 1996b, 2000a, 2000b). The historical trend toward population aging in developed nations is being echoed in less developed nations, and United Nations projections point to a global convergence in 50 years (Hayward and Zhang 2001; Kinsella 2000; Kinsella and Velkoff 2001; United Nations 1996a, 1996b). Population aging is a worldwide demographic phenomenon.

The aging of populations' age structures, particularly because of dramatic declines in mortality at older ages, has influenced demographers' investigations of recent trends in population health—particularly the linkages between mortality, morbidity, and disability at older ages (Manton 1990). A key question has been whether declining mortality rates in the older population also signal declining morbidity and disability rates. The answer to this question has substantial implications for whether the sizeable gains in *life expectancy* at older ages are accompanied by an increase in *healthy life expectancy*, i.e., the expected number of years in good health. Investigations of the linkages between mortality, morbidity, and disability lie at the heart of anticipating an aging population's demands on health care systems and health care costs (Manton, Stallard, and Corder 1995, 1998; Murray and Lopez 1996; Robine and Romieu 1998; Waidmann and Manton 2000; World Health Organization 2000). Health expectancies provide information that allows the development of health policies targeted at improving the quality of life rather than simply improvements in the overall length of life. Health expectancies also are useful policy tools in monitoring trends in population health, evaluating disparities across major subgroups within a population, targeting health care policies where they are most needed, and identifying the effects of major interventions and policy changes on both the length and quality of life (Crimmins 2002).

Demographic research on the linkages between mortality, morbidity, and disability has led to new ways of modeling the interaction of these processes and new ways of conceptualizing population health. This research makes clear that while disability, morbidity, and mortality are related, they are not isomorphic concepts. Moreover, changes in these individual-level processes sometimes combine in complex ways to generate changes in population health. Understanding population health necessarily involves understanding the interaction of these major health processes.

Our purpose in this chapter is to provide a conceptual overview of the demographic framework used to examine the linkages between mortality, morbidity, and disability (i.e., the healthy life expectancy framework) and to describe the measures and methods used in modeling these linkages—and, implicitly, population health.[1] We emphasize conceptual underpinnings to better evaluate the major gaps in current knowledge as well as current and *potential* complementarities across key lines of research. We show how demographic models of healthy life expectancy are powerful tools in understanding population health, and we discuss how demographic models might inform individual-level analyses of health disparities within a population. We begin by reviewing the conceptual issues underlying research on the association between mortality change and population health.

IMPLICATIONS OF MORTALITY DECLINES FOR POPULATION HEALTH

Between 1950 and 1955 and 1990 to 1995, the world experienced dramatic improvements in mortality rates (Hayward and Zhang 2001). The infant mortality rate fell from 156.0 to 62.0. Life expectancy improved from 45.1 to 62.2 years for males and 47.8 to 66.5 years for females. Mortality declines were most dramatic in less developed regions of the world due to the high levels of mortality observed from 1950 to 1955.

---

[1] A number of recent reviews are available elsewhere that provide in-depth summaries of health expectancy research findings and methods (Crimmins 1996, 1998; Hayward and Zhang 2001; Kinsella 2000; Kinsella and Velkoff 2001; Laditka and Hayward 2003; Waidmann and Manton 2000).

Improvements in mortality rates, particularly in developed nations, have spawned a range of scientific activities designed to gauge the implications of mortality declines for the health and functioning of the surviving populations. The United Nations recognized the importance of this issue in its *Principles for Older Persons*, stating that the goal of scientific advancement must be "to add life in the years that have been added to life" (United Nations 1991). Does declining mortality over a lengthy historical period signify that the members of a population are living longer, healthier lives, i.e., is morbidity being compressed in the life span (Fries 1983)? Or, do mortality rate improvements lead to the lengthening of poor health prior to death?

These questions are at the center of an ongoing debate since the 1980s, in part fueled by contradictory empirical evidence. During the 1970s and into the early 1980s in the United States, reported disability prevalence increased at the same time that mortality rates declined (Crimmins, Saito, and Ingegneri 1989; Verbrugge 1984). An exception to this overall pattern was for persons aged 75 years and older, for whom disability prevalence was relatively stable. Evidence based on the National Long-Term Care Survey for the 1980s and 1990s, however, pointed to an overall decline in disability prevalence for the U.S. population aged 65 years and older (Manton, Corder, and Stallard 1993; Manton, Stallard, and Corder 1995, 1998). Although overall disability prevalence declined during the 1980s and early 1990s, the NLTCS data also showed that changes in specific types of disability prevalence were not consistent (Crimmins, Saito, and Reynolds 1997). Patterns of disability onset and improvement in the 1980s, the transition forces determining disability prevalence, were also inconsistent, clouding whether the changes reflected a historical trend toward improving health (Crimmins, Saito, and Reynolds 1997).

Building on Manton's work using the National Long-Term Care Survey, Crimmins, Saito, and Reynolds (1997) analyzed data from the Longitudinal Study on Aging and the National Health Interview Survey from 1982 to 1993 for persons 70 years of age and older. Their work provided additional evidence of declining disability prevalence in the 1980s, although they found less support for the idea that this was part of an overall trend toward improved health. Schoeni, Freedman, and Wallace (2001) extended Crimmins' analysis of the NHIS data to 1996. They reported declines in disability prevalence between 1982 and 1986 but did not observe additional improvements between 1986 and 1992. Disability prevalence then fell slightly between 1992 and 1996. Schoeni and his colleagues (2001) also noted that disability prevalence improvements, when observed, occurred for people needing help with routine care activities (mild disability) rather than people needing help with personal care, an indicator of more severe disability. Moreover, much of the improvement in disability was concentrated among well-educated persons.

An important confound in this debate is the lack of consistent, high quality, and nationally representative data for a lengthy time period (Hayward and Zhang 2001). The National Health Interview Survey for the United States is the longest available time series of morbidity and disability data. However, design and measurement changes make it challenging to use the NHIS data to make strong inferences about historical trends in disability and morbidity. Comparable time series data sets documenting trends are not available outside the United States. United States–based longitudinal panel studies such as the Longitudinal Study of Aging, the National Long-Term Care Survey, the Survey of Income and Program Participation, and the Health and Retirement Survey have also been used to assess recent changes in morbidity and disability. Survey differences in measurement and design again frustrate researchers who try to reconcile differences in results. A recent study by Freedman, Martin, and Schoeni (2002) presented an evaluation of the quality of eight American data sources used in recent studies of population-level trends in disability. Based on a variety of criteria, the surveys were rated as good (2), fair (4) and poor or mixed (2) for assessing trends. Based only on those surveys rated fair or good, the surveys varied substantially in their estimates of the percentage declines in disability. For example, when disability was defined using self-reported activities of daily living, estimates of disability change ranged from -1.38% to $+1.53\%$ per year.

While methodological challenges make it difficult to ascertain trends in population health, this is only one source of confusion. Conceptually, the association between mortality changes and health changes in the surviving population is not as straightforward as one might think (Crimmins 1996; Crimmins, Hayward, and Saito 1994), and this partially accounts for the lack of clarity in the research literature. If mortality improvements occur primarily among persons already beset by health problems, a greater number of people will survive in poor health. This will lead to higher rates of prevalence of a health problem in a population (e.g., disability), and it will lengthen the years of life with the health condition. However, if mortality rate improvements occur because of delays in the onset of diseases and functional problems, then population health will improve. Thus, prevalence rates and life expectancy with a health condition will decline.

The mixture of fatal and nonfatal conditions in the population adds additional complexity to this relationship. For example, a substantial portion of functional problems in the older population is due to arthritis, a nonfatal condition, while cardiovascular diseases are also an important precursor of functional problems (Verbrugge and Patrick 1995). Improvements in cardiovascular mortality would potentially reduce related functional problems but would have little direct impact on functional problems due to arthritis (Hayward, Crimmins, and Saito 1998). Understanding how mortality change is likely to influence population health thus necessitates knowledge of where in a major disease process health improvements are occurring, as well as the changing mix of fatal and nonfatal disease conditions in the population. Further, progress in fighting some diseases may be more advanced than for others. Indeed, this is to be expected given national health care and research priorities and uneven scientific advances across the range of disease conditions. These factors, in addition to changes in the social and economic characteristics of populations, contribute to uneven changes in disease and disability prevalence—change that need not be uniformly downward (Bonneux et al. 1994; Crimmins 1996; Hayward, Crimmins, and Zhang, in Press). As Crimmins (1996: S224) argues, when mortality rate improvements occur, an increase in disability prevalence is an:

> expected epidemiological stage that can occur when increases in life expectancy are greater than reductions in the incidence of health problems. In addition, at any one time we are likely to see improvements in some indicators of health and not others, and improvements in some age groups and not others.

A Conceptual Framework of Population Health

Under the auspices of the World Health Organization, a conceptual framework of population health was proposed that integrates the concepts of morbidity, disability, and mortality (Manton and Soldo 1985; World Health Organization 1984). The framework is based on a life table survival model where the overall survivorship in a life table cohort is decomposed into the proportion of a cohort that survives without one of three basic health events occurring—morbidity, disability, or death. Figure 27.1 shows the life table framework for a hypothetical population.

The vertical axis in Figure 27.1 identifies the probability of surviving (expressed in terms of a standard population) to a given age without one of the three basic health problems occurring. The areas in the figure refer to the average probability of being in a given health state at a given age. For example, the area beneath the morbidity curve (A) represents the probability of being free of morbidity at each age. By definition, the areas also describe the person-years spent in each health state by a life table cohort. Area C, for example, represents the person-years spent disabled while the combined areas of A and B represent disability-free person-years. Areas B and C combined represent the person-years lived with a chronic condition (morbidity and disability), while area A represents disease-free person years.

Using this life table model, demographers have developed a general summary measure of population health (i.e., healthy life expectancy) that explicitly integrates the mortality and disability (or morbidity) experiences of the population. Conceptually, the measure refers to the length of time that an average individual can expect to be healthy (according to some set of criteria) or unhealthy over the life cycle. This measure captures the *life cycle* burden of a health condition for a population (or population subgroup), i.e., the health-related quality of life for the average person in a population in relation to the overall length of life. In the context of the model shown in Figure 27.1, three indicators make up a family of population health indicators: total life expectancy, disease-free life expectancy, and disability-free life expectancy. The indicators can be interpreted independently of each other, e.g., how disease-free life expectancy or disability-free life expectancy is changing in the population. This type of interpretation responds, for example, to questions about the implications of public health policies or new medical interventions for enhancing specific aspects of population health. The measures can also be interpreted together, e.g., how disease-free life expectancy and disability-free life expectancy change as total life expectancy grows. In this way, investigators can assess whether declines in mortality rates lead to the compression of morbidity and disability

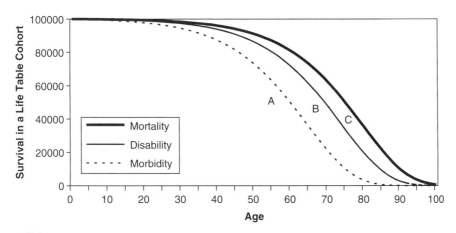

FIGURE 27.1.

during particular time periods and whether different population groups have similar overall survival but differ in terms of life cycle morbidity and disability experiences.

This conceptual framework offers a number of advantages for examining trends in population health, particularly in comparison to examining trends in disability prevalence as described above. Descriptively, the life table approach provides a means to compare population groups' health while controlling for differences in age composition. The framework also provides the means to explicitly address the question of whether declining mortality results in the expansion or compression of the period of life with disability and morbidity. Overall survival curves can be compared across historical periods, as can changes in the person-years of morbidity and disability. By extension, researchers can compare population groups' trends in health and identify the demographic conditions and trends underlying those changes.

The life table measure of healthy (and unhealthy) life expectancy differs from a prevalence rate of health conditions that captures the percentage of a population experiencing a health problem at a point in time. Prevalence reflects not only current experience but also captures health experiences at younger ages that have left their mark on the surviving population (Freeman and Hutchinson 1980; Hayward et al. 2000a; Schoen 1988). For example, blacks' higher prevalence of hypertension during middle age compared to whites' prevalence indicates a higher rate of onset among blacks prior to middle age (Hayward et al. 2000). Prevalence rates also benchmark the *societal* (or a group's) burden of disease at a particular time point, because prevalence rates are inherently properties of groups and not individuals.[2]

MEASURING THE HEALTH OF THE POPULATION

Health is a complex concept denoting compromised well-being stemming from disability and disease, and mental, physical, and emotional problems (Murray and Chen 1992). The main ways in which demographers measure health in the life table model of population health are primarily based on concepts from the World Health Organization's 1980 *International Classification of Impairments, Disabilities, and Handicaps* (ICIDH) (World Health Organization 1980) and Nagi's schemes (1989; 1991; Verbrugge and Jette 1994), adopted by the Institute of Medicine.[3] Conceptually, the WHO and Nagi schemes overlap significantly (Verbrugge and Jette 1994). The ICIDH and Nagi

[2] The individual analogue of a prevalence rate is whether a person has a health condition. Associations between the presence of a health condition and a predictor variable by definition summarize the historical relationship between some predictor variable (e.g., socioeconomic status) and the presence of a health condition prior to the time of observation.
[3] The World Health Organization introduced the *International Classification of Functioning, Disability, and Health* (ICF) in 2001 (World Health Organization 2001). The ICF's changes in terminology make it difficult to explicitly compare to Nagi's scheme and Verbrugge and Jette's disablement process, although the ICF's conceptual framework embraces Verbrugge and Jette's ideas of how extra- and intraindividual factors influence environmental demands and individuals' capabilities. The ICF uses two umbrella terms, functioning and disability. Functioning encompasses body functions, activities executed by the individual, and participation in a life situation. Disability refers to the impairment of physiological functions, organ systems, activity limitation, and participation restriction. Because demographers have relied almost exclusively on the earlier classification schemes, our discussion focuses on these health concepts.

schemes are the basis of Verbrugge and Jette's (1994: 3) framework of disablement which shows:

> the impacts that chronic and acute conditions have on the functioning of specific body systems and on people's abilities to act in necessary, usual, expected and personally desired ways in their society.

Roughly hierarchical, disablement typically begins with the onset of a chronic disease that may have a cascading effect so that a loss of physical or mental function occurs (e.g., impaired mobility, restrictions in body actions that involve various motions or strength, the loss of short-term memory). If functional problems make it difficult or impossible to perform normal social activities, then disability results. At the individual level, this pathway is neither unidirectional or deterministic. Changes in the family, social, community, and health care environments can alter the disablement experience. Persons with a chronic disease, for example, might regain functional abilities through medical treatment. Disabled persons could become nondisabled through the introduction of devices that provide assistance. Conversely, persons with a functional problem might experience hastened disability through the loss of their spouse—the spouse may have made it possible for a person with a functional problem to perform normal social activities.

This conceptualization corresponds roughly to the idea in the gerontological literature that individual aging refers to changes in structure and function. An important feature of this conceptualization is the lack of direct correspondence between disablement and mortality. Mortality *reflects* the aging process of "changes in structure and function" but it does not *define* the aging process. One way to think about the lack of direct correspondence is the sensitivity of mortality to temporal and environmental conditions versus aging processes. For example, how long persons with heart disease live is highly contingent on temporal and proximate conditions such as the availability of emergency services, scientific innovation in the treatment of heart disease, and the differential application of medical procedures, say, across race or sex groups.

Demographers' use of the ICIDH or disablement framework has resulted in a class of measures describing the health of the population.[4] *Disease-free life expectancy* is the expected number of years the average person in a population would expect to live free of disease (or a specific disease depending on the model) if current patterns of morbidity and mortality were to continue over time. Peeters and colleagues (2002), for example, calculated the number of years of life free of coronary heart disease (and with the disease) for the Framingham Heart Study cohort. Calculations for heart disease life expectancy show that life with heart disease can be quite lengthy—about six [D1]years for men aged 50. Other applications of this population health measure include the expected number of years lived with dementia in the Dutch population (Witthaus et al. 1999) and lung cancer expectancies for the U.S. population (Manton and Stallard 1988).

Disability-free life expectancy is the expected number of years of life free of a chronic health condition that limits the normal social activities of life. A number of studies focus on disability defined in terms of household management (measured by instrumental activities of daily living or IADLs) and the ability to provide self-care (measured by activities of daily living or ADLs) (Crimmins, Hayward, and Saito

---

[4] European demographers use a slightly different classification scheme, but the terminology is similar.

1994; Katz 1983; Katz et al. 1983).[5] IADLs refer to problems such as managing money, using the telephone, preparing one's own meals, and doing light housework. ADLs refer to self-care problems such as toileting, bathing, dressing, eating, and getting in and out of bed. Although item wording varies across survey instruments, ADLs and IADLs are among the main ways that health surveys measure disability. Disability-free life expectancies have been calculated for the United States elderly population (Crimmins, Hayward, and Saito 1994; Rogers, Rogers and Branch 1989; Rogers, Rogers, and Belanger 1989), as well as for key population subgroups defined by race, sex, and education (Crimmins, Hayward, and Saito 1996; Hayward, Crimmins, and Saito 1998).

Other studies reference disability in terms of the ability to perform major social roles (e.g., work and school) or normal activities. These measures have been used to document disability-free life expectancy for a number of countries around the world (Robine and Romieu 1998; Robine et al. 1995; Robine, Romieu, and Jee 1998), trends in disability-free life expectancy in the United States (Crimmins and Saito 2001; Crimmins, Saito, and Ingegneri 1997) and OECD countries (Robine, Romieu, and Jee 1998), race/ ethnic, educational and gender differences in disability-free life for the U.S. population (Crimmins and Saito 2001; Hayward and Heron 1999), and social inequality in disability-free life for France (Cambois, Robine, and Hayward 2001), to name only a few studies. Crimmins and Cambois (2002) recently reviewed a range of studies that addressed socioeconomic differentials in healthy life expectancy in European countries, Canada, and the United States. A common finding was that socioeconomic differentials in healthy life expectancy exceeded differentials in total life expectancy.

Health Adjusted Life Expectancy measures health by adjusting life expectancy according to weights assigned to particular health states (Mathers, Robine, and Wilkins 1994; Wolfson 1996). The measure is intended to identify the gap between life in perfect health and life where individuals are beset by ill health. Weights for health states typically range from zero (dead) to one (perfect health). Weighting systems are frequently controversial (Barendregt, Bonneux, and Van der Maas 1996; Mathers, Robine, and Wilkins 1994; Waidmann and Manton 2000). What does perfect health mean? Who judges the assignment of values to particular health problems? Do the values reflect a theoretical premise, empirical evidence, or expert opinion? Given these questions, health-adjusted life expectancies have been less frequently examined in the scientific literature.

This class of measures, however, has become a useful policy tool in evaluating the burden of disease internationally. For example, health-adjusted life expectancies have been used to gauge the burden of illness consequences of eliminating particular diseases from the population (Manuel et al. 2003; Manuel and Schultz 2004; Nolte and McKee 2003). For example, what are the expected years of life if diabetes was eliminated as a health problem? The World Health Organization's Global Programme for Evidence on health policy estimates disability-adjusted life expectancy (DALE) to identify a country's expected years of healthy life. The DALE is calculated by weighting the years of ill health according to severity and then subtracting this figure from the total expected life expectancy. The difference is the equivalent years of healthy life. The World Health Organization ranks countries based on these measures, showing, for example, that the years lost to disability are substantially higher in poorer countries rather than developed

---

[5] Studies that define disability in terms of IADLs and ADLs often refer to disability-free life expectancy as active life expectancy (Crimmins, Hayward, and Saito 1994; Crimmins, Hayward and Saito 1996; Hayward, Crimmins, and Saito 1998). Some researchers reserve the term disability-free life expectancy for health problems that curtail activities in major social roles such as work and school.

countries. This pattern is due to the fact that limitations such as injury, blindness, paralysis, and the functional consequences of tropical diseases such as malaria affect children and young adults. A recent study reported that people in developed parts of the world lose only about 8% of their lives to disability compared to 18% for persons living in the poorest countries (Mathers et al. 2001).

MEASUREMENT AND METHODOLOGICAL ISSUES IN MODELING HEALTHY LIFE EXPECTANCY

Systematic comparisons of health expectancies across studies are challenged by the quality of the health measures and study designs (Freedman et al. 2002; Hayward and Zhang 2001), the operational definitions of the health measures (Crimmins 1996), and the various methods used to calculate health expectancies (Laditka and Hayward 2003). Not surprisingly, this makes it difficult to obtain consistent estimates of the expected years of healthy (and unhealthy) life in a population.

Because estimates of healthy life expectancy reflect assumptions about measurement and modeling, they should be treated as *indicators* of population health rather than an accurate accounting of health experience. As noted earlier, a life table *model* generates health expectancies and thus the expectancies are subject to the model's constraints and assumptions. This makes it difficult to compare exact numerical estimates of healthy life expectancy across studies. Frequently, researchers focus on the relative proportion of life that is healthy (or unhealthy) or the consistency of group (e.g., sex, race, or period) differences in healthy life expectancy.

Efforts to harmonize measures and methods have been promoted by the International Network on Healthy Life Expectancy (known by its French acronym of REVES—Réseau Espérance de Vie en Santé). Recognized by the World Health Organization, REVES is a grassroots scientific organization dedicated to promoting international consistency in the design, measurement, and calculation of health expectancy measures used in monitoring population health (http://www.prw.le.ac.uk/reves/). Illustrative of these efforts is the REVES project begun in 1997 under the auspices of the European Health Monitoring Programme and supported by the European Commission. The project's aim has been to set up a coherent set of instruments to measure health expectancies for the European Union. Seven research teams representing six countries and many academic disciplines have been involved in this effort (Robine, Jagger, and Egidi 2000). The project teams have made preliminary recommendations on 10 instruments documenting chronic morbidity, functional limitations (physical, sensory, and cognitive), disability, self-perceived health, and mental health. The REVES report is under review for comment by European policymakers.

Efforts such as those by REVES and the World Health Organization's Global Burden of Disease project (Mathers et al. 2002; Murray and Lopez 1996) are particularly important for the ongoing monitoring of population health. Cross-sectional surveys fielded repeatedly over some period typically provide the monitoring data. The National Health Interview Survey for the United States, for example, provides annual health data for the population since 1969. Similarly, the National Long-Term Care Survey provides information about the health of Medicare-enrolled Americans aged 65 years and older for 1982, 1984, 1989, 1994, and 1999.

Increasingly, however, researchers are utilizing longitudinal panel data to develop healthy life expectancy measures reflecting the complexity of age-related *changes* in health. Longitudinal panel data reveal that as persons age, they not only experience the onset of disability but they also recover from disability (Crimmins, Hayward, and Saito 1994; Land, Guralnik, and Blazer 1994; Rogers et al. 1989).[6] Onset and recovery are typically inferred from respondents' reports of current disability measured at multiple times in the course of the panel study. For example, a respondent may report being disabled at the time of a baseline interview but then report being nondisabled at a subsequent interview—and perhaps being disabled again at some future date.

An issue not well addressed in the literature is that some of the traditional health measures, particularly measures of disability (e.g., ADLs, IADLs, and work and domestic disability), do not translate well in a conceptual sense to a longitudinal design or longitudinal analysis (Crimmins 1996; Crimmins and Hayward 1997). At any particular survey wave, for example, reported disability is not exclusively the outcome of a biomedical process, but it is also an outcome of dysfunction (organ system or bodily function) *and* the environmental demands on functioning. Changes in a person's reports of disability across interview waves may reflect differences in the level of social and environmental support as well as changes in physical or mental functioning. For example, marital status changes or the addition of technology can result in changes in individuals reporting that they need or get less help with tasks without improvements in the underlying biomedical process.

This uncertainty points to the importance of differentiating functional changes from environmental changes in longitudinal health surveys in order to understand how changes in healthy life expectancy occur (Crimmins and Hayward 1997). For example, a decline in the years of disabled life could be a consequence of reductions in disabling diseases such as cardiovascular diseases and arthritis. Declines might also be attributable to the reduction of environmental challenges and the introduction of new technologies and medications. In the latter case, reductions in the expected years with disability are not a reflection of changes in health as we typically think of them. Rather, such declining disability reflects changes in the ability to cope with poor health.

Another factor contributing to difficulties in making cross-study comparisons of healthy life expectancy is the types of life table approaches used in modeling healthy life (see Laditka and Hayward [2003] for a review of the life table approaches' underlying assumptions, data requirements, and comparative advantages). A large number of studies of trends in healthy life expectancy rely on a prevalence-based life table method, often referred to as the Sullivan method (Sullivan 1966, 1971). Much of the impetus for using the Sullivan method to monitor trends in population health stems from its relatively straightforward data requirements—prevalence rates of health conditions and mortality rates for the population. Mortality rates are typically obtained from a country's statistical agency charged with providing information about the vital statistics of the population. Prevalence rates of health conditions are usually obtained from cross-sectional health surveys. These surveys are increasingly common around the world, and they are relatively inexpensive to field (compared to longitudinal panel surveys). The sample sizes of these surveys also yield highly reliable prevalence estimates. Robine and

---

[6] This has led to the use of multistate life table methods in calculating healthy life expectancy, because this approach explicitly allows for age-related declines and improvements in health (Laditka and Hayward 2003).

collaborators (1995) report that a growing number of countries are using the Sullivan method to monitor changes in population health.

However, a potential problem using the Sullivan method for examining changes in population health is its insensitivity to dramatic swings in disability and mortality. During periods of rapidly improving survival, for example, the Sullivan method underestimates improvements in healthy life expectancy (Barendregt, Bonneux, and Van der Maas 1994) relative to overall gains in survivorship. However, when changes in health and mortality are relatively smooth, a situation that is characteristic of more recent shifts in population health, the Sullivan method appears to provide realistic scenarios of long-term trends (Mathers and Robine 1997).

With the increased availability of longitudinal data on health changes, researchers have begun to use multistate life tables (and most recently microsimulations) to model the interactions of morbidity, disability, and mortality (Crimmins, Hayward, and Saito 1994; Laditka and Wolf 1998; Land, Guralnick, and Blazer 1994; Rogers, Rogers, and Branch 1989; Rogers, Rogers, and Belanger 1989). Estimates of healthy life calculated by the Sullivan method and the multistate model are difficult to compare directly because of the models' assumptions and the fact that they often use different sources of data (e.g., cross-sectional surveys compared panel studies). An advantage of the multistate model, however, is that it can be used to better assess the underlying causes of changes in healthy life expectancy and the prevalence of health conditions in the population. For example, Crimmins, Hayward, and Saito (1994) used a multistate life table model to demonstrate how healthy life expectancy (defined in terms of ADL and IADL disability) and prevalence respond to changes in the incidence rates governing declines and improvements in health, as well as changes in health-specific mortality. Hayward, Crimmins and Saito (1998) used a similar approach to show how healthy life expectancy is affected by the elimination of several major causes of death.

Although the multistate model has many desirable properties compared to the Sullivan method (Laditka and Hayward 2003), a potential drawback of the multistate method for monitoring trends in population health is its reliance on longitudinal data as inputs to the life table. The limited amount of longitudinal data for lengthy historical periods has clearly inhibited the use of the multistate method to investigate population health trends. Even if such data were available, however, potential methodological problems warrant serious consideration. For example, because longitudinal data are typically obtained from panel surveys, the reliability of the incidence rates of health change—the inputs for the multistate model—are potentially problematic because of the sparse numbers of health events at certain ages and for some population subgroups. The implications of sample attrition for incidence rates are also poorly understood, especially given that attrition may be related to largely unmeasured biomedical processes. Additional methodological research is needed to understand the sensitivity of the multistate model to design and measurement limitations of longitudinal panel surveys.

SOME IMPORTANT LESSONS OF DEMOGRAPHIC MODELS OF POPULATION HEALTH

An important outcome of demographers' investigations of population health has been the understanding that mortality, morbidity, and disability are related but not isomorphic concepts. An individual may contract a fatal disease condition, for example, but need not die from that cause (Manton and Stallard 1988). Moreover, for some diseases such as heart disease, individuals may live with the disease for many years before death (Peeters et al. 2002). Disability is not necessarily a permanent condition nor is it a condition that inevitably precedes death in the older population (Crimmins, Hayward, and Saito 1994, 1996; Rogers, Rogers, and Branch 1989a; Rogers, Rogers, and Belanger 1989b). Moreover, disability is associated with both fatal and nonfatal chronic conditions, so severe disability is not necessarily the final stage of poor health prior to death (Crimmins, Hayward, and Saito 1994; Verbrugge and Patrick 1995). The key point is that death is not always the outcome of an evolutionary process wherein individuals contract a fatal condition, the condition induces functional problems and disability, and when advanced, the condition results in death. The process can be fairly complex and is not obvious.

This complexity carries over to population subgroup differences in the processes defining population health. Crimmins et al. (1996) showed, for example, that men aged 70 years and older were more likely than women to die across the full range of functioning problems (although high levels of chronic health problems attenuated the sex effect somewhat). Men were also more likely to recover from functioning problems than were women. Women, however, experienced drastically higher rates of functional decline than did men. Sex appears to affect mortality and disability in the opposite directions in that women live longer than men, but they also live more years with functional problems.

At present, attention to subgroup differences in population health processes is restricted largely to race and sex groups. A handful of studies have also documented educational differences in population health processes (Crimmins, Hayward, and Saito 1996; Hayward, Crimmins, and Zhang, in Press; Land, Guralnick, and Blazer 1994; Zimmer et al. 1998). Generally, poorly educated persons appear to have higher rates of disability onset, as well as higher rates of death among persons without functioning problems. Once functioning problems occur, however, there is less evidence of an educational effect on mortality. The consequences of education's effects on the transitions making up the process are that education is associated with an increase of both total life and disability-free life and a compression of the period of life with functional problems.

In many ways, demographic models of population health are important starting points for explanatory analyses of health and mortality (e.g., see the demography of health chapter 26, "Health Demography," chapter 10, "Adult Mortality," in this *Handbook*). At a basic level, demographic models illustrate the difficulties confronting cross-sectional studies of health in making strong inferences about causal associations. For example, the association between education and respondents' reports of disability in a cross-sectional survey could reflect (prior) educational differences in the onset of disability, recovery from disability, and survival with (and without) disability that have left their mark on the surviving population (Hayward et al. 2000). Without understanding how education is associated with each of the transitions constituting the underlying process, interpretation of the cross-sectional association is ambiguous by definition.

This problem points to the need for longitudinal panel [D2]studies of health that take into account the underlying processes generating the observed health measure. Ideally, researchers should directly model the associations between explanatory variables and each of the transitions, but data limitations (the lack of longitudinal data, sparse data problems) necessarily limit the feasibility of this argument—hence the frequent reliance on cross-sectional data. In the face of data limitations, a more careful conceptualization of the health process is called for to aid in interpreting the cross-sectional associations between predictor measures and the health outcome.

Despite the difficulty of approaching population health via individual-level health processes, a growing number of individual-level studies are examining health transitions. However, these studies are typically restricted to subsets of transitions (e.g., the onset of a health condition) (Freedman and Martin 1999; Hayward et al. 2000) and rarely focus on the full set of transitions defining the interplay between morbidity, disability and mortality (a recent exception is Zimmer et al. [1998]). A number of individual-level explanatory studies of health transitions have focused on the ultimate health event—mortality. Morbidity is not considered explicitly, and the assumption of isomorphism between morbidity and mortality is implicit. This results in potentially ambiguous interpretations of how explanatory variables are associated with the process leading to death. For example, as noted above, demographers have documented that education is negatively associated with the onset of functional problems and negatively associated with recovery but does not appear to have a strong association with mortality among persons with functioning problems. This suggests that education's frequently documented association with mortality largely reflects its association with the onset of health problems but has less to do with the mitigation of the fatal consequences of a health problem.

Demographic models of population health, therefore, are an important first step in laying the groundwork for explanatory models of health. Demographic models are useful in identifying health trajectories that are made up of morbidity, disability, and mortal events. These models also are important in evaluating key subgroup differences in population health and how specific morbidity, disability, and mortality experiences give rise to overall differences. The demographic models, in turn, help to ground the development of theoretical models and explanatory analyses that closely articulate with the interplay of morbidity, disability, and mortality.

CONCLUSIONS

Demographic models of population health combining morbidity, disability, and mortality are a scientific response to post-World War II trends in population aging in developed nations. Population aging has brought about greater demands for health care and old age Social Security as proportionately larger numbers of older persons make up the population. Not surprisingly, concerns about whether longer life signals better or worse health have led to population health monitoring systems and an ever expanding body of research.

Sullivan (1971) provided the first calculations of healthy life expectancy in 1971. Since that time, health expectancies have been calculated for numerous countries—both developed and developing—and the methods, and measures, as well as the associated scientific debates, have become increasingly sophisticated. Recently, the International Network on Healthy Life Expectancy (REVES) published a book, *Determining Health Expectancies* (Robine et al. 2003), which provides a detailed look at how health expectancy research and methods have evolved in the scientific community.

Health expectancy research has contributed significantly to the current understanding of the recent trends in population health. For example, this research has clarified that different components of morbidity—disease, disability, and self-perceived health—need not move in the same direction at the same time (Crimmins, Saito, and Reynolds 1997; Freedman and Martin 1998; Manton, Corder, and Stallard 1993). As Crimmins

(1996) notes, some of these indicators may rise during periods of falling mortality, a natural (although not necessarily inevitable) part of the epidemiological transition. Rising disability is not necessarily a signal of the failure of policies aimed at enhancing population health. Rather, this trend may be a sign of success. Although the evidence must still be verified, health expectancy research suggests a shift in the United States in the distribution of disability levels toward the less severe problems that accompanied the decline in old age mortality in recent decades.

Furthermore, health expectancy research has begun to clarify how major population subgroups differ in their morbidity, disability, and mortality experiences. Frequently population subgroups' health experiences differ in unexpected ways and may be masked by using prevalence rates of health and mortality rates as benchmarks. Demographic models' superior descriptions of how health problems unfold in population subgroups are particularly useful in helping refine theoretical arguments underlying health disparities. Health expectancy research points to the importance of carefully delineating the fundamental transitions defining population health, evaluating where in a given process groups differ, and then bringing multivariate techniques to bear in analyzing these transitions to understand the causal factors involved. This articulation between demographic models and individual-level explanatory models holds considerable promise for a more sophisticated understanding of the fundamental causes of population-level health disparities.

Health expectancy research has considerable scientific momentum. Globally, policymakers and researchers are engaged in new partnerships aimed at monitoring population health. This has led to an increase in the number of countries fielding health surveys and a sustained commitment within countries to field health surveys over time to monitor health trends. Within the scientific community, demographers and other health scientists are engaged in informative scientific debates over health expectancy methods and measures, investigating how different facets of morbidity interact and change over time, and assessing disparities in the health experiences of their nation's population. These activities are frequently collaborative, involving teams of researchers from multiple disciplines and from multiple countries.

Health expectancy research has come a long way since Sullivan first calculated an index of population health in which morbidity and mortality were integrated. Clearly, however, the scientific fervor surrounding substantive and methodological debates points to additional future advances in understanding the sources of change in population health and the extent to which these changes are shared within a population. This research will take place against a demographic backdrop of global population aging, scientific and technological improvements in combating disease, improvements in educational attainment, and the social capacity for good health in populations—factors that are likely to make population health a moving target. Thus, the epidemiological transition associated with population aging is far from complete, making it difficult to anticipate future changes in the burden of disease.

REFERENCES

Barendregt, J. J., L. Bonneux, and P. J. Van der Maas. 1994. Health expectancy: An indicator for change? Technology Assessment Methods Project Team. *Journal of Epidemiology and Community Health* 48(5):482–487.

Barendregt, J. J., L. Bonneux, and P. J. Van der Maas. 1996. DALYs: The age-weights on balance. *Bulletin of the World Health Organization* 74(4):439–443.

Bonneux, L., J. J. Barendregt, K. Meeter, G. J. Bonsel, and P. J. Van der Maas. 1994. Estimating clinical morbidity due to ischemic heart disease and congestive heart failure: The future rise of heart failure. *American Journal of Public Health* 84:20–28.

Cambois, E., J. M. Robine, and M. D. Hayward. 2001. Social inequalities in disability-free life expectancy in the French male population, 1980–1991. *Demography* 38(4):513–524.

Crimmins, E. M. 1996. Mixed trends in population health among older adults. *Journal of Gerontology: Social Sciences* 51B:S223–S225.

Crimmins, E. M. 1998. Is disability declining among the elderly? Defining disability and examining trends. *Critical Issues in Aging* 2:10–11.

Crimmins, E. M. 2002. The relevance of health expectancies: Introduction. In *Determining health expectancies*. Edited by J. M. Robine, C. Jagger, C. D. Mathers, E. M. Crimmins, and R. M. Suzman. Chichester, West Sussex, England: John Wiley @ Sons.

Crimmins, E. M., and E. Cambois. 2002. Social inequalities in health expectancy. In *Determining health expectancies*. Edited by J.-M. Robine, C. Jagger, C. D. Mathers, E. M. Crimmins, and R. M. Suzman. Chichester, West Sussex, England: John Wiley & Sons.

Crimmins, E. M., and M. D. Hayward. 1997. What can we learn about competence at older ages from active life expectancy. In *Social structural mechanisms for maintaining competence in old age*. Edited by K. W. Schaie, S. Willis, and M. D. Hayward, 1–22. New York: Springer.

Crimmins, E. M., M. D. Hayward, and Y. Saito. 1994. Changing mortality and morbidity rates and the health status and life expectancy of the older population. *Demography* 31:159–175.

Crimmins, E. M., M. D. Hayward, and Y. Saito. 1996. Differentials in active life expectancy in the older population. *Journal of Gerontology: Social Sciences* 51B:S111–S120.

Crimmins, E. M., and Y. Saito. 2001. Trends in healthy life expectancy in the United States, 1970–1990: Gender, racial, and educational differences. *Social Science and Medicine* 52:1629–1641.

Crimmins, E. M., Y. Saito, and D. Ingegneri. 1989. Changes in Life expectancy and disability-free life expectancy in the United States. *Population and Development Review* 15:235–267.

Crimmins, E. M., Y. Saito, and D. Ingegneri. 1997. Trends in disability-free life expectancy in the United States. *Population and Development Review* 23:555–572.

Crimmins, E. M., Y. Saito, and S. L. Reynolds. 1997. Further evidence on recent trends in the prevalence and incidence of disability among older Americans from two sources: The LSOA and the NHIS. *Journal of Gerontology: Social Sciences* 52(2):S59–71.

Davis, K., M. S. Bernstam, and R. Ricardo-Campbell. 1987. *Below-replacement fertility in industrial societies*. New York: Cambridge University Press.

Freedman, V. A., and L. G. Martin. 1998. Understanding trends in functional limitations among older Americans. *American Journal of Public Health* 88:1457–1462.

Freedman, V. A., and L. G. Martin. 1999. The role of education in explaining and forecasting trends in functional limitations among older Americans. *Demography* 36:461–473.

Freedman, V. A., L. G. Martin, and R. F. Schoeni. 2002. Recent trends in disability and functioning among older adults in the United States: A systematic review. *Journal of the American Medical Association* 288(24):3137–3146.

Freeman, J., and G. B. Hutchinson. 1980. Prevalence, incidence, and duration. *American Journal of Epidemiology* 112:707–723.

Fries, J. F. 1983. The compression of morbidity. *Milbank Memorial Fund Quarterly* 61:397–419.

Hayward, M. D., E. M. Crimmins, T. P. Miles, and Y. Yu. 2000. The significance of socioeconomic status in explaining the racial gap in chronic health conditions. *American Sociological Review* 65:910–930.

Hayward, M. D., E. M. Crimmins, and Y. Saito. 1998. Cause of death and active life expectancy in the older population of the United States. *Journal of Aging and Health* 10:192–213.

Hayward, M. D., E. M. Crimmins, and Z. Zhang. 2000. The racial burden of chronic disease: A life cycle model of heart disease experience. Paper presented at the Annual Meetings of the Population Association of America, Los Angeles.

Hayward, M. D., E. M. Crimmins, and Z. Zhang. In press. Consequences of educational change for the burden of chronic health problems in the population. In *The distribution of private and public resources across generations*. Edited by A. H. Gauthier, C. Chu, and S. Tuljapurkar. New York: Oxford University Press.

Hayward, M. D., and M. Heron. 1999. Racial inequality in active life among adult Americans. *Demography* 36:77–91.

Hayward, M. D., and Z. Zhang. 2001. The demographic revolution in population aging: A century of change, 1950–2050. In *Handbook of aging and the social sciences, 5th ed.* Edited by R. K. Binstock and L. K. George, 69–85. New York: Academic Press.

Katz, S. 1983. Assessing self-maintenance: Activities of daily living, mobility, and instrumental activities of daily living. *Journal of the American Geriatrics Society* 31(12):721–727.

Katz, S., L. G. Branch, M. H. Branson, J. A. Papsidero, J. C. Beck, and D. S. Greer. 1983. Active life expectancy. *New England Journal of Medicine* 309(20):1218–1224.

Kinsella, K. 2000. Demographic dimensions of global aging. *Journal of Family Issues* 21:541–558.

Kinsella, K., and V. A. Velkoff. 2001. *An aging world.* Washington, D.C.: U.S. Government Printing Office.

Laditka, S. B., and M. D. Hayward. 2003. The evolution of demographic methods to calculate health expectancies. In *Determining health expectancies.* Edited by J. M. Robine, C. Jagger, C. D. Mathers, E. M. Crimmins, and R. M. Suzman, 221–234. Chichester, West Sussex, England: John Weley & Sons.

Laditka, S. B., and D. A. Wolf. 1998. New methods for analyzing active life expectancy. *Journal of Aging and Health* 10:214–241.

Land, K., J. Guralnik, and D. Blazer. 1994. Estimating increment-decrement life tables with multiple covariates from panel data: The case of active life expectancy. *Demography* 31:289–319.

Manton, K. G. 1990. Mortality and morbidity. In *Handbook of aging and the social sciences, 3rd ed.* Edited by R. K. Binstock and L. K. George, 64–90. New York: Academic Press.

Manton, K. G., L. S. Corder, and E. Stallard. 1993. Estimates of change in chronic disability and institutional incidence and prevalence rates in the U.S. elderly population from the 1982, 1984, and 1989 National Long Term Care Survey. *Journal of Gerontology* 48(4):S153–166.

Manton, K. G., and B. Soldo. 1985. Dynamics of health changes in the oldest old: New perspectives and evidence. *Milbank Memorial Fund Quarterly* 63:206–285.

Manton, K. G., and E. Stallard. 1988. *Chronic disease modelling: Measurement and evaluation of the risks of chronic disease processes.* New York: Oxford University Press.

Manton, K. G., E. Stallard, and L. S. Corder. 1995. Changes in morbidity and chronic disability in the U.S. elderly population: Evidence from the 1982, 1984, and 1989 National Long Term Care Surveys. *Journal of Gerontology: Social Sciences* 50B:S194–S204.

Manton, K. G., E. Stallard, and L. S. Corder. 1998. The dynamics of dimensions of age-related disability 1982 to 1994 in the U.S. elderly population. *Journals of Gerontology: Medical Sciences* 53(1):B59–70.

Manuel, D. G., W. Luo, A. M. Ugnat, and Y. Mao. 2003. Cause-deleted health-adjusted life expectancy of Canadians with selected chronic conditions. *Chronic Diseases in Canada* 24(4):108–115.

Manuel, D. G., and S. E. Schultz. 2004. Health-related quality of life and health-adjusted life expectancy of people with diabetes in Ontario, Canada, 1996–1997. *Diabetes Care* 27(2):407–414.

Mathers, C. D., C. J. Murray, A. D. Lopez, R. Sadana, and J. A. Salomon. 2002. Global patterns of healthy life expectancy for older women. *Journal of Women and Aging* 14(1–2):99–117.

Mathers, C. D., and J. M. Robine. 1997. How good is Sullivan's method for monitoring changes in population health expectancies? *Journal of Epidemiology and Community Health* 51(1):80–86.

Mathers, C. D., J. M. Robine, and R. Wilkins. 1994. Health expectancy indicators: Recommendations for terminology. In *Advances in health expectancies.* Edited by C. D. Mathers, J. McCallum, and J. M. Robine, 34–41. Canberra, Australia: Australian Institute of Health and Welfare.

Mathers, C. D., R. Sadana, J. A. Salomon, C. J. Murray, and A. D. Lopez. 2001. Healthy life expectancy in 191 countries, 1999. *Lancet* 357(9269):1685–1691.

Murray, C. J. L., and L. C. Chen. 1912. Understanding morbidity change. *Population and Development Review* 18:481–503

Murray, C. J. L., and A. D. Lopez. 1996. *The global burden of disease.* Cambridge, Mass.: Harvard University Press.

Nagi, S. Z. 1989. The concept and measurement of disability. In *Disability policies and government programs.* Edited by E. D. Berkowitz, 1–15. New York: Praeger.

Nagi, S. Z. 1991. Disability concepts revisited: Implications for prevention. In *Disability in America: Toward a national agenda for prevention.* Edited by A. M. Pope and A. R. Tarlov, 309–327. Washington, D.C.: Institute of Medicine, National Academies Press.

Nolte, E., and M. McKee. 2003. Measuring the health of nations: analysis of mortality amenable to health care. *British Medical Journal* 327(7424):1129.

Peeters, A., A. A. Mamun, F. Willekens, and L. Bonneux. 2002. A cardiovascular life history. A life course analysis of the original Framingham Heart Study cohort. *European Heart Journal* 23(6):458–466.

Robine, J. M., C. Jagger, and V. Egidi. 2000. *Selection of a coherent set of health indicators: A first step towards a user's guide to health expectancies for the European Union.* Montpellier, France: Euro-REVES.

Robine, J. M., C. Jagger, C. D. Mathers, E. M. Crimmins, and R. M. Suzman. 2003. *Determining health expectancies.* Chichester, West Sussex, England: John Wiley & Sons.

Robine, J. M., and I. Romieu. 1998. Healthy active ageing: Health expectancies at age 65 in the different parts of the world. Presented at World Health Organization Expert Committee on Determinants of Healthy Ageing, 1998, Geneva, Switzerland.

Robine, J. M., I. Romieu, E. Cambois, H. P. A. Van de Water, H. C. Boshuizen, and C. Jagger. 1995. Global assessment in positive health, contribution of the Network on Health Expectancy and the Disability Process to the World Health Report 1995: Bridging the Gaps.

Robine, J. M., I. Romieu, and M. Jee. 1998. Health expectancies in OECD countries. Montpellier, France: REVES.

Rogers, R. G., A. Rogers, and A. Belanger. 1989. Active life among the elderly in the United States: Multistate life-table estimates and population projections. *The Milbank Quarterly* 67(3–4):370–411.

Rogers, A., R. G. Rogers, and L. G. Branch. 1989. A multistate analysis of active life expectancy. *Public Health Reports* 104(3):222–226.

Schoen, R. 1988. *Modeling multigroup populations.* New York: Plenum Press.

Schoeni, R. F., V. A. Freedman, and R. B. Wallace. 2001. Persistent, consistent, widespread, and robust? Another look at recent trends in old-age disability. *Journal of Gerontology: Social Sciences* 56(4):S206–218.

Sullivan, D. F. 1966. Conceptual problems in developing an index of health. *Vital Health Statistics 1* 2(17): 1–18.

Sullivan, D. F. 1971. A single index of mortality and morbidity. *HSMHA Health Reports* 86(4):347–354.

United Nations. 1991. United Nations principles for older persons. New York: United Nations.

United Nations. 1996a. *World population prospects: The 1996 revision. Annex I: Demographic indicators.* New York: Department for Economic and Social Information and Policy Analysis, Population Division.

United Nations. 1996b. *World population prospects: The 1996 revision. Annex II and III: Demographic indicators by major area, region, and country.* New York: Department for Economic and Social Information and Policy Analysis, Population Division.

United Nations. 2000a. Replacement migration. New York: United Nations.

United Nations. 2000b. United Nations expert group meeting on policy ageing and population decline. New York: United Nations.

Verbrugge, L. M. 1984. Longer life but worsening health? Trends in health and mortality of middle-aged and older persons. *Milbank Memorial Fund Quarterly* 62(3):475–519.

Verbrugge, L. M., and A. M. Jette. 1994. The disablement process. *Social Science and Medicine* 38(1):1–14.

Verbrugge, L. M., and D. L. Patrick. 1995. Seven chronic conditions: Their impact on U.S. adults' activity levels and use of medical services. *American Journal of Public Health* 85:173–182.

Waidmann, T. A., and K. G. Manton. 2000. Measuring trends in disability among the elderly: An international review. Washington, D.C.: Urban Institute.

Witthaus, E., A. Ott, J. J. Barendregt, M. Breteler, and L. Bonneux. 1999. Burden of mortality and morbidity from dementia. *Alzheimer Disease Association Disorders* 13(3):176–181.

Wolfson, M. C. 1996. Health-adjusted life expectancy. *Health Reports* 8(1):41–46 (English); 43–49 (French).

World Health Organization. 1980. *International classification of impairments, disabilities, and handicaps.* Geneva, Switzerland.

World Health Organization. 1984. The uses of epidemiology in the study of the elderly: Report of a WHO Scientific Group on the Epidemiology of Aging. Geneva, Switzerland: WHO (Technical Report Series 706).

World Health Organization. 2000. *The World Health Report 2000.* Geneva, Switzerland: World Health Organization.

World Health Organization. 2001. *International classification of functioning, disability, and health.* Geneva, Switzerland.

Zimmer, Z., X. Liu, A. Hermalin, and Y. L. Chuang. 1998. Educational attainment and transitions in functional status among older Taiwanese. *Demography* 35(3):361–375.

CHAPTER 28

Population Policy

John F. May[*]

This chapter examines the development of population policies over the last half-century, and their potential role in the foreseeable future, from the standpoint of demographic transition theory. First, it addresses population issues during each phase of the demographic transition, including those defined by fertility (high or low) and others linked to mortality, migration (national and international), and population aging. Second, the chapter covers both more- and less-developed countries. Finally, it focuses on programs and interventions.

Three sets of issues dominated the global population policy agenda during most of the last half of the 20th century. In the less-developed countries, population policies focused on the economic, social, and environmental impacts of rapid population growth and on measures to reduce high fertility rates that had failed to adjust to falling and sometimes rather low mortality rates. In the more-developed countries, policy was focused on immigration and population aging that resulted from fertility declines and, in some countries, the implications of subreplacement fertility. In the final decade of the century, policy attention was also drawn, particularly in sub-Saharan Africa, to the demographic, economic, and social implications of the HIV/AIDS pandemic and the resurgence of tuberculosis and malaria.

As the century entered its last decade the political climate for population policy also changed. A series of international conferences, most notably the International Conference on Population and Development (ICPD) held in Cairo in 1994, called for a shift from macrolevel approaches to population issues to ones that emphasized the

[*] The findings, interpretations, and conclusions expressed herein are those of the author and do not necessarily reflect the views of the Board of Executive Directors of the World Bank or the governments they represent. The author wants to thank the Editors of the Handbook on Population for their invaluable guidance as well as Dr. Thomas W. Merrick, the World Bank, for his advice and help when preparing this chapter. Insightful comments on earlier drafts and suggestions for improvement were also received from Dr. Jean-Claude Chesnais, Dr. Henry P. David, Dr. Enéas Gakusi, Dr. Léon Gani, Dr. Thomas Goliber, Dr. Ok Pannenborg, and Dr. Marcel Vekemans.

health and welfare of individuals. This new focus helped supersede top-down population interventions that were perceived to be adversely undermining human rights and
gender equity. The demographic and epidemiological conditions that generated earlier
policy responses had also changed. Many regions (with the exception of most of sub-
Saharan Africa and some countries in the Middle East) were well on their way to
completing the transition to low fertility and population growth rates. In sub-Saharan
Africa, HIV/AIDS and the persistence of high fertility levels (above five children per
woman on average) continue to undermine efforts to reduce poverty.

The chapter begins with a review of substantive issues, including rationales for and
definitions of population policies, as well as their modes of operation. Then it presents
research findings on population policies, especially as they pertain to the relationships
between demographic variables and socioeconomic development and the ongoing debate about whether and how to influence demographic change. This is followed by a
review of implementation approaches, including discussion of the various stages of
policy design, implementation, and assessment. Finally, the chapter concludes with
observations about prospects for further development of population policies.

SUBSTANTIVE ISSUES

Population Policy Rationales and Definitions

The current situation of world population is the result of the demographic transition, a
transformation process that began 300 years ago. This process started at the beginning
of the 18th century in Britain and France, then spread to the rest of Europe and the
territories of European settlement, and finally to the other continents. These shifts of
demographic regime have brought profound changes, the most important being the
decline of mortality (the first phase of the demographic transition) that in turn triggered
a population upsurge that also began in the 18th century. This was followed by the onset
of fertility decline at the end of the 19th century (the second phase of the demographic
transition). This second phase is still underway in some developing countries, particularly in sub-Saharan Africa, where completion of the transition is also affected by the
expansion of the HIV/AIDS epidemic.

The demographic transition often creates temporary imbalances due to rapid
increases in the rate of population growth. When the demographic transition is completed, countries may experience other types of imbalances, for example, when fertility
drops to subreplacement levels that can lead to negative population growth and other
consequences (e.g., hyperaging). Below-replacement fertility currently affects 43% of the
world population, primarily because of the large size of China's population, which is
below replacement levels (Population Reference Bureau 2003).

Population policies are designed to regulate and, if possible, mitigate these problems by adjusting population size and structure to the needs and aspirations of the
people. Population policies can be defined as direct or indirect actions taken in the
interest of the greater good by public authorities in order to address imbalances between
demographic changes and other social, economic, and political goals.[1]

---

[1] This definition, which proposed, is an attempt to summarize numerous definitions of population policies
(see, for instance, Anonymous 1983; Demeny 2003a).

There is an ongoing debate about whether and how public authorities should intervene in order to accelerate the demographic transition and, by implementing population policies, correct imbalances caused by the increase or decrease of populations and changes in demographic structure. Alternatively, some contend it might be better to let natural, self-regulatory mechanisms, if any, do their work (Demeny 1986, 2003a). These are difficult questions. In the case of mortality reduction, there has always been a large consensus in favor of interventions. Furthermore, recent decades have also seen the strengthening of arguments in favor of fertility reduction and family planning. In contrast, there is much less consensus regarding the desirability and effectiveness of population distribution policies. In industrialized countries, public authorities have often been reluctant to implement pronatalist policies.

Demographic trends are essentially the result of decisions people make as individuals or as couples, the overall aim being the achievement of individual or family-level goals. At the societal level, however, these personal decisions can have adverse effects, which economists have labeled "negative externalities." Externalities result when societal costs and benefits are out of line with those that are taken into account by individuals, so that the costs to society are greater than those borne by individuals (with similar considerations on the benefit side). For example, high fertility levels may bring wealth and power for some families but jeopardize the well-being of the community and its physical environment by depleting natural resources, causing deforestation in the case of agrarian societies, or aggravating unemployment, poverty, or anarchic urbanization (Pebley 1998). The presence of such externalities was one of the principal rationales that led governments and donor agencies to promote and frequently adopt population policies aimed at reducing fertility rates in poor countries. A critical question has been how to balance individual and societal freedoms, rights, and responsibilities, i.e., whether the adverse societal consequences are serious enough to warrant an abridgement of individual rights and freedoms. (In this regard, China's policy is a noteworthy case.)

In addition to the argument about negative externalities, two other economic considerations have been used to justify interventions in the area of population. The first encompasses what might be labeled "social compacts" in the sense that a society may decide, for reasons of equity and fairness, that every person should have access to certain goods or basic needs (e.g., the survival of children), regardless of his or her capacity to pay for them. Second, the concept of wealth redistribution, in particular through sales and income taxes, can also be advocated as a way of ensuring access to these goods. These arguments go beyond economics and involve political, ethical, philosophical, and human rights considerations.

Nation-states are generally the prime actors that implement population policies. Their legitimacy derives from the obligation to pursue the common well-being of citizens. In addition, only the nation-state can safeguard human rights and the principles of equity. The state may wish to act in order to reduce mortality and/or to adapt to the effects of population growth either by reducing that growth or by stimulating it when necessary (e.g., through interventions to increase fertility). Consequently, population policies have usually been designed at the national level.

Development agencies, multilateral as well as bilateral, have often assisted states in the development and implementation of population policies, particularly in the less-developed countries. Recently, it has also become clear that interventions in the social sectors are necessary to foster economic growth. The task has thus been for international organizations to promote the availability of these publicly provided goods in order to improve human development outcomes (namely education, health, nutrition, reproductive health, and social protection).

In conjunction with the efforts of the public sector, the private sector can also play an important role in the implementation of population policies. Nongovernmental organizations (NGOs) have contributed greatly to population programs and population research, as have community-based organizations, private commercial enterprises, and volunteer associations (McNicoll 1975). Community-based systems and social marketing methods have been used successfully to distribute health products such as oral rehydration salts, contraceptives, and impregnated bed-nets (to prevent malaria) by making them available on the market just like any other consumer good.

The priorities and methods adopted by nation-states to reach policy goals (whether designed and implemented with or without the help of the private sector) have changed markedly over recent decades. Following the end of the Second World War, a global, macrodemographic strategy prevailed. Its aim was to reach rapidly global quantitative objectives, mostly by curbing fertility. At that time, the field of demography experienced a marked shift from a social science to a policy-oriented science (Hodgson, 1983). This interventionist streak was thereafter reinforced by the emergence of the so-called *Population Movement* in the United States during the 1960s (Donaldson 1990; Harkavy 1995). However, the overall approach advocated by states and international organizations was later viewed to have neglected the rights and aspirations of individuals and couples (United Nations 1995).

Considerations about individual rights and needs were reasserted during the 1994 International Conference on Population and Development (ICPD) in Cairo. ICPD stressed the importance of individual choices and the necessity to further empower women. Subsequent international conferences shared this preoccupation, and it was the main theme of the ICPD+5 process, the follow-up to the ICPD, which included a major meeting in The Netherlands and a meeting of the UN General Assembly in 1999. The Cairo Conference reframed population issues in terms of global development and the fight against poverty, advocating a multisectoral approach. It also integrated family planning into the larger context of reproductive health, which encompasses actions to improve reproductive and sexual health, decrease maternal mortality levels, and slow the spread of the HIV/AIDS epidemic (including sexually transmitted infections). Since it favored a bottom-up approach, this new focus on reproductive health called for a more active role by communities, NGOs, and the private sector. It is complemented by a concern for fundamental human rights (including access to services) and efforts to improve the status of women and reduce gender inequality, and by a greater recognition of the needs of adolescents (United Nations 1995).

The Population Policy Process

This section addresses four fundamental questions: What is the nature of the population policy process? Who are the various policy actors? Which demographic variables are amenable to interventions? And, finally, what are the policy levers and the instruments available to implement population policies?

The *population policy process* consists of the conditions, events, and products that connect the initial idea for a population policy to its ultimate development and implementation. In principle, the process is comprehensive, sequential, and logical, one step leading to the next. In fact, the course of population policy development varies widely from one country to the next. Several paradigms have been developed for describing generic features of the policy development process (e.g., Berelson 1977; Micklin 1994). Generally, the process begins with recognition that demographic issues exist and need to be addressed. The stages that follow may include some or all of the following: creation of political and/or popular support, policy formulation, adoption, and implementation. Finally, the impact of the population policy needs to be evaluated and, depending on the results achieved, policy reformulation may begin the process all over again. Efforts to develop typologies of the population policy process are useful for analytic purposes, but the actual experience of few countries corresponds well to any such model.

Typically, the population policy process is not a smooth and highly coordinated sequence of events. Sometimes policy innovation or reform can be achieved only when there is convergence between the perception of population problems, routine political processes (politics), and the organization of interest groups whose principal aim is to promote population policy. Consequently, demographic issues tend to be identified and addressed according to timetables that differ from those that govern routine daily politics. Other policy reforms are often considered according to their own criteria, regardless of their relevance to the demographic issues at hand and/or the influence of the policies adopted previously. Moreover, the population policy process is often antagonistic, for example, in the policy dialogue between sovereign states and development agencies. Likewise, the policy reforms proposed by governments can be opposed by some national constituencies (e.g., citizens, lobbies, or communities). In short, one can identify a variety of social and political barriers that impede the development of national, let alone regional or global, population policies.

High-level political commitment appears to be indispensable to the generation of effective population policies (Warwick 1982). To be efficient, policy reform must go beyond the recommendations of experts and technicians (sometimes already partisans of the policy reform) and appeal to political leaders. Population policies that have been pushed on countries by donors and outside agencies have generally met with little success because they seldom engaged concerned constituencies whose participation was key to success of the policy. For example, the efforts in Ghana to address population concerns, as spelled out in the 1969 population policy, were to a large extent introduced from outside using a top-down approach and had little impact. Eventually, the Ghana policy was revised in 1994 to take into account the needs and aspirations of the population. The genuine involvement of the ultimate policy beneficiaries proved to be the only sensible way forward (Benneh, Nabila, and Gyepi-Garbrah 1989; Population Impact Project 1995).

Various *policy actors* participate in the different stages of the population policy process. First of all, the regulatory answers to population pressure come directly from individuals, households, and specific social and/or geographical groups. These regulatory measures comprise individuals' or households' decisions to seek new economic opportunities (for instance, cultivate new or marginal land), to migrate internally or externally, and to marry later and even choose celibacy (or choose not to have offspring). These varied responses (demographic as well as nondemographic) are said to be *multiphasic* because they are applied simultaneously or in sequence (Davis 1963). They might also include, for instance, additional savings to increase pension revenues in aging populations. All these answers are social adjustments to population pressure and do not strictly belong to the domain of population policy, even though they might be encouraged by the state.

Public sector responses to demographic problems may take the form of population policies or at least social regulations. As already mentioned, population policies are conscious actions by the state to address, in the interest of the public good, problems ascribed to imbalances between demographic variables and societal goals. Public authorities may or may not consider population issues to be their responsibility. The authorities can also consider that the demographic variables are not likely to be modified by deliberate interventions. In fact, policy responses to population issues are motivated by a truly interventionist approach: it is considered possible to act, directly or indirectly, on demographic trends. Population policies that aim to decrease fertility are called *antinatalist*, while those that attempt to increase fertility are called *pronatalist*; policies whose objectives are to increase population through means other than higher fertility, for example through immigration, are called *populationist* (Van De Walle 1982).

As mentioned above, the state may wish to implement measures to adapt to the effects of population growth, reduce population growth itself, or stimulate a low or even a negative rate of demographic growth. However, it is important to assess whether actions in this area should be undertaken by governments at the national level, in a strong and direct way, or at the local level, more discreetly, using private and nongovernmental organizations. The widespread intervention of the private commercial and noncommercial sector can lead to a loss of influence for states' policies, as happened for instance in Haiti. The problem of citizens' refusal to adhere to population policy measures, when these are considered too much of a constraint, must also be considered. It is important that population policies and programs be endorsed by the general public as well as the target populations and supported by efficient levels of intervention (centralized or decentralized), with responsibilities clearly defined and shared among the public and private sectors (Hyden 1990).

When it comes to the *demographic variables amenable to intervention*, it is useful to distinguish between passive and active measures. The former are a mere adaptation to the effects of population growth, for example, through the promotion of education and employment or development of housing schemes and other infrastructure strategies. Active measures address the causes of the population problems and are intended to influence basic demographic conditions and trends. Migratory measures and policies pertaining to the movement of populations belong to this second category. Countries may encourage immigration, as in Canada and the United States, or organize emigration, as the Philippines or Pakistan have done toward Middle East countries. Other countries have expelled large numbers of immigrants (as in Ghana in 1969 and Nigeria in 1983 and 1985). These migratory movements can be spontaneous or organized (for instance, voluntary population redistribution or transmigration programs as in Indonesia). Repatriation programs have also been organized, however without much success, to entice immigrants to return to their country of origin (e.g., Germany, France, and Switzerland).

The choice of policy responses to population issues depends on the values of the decision makers. Certain courses of action are never proposed by governments, development agencies, and nongovernmental organizations (NGOs), because they are considered immoral and, moreover, would never be accepted by the public. Examples are proposals to slow or even halt the decline of mortality. A controversy was stirred by Maurice King (1990) in the medical journal *The Lancet* when he proposed to slow down the decrease of infant and child mortality to avoid seeing some countries fall into the Malthusian trap, defined as the incapacity of a country to feed its population without outside help. This proposal goes against the desire for survival rooted in human nature, not to mention the insurmountable equity problems it poses.

Actually, the first policy interventions to be put in place are usually focused on mortality. Experience has often been shown that fertility reduction requires prior reductions in mortality, particularly infant and child mortality. Driven by the fear that several of their offspring might die in young age, many couples have a large number of children only to ensure the survival of a few. Therefore, a synergy may exist between the decline in mortality and fertility (Cleland 2003). However, family planning programs have been focused mostly on the reduction of fertility, sometimes isolating it from its larger socioeconomic context.

Fertility is the other major demographic variable in which interventions have been tried. This variable remains crucial in numerous countries that have not completed their demographic transition (Bulatao 1984). In particular, youthful age structure and above-replacement levels of fertility are recognized as being key to the future of population growth. John Bongaarts (1994) has refined this analysis by disentangling the effects of unwanted fertility and the desire for a large family size (more than two children). This distinction has the advantage of being operational because it addresses, first, unwanted fertility by reinforcing family planning programs and, second, the desire for a large family by expanding information, education, and communication (IEC) programs and behavioral communication for change (BCC) campaigns. Finally, sound actions on fertility also require distinctions among the proximate determinants of fertility (biological and behavioral variables such as union patterns, breastfeeding, postpartum abstinence, and sterility), the intermediate determinants (e.g., education and socioeconomic variables), and relevant contextual factors (for example, cultural norms, communications, and infrastructures).

The choice of *policy levers and instruments to implement population policies* is also important. If one admits that population policies can influence the different components of population change, especially fertility, then some actions can be more effective than others. Policies can simply facilitate changes in reproductive behavior by making available family planning services. However, the state may also try to modify reproductive behavior by using explicit measures, specifically designed to modify demographic variables, or implicit measures, which comprise public sector activities that could influence these variables, whether or not the state desires to do so (Johansson 1991).

Population policies can be used to intervene only on certain levers (in both public and private sectors); these focused interventions include four instruments: information availability, laws and regulations, taxation and subsidy mechanisms, and direct investments (including the offer of services) (Mosley, Jamison, and Henderson 1990). According to these levers, fertility is regulated in part by making available family planning information. Governments can also enact normative laws and regulations (Heckel 1986) or adopt institutional reforms (McNicoll 1982) in an attempt to influence fertility. Taxes and subsidies, for instance in the form of tax exemptions for child care costs, are available in some countries (e.g., the United States). Incentives (e.g., money given to accept sterilization) also fall in this category.

Although direct investments in the health system and the organization of family planning services appear to be among the most efficient means available to governments to intervene directly in fertility, several indirect interventions may also be used successfully beyond family planning, such as investments in education, incentives programs, and enhanced female participation in the labor force (Berelson 1969). Of course, there are links among the four areas listed by Mosley and colleagues: for example, making family planning services available (direct investments) will be easier if advertising for contraceptives is authorized (laws and regulations). In addition, policies geared at lowering fertility must choose optimally between the various paths to fertility reduction according to their acceptability, feasibility, and effectiveness (Berelson 1977).

Finally, the implementation of national population policy reforms by the public sector can take three forms: efforts to plan socioeconomic development, implementation of family planning programs, and/or adoption of formal national population policies. Development planning is an administrative process by which governments define their economic and social development goals for the different sectors. These plans focus on the implementation of adaptive responses to the effects of population growth, particularly by increasing the rate of economic growth. Family planning programs are a second type of action, which act directly on fertility to reduce population growth. Often, family planning interventions have focused more on the supply of services than the creation of demand, although both approaches are complementary and work in synergy (Demeny 1992; Phillips and Ross 1992). The third type of action, namely comprehensive national population policies, addresses demographic variables across all economic and social sectors. Social development policies (e.g., education, health, housing, and infrastructures) are typically included in population policies as they also contribute to changes in demographic variables. For instance, fertility declines in Sri Lanka, Kerala, and Tamil Nadu—their total fertility rate (TFR) was about 2.0 in mid-2003—were triggered essentially by such policies. In industrialized countries, population policies are also frequently implemented through social policies, explicit or implicit.

This review of rationales, definitions, and processes of population policies has shown the very large range of issues covered in this specific area. Diverse rationales (economic, ethical, and equity-driven) justify public interventions that attempt to modify population trends. Such interventions are best initiated, implemented, and monitored by nation-states, with the help of other actors from the private sector and international development agencies and transnational lobbies. Finally, the population policy process itself encompasses a wide spectrum of approaches, actors, policy levers, and instruments.

RESEARCH FINDINGS

Ideological and political views on demographic issues have always been polarized. During the 19th century, Malthusians and Marxists disagreed vigorously on the nature and even the existence of demographic problems. In *The Conditions of Agricultural Growth* (1965), Ester Boserup challenged the Malthusian linkage between individuals and production by reassigning to the former the role of the independent variable of the system. In her later works, she widened her analysis to take into account the evolution of technology and the improvement of woman's status (Boserup 1970, 1981).

The focus on ideational changes affecting fertility has added a new dimension to the debate by reaffirming the importance of individual preferences and behavior (the process of diffusion and innovation), as opposed to the concept of adaptation and modernization (Cleland and Wilson 1987). It was also recognized that an economic crisis (defined as the worsening of economic conditions after an initial improvement) could trigger a fertility decline because couples may wish to preserve their previous standard of living by limiting the number of offspring.

With respect to environmental concerns, the chasm between optimists and pessimists has always existed and remains to this day, as illustrated by the debate between Paul Ehrlich, author of *The Population Bomb* (1968) and *The Population Explosion* (1990), and Julian Simon, author of *The Ultimate Resource* (1981) (on this debate, see Simon 1996).

Since publication of Malthus' *Essay*, the relationships between socioeconomic variables and population growth have been debated, especially for developing countries (Kelley 1988; Blanchet 1991). For instance, India was used as a case study in the seminal volume by Coale and Hoover (1958), who asserted that a country that experiences a decline in fertility would achieve an increase in income. Other authors, however, have denied any major impact of demographic variables on socioeconomic development and "saw population growth as a fairly neutral factor in development performance" (McNicoll 2003; see also U.S. National Academy of Sciences 1986). These issues are discussed in some detail in Micklin's chapter in this Handbook.

Economists have been particularly skeptical regarding the usefulness of family planning programs to reduce fertility. This position is exemplified by Pritchett (1994), who stressed that changes in demand (i.e., in desired fertility) trigger fertility declines to a much greater extent than large-scale family planning programs. In fact, such analyses should be complemented by a closer look at the way social change actually takes place. Several phenomena, such as the diffusion of new cultural models, the role of the mass media (Westoff and Rodriguez 1995), the emergence of community empowerment, social interactions between various groups, and the rise of women's rights are factors that challenge the economists' classic approach and conventional wisdom. In this respect, proponents of social change cite the example of Bangladesh, where the decrease in fertility occurred in the mid-1970s and the 1980s, despite the persistence of mass poverty. In Bangladesh, improved education of women as well as their larger participation in the monetary economy could have brought about a first-stage drop in fertility, even without important economic gains (the fertility decline seems to have stalled in the late 1990s) (Adnan 2002). However, changes in demand can themselves be influenced by the implementation of family planning programs; other authors stress supply side factors (i.e., acceptability of and access to birth control) as the main cause of the fertility decline in Bangladesh (Cleland et al. 1994).[2]

Notwithstanding these controversies, which often appeared to be more ideological than based on research and solid evidence, a significant consensus has emerged around the idea that *rapid* population growth exerts some severe constraints on countries and regions at low levels of socioeconomic development (Kelley 1988; Birdsall, Kelley, and Sinding 2001). One important constraint is captured by the notion of *population pressure*, i.e., the number of people in relation to the natural and financial resources of a given territory.[3] A population that is too large or growing too rapidly is viewed as out of balance with its capacity to achieve socioeconomic development.[4] However, it is difficult to measure population pressure with precision, although population densities in

---

[2] Pakistan's total fertility rate (estimate of 4.8 in mid-2003) declined later than Bangladesh's (estimate of 3.6, same date; Population Reference Bureau, 2003). Since the two countries are culturally quite similar and were politically united until 1971, the contrast in their fertility transitions appears to be linked to large-scale family planning efforts that have taken place in the latter but not in the former.

[3] Once again, the case of Bangladesh is a vivid illustration of the pressure on land (the population density exceeds 2,600 inhabitants per square mile; Population Reference Bureau 2003).

[4] Population growth is believed to be "optimal" when it does not exceed these limits.

relation to total or usable land areas and rates of unemployment have been used as proxy measures.

A second constraint, which goes beyond the number of inhabitants, is the *rate* of population growth. On the basis of empirical findings, the World Bank (1994) estimated that a population growth rate above 2% per year could slow the increase of incomes in poor countries. A third constraint is seen in the effects of rapid population growth on the mobilization of human capital investments and exacerbation of the social demand (demand for services). In a situation of rapid population growth, efforts made to meet demographic investments must be constantly accelerated just to preserve the status quo (a "treadmill" effect). Rapid population growth can also threaten the macroeconomic stability of a country, because considerable financial resources need to be mobilized for human capital investments. The fourth of these demographic constraints stems from the effects of changes in population age structure and dependency ratios on economic development.

Arguably this last phenomenon is the most important element that has been highlighted by recent economic research (Birdsall, Kelley, and Sinding 2001). The situation of East Asian countries has shed light on the impact of sharp fertility declines on economic performance before the crisis of 1997 to 1998 (this has been called the demographic bonus or demographic dividend). By diminishing the relative proportion of youth, a rapid decline in fertility reduced the dependency ratios between generations and boosted the share of the potential labor force. This in turn enabled governments to raise investment levels for health and education and also to increase their economic investments. However, changes in the age structure can only be exploited when they are accompanied by adequate investments and sound public policies. Moreover, the demographic dividend is not a permanent state. Rather, it is an opportunity that must be seized over a relatively short term before population aging sets in (Bloom, Canning, and Sevilla 2003).[5]

Conversely, situations of prolonged declines in fertility, demographic aging, and depopulation can have negative consequences for the economy. The financing of retirement schemes, both pay-as-you-go plans and capitalization systems (as the case of Chile), becomes a problem when the proportion of workers diminishes compared to that of the retired population. Health expenditures also grow more rapidly in aging populations. Another, less well-known aspect is the slowing down of the economy that could be caused by prolonged subreplacement fertility (Chesnais 1995). The relatively higher unemployment levels in Europe and Japan could be explained in part by the decrease in fertility, its related negative impact on investments (housing, equipment, infrastructures, etc.), and the lack of consumers that depresses certain sectors of the economy (e.g., education, leisure). This could also, over the long term, jeopardize the stability of fiscal systems (Faruqee and Mühleisen 2001) and create an explosion of public debt.

The classic debate on relationships between demographic variables and socioeconomic development has also recently been complemented by a reexamination of the links between demographic trends, on the one hand, and efforts to reduce poverty and inequality, on the other. Family planning alone will not necessarily reduce poverty in developing countries, but neither will many of the current strategies of economic development. In fact, a slower rate of population growth, especially when combined

---

[5] As industrialization proceeds, it could be argued that the positive effects of the demographic bonus might be eroded because of the rising costs of children.

with equitable economic development, gender inequality reduction, and human rights enhancement, may help reduce poverty and unemployment levels, especially in a context of accelerated globalization. Therefore fertility reduction and family planning do matter, both for poor households and for poor countries, although they are not the only, or even the most important, factors in poverty reduction (Merrick 2002).

Beyond this purely economic debate, proponents of *laissez-faire* policies clashed during the 1970s with those favoring interventions to control demographic variables in developing countries before the Cairo Conference process was initiated. Again, these discussions in developing countries have been admittedly more ideological than substantive because firm evidence was not always available. Moreover, the concerned populations have often reacted on their own to the evolution of demographic trends (e.g., through regulation responses).

More recently, the traditional scope for policy interventions has become even wider as new challenges have emerged, such as rapid urbanization that often results in very large cities and/or slums, the new threats posed by HIV/AIDS, tuberculosis, and malaria, and the need for policies geared to women and adolescents. In some countries (e.g., China), the population will continue to grow, despite very low levels of fertility, because of the young age structure (population momentum). Furthermore, the actors active in the policy arena have also multiplied, in addition to the role played traditionally by the nation-states. These phenomena have led to a period of competitive pluralism (Finkle and Crane 1990) that will be discussed below.

Turning to industrialized countries, and particularly to Europe, one notes the lack of solid research on population policies and hence the absence of a rational debate on population issues. Indifference and lack of concern about demographic issues have often prevailed (Demeny 2003b). This has been reinforced by Malthusian attitudes, individualistic values, and occasional excesses of feminist and conservationist ideologies (Chesnais 1995). Indeed the question as to whether to address, and how to address, posttransitional imbalances remains delicate. This debate, when is has occurred, has led in Europe to confrontations along the traditional Left-Right divide. The political Right has often been considered to be populationist, even pronatalist, while the Left is seen to be in favor of free choice or simply *laissez-faire* attitudes (Teitelbaum and Winter 1998). In fact, Europe's history has seen regimes both on the Right (Hitler's Germany, Franco's Spain, and Mussolini's Italy) and the Left (Stalin's Russia and Ceausescu's Romania) take interest in population issues and try to slow depopulation, for example, through very restrictive abortion policies. Other, more neutral, regimes have also advocated pronatalist policies, such as Social Democrat Sweden in the 1930s, Britain in 1944, and Gaullist France after the Second World War. However, pronatalist policies designed by fascist regimes remain vivid memories in Europe and these are often referred to when demographic issues are debated publicly.

To conclude, it must be stressed that demographic issues are currently not addressed in industrialized countries, particularly in Europe, in a manner that is free of political or ideological agendas. The traditional polarization between the Left and the Right makes the debate even more difficult. The somewhat less polarized American political scene has probably contributed to a more objective and less passionate approach to demographic issues in the United States (with the exception of the abortion debate), as have the long-standing tradition of receiving immigrants and higher fertility levels (TFR of 2.0 in the United States and 1.4 in Europe; see Population Reference Bureau 2003).

IMPLEMENTATION OF POPULATION
POLICIES

Implementation Approaches

The medical discoveries of Jenner, Pasteur, and Fleming that contributed to the *reduction of mortality* in Western Europe have also helped to bring a survival revolution to the territories of European settlement and to the other continents. Before the Second World War, colonial powers as well as independent governments in Latin America and Asia had enacted public health measures, launched sanitation and disease vector control programs, and organized targeted campaigns to bring down high mortality levels, notably in cities. For example, specific programs were organized to eradicate malaria, as was done successfully in Sri Lanka in the 1940s through the use of DDT, with strong international support (Livi-Bacci 1992).

Later, these interventions were reinforced through the distribution of antibiotics and vaccines in the 1950s and the introduction of simple medical techniques, such as oral rehydration salts introduced in Bangladesh in the late 1970s. Vaccines have been used systematically in the context of the Expanded Program on Immunization (EPI) established by the World Health Organization (WHO) since 1974 and reinforced since with the help of UNICEF. The EPI was designed to protect children in their first year against six major diseases: tuberculosis, tetanus, poliomyelitis, whooping cough, measles, and diphtheria. The eradication of smallpox, achieved in 1977, was the result of a worldwide coordinated effort, unprecedented in the history of public health (Khlat and Le Cœur 2002).

Despite new threats such as the HIV/AIDS epidemic, all these efforts have considerably reduced mortality levels. This, in turn, contributed to an increase in population growth rates that lasted until 1965–1970, making more compelling the need to address population issues, for example, by initiating family planning programs to reduce fertility. Finkle and Crane (1990) developed a typology of the efforts made by sovereign states to address such issues, identifying three essential phases. First, between 1965 and 1974, the debate was dominated by the desire to control population pressure, with governments trying to reduce population growth through the implementation of family planning programs. Then, from 1974 to 1981, came the demographic variable planning phase, by which the reduction of fertility is associated with larger development planning goals. Finally, the period from 1981 to date is called the time of competitive pluralism: centralized governmental activities are neglected in favor of decentralization, community participation (including in the formulation of population policies), and strategies geared at program users.

Several countries, such as Japan, India, and Egypt, had addressed the issue of *fertility reduction* and consequently implemented family planning programs as early as the late 1940s for Japan and the 1950s in the cases of India and Egypt. Japan shifted in 1948 from a pronatalist to an antinatalist policy, which enabled a rapid rise in the use of fertility regulation, mostly condoms (the pill was long opposed by the medical profession). In 1948, the national eugenic law allowed the use of induced abortion in order to protect the life and health of mothers. These interventions brought a spectacular decline in fertility in only a decade, which proves the efficacy of the policy.

In 1952, India joined the small group of countries seeking to address demographic problems. Interventions were embedded in national development plans, and the policy tool adopted was the expansion of family planning services. Initial results were slow to come, and fertility regulation spread only to certain states, among privileged social classes, and in cities. In 1976, the Indira Gandhi government decided to accelerate the process and launched forced sterilization campaigns. This created a backlash that led to the Congress Party's defeat in the elections of March 1977.

In 1954, Egypt established a Committee on Population Affairs, and several experimental family planning clinics were created by NGOs. In 1961, President Nasser's government endorsed the use of family planning to slow population growth. Population institutions continued to evolve during the following decades and, since 1996, the Ministry of Health and Population has been in charge of the program (Jain 1998). Notwithstanding initial successes, the decline of fertility has slowed during the last decade, especially in rural Upper Egypt. The government has also created new cities in the desert in an attempt to absorb population growth, but the results have been mixed.

China launched its program in earnest in 1971, after a period of considerable hesitation caused by prior Marxist attitudes vis-à-vis population issues. Although the 1953 Census results had demonstrated that the country's population was 100 million larger than expected, the pronatalist policy was only slowly modified in favor of more pragmatic measures (two previous attempts to launch family planning activities, in 1953 to 1957 and 1962 to 1965, had failed because of sudden policy changes).

Thereafter China embarked on a rapid and forced march to demographic transition. The strictly enforced family program reduced fertility by half between 1971 and 1979. Birth quotas and pregnancy authorizations were instituted in 1979. The one-child policy was imposed in 1978 on the entire population, with the exception of the non-Han Chinese minority groups (6% of the population). This policy, designed to accompany the economic modernization reforms of 1978, was successful in cities[6] (easier to control) but failed in the rural areas (64% of the population) (Banister 2003; Scharping 2003).

On the whole, the Chinese population and family planning policy accelerated the demographic transition and probably alleviated some effects of the strong population pressure. However, the population policy also precipitated population aging before an adequate social protection system could be organized.

Despite initial resistance, family planning programs in Latin America started on a large scale in the early 1970s. Programs were either sponsored by the state (e.g., Mexico) or launched through private sector initiatives (as in Colombia and Brazil). Some large countries, such as Indonesia, achieved remarkable successes in the supply of family planning services. Small insular countries (e.g., Mauritius) usually achieved very rapid fertility declines. Eventually, the family planning revolution spread throughout the developing world, including the Islamic countries (e.g., Iran[7]). However, contraceptive prevalence rates remain low in Western sub-Saharan and particularly Central sub-Saharan Africa

---

[6] The policy has indirectly led to female infanticide and/or female infant neglect when parents had fancied to have a male child. In the same vein, the availability of techniques to determine the gender of fetuses has led in some countries to gender-selective induced abortions (e.g., India).

[7] In Iran, the acceleration of the decline of fertility during the late 1980s had preceded by a few years the widespread distribution of family planning methods. This rapid change can be attributed to profound social and economic transformations, including the adoption of an important agrarian reform. In addition, female education levels increased dramatically and females attitudes to parenthood changed as well. The sense of responsibility on the part of men increased also, fostered to some extent by the religious establishment (Ladier-Fouladi 2003).

(Guengant and May, forthcoming), where remnants of French noninterventionist attitudes vis-à-vis population issues (e.g., the French 1920 Law repressing abortion and
contraception) can still be found. In these regions, the contraceptive use gap between
urban and rural areas also remains important.

Family planning programs are generally large-scale endeavors encompassing many
components, including program design and planning, information, education and communication campaigns (IEC), training of service providers, building of health infrastructures, contraceptive logistics, mobilization of financing and support mechanisms,
and monitoring and evaluation. Originally family planning programs had been organized "vertically" (services being offered independently from other medical services), but
the current approach favors integrated approaches (services being made available with
other health interventions, e.g., maternal and child care services). In 1961, Tunisia had
chosen a vertical program and had also discouraged polygamy and promoted the
instruction of women, but later Tunisia integrated family planning with primary health
care. In contrast, Morocco opted to begin with an integrated program. Another strategic choice is between the public and private sectors for the provision of family
planning services. However, the efficiency of different strategies depends on the country's specific context and the degree of maturity of its program. Other considerations in
program design are the method mix (the choice of methods to be offered), which has
implications for budgets (some methods are more expensive) and outcomes (some
methods are more efficient). Finally, it might also be necessary to explore alternative
contraceptive distribution strategies such as over-the-counter sales in pharmacies, community-based distribution, and/or social marketing techniques.

The second period identified by Finkle and Crane, the demographic variable
planning phase between 1974 and 1981, addressed the reduction of fertility in association with larger development planning goals. This echoed the 1974 Bucharest Conference and the positions of the Group of 77, inspired by socialist countries such as the
USSR and China (see discussion below). The goal was to achieve fertility declines
through development plans that attempted to establish quantified economic and social
objectives for the country and its geographical and administrative subdivisions. As
mentioned above, such plans focus on adaptive responses to the effects of population
growth, essentially by promoting economic growth. Rapid population growth can lead
public authorities to integrate demographic variables directly into development plans,
for example, in the education, labor force, or urbanization sectors (Stamper 1977).

However, development plans were often quickly overtaken by the speed of population growth, making this approach less efficient. Moreover, the classic opposition
between capitalists and socialists, quite strong at Bucharest, became less relevant.
Socialist policies of autonomous development and import substitution, that were hostile
to family planning (these were widespread in Latin America and Africa), achieved poor
results. In contrast, liberal policies based on private initiative, international commerce,
and foreign investments, which were more accepting of family planning (with subsidized
commodities), achieved great successes in East Asia.

Formal and official population policies were also enacted during this phase in the
form of comprehensive declarations endorsed by high-ranking authorities (e.g., the
President or National Assembly). Governments around the world were invited by the
United Nations to report about their perceptions and policies regarding demographic
trends in their respective countries. Such enquiries, covering population growth and age
structure, fertility and family planning, health and mortality, spatial distribution, and

international migration, were initiated in 1976 and repeated in 1986, 1996, and 2001 (United Nations 2002).

The *transmigration or resettlement* (Hugo 2003) efforts in Indonesia also belong to this planning phase. Transmigration or spatial redistribution programs consist of relocating populations in order to reduce population pressure in the regions of origin. These programs are complemented by regulatory and financial measures to enable a smoother reinsertion of the migrants. From 1974 to 1994, the Indonesia program resettled a total of 650,000 families or three million people from Java to Sumatra, Kalimantan, and Sulawesi (resettlements were part of successive development plans). However, the influx of Javanese created political tensions in receiving regions. Moreover, such relocation programs are difficult to implement, and they are also controversial because they disrupt traditional living conditions of the populations affected. They can have a negative political connotation (coercion, lack of equity, and violations of cultural and religious freedom) and also be harmful to the environment. From a demographic perspective, the Indonesian plan had a modest impact by absorbing only 15% of Java's population growth. Tangible results were limited, compared to initial objectives, and more importantly, the huge number of Javanese (World Bank 1988). On its own, spatial redistribution is not a viable solution to rapid population growth.

The third period highlighted by Finkle and Crane is the era of competitive pluralism, from 1981 to the present. This last phase, which departs markedly from the previous two, favors decentralized and bottom-up approaches. It aims at empowering communities and addresses the needs of the users. The sphere of activity of population policies has also grown to take into account new challenges such as reproductive health, environmental protection, improvement of the status of women, reduction of maternal mortality,[8] the needs of the adolescents, and the fight against poverty. This phase is dominated by the influence of international public health circles, the international family planning network, and the environmentalists (whose main goal is to reduce population growth). These lobbies have sometimes been criticized by right-to-life activists hostile to family planning methods and abortion. They have also attracted some religious opposition, for example, from the Catholic Church and from some quarters of fundamentalist Islam. These oppositions have on occasion found additional support in the traditional values of societies shaken by modernity and worried about the global Westernization of lifestyles.

After the Second World War, a vast network of international organizations specialized in family planning and population issues emerged, to a large extent under the impulse of the *Population Movement* in the United States.[9] The United Nations Population Commission was established in 1946, and the United Nations Population Fund (UNFPA) was created in 1969. The specialized United Nations agencies, the World Bank, and regional development banks also became involved in population programs.[10]

---

[8] The maternal mortality ratio, i.e., the number of women who die from maternal death per 100,000 live births, is the health indicator that shows the widest variations across world regions. In 1995, the lifetime risk of maternal death was a staggering 1:16 in Africa, but only 1:3,500 in northern America (Maine and Stamas 2003).

[9] The United States' position in the international debate on population issues has been considerably weakened by domestic abortion politics. This has led to periodic defunding of agencies such as UNFPA and the International Planned Parenthood Federation (IPPF).

[10] The first World Bank loan, of 2 million US dollars, was granted to Jamaica in 1970 for strengthening the delivery of contraceptives. The World Bank is currently one of the largest financiers of population and reproductive health activities for countries with low or medium incomes (World Bank 2000).

Important bilateral funding and technical contributions complemented these efforts, especially from the United States Agency for International Development (USAID), Japan, and several European countries such as the Nordic countries, the United Kingdom, The Netherlands, and Germany (the absence of France is noteworthy). All these multilateral and bilateral organizations were rallied by numerous specialized NGOs (often funded with public money), of which the most important is the International Planned Parenthood Federation (IPPF), founded in London in 1952. Finally, the numerous and influential American NGOs, women's coalitions, and foundations also deserve mention (several, such as the Bill and Melinda Gates Foundation, are also active in the areas of HIV/AIDS and immunization programs). Most of these international institutions are active around the world.

Within a few decades, population and family planning issues had become an international concern. This is illustrated by the periodic organization of *regional and global conferences* devoted to population issues (Chasteland 2002). The first intergovernmental conference on population was organized in Bucharest in 1974 and resulted in adoption of the World Population Plan of Action. It had been preceded by several technical conferences in Geneva and London (1927), Rome (1954), and Belgrade (1965). The Bucharest Conference was followed by the Conference of Mexico in 1984. The last world population conference, the ICPD, was held in Cairo in 1994 (United Nations 1995).[11]

These gatherings were initially of a scientific nature but, since Bucharest, progressively became political meetings. The Bucharest Conference took place in the context of the Cold War and amidst concerns over the rapid demographic growth in Asia. This led to confrontations between the advocates of development as a remedy for rapid demographic growth (essentially the nonaligned countries, led by Algeria and joined by the Holy See) and the advocates of family planning programs to curb fertility (essentially led by the United States, Japan, and some European countries). In Mexico, the debate was clouded by the reversal of the American position, triggered by the newly elected Republican Administration, which opposed abortion and promoted the role of the private sector. Finally, in Cairo, an almost global consensus emerged, although some Islamic countries voiced opposition, joined by the Holy See, on induced abortion and the further empowerment of women (Chasteland 2002).

The population conferences dealt with most areas of development because demographic dynamics impinge on multiple sectors (e.g., health, nutrition, education, labor force, status of women, gender issues, urbanization, and environment). The prominent role of the state was emphasized in the conferences as the state was requested to intervene in all sectors of activity evoked in the conferences' recommendations. The conferences were covered by the media, popularizing population concerns among a very wide public. Themes debated at the conferences were further spread by the proliferation of NGOs active in the area of population and family planning. The conferences also contributed to the globalization of population discourse and proved to be an important vehicle to disseminate new ideas and approaches while enhancing the convergence of opinions, achieved in Cairo, and facilitating the collective learning process. Still, one should not forget the gap between the conferences' resolutions and the actual policies implemented at the country level: the conferences' recommendations were adopted in a specific, often euphoric context, more like declarations of principle than concrete

---

[11] No new major population conference was scheduled, either to mark the 10th anniversary of the Cairo Conference or to take place in the foreseeable future after 2004.

engagements. They were also far from involving all countries and continents in the same way. Assurances for funding made in Cairo have not yet been backed by concrete actions.

In *industrialized countries*, policies adopted to address posttransitional imbalances have taken the form of efforts to increase fertility levels in some countries and to design immigration policies, depending on the country status as active immigration seeker or not. More frequently, population policy interventions in industrialized countries have been implicit rather than explicit. In fact, whereas population policies in developing countries are generally well defined and focused on a few key interventions (e.g., family planning programs), the situation is different in industrialized countries, which have complex systems of social policies that are more difficult to adjust to fit new orientations. In this context, it is difficult to coordinate population policy measures since they take the form of an array of socioeconomic regulations that must be implemented by many different agencies.

Notwithstanding these difficulties, there are some examples of successful *fertility policies*; the case of France is of particular interest. The French pronatalist tradition reached its peak with the adoption of the Family Code (*Code de la famille*) in 1939. Through incentives rather than coercion (as was the case with the 1920 law), the family policy triggered a fertility increase as soon as the early 1940s. In 1945, the generous Social Security system complemented the Family Code and, around 1950, help for families culminated at 45% of public social expenses. Just after the Second World War, France's TFR was 0.5 child higher than the TFR of her European neighbors. The result of financial incentives for children (*allocations familiales*) was undeniable. By largely offsetting the expenses involved with large families, such payments ensured a longer and more sustained baby boom than in other European countries. However, the impact of the policy was gradually undermined when the incomes of families were being complemented by the earnings of women. Since mothers had to abandon their jobs, at least temporarily, the loss of revenues for larger families could not be substituted with corresponding social contributions.

Other countries, like Singapore, reverted to pronatalist policies after successful antinatalist programs. The initial effort on family planning combined with demographic investments (health, education, etc.) and other productive investments have probably accelerated the transformation of Singapore into a new industrialized country (fertility had dropped to subreplacement levels in 1986). Since 1984, however, authorities have tried to correct some of the excessive results of the antinatalist policy. The main goal was to encourage fertility among Chinese couples with the highest education levels (Saw 1990). The new policy in favor of higher fertility has not yet shown conclusive results.

In Northern and Western Europe, the TFR is 1.6, although the large majority of couples want to have two children. The key difficulty, especially for women, appears to be reconciling family life with professional careers. Only one European country, Sweden, appears to have succeeded in raising fertility in the mid-1980s.[12] The first lesson is what can be called the feminist paradox. More freedom does not enable women to juggle modern life and replacement fertility levels. To achieve this, they need more autonomy as well as a better recognition of their role in society. The second lesson is the impact of public assistance, which enables women to take advantage of their new

---

[12] Later, fertility declined again in Sweden because it had to cut its public expenditures, as required by Brussels, to be admitted in the European Union.

autonomy. In the case of Sweden, the state's assistance, together with new trends of postmodern societies (rejection of materialism, return to traditional values, etc.) have encouraged a rise in fertility (Chesnais 1996).

Immigration is another measure occasionally advocated for industrialized countries to address low fertility levels and population aging.[13] The first issue regarding immigration policies is the number of immigrants to be accepted[14] or needed to offset fertility decline and meet the increasing demand for age-related services. Hypothetical computations on replacement immigration covering the period 2000 to 2050 have been proposed for several industrialized countries by the United Nations (United Nations 2000). Their main goal was to estimate the number of immigrants necessary every year to maintain the populations of industrialized countries in terms of number (the total population does not change) and structure (either the 15 to 64 age group stays the same or the ratio of the 15 to 64 to the 65+ age groups remains constant). The results are sobering. For example, for the European Union (EU) as a whole: 949,000 immigrants would be necessary every year to keep the EU population constant; 1.5 million would be needed annually to maintain constant the 15 to 64 age group, and 13.5 million would be needed every year to maintain a constant ratio of the 15 to 64 to the 65+ age groups. These results caused a shock in Europe (especially in Germany and France) and highlighted both the discomfort caused by replacement immigration and the urgency to address fertility issues as well.

The second issue is the integration of immigrants. The notion of integration implies assimilation, e.g., learning the language of the receiving country, naturalization for many immigrants, inclusion in the economy with minimal discrimination and adoption of the customs and political mores of the host country. Integration occurs through institutions such as schools, professional groups, and community and neighborhood associations. If immigrants are more numerous than native populations, these institutions no longer serve as efficient tools of the melting pot. If immigrants stay isolated culturally, socially, or religiously and/or do not mingle geographically with the inhabitants of the receiving country (ghettos), the melting pot does not work either. For religious reasons, some immigrant communities experience difficulties in adopting the secular and democratic values of the receiving countries. In this respect, Europe and Japan appear to face more problems in addressing the issue of immigration than long-standing receiving countries such as the United States, Canada, and Australia. Finally, immigration policies have been revised in some countries to attract highly qualified immigrants needed for the economy.

Implementation Results

One approach to measuring the efficacy of population policies is to focus on specific results, using such performance or impact indicators as the infant mortality rate, the under five mortality rate, the expectancy of life at birth, and the contraceptive prevalence rate. Evaluation of population policies could also be done through qualitative

---

[13] It is estimated that there were in 2000 around 175 million international migrants in the world, i.e., persons living outside their countries of birth (Massey 2003).

[14] Unlike the United States, European countries (with the exception of Italy) do not have immigration quotas nor do they discuss such quotas during immigration policy debates.

studies, in the form of field surveys using participatory and community-based methods (e.g., interviews with beneficiaries). Finally, the effectiveness of population policies could be calculated by estimating the costs and benefits of proposed actions, enabling policy makers to choose the most cost-effective approach for the desired results.

Efforts to reduce mortality in the second half of the 20th century have brought about significant improvements in life expectancy at birth. In the developing countries in particular, this indicator has progressed considerably: it was between 35 and 45 years in 1950 to 1955 (far behind industrialized countries), but reached the 60 to 70 years bracket in 1990 to 1995 (reducing the gap with more advanced countries) (Meslé and Vallin 2002). However, the progression of the HIV/AIDS pandemic and the resurgence of old killers like tuberculosis (linked to HIV/AIDS) and malaria appear to be reversing the gains achieved in mortality reduction, especially in sub-Saharan Africa. In many cases (e.g., in Southern Africa), the HIV/AIDS epidemic will deplete the numbers of productive workers, create large numbers of widows and orphans, weaken the economies, and possibly cause HIV/AIDS-related famines. In the most affected countries, the HIV/AIDS crisis has shortened the life span and will modify perhaps the classic model of the demographic transition.

With regard to fertility, the use of modern contraceptive methods by hundreds of million of couples throughout the world testifies to the remarkable success that has been achieved in addressing fertility issues since the end of the Second World War. In 2002, the world contraceptive prevalence rate (the percentage of women married or in a union, aged 15 to 49, using a modern or traditional contraceptive method) was 61% (68% in industrialized countries and 49% in developing countries, excluding China). Globally, 9 out of 10 users rely on a modern method. However, 120 million couples still do not have access to services (World Bank 2000). Female sterilization, IUDs, and the pill represent more than two-thirds of the use of modern contraception worldwide. Contraceptive prevalence remains the lowest in sub-Saharan Africa (only one couple out of five uses a method, traditional or modern). In the developing world, the widest gap is between sub-Saharan Africa and Latin America and the Caribbean (70% use for the latter region). Differences in the use of contraception are less marked in more developed countries (Population Reference Bureau 2002). Induced abortion remains widely used, particularly in Vietnam, Romania, Cuba, and Russia.[15] An estimated 50 million women resort to it every year: approximately 40% are performed illegally and 78% occur in developing countries (United Nations 2001).

As developing countries have reduced considerably their mortality and fertility levels,[16] it remains particularly challenging to measure the specific contribution of population interventions to these changes. The strict state policy of China definitely accelerated the demographic transition. Elsewhere, fertility declines were essentially triggered by the diffusion of modern family planning methods. However, the latter process itself should probably be attributed more to external factors than to family planning programs alone. Major changes have occurred over the last 50 years in the areas of socioeconomic development, urbanization, education, the status of women, and

---

[15] Although the abortion rate per 1,000 women aged 15 to 44 is much lower in China than in these four countries, the demographic weight of China leads to a large number of induced abortions: China, India, and Vietnam account for almost *all* of the legal abortions in the developing countries (Henshaw 2003).

[16] The TFR in all developing countries dropped from 6.1 from 1960 to 1965 to 3.9 from 1985 to 1990 (Sinding 2003).

the revolution of information. In addition, profound changes in attitudes regarding reproduction and sexuality have taken place concomitantly in many countries. These changes were accelerated by the youthfulness of the population pyramid, especially in developing countries,the circulation of new ideas, and the role of the mass media. The international family planning movement also helped to spread ideas and facilitate access to family planning technical know-how. Overall, it appears that population policy efforts have to a large extent benefited from favorable socioeconomic conditions.[17]

The specific impact of formal and official population policies is probably even harder to assess, as illustrated by the example of Kenya. Kenyan authorities had innovated in the sub-Saharan context when they decided, as early as 1967, to reduce fertility levels. Official support for this policy came during the 1970s and was reasserted formally in 1984 (Parliament Sessional Paper No. 4). Despite important investments in family planning, fertility did not decrease until the beginning of the 1980s (the TFR had peaked at 8.1 in the early 1970s). Consequently, several specialists considered the population policy to be a failure (Frank and McNicoll 1987). In fact, interventions had focused initially on the promotion of family planning services through the strengthening of the health system. The establishment of numerous health facilities, which were made more accessible by a network of new roads, took a long time and the results were not perceived immediately. Fertility eventually started to decline because of an array of other factors: increase in female literacy levels, decrease in infant and child mortality rates and, more importantly, increase of the cost of education (schooling fees, uniforms, and school supplies), which prompted parents to opt for smaller families (Kelley and Nobbe 1990). Nevertheless, the support provided by the policy was probably necessary and useful during the program build-up phase (Jain 1998).

The efficiency of interventions on fertility in industrialized countries is also hard to assess. If the example of France already mentioned seems to indicate a positive link between pronatalist interventions (through family policy) and the increase in fertility, other cases are less clear-cut. However, the experience of the Saar might offer *au contraire* an example of an effective intervention. This German region, which was under French administration from 1945 to 1956, benefited during a decade from the French family policy which was at the time in its most generous phase. During this period, the Saar had the highest TFR of all German regions. When the Saar returned to Germany, its fertility fell within a few years to become one of the lowest in Germany. The probable explanation is that families had lost a substantial portion of their purchasing power (since they did not benefit any more from French financial incentives for large families) and had reduced their fertility as a consequence (Schwarz 1989). Other attempts to raise fertility in industrialized countries have also been successful, but only over a limited number of years (as in the case of Sweden, already mentioned).

It must also be stressed that population policies do not always bring the desired results and can be relatively imprecise. In the former German Democratic Republic (GDR), the policy designed to increase fertility provided incentives for couples to marry at a younger age and have children early but led only to a temporary increase of the

---

[17] Several researchers have attempted to separate analytically the effects of population policies/programs and socioeconomic conditions on population change (usually, fertility decline). Although these authors recognize the methodological difficulties in measuring such factors, they appear to conclude that there are small-to-moderate associations between family planning program efforts and declines in fertility, additive to the contributions of socioeconomic improvements and ideational influences (see Hernandez 1984; Mauldin 1982; Mauldin et al. 1978; Mauldin and Ross 1991; and Ross and Mauldin 1996).

crude birth rate (Dorbritz and Fleischhacker 1999).[18] Singapore, as already mentioned, designed a policy to reduce fertility that was at first very successful but that eventually went too far, hence the pronatalist turn-around of the authorities. Arguably it is much more difficult to increase fertility when it is low than to decrease it when it is high. Furthermore, the fine-tuning of population policies to obtain very precise levels of fertility, for instance replacement fertility, seems virtually impossible. Couples in many industrialized countries have opted for low fertility regimes because of the change in values and women's roles (now often more educated than their male counterparts) and the economic crisis and structural unemployment. It is difficult for policy interventions to overcome these trends, particularly as measures to increase fertility require that actions be taken concomitantly in many different areas: fiscal adjustments, family subsidies, urban planning to accommodate larger families, construction of day-care centers and social equipments, and regulations to increase the flexibility of the labor market in favor of women with children.

Turning to immigration, policies in industrialized countries are driven by an economic, rather than demographic, rationale. Most often, such policies are designed to respond to specific shortages of unskilled and/or skilled workers. These countries, however, find it much more difficult to address the issue of replacement immigration. First, one often notes a lack of consensus on the number of immigrants needed, because this number depends on the policy's goals: is it just workers that are needed or should the population be kept identical in numbers *and* structure? The decision pertaining to the age of immigrants must take into account the practical difficulties in finding immigrants of a specific age group and the impossibility of welcoming parents without their children or children without their parents. Most often, receiving societies are not ready to welcome numerous immigrants (except in traditional immigration countries) because these trends directly challenge their conception of national identities (Teitelbaum and Winter 1998).

THE WAY FORWARD

At present, the world appears to be more demographically diverse than ever (World Bank 2000). The variation of demographic patterns and trends ranges from very high fertility to subreplacement fertility situations, from very young to aging populations, and from immigration-open to immigration-adverse societies. Furthermore, new challenges for population policy have emerged, such as the HIV/AIDS epidemic, which could change the course of the demographic transition in the most affected countries. The diversity regarding the completion of the demographic transition among continents, regions, and countries has also changed the context in which population policies must operate. Arguably, population policies are now confronted with a much larger range of demographic issues than before and forced also to reassess their priorities and sharpen their intervention strategies. Therefore, it is timely to reemphasize the relevance of population policies for both developing and industrialized countries.

As far as fertility is concerned, sub-Saharan Africa still faces very high fertility. Since the broad reproductive health agenda might not be efficient in situations of

---

[18] However, the TFR dropped even further in the former GDR after the reunification of Germany, which might be interpreted *au contraire* as a proof of the impact of earlier pronatalist policies.

incipient fertility decline, population policies in this part of the world may have to focus specifically on family planning services. A detailed analysis of the proximate determinants of fertility for sub-Saharan Africa has demonstrated that birth rates will not decrease rapidly unless major programmatic efforts are put into place to boost contraceptive prevalence rates and bring about a significant shift toward modern contraceptive methods (Guengant and May, forthcoming). Fertility policies in sub-Saharan Africa will also need to be complemented with programs geared to the survival of mothers and children. Such policies will be compelled to explore linkages and find synergies with HIV/AIDS programs, particularly with regard to the supply of condoms and the prevention of mother-to-child infection. The HIV/AIDS crisis shows the difficulty of organizing preventive programs and designing effective interventions to change behavior. It also highlights the need for drugs and possibly vaccines to reduce the viral charge of infected persons and slow the transmission of the virus. The effect of population growth on the environment in some countries also creates new types of problems as the physical limits caused by overpopulation might have already been reached in some countries. These could be faced with situations of demographic fatigue (Brown, Gardner, and Halweil 2000) and even destabilization (Kaplan 2000).

In countries where fertility rates have fallen to between five children per woman and the replacement level, efforts to complete the fertility transition should be complemented with parallel public health and social development interventions. In addition, population policies might benefit in some countries from linkages with public health interventions in order to mitigate the mortality caused by alcohol, drugs, and addiction to smoking.

Industrialized countries are dealing with subreplacement fertility, population aging, and immigration. Estimates for France show that between 1946 and 2051 the decline of mortality, in a scenario of low fertility, would account for only a third of the population aging (as measured by the proportion of the people aged 60 and over; see Calot and Sardon 1999). Therefore, industrialized countries will have to give higher priority to fertility interventions. They will also need to define and implement comprehensive migration policies devoid of nationalist or xenophobic passions, while remaining in line with the democratically defined national interest. The more-developed countries have already taken several—sometimes rather different—steps in these various areas. For example, the United States is planning to increase the retirement age. Many European countries are currently designing pension reforms. Some countries, such as those in the Nordic region and The Netherlands, have pioneered part-time working arrangements and brought about changes in gender roles to allow more flexibility for child and elderly care. Other countries have also enacted measures to address their specific labor-market needs through targeting highly skilled and/or less skilled immigrants. The challenge will be to intervene in a comprehensive way through many policy levers in order to bring the desired societal and demographic changes.

The greatest challenge of all, however, will be to develop a more effective approach to institutionalizing population policies. Initially, this objective could be pursued through five related efforts. First, policymakers could seek the largest possible public consensus to support the goals of population policies. This goal might be approached by identifying the most common denominator to justify a policy, (e.g., achievement of a stationary population or the fertility desires of the couples). Second, policies could be organized around a few dynamic concepts such as the principle of equity or the fight against poverty. Third, new policies will have to be more participatory and consider the increased number of actors and stakeholders. This will call for an improvement of policy coordination mechanisms. Fourth, additional data must be collected, particularly on equity issues and international migration patterns. And, fifth, the implementation of the new policies will have to integrate the results of ongoing analytical research.

Population policies, or the lack thereof, will determine to a large extent the demographic evolution of human societies. For instance, the fulfillment of the Millennium Development Goals (MDGs), of which several pertain specifically to population and reproductive health issues (United Nations 2003), will depend on successful interventions to change demographic patterns and trends, which in turn will affect efforts to eradicate poverty and reduce other social inequities. The attainment of global food security goals will also be influenced largely by the success of population policies, as these targets are based on the assumption of declining fertility levels. Therefore, far from being outmoded or old-fashioned, population policies appear to be as relevant as ever.

REFERENCES

Adnan, S. 2002. Dilatation démographique, pression sur les terres et changement social. Une baisse de la fécondité en situation de pauvreté absolue: Le Bangladesh. In *La population du monde. Géants démographiques et défis internationaux*, les cahiers de l'INED N° 149, 2d ed. Edited by J. C. Chasteland and J. C. Chesnais, 63–106. Paris: Institut national d'études démographiques.

Anonymous. 1983. Recueil de définitions des politiques démographiques. In *Politiques de population. Etudes et documents*, pp. 63–82. Paris : Departments of Demography of the Universities of Louvain and Montreal and the Institut national d'études démographiques.

Banister, J. 2003. One-child policy. In *The encyclopedia of population*, *Vol. 2*. Edited by P. Demeny and G. McNicoll, 707–710. New York: Macmillan Reference USA.

Benneh, G., J. S. Nabila, and B. Gyepi-Garbrah. 1989. *Twenty years of population policy in Ghana*. Legon: University of Ghana.

Berelson, B. 1969. Beyond family planning. *Studies in Family Planning* 38:1–16.

Berelson, B. 1977. Paths to fertility reduction: The "policy cube." *Family Planning Perspectives* 9 (5): 214–219.

Birdsall, N., A. C. Kelley, and S. W. Sinding, eds. 2001. *Population matters: Demographic change, economic growth, and poverty in the developing world*. New York: Oxford University Press.

Blanchet, D. 1991. On interpreting observed relationships between population growth and economic growth: A graphical exposition. *Population and Development Review* 17:105–114.

Bloom, D. E., D. Canning, and J. Sevilla. 2003. *The demographic dividend. A new perspective on the economic consequences of population change*. Santa Monica, Calif.: RAND.

Bongaarts, J. 1994. Population policy options in the developing world. *Science* 263 (5148):771–776.

Boserup, E. 1965. *The conditions of agricultural growth: The economics of agrarian change under population pressure*. London: Allen & Unwin.

Boserup, E. 1970. *Women's role in economic development*. New York: St. Martin's Press.

Boserup, E. 1981. *Population and technological change: A study of long-term trends*. Chicago: University of Chicago Press.

Brown, L. R., G. Gardner, and B. Halweil. 2000. *Beyond Malthus: Nineteen dimensions of the population challenge*. New York–London: W.W. Norton.

Bulatao, R. A. 1984. Reducing fertility in developing countries. A review of determinants and policy levers. *World Bank Staff Working Papers* 680. Washington, D.C.: International Bank for Reconstruction and Development.

Calot, G., and J. P. Sardon. 1999. Les facteurs du vieillissement démographique. *Population* 54(3): 509–552.

Chasteland, J. C. 2002. De 1950 à 2000: La communauté internationale face au problème de la croissance de la population mondiale. In *La population du monde: Géants démographiques et défis internationaux*, les cahiers de l'INED N° 149, 2d ed. Edited by J. C. Chasteland and J. C. Chesnais. Paris: Institut national d'études démographiques.

Chesnais, J. C. 1995. *Le crépuscule de l'occident. Démographie et politique* (717–753). Paris: Robert Laffont.

Chesnais, J. C. 1996. Fertility, family, and social policy in contemporary Western Europe. *Population and Development Review* 22: 729–739.

Cleland, J. 2003. Mortality-fertility relationships. In *The encyclopedia of population, Vol. 2*. Edited by P. Demeny and G. McNicoll, 668–672. New York: Macmillan Reference USA.

Cleland, J., J. F. Phillips, S. Amin, and G. M. Kamal. 1994. *The determinants of reproductive change in Bangladesh: Success in a challenging environment*. World Bank Regional and Sectoral Studies. Washington, D.C.: International Bank for Reconstruction and Development.

Cleland, J., and C. Wilson. 1987. Demand theories of the fertility transition: An iconoclastic view. *Population Studies* 41(1): 5–30.

Coale, A. J., and E. M. Hoover. 1958. *Population growth and economic development in low-income countries*. Princeton, N.J.: Princeton University Press.

Davis, K. 1963. The theory of change and response in modern demographic history. *Population Index* 29: 345–366.

Demeny, P. 1986. Population and the invisible hand. *Demography* 23: 473–487.

Demeny, P. 1992. Policies seeking a reduction of high fertility: A case for the demand side. *Population and Development Review* 18: 321–332.

Demeny, P. 2003a. Population policy. In *The encyclopedia of population, Vol. 2*. Edited by P. Demeny and G. McNicoll, 752–763. New York: Macmillan Reference USA.

Demeny, P. 2003b. Population policy dilemmas in Europe at the dawn of the twenty-first century. *Population and Development Review* 29: 1–28.

Donaldson, P. J. 1990. *Nature against us: The United States and the world population crisis, 1965–1980*. Chapel Hill–London: The University of North Carolina Press.

Dorbritz, J., and J. Fleischhacker. 1999. The former German Democratic Republic. In *From abortion to contraception: A resource to public policies and reproductive behavior in Central and Eastern Europe from 1917 to the present*. Edited by H. P. David, 121–143. Westport, Conn.: Greenwood Press.

Ehrlich, P. R. 1968. *The population bomb*. New York: Ballantine Books.

Ehrlich, P. R., and A. H. Ehrlich. 1990. *The population explosion*. London: Hutchinson.

Faruqee, H., and M. Mühleisen. 2001. *Population aging in Japan: Demographic shock and fiscal sustainability*. IMF Working Paper WP/01/40. Washington, D.C.: International Monetary Fund.

Finkle, J. L., and B. B. Crane. 1990. The politics of international population policy. In *International transmission of population policy experience: Proceedings of the Expert Group Meeting on the International Transmission of Population Policy Experience, New York City, 27–30 June 1988*, pp. 167–182. New York: United Nations, Department of International Economic and Social Affairs.

Frank, O., and G. McNicoll. 1987. An interpretation of fertility and population policy in Kenya. *Population and Development Review* 13: 209–243.

Guengant, J. P., and J. F. May. Forthcoming. Impact of the proximate determinants on the future course of fertility in sub-Saharan Africa. In *The future of high fertility. Population Bulletin of the United Nations*. Special Issue Nos. 46/47.

Harkavy, O. 1995. *Curbing population growth: An insider's perspective on the population movement*. New York: Plenum Press.

Heckel, N. I. 1986. Population laws and policies in sub-Saharan Africa: 1975–1985. *International Family Planning Perspectives* 12: 122–124.

Henshaw, S. K. 2003. Induced abortion: Prevalence. In *The encyclopedia of population, Vol. 2*. Edited by P. Demeny and G. McNicoll, 529–531. New York: Macmillan Reference USA.

Hernandez, D. J. 1984. *Success or failure? Family planning programs in the Third World*. Westport, Conn.: Greenwood Press.

Hodgson, D. 1983. Demography as social science and policy science. *Population and Development Review* 9: 1–34.

Hugo, G. 2003. Resettlement. In *The encyclopedia of population, Vol. 2*. Edited by P. Demeny and G. McNicoll, 854–857. New York: Macmillan Reference USA.

Hyden, G. 1990. Local governance and economic-demographic transition in rural Africa. In *Rural development and population: Institutions and Policy, Population and Development Review, A Supplement to Vol. 15*. Edited by G. McNicoll and M. Cain, 193–211. New York: Oxford University Press.

Jain, A., ed. 1998. *Do population policies matter? Fertility and politics in Egypt, India, Kenya, and Mexico*. New York: The Population Council.

Johansson, S. R. 1991. Implicit policy and fertility during development. *Population and Development Review* 17: 377–414.

Kaplan, R. D. 2000. *The coming anarchy: Shattering the dreams of the post Cold War.* New York: Random House.

Kelley, A. C. 1988. Economic consequences of population change in the Third World. *Journal of Economic Literature* 26:1685–1728.

Kelley, A. C., and C. E. Nobbe. 1990. *Kenya at the demographic turning point? Hypotheses and a proposed research agenda.* World Bank Discussion Papers 107. Washington, D.C.: International Bank for Reconstruction and Development.

Khlat, M., and S. Le Cœur. 2002. La santé: Anciennes et nouvelles maladies. In *La population du monde: Géants démographiques et défis internationaux*, les cahiers de l'INED N° 149, 2d ed. Edited by J. C. Chasteland and J. C. Chesnais, 497–525. Paris: Institut national d'études démographiques.

King, M. 1990. Health is a sustainable state. *The Lancet* 336: 664–667.

Ladier-Fouladi, M. 2003. *Population et politique en Iran: De la monarchie à la République Islamique.* Les Cahiers de l'INED N° 150. Paris: Institut national d'études démographiques.

Livi-Bacci, M. 1992. *A concise history of world population.* Cambridge, Mass., & Oxford, UK: Blackwell.

Maine, D., and K. Stamas. 2003. Maternal mortality. In *The encyclopedia of population, Vol. 2.* Edited by P. Demeny and G. McNicoll, 628–631. New York: Macmillan Reference USA.

Massey, D. S. 2003. International migration. In *The encyclopedia of population, Vol. 2.* Edited by P. Demeny and G. McNicoll, 548–553. New York: Macmillan Reference USA.

Mauldin, W. P. 1982. The determinants of fertility decline in developing countries: An overview of the available empirical evidence. *International Family Planning Perspectives* 8: 116–121.

Mauldin, W. P., B. Berelson, et al. 1978. Conditions of fertility decline in developing countries, 1965–75. *Studies in Family Planning* 9: 90–147.

Mauldin, W. P., and J. A. Ross. 1991. Family planning programs: Efforts and results, 1982–89. *Studies in Family Planning* 22: 350–367.

McNicoll, G. 1975. Community-level population policy: An exploration. *Population and Development Review* 1: 1–21.

McNicoll, G. 1982. Institutional determinants of fertility change. In *Determinants of fertility trends: Theories re-examined. Proceedings of a Seminar held in Bad Homburg (F. R. Germany), 14–17 April 1980, International Union for the Scientific Study of Population.* Edited by C. Höhn and R. Mackensen, 147–168. Liège: Ordina Editions.

McNicoll, G. 2003. Population and development. In *The encyclopedia of population, Vol. 1.* Edited by P. Demeny and G. McNicoll, 226–234. New York: Macmillan Reference USA.

Merrick, T. W. 2002. Population and poverty: New views on an old controversy. *International Family Planning Perspectives* 28: 41–46.

Meslé, F., and J. Vallin. 2002. La mortalité dans le monde: Tendances et perspectives. In *La population du monde: Géants démographiques et défis internationaux*, les cahiers de l'INED N° 149, 2d ed. Edited by J.-C. Chasteland and J. C. Chesnais, 527–546. Paris: Institut national d'études démographiques.

Micklin, M. 1994. Population policies in the Caribbean: Present status and emerging issues. *Social and Economic Studies* 43: 1–32.

Mosley, W. H., D. T. Jamison, and D. A. Henderson. 1990. The health sector in developing countries. Problems for the 1990s and beyond. *Annual Review of Public Health* 11: 335–358.

Pebley, A. R. 1998. Demography and the environment. *Demography* 35: 377–389.

Phillips, J. F., and J. A. Ross, eds. 1992. *Family planning programmes and fertility.* Oxford: Clarendon Press.

Population Impact Project. 1995. *Introducing Ghana's revised population policy.* Legon: University of Ghana, Department of Geography and Resource Development, Population Impact Project (PIP/Ghana).

Population Reference Bureau. 2002. *Family planning worldwide: 2002 data sheet.* Washington, D.C.: Population Reference Bureau.

Population Reference Bureau. 2003. *2003 world population data sheet.* Washington, D.C.: Population Reference Bureau.

Pritchett, L. H. 1994. Desired fertility and the impact of population policies. *Population and Development Review* 20: 1–55.

Ross, J. A., and W. P. Mauldin. 1996. Family planning programs: Efforts and results, 1972–94. *Studies in Family Planning* 27: 137–147.

Saw, S. H. 1990. *Changes in the fertility policy of Singapore.* IPS Occasional Paper N° 2. Singapore: Times Academic Press for Institute of Policy Studies.

Scharping, T. 2003. *Birth control in China 1949–2000: Population policy and demographic development.* London: Routledge-Curzon.

Schwarz, K. 1989. Les effets démographiques de la politique familiale en RFA et dans ses Länder depuis la Seconde Guerre Mondiale. *Population* 44: 395–415.

Simon, J. 1981. *The ultimate resource.* Princeton, N.J.: Princeton University Press.

Simon, J. 1996. *The ultimate resource 2.* Princeton, N.J.: Princeton University Press.

Sinding, S. W. 2003, Family planning programs. In *The encyclopedia of population, Vol. 1.* Edited by P. Demeny and G. McNicoll, 363–371. New York: Macmillan Reference USA.

Stamper, B. M. 1977. *Population and planning in developing nations. A review of sixty development plans for the 1970s.* New York: The Population Council.

Teitelbaum, M. S., and J. M. Winter. 1998. *A question of numbers: High migration, low fertility, and the politics of national identity.* New York: Hill and Wang.

United Nations. 1995. *Report on the International Conference on Population and Development. Cairo, 5–13 September 1994.* N° A/CONF.171/13/Rev. 1. New York: United Nations, Department of Economic and Social Affairs, Population Division.

United Nations. 2000. *Replacement migration: Is it a solution to declining and ageing populations?* ESA/P/WP.160. New York: United Nations, Department of Economic and Social Affairs, Population Division.

United Nations. 2001. *Abortion policies: A global review.* Vol. 1. *Afghanistan to France.* ST/ESA/SER.A/187. New York: United Nations, Department of Economic and Social Affairs, Population Division.

United Nations. 2002. *National population policies 2001.* ST/ESA/SER.A/211. New York: United Nations, Department of Economic and Social Affairs, Population Division.

United Nations. 2003. *Human development report 2003. Millennium development goals: A compact among nations to end human poverty.* New York–Oxford: Oxford University Press for the United Nations Development Programme (UNDP).

U.S. National Academy of Sciences. 1986. *Population growth and economic development: Policy questions.* Report of the Working Group on Population Growth and Economic Development, National Research Council. Washington, D.C.: National Academy Press.

Van De Walle, E. 1982. *Multilingual demographic dictionary*: International Union for the Scientific Study of Population. Liège: Ordina Editions.

Warwick, D. P. 1982. *Bitter pills: Population policies and their implementation in eight developing countries.* New York: Cambridge University Press.

Westoff, C. F., and G. Rodriguez. 1995. The mass media and family planning in Kenya. *International Family Planning Perspectives* 21: 26–36.

World Bank. 1988. *Indonesia. The transmigration program in perspective.* Washington, D.C.: International Bank for Reconstruction and Development.

World Bank. 1994. *Population and development. Implications for the World Bank.* Washington, D.C.: International Bank for Reconstruction and Development.

World Bank. 2000. *Population and the World Bank: Adapting to change*, rev. ed. Washington, D.C.: International Bank for Reconstruction and Development.

Epilogue: Needed Research in Demography

Dudley L. Poston, Jr., Amanda K. Baumle and
Michael Micklin

What is the future of the research enterprise in demography? What are the demographic questions and topics requiring attention in the years ahead?

This chapter has three parts. The first sets the stage for the second and third. It consists of a review of Hauser and Duncan's *The Study of Population* and the research priorities articulated by their chapter authors in 1959. Most of the needed research articulated by the chapter authors of *The Study of Population* has been addressed in the 45-year period between its publication and the publication of the present *Handbook*. The second section summarizes the research priorities proposed by many of the authors of this *Handbook*. The last section sets forth and discusses a few research challenges that we deem to be particularly relevant and important for demographic research in future years.

RESEARCH PRIORITIES OF *THE STUDY OF POPULATION*

In *The Study of Population*, editors Philip M. Hauser and Otis Dudley Duncan wrote the first chapter, which set out the book's overview and conclusions. They also wrote Part I, "Demography as a Science," which consists of four chapters dealing with the nature of demography, its data and methods, demography as a body of knowledge, and demography as a profession. In these five chapters they do not address directly the research priorities of demography, but they do make several observations about the research requirements and needs of demography. In their discussions of the knowledge base of demography and the need for theory development, they note that it is not possible to deal conclusively with matters raised about the major foci of the field. To resolve these issues "would be to anticipate accurately the future course of the discipline" (Hauser and Duncan 1959: 16). They continue that although "nothing in demography, any more than in any other science, is ever 'finished,' " it would be good for demography to cast its theories "at least partly in historical terms" (1959: 16). This remains an important objective.

Regarding data requirements, they note the rather obvious need of all countries and territories and their geographical subdivisions for good censuses and registration systems, the two pillars claimed by Walter F. Willcox, the "dean of American demography in his day," that support the "arch" of demography (1959: 53). These data need to be made available both backward and forward in time (1959: 53–54). They also report on needed developments in data processing and delivery. Some of the discussions in the Prologue to this *Handbook* note that many of these data requirements have been addressed rather satisfactorily since 1959.

In an early section outlining the issues they had asked chapter authors to address, Hauser and Duncan state that chapter authors writing about the status of demography in a particular country or geographical area could consider "aspects of demography that should be emphasized or developed further in future research," as well as "the most pressing subjects on which research should be done in the near future" (1959: 24–25). The chapter authors writing about elements of demography were asked to consider the "next steps" in research as well as any obstacles that might hinder these research advances (1959: 25). Some of the chapter authors chose to address these issues, others did not.

In his brief discussion of the development of demography in France, Sauvy writes that demographers need to do a better job in their studies of penetrating the "social complex" of the demographic processes of fertility, mortality, and migration. These "must be studied more and more by relating them to social factors" (Sauvy 1959: 186). And since "these social factors cannot always be comprehended by the too rigid and costly classic statistics (censuses and vital statistics), local inquiries [that is surveys] must be multiplied" (Sauvy 1959: 186). If anything, demography has been characterized since 1959 by a proliferation of fertility and health surveys, both international and country-specific. Moreover, the several chapters in this *Handbook* on population and the social sciences show that demographers in the past 45 years have indeed followed Sauvy's advice.

Grebenik's chapter on the development of demography in Great Britain concludes with the observation that future research is needed that "lies on the borders of demography proper and sociology, social psychology, and allied disciplines" (Grebenik 1959: 201). Once again, many of the chapters in this *Handbook*, particularly those dealing with population and the social sciences, point to significant advances in this regard since 1959.

After reviewing the current status of demography in Germany, Schubnell writes more than two pages on future prospects. He outlines many issues that must be addressed by social scientists in Germany, including the "social equalization of family burdens," the "sociopolitical and labor market effects of rearmament," the "course of the trade cycle," and the "special problems of the process of aging" (Schubnell 1959: 212). Although demography needs to make substantial contributions in all these arenas, he notes that among the most pressing problems that need to be addressed by German demographers are "the structure of families and households," "population mobility and its connection with sifting and selection processes," the "sociopolitically requisite equalization of family burdens," and the "need for the replacement and provision for the population in the various areas of the economy" (Schubnell 1959: 213). Many of these issues are covered in several of this *Handbook's* chapters. One that requires continued research pertains to issues and implications of below-replacement fertility. See in particular the discussions in Morgan and Hagewen's chapter in this *Handbook*.

In their chapters on demography in Brazil and in India, both Mortara (1959) and Chandrasekaran (1959) point to the fact that future research in their countries depends significantly on "adequate demographic data," especially in the case of Brazil, "an efficient organization for the registration of births, deaths, and marriages" (Mortara 1959: 245). The censuses in both countries, the authors write, have become efficient and timely. Even today, many countries have better censuses than they do registration systems. This problem, mentioned in 1959, remains.

In Taeuber's chapter on demographic research in the Pacific area, she correctly writes that in the late 1950s "the greatest of the research fields in the Pacific, and the least cultivated, is that of China and the Chinese" (Taeuber 1959: 274). She observes in some detail the paucity of demographic knowledge and data about China and the Chinese. In 1959, indeed, little was known in and outside China about the country's demography. While today there are still many important demographic research questions that need to be addressed about China, the knowledge base and data on the demography of China have increased tremendously since 1959. Many of these developments are mentioned in several chapters in this *Handbook*. Other treatments are those of Banister (1987), Poston and Yaukey (1992), and Peng and Guo (2000).

In Bogue's chapter on population distribution, he observes that demographers are devoting considerable effort addressing the question of "*how* fluctuations in fertility occur" (Bogue 1959b: 398). He suggests that a major research requirement involves also addressing the question of why, sociologically and socioeconomically, fertility changes occur. "An intensive distributional analysis of interarea variation in fertility and of interarea change in differences in fertility should throw considerable light on this subject" (Bogue 1959b: 398). There has been development in this regard since the publication of Bogue's chapter. See the discussions in Chapter 20, "Ecological Demography," in this *Handbook*.

In his chapter on fertility, Ryder focuses on many areas in which research is needed. He characterizes as insufficient the state of knowledge in the late 1950s pertaining to "quantitative materials concerning the parameters of procreation and their statistical relationship with demographic and socioeconomic variables" (Ryder 1959: 434). Research, he writes, is also needed "in the area of the immediate causes of fertility variation: fecundity, copulation, and contraception. Improvements in the diagnosis of sterility would be of considerable assistance" (Ryder 1959: 434). Discussions in chapter 8, "Fertility," and chapter 24, "Fertility Planning," in this *Handbook*, among others, report some of the advances since the 1950s in social demographic analyses of fertility and investigations of the proximate determinants of fertility.

Dorn (1959) proposes several areas of needed research in his chapter on mortality. Aside from data improvements and methodological advances, he also mentions the need for certain kinds of analytical studies. Referring specifically to the United States, he calls for detailed investigations of urban-rural differences in mortality, studies of metropolitan and nonmetropolitan mortality, mortality analyses focusing on occupation and socioeconomic groups, fetal mortality, the sex differential in mortality, and old age mortality. These topics have received considerable attention since the late 1950s as evidenced in chapter 9, "Infant Mortality," and chapter 10, "Adult Mortality," in this *Handbook* (see also Rogers, Hummer, and Nam 2000).

Bogue's chapter on internal migration ends with the recommendation that demographers "stop oversimplifying the migration situation and underestimating its variability from place to place and over time" (Bogue 1959a: 505). He holds that the following lines of research are needed: demographers must exploit the "existing data relating to migration streams and selective migration." They must estimate multivariate models of migration because "migration, perhaps more than most topics in demography, demands research designs that take into account several variables simultaneously" (Bogue 1959a: 506). And comparative and international studies of internal migration are needed. There have been significant advances along these lines since the 1950s, as may be evidenced by discussions in chapter 11, "Internal Migration," and chapter 20, "Ecological Demography," in this *Handbook*.

In the chapter by Thomas on international migration, the author holds that future research "will be much improved if the most glaring deficiencies of the primary data are eliminated in the developed countries and if the lessons of the past are borne in mind where new records are introduced in underdeveloped countries" (Thomas 1959: 534). Thomas then presents a list of some 30 specific topics that "are aspects of the migration process in the era of unrestricted movement which would well repay intensive analysis" (Thomas 1959: 537). They will not be repeated here, but it is of interest to note that since the publication of Thomas's chapter, many, if not most, of these topics have been satisfactorily addressed by international migration researchers. See the discussions of some of these topics in chapter 12, "International Migration," in this *Handbook* and in the *Handbook of International Migration* edited by Hirschman, Kasinitz, and Dewind (1999).

Glick's chapter on family statistics raises a number of issues that need to be addressed for this area of demography to prosper in the coming years. He first calls for more detailed data on the current status and changing characteristics of family composition. He identifies specific kinds of questions that could be added to the decennial census and to other government surveys. It turns out that many of them have found their way onto survey and census instruments in past decades. Glick also calls for advances in punch card technology so that person characteristics could be cross-classified with characteristics of the family (Glick 1959: 599). The kinds of cross-tabulations wished for by Glick in 1959 are now easily obtained, given the computer technology developed since the 1950s and electronically available government and private surveys and public use samples from the censuses of the U.S. and many other countries.

One of the most important questions for future research raised by Jaffe in his chapter on the workforce is the following: "Will women who take full-time jobs outside the home have smaller completed families than if they had not taken such jobs? Or does it work in reverse? . . . Or are both variables (size of completed family and working-force behavior of the woman) the resultants of other socioeconomic factors?" (Jaffe 1959: 615). This question has generated a great deal of research activity since the 1970s, some of which is discussed in chapters 3, 7, and 8 in this *Handbook*.

The Study of Population contains two chapters dealing with ecology, namely, Frank's (1959) chapter on general ecology, and Duncan's (1959) on human ecology. Both are concerned with the extent to which ecology may provide a framework or perspective for demographic analysis. This is likely the most important contribution of ecology to demography. Indeed Frank notes that "if ecology has anything to offer the demographer, it must be looked for along theoretical lines" (Frank 1959: 672). And Duncan writes that "the ecological framework provides one means of ordering demographic data intelligibly" (Duncan 1959: 710). The major theoretical statement of human ecology was written more than 50 years ago by Amos Hawley in his *Human Ecology: A Theory of Community Structure* (1950). His ideas have led to an abundance of empirical analyses. Many of those focusing on demographic processes are discussed and referenced in chapter 20, "Ecological Demography," in this *Handbook*. Many of those dealing with organizations and corporations are discussed in chapter 15, "Organizational and Corporate Demography." But these are mainly empirical manifestations and extensions of Hawley's (1950) theory of human ecology. Theoretical advances in this field since 1950 have been limited.

In Ackerman's chapter on geography and demography, he mentions several areas requiring research attention. He focuses particular attention on the need to study "the technological element in settlement influences and sustenance patterns as they affect population characteristics" (Ackerman 1959: 724). This has been a major concern of human ecologists since the publication of Hawley's (1950) *Human Ecology*, Duncan's (1959) chapter in *The Study of Population*, and other conceptual and theoretical treatments by Duncan (1961, 1964), Gibbs and Martin (1959), and Schnore (1958, 1961). See the discussions of much of this work in chapter 20, "Ecological Demography," in this *Handbook*, as well as in publications of Namboodiri (1988, 1994), Micklin (1973), Poston, Frisbie, and Micklin (1984), Micklin and Poston (1998), Micklin and Sly (1998), and Poston and Frisbie (1998), among others.

In the chapter on economics and demography, Spengler lays out several areas where future research is needed. Since "population problems deal with the behavior of groups and subgroups of individuals through time … it appears to be essential, if dynamic process analysis is resorted to, that social-psychological considerations be taken into account as well as those of an essentially economic or demographic order" (Spengler 1959: 816). Among the other areas where future research is needed, Spengler calls for more extensive multivariate analyses and the use of time lags in dynamic models. He also suggests the need to inquire into the nature and causes of the apparent appeal made by Marxian views on population to public spokesmen and policymakers. And he recommends longitudinal analyses of the impact of acquisition of consumption on age-specific fertility, as well as the interrelations of the trade-cycle and age-specific fertility. Many of the areas outlined by Spengler in 1959 have been addressed in the past 45 years. See discussions in Chapter 18, "Economic Demography," in this *Handbook* and in Rosenzweig and Stark's (1997) *Handbook of Population and Family Economics*.

In Moore's chapter on sociology and demography, he does not refer explicitly to "future research areas" or "next steps," as did many other authors of chapters in *The Study of Population*. But he does mention a few areas deserving more attention. For instance, he states "that it is probably safe to say that the relation of fertility to the social and psychological aspects of mobility is the most promising lead to part of the 'intervening links' between 'structural' characteristics and fertility behavior" (Moore 1959: 848). He also notes the need to treat mortality and migration as dependent variables and not to focus only on biological and economic explanations. The sociological context must play a role in these models. Several chapters in this *Handbook*, especially Chapter 14, "Sociological Demography," provide considerable evidence of the many accomplishments of social demography in the past 45 years. Some of these were mentioned by Moore in 1959, but many were not.

This section has summarized many of the discussions of future research needs that were articulated by contributors to *The Study of Population*. As noted earlier, most of these research areas have been addressed by demographers in the 45-year period since the publication of Hauser and Duncan's inventory. This Epilogue now turns to summaries of the areas of future research set forth by many of the authors of chapters in this *Handbook*.

RESEARCH PRIORITIES OF THE
HANDBOOK OF POPULATION

Age and Sex

In his chapter on age and sex in this *Handbook*, Poston identifies two major areas in which future age and sex research should focus. He first highlights the possible implications of the unbalanced sex ratios at birth in China, South Korea, Taiwan, and India. In contrast to normal sex ratios at birth (SRBs) of approximately 105, the SRBs in these four countries fell close to 120 in the year 2000. The unbalanced sex ratios have been attributed primarily to a preference for sons in a time when declining fertility and family planning policies limit an individual's opportunities to have a son. Researchers have theorized that individuals in these countries have turned to measures to ensure that they have at least one son, most likely employing sex-selective abortion.

The decline of female births in China, South Korea, and Taiwan could result in a number of long-term problems. When reaching marriage age, many men will find themselves unable to find a wife due to the shortage of women (Poston and Glover 2005). Likely outcomes of this "bride shortage" include employing unmarried young men in public works projects or war, importing new brides from other countries, and the establishment of "bachelor ghettos."

Poston also contends that future research should be directed at the process of demographic aging (see Poston and Duan 2000; Poston 2002). Many countries in Asia and Latin America have experienced significant declines in fertility which will ultimately increase the elderly populations in the years to come. The huge increase in the older population will likely impact the ability of the younger population to support the older population, both economically and emotionally. Further, the role of the government in providing support to the older population will have to be reassessed as the older population increases and the number of younger individuals available to provide support decrease.

Thus, policymakers will need to develop possible methods of caring for the older population, and demographers could play a vital role in this process. Future research in this area could provide guidance to countries on methods to increase support for the older population, including increasing international migration for demographic replacement or raising the retirement age.

Population Distribution and Suburbanization

Guest and Brown's chapter in this *Handbook* notes that suburbanization has influenced significantly the way populations are distributed in the U.S. and throughout the world.

They suggest that the continued outward movement of populations will be one of the most significant demographic trends of the 21st century, dependent in part on transportation developments, which increase the ability of individuals to traverse long distances in shorter time frames. In addition, they note that future suburbanization will also depend on improvements in electronic communication, which will decrease the necessity for daily interactions between individuals, thereby permitting persons to work from their homes.

Due to the likelihood of this continuing trend, Guest and Brown suggest that researchers should focus future research on developing more sophisticated models that have the capacity to explain suburbanization across metropolitan areas and countries. Contextual characteristics could influence the rate of suburbanization, including changing physical boundaries, community amenities, ethnic composition, immigration, and employment patterns. It is these areas that should be the focus of future studies in population distribution and suburbanization.

Marriage and Family

Explanatory models of marriage and the family are evolving in postindustrial societies. There are many issues pertaining to marriage and the family requiring future research. Waite observes in her chapter in this *Handbook* that the notion of what constitutes a family and a marriage is changing with increased cohabitation and the rising recognition of the partnerships of homosexual couples. These developments challenge accepted definitions of what constitutes a family, i.e., must the family be based on a blood relationship or a legal bond? If the response is in the affirmative, cohabiting couples, both heterosexual and homosexual, cannot constitute a family. Many would claim otherwise, especially if children are involved.

In recent years, some U.S. states, and some other countries, have recognized legal rights for homosexuals in the areas of marriage and family. These changes in the legal definition of marriage could affect the social, political, and economic lives of homosexual individuals owing to the rights and benefits carried by marriage (emotional, physical, and economic). This area will likely be a focus of new work in the years ahead.

In addition to changing definitions of marriage and family connected with cohabitation and homosexuality, Waite notes that future research should focus on racial disparities in family patterns. Black men and women have not experienced the same patterns in age at marriage as whites, resulting in blacks having lower ages at marriage than whites (Fitch and Ruggles 2000). In addition, whites marry at approximately twice the rate of blacks (Waite 1995), with the rates of black women predicted to decline and those of white women to remain high (Goldstein and Kenney 2001). In addition to marital differences, the birth rate of unmarried women is three times higher for blacks than for whites (Martin et al. 2002). Future research should be directed toward explaining these differences between marriage and family patterns of blacks and whites.

Demography of Gender

Since the publication of Hauser and Duncan's *The Study of Population* in 1959, research on the demography of gender has increased almost exponentially. Riley notes in her chapter in this *Handbook* that the amount of research incorporating gender indicates that demographers are accepting the significant influence of gender on social and demographic processes.

Although demographers have increasingly incorporated gender into their studies, Riley notes that theoretical and methodological weaknesses in demography result in a failure to truly capture the complex effects of gender. She suggests that the field might benefit from incorporating theoretical and methodological perspectives on gender from other disciplines. By incorporating gender perspectives from feminist studies, for instance, demographers might be able to develop new approaches to the understanding of gender's role in population studies.

Demography of Aging

Drawing on a study conducted by the National Research Council (2001), Uhlenberg notes in his chapter that there are five primary areas in which future research on aging is likely to develop. First, Uhlenberg encourages multidisciplinary research on aging that explores connections among the social sciences; in this manner, policy recommendations would incorporate a more complete picture of the aging process. Second, he emphasizes the importance of collecting longitudinal data. Only longitudinal data are adequate for drawing causal conclusions about aging. Uhlenberg's third proposed area of research involves conducting comparative analyses of aging across countries in order to expand the knowledge base about cross-country similarities and variance in the aging process.

Fourth, computer technology allows the development of databases and the implementation of advanced statistical methods leading to more sophisticated analyses of aging. Data from administrative records may be linked with survey information to increase available information, geographical information can be added to analyses, and multilevel analyses can be undertaken. Finally, Uhlenberg suggests that one of the major theoretical challenges facing demographers in the coming years is to better understand the manner in which societies will change and adapt as their populations grow increasingly older.

Demography of Race and Ethnicity

Much like demographic studies of gender, race and ethnicity have mainly been incorporated into demographic analyses as important, if not essential, controls. Nonetheless, Saenz and Morales argue in their chapter that further development of the demography of race and ethnicity is necessary in the coming years. Just as Riley posits that gender demography could benefit from incorporating outside theories and methodology, Saenz and Morales suggest that demographers should broaden their understanding of the meaning of race and ethnicity. They contend that in the future, demographers should be cognizant of theories of race and ethnicity in sociology and related disciplines in order to gain insight into the manner in which race and ethnicity can be successfully incorporated into demographic research. By understanding the history and context of racial and ethnic groups and related stratification, demographers will be better able to comprehend the manner in which these groups affect and are affected by demographic processes.

Morales and Saenz also identify some specific areas where studies of the demography of race and ethnicity should be focused. Due to the ability of individuals to identify multiple racial identities on the 2000 U.S. census, demographers will now be able to incorporate more fine-tuned distinctions of race and ethnicity into their analyses. Research on multiracial persons could center on the effect of multiracial identity on social and economic circumstances, marriage patterns, racial and ethnic identification of the children of multiracial individuals, and the incorporation of multiracial persons into population projections. Saenz and Morales also suggest that future research should distinguish between immigrant populations based on country of origin, rather than treating Latino and Asian groups as a whole, since group traits and experiences vary by country of origin. Further, researchers should delineate between native-born and foreign-born members of groups because research has indicated that native-born minorities often possess characteristics and degrees of success that differ from those of foreign-born members.

Finally, Saenz and Morales contend that the effects of race and ethnicity on stratification and inequality must be considered in conjunction with other traits that play a role in inequality, such as nativity, gender, class, sexuality, and the color of one's skin. They note that there are few studies which have attempted to incorporate all of these characteristics and argue that future research should attempt to create models which integrate these aspects of inequality.

Labor Force

Labor force demography continues to play an important role in demographic research because the size, structure, and changes of the labor force have a significant effect on the population processes, particularly fertility and migration. In her chapter in this *Handbook*, Sullivan notes that early retirement in developed countries, coupled with declining mortality rates, has resulted in workers in developed countries spending many more years of their lives out of the labor force. In order to provide for the care of these individuals, Sullivan suggests that demographers in the coming years will continue to explore the demographic patterns of retirement in an attempt to provide estimates of future retiring populations. The lack of a mandatory retirement age makes the process of predicting retirement age a challenging one and, as a result, will render the insight of demographers in this area increasingly valuable.

In addition to retirement age, Sullivan suggests that the manner in which young individuals become attached to the labor force will be an area of research focus in the coming years. Research has indicated that the way youths are involved in the labor force during their early years affects future labor force participation, income, completion of college, and criminal activity (Carr, Wright, and Brody 1996; Crutchfield and Pitchford 1997). Further, youth labor force attachment varies between the sexes and among racial and ethnic groups (Deseran and Keithly 1994). Sullivan predicts that this area will continue to be of interest to demographers in the future, as factors influencing youth labor force attachment are likely to differ for future generations.

Finally, Sullivan contends that a continuing issue of import in the area of labor force demography will concern the composition of the labor force following the completion of the demographic transition and the movement from agriculture to industry to service economies. The aging of the labor force, movement toward professional and/or knowledge-based occupations, and the impact of future technological improvements could all play a role in altering the labor force in the coming years.

Fertility

In their chapter in this *Handbook*, Morgan and Hagewen note that fertility is an advanced field of demographic study, boasting uniform methods of measurement and analysis, common interpretations and organizations of data, and some consensus regarding the explanations for a variety of observed events and trends. Despite this development, fertility, like the other demographic processes, is constantly altering and will be an important area of research in both developing and developed countries.

Although common patterns have been observed in many countries in the transition from high to low fertility, there is no guarantee that the same determinants will play a role in the fertility declines for countries undergoing the transition now or in the future. Morgan and Hagewen remark that new phenomena could dramatically alter the transition process, rendering past theories of fertility decline inadequate for explaining current or future declines. Already, countries experiencing recent fertility transitions have exhibited signs of being affected by the infusion of ideas and technology from developed countries, which in turn has resulted in more rapid fertility declines (Bongaarts and Bulatao 2000: 76–77; Bongaarts and Watkins 1996). Thus, future declines are likely to be affected not only by the experiences of countries that have already completed the transition but by perhaps unforeseen political, economic, or social phenomena.

In addition to future research concerning the causes of fertility decline, Morgan and Hagewen note that the world is entering a stage in which fertility in many countries has not only declined but has reached below-replacement levels. In the coming years, these countries will likely be the focus of extensive fertility research, as demographers and policymakers explore how low fertility will decline and whether governments could or should offer effective incentives to raise fertility levels.

Technological developments are also likely to play a role in future fertility developments and, thus, future research. Morgan and Hegewen write that technological developments could result in the ability to safely postpone childbirth, as well as to genetically engineer children. Such developments could affect fertility decisions and their implications, as well as their likely use.

Infant Mortality

In his chapter, Frisbie predicts that future research in the area of infant mortality will continue to explore the relationship between deviations from birth outcome survival optimums and their effects on infant mortality. He suggests that gaining insights about these interrelationships could assist in gaining a better understanding of the variation in perinatal health.

Further, Frisbie contends that the disparity between black and white infant mortality continues to be a pressing issue for research. In particular, he suggests that nationally representative studies need to be conducted exploring the linkages between the decline of the black survival advantage at short gestations and low birth rates connected in part to the manner in which pulmonary surfactant therapy differentially affects neonates with RDS.

Lack of adequate data, however, restricts studies in many areas of infant mortality. Frisbie suggests that the area of infant mortality could benefit from an increase in contextual research, but observes that there is a need for data sets designed specifically for multilevel analysis. In addition, he notes that utilizing random effects models would permit the determination of whether individual-level effects vary by area.

Finally, Frisbie emphasizes that demographers studying infant mortality must collaborate with social epidemiologists and medical researchers to assess the biological factors, as well as the social factors, that act upon infant mortality.

Adult Mortality

Just as in the area of infant mortality, research on adult mortality will benefit from multidisciplinary work that incorporates information from epidemiology, medicine, and biology, as well as from sociology, demography, economics, geography, and history. In their chapter in this *Handbook*, Rogers, Hummer, and Krueger suggest that future research on adult mortality is likely to focus on factors limiting further gains in longevity. In particular, the rise in obesity impacts mortality by increasing the occurrence of diabetes, heart disease, and some types of cancer. In addition, despite warnings regarding the risk of cigarette smoking, a large number of individuals begin smoking every year, and one quarter of the adult population in the U.S. continues to smoke. Rogers and his colleagues note that these trends warrant further study, as they could offset the positive effect on longevity of increased education and public health efforts; further, these trends disproportionately impact racial and ethnic minorities.

The authors suggest that future research on adult mortality should also explore the impact of social and contextual factors on mortality; some research has explored the impact of the marriage and family structure on mortality (Lillard and Waite 1995; Rogers 1995), but future research could examine mortality patterns within households, neighborhoods, and regions.

Internal Migration

In their chapter, White and Lindstrom identify future developments needed in the areas of data, methods, and theory to advance research in internal migration. They observe that the increase in available data, most notably in microdata surveys, has played an important role in developing research in demography as a whole. They predict that data collection will remain a priority in the coming years in order to provide resources for researchers interested in developing behavioral modeling. In particular, they note that longitudinal or event-history information is particularly important for future research on internal migration, as life histories regarding mobility are needed to explore migration in depth.

White and Lindstrom also note that geographic information systems (GIS) technology will likely play a large role in future research on migration. GIS technology permits researchers to no longer be bound by geographical units contained in government data sets, such as states, cities, or tracts. Instead, the researcher can organize information into units that are defined by other characteristics, such as households or employment sites. The technical complexity of GIS, as well as the manner in which notions of space will be redefined, will likely result in future challenges to researchers of migration.

White and Lindstrom further suggest some new directions for research in the area of internal migration. The impact of migration on the labor force, as well as the effect of migration on the provision of government resources, will likely remain areas of focus in the years to come. In addition, White and Lindstrom predict that future improvements in data quality will aid research on the relationship between migration and other demographic factors, including family structure. Further, the development of longitudinal data could aid in studies of migrant adaptation, such as the manner in which migrants adapt to moves between rural and urban settings. Contextual models will also likely play a role in future internal migration studies, incorporating the manner in which characteristics of the place of origin, as well as the destination influence migration behaviors.

Finally, White and Lindstrom suggest that future research is likely to integrate theories in various areas of migration research. For instance, studies of internal migration might be merged with those of local mobility and international migration. In addition, the study of migration of developing countries might be integrated with those of developed countries. Many of the studies in these areas have taken different theoretical paths, but White and Lindstrom suggest they could benefit from incorporating theories from related literature.

International Migration

In the conclusion of their chapter in this *Handbook*, Brown and Bean identify a number of areas for future research in international migration. Low fertility and the rise in longevity have resulted in the aging of populations in many developed countries. One possible solution to the challenges posed by aging populations would be for advanced countries to increase the number of working-aged immigrants. An influx of working-aged immigrants could stall the economic costs associated with an older population. In many countries with aging populations, however, unemployment remains high. As a result, an influx of working-aged immigrants could impact unemployment and other market outcomes, and these costs would need to be balanced with the possible benefits associated with increasing immigration.

Brown and Bean also suggest that future research on international migration will likely concern the manner in which immigrants will be incorporated into countries of destination, as well as the way in which the destination countries will react to ethnically diverse immigrants. Immigrants from less developed countries might not possess the educational background to incorporate themselves into the economies of their destination countries. Definitive findings on the manner in which immigrants are incorporated into destination countries cannot be discerned for some time. Thus Brown and Bean emphasize that theoretical models of incorporation will be necessary in the coming years to guide research and policy. An associated concern is the manner in which the ethnic diversity resulting from immigration will impact destination countries. Such diversity could increase social tension and perhaps prevent the incorporation of immigrants. On the other hand, increasing ethnic diversity may serve to increase ethnic tolerance.

Demography of Social Stratification

Sakamoto and Powers suggest that research in the demography of social stratification should move away from the intensive descriptive analysis that has dominated the area in the past, and focus more on the development of analytical models. They suggest incorporating both exogenous and endogenous variables from demography and stratification to create broader models of social stratification.

In addition to expanding the variables incorporated in social stratification models, Sakamoto and Powers also suggest that future research should focus on understanding commonalities in mobility and inequality between nations. In so doing, researchers are able to determine whether there are any similarities that are perhaps repeatedly present in social stratification, despite varying contexts, thereby expanding upon the theoretical understanding of social stratification.

Social Demography

Hirschman and Tolnay highlight a number of elements of social demography that have characterized, and will likely continue to characterize, the field. Social demography pays particular attention to the role of cohorts in effecting social change. The interpretation of cohort effects is inhibited, however, by the difficulty in separating cohort effects from those of age and period. Nonetheless, Hirschman and Tolnay note that the cohort continues to play an important role in social demography and will doubtless influence future studies in the area.

In addition to the cohort perspective, Hirschman and Tolnay write that studies in social demography have been characterized by the logic of decomposition. Many of the demographic processes are composed of a number of related components; decomposition permits the demographer to focus on each of these components in order to arrive at a better understanding of social phenomena. Social demography will likely continue to use the logic of decomposition to gain further insights into the parts that make up demographic phenomena.

Hirschman and Tolnay also observe that social demography is characterized by its interdisciplinary approach. By incorporating theories, data, and methods from multiple disciplines, social demographers are better able to take unique approaches to their studies. Hirschman and Tolnay posit that future research in social demography will benefit from this interdisciplinary approach as research issues become more complex.

Organizational and Corporate Demography

Carroll and Khessina summarize in their chapter the future of organizational and corporate demography within theory fragments, across theory fragments, and within conceptual frameworks. Although they indicate that future research is likely to occur with respect to all of the theory fragments, Carroll and Khessina note that the density dependence fragment might pose fertile ground for future research because of the challenges in incorporating an explanation of late-stage population declines and resurgences. Further, they suggest that future research should incorporate a more global perspective, comparing findings cross-nationally in an attempt to explain variations in the timing and levels of density-dependent population evolution.

Carroll and Khessina also suggest that future research could occur across theory fragments. In particular, they suggest that corporate demography could benefit from additional research on the cumulativity in model specifications. Further, they suggest that empirical integration should be a focus in the area, as should the attempt to unify theories in the discipline.

Finally, Carroll and Khessina note that new work in organizational and corporate demography could continue the practice of unifying some of the themes of this area with other demographic research. For instance, connecting corporate demography with that of workforce demography, or corporate demography and internal organizational demography, would be especially appropriate. They posit that new research in the area of organizational and corporate demography will continue this trend.

Urban and Spatial Demography

In his chapter, Fossett explores the tension between traditional perspectives on urban and spatial distribution (urban economics, human ecology, and urban geography) and new perspectives (critical, political, postmodern, and sociocultural). Although some argue that the new perspectives should supplant the traditional perspectives in future research, Fossett argues that traditional demographic perspectives are a necessary part of studies of urban and spatial distribution. He notes that the new perspectives contend that culture plays an important role in spatial distribution, but argues that these perspectives do not effectively generalize in order to explain spatial distribution in any overarching way. Although there has not been a large movement to combine traditional and new perspectives, Fossett suggests that future research might benefit most from an attempt to synthesize these two fields in order to develop a more comprehensive picture of urban and spatial patterns.

Anthropological Demography

Only within the past 20 or so years has anthropological demography been formally recognized as a specialty within either anthropology or demography. As noted by Kertzer in his chapter in this *Handbook*, the two fields have been both methodologically and theoretically at odds. Anthropologists have viewed the quantitative, positivist approach of demographers with some skepticism, and demographers have questioned the utility of the deconstructionist, ethnographic approach of anthropologists. Despite the disparity, historically anthropologists have explored many demographic topics, such as fertility, mortality, and migration. The renewed focus of anthropology on demographic topics has resulted in large part from an acknowledgment that demographic studies could benefit from anthropological theory and methods.

As a result, Kertzer predicts that future research in the area of anthropological demography will likely unite demographic studies with anthropological theories concerning culture and symbolism, providing new insights into demographic processes by recognizing the importance of culture. Further, the incorporation of anthropological survey and ethnographic techniques are likely to expand and richen future demographic research.

Economic Demography

Mason predicts that future research in economic demography will be guided by technological advancements and access to information, as well as by a variety of population changes that have occurred or are expected to occur in the coming years. He observes that technological improvements in the ability to store, share, and analyze data have advanced the field by enabling economic demographers to propose and work with increasingly complex models, including complicated microsimulation models and macrosimulation models. Further, the ability to easily and cheaply analyze and share large amounts of data has enabled economic demographers to explore new issues and to collaborate on a global level. Mason writes that as a result of these technological advancements, future research can involve large international collaborative efforts which will provide new insights into the manner in which cultural, historical, social, and economic differences impact economic demography.

Coupled with the impact of technological advancements, Mason argues that future research in economic demography will likely focus on the influence of the aging of populations. First, he contends that the rapid aging of populations in developing countries will likely result in difficulties in obtaining economic security for the elderly. To obtain economic security, developing countries must first establish stable economic and political institutions so that reliance on public pension programs, as well as private savings, becomes a less risky and uncertain prospect. Further, Mason suggests that as population aging becomes a global phenomenon, its impact will be widely felt. For example, the aging of western workers has been moderated by turning toward other nations for production. The impact of global aging, therefore, is likely to be a fertile ground for research for economic demographers as this trend expands.

Finally, Mason suggests that economic demographers are likely to explore the relationship between regional population differences and globalization. The proportion of the world's population located in the more developed regions (i.e., Europe, North America, Australia, New Zealand, and Japan) is shrinking, and, perhaps most notably, its share of the working-age population will shrink, while that of the less developed regions will grow. The impact of such shifts on globalization in the coming years will likely be of interest to economic demographers.

Historical Demography

Assessing "the future" of historical demography poses some limitations since, as van de Walle observes, future research is limited by the existing data, much of which has already been discovered and explored. Historical demography will nonetheless be aided by advancing statistical methodologies and by developing interdisciplinary ties with historical demography and mainstream demography, permitting methods and findings of past studies to influence future ones, and vice versa.

Although van de Walle notes that it is difficult to predict what future discoveries will be made in historical demography, he does suggest some possible directions for future research. He first contends that research will expand into different countries, and extensions of demographic variables back in time will likely be attempted in order to formulate notions of the historical composition of these populations. In addition, he suggests that future research will include the recent trends in historical demography of incorporating comparative approaches and of focusing on substantive issues, rather than the more monographic studies of the past.

Political Demography

Teitelbaum observes in his chapter that future work in political demography will likely focus on four issues: population size, age structure, population composition, and the interactions between immigration and fertility. Population size has been traditionally equated with power. Accordingly, many countries have advocated the notion of increased population size in their pursuit of political power. Although evidence supporting a correlation between size and power is mixed, with fertility declines this issue is likely to be the subject of future research.

Research in political demography is also likely to focus on the political repercussions of population age. With the increased aging of populations that accompanies fertility and mortality declines, some contend that countries with older populations will lose political vigor, as well as military and economic strength. Countries with younger populations, in turn, are viewed as the source of more political turmoil. The manner in which population aging affects the political atmosphere of nations will thus likely be a focus of political demographers.

Teitelbaum also posits that population composition in terms of ethnic, socioeconomic, and geographical groups will likely be the subject of future research, as variations in these groups are thought to impact the distribution of political power. Population composition is intricately connected with immigration and fertility. Thus, Teitelbaum argues that future research in political demography will focus on the impact of immigration and declining fertility on population composition and, in turn, political power.

Fertility Planning

Despite significant advances in fertility planning, Potter and Mundigo observe that a number of areas remain ripe for improvement. The quality of contraceptive services and the use of such services remain stratified in many parts of the world, with the most disadvantaged less likely to use contraceptives, to receive quality services, or to have a variety of contraceptive choices. In addition, unwanted teenage pregnancy remains an issue of concern in many countries where adolescents lack access and/or information to fertility planning services.

In addition to these two widely publicized issues upon which future research should be focused, Potter and Mundigo contend that demographers should also focus on two other reproductive issues where the outcomes are perhaps less clear cut. Below-replacement-level fertility is occurring in European countries and in many East and Southeast Asian countries; there is no consensus, however, as to the cause of this phenomenon or whether it is a threat to the welfare of these countries. Potter and Mundigo thus see below-replacement-level fertility as an important area for future fertility planning research. Second, Potter and Mundigo recommend that future research focus on the dilemma confronting sub-Saharan Africa brought about by rapid population growth due to high fertility and large increases in mortality resulting from the HIV/AIDS epidemic. They suggest that the role of family planning programs in affecting reproductive patterns and treating and preventing HIV/AIDS should be a significant focus of fertility planning research in the coming years.

Small-Area and Business Demography

Smith and Morrison argue that the future of small area and business demography will be directed by a few recent developments in these fields. They first note that the increase of small-area data in the form of administrative records and sample surveys has played a large role in developing the field of small-area demography, as analyses in this field were previously limited by the available data. In addition, businesses have maintained data registries for customers that have created new data sources for studies in business demography. In particular, databases containing customer characteristics have permitted businesses to target consumers. Smith and Morrison note, however, that consumer privacy concerns might result in restrictions on the collection and sharing of such data in the future.

In addition to data developments, increased computer power has permitted the collection, storing, matching, and analysis of data that was once impossible or too costly for most researchers. The development of geographical information systems (GIS) has also aided in the collection and analysis of spatially referenced data, which Smith and Morrison contend is the most significant development in small-area and business demography.

Finally, Smith and Morrison note that business demography does not always focus on small areas; rather, global markets have resulted in new consumer markets all over the world, of which little is known about consumer behavior. Thus, business demographers will likely develop research on these new consumers in the coming years.

Health Demography

Kawachi and Subramanian suggest future areas of research in health demography. They note that future research will continue to develop linkages between the areas of demography and epidemiology. Techniques and measures that were once exclusively used by epidemiologists are now being incorporated into the research of demographers, including collecting biological specimens in longitudinal research and engaging in specific diagnoses of diseases in population surveys (Goldman 2001).

Epidemiologists, in turn, have increasingly looked to population-based samples, rather than clinical samples, and have incorporated social determinants of disease into their studies. Kawachi and Subramanian suggest that cross-disciplinary research will be increasingly important over the coming years, with the AIDS pandemic, population aging, and the increasing disparities between rich and poor countries.

Kawachi and Subramanian further suggest that health demographers will work toward improving methods of measuring, monitoring, and forecasting mortality and morbidity, perhaps focusing particularly on developing the measurement of morbidity and the health transition. In addition, they contend that health demographers will continue to attempt to refine models assessing the determinants of health, including incorporating contextual influences and a time dimension, i.e., health over the life course.

Demography of Population Health

In their chapter in this *Handbook*, Hayward and Warner observe that it is not a simple task to predict the manner in which disease will burden a population in future years because the epidemiological transition is ongoing. The transition is influenced by world-wide population aging, scientific and technological advancements in fighting disease, and advances in educational attainment and health knowledge. These forces will influence not only the epidemiological transition, but also the course of future research in population health, leading to both substantive and methodological advances in the field.

Population Policy

May notes in his chapter that the current demographic diversity of the world will play an important role in the future of population policy. Fertility ranges from very high to below replacement; populations are both young and, increasingly, aging; immigration is welcome in some countries and opposed in others; and countries fall at varying stages of the demographic transition, while the notion of the transition itself is challenged by forces such as the HIV/AIDS epidemic. Population policy will be an important factor in future decades, as the world confronts variation in demographic patterns and attitudes.

To emphasize the impact of diverse demographic patterns on population policy, May highlights the varying policies required by countries with different levels of fertility. In areas with high fertility, he suggests that population policies might need to focus primarily on family planning services. When fertility rates are between five children per woman and the replacement level, May contends that public health and social development interventions should complement the fertility transition. In many industrialized countries, where fertility has fallen below replacement levels, May suggests that a high priority will need to be placed on fertility, emphasizing migration policies in order to offset the aging effect of fertility and mortality declines.

In this way, May demonstrates the continuing importance of population policies, contending that population policy will be most effective with public consensus, a focus on dynamic concepts like equity, a participatory framework, and the incorporation of new data and research.

THREE ADDITIONAL AREAS REQUIRING ATTENTION

After reviewing and reporting the recommended directions for future research suggested by many of the *Handbook* chapter authors, we will now discuss the three areas we deem particularly relevant and important for demographic research in future years. These are areas that to date have received insufficient attention by demographers and, moreover, are areas considered to be preeminent in terms of their actual or potential contribution to the state of demographic knowledge: (1) male fertility; (2) biosocial models of demography; and (3) sexual orientation. This is a short, selective, and perhaps idiosyncratic listing. But these are areas that have impressed us as important, relevant, and challenging. It is not known whether other demographers will agree with the selection. Most probably will not.

Male Fertility

Why are males not included in the study of fertility? In discussions in both the scholarly and popular literatures, the methods and numbers pertaining to fertility rates almost always apply only to females but are referred to as fertility rates and fertility numbers, not as female fertility rates and female fertility numbers. In the development and testing of fertility theories in the demographic and social science literatures, the explanations are implicitly based on females but are referred to as fertility theories, not as female fertility theories.

But as everyone knows, biology dictates that females and males must both intimately be involved in the production of children. Fertility is not a process that only involves women. So, why are males ignored in conventional demographic studies of fertility? The answer is not because female and male fertility rates are the same. Although common sense suggests they should be, in fact they are not, and this is shown below.

Until the past few years virtually all conventional demographic research on fertility has been devoted to analyses of women. Until recently, meetings of the Population Association of America (PAA) and the International Union for the Scientific Study of Population (IUSSP) seldom included sessions on the male side of fertility. Indeed it has only been since the late 1990s that articles and book chapters on male fertility have started to appear in the demographic literature. In 1998 the journal *Demography* published a special issue on the topic of male reproduction. In 2000, a major paper appeared in the journal *Population and Development Review* (Greene and Biddlecom 2000) that evaluated current research and suggested directions for future research on male reproductive roles. Also in 2000, a monograph was published on *Fertility and the Male Life-Cycle in the Era of Fertility Decline* (Bledsoe, Lerner, and Guyer 2000), based in large part on the papers presented at a 1995 conference of the IUSSP.

POPLINE was recently consulted for a review of the literature on the topic of fertility. The POPLINE search reported over 75,000 fertility studies conducted between 1950 and 2000. Of these, only 381 dealt with fertility and reproduction behaviors involving males, two-thirds of which were biological and medical in orientation, focusing on such issues as spermatogenesis (e.g., Aitken et al. 1986) and medical and biological aspects of fertility regulation (Singh and Ratnam 1991). The other one-third was mainly comprised of papers investigating family planning policies (e.g., Adamchak and Adebayo 1987) and fertility regulation (Mbizvo and Adamchak 1992), male attitudes toward fertility and family planning, and economic considerations and cultural factors that shape male fertility (Muvandi 1995). Most of the fertility analyses uncovered in the POPLINE search that included males (often along with females) were published in the last decade.

So why has conventional demographic research in fertility concentrated largely if not exclusively on women? Seven specific reasons have been proposed to justify excluding males from fertility studies (Poston and Chang 2005). First, Greene and Biddlecom (2000: 83) write that the "most important barrier to the inclusion of men in demographic research was normative and reflected the socialization of influential demographers and the research course they set." Men were regarded principally as breadwinners, and "as typically uninvolved in fertility except to impregnate women and to stand in the way of their contraceptive use" (Greene and Biddlecom 2000: 83). This is a gender-related reason and focuses significantly on the social construction of the male gender role. This is not a biological reason but a sociological one. This is hardly a satisfactory reason for ignoring males in fertility studies.

Keyfitz (1977) notes (although does not necessarily endorse) four more reasons. Two of them are (1) data on parental age at the birth of a child are more frequently collected on registration certificates for the mothers than for the fathers and (2) when such data are obtained for mothers and fathers, there are more instances of unreported age data for fathers, especially for births occurring outside marriage.

While it is true that demographic surveys have tended to focus more on women than on men, this situation has improved significantly in recent years. Also, birth registration certificates, particularly in the developed world, now typically include data on both parents. Certificates for births occurring outside marriage, however, occasionally still omit data on fathers. Finally, Coleman (2000: 43) notes that as of 1995, 15 countries in the industrialized world have published, at one or more times in recent years, data and/or rates on male fertility in their demographic yearbooks or related publications.

The next two reasons mentioned by Keyfitz are (3) the fecundity, and hence, the childbearing years of women occur in a more sharply defined and narrower range (15 to 49) than they do for men (15 to 79); and (4) "both the spacing and number of children are less subject to variation among women; a woman can have children only at intervals of 1 or 2 years, whereas a man can have hundreds" (1977: 114). The third point is true theoretically, and indeed "in polygamous populations a man's fertility can remain high well into his fifties and sixties; ... [however], in controlled fertility societies, it peaks ... with a mode in the mid-twenties" (Coleman 2000: 41). This is due in part to low fertility norms in Western societies, as well as to a small average age difference of about two to three years between men and women in first marriages. Regarding the fourth point, Guyer (2000) observes that although biologically a man has the potential for siring dozens more children than a woman, this large difference in number of children ever born only occurs in a few societies and "amongst a tiny minority of the population" (2000: 64).

A fifth reason is that female fertility rates are thought to be more fundamental because they are more physiological; that is, they are more bound by biological limitations, and hence are more influenced by the proximate determinants than are male rates. Indeed several of the proximate determinants are virtually "man-free" (Coleman 2000: 31) and thus less traceable. Also "mothers remember events such as miscarriages and deaths in early childhood more clearly than fathers do, and there is no ambiguity as to whether a child is theirs or not" (Greene and Biddlecom 2000: 85). The fact that births are more traceable to mothers than to fathers cannot be ignored. But this fact makes it all the more necessary to include males in fertility studies, if only because by including males one would then be able to estimate the degree of false paternity in a population, a subject about which little is known. Moreover, Greene and Biddlecom (2000: 85) observe that "since demographers do not limit themselves to counting but also attempt to explain and predict fertility behavior, this methodological justification is patently weak."

A seventh reason proposed to justify the exclusion of men in studies of fertility is the incompatibility of male and female fertility rates. Unless the population is closed and has a stable age distribution, the rates will likely be different. The differential rates are due to a host of causes that are well known to demographers, some of which are that more males are born than females, males have higher age-specific death rates than

TABLE 1. Male and Female Total Fertility Rates: 1994

Country	Male TFR	Female TFR
Australia	1809	2724
Bulgaria	1306	1060
Canada	1567	1539
Denmark	1724	1770
Estonia	1258	1175
Hong Kong SAR	1252	1198
Hungary	1599	1476
Israel	3048	2815
Macao SAR	1655	1390
Mauritius	2243	2034
Panama	2899	2225
Poland	1722	1670
Puerto Rico	2248	1754
Romania	1433	1193
Singapore	1732	1764
Spain	1221	1171
Trinidad & Tobago	1951	1662
Tunisia	3391	2768
United States	1829	2030

females, males marry at older ages than females, males remarry more quickly than females, and emigration and immigration both are usually sex-selective. These and other factors act together to produce male and female fertility rates that are not the same.

The United Nations (2002) has assembled a natality database that includes age-specific fertility rates (ASFRs) for males and females for various years in the 1990s. Table 1 reports male and female total fertility rates for 1994 calculated for the 19 countries with male and female data. Figure 1 graphs these male and female TFRs. Most countries have male TFRs that are larger than their female TFRs. Tunisia and Panama show male TFRs that are 623 and 674 births, respectively, larger than their female TFRs. Among those few countries with larger female TFRs than male TFRs, Australia and the U.S. show the greatest differences, with female TFRs that are 915 and 201 births, respectively, larger than their male TFRs. Only a few countries, namely, Singapore, Canada, and Denmark, have male and female TFRs that are nearly equal (see Poston and Chang [2005] for a similar analysis of the counties of Taiwan).

The fact that male and female fertility rates are not the same makes it all the more important and necessary to analyze male fertility along with female fertility. The factors causing the differentials vary over time in their magnitude and effects on the male and female fertility rates. In some cases they may well be sex-specific and will not be realized or understood empirically unless both male and female rates are investigated.

Biosocial Models of Demography

This section is a review and commentary on what may be referred to as biosocial models of demography, i.e., the development of demographic models of human behavior that combine biological variables (for instance, hormonal levels and genetic factors, among other variables) with social variables to predict demographic outcomes, in particular,

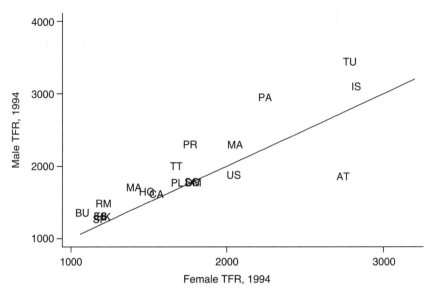

FIGURE 1. Male and female total fertility rates, 1994.

those outcomes or processes that are biological, viz., fertility and mortality. In chapter 21, BioDemography, Carey and Vaupel term this a subfield of what they call biomedical demography.

Aside from demographic studies of the proximate determinants of fertility, the incorporation of biological variables into explanatory models of demographic processes is not an activity to which demographers have devoted even a modest amount of attention. It is likely that there are proportionally more sociologists than demographers developing and testing biosocial models of human behavior. For whatever reasons, demographers have avoided such developments.

Casterline, one of a handful of demographers who recognize the importance of incorporating biological thinking into our theories of demography, observes that demographers "can no longer run away from biosocial models. ... It requires either extraordinary blindness or exceptional stubbornness to fail to recognize that fertility and mortality ... are determined in part by biological variables" (1995: 359).

It is Casterline's belief that after 1994, the "passive avoidance of biosocial models [among demographers] is no longer an option ... [owing to Richard Udry's presidential address in 1994 to the Population Association of America] challenging demographers to take biosocial models seriously" (1995: 360). In his address, Udry reported research showing that "one-fourth of the variance in women's 'gendered' behavior" is accounted for by a model comprised of "prenatal and adult androgen measures and their interaction" (Udry 1994: 570). This research (Udry, Morris, and Kovenock 1995: 367) concludes that "gendered behavior is not entirely socially constructed, but partly built on a biological foundation."

A recent review of the demographic literature found very few examples of empirical research incorporating biological and social variables in models of demographic processes. Carey and Vaupel's chapter in this *Handbook* supports this observation.

Udry is a demographer who over the years has developed and tested biosocial models of demographic outcomes. He has published several papers introducing "biosocial models of adolescent sexuality that combine traditional sociological models with models derived from a biological theory of hormone effects" (1988: 709; see also Udry, Talbert, and Morris 1986). Weller (1995) notes that just because Udry claims that a "behavior has biological foundations [does not mean he believes] it does not also have social foundations" (1995: 281).

Here is a hypothetical equation, proposed by Casterline (1995: 360):

$$D_i = hB_i + sS_i + c(B_i * S_i) + e_i$$

where D is some demographic outcome, B is a vector of biological variables, S is a vector of social variables, h and s are vectors of parameters to be estimated indicating the effects of the biological and social variables, e is a disturbance, and the subscript i refers to individuals.

In the first place, much of demography assumes the parameter h not to be significantly different from zero. Casterline (1995: 361) states that the "denial of the existence of parameter h ... [is] now amply refuted by empirical scientific evidence ... Scientists ... must acknowledge that a substantial and solid body of evidence supports the proposition that individual variation in many behaviors is biologically driven.... The challenge for scientists is to determine the magnitude of parameter h."

In Casterline's equation, the biological and social variables may be considered as additive and as interacting. The $B_i * S_i$ interaction would posit that the "effect of biological variables is conditioned by the level of social variables" (Casterline 1995: 361), a point made also by Udry (1994; see also Udry 1995).

Casterline (1995) and Udry (1994, 1996) both admit that biosocial models will possibly have no role in many demographic studies. Casterline (1995: 368) observes that "a large fraction of the central research questions in social demography concerns secular change and/or macro/societal variation, and hence it is not clear that much attention need be given [in such analyses] to biological variables." The role of biosocial models in demography thus depends greatly on the demographic outcome being investigated. Given the results of Udry and several others regarding the empirical importance of biological variables as predictors of certain types of demographic outcomes, it is concluded that demographers can no longer afford to ignore the potential of biological predictors of them.

Sexual Orientation

Policymakers are increasingly focusing attention on issues concerning the gay and lesbian community. This recent surge in interest may be attributed partly to judicial decisions seen as victories for homosexuals, including the Supreme Court's decision striking down the Texas law against same-sex sodomy and the Massachusetts Supreme Court's ruling that the state constitution requires the state to give same-sex couples marriage rights equal to those of opposite-sex couples (*Lawrence et al. v. Texas* 2003; *Goodridge et al. v. Department of Public Health* 2003). In the coming years, policymakers are likely to look to demographers and other social scientists to provide information on the homosexual community to aid them in constructing arguments for or against certain policies. At the present time, however, little demographic work has been done in the area of sexual orientation. Many questions are just beginning to be explored and some remain virtually untouched.

The demography of sexual orientation remains underdeveloped due in large part to a lack of representative datasets with samples of sufficient size to answer many of the questions that researchers would like to ask about the homosexual community. Many of the larger surveys conducted of the homosexual population were surveys of convenience, such as those drawn from readership of magazines or newspapers (see the discussion of Black et al. [2000]). Thus, U.S. researchers seeking representative samples of the gay and lesbian population have turned predominantly to the General Social Survey (GSS), the National Health and Social Life Survey (NHSLS), and the census to explore research questions. Studies conducted using either the GSS or the NHSLS are limited due to the small number of individuals captured in these surveys who either identify as homosexual or who report having engaged in sexual activity with a same-sex partner. In the NHSLS, for instance, the sample consists of 3,432 American men and women but includes only 12 women and 27 men who identify as homosexual. And it includes only 32 women and 45 men who either identify as homosexual and/or had exclusively same-sex sex partners in the past year. Sample sizes such as these are far too small to conduct many analyses of the homosexual population of interest to demographers, such as their distributions across cities, states, or occupations.

Beginning in 1990, however, the U.S. Census Bureau introduced a change on the long-form questionnaire that resulted in the creation of a large dataset of same-sex individuals. The Bureau offered respondents the option of identifying individuals living in the household as unmarried partners after studies indicated the increasing number of opposite-sex and same-sex individuals living in marriage-like relationships in the United States (Black et al. 2000). The unmarried partner category permits unmarried heterosexual and homosexual couples to identify themselves as a couple. In the 2000 Census, 1,188,782 individuals identified themselves as being in same-sex unmarried partner households on the census, 605,052 being male and 586,730 being female (Simmons and O'Connell 2003). The addition of this category to the census has opened the door for social scientists to explore a number of issues relating to homosexuals that were previously out of reach due to the paucity of data.[1]

Surprisingly, however, little research has been conducted in this area to date, despite the availability of the census data for both 1990 and 2000. And the work that has been done has been dominated by economists rather than demographers. There are a number of important areas of research in the area of sexual orientation, however, in which demographers and other social scientists can and should play an important role in the coming years.

One of the primary concerns of policymakers in both formulating policy goals and determining their impacts will center on the places in which gays and lesbians are located within the country. Data from the 1990 and 2000 U.S. censuses indicate that there are concentrations of gays and lesbians in virtually all the metropolitan areas of the country. However, with but a few exceptions (Black et al. 2000, 2002; Walther and Poston 2004; Poston, Gu, and Walther 2003; Gates and Ost 2004), there has been little

---

[1] Findings based on census data are limited, however, in that only individuals who choose to identify as unmarried partners on the census are captured; thus, individuals who prefer not to self-identify are not counted. Further, the census question allows data to be collected only on partnered homosexuals living in the same household, leaving homosexuals who are single unaccounted for. Nonetheless, the advantages of the census data over other data sources render the census an attractive source for research on homosexuals, and studies attempting to quantify the extent of possible bias have concluded that the problem is not so severe as to warrant abstaining from using census data.

effort among social scientists at indexing these concentrations among the metropolitan areas of the U.S. and examining the extent to which the indexes are associated with the social, ecological, and political characteristics of the areas. Preliminary research using 2000 data indicate that in most metropolitan areas the levels of concentrations of partnered lesbians are higher than those of partnered gays. San Francisco is an outlier, with many more partnered gays per 1,000 never married males than partnered lesbians per 1,000 never married females. Most metropolitan areas show the opposite. Limited research also indicates that ecological characteristics of metropolitan areas reflecting amenities of interest to both homosexuals and heterosexuals are more associated with the levels of homosexual prevalence than are characteristics pertaining to factors important only for homosexuals (Black et al. 2002; Poston, Gu, and Walther 2003). Even less quantitative research has been undertaken regarding the differential concentration of partnered gays and lesbians in the nonmetropolitan and rural areas of the U.S. (Poston and Gu 2004).

Another area of homosexual demography in which there is a major research void is residential segregation. Demographers have paid virtually no attention to patterns of residential segregation of homosexuals from married and unmarried heterosexuals (Compton and Poston 2004). Preliminary research indicates that levels of segregation of homosexuals (gays and lesbians treated separately) from unmarried and married heterosexuals are sizable, that lesbians are less segregated from heterosexuals than are gays, and that gays and lesbians are segregated from each other. Extensive demographic research on racial residential segregation of black and Hispanic minorities from the white majority indicates that the segregation is largely involuntary. Early research on the segregation of homosexuals from heterosexuals suggests that the segregation may be both involuntary and voluntary, but considerable work remains sorting out these differences and estimating statistical models to explain them.

For decades, U.S. politicians have been proposing the adoption of a federal law prohibiting discrimination in employment on the basis of sexual orientation. Policy-makers might turn to social science research to answer important questions in assessing whether such a law is necessary: Do homosexuals earn less than heterosexuals? Are homosexuals segregated into different occupations than heterosexuals? The majority of studies examining homosexuality and work have focused on the relationship between sexual orientation and income. Once controls are introduced for individual characteristics, most research finds that gay men earn less than heterosexual men (Badgett 1995; Klawitter and Flatt 1998; Black et al. 2003). Findings about the earnings of lesbians are mixed, with some studies indicating lesbians earn less than heterosexual women, and others finding little or no difference (Badgett 1995; Klawitter and Flatt 1998). Research is ongoing concerning income differences between homosexuals and heterosexuals, but there is no clear consensus as to the cause of the income differences if they do exist.

Badgett (1995) finds that occupational differences account for some of the income differences between homosexuals and heterosexuals. Occupational segregation, therefore, is another area in which future research needs to be conducted in assessing whether inequalities exist in the workplace between homosexuals and heterosexuals. Baumle (2004) has explored the manner in which homosexuals and heterosexuals are segregated in professional occupations. She finds that partnered homosexuals are overrepresented in the professions as a whole, and appear to be concentrated within fields that are focused on creativity, psychology/counseling, and law/social work. Partnered homosexuals are underrepresented primarily in the engineering and teaching professions.

Additional research needs to be conducted to determine the cause of such occupational segregation, as well as to examine segregation in occupations outside of the professions.

Finally, the debate concerning the legal right of homosexual couples to marriage is one that is virtually global (Merin 2002). There are few places in which homosexuals have been granted marriage rights equal to those of heterosexuals, and family rights vary widely both within and between countries. In order to provide guidance to legislators in formulating marriage and family laws, demographers must develop a literature about the family practices of homosexuals. What is the average length of a homosexual relationship? How prevalent is childrearing among lesbian and gay couples? Do lesbian and gay couples predominantly adopt or raise their own children? These questions, and others, are important to address if demographers and policy makers are to understand the manner in which laws and social policies are to be constructed to address the needs of the homosexual population.

In the above and last section of this Epilogue, three broad areas of demographic research have been proposed requiring major conceptual and methodological advances. They represent challenges to demographers in that strictly speaking they are not mainstream. They require demographers to not undertake fertility analyses that are only based on females, to not estimate demographic models that are only based on social variables, and to not restrict their investigations, implicitly or explicitly, to heterosexuals. According to Horton (1999: 365), an important characteristic of "critical demography," as opposed to "conventional demography," is the posing of "questions that challenge the prevailing social order." In some ways demographic research in the areas outlined above may well challenge existing demographic paradigms.

Finally, the areas and topics presented here comprise a short and very selective list. There are certainly other areas of research requiring the future attention of demographers. Many of them have been discussed in the chapters of this *Handbook* and summarized in an earlier section of this Epilogue.

It was noted earlier in this Epilogue that most of the needed research areas identified in 1959 by the authors of chapters in *The Study of Population* have indeed been addressed in the intervening 45 years. It will be of interest to see several decades from now whether the authors of chapters in this *Handbook* have been as prescient.

REFERENCES

Ackerman, E. A. 1959. Geography and demography. In *The study of population: An inventory and appraisal.* Edited by P. M. Hauser and O. D. Duncan, 717–727. Chicago: University of Chicago Press.

Adamchak, D. J., and A. Adebayo. 1987. Male fertility attitudes: A neglected dimension in Nigerian fertility research. *Social Biology* 34: 57–67.

Aitken R. J., S. Irvine, J. S. Clarkson, and D. W. Richardson. 1986. Predictive value of in vitro sperm function tests. In *Male contraception: Advances and future prospects.* Edited by G. I. Zatuchni, A. Goldsmith, J. M. Spieler, and J. J. Sciarra, 138–151. Philadelphia: Harper & Row.

Badgett, M. V. L. 1995. The wage effects of sexual orientation discrimination. *Industrial and Labor Relations Review* 48: 726–739.

Banister, J. 1987. *China's changing population.* Palo Alto, Calif.: Stanford University Press.

Baumle, A. K. 2004. Sexual orientation and the professions: Occupational segregation and the effect of state antidiscrimination laws. Paper presented at the annual meeting of the Southwestern Sociological Association, Corpus Christi, Texas, March 17–20.

Black, D., G. Gates, S. Sanders, and L. Taylor. 2000. Demographics of the gay and lesbian population in the United States: Evidence from available systematic data sources. *Demography* 37: 138–154.

Black, D., G. Gates, S. Sanders, and L. Taylor. 2002. Why do gay men live in San Francisco? *Journal of Urban Economics* 51: 54–76.

Black, D., H. R. Makar, S. Sanders, and L. Taylor. 2003. The earnings effects of sexual orientation. *Industrial and Labor Relations Review* 56: 449–469.

Bledsoe, C., S. Lerner, and J. I. Guyer, eds. 2000. *Fertility and the male life-cycle in the era of fertility decline.* New York: Oxford University Press.

Bogue, D. J. 1959a. Internal migration. In *The study of population: An inventory and appraisal.* Edited by P. M. Hauser and O. D. Duncan, 486–509. Chicago: University of Chicago Press.

Bogue, D. J. 1959b. Population distribution. In *The study of population: An inventory and appraisal.* Edited by P. M. Hauser and O. D. Duncan, 383–399. Chicago: University of Chicago Press.

Bongaarts, J., and R. A. Bulatao, eds. 2000. *Beyond six billion: Forecasting the world's population.* Washington, D.C.: NAS Press.

Bongaarts, J., and S. C. Watkins. 1996. Social interactions and contemporary fertility transitions. *Population and Development Review* 22: 639–682.

Carr, R. V., J. D. Wright, and C. J. Brody. 1996. Effects of high school work experience a decade later: Evidence from the National Longitudinal Survey. *Sociology of Education* 69: 66–81.

Casterline, J. B. 1995. Biosocial models: Can demographers ignore them? *Population Research and Policy Review* 14: 359–371.

Chandrasekaran, C. 1959. Survey of the status of demography in India. In *The study of population: An inventory and appraisal.* Edited by P. M. Hauser and O. D. Duncan, 249–254. Chicago: University of Chicago Press.

Coleman, D. A. 2000. Male fertility trends in industrial countries: Theories in search of some evidence. *Fertility and the male life-cycle in the era of fertility decline.* Edited by in C. Bledsoe, S. Lerner, and J. I. Guyer, 29–60. New York: Oxford University Press.

Compton, D., and D. L. Poston, Jr. 2004. The residential segregation of homosexuals from heterosexuals in American cities in 2000. Paper presented at the annual meeting of the American Sociological Association, San Francisco, August 14–17.

Costanzo, A. 1959. Contributions of Italy to demography. In *The study of population: An inventory and appraisal.* Edited by P. M. Hauser and O. D. Duncan, 217–234. Chicago: University of Chicago Press.

Crutchfield, R. D., and S. R. Pitchford. 1997. Work and crime: The effects of labor stratification. *Social Forces* 76: 93–118.

Deseran, F. A., and D. Keithly. 1994. Teenagers in the U.S. labor force: Local labor markets, race, and family. *Rural Sociology* 59;4 (Winter): 668–692.

Dorn, H. F. 1959. Mortality. *The study of population: An inventory and appraisal.* Edited by P. M. Hauser and O. D. Duncan, 437–471. Chicago: University of Chicago Press.

Duncan, O. D. 1959. Human ecology and population studies. In *The study of population: An inventory and appraisal.* Edited by P. M. Hauser and O. D. Duncan, 678–716. Chicago: University of Chicago Press.

Duncan, O. D. 1961. From social system to ecosystem. *Sociological Inquiry* 31: 140–49.

Duncan, O. D. 1964. Social organization and the ecosystem. In *Handbook of modern sociology.* Edited by R. E. L. Faris, 37–82. Chicago: Rand-McNally.

Fitch, C. A., and S. Ruggles. 2000. Historical trends in marriage formation: The United States 1850–1990. In Ties that bind: Perspectives on marriage and cohabitation. Edited by L. Waite, C. Bachrach, M. Hindin, E. Thomson, and A. Thornton, 59–90. New York: Aldine de Gruyter.

Frank, P. W. 1959. Ecology and demography. In *The study of population: An inventory and appraisal.* Edited by P. M. Hauser and O. D. Duncan, 652–677. Chicago: University of Chicago Press.

Gates, G. J., and J. Ost. 2004. *The gay and lesbian atlas.* Washington, D.C.: The Urban Institute Press.

Gibbs, J. P., and W. T. Martin. 1959. Toward a theoretical system of human ecology. *Pacific Sociological Review* 2: 29–36.

Glick, P. C. 1959. Family statistics. In *The study of population: An inventory and appraisal.* Edited by P. M. Hauser and O. D. Duncan, 576–603. Chicago: University of Chicago Press.

Goldman, N. 2001. Social inequalities in health. Disentangling the underlying mechanisms. In *Population health and aging: Strengthening the dialogue between epidemiology and demography.* Edited by M. Weinstein, A. I. Hermalin, and M. A. Stoto, 118–139. Annals of the New York Academy of Sciences, Vol. 954.

Goldstein, J. R., and C. T. Kenney. 2001. Marriage delayed or marriage forgone? New cohort forecasts of first marriage for U.S. women. *American Sociological Review* 66: 506–519.

Goodridge et al. v. Department of Public Health, 798 N. E. 2d 941 (Mass. 2003).

Grebenik, E. 1959. The development of demography in Great Britain. In *The study of population: An inventory and appraisal*. Edited by P. M. Hauser and O. D. Duncan, 190–202. Chicago: University of Chicago Press.

Greene, M. E., and A. E. Biddlecom. 2000. Absent and problematic men: Demographic accounts of male reproductive roles. *Population and Development Review* 26: 81–115.

Guyer, J. I. 2000. Traditions of studying paternity in social anthropology. In *Fertility and the male life-cycle in the era of fertility decline*. Edited by C. Bledsoe, S. Lerner, and J. I. Guyer, 61–90. New York: Oxford University Press.

Hauser, P. M., and O. D. Duncan, eds. 1959. *The study of population: An inventory and appraisal*. Chicago: University of Chicago Press.

Hawley, A. H. 1950. *Human ecology: A theory of community structure*. New York: Ronald Press.

Hirschman, C., P. Kasinitz, and J. Dewind, eds. 1999. *The handbook of international migration*. New York: Russell Sage Foundation.

Horton, H. D. 1999. Critical demography: The paradigm of the future? *Sociological Forum* 14: 363–367.

Jaffe, A. J. 1959. Working force. In *The study of population: An inventory and appraisal*. Edited by P. M. Hauser and O. D. Duncan, 604–620. Chicago: University of Chicago Press.

Keyfitz, N. 1977. *Applied mathematical demography*. New York: John Wiley & Sons.

Klawitter, M. M. 1998. The determinants of earnings for women in same-sex and different-sex couples. Paper prepared for presentation at Allied Social Science Associations meetings, Chicago, January 1998.

Klawitter, M. M., and V. Flatt. 1998. The effects of state and local antidiscrimination policies on earnings for gays and lesbians. *Journal of Policy Analysis and Management* 17: 658–686.

Lawrence et al. v. Texas, 123 S. Ct. 2472 (2003).

Lillard, L. A., and L. Waite. 1995. Til death do us part: Marital disruption and mortality. *American Journal of Sociology* 100(Mar): 1131–1156.

Martin, J. A., B. E. Hamilton, S. J. Ventura, F. Menacker, and M. M. Park. 2002. Births: Final data for 2000. *National Vital Statistics Reports*. Vol. 50, No. 5. Hyattsville, Md.: National Center for Health Statistics.

Mbizvo, M. T., and D. J. Adamchak. 1992. Male fertility regulation: A study on acceptance among men in Zimbabwe. *Central African Journal of Medicine* 38: 52–57.

Menn, Y. 2002. Equality for Same-Sex Couples: The Legal Recognition of Gay Partnerships in Europe and the United States. Chicago, IL: University of Chicago.

Micklin, M. 1973. Introduction: A framework for the study of human ecology. In *Population, environment and social organization: Current issues in human ecology*. Edited by M. Micklin, 2–19. Hinsdale, Il.: Dryden Press.

Micklin, M., and D. L. Poston, Jr., eds. 1998. *Continuities in sociological human ecology*. New York: Plenum Press.

Micklin, M., and D. F. Sly. 1998. The ecological complex: A conceptual elaboration. In M. Micklin and D. L. Poston, Jr., eds. *Continuities in sociological human ecology*. New York: Plenum Press.

Moore, W. E. 1959. Sociology and demography. In *The study of population: An inventory and appraisal*. Edited by P. M. Hauser and O. D. Duncan, 832–851. Chicago: University of Chicago Press.

Mortara, G. 1959. Demographic studies in Brazil. In *The study of population: An inventory and appraisal*. Edited by P. M. Hauser and O. D. Duncan, 235–244. Chicago: University of Chicago Press.

Muvandi, I. 1995. Determinants of male fertility and sexual behaviour in Kenya. Centre for African Family Studies [CAFS], *CAFS Research Reports*, Series No. 2.

Namboodiri, K. 1988. Ecological demography: Its place in sociology. *American Sociological Review* 53: 619–633.

Namboodiri, K. 1994. The human ecological approach to the study of population dynamics. *Population Index* 60: 517–539.

National Research Council. 2001. *Preparing for an aging world: The case for cross-national research*. Washington, D.C.: National Academies Press.

Peng, X. Z., and Z. G. Guo, eds. 2000. *The changing population of China*. Malden, Mass.: Blackwell.

Poston, D. L., Jr. 2002. South Korea's demographic destiny: Marriage market and elderly support implications for the 21st century. In *International conference on the longevity and social, medical environment of the elderly*, 69–83. Taegu, South Korea: Institute of Gerontology, Yeungnam University.

Poston, D. L., Jr., and C. F. Chang. 2005. Bringing males in: A critical demographic plea for incorporating males in methodological and theoretical analyses of human fertility. *Critical Demography*, forthcoming.

Poston, D. L., Jr., and C. C. Duan. 2000. The current and projected distribution of the elderly and eldercare in the People's Republic of China. *Journal of Family Issues* 21: 714–732.

Poston, D. L., Jr., and W. P. Frisbie. 1998. Human ecology, sociology and demography. In *Continuities in sociological human ecology*. Edited by M. Micklin and D. L. Poston, Jr., 27–50. New York: Plenum Press.

Poston, D. L., Jr., W. P. Frisbie, and M. Micklin. 1984. Sociological human ecology: Theoretical and conceptual perspectives. In *Sociological human ecology: Contemporary issues and applications*. Edited by M. Micklin and H. M. Choldin, 91–123. Boulder, Cols.: Westview.

Poston, D. L., Jr., and K. S. Glover. 2005. China's demographic destiny: Marriage market implications for the 21st century. In *Fertility, family planning and population policy in China*. Edited by D. L. Poston, Jr., C. Lee, C. Chang, S. L. McKibben, and C. S. Walther. London: Routledge Publishers, forthcoming.

Poston, D. L., Jr., and Y. Gu. 2004. Patterns of homosexuality in the nonmetropolitan areas of the United States in 2000. Paper presented at the annual meeting of the Rural Sociological Society, Sacramento, August 12–14.

Poston, D. L., Jr., Y. Gu, and C. S. Walther. 2003. The ecology of homosexuality. Paper presented at the annual meeting of the Southern Demographic Association, Washington, D.C., October 23–25.

Poston, D. L., Jr., and D. Yaukey, eds. 1992. *The population of modern China*. New York: Plenum Press.

Rogers, R. G. 1995. Marriage, sex, and mortality. *Journal of Marriage and the Family* 57(2): 515–526.

Rogers, R. G., R. A. Hummer, and C. B. Nam. 2000. *Living and dying in the USA: Behavioral, health, and social differentials of adult mortality*. San Diego, Calif.: Academic Press.

Rosenzweig, M. R., and O. Stark. 1997. Handbook of population and family economics. In *Handbooks in economics*. Edited by K. J. Arrow and M. D. Intriligator. Amsterdam: Elsevier.

Ryder, N. B. 1959. Fertility. In *The study of population: An inventory and appraisal*. Edited by P. M. Hauser and O. D. Duncan, 400–436. Chicago: University of Chicago Press.

Sauvy, A. 1959. Development and perspectives of demographic research in France. In *The study of population: An inventory and appraisal*. Edited by P. M. Hauser and O. D. Duncan, 180–189. Chicago: University of Chicago Press.

Schnore, L. F. 1958. Social morphology and human ecology. *American Journal of Sociology* 63: 620–634.

Schnore, L. F. 1961. The myth of human ecology. *Sociological Inquiry* 31: 128–139.

Schubnell, H. 1959. Demography in Germany. In *The study of population: An inventory and appraisal*. Edited by P. M. Hauser and O. D. Duncan, 203–216. Chicago: University of Chicago Press.

Simmons, T., and M. O'Connell. 2003. Married couple and unmarried-partner households: 2000. *Census 2000 Special Reports*. CENSR-5. Washington, D.C.: U.S. Census Bureau.

Singh, K., and S. S. Ratnam. 1991. New developments in contraceptive technology. *Advances in Contraception* 7: 137–157.

Spengler, J. J. 1959. Economics and demography. In *The study of population: An inventory and appraisal*. Edited by P. M. Hauser and O. D. Duncan, 791–831. Chicago: University of Chicago Press.

Taeuber, I. B. 1959. Demographic research in the Pacific area. In *The study of population: An inventory and appraisal*. Edited by P. M. Hauser and O. D. Duncan, 259–285. Chicago: University of Chicago Press.

Thomas, B. 1959. International migration. In *The study of population: An inventory and appraisal*. Edited by P. M. Hauser and O. D. Duncan, 510–543. Chicago: University of Chicago Press.

Udry, J. R. 1988. Biological predispositions and social control in adolescent sexual behavior. *American Sociological Review* 53: 709–722.

Udry, J. R. 1994. The nature of gender. *Demography* 31: 561–573.

Udry, J. R. 1995. Policy and ethical implications of biosocial research. *Population Research and Policy Review* 14: 347–357.

Udry, J. R. 1996. Biosocial models of low-fertility societies. In Fertility in the United States: New patterns, New theories. Edited by J. B. Casterline, R. D. Lee, and K. A. Foote, 325–336. *Population and Development Review* 22 (Supplement).

Udry, J. R., N. M. Morris, and J. Kovenock. 1995. Androgen effects on women's gendered behavior. *Journal of Biosocial Science* 27: 359–368.

Udry, J. R., L. M. Talbert, and N. M. Morris. 1986. Biosocial foundations for adolescent female sexuality. *Demography* 23: 217–230.

United Nations. 2002. *Demographic yearbook, natality statistics*. CD-ROM Special Topic, DYB-CD, No. E/F.02.XII. 6. New York: United Nations.

Waite, L. J. 1995. Does marriage matter? *Demography* 32:483–508.

Walther, C. S., and D. L. Poston, Jr. 2004. Patterns of gay and lesbian partnering in the larger metropolitan areas of the United States. *Journal of Sex Research* 41: 201–214.

Weller, R. 1995. Biosocial models of demographic behavior: An introduction. *Population Research and Policy Review* 14: 277–282.

Name Index

Abbott, A., 2n.4, *13*
Abiodun, J. O., 482, 487, 488, 490, 493, 494, 499, 501, *515*
Abler, R. F., 482, *515*
Abrahamse, A. F., 763, 774, 775, *782, 783*
Abrahamson, M., 501, *515*
Abrahamson, P. R., 440, *442*
Abraido-Lanza, A. F., 178, *198*
Abrams, B., 270, *279*
Acevedo-Garcia, D., 798, *805*
Ackerman, E. A., 417, *418*, 857, *878*
Adamchak, D. J., 871, *878, 880*
Adams, J. S., 482, 515, *515*, 633, *650*
Adebayo, A., 871, *878*
Adelman, R. M., 437, *448*
Adelstein, A. M., 266, 270, *280*
Adler, E. S., 211, 220, *222*
Adler, N. E., 294, 295, *305*
Adnan, S., 835, *849*
Aguayo, S., 723, *730*
Aguirre, B. E., 172, 183, 184, 192, *202, 204*
Ahlburg, D. A., 6, *13*, 162, *166*, 408, *410*, 563, 564, *571, 573*
Aitken, R. J., 871, *878*
Akerman, S., 581, *596*
Alba, F., 750, 751, *757*
Alba, R. D., 182–183, 186, *199, 202*, 385, *410*, 433, 434, 440, *442, 445, 446*, 506, *515*
Alberts, S. C., 627, *650*
Albrecht, S. L., 270, *277*
Alcoff, L., 130, *135*
Alderson, A. S., 211, *224*, 408, *414*
Alexander, G. R., 259, 272–273, *277*
Alexandersson, G., 488, *515*

Alihan, M. A., 602, *619*
Alker, H. A., Jr., 797, *805*
Allen, W., 174, *199*
Allison, P. D., 685, *712*
Allman, K. M., 173, *199*
Almeida, C., 802, *805*
Almgren, G., 262, *279*, 438, *445*
Alonso, W., 480, *515, 518*
Alter, G., 581, *596*
Altmann, J., 627, *650*
Altonji, J. G., 399, *410*, 552, 554, *571*
Alva, S., 119, *136*
Alvirez, D., 194, *204*
Alwin, D. F., 439, *445*
Amburgey, T. L., 458, 466, *473*
Amey, C., 295, *309*
Anas, A., 480, 492, 508, *515*
Anderson, B., 585, *597*
Anderson, B. A., 174, 177, *199*
Anderson, E., 501, *515*
Anderson, G. F., 158, *164*
Anderson, J. E., 738, *757*
Anderson, M., 585, *596*
Anderson, M. J., 423, *442*, 723, *729*, 767, *782*
Anderson, R. N., 184, *199*, 285, 292, 293, 303, *305*
Anderton, D. L., 581, 588, *596*
Andreas, P., 354, *378*
Andrews, P., 646, *656*
Andrews, W. W., 267, *279*
Anker, R., 123, *135*
Aparicio, R., 750, *757*
Appelbaum, M., 17, *18*
Appelbaum, R. P., 358, *378*
Appleby, A. B., 582, *596*

Appold, S. J., 211, *222*, 490, *516*
Arel, D., 21, *57*, 532n, *545*
Arias, E., 177, 178, *199*
Armer, J. M., 439, *447*
Armstrong, J. S., 773, *782*
Armstrong, R. J., 291, *305*
Arno, P. S., 159, *164*
Arnold, F., 51, *55*
Arnott, R., 480, 492, 508, *515*
Arriaga, E. E., 33, 38, 44, *55*
Arrizabalaga, J., 589, *596*
Arthur, W. B., 690, *712*
Artis, J. E., 160, *166*
Arum, R., 383–384, *413*
Ashenfelter, O., 399–400, *410–411*
Askew, I., 756, *757*
Attanasio, O. P., 552, *571*
Audia, P. G., 466, *477*
Auerbach, A. J., 551–552, 556, *571*
Ault, A. B., 800, *806*
Austad, S. N., 628, 646–647, *650*
Avakame, E. F., 212, *221*
Averitt, R. T., 356, *378*
Axinn, W. G., 94, 101, *105*
Axtell, R., 498n, 508, *517*
Aykan, H., 157, *165*

Baccaini, B., 313, 314, *342*
Bacci, A. L., 628, *650*
Bach, R. L., 357, *380*
Bachi, R., 38, *55*
Bachrach, C., 91, 92, *105*, 113, 130, *135*, 627, *650*
Back, K., 7, *14*
Backlund, E., 383, *413*
Badgett, M. V. L., 877, *878*
Bagnall, R. S., 583, *596*

Bahr, H. M., 502, *515*
Bailey, M., 273, *282*
Bailey, S., 354, *379*
Bailey, T., 356, *378*
Balakrishnan, T. R., 100, 102, *108*
Balcazar, H., 258, *277*
Baldassare, M., 77, *84*
Balk, D., 114, 115, 124, *135*
Banaszak-Holl, J., 466, *475*
Bane, M. J., 404, 405n, *411*
Banerjee, B., 325, *342*
Banfield, E., 404, *411*
Banister, J., 51, *55*, 839, *849*, 855,
    878
Banja, F., 542, *543*
Banks, J. E., 629, *656*
Barber, J. S., 94, *105*
Barcikowski, R. S., 797, *805*
Barclay, G. W., 13, *13*
Bardet, J. P., 580, 595, *596*
Barendregt, J. J., 816, 819, *822*
Barker, D. P. J., 627, *650*
Barley, S. R., 220, *224*
Barnett, W. P., 453–455, 457, 458,
    458n, 459, 464–466, *473, 476*
Baron, J. N., 453, 454, 457, 468, *473*
Barrett, M., 116, 129, 130, *135*
Barro, R. J., 553, 557, *571*
Barron, D. N., 458n, 459, 471, *473,
    474*
Barth, E. A. T., 502, *515*
Bartholomew, G. A., 626, *650*
Barton, N. H., 635, *655*
Basch, L., 539, *544*
Basu, A., 120, *136*
Basu, K., 120, *136*
Batliwala, S., 117, *141*
Battaglia, F. C., 258, *277*
Bauer, J., 211, *221*
Baum, C. L., 218, *221*
Baum, J. A. C., 466, *474*
Bauman, K. J., 384, *411*
Baumer, E. P., 437, 438, *442*
Baumle, A. K., 877, *878*
Bawah, A., 112, *136*
Baydar, N., 315, *342*
Bayer, P., 507, *515*
Beaglehole, R., 800, *805*
Beale, C. L., 606, 613, *619, 620*
Bean, F. D., 151, *164*, 183, 186, *199*,
    205, 347n, 354, 361, 363–365,
    369–372, 377, *378, 379, 382*
Bean, L. L., 581, 588, *596*
Bean, R., 356, *381*
Beck, E. M., 356, *381*, 502, *515, 524*
Becker, C. M., 295, *305*, 312, *342*
Becker, G., 531, *543*

Becker, G. S., 90, *105*, 355, *378*, 550,
    553–556, *571*
Beeson, P. E., 762, *782*
Begon, M., 628, *650*
Behrman, J. R., 383, *414*
Behrman, R. E., 273, *282*
Belanger, A., 816, 819, 820, *825*
Bell, F. C., 160, *164*
Bell, G., 628, 636, *650*
Bell, M., 329, *342*
Bell, W., 501, 507, *515, 523*
Bell-Rose, S., 365, *378*
Ben-Porath, Y., 554, *571*
Ben-Shlomo, Y., 793, *805, 806*
Bendix, R., 386, 391, *414*
Bener'ia, L., 215, *221*
Bengtsson, T., 581, *596*
Benitez-Zenteno, R., 750, *757*
Benneh, G., 831, *849*
Bennett, J. W., 527, *543*
Bennett, N. G., 101, *105*, 267, *278*,
    695, 697, 698, *712, 716*
Berelson, B., 744, *757*, 831, 833, 834,
    849
Berer, M., 756, *757*
Berg, E. J., 325, *342*
Berg, R. R., 183, *199*, 363, *378*
Bergmann, B. R., 406, *411*
Berhanu, B., 124, *138*
Berkman, L. F., 298, *305*, 787–792,
    796, 804, *805, 806*
Berkson, J., 684, *712*
Bernadelli, H., 685, *712*
Bernhardt, E. M., 17, *18*
Bernheim, B. D., 557, *571*
Bernstam, M. S., 809, *823*
Berry, B. J. L., 481–482, 487, 488,
    490, 493–495, 499, 501, 502,
    511, *515*, 602, 615, *619*
Bertazzi, P. A., 762, *782*
Berube, A., 67, *85*
Bhopal, R., 254, *278*
Bianchi, S., 112, *136*, 217, *222*
Biblarz, T. J., 93, *107*
Biddlecom, A. E., 112, *137*, 871,
    872, *880*
Bideau, A., 588, *599*
Bielby, W. T., 402, *411*
Bigelow, L. S., 464, *474*
Billari, F. C., 243, *247*, 755, *758*
Billy, J. O. G., 387n, *414*
Bilsborrow, R. E., 318, 319, 323,
    325, *342*
Binkin, N. J., 269, *282*
Biraben, J. N., 582, 589, *596*
Birch, L. C., 645, *650*
Bird, A., 454, *477*

Bird, C. E., 277, *279*
Birdsall, N., 835, 836, *849*
Birke, L., 110, *136*
Black, D., 103, *105*, 480, *515*, 876,
    877, *878–879*
Black, W. C., 627, *650*
Blake, J., 230, *247*
Blalock, H. M., Jr., 184, *199*, 432,
    437, 438, *442–443*, 502, *516*
Blanc, A. K., 101, *105*, 113, 122,
    123, *136, 139, 141*
Blanc-Szanton, C., 539, *544*
Blanchard, K. S., 260, *278*
Blanchet, D., 835, *849*
Blank, R. M., 219, *222*
Blau, D. M., 383, *411*
Blau, F. D., 216, *222*
Blau, P. M., 17, *18*, 184, *199*, 385,
    386, 388, 390, 402, *411*, 420,
    432, 436, *443*
Blauner, R. A., 183, *199*
Blayo, Y., 582, *596*
Blazer, D. G., 215, *224*, 685, *714*,
    818–820, *824*
Bledsoe, C., 529–531, 535, 542, *543*,
    871, *879*
Blinder, A. S., 557, *571*
Bloch, F., 120, *140*
Bloch, S., 159, *166*
Bloom, D. E., 101, *105*, 560, 563,
    564, *571–572*, 745, *757*, 836,
    849
Bloom, S., 118, 121, *136*
Blossfeld, H.-P., 391–392, 402, 410,
    411, 415
Blumen, I., 394, *411*
Bobo, L., 500, 506, *524*
Bogue, D. J., 17, *18*, 19, 22, *55*, 227,
    228, 256, *278*, 311, *342*, 489,
    490, *516*, 731, *732*, 735, 753,
    757, 759, 855, 856, *879*
Boisjoly, J., 384, *412*
Boldrin, M., 155, *165*
Bolger, N., 218, *224*
Bollen, K. A., 211, *222*, 490, *516*
Bolton, N. M., 774, *782*
Bommier, A., 552, *572*
Bonacich, E., 357, *378*
Bond Huie, S. A., 293, 295, 298, *305*
Bongaarts, J., 103, *108*, 160, *167*,
    229, 230, 233, 237, 239–241,
    243, 245, 246, *246*, 627, *650*,
    684, 707, 707n, 708, 709n, *712*,
    738, 743, 753, 755, *757*, 772,
    782, 833, *849*, 862, *879*
Bonilla-Silva, E., 171, 173, 185–186,
    196, *199, 200*, 255n, *278*

Bonita, R., 800–803, *805*
Bonneuil, N., 583, *596*
Bonneux, L., 812, 816, 819, *822, 823*
Boone, C., 455, 465, *474*
Booth, A., 91, 101, 104, *105*
Booth, H., 702, *712*
Booth, K., 321, *346*
Borchert, J. R., 488, *516*
Borchigud, W., 171, *199*
Borg, M. O., 383, *411*
Borgatta, E. F., 488, *519*
Borgerhoff-Mulder, M., 530, *543*
Borjas, G. J., 212, *222*, 354, 364,
    373, 374, *378, 379*, 385, *411*
Borrotto, R. J., 762, *782*
Boserup, E., 561, *572*, 834, *849*
Boucekkine, R., 551, *572*
Boulier, B. L., 408n, *411*
Bound, J., 212, *222*
Bourne, L. S., 64, 65, *84*, 482, *516*
Bouvier, L. F., 227, *228*
Bowles, G. K., 606, *619*
Boyd, M., 338, *342*
Boyle, P., 383, *411*
Bradburn, N. M., 93, *105*
Bradley, C., 532, *543*
Bradshaw, B. S., 606, *619*
Brambila, C., 752, *757*
Bramlett, M. D., 100, 102, *105*
Branch, L. G., 683, *716*, 816, 819,
    820, *825*
Brass, W., 6, *13*, 702, 706, *712*
Bravo, J., 558, *572*
Bravo-Ureta, B. E., 325, *342*
Brea, J. A., 325, *342*
Breckenridge, R. S., 466, *477*
Breen, R., 402, 410, *411*
Brenner, W., 275, *278*
Breslow, L., 298, *305*
Bresnahan, M., 789, 803, *807*
Brettell, C., 321, *342*, 537, *543*
Brewer, B., 490, *516*
Brewster, K. L., 128, *140*, 217, *222*,
    225, 234, *248*, 437, *443*
Brien, M. J., 92, 102, *105, 106*
Briggs, R., 613, *619*
Brines, J., 91, *105*
Brinton, M. C., 217, *222*
Bröchler, V., 465, *474*
Brockerhoff, M., 319, *342*
Brodie, J. F., 588, *596*
Brody, C. J., 221, *222*, 861, *879*
Brooks, C., 212, *224*
Brooks-Gunn, J., 212, *223*, 437, *443*
Brostrom, G., 702, *712*
Brown, D., 183, *200*
Brown, D. L., 63, *85*, 606, *619*

Brown, J. C., 585, 588, *596*
Brown, J. R., 552, *572*
Brown, J. W., 158, *165*
Brown, L. A., 323, *342*
Brown, L. R., 848, *849*
Brown, P., Jr., 173, *200*
Brown, S. L., 91, 104, *105*
Brown, W., 130, *136*
Browne, I., 213n, 218, *222, 225*
Browner, C. H., 125, *136*, 531, *543*
Brubaker, R., 723, *729*
Brüderl, J., 459, *474*
Brueckner, J. K., 495, *516*
Brumback, B., 796, *805*
Brumberg, R., 562, *574*
Bryan, K. N., 766, *782*
Bryan, T., 769, 771, *782*
Bryk, A. S., 438, *443*, 798, *805*
Bucher, H., 339, *342*
Bulatao, R. A., 229, 232, 245, *246,
    247*, 627, 634, *650, 657*, 772,
    782, 833, *849*, 862, *879*
Bulusu, L., 266, 270, *280*
Bulut, A., 740, *757*
Bumpass, L. L., 91, 97, 98, 100–102,
    105, 107, 233, 245, *247, 249*,
    403, *411*, 421–422, 427, *443*,
    448
Bunting, J., 803, *805*
Burch, T. K., 88, *105*
Burgess, E. W., 420n, 432, *447*, 481,
    492, 494, 496–498, *516, 522*,
    602, *622*
Burner, S. T., 158, *165*
Burns, M. A., 626, *650*
Burr, J. A., 220, *222*, 502, *516*
Burstein, L., 797, *807*
Burt, R. S., 213, *224*, 459, *474*
Burtless, G., 384, *414*
Burton, M. D., 457, 468, *473*
Buss, T. F., 215, *222*
Butters, R. D., 507, *516*
Byers, E., 580, *597*

Cabral, H., 270, *278*
Cabrera, G., 750, *757*
Caces, F., 325, *342*
Cafferty, P., 371, *379*
Cain, M. T., 114, 122, *136*, 232, *247*
Calavita, K., 359, 369, *379*
Caldwell, D., 455, *476*
Caldwell, J. C., 5, 5n.6, *13*, 88, *105*,
    110, 119, 121, *136*, 156, *165*,
    231, 233, 240, *247*, 251, 263,
    278, 437, *443*, 528, *543*, 627,
    650, 738, 756, *757*, 790, 800,
    801, *805*

Caldwell, P., 88, *105*, 240, *247*, 756,
    757
Calot, G., 848, *849*
Camacho, T., 298, *306*
Cambois, E., 383, *411*, 683, *712*,
    816, *823*
Cameron, J. L., 627, *651*
Campbell, A., 420, *444*
Campbell, A. A., 244, *247*
Campbell, B., 627, *651*
Campbell, C., 581, *598*
Campbell, P. R., 370, *379*
Cancian, M., 406–407, *411*
Canning, D., 564, *571*, 745, *757*,
    836, *849*
Carey, J. R., 253, 255, *278*, 291, *305*,
    628–630, 634, 637–642, 647,
    649, *651, 653, 656*
Carlson, E., 214, *222*
Carnes, B. A., 162, *166*, 288, 290,
    308
Carnevale, S., 762, 775, *785*
Carpenter, N., 424, *443*
Carr, R. V., 221, *222*, 861, *879*
Carrasco, R., 217, *222*
Carrier, N. H., 38, *55*
Carrigan, J. A., 287, *308*
Carrington, W., 324, *342*
Carroll, G. R., 452, 453n, 454n, 455,
    456n, 457–458, 458n, 459–462,
    462n, 463–468, 468n, 469,
    469n, 470–472, *473–477*
Carter, A. T., 528, 530, *543*
Carter, M., 183, *199*
Carver, K. P., 170, *205*, 265, 265n,
    267, 274, *281*
Casper, L. M., 91, 98–99, *106, 107*
Cassel, C., 290, *308*
Cassidy, M. L., 52, *55*
Cassidy, R. C., 187, *201*
Castells, M., 483, *516*, 602, *619*
Casterline, J. B., 123, *141*, 147, *165*,
    437, *443*, 627, *650*, 874, 875,
    879
Casti, J. L., 660, 662, *712*
Castles, S., 357, *379*
Castro Martin, T., 122, 123, *136*
Caswell, H., 628, 629, *651*
Cavalli-Sforza, L. L., 627, *651*
Cayton, H. R., 170, *200*
Cecil, R., 530, *543*
Cerrutti, M., 216, *222*
Cervantes, A., 270–271, *278*
Chafetz, J. S., 123, *136*
Chai, K. J., 506, *517*
Chaloupka, F. H., 304, *306*
Champion, A. G., 313, 341, *342, 343*

Chand, S. K., 155, *165*

Chandrasekaran, C., 855, *879*

Chang, C.-F., 22, *57*, 112, *140*, 183, *199*, 607, *622*, 871, 873, *880*

Chang, G., 134, *137*

Charbonneau, H., 580, *597*

Charles, C. Z., 500, 506, *516*

Charles, M., 210, 217, *222*, 384, 403, *410*, *411*

Charlesworth, R., 629, 635, 636, *651*

Chase-Dunn, C. K., 490, *516*

Chasteland, J. C., 842, *849*

Chatterjee, N., 131n, *136*

Chattopadhyay, A., 328, *342*

Chavez, L. R., 538, *544*

Chen, L. C., 119, *139*, 253, *280*, 814, *824*

Chen, M.-H., 685, *714*

Chen, M-J., 454, *475*

Chen, N., 316, 317, 338, *342*

Chen, Y. P., 155, *165*, 332, *344*

Cheng, L., 358, *379*

Cherlin, A. J., 98, *105*, 242, *247*, 427, 440, *443*

Chesnais, J. C., 128, *136*, 147, *165*, 588, *597*, 836, 837, 844, *850*

Cheung, P. P., 402, *415*

Cheung, W. Y., 273, *278*

Chevan, A., 384, *411*, 501, *516*

Chew, K. S. Y., 173, *199*

Chiang, C.-L., 676, 682, *712–713*

Chiswick, C. U., 102, *106*

Cho, N., 51, *57*

Cho, T. S., 454, *475*

Cho, Y., 270, *279*

Choe, M. K., 383, *414*

Choldin, H. M., 436, *446*, 501, *522*

Chomitz, V. R., 273, *278*

Chorley, R. J., 482, *516*

Christaller, W., 480, *516*

Christian, M., 173, *199*

Chu, C. Y. C., 552, *572*

Chu, J., 25, 51, *56*, *57*

Chuzhu, Z., 748, *758*

Clark, A. L., 604n, *619*

Clark, C., 493, 493n, 506, *516*

Clark, R., 211, 220, *222*

Clark, W., 337, *342*, 636, *651*

Clark, W. A. V., 494, 514, 515, *516*

Clarkberg, M., 91, 101, 102, *105*

Clarke, C. J., 611, *620*

Clarke, G. M., 629, *657*

Clarke, J. I., 43, *56*

Clay, J. W., 319, *342*

Cleland, J., 6–7, *13*, 110, 119, 122, *136*, *138*, 233, *247*, 527, *544*, 763, 766, 767, *782*, 833–835, *850*

Cleland, J. G., 738, *757*

Cliggett, L., 537, *544*

Clingman, E. J., 269, *282*

Clive, J., 685, *717*

Clogg, C. C., 216, *222*, 397, *411*

Clutton-Brock, T. H., 628, *651*

Clyburn, S., 269, *282*

Coale, A. J., 2, 6, *13*, 23–24, *56*, 98, *105*, 144, 145, *165*, 233, 241, *247*, 527, 562, *572*, 583, 585, 587, 588, 590, *597*, 677, 695–700, 702, 705–706, *713*, 716, 734, 743, *757*, 835, *850*

Cobas, J. A., 270, *278*

Cochrane, S., 122, *136*

Cohen, B., 628, 645, *654*

Cohen, J. E., 629, 633, *651*, 690, *713*

Cohen, L. E., 472, *476*

Cohen, P. N., 438, *443*

Cohen, S. E., 82, *84*

Cohen, Y., 194, *204*, 495, *515*

Colberg, E., 606, *623*

Cole, J., 538, *544*

Cole, L. C., 629, 645, *651*

Cole, S., 462n, *474*

Cole, W. E., 325, *342*

Coleman, C., 771, *783*

Coleman, D. A., 2, *13*, 22, *56*, 220, *222*, 872, *879*

Coleman, J., 439, *443*

Coleman, J. S., 472, *474*, 684, *713*

Coleman, S., 741, *757*

Collier, J., 111, *141*

Collins, C., 794, *808*

Collins, F. S., 626, *651*

Collins, J. L., 325, *342*

Collins, J. W., 262, 263, *278*

Compton, D., 877, *879*

Congdon, P., 329, *346*

Conley, D., 263, 267, *278*

Cook, J., 116, *137*

Cook, K., 213, *224*

Cook, R., 112, *136*, 745, *758*

Cooley, C. H., 486, *516*, 612, *619*

Cooper, R. S., 295, *306*

Corder, L. S., 685, *715*, 810, 811, 821, *824*

Cordero-Guzman, H., 213, *225*

Coreil, J., 178, *202*, 266, 269, 270, *280*, 294, *307*

Cornelius, D., 260, *280*

Coronado, J. L., 557, *572*

Corzine, J., 502, *516*, *517*

Corzine, L., 502, *516*

Costa, D. L., 304, *306*

Costner, H., 432, *443*

Cotter, D. A., 214, 217, *222*

Cotton, J., 194, *199*

Cottrell, W. F., 510n, *516*

Cowgill, D. O., 501, *517*

Cox, D. R., 285, 286, *305*, 554, *572*, 684–685, *713*

Cox, O. C., 170, *199*

Cox, P. R., 13, *13*

Cramer, J. C., 252–253, 265, 266, 270, 273, *278*

Crane, B. B., 744, 745, *758*, 837, 838, *850*

Crane, J., 437, 439, *443*

Crank, J., 270, *281*

Cready, C. M., 184, *199*, 482, 502, *518*

Creech, J. C., 502, *516*, *517*

Crenshaw, E. M., 82, *85*, 480n, 490, 491, 504, 515, *520*

Cressey, P. F., 496, 497, 500, 502, *517*

Crews, J. E., 628, *654*

Crimmins, E. M., 5, *13*, 233, *247*, 255, 276, *282*, 385, *411*, 626, 628, *651*, 683, *713*, 810, 810n, 811–812, 815–816, 816n, 817–821, *823*

Crouse, J., 390, *413*

Crowder, K. D., 433, 437, 438, *443*, *447–448, 506, 517*

Crown, W., 160, *165*

Crutchfield, R. D., 221, *222*, 861–862, *879*

Cruz-Janzen, M., 172, *200*

Cunha, J. M. P. D., 318, 319, *343*

Curran, S. R., 159, *165*, 338, *343*

Curtin, S. C., 362, *382*

Curtsinger, J. W., 626, *651*

Cutler, D. M., 551, *572*

Dacin, T., 466, *473*

Daly, M., 91, *106*

Daniels, M., 794, *806*

Danziger, S., 383, 404, 406, 407, *411*

Darity, W. A., Jr., 194, *200*

Darwin, C., 632, *651*

Das Gupta, M., 118, 121, *136*, 541, *544*

DaVanzo, J., 753, *759*

Davey Smith, G., 793, *805*

David, R. J., 254, 262, *278*

Davila, A., 329, *345*

Davis, H. C., 772, *782*

Davis, K., 1n.2, *13*, 17, *18*, 19, *56*, 60, 61, *84*, 230, *247*, 419–421, *443*, 604, 607, *620*, 731, *732*, 738, *758*, 809, *823*, 831, *850*

Davis, S. T., 771, *782*
Davis-Lloyd, R., 530, *544*
Day, J. C., 145, 146, 150, *165*
Day, K. M., 762, *783*
de Certeau, M., 133, *136*
De Graaf, P. M., 402n, *411*, *412*
de la Cadena, M., 172, *200*
de la Croix, D., 551, *572*
de Lattes, Z. R., 326, *343*
de Moivre, A., 673, *713*
De Vita, C. J., 266, *278*
DeAnda, R. M., 219, *222*
Dear, M. J., 485, *517*
DeAre, D., 617, *620*
DeAre, F., 314, *344*
Deaton, A. S., 384, *411*, 552, 562, *572*
Debpuûr, C., 754, *758*
Debre, R., 727, *729*
Deevey, E. S. J., 628, *651*
DeJong, D. N., 762, *782*
DeJong, G. F., 219, *222*, 323, 325, 326, 338, *343*, *345*, 421, *444*, 606, *623*
Delacroix, J., 457, 459, *474*
Delaney, C., 532, *544*
DeLargy, P. F., 319, *342*
DellaPergola, S., 186, *200*
Demeny, P., 6, *13*, 24, *56*, 145, *165*, 376, *379*, 417, *418*, 677, 705, *713*, 753, 755, *758*, 828n, 829, 834, 837, *850*
Demos, J., 582, *597*
Den Boer, A., 53, *56*
DeNavis-Walt, C., 427, *443*
Denton, N. A., 185, 192, *202*, 433, *446*, 496, 499, 500, 502, *521*
DeRousseau, J. C., 628, *651*
Desai, S., 112, 119, 120, 123, *136*, 218, *222*, 731, *732*
Deseran, F. A., 221, *222*, 862, *879*
Detragiache, E., 324, *342*
DeTurk, P. B., 285, 292, 293, *305*
Deurloo, M., 337, *342*
DeVaro, J. L., 196, *200*
Devine, J., 771, *783*
DeVore, I., 527, *545*
Devos, I., 590, *597*
Dewind, J., 856, *880*
Diamond, J., 642, *651*
Dickinson, R. E., 613, *620*
Dicks-Mireaux, L., 557, *572*, *573*
Dieleman, F., 337, *342*
Diez-Roux, A. V., 261, 277, *278*, 792, *805*
DiGregorio, D. A., 506, *523*
Dikotter, F., 171, *200*

DiMaggio, P., 11, *14*
DiPrete, T. A., 218, *223*, 384, 388, 400–402, *411*, *412*, 438, *443*
Disney, R., 154, 155, *165*
Dixon, J., 787, *805*
Dixon, R., 123, *136*
Dixon-Mueller, R., 112, 114, 117, 135, *136*, 745, *758*
Doane, A. W., 173, *200*
Dobrev, S. D., 464–465, 471, *474*
Dobzhansky, T., 645, *651*
Doeringer, P. B., 453, *475*
Dogan, M., 480n, 490, *517*
Doll, R., 796, *805*
Dominguez, K. M., 562, *572*
Donahoe, D. A., 215, *223*
Donaldson, L., 254, *278*
Donaldson, P. J., 830, *850*
Donato, K. M., 213, *225*, 320, 335, *343*, 358, *379*
Doodoo, F. N., 194, *200*
Dooley, M., 407, *412*
Dorbitz, J., 847, *850*
Dorn, H. F., 227, *228*, 283, *305*, 855, *879*
Doty, P., 160, *165*
Douglas, B., 787, *805*
Downey, D. B., 384, *415*
Downey, G., 218, *224*
Downs, B., 159, *165*
Doyle, P., 782, *783*
Drake, S., 170, *200*
Drentea, P., 295, *305*
Drever, F., 803, *805*
Dreze, J., 212, *224*
Du Bois, W. E. B., 170, *200*
Du Pasquier, L. G., 682, *713*
Duan, C. C., 53, *57*, 858, *880*
Dudley, S., 421, *443*
Duleep, H. O., 217, *223*, 383–384, *412*
Duncan, B., 71, *84*, 420, 427, 432, 433, *443*, *444*, 490, 498, 502, 506, *517*, 617, *620*
Duncan, C., 792, 797, 798, 798n, 799, *807*
Duncan, C. J., 583, *599*
Duncan, G. J., 384, *412*
Duncan, O. D., 1–2, 5, 6, *14*, 19–20, 48, *56*, 170, *201*, 227, *228*, 384– 385, 385n, 386, 386n, 388, 390, 393, 396, 400, 402, *411–413*, *415*, 417, *418*, 420–422, 424, 425, 427, 428, 430–433, 436, *443–445*, 452, *475*, 481, 490, 498, 502, 506, *517*, 577–579, 594, *597*, 601–604, 608,

611–612, *620*, 630, 632, 635, *652–653*, 853, 854, 856, 857, 859, *879*, *880*
Dunn, T., 399, *410*
Dupâquier, J., 595, *596*
Durand, J., 358, 363, *379*, *380*
Durden, G. C., 194, *200*
Durfy, S. J., 96, *106*
Durkheim, É., 292, 296, *305*, 608, *620*
Durrant, V., 120, 121, 124, *137*
Dwyer, J. H., 265, 270, *282*

Easterlin, R. A., 233, *247*, 373, 374, *379*, 435, *444*
Eaton, J., 239, *247*
Eberstadt, N., 51–52, *56*, 156, *165*
Eberstein, I. W., 265, 266, 273, *278*, *280*, *282*, 490, 503, *517*, 608, *620*
Echevarria, S., 178, *200*, 276, *278*, *279*
Eckersley, R., 787, *805*
Edelman, D., 275, *278*
Edin, K., 217, *223*
Edmonston, B., 74, *86*, 186, *200*, 365, 367, 369, 373, *378*, *380*, 495, *517*, 767, *783*
Edwards, L. N., 218, *223*
Edwards, S., 155, *165*
Eggars, M. L., 500, *521*
Eggebeen, D. J., 173, *199*
Egidi, V., 817, *825*
Egolf, B., 298, *305*
Ehrlich, P. R., 744, *758*, 834, *850*
El Dawla, A. S., 112, *137*
Elandt-Johnson, R. C., 671, 677, 682, *713*
Eliason, S. R., 216, *222*
Ellaway, A., 791, 792, *806*
Ellis, D. R., 762, 769, *784*
Ellison, C. G., 296, *305*
Ellison, P. T., 526, *544*, 629, *652*
Ellsberg, M., 121n, *138*
Elo, I. T., 294–295, 299, 304, *305–306*, 308
Emerson, M., 506, *517*
Emigh, R. J., 96, *106*
Enchautegui, M. E., 213, *223*
England, P., 438, *446*
Entwisle, B., 438, 439, *444*, *446*
Epstein, J. M., 498n, 508, *517*
Erikson, R., 401, 402n, 409–410, *412*
Erli, Z., 749, *758*
Errington, S., 115, *137*
Ervin, D. J., 606, *620*

Eschbach, K., 172, 177–178, *200*, 354, *379*, 501, *517*

Escobar Latapi, A., 355, *381*

Espenshade, T. J., 369, *379*

Esping-Andersen, G., 234, *247*

Espino, R., 174, *200*

Espinosa, K. E., 358, *380*

Ettner, S. L., 218, *223*

Euler, L., 23, *56*

Evandrou, M., 160, *165*

Evans, J., 220, *224*

Evans, M., 130, *137*

Evans, M. D. R., 213, *223*

Ewbank, D. C., 96, *106*, 626, 629, 646, 649, *652*

Fair, R. C., 562, *572*

Falaris, E., 325, *343*

Falkingham, J., 160, *165*

Fang, D., 183, *200*

Fansler, D. A., 495, *516*

Farkas, G., 438, *446*

Farley, R., 78, *84*, 186, *200*, 383, *412*, 423–424, 440, *444*, *445*, 496, 498, 502, 506, *517*

Faruqee, H., 836, *850*

Fausto-Sterling, A., 21, *56*

Feagin, J. R., 171, 173, 185, *200*, 483, 501, 511, *517*, *519*, *523*

Fearnside, P. M., 319, *343*

Featherman, D. L., 385, 386, 388, 400, 402, *412*, *413*, 420, 430, *444*, *445*

Feder, M. E., 627, *652*

Federici, N., 111, *137*

Feeney, D., 770, *783*

Feeney, G., 243, *246*, 707, 707n, 708, 709n, *712*

Fei, J. C., 324, *345*

Feldstein, M., 155, *165*, 557, *572*

Felitti, V. J., 793, *805*

Feller, W., 688, *713*

Feng, W., 232, *247*, 595, *598*

Fennelly, K., 92, *106*

Ferber, M. A., 216, *222*

Ferguson, J., 538, *544*

Ferrante, J., 173, *200*

Ferree, M. M., 110, 130, *137*

Fichman, M., 459, *475*

Field, J., 213, *223*

Fielding, E. L., 496, *518*

Fields, J., 98–99, *106*

Fienberg, S. E., 441, *446*, 723, *729*, 767, *782*

Finch, C. E., 96, *106*, 626, 629, 630, 634, 640, 648, 649, *652*, *657*, 712, *713*, *717*

Findley, S. E., 323, *343*

Finkelstein, S., 455, *475*

Finkle, J. L., 112, *139*, 744–745, *758*, 837, 838, *850*

Firey, W., 484, *518*, 602, *620*

Firth, R., 526, *544*

Fiscella, K., 267, *278*

Fischer, C., 62, *84*

Fisher, A., 738, *758*

Fisher, K., 594, *597*

Fisher, R. A., 645, *652*

Fitch, C. A., 94, 96, 98, 99, 104, *106*, 859, *879*

Fix, E., 682, *713*

Fix, M., 355, 357, 370, 375, *378*, *379*, *381*

Flatau, E., 21, *56*

Flatt, S., 454, *475*

Flatt, V., 877, *880*

Fleischhacker, J., 847, *850*

Fleury, M., 577, *597*

Flieger, W., 19, *57*, 672, 691n, 692, *714*

Flinn, M., 593, *597*

Flotow, M., 771, *784*

Flowerdew, R., 321, *343*

Flusty, S., 485, *517*

Fogel, R. W., 88, *106*, 304, *306*

Folbre, N., 121, 124, 128, 134, *137*

Foley, R. A., 628, 642, *652*

Follett, R. S., 196, *200*

Foner, N., 538, *544*

Fong, M. S., 682, 683, *713*

Fonow, M., 116, *137*

Forbes, D., 178, *200*, 252, 256, 257, 260, 261, 270, 271, 275, *278–279*

Forcey, L. R., 134, *137*

Ford, K., 183, *200*

Ford, L., 83, *85*

Ford, R. G., 500, *518*

Ford, T. R., 421, *444*

Forrest, J., 194, *202*

Forristal, J., 438, *443*

Fortes, M., 526, *544*

Fossett, M. A., 184, *201*, 438, *444*, 482, 502, 508, *516*, *518*

Foster, C., 631, 643, *652*

Foucault, M., 130, 133, *137*

Francese, P., 221, *223*

Frank, O., 846, *850*

Frank, P. W., 417, *418*, 601, *620*, 632, *652*, 856, 857, *879*

Frank, R., 254, 255, 267, 275, *278*

Frankenberg, E., 552, 554, *572*

Frankenberg, R., 173, *201*

Franklin, S., 134, *137*

Franz, M. M., 174, *200*

Frauenthal, J. C., 676, 700, *713*, *714*

Frazier, E. F., 170, *201*

Freedman, D., 94, *106*

Freedman, L. P., 112, *137*

Freedman, R., 420, 437, *444*

Freedman, V. A., 157, *165*, 811, 812, 817, 821, *823*, *825*

Freeman, D. H., 274n, 275, *280*

Freeman, H. P., 298, *307*

Freeman, J., 452, 456n, 457–459, 466, 468, 471, *475*, 813, *823*

Freeman, L. C., 508, *518*

Freeman, R. B., 560, *572*

Freese, J., 643, *652*

Fremont, A. M., 277, *279*

French, R., 589, *596*

Frenk, J., 260, *279*

Frey, W. H., 65, 67, *85*, 315, 324, 332, *343*, *346*, 441, *444*, 495–496, 502, 508, 510, *517–518*

Fricke, T. E., 88, 92–93, *107*, 132, 133, 135, *138*, 234, *247*, 526n, 527, *544*, *545*

Fridlizius, G. G., 581, *596*

Friedberg, L., 89, *106*

Friedlander, D., 607, *620*

Friedman, D., 17, *18*

Friedmann, J., 480, *518*

Frier, B. W., 583, *596*

Fries, J. F., 289, 291, *306*, 811, *823*

Frisbie, W. P., 178, 184, *200*, *201*, 252, 252n, 254, 256–258, 258n, 260, 261, 265–267, 270, 271, 273, 275, 276, *278–279*, *282*, 436, 438, *444*, *445*, 481, 490, 493, 494, 496, 499, 502, 503, 505, *517–518*, *522*, 602, 603, 605–606, 608, 608n, 609–611, 613, 614, 617, *620–622*, 857, *880*, *881*

Fu, H., 244, *247*

Fuchs, V. R., 98, *107*, 297, *306*

Fuentes-Afflick, A. T., 264, *279*

Fuguitt, G. V., 63, 70, *85*, 313–314, *344*, 430, *446*, 606, 613, 617, *620*, *621*

Fujita, M., 480, 487, 492, 494, 508, *518*

Fullerton, H. N., Jr., 214, *223*

Fullilove, M. T., 254, *279*

Funck-Jensen, U., 685, *713*

Furedi, F., 131, *137*

Furtado, C., 357, *379*

Futuyma, D. J., 629, *654*

Gage, R. P., 684, *712*

Gage, T. B., 254, 258, 259, *279*, 526, *544*, 628, *652*

Gaile, G. L., 781, *783*

Gaillard, J.-M., 629, *652*

Galdi, D., 771, *783*

Gale, W. G., 557, *572*

Gallagher, M., 89–90, 101, *107*, 296, *309*

Galle, O. R., 489–490, 502, *516–519*

Galloway, P. R., 583, 585, 588, *597*

Gangestad, S. W., 627, *652*

Gans, H., 172, *201*

Ganzeboom, H. B., 387n, 401, 402, 402n, 410, *411–412*, 416

Gardner, G., 848, *849*

Garenne, M., 301, *308*

Garfinkel, I., 406, *412*

Garnier, M. A., 402, *412*

Garreau, J., 64, *85*

Garrett, P., 213, *225*

Garrison, H., 325, *343*

Garrison, W. L., 482, *519*

Gates, G. J., 876, *879*

Gatson, S. N., 173, *201*

Gatzweiler, H.-P., 339, *342*

Gauthier, H. L., 613, *620*

Gautier, E., 577, *597*

Gavrilov, L. A., 628, *652*

Gavrilova, N. S., 628, *652*

Gaynor, P. E., 194, *200*

Gee, E. M., 156, 158, *165*

Gendell, M., 220, *223*

George, L., 150, 158, *167*

George, R., 766, *782*

Gerdes, L. U., 649, *652*

Gereffi, G., 358, *378, 379*

Germain, A., 114, 117, 135, *136*

Geronimus, A. T., 266, *279*

Geschwender, J. A., 217, *223*

Gettys, W. E., 602, *620*

Getz, W. M., 629, *652*

Ghimire, D. J., 94, *105*

Ghosh, M., 768, *783*

Ghuman, S., 116, *137*

Gibbs, J. P., 481, 502, *515, 519*, 602, 606–609, *620*, 857, *879*

Giddens, A., 17, *18*

Giesen, D., 91, *107*

Gillaspy, R. T., 770, *783*

Gille, H., 738, *758*

Gilpin, R., 362, *379*

Ginsburg, F. D., 126, 130, *137*, 532, *544*

Gittleman, M., 384, *412*

Gladney, D. C., 171, *201*

Gladwell, M., 736, *758*

Glaeser, E. L., 495, 495n, 508–509, *519*

Glass, D. V., 393, 394, *412*, 734, *758*

Glass, J. L., 218, *223*

Glazer, N., 173, *201*

Glenn, E. N., 134, *137*

Glick, P. C., 17, *18*, 856, *879*

Glick, W. H., 455, *475*

Glick-Schiller, N., 539, *544*

Glover, K. S., 51, *57*, 858, *881*

Gmelch, G., 537, 539, *544*

Gmelch, S., 539, *544*

Gobalet, J. G., 766, 776, *783*

Goetz, A. R., 323, *342*

Gokhale, J., 552, 556, *571, 572*

Goldberg, H. I., 740, *758*

Goldblatt, P. O., 292, *306*

Golden, R. M., 76, 78, *85*

Goldenberg, R. L., 267, *279*

Goldenweiser, E. A., 424, *445*

Goldin, C., 563–566, *572*

Goldman, N., 790–791, 794, 795, 804, *805*, 869, *879*

Goldscheider, C., 22, *56*, 98, 101, *106*, 338, *343*, 422, *445*

Goldscheider, F., 112, *137*

Goldstein, D., 646, *655*

Goldstein, H., 798, 799n, *805, 806*

Goldstein, J. R., 98, 102, 104, *106*, 627, 628, *654*, 700, 701, *713*, 859, *879*

Goldstein, S., 227, *228*, 332, *346*

Goldthorpe, J. H., 401–402, 402n, 409–410, *411–412*

Gomez, C., 172, 174, *200, 201*

Gompertz, B., 637, *652*

Gonul, F., 215, *223*

Gooderham, M., 725, *729*

Goodkind, D., 51, 52, *56*

Goodman, L. A., 394–396, *412*

Goody, J., 535, *544*

Gordon, D., 483, *519*

Gordon, L., 130, *137*

Gordon, M., 182, *201*, 432, 433, *445*

Gordon, P., 495, *519*

Gordon, R. H., 557, *571*

Gorman, B., 178, *202*, 270, *280*

Gortmaker, S. L., 251, 254, 265, 274, *279*, 383, *412*

Gotcher, D. J., 616, *622*

Gottdeinner, M., 481, 483, 486, 494–495, 501, 511, *519*

Gottemoeller, M., 121n, *138*

Gottschalk, P., 404, 406–407, *411, 412*

Gould, J. B., 762, *783*

Gould, P. R., 482, *515*

Grady, W. R., 220, *223*, 685, *713*

Grambsch, P. M., 685, *717*

Gramsci, A., 133, *137*

Granovetter, M. S., 358, *379*

Grant, L., 154, *165*

Grasmuck, S., 354, 355, *379*

Graunt, J., 789, *805*

Graves, P. E., 337, *344*, 616, *620*

Grebenik, E., 854, *880*

Green, A., 321, 330, *345*

Greene, M. E., 112, *137*, 871, 872, *880*

Greene, R., 131n, *137*

Greenhalgh, S., 110, 116, 127, 129n, 131, 131n, 132, 133, *137*, 240, *247*, 527, 529, 532–533, 541n, 542, *544*, 747–748, *758*

Greenland, S., 796, 797n, *805, 807*

Greenwood, M. J., 311, 332, *343*

Greville, T. N. E., 676, *713*

Grey, D. W., 647, *656*

Grieco, E., 187, *201*

Griffin, E., 83, *85*

Griffiths, C. J., 316, *344*

Griliches, Z., 398, 399, *412*

Grimes, P., 490, *516*

Groeneveld, L. P., 685, *717*

Gronau, R., 408, *412*

Gross, A. B., 183, *201*

Grossman, G., 561, *572*

Grossman, M., 295, 304, *306*

Gruenfelder, C., 628, *651*

Gruenwald, P., 258, *279*

Grusky, D. B., 384, 388, 400, 402, 403, *410–412*

Gryn, T. A., 11, *14*

Gu, B. C., 51, *56*, 617, *622*

Gu, D., 683, 684, *717*

Gu, X., 157, *166*

Gu, Y., 332, *344*, 616, *622*, 876, 877, *881*

Gualtieri, S., 172, *201*

Guendelman, S., 270, *279*

Guengant, J. P., 840, 848, *850*

Guest, A. M., 62, 70–71, 76, 78, *85*, 262, *279*, 433, 438, *445*, 485, 499, 501, *519*, 617, *620*

Guest, P., 437, *445*

Guillard, M., 645, *652*

Guillemard, A., 220, *223*

Guillot, M., 13, *14*, 97, *107*, 144, *166*, 227, *228*, 235, 236, *248*, 285, 286, *308*, 429, *447*, 664, 699, *716*, 797n, *807*

Guilmoto, C. Z., 338, *343*

Guinnane, T. W., 585, 588, *596*

Guio, A., 212, *224*

Gullason, E. T., 557, *572*
Gunnell, D., 793, *805*
Guo, G., 212, *223*, 319, *346*, 384, 399n, *412*
Guo, Z. G., 855, *880*
Gurak, D. T., 217, *223*
Guralnik, J. M., 215, *224*, 685, *714*, 818–820, *824*
Gustaffson, S. S., 218, *223*
Guterbock, T. M., 495, *517*
Gutman, G. M., 156, 158, *165*
Gutman, R., 5, *14*
Guyer, B., 269, 272, 274–275, 277, *279*
Guyer, J. I., 531, 535, *543*, *544*, 871, 872, *879*, *880*
Guzzo, K. B., 234, *248*
Gyepi-Garbrah, B., 831, *849*

Haag, G., 329, *343*, *346*
Haan, M., 298, *306*
Haberland, N., 746, *758*
Hack, M., 252, *279*
Hackenberg, R., 83, *85*, 800, *807*
Hadden, J. K., 488, *519*
Hadden, K., 607, *621*
Haeckel, E., 602, *620*
Hagan, J. M., 354, 357, 358, *379*
Haggett, P., 482, *516*, *519*
Hahn, R. A., 287, *306*
Hahn, S., 626, *653*
Haight, R. G., 629, *652*
Hailemaria, M., 124, *138*
Haines, M. R., 95, *106*, 260, *281*, 584, 585, 589, *597*, *599*
Hajnal, J., 52, *56*, 590, *597*
Hall, R., 174, *201*
Hall, T. D., 490, *516*
Haller, A. O., 390, *415*
Halli, S. S., 13, *14*, 20, *56*, 177, *201*
Halter, J. B., 626, 627, *652*
Halweil, B., 848, *849*
Hambrick, D. C., 454, 455, *475*
Hamilton, B. E., 176, *201*
Hamilton, D., 196, *201*
Hamilton, W. D., 636, *652*
Hamm, R. R., 763, 770, 775, *784*
Hammel, E. A., 527, 529, 534, *545*, 585, 588, *597*
Hammer, M., 642, *652*
Hammerslough, C., 685, *717*
Hamvas, A., 274, 275, 277, *279–280*
Han, J., 466, *475*
Han, S., 220, *223*
Han, W. J., 218, *223*
Handwerker, W. P., 533, *545*
Hankins, M., 495, *523*

Hannan, M. T., 392, *416*, 452, 456n, 457–458, 458n, 459–462, 462n, 463, 464, 466–468, 468n, 469, 469n, 470–472, *473–477*, 482, 502, *519*, 685, *717*
Hannum, E., 384, *413*
Hansen, M. T., 465, 466, *473*
Haraway, D., 131, *137*
Harding, S., 130, 131, *137–138*
Hardoy, J., 317, *343*
Hardy, M., 220, *224*
Hargens, L. L., 456, 468n, *475*
Harkavy, O., 830, *850*
Härm, E., 585, *597*
Harpending, H., 627, 646, *652*
Harper, G., 771, *783*
Harper, S., 82, *85*
Harris, C., 488, 494, *519*, *524*
Harris, J. R., 324, *343*, 354, *379*
Harris, K. M., 212, 216, 217, *223*, 384, *412*
Harris, M., 527, *545*
Harrison, J. R., 454n, 455, *474*
Harrison, S., 629, *652*
Harshman, L. E., 626, 645, *652*
Hartling, H., 64, *85*
Hartouni, V., 134, *138*
Harvey, D., 482, 483, *519*
Harvey, J., 781, *783*
Hassan, F. A., 526, *545*
Hastings, A., 629, *652*
Hatch, L. R., 220, *223*
Hathaway, D. E., 617, *621*
Haub, C., 260, *280*
Hauser, P. M., 1, 2, 5, 6, *14*, 19–20, 48, *56*, 170, *201*, 227, *228*, 294, 295, *306*, 384, *413*, 420–422, 427, *445*, 452, *475*, 577–579, 594, *597*, 601, 630, 632, 635, *652–653*, 731, *732*, 853, 854, 859, *880*
Hauser, R. M., 385, 386, 388, 388n, 393, 395, 396, 399–402, *412–413*, *416*, 428, 430, 439, *445*
Haveman, H. A., 453n, 457, 472, *474*, *476*
Hawkes, K., 642, *653*
Hawley, A. H., 17, *18*, 20, 22–23, *56*, 61–62, *85*, 262n, *280*, 420, 436, *445*, 481, 482, 486, 489, 494, 499, 502, 602–605, 608, 612, 614, 616, 617, *621*, 857, *880*
Hayami, Y., 561, 562, *573*, 581, 595, *597*
Hayashi, F., 552, 554, *571*
Hayes-Bautista, D. E., 178, *201*
Hays, S., 134, *138*

Hayward, M. D., 220, *223*, 294, *307*, 383, *411*, 683, 685, *712–713*, 809, 810, 810n, 811–813, 815–816, 816n, 817–818, 818n, 819–821, *823–824*
Hechter, M., 17, *18*
Heckel, N. I., 833, *850*
Heckman, J. J., 398, *413*, 507, *520*
Hedstrom, P., 452n, *476*
Heer, D. M., 502, *520*
Heigl, A., 684, *713*
Heise, L., 121n, *138*
Helfand, S. L., 626, *653*
Helpman, E., 561, *572*
Helson, R., 219, *225*
Hemley, D., 295, *305*
Henderson, D. A., 833, *851*
Henderson, J., 589, *596*
Henderson, J. V., 480, 492, *520*
Henderson, V., 480, *515*
Hendricks, C., 275, *278*
Hendry, E. F., 218, *223*
Henripin, J., 580, *597*
Henry, L., 23, *56*, 231, 239, *247*, 577, 578, 580, 587, *597*, *598*
Henshaw, S. K., 244, *247*, 845n, *850*
Herdt, G., 536, *545*
Herlihy, D., 583, *597*
Hermalin, A. I., 303, *309*, 439, *444*, 552, *573*, 789, 804, *807*
Hernandez, D. J., 846n, *850*
Hernes, G., 98, *106*
Heron, M., 816, *824*
Herring, C., 174, 185, *201*, *202*
Herrnstein, R. J., 388, 400n, *413*
Herskind, A. M., 640, *653*
Hertel, B. R., 174, *202*
Herting, J. R., 315, 333, *343*
Hertz-Picciotto, I., 254, *280*
Hertzman, C., 793–794, *805*, *806*
Hess, B., 110, *137*
Hessol, N. A., 264, *279*
Heuveline, P., 13, *14*, 97, *107*, 144, *166*, 227, *228*, 235, 236, *248*, 285, 286, 298, *306*, *308*, 429, *447*, 664, *716*, 797n, *807*
Hibbs, J., 770, *783*
Higginbotham, E. B., 130, *138*
Higgins, M., 562, *575*
Hill, A., 528, 542, *543*
Hill, A. B., 796, 801, *805*
Hill, A. G., 528, 541n, *545*
Hill, E. T., 212, *223*
Hill, J. A., 424, *445*
Hill, K., 629, 629, *653*
Hill, M. E., 174, *201*, 286, 294, *306*
Hill, R., 7, *14*

Hill, R. C., 483, *520*
Himes, J. H., 273, *277*
Hinde, A., 13, *14*, 24, *56*
Hirsch, J. S., 539, *545*
Hirschl, T. A., 606, *621, 622*
Hirschman, C., 5n.6, *14*, 110, *138*, 186, *201*, 298, *306*, 384, *413*, 430, 434, 437, 438, 440, *445*, 856, *880*
Hirsh, M., 130, *138*
Hobbs, F., 20, 33, 34, 37, 38, 48, *56*, 63, *85*
Hobcraft, J. N., 627, *653*
Hobroft, J., 7, *13*
Hoch, S. L., 582, *597*
Hodge, R. W., 394, *413*, 428, *445*
Hodgson, D., 234, *247*, 735, 755, *758*, 830, *850*
Hodson, R., 219, *223*
Hoem, J. M., 398, *413*, 682, 683, 685, 691, *713*
Hogan, D. P., 124, *138*, 534, *545*
Holford, T. R., 391n, *413*
Hollifield, J. F., 359, *379*
Hollingsworth, T. H., 578, 581, *597*
Hollos, M., 540, *545*
Holzgreve, W., 626, *653*
Holzmann, R., 557, *573*
Hondagneu-Sotelo, P., 354–355, *379*
Hoover, E. M., 71, 78, *85*, 480, *520*, 562, *572*, 743, *757*, 835, *850*
Hope, K., 402, *413*
Hopkins, D. R., 586, 589, *597*
Horan, P. M., 356, *381*
Horiuchi, S., 19, *56*, 291, *306*, 628, *653*, 695, 697, *712*
Horton, F. E., 482, 487, 488, 490, 493, 494, 499, 501, *515*
Horton, H. D., 185, 197, *201*, 878, *880*
Hosmer, D. W., 685, *713*
Houdaille, J., 580, *597, 598*
Hough, G. C., Jr., 683, *714*
House, J. S., 295, 296, *307, 308*
House, R. J., 459, *477*
Hout, M., 185, *202*, 383–384, 388, 396, 400, 400n, 401–403, 410, *413, 415*
Hovy, B., 361, *379*
Howell, N., 239, *247*
Hoyert, D. L., 293, *306*
Hoynes, H. W., 552, *571*
Hoyt, H., 494, 498, 499, *520*
Hsueh, J. C.-T., 383, *415*
Hsueh, S., 219, *223*
Huang, C., 581, 595, *600*
Huang, M.-H., 388, *413*

Hubbard, R. G., 557, *573*
Huber, G. P., 455, *475*
Hudson, V. M., 53, *56*, 490
Huff-Corzine, L., 502, *517*
Hughes, M., 174, *202*
Hugo, G., 320, 325, 341, *343*, 841, *850*
Hui, S., 438, *449*
Hull, T. H., 51, *56*
Hullen, G., 684, *713–714*
Hulsey, T. C., 274, *280*
Hummer, A. R., 285, 291, 292, 295, 296, 298, 299, *308*, 856, 862, *881*
Hummer, R. A., 173, 178, *202*, 258, 265–266, 269–274, *278–281*, 293–296, 299, 303, *305–307*
Hunter, A. A., 501, *520*
Hunter, L., 341, *343*
Hunter, M. L., 174, *199, 202*
Huntington, S., 723, *729*
Hurd, R. M., 494, *520*
Huriot, J., 480, 492, *520*
Hurtado, A. M., 629, *653*
Hussey, J. M., 262, *279*, 438, *445*
Hutchinson, G. B., 813, *823*
Hutchinson, R., 481, 486, 494–495, 501, 511, *519*
Hwang, S., 183, 184, 192, *202, 204*, 770, *784*
Hyden, G., 832, *850*

Iachine, I. A., 650, *657*, 712, *717*
Ibrahim, B., 115, *139*
Ibrahim, J. G., 685, *714*
Iceland, J., 192, 193, *202*, 384, 404, 405, *413*
Ignatiev, N., 172, *202*
Illeris, S., 313, *343*
Ingegneri, D., 683, *713*, 811, 816, *823*
Ingoldsby, B. B., 239, *247*
Ingram, P., 456n, *476*
Inhorn, M. C., 134, *138*, 531, *545*
Inouye, S. K., 626, *653*
Irwin, M., 613, *621*
Isaacs, S., 112, *137*
Isard, W., 480, *520*
Ishida, H., 402, *413*

Jackson, K. T., 66, 71, *85*
Jackson, M. E., 160, *165*
Jacobsen, J. P., 217, *223*
Jacquard, A., 633, *653*
Jaeger, A., 155, *165*
Jaffe, A. J., 17, *18*, 209, *224*, 856, *880*
Jaffee, J., 465, *476*

Jagger, C., 817, *825*
Jain, A., 839, 846, *850*
Jain, D., 120, 123, *136*
James, D. R., 507, *520*
Jamison, D. T., 833, *851*
Jannetta, A. B., 582, 595, *598*
Jaret, C., 483, *520*
Jargowsky, P. A., 498, 500, 501, *520*
Jayaratne, T., 116, *138*
Jee, M., 816, *825*
Jejeebhoy, S., 120–122, 124, 128, 129, 132, 133, *138*
Jencks, C., 390, 399, 402, *413*
Jenny, A. M., 276, *280*
Jensen, A., 111, 123, *139*
Jensen, E. R., 563, *571, 573*
Jensen, L., 357, *380*, 439, *447*
Jensen, R., 173–174, *202*
Jette, A. M., 814–815, *825*
Jetter, A., 134, *138*
Jia, Z., 617, *622*
Jiang, L., 158, *165*, 684, *714, 716*
Jiobu, R. M., 502, *520, 521*
Johansson, S. R., 51, *56*, 833, *850*
Johnson, D., 101, *105*
Johnson, D. G., 564, *573*
Johnson, G. C., 610, *622*
Johnson, K. M., 775, *783*
Johnson, N. E., 52, *56*, 294, *306*
Johnson, N. J., 383, *413*
Johnson, N. L., 671, 677, 682, *713*
Johnson, T. E., 626, 628, *653*
Johnston, R., 194, *202*
Jones, C. I., 561, *573*
Jones, D. L., 466, *477*
Jones, D. R., 292, *306*
Jones, J. R., 319, *344*
Jones, K., 791, 792, 797, 798, 798n, 799, *805, 807*
Jones, K. E., 627, *656*
Jonsson, J. O., 402n, *414*
Jonsson, S. H., 699, 700, *716*
Joppke, C., 352, *379*
Jordan, C. W., Jr., 659, 664, 669, 682, *714*
Jovanovic, B., 392, *414*
Joyce, M., 384, *412*
Joyner, K., 91, *105*
Judd, K. L., 557, *573*
Judge, D. S., 628, 634, 639, 641, 642, 651, *653*
Juster, T. F., 287, *306*

Kabeer, N., 112, 115, *138*
Kahl, J. A., 393, *414*
Kahn, M. E., 495, 495n, *519*
Kaining, Z., 749, *758*

Kalbfleisch, J. D., 685, *714*
Kallan, J. E., 258, 266, 267, 273–274, *280*
Kalleberg, A., 220, *224*
Kallmann, F. J., 417, *418*, 632, *653*
Kalmijn, M., 184, *202*
Kandel, W., 528, *545*
Kannisto, V., 639, 643, *653*, 702, *717*
Kantrow, L., 581, *598*
Kaplan, G. A., 298, *306*, 794, *806*
Kaplan, H. S., 232n, *247*, 566, *573*, 627–629, 645, *653*
Kaplan, R. D., 848, *851*
Karageorgis, S., 357, *379*
Karoly, L. A., 384, *414*
Karp, H. H., 616, *621*
Kasarda, J. D., 82, *85*, 387n, *414*, 480n, 481, 482, 486, 490, 491, 493–496, 499, 501, 502, 504, 508, 510, 515, *515*, *517*, *518*, *520*, 607, 609, 613, 615, 618, *619*, *621*
Kasinitz, P., 856, *880*
Kass, R., 488, *520*
Katkin, W., 182, *202*
Katz, E., 325, *344*
Katz, L. F., 563–566, *572*
Katz, S., 683, *714*, 816, *824*
Kaufman, G., 112, *137*
Kaufman, J. S., 295, *306*, 749, *758*
Kaufmann, C., 723, *729*
Kaufmann, G., 119, *138*
Kavee, A. L., 217, *225*
Kawachi, I., 295, *306*, 787–792, 796, 804, *805–806*
Kawano, Y., 490, *516*
Kay, G., 319, *344*
Kearney, M., 539, *545*
Kearns, R. A., 791, *806*
Keck, S. L., 454, *476*
Keely, C. B., 364, *378*
Keilman, N., 162, *165*, 707–708, *714*, *717*
Keith, L., 270–271, *278*
Keith, V. M., 174, *202*
Keithly, D., 221, *222*, 862, *879*
Keller, E. F., 116, 130, *138*
Kelley, A. C., 561n, 562–564, *571*, *573*, 835, 836, 846, *849*, *851*
Kelley, J., 213, *223*
Kelly, D., 458, 466, *473*
Kelly, J., 130, *138*
Kelly, K. D., 616, *621*
Kelly, S., 794, *806*
Kennedy, B. P., 295, *306*, 804, *806*
Kennedy, L., 590, *597*
Kennedy, P., 723, *729*

Kenney, C. T., 98, 104, *106*, 859, *879*
Kenyon, C., 626, *653*
Kerckhoff, A. C., 219, *224*
Kertzer, D. I., 21, *57*, 132, 133, 135, *138*, 234, *247*, 526n, 527, 529, 532n, 533, 534, 540, *545*, 586, *598*
Kessel, S. S., 266, *280*
Kestenbaum, B., 293, *307*, 774, *783*
Keyfitz, N., 6, *14*, 19, 23, *57*, 144, *165*, 303, *306*, 394, *414*, 451, 452, *476*, 486, *520*, 628, 632–633, *653*, 659, 662, 664, 672, 675, 675n, 676, 677, 682, 686, 690, 691, 691n, 692, 699–701, 706, *714*, *716*, 872, *880*
Khan, A., 171, *202*
Khanam, S., 122, *136*
Khlat, M., 838, *851*
Kiecolt, K. J., 184, *201*, 502, *518*
Kiely, J., 252, *280*
Kiernan, K., 92, 94, 98, 99, 101, *106*
Killingsworth, M. R., 196, *202*
Kim, D., 51, *57*
Kim, S., 490, *520*
Kim, T-Y., 465, 471, *474*
Kim, Y. J., 699–701, 708, *714*, *716*
King, D., 490, *520*
King, M., 832, *851*
King, M. A., 557, *572*, *573*
King, M.-C., 627, *655*
King, R. B., 234, 246, *247–248*
Kingson, E. R., 155, *166*
Kington, R. S., 293, 295, *306*, *309*
Kinsella, K., 147, 162, *166*, 552, *573*, 629, *652*, 712, *713*, 809, 810n, *824*
Kintner, H. J., 763, 765, 772, 778, *783*
Kippen, R., 363, *380*
Kirby, J. B., 160, *167*
Kirk, D., 5, 5n.5, *14*, 227, *228*
Kirkwood, T. B. L., 635, *653*
Kiser, C. V., 7, *14*
Kishor, S., 113, 115, 120, 124, *138*, *139*, 210, 212, *224*, *225*
Kitagawa, E. M., 294, 295, *306*, 427, *445*
Kitamura, Y., 556, *575*
Klaff, V. Z., 70, *85*
Klapisch-Zuber, C., 583, *597*
Klawitter, M. M., 877, *880*
Klein, J. P., 685, *714*
Klein, N. K., 252, *279*
Kleinman, J. C., 266, *280*
Klerman, J. A., 218, *224*
Kligman, G., 126, *138*, 534, *545*

Kline, J., 252, 257, 274, *280*
Klohnen, E. C., 219, *225*
Knight, J., 159, *166*
Knodel, J. E., 24, *58*, 232–233, *247*, *248*, 435, 440, *445*, *448*, 527, *545*, 581, 585, 587, 591–593, *598*
Knox, P., 480n, *520*
Kochanek, D. A., 268, *280*
Koenig, H. G., 297, *307*
Koenig, M. A., 753, *758*
Kogan, M. D., 273, *277*, 394, *411*
Kohler, H.-P., 243, *247*, 383, *414*, 627, 649, *654*, 708, *714*, 755, *758*
Kohlhase, J., 495, 508, 509, *519*
Kohn, M. L., 219, *224*
Kollek, R., 628, *654*
Kolluri, B. R., 557, *572*
Korenman, S. D., 266, *279*
Kotelchuck, M., 272, 273, *277*, *280*
Kotlikoff, L. J., 551–552, 554, 556, *571*, *573*
Koufopanou, V., 628, *650*
Kovar, M. G., 287, *308*
Kovenock, J., 874, *881*
Kraly, E., 438, *445*
Kramer, M. S., 258, *280*
Kreager, P., 529, *545*, 731, *732*
Kreider, B., 215, *224*
Krieger, N., 294, *307*, 793, *806*
Kritz, M. M., 217, *223*, 324, *344*
Krivo, L., 617, *621*
Krout, J. A., 606, *621*
Krueger, A., 400, *410*
Krueger, D., 557, *573*
Krueger, P. M., 285, 295, 299, *307*, *308*
Krugman, P., 480, 487, 498n, 508, *518*, *520*
Kubler, F., 557, *573*
Kuh, D. L., 793, *806*
Kuhlthau, K., 218, *224*
Kuijsten, A., 684, *714*
Kulczycki, A., 183, *202*
Kumar, A., 495, *519*
Kunda, G., 220, *224*
Kung, H.-C., 293, *306*
Kupiszewski, M., 767, *784*
Kutscher, R. E., 217, *224*
Kuznets, S., 491, *520*
Kwong, P., 53, *57*

Lacker, J. M., 196, *200*
Ladanyi, J., 194, *202*
Ladier-Fouladi, M., 839n, *851*
Laditka, S. B., 810n, 817, 818, 818n, 819, *824*

Laird, N., 391n, *414*
Lam, D., 627, *654*
Lancaster, J., 629, 645, *653*
Land, K. C., 215, *224*, 424, 425, *445*, 660, 663, 673, 677, 681–685, 708–710, *714–717*, 818–820, *824*
Landale, N. S., 92, *106*, 172, 178, 183, *202*, 270, 273, 276, *280*, 383, *415*
Landau, R., 371, *379*
Landsman, N., 182, *202*
Lapkoff, S., 566, *573*
Larson, D. B., 297, *307*
Larson, E. L., 451n, *476*
Laslett, P., 578, 582, 584, 591, *598*, *599*
Lather, P., 116, *138*
Lattes, A., 341, *343*
Laub, J. H., 53, *58*
Lauby, J., 326, 338, *344*
Lauderdale, D. S., 293, *307*, 774, *783*
Laumann, E. O., 90, 103, *106*
Lavrakas, P. J., 295, *305*
Lawless, J. F., 685, *715*
Lawrence, B. S., 454n, *476*
Lawson, V. A., 53, *58*
Layard, R., 408, *414*
Lazear, E. P., 552, *573*
Le Cœur, S., 838, *851*
LeClere, F. B., 298, *307*
Lee, C., 220, *224*
Lee, E. S., 329, *344*
Lee, G. R., 52, *55*
Lee, H., 116, *137*
Lee, I-Min, 299, *307*
Lee, J., 377, *379*
Lee, J. Z., 232, *247*, 581, 595, *598*
Lee, R. B., 527, *545*
Lee, R. D., 5, *14*, 238, *247*, 551–552, 558, 560, 561n, 562, 564, 566, 567, *572–574*, 583, 585, 588, *597*, *598*, 627–629, 636, 644, *654*
Lee, S. M., 186, 187, *200*, *202*
Lee, Y., 217, *222*
Lee, Y.-J., 554, *574*
Leff, N. H., 562, *574*
Legazpi Blair, M. C., 325, *343*
Lehrer, E., 102, *106*
Leibfritz, W., 552, 556, *571*
Leibowitz, A., 218, *224*
Leimer, D. R., 557, *574*
Lein, L., 217, *223*
Leinberger, C. B., 64, *85*
Lemeshow, S., 685, *713*
Lenski, G. E., 611, *621*

Léridon, H., 239, *247*, 633, *654*
Lerman, R. I., 217, *224*, 409, *414*
Lerner, S., 531, *543*, 871, *879*
Leslie, P. H., 394, *414*, 685, *715*
Lesnoy, S., 557, *574*
Lesthaeghe, R. J., 88, *106*, 233, 234, *247*, 585, *598*
Leung, S., 183, *202*, 433, *446*
LeVay, S., 53, *57*
Levhari, D., 325, *346*
Levin, C. E., 219, *224*
Levin, D., 582, *600*
Levin, L., 557, *571*
Levin, M. H., 782, *784*
Levine, C., 159, *164*
Levine, D., 590, *598*
Levine, N., 535, *545*
Levinthal, D. A., 459, *475*
Levitt, B., 459, *476*
Lévy, C., 580, *598*
Levy, F., 371, *379*, 424, *445–446*
Levy, M. B., 325, *344*
Lewin, E., 134, *139*
Lewin-Epstein, N., 194, *202*
Lewis, D. T., 731, *732*
Lewis, E. L., 685, *715*
Lewis, O., 404, *414*
Lewis, W. A., 324, *344*
Lewontin, R. C., 633, 645, *654*
Leyland, A. H., 798, 799n, *806*
Li, J., 110, 116, 127, 129n, 131, 131n, 132, 133, *137*, 240, *247*
Li, N., 383, *414*
Li, N., 700, 701, *715*
Li, V. C., 748, *758*
Liang, Z., 317, 324, 332, 339, *344*, *346*
Licandro, O., 551, *572*
Lichter, D. T., 183, *204*, 313–314, *344*, 406, *414*, 613, *621*
Lieberman, E., 273, *278*
Lieberson, S., 192, *202*, 420, 424, 428, 430, 432–435, *446*, 490, 502, *517*, *520*
Light, I., 357, *379*
Lii, D. T., 184, *205*, 438, *448*
Lillard, L. A., 92, 102, *105–107*, 296, 303, *307*, 552, 554, *572*, *574*, 863, *880*
Lin, G., 315, 333, *344*
Lin, H., 422, *448*
Lin, N., 213, *224*
Lindstrom, D. P., 319, 320, *344*
Lindstrom, M. J., 64, *85*
Lines, W. J., 724, *729*
Link, B. G., 294, 300, *307*
Lipset, S., 386, 391, *414*

Liu, B. C., 617, *621*
Liu, T., 581, *598*
Liu, Z., 51, *55*
Livi-Bacci, M., 581, 582, 585, 589, 595, *598*, 633, *654*, 838, *851*
Llanes, D., 183, *202*
Lloyd, C., 115, 122, 123, *139*, *141*
Lloyd, C. B., 563, *574*
Lo, C. P., 781, *783*
Lo, F., 480n, 490, *521*
Lobo, A. P., 183, *202*
Lochner, K., 798, *805*
Lockwood, C., 64, *85*
Logan, J. R., 76, 78, *85*, 89, *106*, 183, 199, *202*, 433, 434, 439, *442*, *446*, 449, 483, 501, 506, 513, 515, *521*, 523, 602, *621*
Logue, B. J., 580, *598*
Loi, V. M., 298, *306*
Lollar, D. J., 628, *654*
London, B., 64, *85*, 490, 515, *521*, 606–607, *621*
Long, J. F., 771, 773, *783*
Long, L., 314, 328, 329, 334, 335, *344*
Longford, N., 798, *806*
Longman, T., 172, *202*
Longva, S., 768, *783*
Lopez, A., 24, *57*, 690, *715*
Lopez, A. D., 810, 817, *824*
Lorber, J., 110, *137*
Lorimer, F., 1, *14*, 419, *446*, 527, *545*
Lotka, A. J., 23, *57*, *58*, 632, 644–645, *654*, 659, 685–687, *715*, *716*
Loucky, J., 357, *379*
Low, B. S., 604, 604n, *619*, *621*
Lowell, L., 371, 372, *378*
Lowry, I. S., 82, *85*
Lozano-Ascencio, F., 355, 356, *380*, *381*
Lu, H.-H., 100, 101, *105*, 422, *443*
Lubchenco, L. O., 258, *277*
Lubkemann, S., 539, *545*
Lucas, R. E. B., 312, 325, *344*, *346*, 561, *574*
Luker, K., 126, *139*
Lundstrom, H., 290, *309*, 639, *657*
Lupton, J., 90, *107*
Lutz, A., 385, *410*
Lutz, W., 6, *13*, 162, 163, *166*
Lye, D. N., 159, *166*
Lynch, J. W., 794, *806*
Lynch, K. A., 595, *600*
Lynch, S. M., 235, *248*, 421, *447*, 663, *715*
Lynn, F. B., 435, *446*

Ma, Z., 339, *344*
MacCormick, C. P., 530, *545*
Macintyre, S., 791, 792, *806*
Mackenbach, J. P., 800n, *806*
MacLeod, D., 183, *203*
Madamba, A. B., 219, *222*
Madans, J. H., 683, *715*
Maine, D., 117–118, *139*, *141*, 841n, *851*
Malaney, P., 745, *757*
Malhotra, A., 115, *139*
Malkki, L. H., 536, *545*
Malloy, M. H., 274n, 275, *280*
Malone, N. J., 363, *380*
Malthus, T. R., 593, 630, 632, *654*, 720–722, 835
Mandell, M., 771, *784*
Mangel, M., 628, *654*
Mankiw, G., 561n, *574*
Manning, W. D., 92, 102, *107*
Mansfield, E., 386, *414*
Manton, K. G., 157, *166*, 286, 290, *307*, 309, 397, *416*, 628, 629, 638, 639, 649, *654*, *656*, 685, *715*, *717*, 810, 810n, 811, 813, 815, 816, 820, 821, *824*, *825*
Manuel, D. G., 816, *824*
Manza, J., 212, *224*
Mao, M. X., 329, 339, *345*, *346*, 505, *521*, 616, *622*
March, J. G., 459, *476*
Mare, R. D., 383, 385n, 389, 394n, 399n, 409, 410, *414*, 427, *446*
Margolis, M. L., 538–539, *546*
Mark, N., 17, *18*
Markides, K. S., 178, *202*, 266, 269, 270, *280*, 294, *307*
Markusen, A. R., 504, 510, 510n, 514, 515, *521*
Marmot, M. G., 266, 270, *280*, 787, *806*
Marshall, B., 111, *139*
Marshall, H. H., Jr., 502, *520*, *521*, 617, *621*
Martin, D., 362, *380*
Martin, E., 130, *139*, 531, *546*
Martin, J. A., 105, *107*, 176, *201*, 268, *280*, 859, *880*
Martin, L. G., 157, 158, *165*, *166*, 812, 821, *823*
Martin, N., 400, *414*
Martin, P. L., 347, 355, 357, 359, *380*, *381*
Martin, T. C., 97, 98, 102, *107*
Martin, W. A., 617, *620*
Martin, W. T., 481, *519*, 602, 608, 610, *620*, *621*, 857, *879*

Martinez-Piedra, R., 762, *782*
Maruszko, L., 354, *381*
Marx, E., 539, *546*
Mason, A., 558–560, 562–564, *573–574*, *772*, *783*
Mason, K. O., 5n.6, *14*, 17, *18*, 111, 114, 115, 119, 121–123, 131, 133, *137*, *139*, 218, *224*, 233, 240, 244–245, *247*, 564, *571*
Mason, W., 439, *444*
Mason, W. M., 438, 441, *446*
Massey, D. S., 183, 185, 192, *201–203*, 338, 341, *344*, 354–356, 358, 363, 369, 372, *379–380*, 383, *414*, 433, 435, 440, 441, *446*, 496, 498–500, 502, *521*, 528, *545*, *546*, 844n, *851*
Massey, J. L., 502, *524*
Mathers, C. D., 801–803, *805*, 816–817, 819, *824*
Matras, J., 393, 394, *414*, 422, *446*
Matthews, B. J., 88, *105*
Matthews, T. J., 362, *382*
Mauldin, W. P., 753, *758*, 846n, *851*
Maxwell, N. L., 212, *224*
May, J. F., 840, 848, *850*
Mayer, A., 239, *247*
Mayer, H. M., 488, *521*
Mayer, K. U., 441, *446*, 627, *656*
Maynard, M., 116, 131, *139*
Mbizvo, M. T., 871, *880*
McCaa, R., 582, *598*
McCain, B., 454, *476*
McCarthy, J., 116–118, 129n, 131, *139*, *140*
McCarthy, K. F., 617–618, *621*
McCarthy, P. J., 394, *411*
McCarton, C., 258, *280*
McCarty, C., 298, *309*
McCauley, W. J., 506, *521*
McClintock, A., 130, *139*
McClure, M. E., 626, *654*
McCollough, M. E., 297, *307*
McCord, C., 298, *307*
McCormick, M. C., 252, *280*
McCreary, L., 438, *446*
McDonald, E., 245, *249*
McDonald, P., 234, *247*, 363, *380*
McDonough, P., 295, *307*, 794, *806*
McEwen, B. S., 627, 628, *654*, 794–795, *806*
McFalls, J. A., Jr., 171, *203*
McFarland, D. D., 690, *715*
Mcfarlane, A., 590, *598*
McGarry, K., 552, 557, *574*
McGee, D. L., 295, *306*
McGee, T. G., 316, *344*

McGue, M., 640, *654*
McIntosh, C. A., 112, *139*
McIntosh, C. L., 745, *758*
McKee, J. B., 502, *521*
McKee, M., 800, 802, *806*, 816, 824
McKendrick, D. G., 456n, 466, *473*, 476
McKenzie, R. D., 481, 489, 490, 496–497, *521–522*, 602, 603, 621
McKeown, T., 589, *598*
McKibben, J. N., 762, 775, *783*
McKowen, T., 259, 260, *280*
McKusick, D. R., 158, *165*
McLanahan, S., 91, *107*, 406, *412*, *414*, 529, *546*
McLaren, A., 588, *598*
McLemore, S. D., 169, 182, *203*
McMillen, M. M., 683, *714*
McNeil, D. R., 98, *105*, 702, 706, *713*
McNeil, W., 586, 589, *598*
McNicoll, G., 134, *139*, 417, *418*, 528, *546*, 830, 833, 835, 846, *850*, *851*
McPherson, M., 466, *476*
McQuillan, K., 596, *598*
Meagher, T. R., 629, *654*
Measham, D., 746, *758*
Meindl, R. S., 526, *546*
Meissner, D., 362, *380*
Mellor, E. F., 216, *224*
Melville, H., 451–452, *476*
Memmott, M. M., 159, *164*
Menken, J. A., 103, *108*, 160, *167*, 685, *715*
Merin, 878, *880*
Merli, G., 698, *715*
Merli, M. G., 383n, *414*
Merrell, M., 676, *716*
Merrick, T. W., 837, *851*
Mertens, W., 9, 9n.8, *14*
Meslé, F., 845, *851*
Messner, S. F., 440, *448*
Meyer, D. R., 489, 490, *522*
Meyer, J. W., 462, *476*
Meyerson, F. A. B., 154, *166*
Mezias, S. J., 466, *474*
Michael, R. T., 98, *107*, 552, *573*
Michelson, W., 615, 616, *621*
Micklin, M., 12, *14*, 193, *204*, 436, *446*, 601–602, 608, *622*, 731, *732*, 831, *851*, 857, *880*, *881*
Mileti, D. S., 298, *307*
Miller, C. C., 455, *475*
Miller, H. P., 424, *446–447*

Miller, J. E., 258, 267, *280*
Miller, M. J., 357, *379*
Miller, M. L., 160, *164*
Miller, P., 400, *414*
Miller, R. E., 391, *416*
Miller, T., 558, 560, 562, *573–574*, 771–772, *783*
Millman, S., 267, 274, *281*
Mills, E. S., 480, *522*
Mincer, J., 392, *414*
Mineau, G. P., 581, 588, *596*
Miniño, A. M., 285, 290, 292, 294, 301, 302, *307*
Minkoff, D. C., 456n, *476*
Mirowsky, J., 90, *107*, 383, *415*
Mishra, U. S., 125, *140*
Mitchell, S., 766, *783*
Modell, J., 357, *378*
Modigliani, F., 562, *574*
Moen, P., 218, 220, *223, 224*
Moeschberger, M. L., 685, *714*
Mohanty, C. T., 130, *139*
Mojarro, O., 752, *759*
Molho, I., 323, *344*
Molla, M. T., 682, 683, *715*
Molotch, H. L., 483, *521, 522*, 602, *621*
Money, J., 21, *57*
Monson, R. R., 294, *307*
Montgomery, M. R., 563, *574*, 628, 645, *654*
Moon, G., 791, 797n, *805, 806*
Moore, D. E., 294, *307*
Moore, H., 130, *139*
Moore, W. E., 2, *14*, 417, *418*, 420, 425, *443, 447*, 857–858, *880*
Morales, R., 357, *380*
Moreno, L., 319, *346*
Morenoff, J. D., 270, *281*, 788, 795, 796, *807*
Morgan, L. A., 453, *476*
Morgan, S. P., 122, *139*, 230, 234, 235, 243, 245, 246, *247–248*, 421, 440, 441, *447*, 663, *715*, 755, *759*
Moriyama, I. M., 643, *654*
Morrill, R., 781, *783*
Morris, A., 185, *203*
Morris, L., 738, *759*
Morris, M., 373, *380*
Morris, N. M., 874, 875, *881*
Morris, S. S., 219, *224*
Morrison, A. R., 312, *342*
Morrison, P. A., 617–618, *621*, 763, 774–777, 780, 782, *782–784*
Mortara, G., 855, *880*
Mosher, W., 100, 102, *105*

Mosley, W. H., 119, *139*, 253, *280*, 833, *851*
Moss, N., 294, *307*
Moss, N. E., 265, 265n, 267, 274, *281*
Mossel, P. A., 399, *413*
Mosteller, F., 439, *447*
Moynihan, D. P., 439, *447*
Mueser, P. R., 328, 336, 337, *344*, *346*, 390, *413*
Mühleisen, M., 836, *850*
Muhuri, P., 123, *139*
Mukherjee, R., 393, *414*
Mulatu, M. S., 295, *307*
Mullen, B. P., 433, *446*, 500, *521*
Müller, H.-G., 628, 649, *654–655*
Mulligan, G. F., 315, 329, *345*, 487, *522*
Mulvey, C., 400, *414*
Mundigo, A. I., 747, *759*
Munnell, A. H., 557, *574*
Muñoz-Franco, E., 320, *344*
Munz, M., 329, *344*
Murdock, G. P., 19, *57*
Murdock, S. H., 762, 763, 769, 770, 775, *784*
Murguia, E., 174, *203, 205*
Murphy, K. M., 555, 556, *571*
Murray, C., 388, 400n, *413*
Murray, C. J. L., 802, 803, *806*, 810, 814, 817, *824*
Murray, S. O., 53, *57*
Murthi, M., 212, *224*
Musgrave, M., 616, *622*
Musick, M. A., 296, *307*
Muth, R., 480, *522*
Muvandi, I., 871, *880*
Myers, R. J., 38, *57*
Myers, S. L., Jr., 194, *200*
Myrdal, G., 727, *729*

Nabila, J. S., 831, *849*
Nagel, J., 502, *522*
Nagi, S. Z., 814, *824*
Nahar, S., 122, *136*
Nam, C. B., 5, *14*, 265–266, 269, *278, 280, 281*, 285, 291, 292, 294–296, 298, 299, 303, *307*, *308*, 312, 329, *345*, 856, 862, *881*
Namboodiri, K., 20, 24, *57*, 61, *85*, 391n, *414*, 420, 436, *447*, 481, *522*, 602, 604n, 608, 611, *622*, 857, *880*
Namboodiri, N. K., 230, *248*
Nan, L., 748, *758*
Nardi, E., 586, *598*

Nathanson, C. A., 291, *307*
Nations, M., 536, *546*
Nattrass, N., 180, *203*
Nawar, L., 115, *139*
Neidert, L., 184, *201*, 438, *444*, 502, *518*
Nelson, C., 172, *203*
Nelson, H., 772, *784*
Nelson, R., 459, *476*
Nemeth, R. J., 490, *523*
Nesbitt, R. E. L., Jr., 255, *282*
Nesse, R. M., 628, *657*
Newell, C., 236, *248*
Newman, A. E., 453, *473*
Neymann, J., 682, *713*
Nguyen, V.-K., 629, *655*
Ni Bhrolchain, M., 242, *248*, 441, *447*
Nichiporuk, B., 723, *729*
Nickens, H. W., 293, *306*
Nielsen, F., 211, 219, *224*, 408, *414*
Niggli, P., 319, *342*
Niraula, B. B., 122, *139*
Nobbe, C. E., 835, 846, *851*
Nock, S. L., 91, 104, *107*
Noel, D. L., 482, 502, *515, 522*
Nogle, J. M., 324, *344*
Nolte, E., 816, *824*
Noonan, J., 586, *598*
Nooteboom, B., 465, *476*
Norwood, J. L., 215, *224*
Notestein, F. W., 231, *248*, 660, *715*, 731, *732*, 800, *806*
Notkola, V., 582, *599*
Noymer, A., 301, *308*
Nucci, A., 314, *344*
Nugent, J. B., 232, *248*
Numan, M., 628, *655*
Nuñez, L., 752, *759*
Nutty, C. L., 506, *521*
Nyden, P., 501, *522*
Nye, J. S., 362, *380*
Nygren, O., 51, *56*

Obach, B. K., 172, *203*
O'Barr, J., 134, *139*
Oberai, A. S., 315, *345*
Obermeyer, C. M., 117, 118, 128, 132, *139*
O'Brien, E., 173, *200*
Obudho, R. A., 317, *345*
O'Campo, P., 261, 276, *281*
O'Connell, M., 243, *248*, 876, *881*
Odland, J., 211, *224*
Oeppen, J., 162, *166*
Offutt, K., 243, *248*
Ogawa, H., 492, 494, *518*

Ogburn, W. F., 510, *522*, 611, *622*
O'Hare, W., 770, *784*
Ohlendorf, G. W., 390, *415*
Ohlsson, R., 581, *596*
Okun, B. S., 588, *599*
Okunishi, Y., 560, *574*
Oliver, D., 391n, *414*
Oliver, M. L., 185, *203*, 293, *308*
Olneck, M. R., 399, *415*
Olshansky, S. J., 162, *166*, 288, 290, 301, *308*, 628, *655*, 800, *806*
Olzak, S., 456n, *476*, 502, *522*
Omer, A., 183, *205*
Omi, M., 173, *203*
Omran, A. R., 260, *281*, 300, *308*, 800, *806*
O'Neill, B. C., 163, *166*, 684, *716*, 772, *784*
Ong, P., 357, *380*
Opitz, W., 772, *784*
Oppenheimer, V. K., 529, *546*
Oppong, C., 123, *139*
O'Reilly, C. A., 454–455, *476*, *477*
Orfield, M., 71, *85*
Orleck, A., 134, *138*
Oropesa, R. S., 92, *106*, 172, 178, 183, *202*, 270, *280*, 383, *415*
Ortega, J. A., 243, *247*, 755, *758*
Orubuloye, I. O., 240, *247*
Orzack, S. H., 628, *655*
Ost, J., 876, *879*
Osterveen, K., 582, *598*
Oucho, J. O., 319–321, *345*
Outlaw, L., 173, *203*
Owen, D., 321, 330, *345*
Owens, K., 627, *655*

Paasch, K., 170, *205*
Page, B. R., 556, *572*
Paget, W. J., 702, *715*
Pagnini, D., 183, *203*
Pahl, R. E., 514, *522*
Paine, R., 526, *546*
Palan, V. T., 17, *18*
Palloni, A., 252, 267, 270, 274, *281*, 628, *655*, 788, 795, 796, *807*
Palmer, G., 391, *415*
Palmer, I., 321, *345*
Palmore, E., 20, *57*
Pampel, F. C., Jr., 214, 220, *224*, 262, 263, *281*, 292, *308*, 408n, *415*, 501, *522*
Panik, M. J., 557, *572*
Papadopoulos, N. T., 628, *655*
Pappas, G., 295, *308*, 803, *807*
Parasuraman, S., 120, *138*
Parcel, T. L., 438, *447*

Parish, W. L., 217, *222*, 554, *574*
Park, C. B., 51, *57*
Park, D., 465, *476*
Park, R. E., 182, *203*, 420n, 432, *447*, 481, 496, 497, *522*, 602, *622*
Parker, J. D., 276, *280*
Parks, W., II, 216, *224*
Parrado, E. A., 217, 220, *225*, 355, *380*
Parrott, B., 762, 775, *785*
Parsons, T., 388, *415*
Partridge, L., 628, 635, *655*
Passel, J. S., 178, 186, *200*, *203*, 365, 367, 369, 370, 373, 375, *378–380*, *382*
Patel, K. V. K., 178, *203*, 271, *281*
Patrick, D. L., 812, 820, *825*
Patrinos, H. A., 194, *203*
Patterson, O., 507, *522*
Pattillo, M., 185, *203*
Pattnayak, S. R., 251, *281*
Pavalko, E. K., 160, *166*
Paxson, C. H., 384, *411*, 562, *572*
Pearce, J. W., III, 217, *223*
Pearl, J., 432, *447*
Pearl, R., 630, 632, *655*
Pebley, A. R., 829, *851*
Pedraza, S., 326, 335, *345*
Peek, C. W., 217, *225*
Peeters, A., 815, 820, *825*
Peiyun, P., 748, *759*
Péli, G., 456n, 457, 465, *476*
Peng, X. Z., 855, *880*
Perkins, A., 438, *449*
Perlmann, J., 21, *57*, 173, 186, *203*, 440, *447*
Perrenoud, A., 589, *599*
Peschard, K., 629, *655*
Pescovitz, O. H., 21, *58*
Pessar, P. R., 354, 355, *379*
Petchesky, R. P., 112, *140*
Peters, H. E., 214, *224*, 408n, *415*
Peters, K. D., 298, *307*
Petersen, T., 453, *476*
Petersen, W., 349, *380*, 723, *729*
Peterson, P. G., 143, 156, *166*
Pfeffer, J., 454–456, 459, 468n, *476*, *477*
Phelan, J., 294, 300, *307*
Phelan, T., 496, *523*
Phelps, C. E., 742, *759*
Philipov, M., 708, *714*
Phillips, A., 116, 129, 130, *135*
Phillips, D., 194, *203*
Phillips, D. A., 805, *807*
Phillips, D. J., 472, *476*

Phillips, J. F., 834, *851*
Phua, V., 192, *203*
Pickard, L., 159, *166*
Pillai, V. K., 262, 263, *281*
Pimental, E. E., 702, *717*
Pinnelli, A., 128, *140*
Piore, M. J., 356, *380*, 453, *475*
Pison, G., 535, *543*
Pitchford, S. R., 221, *222*, 861–862, *879*
Pittenger, D. B., 772, *784*
Plane, D., 315, 329, *345*
Podolny, J. M., 459, 465, 466, *476*, *477*
Pol, L. G., 764, 765, *784*, 787, 789, 804, *807*
Polednak, A. P., 262, *281*
Pollak, R. A., 628, *655*
Pollard, A. H., 13, *14*, 23, *56*
Pollard, G. N., 13, *14*
Pollard, J. H., 703, *715*
Pólos, L., 456n, 457–458, 461, 464, 471–472, *475–477*
Pope, D., 134, *139*
Portes, A., 183, *203*, 357, 373, *380*, *382*, 434, 439, *447*
Post, J. D., 582, *599*
Post, W., 581, *599*
Poston, D. L., Jr., 20, 22, 25, 37, 51, 53, *57*, 112, *140*, 174, 178, 193, 194, *204*, 227, *228*, 256, *281*, 329, 339, *345*, 436, *445*, *446*, 481, 490, 505, *522*, *523*, 602–608, 608n, 609–611, 613, 614, 616–617, *620–623*, 855, 857–858, 871, 873, 876–877, *879–881*
Poterba, J., 552, *574*
Potter, E., 130, *135*
Potter, J. E., 7, *15*, 742, 743, 750–752, *757*, *759*
Potter, R. G., 230, 239, 240, *246*
Potts, M., 232n, *248*
Poulain, M., 313, 330, 335, 336, *345*
Poulsen, M., 194, *202*
Powell-Griner, E., 299, *309*
Powers, D. A., 383, 399n, *415*
Prais, S. J., 394, *415*
Prentice, R. L., 685, *714*
Pressat, R., 634, *655*
Presser, H. B., 111, 112, *140*, 210, *225*
Preston, S. H., 13, *14*, 19, 23, *56*, *57*, 97, *107*, 144, *166*, 227, *228*, 235, 236, *248*, 252, 259–260, *281*, 285–286, 294–295, 298, 299, 304, *305–306*, *308*, 420, 422, 427, 429, 435, 441, *447*, 555,

574, 584, 589, *599*, 628, 631, *655*, 664, 671, 675–677, 682, 695–699, *715–716*, 797n, *807*
Pribesh, S., 384, *415*
Price-Spratlen, T., 62, 71, 76, *85*
Pritchett, L. H., 753, *759*, 835, *851*
Protash, W., 77, *84*
Prskawetz, A., 684, *716*
Pullum, S. G., 252, 254, 257, 258, 258n, 267, 270, 271, 275, *278*, *279*, *282*
Pumain, D., 313, 314, *342*
Pursell, D. E., 606, *622*
Purvis, J., 116, *139*

Qian, Z., 183, *204*
Quétel, C., 589, *599*
Quiroga, R. E., 325, *342*

Rabino, G., 329, *344*
Radcliffe, C., 217, *224*
Radcliffe-Brown, A. R., 526, *546*
Rafalimanana, H., 252, *281*
Raffalovich, L. E., 402, *412*
Rager, F. A., 726, *729*
Rahman, M., 753, *759*
Rainer, J. D., 417, *418*, 632, *653*
Rainwater, L., 404, 406, *415*
Rajan, S. I., 125, *140*
Raley, R. K., 100, 101, *107*
Ramachandran, K. V., 38, 48, *57*
Ramanathan, M., 125, *140*
Ramsbey, T. W., 211, 220, *222*
Ranganathan, D. S., 275, *281*
Ranger-Moore, J., 466, *475*, *477*
Ranis, G., 324, *345*
Rao, J. N. K., 762, 768, *783*, *784*
Rao, K. V., 13, *14*, 20, *56*
Rao, V., 120, *140*
Rapp, R., 134, *140*, 532, *544*
Rappaport, J., 510, *522*
Ratnam, S. S., 871, *881*
Raudenbush, S. W., 438, *443*, 798, *805*
Ravenstein, E. G., 329, *345*
Razin, A., 555, *574*
Razzaque, A., 753, *759*
Redburn, F. S., 215, *222*
Reddy, P. H., 88, *105*
Reder, M. W., 408, *415*
Redfern, P., 768, 782, *784*
Redfield, R., 537, *546*
Reed, D., 383, 407, *411*, *415*
Reed, J. S., 502, *522*
Reed, L. G., 676, *716*
Rees, P. H., 313, 327, 329, *345*, 493, 499, *522*, 602, *619*, 767, *784*

Regan, M. C., Jr., 89, *107*
Regets, M. C., 384, *412*
Reher, D. S., 583, 588, 595, *599*
Reich, D., 646, *655*
Reimers, D. M., 359, 364, 372, *381*
Rein, M., 159, *166*, 220, *223*, 406, *415*
Reindl, M., 293, *306*
Reinhardt, U. E., 157, *166*
Reinharz, S., 116, *140*
Reiss, A. J., Jr., 424, *444*
Renne, E. P., 126, *140*, 531, 533, *546*
Repak, T. A., 357, *381*
Repetti, R., 793, *807*
Reuben, D. B., 626, 627, *652*
Reynolds, S. L., 811, 821, *823*
Reznick, D. N., 628, 647, *655*
Ricardo-Campbell, R., 809, *823*
Rich, A., 130, *140*
Richards, T., 496, *517*
Richardson, H. W., 487, 495, *519*, *522*
Riche, M. F., 173, *204*
Richter, K., 314, *345*
Ricklefs, R. E., 629, 645, *655*
Riddle, J. M., 588, *599*
Rigdon, S. M., 748, *759*
Riley, J. C., 156, *166*
Riley, L., 218, *223*
Riley, N. E., 110, 115–116, 123, 129n, 130, 131, 131n, 133, *136*, *140*
Rindfuss, R. R., 92, *107*, 128, *140*, 217, *222*, *225*, 230, 234, 237, 243, *248*, 336, *345*, 427, 435, 440, *443*, *447*
Rives, N. W., 765, 768, *784*
Roach, D. A., 629, 647, *655*
Robert, S. A., 262, *281*, 294, 295, 298, 304, *308*
Roberts, B. R., 355, 356, *381*, 480n, *522*
Roberts, B. W., 219, *225*
Roberts, K. D., 325, 330, *345*
Roberts, K. H., 797, *807*
Robin, J., 584, 591, *599*
Robine, J.-M., 383, *411*, 629, *655*, 657, 683, *712*, 810, 816–819, 821, *823–825*
Robins, P. K., 383, *411*
Robinson, R., 213n, *225*
Robinson, S., 792, *807*
Robinson, W. S., 603, *623*
Robson, A., 645, *653*
Rockett, I. R. H., 788, *807*
Roderick, G. K., 629, 629, *655*

Rodgers, J. L., 627, 649, *654*
Rodriguez, C. E., 172, *204*
Rodriguez, G., 122, *136*, 398, 399n, *412*, *416*, 835, *852*
Rogers, A., 23, *57*, 329, 333, 335, *345*, 628, 629, *655*, 682–684, 702, 704, *715*, *716*, 816, 818–820, *825*
Rogers, A. R., 627, *652*
Rogers, C. C., 243, *248*
Rogers, R., 383, *415*
Rogers, R. G., 256, 266, 269, 270, *279*, *281*, 285, 287, 291–293, 295, 296, 298–299, 303, *305–309*, 683, *716*, 800, *807*, 816, 819–820, *825*, 856, 862, *881*
Rogoff, N. R., 393, 393n, *415*
Rohwer, G., 392, *411*
Rollet-Echalier, C., 589, *599*
Romer, D., 561, 561n, *574*
Romieu, I., 810, 816, *825*
Romo, H. D., 169, 182, *203*
Roof, W. C., 502, *522*, *524*
Root, B. D., 338, *345*
Root, M. P. P., 173, *204*
Rose, G., 262, *281*, 791, *807*
Rose, M. R., 628, 635, *653*, *655*
Rosenberg, H. M., 287, 293, *309*
Rosenbloom, J. L., 217, *223*
Rosenfeld, R. A., 216, *225*
Rosenfield, A., 118, *139*
Rosenwaike, I., 286, 294, *306*, *309*
Rosenzweig, M. R., 273, *281*, 550, *574*, 857, *881*
Ross, C., 627, *656*
Ross, C. E., 90, *107*, 383, *415*
Ross, E. B., 527, *545*
Ross, J. A., 753, *758*, 834, 846n, *851*
Ross, K., 178, *204*
Rossi, A. S., 95, *107*
Rossi, P. H., 95, *107*, 337, *345*, 428, *445*
Rothman, B. K., 130, *140*, 792, 797n, *807*
Rouse, C., 400, *410–411*
Rouse, D. J., 267, *279*
Rowan, B., 462, *476*
Rowe, D. C., 254, *282*
Rowland, D. T., 13, *14*
Roy, K., 51, *56*
Rubin, L. B., 95, *107*
Ruef, M., 456n, 471, *477*
Ruel, M. T., 219, *224*
Rueppell, O., 629, *656*
Ruggles, S., 94, 96, 98, 99, 104, *106*, 437, *447*, 552, 575, 584, *599*, 859, *879*

Rumbaut, R. G., 183, *203*, 270, *281*, 373, *380*, 434, *447*
Russell, C., 764, *784*
Russell, I. T., 258–259, 274, 275, *282*
Russell, K. F., 526, *546*
Russell, S. S., 723, *729*, *730*
Rutenberg, N., 127, *141*
Rutstein, S., 123, *139*
Ruttan, V. W., 561, *573*
Rutter, M. L., 627, *656*
Ryder, N. B., 1n.1, *14*, 17, *18*, 227, 228, 231, 237, 242, 244, *248*, *249*, 427, 440, *447*, 707, 710–711, *716*, 734, *759*, 855, *881*
Ryff, C. D., 628, *656*
Rytina, S., 388, *415*

Sabagh, G., 71, *84*, 243, *248*, 432, *443*, 617, *620*
Sacher, G. A., 639, *656*
Sachs, J. D., 510, *522*
Sadka, E., 555, *574*
Saenz, R., 172–174, 183–184, 192, *199*, *202–204*, 329, *345*, 606, *623*
Sagi, P., 7, *15*
Saito, Y., 629, *651*, *655*, 683, *713*, 811–812, 815–816, 816n, 818–821, *823*
Sakai, A. K., 629, *656*
Sakamoto, A., 185, 196, *204*, 388, *415*
Salancik, G. R., 459, *476*
Salt, J., 359, *381*
Salzman, H., 159, *166*
Sampson, R. J., 53, *58*
Samuelson, P., 551, *575*
Samwick, A., 557, *572*
Sandefur, G. D., 337, *345*, 406, *414*
Sanders, J. M., 212, *225*
Sanders, R. D., 325, *342*
Sanders, S., 217, *223*
Sane, K., 21, *58*
Santow, G., 117, *140*, 734, *759*
Sanz-Gimeno, A., 583, *599*
Sardon, J. P., 848, *849*
Sargent, C. F., 530, *544*
Sarma, P. S., 699, *714*
Sassen, S., 357, 358, 362, *381*, 480n, *522*
Sathar, Z. A., 120–122, 124, 128, 129, 132, 133, *137*, *138*, *140*
Satterthwaite, D., 317, 319, *343*, *346*
Sauvy, A., 727, *729*, 854, *881*
Saw, S. H., 843, *851*
Sawyers, L., 483, *523*
Schaeffer, P. V., 325, *346*

Scharping, T., 839, *851*
Schelling, T. C., 498n, 508, *522–523*
Scheper-Hughes, N., 116, 132, *140*, 536, 541, *546*
Scheuerlein, A., 629, 645, *655*
Scheuren, F., 768, 782, *784*
Schick, F. L., 269, 272, *281*
Schick, R., 269, 272, *281*
Schlesinger, E. R., 255, *282*
Schmidt, R. M., 561n, 562, 563, *573*
Schneider, J., 533, *546*, 734, *759*
Schneider, M., 496, *523*
Schneider, P., 533, *546*, 734, *759*
Schneider, S. H., 663, *715*
Schnore, L. F., 62, 64, 67, 83, *85–86*, 431, 432, 436, *444*, *447*, 499, *523*, 602, 615, 617, *623*, 857, *881*
Schoen, R., 23, *58*, 244, *248*, 333, *346*, 664, 673, 677, 678, 680n, 681–684, 699–701, 712, *715–716*, 813, *825*
Schoenbaum, M., 212, *222*
Schoendorf, K. C., 265, 276, *280*, *282*
Schoeni, R. F., 157, *165*, 552, 557, *574*, 811, 812, *823*, *825*
Schofield, H., 159, *166*, 578, 593
Schofield, R. S., 2, *13*, 582, 583, 588–590, 593, 595, *599*, *600*
Schooler, C., 295, *307*
Schubnell, H., 854–855, *881*
Schultz, D. A., 404, *415*
Schultz, S. E., 816, *824*
Schultz, T. P., 273, *281*, 325, *346*
Schultze, C., 767, *783*
Schulz, R., 159, *166*
Schüssler, R., 459, *474*
Schwab, W. A., 488, *523*
Schwartz, J. E., 184, *199*
Schwartz, S., 791, 792, *807*
Schwarz, K., 846, *852*
Schwethelm, B., 265, *282*
Schwirian, K. P., 495, *523*
Scott, A., 483, *523*
Scott, C., 7, *13*
Scott, J. W., 126, 127, 130, 131, 133, *141*
Scott, S., 583, *599*
Scott, S. R., 98, *107*
Scott, W. J., 337, *345*
Scribner, R., 252, 265, 270, *282*
Scrimshaw, S., 530, *546*
Secombe, K., 295, *309*
Seekings, J., 180, *203*
Seeman, T., 626, *651*, 793, *807*
Seeman, T. A., 255, 276, *282*

Seeman, T. E., 795, *807*
Seeman, T. S., 794–795, *806*
Seever, P. M., 782, *784*
Séguy, I., 580, 582, *599*
Seltzer, J. R., 745, 747, *759*
Semyonov, M., 194, *202*, 204
Sen, A., 403, *415*, 801, *807*
Sen, G., 111, 117, *140*, *141*
Serbanescu, F., 740, *758*
Serow, W. J., 312, 329, *345*, 762, *784*
Setel, P., 531, *546*
Settersten, R. A. J., 627, *656*
Severeide, P. I., 768, *783*
Sevilla, J., 564, *571*, 836, *849*
Sewell, W. H., 390, 399, *413*, *415*, 439, *445*, 447
Shah, N. M., 211, *225*
Shahidullah, M., 771, *784*
Shai, D., 251, *281*
Shapiro, J. M., 508, 509, *519*
Shapiro, S., 255, *282*
Shapiro, T. M., 185, *203*, 293, *308*
Sharpe, F. R., 23, *58*, 685, 686, *716*
Shavit, Y., 402, 410, *415*
Sheldon, E. B., 425, *447*
Shema, S. J., 794, *806*
Shen, Y., 437, *448*
Shevky, E., 501, *523*
Shin, E. H., 490, *520*, 606, *623*
Shiono, P. H., 273, *282*
Shirey, L., 159, *166*
Shlay, A. B., 506, *523*
Shoen, R., 699, 708, *714*
Shonkoff, J. P., 805, *807*
Shook, D. R., 628, *653*
Shorter, E., 233, *248*
Shryock, H. S., 13, *14*, 21, 22, 33, 34, 37, 38, 40, 42–44, 48, *58*, 256, 257, *282*, 360, *381*, 384, *415*, 426, *447*, 628, *656*, 675, *716*
Shu, J., 174, *204*
Shulman, S., 196, *204*
Siahpush, M., 287, *309*
Sickles, R. C., 293, 295, 304, *309*
Siebert, H., 155, *165*
Siebert, M. T., 184, *201*, 502, *518*
Siegel, J. S., 2, 6, 12–13, *14*, 21, 22, 33, 34, 37, 38, 40, 42–44, 48, *58*, 256, 257, *282*, 360, *381*, 384, *415*, 426, *447*, 628, *656*, 675, *716*, 731, *732*, 761, 765, 766, 769, 771, *784*
Siegel, P., 428, 430, *445*, *447*
Siegelman, P., 507, *520*
Sigle-Rushton, W., 529, *546*
Siiskonen, H., 582, *599*
Sikes, M. P., 185, *200*

Silk, J., 535, *545*
Silver, B. D., 174, 177, *199*
Silver, L. M., 246, *248*
Silverman, A., 432, *446*
Simkus, A. A., 498, *523*
Simmons, A. B., 321, *346*
Simmons, J. W., 482, *516*
Simmons, T., 876, *881*
Simon, J. L., 373, *381*, 725, *729*, 835, *852*
Simons, T., 456n, *476*
Simpson, S., 769, *784*
Sincich, T., 773, *784*
Sinding, S. W., 835, 836, 845n, *849*, *852*
Singer, B., 398, *413*
Singer, B. H., 628, *656*, 685, *715*
Singer, J. D., 685, *716*
Singh, G. K., 287, *309*
Singh, J. S., 744, 745, *759*
Singh, J. V., 459, 466, *474*, *477*
Singh, K., 871, *881*
Singh, S., 123, *141*, 266, 270, *282*
Sinha, D., 685, *714*
Sirken, M. G., 243, *248*
Sjoberg, G., 60, *86*, 611, *623*
Skeldon, R., 320, *346*
Skerry, P., 767, *784*
Skidmore, T. E., 171, *204*
Skinner, C., 194, *204*
Skinner, G. W., 530, 536, *546*
Sköld, P., 581, 589, *599*
Skolnick, M., 581, *599*
Slatkin, M., 629, *656*
Sly, D. F., 312, 329, *345*, 601, 602, 605, 606, 612, *622*, *623*, 857, *880*
Small, K. A., 480, 492, 508, *515*
Smeeding, T., 384, 406, *412*, *415*
Smith, B. L., 178, *199*
Smith, D., 659, *716*
Smith, D. A., 483, 489n, 490, 504, 511, 515, *521*, *523*
Smith, D. P., 13, *14*, 38, 40, 47, *58*
Smith, H., 116, *137*
Smith, H. L., 114, 122, *139*, *141*, 245, *247*, 402, *415*, 437, *447*
Smith, J. P., 74, *86*, 90, *107*, 295, *309*, 338, *346*, 405n, *415*
Smith, K. G., 455, *477*
Smith, K. R., 296, *309*
Smith, M., 483, *523*
Smith, R. M., 582, 590, *598*, *599*
Smith, S. K., 298, *309*, 766, 767, 769, 771–773, 777, *784*
Smith, T. C., 530, *546*
Smith, T. W., 93, *107*

Smock, P. J., 91, 92, 102, *107*, 496, *523*
Snipp, C. M., 173, 178, 187, *204*
Sobek, M., 437, *447*
Sobel, M. E., 216, *225*, 396, 400, *415*
Sogner, S., 111, *137*
Soja, E. W., 485, *523*
Soldo, B., 813, *824*
Solis, P., 254, 258, 258n, 275, *282*
Solow, R. M., 218, *225*, 560, *575*
S?rensen, A. B., 388, 391, *416*, 454n, 455, 461, 472, 473, *477*
Sorenson, O., 466, *473*, *477*
Sorlie, P. D., 294, *309*, 383, *413*
Soule, M. E., 629, *656*
South, S. J., 19, *58*, 217, *225*, 433, 437–438, 440, *442*, *447–448*, 490, 506, *523*
Speare, A., Jr., 332, *346*, 495, *518*
Spelman, E., 130, *141*
Spengler, J. J., 2, *14*, 417, *418*, 549, *575*, 734, *759*, 857, *881*
Spickard, P. R., 173, *204*, *205*
Spiegelman, M., 13, *14*, 38, *58* ·
Spilerman, S., 390, 391, *416*, 425, *445*
Spitze, G. D., 89, *106*
Spivak, A., 554, *573*
Springer, K. W., 263, *278*
Spuhler, J. N., 417, *418*, 632, 646, *656*
Squires, G. D., 64, *86*
Stacey, J., 93, 95, *107*
Stack, C., 404, *416*
Stahura, J. M., 496, *523*
Stallard, E., 286, 290, *307*, *309*, 397, *416*, 628, 629, 638, 639, *654*, *656*, 685, *715*, 810, 811, 815, 820, 821, *824*
Stamas, K., 841n, *851*
Stamper, B. M., 840, *852*
Standing, G., 17, *18*
Stark, J. D., 629, *656*
Stark, O., 325, 326, 338, *344*, *346*, 349, 355, *381*, 550, *574*, 857, *881*
Starsinic, D. E., 770, *784–785*
Stearns, L. B., 501, *521*, *523*
Stearns, S. C., 629, *656*
Steckel, R. H., 585, *597*
Stecklov, G., 700, *713*
Stein, Z., 252, 257, 274, *280*
Steingraber, S., 319, *342*
Steinmetz, E., 192, *202*
Stellar, E., 627, 628, *654*
Stephen, E. H., 183, *205*
Stepick, A., 357, *380*, *381*

Stern, R., 490, *519*
Sternlieb, G., 62, *86*
Stevens, G., 347n, 377, *378*
Steward, J. H., 527, *546*
Stewart, A., 116, *138*
Steyn, M., 173, *205*
Stier, H., 214, *225*
Stillwell, J., 329, *346*
Stinchcombe, A. L., 459, *477*
Stinebrickner, T. R., 218, *225*
Stinner, W. R., 606, *623*
Stokes, R., 384, *411*
Stolnitz, G. J., 5n.6, *15*
Stolzenberg, R. M., 91, 101, *105*
Stone, L. O., 22, *58*
Stone, R. I., 159, *166*
Stoops, N., 63, *85*
Stoto, M. A., 303, *309*, 789, 804, *807*
Stratton, L. S., 213, *225*
Streicker, J., 172, *205*
Stringer, C. B., 646, *656*
Strong, M., 682, *716*
Stroup, D. F., 287, *306*
Stuart, T. E., 453, 454, 461, 466, *473*, *477*
Sturrock, J. R., 556, *572*
Stycos, J. M., 7, *14*, *15*, 417, *418*, 732, *732*, 745, *759*
Subramanian, S. V., 792, 797, 798, 798n, 799, *807*
Suchindran, C. M., 391n, *414*
Sudman, S., 93, *105*
Suhrke, A., 723, *730*
Sullivan, D. F., 683, *716*, 818, 821, *825*
Sullivan, T., 440, *448*
Sullivan, T. A., 187, *205*, 216, 219, 222, 223, *225*
Summer, L., 159, *166*
Summers, A. A., 82, *86*
Sunshine, M. H., 508, *518*
Suro, R., 364, *381*
Susser, E., 789, 791, 803, *807*
Susser, M., 252, 257, 274, *280*, 791, *807*
Sutker, S. S., 490, *524*, 617, *623*
Suttles, G., 603, *623*
Sutton, P. D., 176, *201*
Suwal, J., 177, *205*
Suzman, R., 287, *306*
Sverdrup, E., 682, *717*
Swagel, P., 555, *574*
Swaminathan, A., 453n, 456n, 457, 464, 465, 471, 472, *474*, *477*
Swanson, D. A., 2, 6, 13, *14*, 763, 765–767, 772, 773, 778, *783*, *784*

Swanson, L. E., 184, *205*
Swedberg, R., 358, *379*
Swedlund, A. C., 580, *599*
Sweeney, M., 422, *448*
Sweet, J. A., 237, *248*, 403, *411*,
      421–422, 427, 435, *447, 448*
Swicegood, C. G., 183, *199*, 230,
      243, *248*, 363, *378*, 440, *447*
Swicegood, G., 438, *444*
Sykes, Z. M., 685, 690, *717*
Szreter, S., 5n.6, *15*, 110, *141*, 588,
      599

Tabb, W. K., 483, *523*
Taeuber, A. F., 62, *86*, 428, 434, *448*,
      507, *523*
Taeuber, I. B., 855, *881*
Taeuber, K. E., 62, *86*, 421–422,
      425, 428, 433, 434, *448*, 507,
      520, 523
Taj, A. M., 122, *139*, 244–245, *247*
Takayama, N., 556, *575*
Takeshita, J. Y., 420, *444*
Takyi, B. K., 194, *200*
Talbert, L. M., 875, *881*
Tanur, J. M., 215, *224*
Tanzi, R. E., 629, 640, *652*
Tarver, J., 606, *623*
Tatar, M., 647, *656*
Tate, R., 797, *807*
Taubman, P., 293, 295, 304, *308*,
      309
Taylor, D., 134, *138*
Taylor, E. E., 355, 357, *381*
Taylor, H. C., 736, *759*
Taylor, H. G., 252, *279*
Taylor, J., 178, *204*
Taylor, J. E., 349, 355, 358, *381*
Taylor, P., 480n, *520*
Taylor, S. E., 793, *807*
Tayman, J., 606, *623*, 762, 766, 767,
      772, 773, 775, *784, 785*
Teachman, J. D., 170, *205*, 229n,
      249, 438, *448*
Teitelbaum, M. S., 171, *205*, 585,
      599, 720, 721, 723–727, *729*,
      730, 837, 847, *852*
Teller, C. H., 269, *282*
Telles, E., 174, *199*, 371, 372, *378*
Telles, E. E., 174, 194, *203, 205*
Temkin-Greener, H., 580, *599*
Thatcher, A. R., 702, *717*
Therneau, T. M., 685, *717*
Thernstrom, A., 507, *523*
Thernstrom, S., 507, *523*
Therriault, G., 254, 259, *279*
Thisse, J., 480, 492, 508, *518*, *520*

Thomas, B., 227, *228*, 856, *881*
Thomas, D., 334, 338, *346*
Thomas, D. W., 617, *620*
Thomas, R. K., 763–766, 776, *783–*
      785, 787, 789, 804, *807*
Thompson, W., 480, 491, *523*
Thompson, W. S., 420, *448*, 731,
      732, 800, *807*
Thomsen, I., 768, *783*
Thomson, E., 244, 245, *249*
Thornton, A., 88, 92–93, 98, 101,
      105–107, 422, *448*
Thrall, G. I., 781, *783*
Thrall, P. H., 629, *656*
Tian, Y., 617, *622*
Tiedje, K., 172, *205*
Tienda, M., 172, 184, 194, *203–205*,
      212–214, 219, *222–223, 225*,
      321, *346*, 372–374, *378, 379*,
      438, *448*
Tigges, L. M., 438, *448*
Tilly, L., 130, *141*
Timaeus, I. M., 582, *599*, 702, *715*
Timberlake, M., 480n, 490, *523*
Timiras, P., 635, *656*
Tobin, G. A., 62, *86*
Tobin, J., 562, *575*
Tobler, W., 22, *58*
Todaro, M. P., 324, *343, 346*, 354,
      379, 381
Toh, M. H., 562, *575*
Tolbert, C. M., 356, *381*
Tolley, H. D., 290, *307*, 685, *715*
Tolnay, S. E., 335, *346*, 422, 437,
      438, *448*, 502, *515, 524*
Tomassini, C., 159, *166*
Tomes, N., 553, *571*
Toossi, M., 214, *223*
Tootle, D. M., 438, *448*
Torrey, B. B., 406, *415*
Townsend, N., 531, *546*
Toyota, M., 172, *205*
Traphagan, J. W., 159, *166*
Treadway, R., 588, 590, *597*
Treas, J., 91, *107*, 406–408, *416*
Treiman, D. J., 387n, 388, 401–403,
      410, *412, 416*, 428, *448*
Trempe, R., 725, *729*
Trent, K., 19, *58*, 437, *448*
Trevarthan, W. R., 628, *656*
Troesken, W., 762, *782*
Trovato, F., 177, 178, *205*
Truesdell, L. E., 424, *445*
Trussel, J., 398, *416*, 685, *717*
Trussell, T. J., 2, *13*, 587, *597*, 700,
      702, 706, *713*
Tsui, A. O., 753, *759*

Tsuya, N., 125–126, *141*
Tuana, N., 110, *141*
Tucker, C. J., 328, 329, *344*
Tucker, D. J., 459, *477*
Tuljapurkar, S., 628, 629, 630, 634,
      644, *651, 656*, 700, 701, *715*
Tuma, N. B., 391, 391n, 392, *416*,
      460, 468, *477*, 685, *717*
Turner, J. H., 17, *18*
Twine, F. W., 172, *205*
Tzeng, J. M., 185, 196, *204*

Udry, J. R., 110, 110n, *141*, 440,
      448, 874, 875, *881*
Uhlenberg, P. R., 155, 159–161, *166*,
      167, 173, *199*, 440, *448*, 860
Uhlmann, E., 174, *205*
Uhrig, S. C. N., 456n, *476*
Ullman, E. L., 487, 488, 494, *519*,
      524
Ultee, W. C., 387n, *412*
Urquidi, V., 751, *759*
Urton, W., 328, 329, *344*
Üstüm, T. B., 802, *807*

Valente, P., 316, 317, 338, *342*
Valentine, C., 404, *416*
Vallin, J., 163, *167*, 588, *599*, 845,
      851
Van Arsdol, M. D., Jr., 71, *84*, 432,
      443, 617, *620*
van de Giessen, H., 243, *249*
van de Kaa, D. J., 5n.6, *15*, 234, *249*
van de Walle, E., 24, *58*, 232, 233,
      247, 249, 527, 531, *545, 546*,
      585, 587, 598, *599*, 832, *852*
van den Berghe, P. L., 602, *623*
Van Den Oord, E. J. C. G., 254, *282*
van der Geest, S., 540, *546*
Van der Maas, P. J., 816, 819, *822*
van Ginneken, J., 119, *136*
Van Hook, J. V. W., 183, *199*, 369,
      382
Van Imhoff, E., 707–708, *714, 717*
Van Kempen, R., II, 194, *205*
Van Landingham, M., 440, *448*
Van Olffen, W., 455, *474*
Van Weesep, J., 194, *205*
van Witteloostuijn, A., 465, *474*
Vance, R. B., 5, *15*, 490, *524*, 617,
      623
VandenHeuvel, A., 92, *107*
Vanderheuvel, A., 215, *225*
Vanneman, A., 115, *139*
Vasselinov, E., 385, *410*
Vaupel, J. W., 6, *13*, 96, *106*, 162,
      166, 286, *307, 309*, 397, *416*,

628–630, 635, 636, 638, 641, 644, *652*, *656*, 684, 702, 712, *713*, *717*

Velkoff, V. A., 53, *58*, 147, 162, *166*, 552, *573*, 809, 810n, *824*

Venables, A. J., 480, 487, *518*

Ventresca, C. A., 495, *523*

Ventura, S. J., 362, *382*

Vera, H., 173, *200*

Verbrugge, L. M., 811, 812, 814–815, 820, *825*

Verdugo, N. T., 194, *205*

Verdugo, R. R., 194, *205*

Vernez, G., 364, *378*

Vernon, R., 71, 78, *85*, 491, 510, *524*

Vines, G., 110, *136*

Vishwanath, T., 324, *342*

Vogler, G. P., 628, *656*

Voland, E., 526, *546*

Volkovics, E. J., 703, *715*

Voss, K., 383–384, *413*

Voss, P. R., 775, *785*

Wachter, K. W., 159, *167*, 440, *448*, 627, 629, 630, 634, 644, *657*, 712, *717*

Wade, J., 456n, *477*

Wadhwa, P. D., 273, *282*

Wadycki, W. J., 325, *344*

Wagener, D. K., 683, *715*

Wagner, W. G., 455, *477*

Wahl, R. J., 216, *222*

Waidmann, T. A., 810, 810n, 816, *825*

Waite, L. J., 89–92, 101–102, 104, *105–107*, 218, *222*, 296, 303, *307*, *309*, 859, 863, *880*, *881*

Waldfogel, J., 218, *223*

Waldinger, R., 356, 357, *378*, *382*

Waldmann, T., 212, *222*

Waldo, D. R., 158, *165*

Waldron, I., 291, *309*

Walker, A., 155, *167*

Wall, R., 584, 591, *598*, *599*

Wallace, R. B., 96, *107*, 626, 629, *657*, 800, *807*, 811, *825*

Wallerstein, I., 357, *382*, 490, *524*

Walters, P. B., 488, *524*

Walther, C. S., 616, *623*, 876, 877, *881*

Walton, J., 483, 514, *524*

Wang, Z., 684, *717*

Wanner, R. A., 490, *524*

Ward, D., 61, *86*

Ward, M. P., 196, *200*

Ward, V., 118, *141*

Wardle, L., 104, *108*

Wardwell, J. M., 63, *86*, 606, *623*

Warner, S. B., 61, *86*

Warren, C., 116, *141*

Warren, E., 440, *448*

Warren, J. R., 385, *416*, 428, *445*

Warren, J. W., 172, *205*

Warren, R., 369–370, *382*

Warwick, D. P., 831, *852*

Waters, M. C., 21, *57*, 172–173, 186, *203*, *205*, 424, 439, 440, *446–449*

Watkins, S. C., 103, *108*, 117, 127, *141*, 160, *167*, 233–234, 241, 245, *246–247*, 249, 383, *414*, 437, *448*, 584, 585, 587, *597*, *599*, 735, 743, 755, *757*, *758*, 862, *879*

Wattenberg, B. J., 725, *729*

Way, A. A., 738, *758*

Weber, A., 480, *524*

Weber, M., 453, *477*

Webster, C. J., 781, *785*

Weeden, K. A., 384, *416*

Weeks, J. R., 20, 22, 34, *58*, 169, *205*, 260, 270, *281*, *282*

Weidlich, W., 329, *346*

Weil, D., 561n, *574*

Weil, P., 723, *729*

Weinberg, D. H., 192, *202*

Weinberger, M. B., 122, *141*

Weiner, M., 719, 723, *730*

Weinstein, M., 96, *108*, 303, *309*, 649, *657*, 789, 804, *807*

Weir, D., 587, *599*

Weisbenner, S. J., 552, *572*, *574*

Weiss, K. M., 646, *657*

Weiss, M. J., 766, *785*

Welch, F., 196, *200*

Weller, R. H., 273, *282*, 875, *881*

Wells, R. V., 95, *108*, 584, *599*

Wenk, D., 213, *225*

West, E., 458n, 459, *474*

Westbrook, J. L., 440, *448*

Westoff, C. F., 7, *15*, 237, 244, *248*, *249*, 738, *759*, 835, *852*

Wheat, L. F., 613, *623*

Whelpton, P. K., 7, *14*, 420, *444*

White, D. R., 490, *523*

White, H., 773, *785*

White, H. C., 394, *416*

White, J., 538, *546*

White, K. M., 162, *167*

White, L., 159, *167*

White, M. J., 183, 192, *203*, *205*, 319, 324, 328, *346*, 494, 498, 501, *524*

White, R., 606, 611, *622*

White, T., 127, *141*

Whiteford, M. B., 321, *346*

Widgren, J., 347, *380*

Wiersema, M., 454, *477*

Wilcox, A. J., 254, 257–259, 274, 275, *282*

Wilcox, J., 502, *524*

Wilkins, R., 816, *824*

Wilkinson, D., 127, *141*

Wilkinson, R. G., 295, *306*, 787, 804, *806*

Willcox, W. F., 854

Willekens, F. J., 214, *225*, 684, *717*

Willet, J. B., 685, *716*

Williams, D. R., 296, *307*, 794, *808*

Williams, G. C., 628, 635, 642, *657*

Williams, M., 501, *523*

Williams, R. L., 258, 269, *282*

Williamson, J. B., 155, *166*, *167*

Williamson, J. G., 562, 563, *572*, *575*, 745, *757*

Willie, C. V., 185, *206*

Willigan, J. D., 595, *600*

Willis, R. J., 96, *108*, 551–552, 554, 567, *572*, 574, *575*, 649, *657*

Wills, G., 737, *759*

Wilmoth, J. R., 290, 291, *306*, *309*, 629, 639, *657*

Wilson, C., 110, *136*, 233, *247*, 527, *544*, 587, *600*, 767, *785*, 834, *850*

Wilson, E. O., 629, 633, 643, *657*

Wilson, F. D., 213, *225*, 315, *346*, 489, 496, *523*, *524*

Wilson, G., 185, *206*

Wilson, K. L., 357, *382*

Wilson, M. I., 91, *106*

Wilson, W. J., 184, *206*

Winant, H., 173, *203*

Winckler, E. A., 749, *759*

Windzio, M., 472, *477*

Winegarden, C. R., 408n, *416*

Winsborough, H. H., 61, *86*, 441, *449*, 493, *524*

Winter, J. M., 171, *205*, 723, 724, 726, *729*, 837, 847, *852*

Winter, S., 459, *476*

Wise, D. A., 154, *167*, 220, *225*

Wise, D. E., 557, *571*

Wise, P. H., 251, 253–255, 274, *279*, *282*, 383, *412*

Witsberger, C., 101, *107*

Witthaus, E., 815, *825*

Wolf, A. P., 581, 595, *600*

Wolf, D. A., 159, *166*, 628, *657*, 819, *824*

Wolf, M., 122, *141*

Wolfson, M. C., 816, *825*

Wong, G. Y., 438, *446*

Wong, M., 194, *206*, 430, *445*
Wong, R. S., 399, *413*
Wongbundhit, Y., 797, *807*
Wood, A. P., 319, 325, *346*
Wood, J. W., 526, *547*
Woodbury, M. A., 685, *715*, *717*
Woodrow, K., 683, *716*
Woods, R., 585, 589, *600*
Worcester, K. W., 424, 425, *449*
Worthman, C. M., 627, *657*
Wright, E. O., 386, 388, *416*
Wright, J. D., 221, *222*, 861, *879*
Wrightson, K., 582, *600*
Wrigley, E. A., 580, 582, 589, 590, 593, 594, *600*
Wrigley, J., 357, *382*
Wu, C.-L., 383, *415*
Wu, H., 196, *204*
Wu, Z., 100, 102, *108*
Wurdock, C., 496, *517*
Wyer, M., 134, *139*
Wypij, D., 118, 121, *136*
Wyshak, G., 270–271, *278*

Xie, Y., 315, 333, *344*, 384, 397, *413*, *416*, 702, *717*
Xu, W., 438, *448*

Yamaguchi, K., 685, *717*
Yamin, A. E., 118, *141*

Yanagisako, S., 111, *141*
Yancy, G., 506, *517*
Yang, C., 684, *717*
Yang, P. Q., 357, *382*
Yang, X., 319, *342*
Yashin, A. I., 397, *416*, 649, 650, *654*, *657*, 712, *717*
Yaukey, D., 855, *881*
Yeates, M., 482, 511, 513–515, *524*
Yerushalmy, J., 257, *282*
Yeung, Y., 480n, 490, *521*
Yinger, J. M., 182, 183, *206*, 507, *524*
Yoshida, H., 556, *575*
Young, A. G., 629, *657*
Young, H. P., 498n, 508, *524*
Young, L. J., 627, *658*
Young, Y., 437, *445*
Young-DeMarco, L., 98, *106*
Yu, S. M., 266, 270, *282*
Yusuf, F., 13, *14*

Zabalza, A., 408, *414*
Zelnick, M., 583, *597*
Zeng, Y., 25, 51, *58*, 150, 158, *167*, 683–684, 701–704, 706, 708–710, *717*
Zenteno, R. M., 217, 220, *225*, 440, *446*, 528, *546*
Zevallos, Z., 172, *206*

Zhai, N. B., 227, *228*
Zhang, K., 52, *56*
Zhang, T., 52, *58*
Zhang, Z., 809–812, 817, 820, *823*, *824*
Zhao, Z., 581, 595, *600*
Zhenming, X., 749, *758*
Zhou, M., 53, *58*, 78, *85*, 183, *203*, 439, *449*, 513, *521*
Zhou, X., 438, *449*
Zhu, J., 317, *346*
Zick, C. D., 296, *309*
Zimmer, Z., 820, 821, *825*
Zimmerman, D., 399, *411*
Zipf, G., 480, *524*
Zlidar, V. M., 738, *759*
Zlotnik, H., 316, 317, 338, *342*, 348–350, 352, 360, *382*
Zolberg, A. R., 352, 367, *382*, 723, *730*
Zorbaugh, H., 603, *623*
Zsembik, B. A., 217, *225*
Zuberi, T., 170, 173, 196–197, *206*, 254, *282*
Zubrinsky, C. L., 500, *524*
Zuckerman, E. W., 456n, *477*
Zwingle, E., 59–60, *86*

Subject Index

Abortion
  difficulty obtaining reliable information from
      women about, 244
  and fertility, 239
Abroad migration rate (AMR), 179
Acculturation, 182; *see also* Assimilation
  language and, 190, 191
Activities of daily living (ADLs), 815–816
Adaptation, 639
Administrative records, as source of data, 330, 361,
      767–768, 770; *see also* Vital statistics
Africa; *see also specific countries*
  fertility, 240–241, 847–848
  sub-Saharan, 847–848
  trajectories of population aging in, 148–149
African Americans; *see also* Black population
  spatial assimilation dynamic for, 500–501
Age
  median, 4, 161
  mortality and, 288–291, 637, 815
  mortality as decelerating at advanced, 637
  percent surviving by, 289, 290
  of stable population, mean, 694
Age accuracy index (AAI), 40, 42, 47
Age-adjusted death rates (AADR) for various racial/
      ethnic groups, 177
Age-adjusted interstate migration rates (AAIMR),
      178–179
Age and sex structure of population, 19–23; *see also*
      Life tables
  methods, measures, and empirical findings, 25
    evaluation of age dependency patterns, 33–34
    evaluation of age structure patterns based on 5-year
      group data, 38, 40–42
    evaluation of age structure patterns based on single
      year of data, 34–38

Age and sex structure of population (*cont.*)
    evaluation of overall age and sex structure patterns,
      44, 47–48
    evaluation of sex structure patterns, 42–44
    population pyramid, 25–32
  research directions, 48–55
  theoretical issues, 23–25
  for various racial/ethnic groups, 174–176
Age categories, ratio of the size of, 161–162
Age composition, 696
  stable, 694
Age heaping, 34
Age profile of mobility, 334–335
Age-ratio score (ARS), 40
Age sex accuracy index (ASAI), 44, 47–49
Age-sex pyramid, 25–32
Age-specific fertility rate (ASFR), 236, 237, 873
Aging, population, 635, 726–727; *see also* Senescence
  demographic determinants of, 144–147
  demography of, 143
  future research directions, 163–164
  health, health care, and, 155–158
  immigration and, 844
  and kinship structure, 158–161
  in Latin America and Asia, 570
  measures, 161–162
    projection uncertainties, 162–163
  migration and, 151–154
  trajectories of, 147–150
Aging index, 162
Agricultural technology, 613–614
AIDS: *see* HIV/AIDS
Alcohol consumption, maternal, 273
Allostatic load, 794–795
American Community Survey (ACS), 768
American Indians, death rates of, 177–178

Antagonistic-pleiotropy model, 635
Anthropological demography, 525–526
    conceptual framework, 526
        history, 526–528
        the problem of culture, 528–529
    future prospects, 542–543
    interpretivist approach, 540–541
    methodological challenges, 540–541
    research exemplars, 541–542
    theoretical models
        fertility, 529–534
        marriage and households, 534–536
        migration, 536–539
        mortality, 536
Antibiotics, 838
Area/place effects (health), 792
Asia, population aging in, 570
    trajectories of, 148–149
Asians: see Race
Assets and Health Dynamics Among the Oldest Old
        (AHEAD), 288
Assimilation; see also Immigrants, integration
    cultural and structural aspects, 182
    defined, 433
    secondary group structural, 433
Assimilation perspective, 182–183
    modification to, 183
Association models, 396
Asylum seekers, 352, 367–368
Atomistic fallacy, 792
Australia, 724
Autonomy, gender and, 115

Bachelors, 52, 53
Bavaria, 592
Below-replacement levels of fertility, 755, 809
Biodemography, 629–630; see also Biological
        demography
    levels and sublevels, 625–629
    workshops on, 633–634
Biodemography of Longevity workshop, 633–634
Biological-demographic paradigm, emerging, 642–643
    levels of specificity, 644
    model system, 643–644
Biological-demographic principles, 634–635
    human primates and, 640–642
    of longevity, 638–641
    of mortality, 637–638
    of senescence, 635–637
Biological-demographic research, emerging areas of
    examples of, 644–647
Biological demography; see also Biodemography
    conceptual framework, 630–631
    contribution to mainstream demography, 631
    historical overview
        convergence of ideas, 632–633
        early history, 632

Biological demography (cont.)
    recent coalescence, 633–634
Biomarkers, 96, 790, 794
    two classes of, 794–795
Biomedical demography, 648–650; see also
        Health demography; Medical demography
Biosocial models of demography, 873–875
Birth-death interactions, 628
Birth intervals, 267
Birth outcomes
    dimensions of, 275
    and infant mortality, 254, 275–276
    measuring, 257–258
Birth planning policies, 51
Birth rate
    crude, 693
    intrinsic, 694
Birth weight, 254, 258; see also Low birth weight
    distribution of, 258–259
    parental, 267
Birth(s), 627
    early: see Preterm birth
    heavy, 275
    identifying wanted vs. unwanted, 238; see also
        Pregnancies, wanted vs. unwanted
    immature: see Intrauterine-growth-retarded
        (IUGR) birth
    late: see Postterm births
    small, 275
Black middle class, 500
    movement into inner-ring suburban neighborhoods,
        500
Black population; see also African Americans
    suburban growth and, 74–76, 81
Black-white gap in life expectancy, 293–294
Blacks; see also Race
    and declining significance of race, 184–185
Body mass index (BMI), 299
Body size and extended longevity, 641
Bongaarts-Feeney (B-F) quantum adjustment formula,
        707–709
Bracero program, 369
Brain size and extended longevity, 641
Break-in-transportation theory, 487, 489
Breast-feeding, 239–240, 274, 592
Burgess-Hoyt sectored zone model, 498–500
Business demography, 761, 764, 781–782
    evolution of the field, 764
    illustrations, 773–780
    practitioners, 764–765
    tools, 765
        computer hardware and software, 766, 781
        data sources, 766–768
        demographic concepts, measures, and techniques,
            765–766
        population estimates, 768–771
        population projections, 768–769, 771–773

Cairo Conference: *see* International Conference on Population and Development
Cambridge Group and social history of England, 593–594
Canada, 724
Capital deepening, 560
Capitalism, 483
Case-fatality ratio, 698
Catholic Church and fertility, 596, 736–737
Causal models, 431–432
Cellular biodemography, 627
Census Bureau
    assumptions of fertility, mortality, and migration for 2050, 146
Census(es), 65, 236, 330, 361, 766–767
    data collected in 2000, 767
    inter- and postcensal estimates, 769
Central place theory, 480, 487–489, 509–510
Centralization, 497, 499
Characteristic equation, 696
Chicago-Berkeley school of demography, 421
Chicago School of Sociology, 420
Chicago School of urban geography, 482, 513
Child care costs, 218
Child morbidity and mortality, 119–121, 591–593
Childbearing age; *see also* Maternal age
    mean, 689, 690, 692
    variance, 692
Childrearing
    marriage, cohabitation, and, 92
Children
    count of own, 236–237
    demand for, 237
    economic value of, 231–232
China, 855
    birth planning policy, 127, 747–750, 752, 839, 845
    demographic aging, 53–55
    fertility decline, 240, 241
    migration and urban growth, 338–339, 505
    sex ratio at birth (SRB), 49–53
    State Family Planning Commission, 749
Church records, 580–583
Cities; *see also* Urban and spatial demography
    processes through which they grow, 486
Citizenship status, 189–191
Class differentials, 402; *see also* Social stratification
Climate, 616–617
Clinical trials, 795–796
Clustering, 499
Cohabitation, 91–92, 100–101
Cohort-component method of population projection, 772–773
Coinsurance, marriage and, 90
Collective effects (health), 792
Colonialism model, internal, 183–184
"Colonized groups," 169
Communication technologies, 491, 495, 766, 781

Comparative approach, 595
Competition, 497, 498, 502
Competitive pluralism, era of, 841
CONAPO, 751, 752
Concentration, 493, 496, 499
Concentric zone model, 498–499
Congestion in cities, 493
Congregation, 497, 498
Consumer markets, population shifts and, 780
Contraception, 124–125, 239, 845; *see also* Fertility planning
    in less developed countries (LDCs), 738–739, 845
    natural fertility and history of, 588
    oral, 736, 737
        and women's career and marriage decisions, 564–566
    percent of married women of reproductive age using, 741–742
Corporate demographic analysis; *see also* Organizational ecology/corporate demography
    logical structure underlying, 455–456
Counterstream (migration), 329
Court records, 586
Covenant marriage, 89
Cox regression models, 684–685
Critical demography paradigm, 197
Critical theory and critical perspectives, 483–484
Cross-classification/cross-tabulation, 392–393
Cross-cultural perspectives, 80–83
Cultural anthropology: *see* Anthropological demography
Cultural assimilation, 182; *see also* Assimilation
Cultural hypothesis (Mexican American infant mortality), 270–271
Cumulative causation, 324, 358
Cumulative model, 794
Current Population Reports (CPR), 426
Current Population Survey (CPS), 426, 427, 768

Darwinism, 635; *see also* Evolutionary demography
Death, 637; *see also* Mortality
    causes of, by age group, 300–302
Death pyramid, 288–289
Death rate, crude, 693
Decentralization, 495, 496
Deconcentration, 496
Delivery (childbirth), complications of, 273
Demographic aging, 53–55
Demographic analysis, 386–387
Demographic and Health Surveys (DHS), 112–113
Demographic change, perceptions of, 722
Demographic dividend, 558–561, 746
Demographic explanations, structure of, 455–456
Demographic index/rate, definition of a, 661, 662
Demographic indicators, 3, 4
Demographic indices, summary, 706

Demographic materials, 6–8

Demographic methods, 2, 6

Demographic model, formal, 660; *see also* Demography, formal

Demographic models and theories, 2, 5–6; *see also* Models

Demographic periodicals, 11

Demographic phenomena and data, nature of, 663–664

Demographic praxis, 2, 12

Demographic relations in stationary, stable, and nonstable populations, 696

Demographic schedules, 702; *see also* Modeling demographic schedules

Demographic transition model, 587, 660

Demographic transition theory, 722

Demography, 1; *see also specific topics*
  applied, 731–732
  assessment of the progress of, 12–13
  critical *vs.* conventional, 878
  definitions, 2, 384, 454, 634
  evolution (1950-2000), 2–12
    development of disciplinary resources, 5–8
  formal, 722; *see also* Demographic model, formal
  infrastructure, 2, 8–12
    affiliated organizations, 9–11
    professional organizations, 9
  schools of, 421
  writings on, 1–2

Demography, 170, 383–384, 595

Density dependence theory, 461–464

Destination uncertainty, 322

Developing countries; *see also* Contraception
  intended parity/desired family size, 245
  labor force, 210
  suburbanization, 82–83

Digit avoidance, 34

Digit preference, 34

Dilution, 776

Diminishing returns, law of, 561

Disability, 812–815, 818

Disability-adjusted life expectancy (DALE), 816

Disability-adjusted life-year (DALY), 802

Discourse analysis, 131

Disease-free life expectancy, 815–816

Diseases; *see also* Health; HIV/AIDS
  etiology, 300
  and mortality, 300–303, 589

"Disposable soma" model, 635

Dissimilarity index, 192–193

Divorce
  legal aspects of, 89
  probability of, 97–98

DNA, 636, 649

Dobe!Kung, 239–240

Domestic violence, 120, 121

Dominance relations, 489, 490, 503

Drug use, maternal, 273

Earnings; *see also* Income; Poverty
  low pay rates, 216
  in private nonagricultural industries, 372
  of women, 407–408

Earnings inequality, 195–196
  measures of, 194–195

Easterlin effect, 214, 408n

Ecological biodemography, 629, 646–647

Ecological complex, 601

Ecological demography, 618–619; *see also* Human ecology
  defined, 604
  demographic processes and, 604–607
  nature of, 602–604

Ecological theory, 436, 498, 501–502; *see also* Organizational ecology/corporate demography

Ecology, defined, 602

Economic demography, 422, 549–550; *see also* Political demography
  conceptual frameworks, 550–551
  future prospects, 568–571
  research exemplars, 564–569
  theoretical models, 551
    intergenerational transfer, 551–558
    methodological challenges, 563–564
    population and development, 558–563

Economic development
  migration, urbanization, and, 338–339

Economic geography, 480–481

Economic principles, neoliberal, 359

Economic theory, neoclassical, 324, 325, 354–355; *see also* Neoclassical growth model

Economically active life, tables of, 214–215

Economy, rural subsistence and urban industrial sectors of, 324

Education
  and fertility, 122, 123, 125, 409
  maternal, 264–265
  race, ethnicity, and, 180
  and reasons for migration, 322
  socioeconomic status (SES) and, 295

Education level, risk of death by, 295, 296

Educational attainment, gender differentials in, 402–403

Egypt, 134, 838, 839

Elderly: *see* Aging

Electric streetcars, 61–62

Electronic communications, 83

Emigration: *see* Immigration; Migration

Empirical force function, 666

Employment; *see also* Jobs; Work
  involuntary part-time, 216

Employment activities in suburban rings, 84
  explosive development of diverse, 64

Employment opportunities, evaluating affirmative action goals for equalizing, 777

Employment rate, 215–216

Empowerment: *see under* Gender
Empty places, 388
England, history of fertility planning in, 735
Environment
  defined, 615
  human ecology and, 615–618
  physical and social/ecumenic dimensions, 616–617
Environmental characteristics and suburban growth, 76
Epidemics, disease, 589; *see also* Diseases; HIV/AIDS
Epidemiological paradox, 294
Epidemiological transition, 260, 588–590, 800–801
Epidemiologists; *see also* Social epidemiologists
  vs. demographers, 791
Epidemiology, 788; *see also* Health demography
Ergodicity, weak, 24
Ethnic diversity, immigration and, 377
Ethnicity; *see also* Race and ethnicity; *specific ethnic
    groups*
  "symbolic," 172
  "voluntary," 172
Ethnographic methods (research methodology), 95
Eurasian Project on the History of Population and
    Family, 595
Europe; *see also specific countries*
  suburbanization, 81–82
  trajectories of population aging in, 149
European Union (EU), 313
  population projections, 152, 153
Event history model, 685
Evolutionary demography, 629, 635, 644–645
Evolutionary models of life history characteristics, 635
EWI ("enter without inspection") immigrants, 368
Expectation of life at birth, 638; *see also* Life expectancy
Expected average future lifetime, 669
Exposure rates, 671

Factorial ecology, 501
Family household momentum, 698–702
Family mode of social organization, 88–89
Family planning: *see* Fertility planning
Family reconstitution on basis of nominal records of
    vital events, 580–581
Family size declines, 233
Family structure(s), 98, 422; *see also* Kinship structure
  alternative, 103; *see also* Gay and lesbian families;
      Sexual orientation
  and fertility, 121–122
  and poverty, 404–406, 409
Family transfer: *see* Intergenerational transfer(s)
Family(ies), 87, 422, 628
  data for the study of, 93–96
  defining the, 87, 88, 93
  female-headed, 406
  gay and lesbian, 92–93, 103; *see also* Sexual
      orientation
  research directions, 104–105
"Fateful triangle" model, 128

Feminism and population debate, 745
Feminist influences in anthropology, 531–532, 536, 542
Feminist movement, 234
Feminist studies, 130
Fertility, 229–230; *see also specific topics*
  anthropological research on, 529–534
  below-replacement levels of, 755, 809
  ecological analysis of, 606–607
  empirical findings, 238–245
  male, 871–873
  methods and measures, 235–238
  natural, 239
  political economy of, 532–533
  reduction of, 838
  research direction, 245–246
  theoretical issues, 230, 245
    analytic frameworks, 230–231
    causal/behavioral theories, 231–235
  timing failure, 238
  timing of, 242–243; *see also* Marriage timing
Fertility behavior, 606; *see also specific topics*
Fertility change, as period *vs.* cohort phenomenon, 242
Fertility delay/postponement, 243
  as antinationalist, 242–243
Fertility expectations/desires/intentions, 237, 238; *see
      also* Intended parity; Pregnancies, wanted *vs.*
      unwanted
  aren't reliable or valid indicators of future fertility,
      244
  as fixed target *vs.* set of sequential intentions, 238
  recollection of, at time of pregnancy, 238
  similarities of men and women's, 244–245
Fertility history(ies)
  collecting women's, 243–244
  retrospective, 237
Fertility literature, "social facts" from, 238–245
Fertility planning, 733–734, 839–840; *see also*
      Population policy(ies)
  evolution of an idea, 734–735
  implementation results, 752–754
  implementation strategies
    case studies, 746–752
    logics for intervention, 743–746
  next steps, 754–757
  pioneers, 735–736
  research findings, 737–743
  technological change, 736–737
Fertility practices, 51
Fertility rate(s); *see also* Total fertility rate
  age-specific, 236, 237, 873
  cohort, 662
  male and female, 873, 874
  period total, 662
Fertility transition model, stages of, 231–233, 241, 242
Fertility transition(s), 231
  continues until fertility reaches levels of about two
      children, 241–242

Fertility transition(s) (*cont.*)
    involves assessment of social conditions and possible
        responses, 241
    social institutions and, 240–241
    theories of: *see* Fertility, theoretical issues
    timing of the onset of, 240
Fertility variability between populations, determinants
    of, 230–231
Fetal death, 257
Fetal growth ratio (FGR), 258
Fetal mortality, 257
Filtering, 491
Fixed-target model, 238
"Floating population," 330
Force of mortality function, empirical/human, 666–667
Foreign-born population, 348, 373; *see also* Immigration
Fox, Vicente, 752
Frailty, 628
France, 580–581, 724, 843
    demography in, 577–578
    Family Code, 843
Functional specialization (spatial systems), 488

Gay and lesbian families, 92–93, 103
Gay and lesbian individuals, 875–878
Gender; *see also* Sex differences; Women
    defining, 110–111
    in demography, increasing attention to, 111–113
    demography of, 109–110, 113, 135; *see also* Age and
        sex structure of population; Racial and ethnic
        groups, age-sex pyramids for
        epistemological approaches to, 130–131
        methods and measures, 113–116, 130–131
        morbidity and mortality, 117–121
        sociocultural context and, 132–133
        theoretical issues, 129–135
    education and, 122, 123, 125, 402–403
    and fertility, 121–125
        role of work, 122–124
    power, empowerment, and, 115–116, 120, 124–127,
        133, 134
    toward broader thinking about, 128–129
Gender change out of demographic change, 128
Gender roles and inequality; *see also* Gender
    and infant and child health, 120
    and maternal health, 118
    resistance to, 126–128
    and women's health, 118
General Motors (GM), 778
Generation, mean length of a, 694
Genetic biodemography, 626, 645–646, 649–650;
        see also DNA
Genomic biodemography, 627, 645–646; *see also* DNA
Geographic boundaries, shifting
    methodological problem of, 763
Geographic information systems (GIS), 340, 505, 776, 781
Geography, 482

German family genealogies, 591–593
Germany, 724, 846, 854–855
    infant mortality (and morbidity), 591–592
Globalization, regional population difference and,
        570–571
Grandparent-grandchild relationships, population aging
        and, 160–161
Group size perspective, relative, 184
Groupings: *see* Segregation
Growth, population: *see* Population growth; Stable
        population theory

Hazard function: *see* Mortality, force of
Hazards regression model, 684, 685
Health; *see also* Mortality; Population health
    positive selection of migration according to, 270
    spatial analysis and public, 776
Health adjusted life expectancy, 816
Health and Retirement Study (HRS), 288
Health benefits, costs of, 777–778
Health care; *see also* Postnatal care; Prenatal care
    population aging, health, and, 155–158
Health demographers: *see* Social epidemiologists
Health demography; *see also* Social epidemiology
    defined, 787
    geographical and contextual perspective, 791–793
    integrating biological markers and psychosocial
        pathways, 794–795
    life course perspective, 793–794
    links between epidemiology and, 787–788, 804
        historical, 788–790
    methodological issues, 795
        multilevel statistical methods, 797–799
        social epidemiology *vs.* social demography, 795–796
    nature of, 787–788
    next steps, 795, 803–805
    population health perspective, 790–791
Health indicators for U.S. older population, 157
Health insurance, 265
Health transition theory, 800
Healthy expectancy research, 821–822
Healthy life expectancy (HALE), 802, 810, 814, 818, 819
    measurement and medical issues in modeling, 817–819
Healthy People 2010, 304
Hegemonic stability, theory of, 359
Hindu women, 129
Hispanics: *see* Latinos/Hispanics
Historical demography, 577–578
    conceptual frameworks, 578–579
    definitions, 578, 579
    future prospects, 594–596
    methodological challenges (sources and techniques),
        585–586
        aggregate analysis of censuses, 584–585
        family reconstitution on basis of nominal records of
            vital events, 580–581
        medical, religious, legal, or literary evidence, 586

Historical demography (*cont.*)
   microdata from censuses, 583–584
   parish records used aggregatively, 582–583
  research exemplars, 591
   macrodemography, 593–594
   microdemography, 591–593
  theoretical models, 586–587
   crises of mortality and the epidemiologic transition,
    588–590
   natural fertility and fertility transition, 587–588
   western European marriage pattern and structure of
    households, 590–591
HIV/AIDS, 300–301, 756, 802, 845
Home buyers, demographic insights to facilitate catering
    to, 773–774
Homosexual marriage, 878; *see also* Gay and lesbian
    families
Homosexuality, 53, 875–878
Household structure and suburban growth, 75, 76
Households, female-headed, 406
Housing unit method of estimating population, 769
Human capital investment, 555, 562–563
Human capital theory, 212–213, 355, 453
Human ecological concepts and analysis
    of migration, 608
  environment, 615–618
  organization, 608–610
  population, 610–611
  technology, 611–615
Human ecology, 436, 481–482, 601–602; *see also*
    Ecological demography
  nature of, 602–603
Human Ecology (Hawley), 602
Human survival function, 664–665
Human sustenance relations, 481
Hutterites, 239–240
Hypersegregation, 499–500

Immature birth: *see* Intrauterine-growth-retarded
    (IUGR) birth
Immigrant groups in countries of destination,
    incorporation of, 376–377
Immigrants, 349, 538
  concentrations of, in various countries, 347
  health, 270–271
  integration, 844; *see also* Assimilation
  number of, 350–353, 364–366, 373
  unauthorized, 368–370
   apprehensions of, 369
Immigration, 52, 347–349, 377–378, 856; *see also*
    Migration
  to address low fertility and population aging, 844
  fertility and, 728
  meaning of the term, 362
  methods and measures, 359–360
   data sources, 360–362
   research directions, 375–377

Immigration (*cont.*)
  and suburban growth, 74–75, 79–81
  theoretical issues, 352, 354–359
   new economic theories, 355–356
  to United States, 362–363
   composition of migration flows, 364–367
   demographic and economic contexts of, 371–375
   kinds of migration flows, 363–364
   reasons it is important, 362–363
   refugees and asylees, 367–368
   unauthorized immigrants, 368–370
Immigration and Naturalization Service (INS),
    legislation administered by, 364, 365
In-group solidarity, 498
In-groups *vs.* out-groups, 498
In-migration, 151, 152
Income; *see also* Earnings; Poverty
  and infant mortality, 260–261
  measurement, 426–427
Independence, model of, 395
India, 838–839, 855
Individualistic fallacy, 792
Inequality
  demographic research on the level of, 403–408
  demography and, 388–389, 423
  in distribution of family income, 406–408
Infant death rate, 256
Infant mortality (and morbidity), 119–121, 251–252, 259
  consequences, 252
  current levels, 260–262
  directions for future research, 276–277
  endogenous *vs.* exogenous, 256, 265
  factors associated with, 251, 252, 262
   behavioral factors, 273
   biological/biomedical factors, 266–267, 272–273
   birth outcomes, 254, 275–276; *see also*
    Birth outcomes
   demographic, 266
   Gross National Income (GNI), 260–261
   macrolevel research findings, 262–263
   microlevel research findings, 263–276
   multilevel findings, 276
   psychosocial factors, 273–275
   race/ethnicity, 267–272
   socioeconomic status (SES), 264–266
  in Germany, 591–592
  historical trends, 259–260
  measuring, 255–257
  methodological issues, 258
   distributional issues, 258–259
   population-specific standards, 259
  peri- *vs.* neo- *vs.* postneonatal, 256, 257
  theoretical issues
   general conceptual approaches, 252–253
   specific, 253–255
Infant mortality rate (IMR), 4, 251, 256, 260, 261, 268,
    269; *see also* Infant mortality

Infant mortality transition, 259–262
Infanticide, female, 51
Infants, sex of, 274
Infectious diseases, 300, 589; *see also* Diseases;
    HIV/AIDS
Innovation and economic growth, 561–562
Instrumental activities of daily living (IADLs),
    815–816
Insurance function of marriage, 90
Intended parity, 238, 244
Interdependence, 490, 491, 503, 609
Intergenerational transfer(s), 551–552
    familial models of, 552–554
    methodological challenges for research on, 563–564
    public policy and, 556–558
    respective roles of family and public sector, 554–556
"Intergenerational Transfers and the Economic Life
    Cycle" (Lee), 566–569
Intergroup relations, nativity and, 198
Intermarriage and assimilation, 190–192
Internal colonialism model: *see* Colonialism model
Internal migration: *see* Migration
*International Classification of Functioning, Disability,
    and Health* (ICIDH), 814n
International Conference on Population and
    Development (ICPD), 745, 746, 749, 827,
    830, 842
International Network on Healthy Life Expectancy
    (REVES), 817
International Union for the Scientific Study of
    Population (IUSSP), 111, 632, 735, 871
Internet, demography and the, 11–12
Interpregnancy interval, 267
Intrauterine-growth-retarded (IUGR) birth, 257,
    262, 267
Invasion, 497
Islam and women, 128–129
Isolation, 499
Isolation index, 192–194

Japan
    marriage timing and fertility in, 125–126
    population projections, 152, 153
Java, 841
Job search models, 323
Jobs; *see also* Employment; Work
    marginal, 219
    occupational prestige, 428

Kenya, 127–128, 532, 846
Kerala, India, 125
Key function, 489
Kinship-level biodemography, 627–628
Kinship structure; *see also* Family structure(s)
    population aging and, 158–161
Kinship system, anthropological research on, 530, 531
Korea, South: *see* Republic of Korea

Labor, macrospatial division of, 490, 491
Labor (childbirth)
    complications of, 273
Labor force, 209
    and country's level of development, 210
    defined, 209
    empirical findings regarding, 217–220
    macro- *vs.* microlevel approaches, 211–212
    methods and measures, 214–216
        longitudinal measures, 216
    in *vs.* out of the, 215
    research directions, 220–221
    theoretical considerations, 212–214
    youth attachment to, 221
Labor force characteristics, 779–780
Labor force growth, population and, 559–560
Labor force participation, women's
    family income and, 407
    fertility and, 214, 217–218, 234, 563, 564–566
Labor force participation rate, 211
Labor market
    formal *vs.* informal, 219
    internal, 453
Labor market discrimination, 213
Labor market segmentation theory, 356–357
Labor migration, 350
Labor supply and demand, 218, 219
Land tenure policy and fertility, 533
Land use, 492–496
Language, acculturation and, 190, 191
Latent effects, 793
Latin America; *see also* Mexicans and Mexican
    Americans
    population aging in, 570
        trajectories of, 148–149
Latinos/Hispanics; *see also* Mexicans and Mexican
    Americans; Race and ethnicity
    mortality rates, 294
        death rates, 177, 178
        distribution by racial group identification/
            classification, 187–189
Legally mandated standards, conforming to, 777
Legitimation (organizations), 461–462
Length of service (LOS) of members of organization,
    454–455
Li-Tuljapurkar relationship, 700, 701
"Liability of adolescence" (organizations), 459
"Liability of newness" (organizations), 459
"Liability of obsolescence" (organizations), 459
"Liability of senescence" (organizations), 459
"Liability of the middle" (organizations), 466
Life course effects, 793
    types of, 793–794
Life course framework, 230, 231
Life-cycle model/theory, 431–432, 562; *see also under*
    Suburban growth, perspectives on
Life endurancy, 638

Life events, stressful, 273
Life expectancy, 4, 285–286, 638, 810; *see also* Life span;
     Life tables; Longevity; Mortality
  by state, 297
Life expectation function, 669
Life history calendar, 332
Life History Calendar (LHC), 94
Life history theory, 645
Life span, 285; *see also* Life expectancy
  heritability of individual, 640
  as indeterminate, 639
  limitless, 639
  median, 638
  record, 638
Life Span (Carey and Tuljapurkar), 634
Life table review, cohort, 669
Life table theory/models, 813–814, 817, 819
  classic single-decrement population, 664–670
  multistate/increment-decrement, and projection,
    682–684, 819
Life tables, 286, 431, 665–666, 705
  estimation of abridged, 675–677
    initiating the abridged table, 677–680
  estimation of complete (unabridged), 672–674
    initiating and terminating complete life table,
      674–675
  estimation of complete (unabridged) and abridged, 670
    considerations in traditional methods of, 670–671
    data available for, 671
  multiple-decrement, 680–682
  prevalence-rate-based, 683
Lifestyle clusters, 766
Longevity, 628; *see also* Biological-demographic
    principles, of longevity; Life expectancy
  as adaptive, 639
Longitudinal studies, hazard regression models and
    survival curves from, 684–685
Lotka integral equation, 686
Low birth weight (LBW), 254, 259, 269; *see also*
    Birth weight
Luo, 127–128

M-curve, loss of the, 217–218
Macroeconomics, 550–551
Manufacturing and suburban growth, 76–77
Marital disruption and union dissolution, 102
Marital fertility, index of, 585
Marital history life tables, 97
Marital status and infant mortality, 266
Market opportunities, spotting hidden, 780
Markov chain theory, 394
Marriage, 87, 89
  age at, 97–99
  among blacks, 104–105
  benefits, 90–91
  vs. cohabitation: *see* Cohabitation
  cross-cultural differences, 98–100

Marriage (*cont.*)
  culture, ethnicity, and, 98–99
  defining, 90–91, 93
  key features of the institution of, 89–90
  legal aspects, 89
  probability of, 97–98
  proportion of people married, 99
  research directions, 104–105
  studying
    data for, 93–96
    historical methods of, 95–96
  union formation, 101–102
Marriage immigration, 52
Marriage systems, anthropology research on, 534–536
Marriage timing, 125–126
  oral contraception and, 565–566
Maternal age; *see also* Childbearing age
  and pregnancy outcomes, 266
Maternal drug use, 273
Maternal education, 264–265
Maternal health, morbidity, and mortality, 117–118,
    265–267
Maternal morbid conditions, 266–267
Maternal mortality, 841
Maternal nativity and pregnancy outcomes, 266
Maternal smoking, 259, 273
Maternal weight gain, 273
Mathematical demography, 659, 711–712; *see also* Life
    tables; Modeling; Stable population theory
Medical demography, 628; *see also* Biomedical
    demography; Health demography
Medical models, 252–253
Membership lists, 586
Men; *see also* Gender
  role of demographic outcomes, 112
Method of expected cases, 429, 430
Metropolitan areas (MAs); *see also* Suburbs
  age of, and growth patterns, 67–69
  historical perspective on, 67–69
  spatial inequality in, 193
Metropolitan Statistical Areas (MSAs), 65, 69
Mexican immigrants, 178
Mexicans and Mexican Americans, infant mortality rate
    of, 261–263, 269–271, 276
Mexico, 125
  fertility planning, 750–752
  National Population Council (CONAPO), 751, 752
Michigan-Wisconsin school of demography, 421
Microeconomics, 550, 551
Migrant adaptation, 318–319, 338
Migrant networks, 338
Migrants, free, 349
Migration, 311–312, 321, 349, 628, 841; *see also* Net
    migration
  age differences in, 22, 334–335
  anthropological studies of, 536–539
  concept and definition, 326–328

Migration (*cont.*)
  data and data sources, 329–333, 339–340
  ecological analysis of, 604–606
  empirical findings, 333–339
  international: *see* Immigration
  "laws" of, 329
  in less developed countries (LDCs), 315–321
    theoretical issues, 324–326
  life cycle and, 323
  methods and measures, 326–332
    aggregate data and analysis, 333
    contextual and multilevel models, 332–333, 341
    distance and point-to-point measures, 328–329
    metropolitan territory and other functional units, 328
  micro-decision-making model, 321–323
  in more developed countries (MDCs), 312–315
    policy concerns, 315
  nature of, 348–349
  psychic costs of, 322, 323
  research directions, 339–340
    geographical information, 340
    theory, concept, and empirical frontiers, 340–341
  sex differences in, 22, 326, 335, 349, 539
  social structure, context, and, 323–324
  sustenance differentiation and, 608–609
  type of move and reasons for, 321, 322
  types of, 336
    circular, 319–320
    forced, 349
    impelled, 349
    interregional, 337
    mass, 349
    replacement, 152
    temporary, 320
    "yo-yo," 539
Migration-defining boundary (MDB), 327, 328
Migration event history, 327
Migration selectivity hypothesis (Mexican American infant mortality), 270, 271
Migration streams, structure of, 315
Mills-Muth model of land use, 493–494
Mining, 610
Mobility: *see* Migration; Social mobility
Modeling demographic schedules, 702–704
Modeling standard schedules and summary demographic indices, 705–707
Models, 662
  descriptive, 661
  deterministic, 665–666
  explanatory, 661
  formal, 660
  in science and demography, 660–662; *see also* Demographic models and theories
  uses, 662–663
Molecular demography, 626, 649
Monkeys, life spans of, 641–642

Monocentric cities and monocentric models, 492–494
Morbidity, 628; *see also* Infant mortality (and morbidity); Mortality
  measurement, 801–802
  trends and differentials in, 799–802
    global, 802–803
Mortality, 283–285, 288, 303–305; *see also* Infant mortality
  age-specific, 637
  anthropological theorizing on, 536
  cause-specific, 300, 301
  crises of, 588–590
  data and methods
    common data sources, 286–288
    conventional methods and techniques, 285–286
  demographic characteristics and, 628
    age, 22, 288–291, 637
    race/ethnicity, 292–294
    sex, 22, 291–292, 637–638
  distal causes, 284
    geographical factors, 297–298
    human-made and environmental hazards, 298
    social relations, 295–297
    socioeconomic status (SES), 294–295
  ecological analysis of, 606–607
  fertility and, 233, 833
  force of, 666–669
  framework depicting factors related to, 284
  mathematical models of, 637
  measurement, 801–802
  proximate factors, 284, 298–299
  reduction of, 838
  as reflecting but not defining the aging process, 815
  research directions, 303–305
  trends and differentials in, 799–802
    global, 802–803
Mortality outcomes, 299–303
Mortality rates, age-specific and age-standardized, 285, 290–291; *see also under* Mortality
Mortality tables: *see* Life tables
Mortality trajectories
  as facultative, 638
  selection as shaping, 638
Motherhood; *see also* Maternal
  employment of young mothers, 217–218
  meaning of, 133–135
Motor vehicles, 61–62, 780
"Mover-stayer" model, 394
Multinucleation, 494
Mutation accumulation model, 636
Myers blended method (MBM), 38, 39

National Center for Health Statistics (NCHS), 287
National Health Interview Survey (NHIS), 287, 811
National identity, 172; *see also* Race and ethnicity
National Long-Term Care Survey (NLTCS), 811
National Longitudinal Mortality Study (NLMS), 287

Native Americans: *see* American Indians
Nativity status, 189–191
Natural areas, 498, 501
Natural fertility, 231, 530, 587
Negative externalities, 829
Neighborhood History Calendar, 94
Neighborhood vehicles (NVs), 780
Neoclassical growth model, 560–561; *see also*
        Economic theory, neoclassical
Neonatal mortality, 256
Neonatal mortality rate (NMR), 263, 268
Net maternity function, 686–687, 691–693
Net migration (NM), 333, 350, 351
  by settlement size, 314
Net reproduction rate (NRR), 692, 697, 699
Network theory, 358–359
Newspaper readership, demographics and, 774
Nigeria, 126, 533, 535
Nongovernmental organizations (NGOs), 830, 842
Nonmetropolitan turnaround, 313–314
Northern America, trajectories of population
        aging in, 149
"Not in the labor force" (NILF), 215

Obesity and mortality, 299
Obsolescence-senescence processes, 459–461
Occupational Changes in Generation (OCG) survey, 430
Occurrence rates, 671
Old age-dependency ratio (Old Age DR), 33, 162
Organ biodemography, 627
Organization for Economic Cooperation and
        Development (OECD), 157–158
Organization in human ecology, 608–610
Organizational change, 456–458
  content *vs.* process of, 457–458
Organizational demography, 451–452
  conceptual frameworks, 452–456; *see also*
        Organizational ecology/corporate
        demography
  internal, 454–455
Organizational ecology/corporate demography, 452,
    455–456
  future prospects, 470
    across conceptual frameworks, 472–473
    across theory fragments, 471–472
    within theory fragments, 470–471
  methodological challenges, 466–467
    data collection, 467–468
    simultaneity, 469–470
    unobservable heterogeneity, 468–469
  theoretical models, 456
    age dependence in organizational mortality rates,
      458–461
    density dependence in vital rates, 461–464
    localized competition, 466
    Red Queen competition, 465–466
    resource partitioning, 464–465

Organizational ecology/corporate demography (*cont.*)
  structural inertia and change, 456–458, 464
Organizational features, core *vs.* peripheral, 458
Organizational mortality rates, age dependence in,
    458–461
Organizations
  founding, growth, and mortality, 461–464
  life-beginning and life-ending events, 469
Out-migration, 151, 152
Own children analysis, 236–237

Pakistan, 34, 36
Pakistani women, 129
Paleodemography, 646
Parent-child relationships, aging parents and, 158–160
Parish records, 580, 581
  used aggregatively, 582–583
Pay-as-you-go (PAYG) pension systems, 154–155, 557
Pennsylvania-Brown school of demography, 421
Pension programs, public, 154–155, 557–558
  "paradigmatic" reform, 155
  "parametric" reform, 155
Perinatal mortality, 257
  weight-specific, 258
Perinatal mortality ratio, 257
Period-cohort tempo equation, 710
Person-years equations, 673, 674
Person-years function, 668–669
Person-years of exposure, 235
Phenotype and race, 171
Physiological biodemography, 627
Piecewise-constant force function, 673
Piecewise-constant force of mortality/piecewise-
    exponential survival function model,
    672–673
Piecewise-hyperbolic force of mortality function, 674
Piecewise-hyperbolic force/piecewise-linear survival
    function model, 673–674, 678
Place stratification model, 433–434
Policy levers, 833
Political demography, 728–729
  conceptual frameworks, 719–720
  defined, 728
  future prospects, 723–728
  impact of interactions between immigration and
    fertility, 728
  impact of population composition, 727–728
  impact of population size, 723–726
  impact of population structure, 726–727
  methodological challenges, 721–723
  research exemplars, 723
  theoretical models, 720–721
Political economy of fertility, 532–533
Political economy theories, 359, 482–484
Political redistricting, 776–777
Polyandry, 52, 535
Polygyny, 534–535

Pontifical Commission on Birth Control, 736–737
POPLINE, 871
Population
  characteristic equation for, 696
  social sciences and, 417–418
  writings on, 1–2
Population and Biology workshop, 633
Population and Development Review (PDR), 426
Population Association of America (PAA), 111, 421,
      632, 871
Population at risk, 235
Population conferences, 744; *see also* International
      Conference on Population and Development
      (ICPD)
  regional and local, 842
Population debate, 745, 835; *see also* Population
      policy(ies)
Population density, 4, 492–496
  and population growth, 77–78, 80
Population diffusion, 312–313
Population distribution
  intrametropolitan, 314–315
  uneven, 499
Population ecology, 601; *see also* Ecological
      demography; Human ecology
Population explosion, 59, 234
Population growth, 4, 743–745; *see also*
      Fertility planning
  rapid, and constraints on countries with low
      socioeconomic development, 835–836
*Population Growth and Economic Development in
      Low-Income Countries* (Coale and Hoover),
      743
Population growth rate, intrinsic, 690
Population health, 821–822; *see also* Health
  conceptual framework for, 812–814
  demography of, 809–810
  implications of mortality declines for, 810–814
  lessons of demographic models of, 819–821
  measuring, 814–817
Population health perspective, 790–791
Population implosion, 59–60
  moves outward, 61–63
  worldwide, 60–61
Population life tables: *see* Life tables
Population momentum, 698–702
  defined, 699
Population Movement in 1960s, 830, 841
Population parameters, trend of, 3–5
Population policy process, 830–834
Population policy(ies), 827–828; *see also* Fertility
      planning
  active *vs.* passive measures, 832
  formal and official, 840–841
  implementation approaches, 838–844
  implementation results, 844–847
  policy actors, 831

Population policy(ies) (*cont.*)
  policy levers and instruments to implement, 833
  pro- *vs.* antinationlist, 832
  rationales and definitions, 828–830
  research findings, 834–837
  the way forward, 847–849
Population pressure, 835–836
Population principles, 628–630
Population Problems (Thompson), 420
Population processes, 227–228
Population projections, 145–147
Population pyramid, 25–32
Population registers, 581
Population structure, 17–18
Population waves, illustration of the wearing off of,
      689
Populationist policies, 832
Postmodern perspective on urban and spatial
      demography, 485
Postnatal care, 274
Postneonatal mortality, 256
Postneonatal mortality rate (PNMR), 268
Postterm births, 275
Potential support ratio (PSR), 54–55, 152–153, 162
Poverty, 743; *see also* Earnings; Income
  demographic factors affecting level of, 403–406
    "culture of poverty" view, 404
    "situational view," 404
  immigration and, 79–80
  race, ethnicity, and, 181
  spatial distribution of urban, 500
  structural perspective on, 185
  and suburban growth, 75, 76, 78–81
Pregnancies, wanted *vs.* unwanted, 273–274; *see also*
      Birth(s), identifying wanted *vs.* unwanted
Pregnancy loss, previous, 266
Pregnancy outcomes; *see also* Infant mortality
  sociodemographic factors and, 255
Premature birth, 257; *see also* Preterm birth
Prenatal care (PNC), 272–273
Prenatal death: *see* Fetal death
Prenatal determination of sex, 51
Preterm birth, 267, 275; *see also* Premature birth
  previous, 266
Primate patterns; *see also under* Biological-demographic
      principles
  post-reproduction expected from, 642
Princeton European project, 585, 587
Princeton school of demography, 421
Product cycle theory, 510
ProFamy multistate family household projection model,
      684, 701, 702
Proportional hazards regression model, 684
Proximate determinants framework, 230–231, 239, 253

Quadratic hyperstable (QH) model, 700, 701
Quantum/tempo adjustment formulas, 707–711

Quasi-independence, model of, 395
Quasi-symmetry, model of, 396

Race and ethnic group identification/classification, 172, 173, 187–191
Race and ethnicity; *see also specific races and ethnic groups*
  demography of, 169–171; *see also* Segregation
    construction of, 171–172
    literature on, 170
    research directions, 197–198
  internal and international migration and, 178–179
  and life chances, 180–182
  methods, measures, and empirical findings
    analytical procedures issues, 196–197
    data issues, 186–187
    measures associated with race/ethnicity and inequality, 187–197
  and mortality, 292–294
  multiracial identities, 173, 189
  politics and, 777
  terminology, 172
  theoretical issues regarding
    assimilation perspective, 182–183
    structural perspectives, 183–186
  whiteness and privilege, 173–174
Racial and ethnic discrimination; *see also* Racism; Segregation
  "incremental," 196
  measurement of, 196
Racial and ethnic groups, age-sex pyramids for, 174–176
Racial and ethnic indicators, 189–191
Racial and ethnic variation in infant mortality, explaining, 254–255
Racial and ethnic variation in sociodemographics, 174
  fertility, 176–177
  mortality, 177–178
  population composition, 174–176
Racialized social system perspective, 185–186
Racism, 171, 197; *see also* Racial and ethnic discrimination
Railways, 61
Randomized clinical trials (RCTs), 795–796
Ratio-Correlation, 770
"Rebound" growth pattern in central cities, 66, 69
Redistricting, political, 776–777
Redmond, Washington, 64
Refugees, 350–352, 367–368
Regional science perspective, 480–481
Religion and fertility, 596, 736–737
Religious involvement and mortality, 296–297
Rents, theory of, 480–481
Replacement Migration (UN report), 152
Reproduction, 627
  as longevity determinant, 640

Reproduction rate
  gross, 692
  net, 692, 697, 699
Reproductive rights activists, 112
Reproductive value, total, 689
Republic of Korea (ROK)
  age ratios by sex, 40, 41
  demographic aging, 53–55
  population pyramid, 25–27
  sex ratio at birth (SRB), 49–53
  sex ratios by age group, 44–46
  single years of age data, 34, 35, 37–39
Research challenges requiring additional attention, 870–878
Research priorities, 858–870; *see also under specific topics*
  of *Study of Population* (Hauser and Duncan), 853–858
Resettlement, 841
Resource-partitioning theory, 464–465
Respiratory distress syndrome (RDS), 274, 277
Retirement, 288
  age structure and, 220
Reurbanization, 314
REVES, 817
Risk factor epidemiology, 788
Rock, John, 736
Rural places of origin, impact of migration on, 320–321
Rural renaissance, 313–314
Rural-rural migration
  and extension of agricultural frontier, 319
  temporary, 320
Rural subsistence sector of economy, 324–325
Rural-urban fertility differentials, 318–319
Rural-urban migration, and growth of megacities, 316–317
Ryder's translation equation, 710
  extension of, 710–711

Salaries: *see* Earnings; Income
Same-sex couples, 92–93
Saving (economics), 562
"School effects," 439
School enrollment, forecasting
  myth *vs.* reality in, 775–776
Secondary outcomes (health), biomarkers of, 794, 795
Sectored zone model, 498–499
Segregation, 427–428; *see also* Social stratification; Spatial assimilation
  dimensions, 499
  methodological challenges, 505–508
  structural perspective on, 185
Segregation patterns
  demand-side dynamics, 498–501
  supply-side dynamics, 498–501, 507
Senescence, 635–637; *see also* Obsolescence-senescence processes
  all sexual organisms senesce, 636–637
  defined, 635

Senescence rate, natural selection as shaping, 635–636

Senior Risk Zones (SRZs), 776

Sex differences; *see also* Gender; Women
  in mortality, 22, 291–292, 637–638

Sex ratio at birth (SRB), 43, 48–53

Sex ratio at conception (SRC), 51

Sex ratio difference (SRD), 43–44

Sex ratio score (SRS), 44, 48

Sex ratio (SR), 43–44

Sex structure of population: *see* Age and sex structure of
      population

Sexual activity
  contraception and, 565–566
  marriage and, 90, 103

Sexual orientation, demography of, 875–878

Sibling models, 399

Silicon Valley, 64

Singulate mean age at marriage (SMAM), 97

Site evaluation and selection, demography and, 774–775

Small-area analysis
  distinctive problems of, 763
  objectives of, 762
    advance knowledge, 762
    informing public policy, 762
    supporting business decision making, 763

Small-area demography, 761, 762, 781–782
  illustrations, 773–780
  tools
    computer hardware and software, 766, 781
    data sources, 766–768
    demographic concepts, measures, and techniques,
        765–766
    population estimates, 768–771
    population projections, 768–769, 771–773

Small-for-gestational-age (SGA) birth, 257–258, 266

Smoke, ambient, 274

Smoking, 299
  maternal, 259, 273

Social area analysis, 501

Social capital, 213, 358

Social class: *see* Class differentials; Social stratification;
      Socioeconomic status

Social demography, 419–423, 440–442
  contextual analysis and, 436–440
  as explanatory sociology, 428–429, 432–435
    from hypothesis testing to causal modeling,
        431–432, 439
    standardization and method of expected cases,
        429–431
  limits to explanatory, 434–435
  and studies of social and spatial assimilation, 432–434

Social distance, 497–499, 502

Social epidemiologists, 788, 789, 791, 796, 804

Social epidemiology, 789–790
  common agenda of demography and, 790

Social expected duration, 356

Social groupings: *see* Segregation

Social indicators movement, 424–425

Social mobility; *see also* Migration; Social stratification
  cross-national studies of, 401–403
  defined, 385
  demographic studies of, 392–393
  demography and, 387–388
  intra- *vs.* intergenerational, 385
  model of perfect, 395
  as probability process, 394–395
  statistical models for mobility tables, 395–397
  studies of heterogeneous populations, 397–398
  in U.S., findings regarding, 400–401

Social mobility rates, across nations and time periods
  similarity in relative mobility rates, 401–402
  variation in, 401

Social models, 252, 253

Social networks and migrant flows, 338

Social organizational characteristics, and health, 792

Social patterns and trends, description of, 423–428

Social Security, 557

Social stratification, demography of, 383–384, 423;
      see also Assimilation; Segregation; Social
      mobility; Socioeconomic status
  definition and scope, 384–387
  findings from cross-national studies, 401–403
  methodological orientation, 386–387
  methods and measures, 389–390
    change processes, 389–390
    methods for individual change, 390–392
    sibling studies, 398–400
    studies of heterogeneous populations, 397–398
  relation to other demographic topics, 387
  research directions, 408–410

Sociocultural anthropology, 526; *see also*
      Anthropological demography

Sociocultural perspective on urban and spatial
      demography, 484–485

Socioeconomic assimilation, 433

Socioeconomic inequality: *see* Inequality

Socioeconomic life cycle, 431; *see also* Life-cycle model/
      theory

Socioeconomic status (SES); *see also* Class differentials;
      Segregation; Social stratification
  health and, 793
  and mortality, 294–295
  multidimensional nature of, 295
  and suburban growth, 75, 76, 78–80

Sociological demography, 422; *see also* Social
      demography

South Korea: *see* Republic of Korea

Spatial assimilation, 433, 434, 497, 500–502; *see also*
      Assimilation; Segregation

Spatial assimilation model, 433, 499

Spatial distribution, 479; *see also* Urban and spatial
      demography

Spatial inequality, measures of, 192–194

Special location theory, 487, 489

Spousal abuse, 120, 121
Stable growth birth trajectory, 690
Stable population theory, 24, 144–145
    classic, 685–686
        net maternity function, 686–687, 691–693
        numerical solution of characteristic equation,
            690–691
        relations under stability, 693–695
        renewal equation and stable growth, 686–690
    nonstable population and variable-r extensions of,
        695–702
Standardization methods, 429–430
    direct, 430–431
    indirect, 429–430
Stationary population, 669–670, 696
    properties, 670
Status: *see* Segregation; Socioeconomic status
Status attainment process in industrialized nations, 402
Status inheritance, 394
Status zones, 498–499
Step migration, and growth of towns and secondary
        cities, 317–318
"Stratified reproduction," 532
Streams of migration, 329
Streetcars, 61–62
Stress, 273
Stress process, mediators of, 794–795
Stressful life events, 273
Structural mobility: *see* Social mobility
Structural models of population projection, 772, 773
Structural perspectives, 183–186
Structuralism, school of new, 438
Study of Population, The (Hauser and Duncan), 1–3, 5, 6,
        12, 17, 170, 417–418, 421, 577–578, 594, 601, 731
    research priorities, 853–858
Suburban development, changing, 63–65
Suburban futures, 83–84
Suburban growth
    immigration and, 74–75, 79–81
    old *vs.* new metropolitan areas, 67–70
    perspectives on, 73–78
        life-cycle perspective, 70–71, 73, 78, 79, 84
    population decline amidst, 70–72
    slowing *vs.* roaring, 65–67
Suburban movement across metropolitan areas, 64
Suburban rings, 64, 69, 70
    population in central cities and, 66
Suburban sprawl, 64
Suburbanization
    population distribution and, 60; *see also* Population
        implosion
    racial dynamics and, 496
Suburbia, population composition of various parts of,
        64–65
Suburbs, 62; *see also* Metropolitan areas
    distance from city and growth of, 72–73, 79, 80
    distance zones used to categorize, 72

Suburbs (*cont.*)
    historical perspective on, 72–78
    how they evolve in status, 78–80
Succession, 497–499
Sullivan method, 818–819
Survey data, 361
    and associated analytical sources, 331–332
Survey methods, 93–95, 237
Surveys, sample, 768
Survival function, 664–665
Sustenance acquisition, technology and, 613, 614
Sustenance differentiation, 608–610
    elements of, 608
Sustenance organization, 606–607
    age and sex structure of population and, 22–23
    dimensions of, 608–610
    efficiency, 610
Sustenance-related pursuits, 610
Symmetry, model of, 396

Taiwan
    demographic aging, 53–55
    sex ratio at birth (SRB), 49–53
Tax Returns method, 770
Tax rolls, 586
Technological reductionism, 494–495
Technology, 83–84, 561, 612–615
    definitions, 611–612
    dimensions, 611–613
    and growth of cities, 486
    reasons for impact on social change and adaptation,
        611
Tempo adjustment formulas, 707–711
Temporal distance trends, 72–73
Theoretical Population Biology (*TPB*), 632
Theories, 662; *see also* Models
Time(age)-inhomogenous stochastic process, 681
Timing failure, 238
Tombstones, 586
Total-dependency ratio (Total-DR), 33–34
Total fertility rate (TFR), 4, 176, 236, 243, 703, 706–711,
        739
    male and female, 873, 874
Transition probability, 391
Transmigration, 841; *see also* Immigration; Migration
Transport systems, transition to decentralized, 495
Transportation technology, 61–62, 83, 491, 494–495,
        508, 612–613; *see also* Motor vehicles
Treiman constant, 401
Trend extrapolation method of population projection,
        772, 773

Underemployment, 215–216
Unemployment rate, 211
United States
    civilian labor force
        immigrants and change in, 373–375

United States (*cont.*)
  unemployment rate and, 374
  nonimmigrant entrants, 370–371
  population aging in
    migration to and, 151–152
    trajectories of, 150
  population by race/ancestry, 365, 367
  Population Movement in 1960s, 830, 841
  population projections, 152, 153
  racial/ethnic groups, 187–189
United States females, stable population parameters and
    indices for, 691
United States males, abridged life tables for,
    677–678
Urban, percent, 4
Urban and spatial demography, 479–480, 485
  conceptual frameworks, 480–486
  future directions of traditional and new perspectives,
    513–515
  future prospects, 511
    appreciation of formal models, 512–513
    approaches to conceptualization and measurement,
      512
    approaches to standards of evidence and
      philosophy of science, 513
    differences in research practices, 512
    orientation to social policy, 513
    problem selection and area agenda, 511–512
  intraurban spatial distribution, 504
    land use and population density, 492–496
    monocentric models, 492–494
    research exemplars, 508–511
    segregation of social groups, 496–503, 505–508
  macrospatial distribution, 487–488
  methodological challenges, 503–508
  success of cities (node and hinterland), 485–486
Urban ecological perspective, 481–482
Urban economics, 480–481
Urban geography, 482
Urban growth rates, percent attributable to internal
    migration/classification, 316–317
Urban hierarchy theory, 492
Urban industrial sector of economy, 324, 325
Urban influence, 618

Urban systems, horizontal and vertical dimensions of,
    489
Urbanization
  and counterurbanization, 313–314
  migration, economic development, and, 338–339

Vaccines, 838
Variable rate-of-growth model, 562
Vignette technique (research methodology), 95
"Visa-overstays," 368
Vital registration, 94
Vital statistics, 767; *see also* Administrative records

Wages: *see* Earnings; Income
"Weak ergodicity," 24
Whipple's method (WM), 37
"White flight," 496
White privilege, 173–174; *see also* Race
Women; *see also* Family(ies); Gender; Labor force
      participation; Motherhood; Sex differences
  autonomy, 115–116
  reasons fertility research has focused on, 871–873
  status; *see also* Gender roles and inequality
    independent- and community-level components of,
      120
Work; *see also* Employment; Jobs
  and fertility, 122–124
  future of, 221
Workers
  discouraged, 215
  marginalization of, 218–220
Workforce demography, 452–454
World Fertility Survey (WFS), 738
World Health Organization (WHO), 801–802, 812
World Population Conference (WPC), 744
World Population Plan of Action (WPPA), 744, 745
World systems theory, 357–358
Worldwide implosion: *see* Population implosion,
    worldwide

Yoruba in Nigeria, 533, 535
Youth-dependency ratio (Youth-DR), 33

Zeng-Land tempo adjustment formula, 709